MOSBY'S
Emergency Dictionary
Quick Reference for
Emergency Responders

MOSBY'S
EMERGENCY
DICTIONARY

Quick Reference for
Emergency Responders

HUNTER

illustrated

17 page full-color atlas

Edited by

James G. Yvorra

The C. V. Mosby Company

ST. LOUIS • WASHINGTON, D.C. • TORONTO   1989

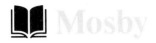

Editor: Richard A. Weimer
Assistant editor: Adrianne Cochran
Project manager: Patricia Gayle May
Book design: Gail Morey Hudson
Publisher: Thomas A. Manning

Copyright 1989 by the C.V. Mosby Company

Printed in the United States of America

The C.V. Mosby Company
11830 Westline Industrial Drive, St. Louis, Missouri 63146

Adapted from Mosby's Medical and Nursing Dictionary, ed 2,
St. Louis, 1986, The C.V. Mosby Co.

Library of Congress Cataloging in Publication Data

Mosby's emergency dictionary.

    1. Emergency medicine—Dictionaries. I. Yvorra,
James G.
RC86.7.M663   1989   616'.025'0321   88-23132
ISBN 0-8016-3525-X

TS/VH/VH 9 8 7 6 5 4 3 2 1

CONTENTS

Contents

JAMES G. YVORRA

This first edition of *Mosby's Emergency Dictionary* is dedicated to James G. Yvorra. On January 29, 1988, as this project was nearing completion, Jim was killed while attempting to provide emergency care to victims of an automobile accident on Washington, D.C.'s Capitol Beltway. At the time of his death, Jim held the rank of Volunteer Deputy Fire Chief with the Prince George's County, Maryland, Fire Department (Berwyn Heights Station).

Jim Yvorra was born in Elwood City, Pennsylvania, in 1952. After graduating from high school, he attended Indiana University of Pennsylvania, where he received his B.A. in English and Journalism. He began his career in 1974 as an EMS education and training coordinator for Pennsylvania's Lycoming, Sullivan, and Tioga counties.

From 1976 to 1978 Jim served as senior instructor with the Maryland Fire and Rescue Institute at the University of Maryland's main campus in College Park. During his tenure, he was responsible for certifying more that 1000 emergency medical technicians throughout the state.

In 1978, Jim joined the Robert J. Brady Company in Bowie, Maryland, where he was executive editor of emergency medical and fire service publications. While at Brady, he worked on an impressive list of projects including *Emergency Care, Trench Rescue,* and *Investigating the Fire Ground.*

In 1983, Jim formed his own publishing company. His first book was Alan Brunacini's highly acclaimed text, *Fire Command.* Other works include the recently published *Hazardous Materials: Managing the Incident.*

Jim was dedicated to the emergency response profession. His friends and coworkers will miss him deeply. We hope that the *Emergency Dictionary* continues Jim's work by providing an additional asset to your response program.

FOREWORD

Dictionaries provide an important tool for students and educators by facilitating communication through standard terminology. Exchanging information with clarity is critical in emergency response work. This first edition of *Mosby's Emergency Dictionary* provides public safety personnel and emergency medical professionals with the first comprehensive quick reference to key terms of the business.

In addition to listing more than 20,000 important terms, the book features valuable appendices containing full-color charts, the rule of nines, signs and symptoms of poisoning, and pediatric CPR. Special emphasis has been placed on hazardous materials emergencies, with charts explaining key marking and identification systems that may be encountered in the field.

The text draws on thousands of terms previously screened by members of the medical and educational communities in *Mosby's Medical and Nursing Dictionary*. New terminology has been researched and edited by James G. Yvorra, resulting in a new, convenient, and important reference book.

Michael S. Hildebrand
Port Republic, Maryland

CONSULTANTS

DONNA C. AGUILERA, Ph.D., F.A.A.N.

Consultant in Clinical Psychology,
Beverly Hills, California

MATT ANDERSON

Training Coordinator
Emergency Medical Services Section
Juneau, Alaska

KATHLEEN G. ANDREOLI, D.S.N., F.A.A.N.

Vice President for Educational Services,
Interprofessional and International Programs;
Professor of Nursing,
The University of Texas
Health Science Center at Houston,
Houston, Texas

MIRIAM G. AUSTRIN, R.N., B.A.

Allied Health Care Consultant;
Past Coordinator-Director,
Medical Assistant Program,
St. Louis Community College,
St. Louis, Missouri

DIANE M. BILLINGS, R.N., M.S.Ed.

Associate Professor of Nursing,
Indiana University School of Nursing,
Indianapolis, Indiana

VIOLET A. BRECKBILL, R.N., Ph.D.

Dean and Professor, School of Nursing,
State University of New York at Binghamton,
Binghamton, New York

CAROLYN H. BROSE, Ed.D., R.N.

President, Nu-Vision, Inc.,
Liberty, Missouri

CHARLENE D. COCO, R.N., M.N.

Assistant Professor of Nursing,
Louisiana State University Medical Center
School of Nursing, Associate Degree Program,
New Orleans, Louisiana

MARY H. CONOVER, R.N., B.S.

Instructor of ECG and Arrhythmia Workshops,
West Hills Hospital,
Canoga Park, California,
and throughout the western United States

HELEN COX

Principal Nurse Educator, School of Nursing,
St. Vincent's Hospital,
Ascot Vale, Victoria,
Australia

JOYCE E. DAINS, R.N., M.S.N.

Assistant Professor of Nursing,
The University of Texas
Health Science Center at Houston,
Houston, Texas

RENE A. DAY, R.N., M.Sc.

Associate Professor, Faculty of Nursing,
University of Alberta,
Edmonton, Alberta,
Canada

PAMELA BAKHAUS doCARMO, MS, REMT/P

Associate Professor, Program Head,
Emergency Medical Services Technology
Northern Virginia Community College
Annandale, Virginia

JAMES J. DILLON, Jr.

Fire/Emergency Ambulance Division
Washington, D.C.

GERALD M. DWORKIN, Consultant

Lifesaving Resources
Springfield, Virginia

CRAIG DUNHAM, MS, EMT-P

Tecumseh, Michigan

CLAIRE M. FAGIN, Ph.D., F.A.A.N.

Dean and Professor,
University of Pennsylvania
School of Nursing,
Philadelphia, Pennsylvania

A. JOLAYNE FARRELL, R.N., M.P.H.

Gerontological Consultant,
Toronto, Ontario,
Canada

WILLIAM F. FINNEY, M.A., R.T.

School of Allied Medical Professions,
The Ohio State University,
Columbus, Ohio

RICHARD D. FLINN

Executive Director, Pennsylvania Emergency Health Services Council
Camp Hill, Pennsylvania

MARILYN E. FLOOD, R.N., Ph.D.

Associate Director of Nursing,
University of California Hospitals,
San Francisco, California

CATHERINE INGRAM FOGEL, R.N.C., M.S.

Associate Professor,
School of Nursing,
Department of Primary Care,
University of North Carolina,
Chapel Hill, North Carolina

ANNE GRAY, M.Ed., B.A., Dip.N.Ed.

Head, Department of Nursing,
Kuring-gai College of Advanced Education,
Lindfield, New South Wales,
Australia

JANET GRAY, B.S.N., M.A.

Nursing Assistant Program, Wascana Institute,
Regina, Saskatchewan,
Canada

SUSAN J. GROBE, R.N., Ph.D.

Associate Professor,
The University of Texas at Austin,
Austin, Texas

MAUREEN W. GROËR, R.N., Ph.D.

Professor of Nursing,
University of Tennessee, Knoxville,
College of Nursing,
Knoxville, Tennessee

JANET A. HEAD, RN, REMT-A

Associate Director for Basic Life Support Programs
Emergency Medical Training Department
Kansas University Medical Center
Kansas City, Kansas

JANE HIRSCH, R.N., M.S.

Assistant Director of Nursing,
Assistant Clinical Professor,
Department of Biodysfunction,
School of Nursing,
University of California,
San Francisco, California

EUGENE M. JOHNSON, Jr., Ph.D.

Professor, Department of Pharmacology,
Washington University Medical School,
St. Louis, Missouri

VIRGINIA BURKE KARB, R.N., M.S.N.

Assistant Professor,
University of North Carolina at Greensboro,
School of Nursing,
Greensboro, North Carolina

JUDITH BELLIVEAU KRAUSS, R.N., M.S.N.

Associate Dean and Associate Professor,
Psychiatric Mental Health Nursing,
Yale University School of Nursing,
New Haven, Connecticut

MAVIS E. KYLE, R.N., M.H.S.A.

Assistant Dean, Associate Professor,
College of Nursing,
University of Saskatchewan,
Saskatoon, Saskatchewan,
Canada

LINDA ARMSTRONG LAZURE, R.N., M.S.N.

Creighton University
School of Nursing,
Omaha, Nebraska

Sgt. ART LONG

California Highway Patrol
Emergency Planning Officer

MAXINE E. LOOMIS, R.N., Ph.D., F.A.A.N.

Professor and Assistant Dean for
Professional Development,
University of South Carolina
College of Nursing,
Columbia, South Carolina

JANNETTA MacPHAIL, R.N., Ph.D., F.A.A.N.

Dean and Professor, Faculty of Nursing,
The University of Alberta,
Edmonton, Alberta
Canada

ANN MARRINER, R.N., Ph.D.

Professor, Graduate Department of Nursing Administration
and Teacher Education,
Indiana University
School of Nursing,
Indianapolis, Indiana

EDWINA A. McCONNELL, R.N., M.S.

Independent Nurse Consultant,
Madison, Wisconsin

JANICE M. MESSICK, R.N., M.S., F.A.A.N.

Consultant,
Laguna Hills, California

PATRICIA A. MICKELSEN, Ph.D.

Associate Director,
Clinical Microbiology Laboratory,
Stanford University Hospital,
Stanford, California

SUSAN I. MOLDE, R.N., M.S.N.

Associate Professor,
Yale University School of Nursing,
New Haven, Connecticut

MARY N. MOORE, Ph.D., R.N.

School of Nursing,
University of Pennsylvania,
Philadelphia, Pennsylvania

HELEN K. MUSSALLEM, O.C., B.N., M.A., Ed.D., O.St.J., LL.D., D.Sc., F.R.C.N., M.R.S.H.

Special Advisor to National and International
Health-Related Agencies;
Former Executive Director,
Canadian Nurses Association,
Ottawa, Ontario,
Canada

SUSAN JENKINSON NEUMAN, R.N., B.A.

Nursing Practice Officer,
College of Nurses of Ontario,
Toronto, Ontario,
Canada

MARIE L. O'KOREN, R.N., Ed.D., F.A.A.N.

Dean, School of Nursing,
The University of Alabama in Birmingham,
Birmingham, Alabama

KATHLEEN DESKA PAGANA, R.N., M.S.N.

Instructor of Nursing,
Lycoming College,
Williamsport, Pennsylvania

ANN M. PAGLIARO, R.N., M.S.N.

Associate Professor, Faculty of Nursing,
The University of Alberta,
Edmonton, Alberta
Canada

ANNE GRIFFIN PERRY, R.N., M.S.N.

ANA-Certified Adult Nurse Practitioner;
Associate Professor,
Graduate Nursing Program — Cardiopulmonary Option,
School of Nursing,
St. Louis University,
St. Louis, Missouri

SUSAN FOLEY PIERCE, R.N., M.S.N.

University of North Carolina,
Chapel Hill, North Carolina

PATRICIA A. POTTER, R.N., M.S.N.

Clinical Director of Surgical Nursing,
Barnes Hospital,
St. Louis, Missouri

JACK D. PRESTON, D.D.S.

Harrington Professor of Esthetic Dentistry;
Director, Advanced Education in Prosthodontics,
University of Southern California
School of Dentistry,
Los Angeles, California

BETTI REIBER, RN

Director of Installation and Training, Clinicom
Denver, Colorado

GINETTE RODGER, R.N., B.ScN., M.N.Adm.

Executive Director, Canadian Nurses Association,
Ottawa, Ontario,
Canada

CHARLOTTE SEARLE, D.Phil., R.N.

Professor and Head, Department of Nursing Science,
University of South Africa,
Pretoria, South Africa

CAROLYN R. SCHMIDT

EMS Administrator/Certification
Office of Emergency Medical Services
Arkansas Department of Health
Little Rock, Arkansas

KAY SEE-LASLEY, M.S., R.Ph.

Medical Editorial Consultant,
Writer/Consultant in Medicine and Christian Literature,
Board Member, Chairman of Missions,
Christian Pharmacy Fellowship International,
Lawrence, Kansas

SUSAN BUDASSI SHEEHY, R.N., M.S.N., C.E.N.

Clinical Nurse Specialist,
Emergency and Ambulatory Services,
St. Joseph Hospital and Health Care Center,
Tacoma, Washington;
Associate Professor of Clinical Nursing,
Department of Physiological Nursing,
University of Washington School of Nursing,
Seattle, Washington

SANDRA L. SIEHL, R.N., M.S.N.,

Oncology Clinical Nurse Specialist,
The Jewish Hospital of St. Louis,
Washington University Medical Center,
St. Louis, Missouri

MARGRETTA M. STYLES, R.N., Ed.D., F.A.A.N.

University of California,
San Francisco, California

MARY ANN TALLEY, BSN, MPA

Program Director of EMS Education
University of South Alabama
Mobile, Alabama

JUNE D. THOMPSON, R.N., M.S.

Assistant Professor of Nursing
The University of Texas
Health Science Center at Houston,
Houston, Texas

FREIDA B. TRAVIS, EMT, MEd

EMS Training Coordinator, State of Florida
Tallahassee, Florida

DIANA M. UHLER, R.N.

Department of Dermatology,
Gundersen Clinic, Ltd.,
La Crosse, Wisconsin

LERMA UNG

Senior Lecturer, Department of Clinical Nursing,
Phillip Institute of Technology,
School of Nursing,
Bundoora Campus,
Bundoora, Victoria,
Australia

MILDRED WELLBROCK, MSc

Instructor Coordinator
EMT Program at Wichita State University
Wichita, Kansas

PAM WEST, RN, MSN

Director, Emergency Medical Services Division
Texas Department of Health
Austin, Texas

LUCILLE WHALEY, R.N., M.S.

Pediatric Nurse Specialist;
Formerly Professor of Nursing,
San Jose State University,
San Jose, California

CASIE WILLIAMS, RN, MEd

Southern Region EMS Council, Inc.
Anchorage, Alaska

BETHANY L. WISE, M.S., M.T.(ASCP)CLS

Instructor, Medical Technology Division,
School of Allied Medical Professions,
The Ohio State University,
Columbus, Ohio

GUIDE TO THE DICTIONARY

A. ALPHABETIC ORDER

The entries are alphabetized in dictionary style, that is, letter by letter, disregarding spaces or hyphens between words:

analgesic	artificial lung
anal membrane	artificially acquired immunity
analog	artificial pacemaker

(Alphabetized in telephone-book style, that is, word by word, the order would be different: **anal membrane / analgesic / analog; artificial lung / artificial pacemaker / artificially acquired immunity.**)

The alphabetization is alphanumeric; that is, words and numbers form a single list, numbers being positioned as though they were spelled-out numerals: **Nilstat / 90-90 traction / ninth nerve** (An example of the few exceptions to this rule is the sequence **17-hydroxycorticosteroid / 11-hydroxyetiocholanolone / 5-hydroxyindoleacetic acid,** which can be found between the entries **hydroxochloroquine sulfate** and **hydroxyl,** not, as may be expected, **17-**. . . in letter "S," **11-**. . . in letter "E" and **5-** . . . in letter "F.")

Small subscript and superscript numbers are disregarded in alphabetizing: **No / N₂O / nobelium**

For the alphabetization of combining forms, see F below.

B. COMPOUND HEADWORDS

Compound headwords are given in their natural word order: **abdominal surgery,** not **surgery, abdominal; achondroplastic dwarf,** not **dwarf, achondroplastic.**

When appropriate, a reference is made elsewhere to the nonalphabetized element; the entry **dwarf,** for example, shows this indirect cross-reference: ". . . Kinds of dwarf include **achondroplastic dwarf,** . . ." (followed by 16 more terms ending in "dwarf").

There are few exceptions to this natural word order; nearly all of these concern formal classifications, for example: "**comfort, alteration in: pain,** a nursing diagnosis accepted by the Fourth National Conference on the Classification of Nursing Diagnoses. . ."

(Note: In this guide, the term "headword" is used to refer to any alphabetized and nonindented definiendum, be it a single-word term or a compound term.)

C. MULTIPLE DEFINITIONS

If a headword has more than one meaning, the meanings are numbered and are often accompanied by an indication of the field in which a sense applies: "**fractionation, 1.** (in neurology) . . . **2.** (in chemistry) . . . **3.** (in bacteriology) . . . **4.** (in histology) . . . **5.** (in radiology) . . ."

Smaller differences in meaning are occasionally separated by semicolons: "**enervation, 1.** the reduction or lack of nervous energy; weakness; lassitude, languor. **2.** removal of a complete nerve or of a section of nerve."

Words that are spelled alike but have entirely different meanings and origins are usually given as separate entries, with superscript numbers: "**aural¹,** of or pertaining to the ear or hearing. . ." followed by "**aural²,** of or pertaining to an aura."

For reference entries that appear in the form of numbered senses, see the example of **hyperalimentation** at E below.

D. THE BOLDFACE ELEMENTS OF AN ENTRY

After the entry headword, which has large boldface type, the following elements may occur in boldface, in this order.

In large boldface:

■ HEADWORD ABBREVIATIONS: **central nervous system (CNS)**

A corresponding abbreviation entry is listed: "**CNS,** abbreviation for **central nervous system.**" (For abbreviation entries, see F below.)

Occasionally the order is reversed: "**DDT (dichlordiphenyltrichloroethane),**" with a corresponding reference entry: "**dichlordiphenyltrichloroethane. See DDT.**" (For reference entries, see E below.)

In smaller boldface (all others):

■ PLURAL OR SINGULAR FORMS that are not obvious.

The first form shown is the more common except when plurals are of more or less equal frequency: "**carcinoma,** *pl.* **carcinomas, carcinomata**"; "**cortex,** *pl.* **cortices**"; "**data,** *sing.* **datum**"

A reference entry is listed only when the terms are alphabetically separated; for example, there are several entries between **data** and "**datum. See data.**"

■ HIDDEN ENTRIES, that is, terms that can best be defined in the context of a more general entry. For example, the definition of the entry **equine encephalitis** continues as follows: ". . . **Eastern equine encephalitis (EEE)** is a severe form of the infection . . . **western equine encephalitis (WEE),** which occurs . . . **Venezuelan equine encephalitis (VEE),** which is common in . . ."

The corresponding reference entries are "**eastern equine encephalitis. See equine encephalitis.**"; "**western equine encephalitis. See equine . . .**"; and so forth. For further reference, from the abbreviations **EEE, WEE,** and **VEE,** see F below.

■ INDIRECT CROSS-REFERENCES to other defined entries, shown as part of the definition and usually introduced by "Kinds of": "**dwarf,** . . . Kinds of dwarfs include **achondroplastic dwarf, Amsterdam dwarf,** . . . , and **thanatophoric dwarf.**"

The entry referred to may or may not show a reciprocal reference, depending on the information value.

■ SYNONYMOUS TERMS, preceded by "Also called," "Also spelled," or, for verbs and adjectives, "Also": "**abducens nerve,** . . . Also called **sixth nerve.**"

A corresponding reference entry is usually given: "**sixth nerve. See abducens nerve.**"

Occasionally the synonymous term is accompanied by a usage label: "**abdomen,** . . . Also called *(informal)* **belly.**"

If a synonymous term applies to only one numbered sense, it precedes rather than follows the definition, to avoid ambiguity: "**algology, 1.** the branch of medicine that is concerned with the study of pain. **2.** also called **phycology.** the branch of science that is concerned with algae." (Whenever a synonymous term *follows* the last numbered sense, it applies to all senses of the entry.)

■ (DIRECT) CROSS-REFERENCES, preceded by "See also" or "Compare," referring to another defined entry for additional information: "**abdominal aorta,** . . . See also **descending aorta.**"

The cross-reference may or may not be reciprocal.

Cross-references are also made to illustrations, to tables, to the color atlas, and to the appendixes.

For cross-references from an abbreviation entry (with "See"), see F below.

■ PARTS OF SPEECH related to the entry headword, shown

as run-on entries that do not require a separate definition: "**abalienation,** . . . — **abalienate,** *v.,* **abalienated,** *adj.*"

E. REFERENCE ENTRIES

Reference entries are undefined entries referring to a defined entry. There, they usually correspond to the boldface terms for which reference entries are mentioned at D above.

However, many of the less frequently used synonymous terms are listed as a reference only; at the entry referred to, the reader's attention is not drawn to them with "Also called."

A reference entry may also refer to a defined entry for other reasons: A particular lightface term in the definition is occasionally referred to: "**motion sickness,** . . . air sickness . . ." — with the reference entry "**air sickness: See motion sickness.**" Or a reference is made to give additional access to a definition or to part of a definition: "**congenital condition. See congenital anomaly.**" — although the latter entry does not literally mention "congenital condition," and is not a synonymous term.

Some reference entries appear in the form of a numbered sense of a defined entry: "**hyperalimentation, 1.** overfeeding or the . . . in excess of the demands of the appetite. **2.** See **total parenteral nutrition.**" The latter entry says "Also called **hyperalimentation.**"

If two or more alphabetically adjacent terms refer to the same entry or entries, they are styled as one reference entry: "**coxa adducta, coxa flexa. See coxa vara.**"

A reference entry that would be derived from a boldface term in an immediately adjacent entry is not listed again as a headword; it becomes a "hidden reference entry": "**acardius amorphus,** . . . Also called **acardius anceps.**" But **acardius anceps** is not listed again as a reference entry because it would immediately *follow* the entry, the next entry being **acariasis.** Likewise: "**acoustic neuroma,** . . . Also called **acoustic neurilemmona, acoustic neurinoma, acoustic neurofibroma.**" But the three synonymous terms are not listed again as reference entries because they would immediately *precede* the entry, the entry ahead being **acoustic nerve.** Therefore:

> If a term is not listed at the expected place, the reader might find it among the boldface terms of the immediately preceding or the immediately following entry.

F. OTHER KINDS OF ENTRIES

■ ABBREVIATION ENTRIES: Most abbreviation entries, including symbol entries, show the full form of the term in boldface: "**ABC,** abbreviation for **aspiration biopsy cytology.**" "**H,** symbol for **hydrogen.**" Implied reference is made to the entries **aspiration biopsy cytology** and **hydrogen** respectively.

Abbreviation entries for which there is no corresponding entry show the full form in italics: "**CBF,** abbreviation for *cerebral blood flow.*" "**f,** symbol for *respiratory frequency.*"

A combination of abbreviation entry and reference entry occurs when the abbreviation is that of a boldface or light-face term appearing under another headword. For example, the hidden entries at D above (in addition to the reference entries shown there), are also referred to in the following manner: "**EEE,** abbreviation for **eastern equine encephalitis.** See **equine encephalitis.**" An example with a light-face term: "**HLA-A,** abbreviation for *human leukocyte antigen A.* See **human leukocyte antigen.**" The latter entry says ". . . They are HLA-A, HLA-B, HLA-C . . ."

■ COMBINING FORMS: For a definition, see the entry **combining form.** The large amount and the nature of combining-form entries are an important feature of this dictionary. Through the combining forms the reader has additional access to the meanings of headwords and the words used in defining them. But the combining forms give also access to thousands of terms that are not included in this dictionary (and, to a large extent, are not found in any other reference work). For example, the combining-form entries **xylo-** and **-phage** (plus **phagia, phago-,** and **-phagy**) may lead to the meaning of "xylophagous," namely, "wood-eating."

Combining-form headwords consisting of variants are alphabetized by the first variant only. For example, "**epi-, ep-,** a combining form meaning 'on, upon'. . ." is followed by **epiblast** (notwithstanding "**ep-**"). The other variant or variants are listed in their own alphabetical place as reference entries referring to the first variant: "**ep-.** See **epi-.**"

■ ENTRIES WITH SPECIAL PARAGRAPHS: Among the entries on diseases, drugs, and procedures, at least 1000 feature special paragraphs. These paragraphs are headed as follows.

For disease entries: "observations," "intervention," and "nursing considerations."

For drug entries: "indications," "contraindications," and "adverse effects."

For procedure entries: "method," "nursing orders," and "outcome criteria."

G. FURTHER COMMENTS

■ ETYMOLOGY is shown only in entries where it contributes immediately to a better understanding of the meaning:

"**lysergide,** . . . Also called **LSD** (an abbreviation of the original German name, *Lyserg-Säure-diäthylamid*), **lysergic acid diethylamide,** *(slang)* **acid.**" "**hangnail,** . . . painful . . . ("Hang" is not related to the verb but is an old English word for pain.) . . ."

■ EPONYMOUS TERMS THAT END IN "SYNDROME" OR "DISEASE" are given with an apostrophe (and "s" where appropriate) if they are based on the name of one person: **Adie's syndrome; Symmers' disease; Treacher Collins' syndrome** (the ophthalmologist Edward Treacher Collins). If they are based on the names of several people, they are given without apostrophe: **Bernard-Soulier syndrome; Brill-Symmers disease.**

■ ABBREVIATIONS AND LABELS IN ITALIC TYPE: The abbreviations are *pl.* (plural), *npl.* (noun plural), *sing.* (singular); *n.* (noun), *adj.* (adjective), *v.* (verb). The recurring labels are *slang, informal, nontechnical, obsolete, archaic; chiefly British, Canada, U.S.*

■ DICTIONARY OF FIRST REFERENCE for general spelling preferences is *Webster's New Collegiate Dictionary;* thereafter: *Webster's Third New International Dictionary.* End-of-line hyphenation of technical terms follows *The Medical & Health Sciences Word Book* (Houghton Mifflin).

H. PRONUNCIATION

■ SYSTEM: See the pronunciation key. The pronunciation system of this dictionary is basically a system that most readers know from their use of popular English dictionaries, especially the major college or desk dictionaries. All symbols for English sounds are ordinary letters of the alphabet with few adaptations, and with the exception of the schwa /ə/ (the neutral vowel).

■ ACCENTS: Pronunciation, given between slants, is shown with primary and secondary accents, and a raised dot shows that two vowels or, occasionally, two consonants, between the slants are pronounced separately:

anoopsia /an′ō•op′sē•ə/
cecoileostomy /sē′kō•il′ē•os′təmē/
methemoglobin /met′hēməglō′bin, met•hē′məglōbin/

Without the raised dot, the second /th/ in the last example would be pronounced as in "thin." (The pronunciation key lists the following paired consonant symbols as representing a single sound: /ch/, /ng/, /sh/, /th/, /*th*/, /zh/, and the foreign sounds /kh/ and /*kh*/ — if no raised dot intervenes.)

■ TRUNCATION: Pronunciation may be given in truncated form, especially for alternative or derived words:

defibrillate /dif ī′brilāt, difib′-/
bacteriophage /baktir′ē•əfāj′, ... —**bacteriophagy** /of′əjē/, *n.*

In the last example, the reader is asked to make the commonsense assumption that the primary accent of the headword becomes a secondary accent in the run-on term:

/baktir′ē•of′əjē/.

■ LOCATION: Pronunciation may be given for any boldface term and may occur anywhere in an entry:

aura /ôr′ə/, **1.** *pl.* **aurae** /ôr′ē/, a sensation . . . **2.** *pl.* **auras,** an emanation of light . . .

micrometer, 1. /mīkrom′əter/, an instrument used for . . . **2.**/ mī′krōmē′tər/, a unit of measurement . . .

Occasionally it is given for a lightface term:

b.i.d., (in prescriptions) abbreviation for *bis in die* /dē′ā/, a Latin phrase meaning . . .

boutonneuse fever . . . , an infectious disease . . . a tache noire /täshnô•är′/ or black spot . . .

■ LETTERWORD VERSUS ACRONYM: For definitions of these terms, see the entries **letterword** and **acronym** in this dictionary. If the pronunciation of an abbreviation is not given, the abbreviation is usually a letterword.

ABO blood groups [read /ā′bē′ō′/, not /ā′bō/]

If the abbreviation is an acronym, this is indicated by pronunciation:

AWOL /ā′wôl/

Some abbreviations are used as both:

JAMA /jä′mä, jam′ə, jā′ā′em′ā′/

■ FOREIGN SOUNDS: Non-English sounds do not occur often in this dictionary. They are represented by the following symbols:

/œ/	as in (French) **feu** /fœ/, **Europe** /œrôp′/; (German) **schön** /shœn/, **Goethe** /gœ′te/
/Y/	as in (French) **tu** /tY/, **déjà vu** /dāzhävY′/; (German) **grün** /grYn/, **Walküre** /vulkY′rə/
/kh/	as in (Scottish) **loch** /lokh/; (German) **Rorschach** /rôr′shokh/, **Bach** /bokh, bäkh/
/kh/	as in (German) **ich** /ikh/, **Reich** /rīkh/ (or, approximated, as in English **fish:** /ish/, rīsh/)
/N/	This symbol does not represent a sound but indicates that the preceding vowel is a nasal, as in French **bon** /bôN/, **en face** /äNfäs′/, or **international** /aNternäsyōnäl/.
/nyə/	Occurring at the end of French words, this symbol is not truly a separate syllable but an /n/ with a slight /y/ (similar to the sound in ''onion'') plus a near-silent /y/, as in **Bois de Boulogne** /bo͞oloͅ′nyə/, **Mal**-gaigne /mälgā′nyə/.

Because this work is a subject dictionary rather than a language dictionary, certain foreign words and proper names are rendered by English approximations. Examples are **Müller** /mil′ər/ (which is closer to German than /mY′lər/),

Niemann /nē′mon/ (which is closer than /nē′män/), **Friedreich** /frēd′ rîsh/ (which is close enough for anyone not used to pronouncing /kh/), or **jamais vu,** for which three acceptable pronunciations are given: /zhämävY′/ (near-French) and the approximations /zhämävē′/ and /zhämävo͞o′/ (/-vē′/ being much closer to French than /-vo͞o′/). Depending on usage, a foreign word or name may be given with near-native pronunciation, with entirely assimilated English pronunciation (as **de Quervain's fracture** /dəkərvānz′/), or with both (as **Dupuytren's contracture** /dYpY•itraNṣ′, dēpē•itranz′/ or **Klippel-Feil syndrome** /klipel′fel′, klip′əlfīl′/).

At any rate, the English speaker should not hesitate to follow whatever is usage in his or her working or social environment.

Many of the numerous *Latin* terms in this dictionary are not given with pronunciation, mainly because there are different ways (all of them understood) in which Latin is pronounced by the English speaker and may be pronounced by speakers elsewhere. However, guidance is given in many cases, often to reflect common usage.

■ LATIN AND GREEK PLURALS: The spelling of Latin and Greek plurals is shown in most instances. However, when the plural formation is regular according to Latin and Greek rules, the pronunciation is usually not included. Therefore, the following list shows the suggested pronunciation of selected plural endings that are frequently encountered in the field of medicine.

NOTE: Notwithstanding the listing of Latin and Greek plurals in this dictionary, and notwithstanding the foregoing examples, in most instances it is acceptable or even preferable to pluralize Latin and Greek words according to the rules of English words. (For certain kinds of entries, both the English and the foreign plurals are given in this dictionary, usually showing the English form first, as, for example, in nearly all **-oma** nouns: **hematoma,** *pl.* **hematomas, hematomata.**)

W.D.G.

PLURAL ENDINGS	EXAMPLES
-a/-ə/	**inoculum,** *pl.* **inocula** /inok′ yo͞olə/
-ae/-ē/	**vertebra,** *pl.* **vertebrae** /vur′təbrē/
-ces /sēz/	**thorax,** *pl.* **thoraces** /thôr′əsēz/
	apex, *pl.* **apices** /ā′pisēz/
-era /-ərə/	**genus,** *pl.* **genera** /jen′ərə/
-ges /-jēz/	**meninx,** *pl.* **meninges** /minin′jēz/
-i /-ī/	**calculus,** *pl.* **calculi** /kal′kyəlī/
	coccus, *pl.* **cocci** /kok′sī/
-ia /-ē•ə/	**criterion,** *pl.* **criteria** /krītir′ē•ə/
-ides /-idēz/	**epulis,** *pl.* **epulides** /ipyo͞o′lidēz/
-ina/-ənə/	**foramen,** *pl.* **foramina** /fəram′ənə/
-ines /-ənēz/	**lentigo,** *pl.* **lentigines** /lentij′ənēz/

PLURAL ENDINGS	EXAMPLES
-omata /-ōʹmətə/	**hemotoma,** *pl.* **hematomata** /hēʹmətōʹmətə/
-ones /-ōʹnēz/	**comedo,** *pl.* **comedones** /komʹədōʹnēz/
-ora /-ərə/	**corpus,** *pl.* **corpora** /kôrʹpərə/
	femur, *pl.* **femora** /femʹərə/
-ses/-sez/	**analysis,** *pl.* **analyses** /ənalʹəsēz/
-udes /-o͞oʹdēz/	**incus,** *pl.* **incudes** /inko͞oʹdēz/
-us /-o͞os/	**ductus** (/dukʹtəs/), *pl.* **ductus** /dukʹto͞os/

PRONUNCIATION KEY

Vowels		**Consonants**	
SYMBOLS	KEY WORDS	SYMBOLS	KEY WORDS
/a/	hat	/b/	book
/ä/	father	/ch/	chew
/ā/	fate	/d/	day
/e/	flesh	/f/	fast
/ē/	she	/g/	good
/er/	air, ferry	/h/	happy
/i/	sit	/j/	gem
/ī/	eye	/k/	keep
/ir/	ear	/l/	late
/o/	proper	/m/	make
/ō/	nose	/n/	no
/ô/	saw	/ng/	sing, drink
/oi/	boy	/ng•g/	finger
/o͞o/	move	/p/	pair
/o͝o/	book	/r/	ring
/ou/	out	/s/	set
/u/	cup, love	/sh/	shoe, lotion
/ur/	fur, first	/t/	tone
/ə/	(the neutral vowel, always unstressed, as in) ago, focus	/th/	thin
		/th/	than
		/v/	very
/ər/	teacher, doctor	/w/	work
		/y/	yes
		/z/	zeal
		/zh/	azure, vision

For /œ/, /Y/, /kh/, /kh/, /N/, and /nyə/,
see FOREIGN SOUNDS, p. xxi.

A

āa, āā, ĀĀ, (in prescriptions) abbreviation for **ana,** meaning equal amounts of each ingredient.

AA, abbreviation for **Alcoholics Anonymous.**

abalienation /abāl′yənā′shən/, a state of physical decline or mental illness.

abarticulation /ab′ärtik′yəlā′shən/, dislocation of a joint.

abasia /əbā′zhə/, inability to walk.

Abbokinase, a trademark for a drug used to dissolve blood clots in deep veins (urokinase).

abdomen /ab′dəmən, abdō′mən/, the part of the body between the chest and the hips. The **abdominal cavity** is the space in the body that holds part of the esophagus, stomach, small intestines, liver, gallbladder, pancreas, spleen, kidneys, and tubes (ureters) that deliver urine from the kidneys to the bladder.

abdominal binder /abdom′ənəl/, a wide bandage or elastic band that is wrapped around the stomach area. A binder is sometimes used after surgery for support and to lessen pain.

abdominal delivery. See **cesarean section.**

abdominal inguinal ring, a part of the muscles in the groin. It is naturally weak, and hernias may occur here.

abdominal pain, pain in the belly that can be sudden or long-term, local or general. It can be an important symptom because surgery or medical treatment may be needed. The most common causes of severe pain are infection, a tear in the abdominal contents, and blockage of the bloodstream, intestine, or kidney. Conditions causing pain that may need surgery include appendicitis, pouches in the intestines (diverticulitis), gallbladder problems, pancreas infection, a bleeding peptic ulcer, blocked intestines, pouches in an artery wall (abdominal aortic aneurysms), and damage to an organ. Other causes of pain that may require surgery include serious pelvic inflammatory disease, a break in an ovarian cyst, and pregnancies outside the uterus. Pain during pregnancy may be caused by the weight of the fetus, or moving the bowels. Contractions during premature labor may cause severe pain. Some diseases that can cause pain include systemic lupus erythematosus, lead poisoning, hypercalcemia, sickle cell anemia, diabetic acidosis, porphyria, tabes dorsalis, and black wid-

ow spider poisoning. An **acute abdomen** is the quick onset of severe pain in the belly. It should be examined right away, because surgery may be needed. Facts about the start, length of time, type of pain, location, and other symptoms are needed so that a correct diagnosis can be made. The nurse or doctor will ask questions about changes in bowel habits, weight loss, bloody stool, diarrhea, color of stool, and what makes the pain better or worse. Constant, increasing pain is often caused by appendicitis or a pouch in the intestines (diverticulitis). However, pain that starts and stops can mean a blockage of the bowel, kidney stones, or gallstones. **Visceral pain** refers to pain caused by any abonormal condition mainly in the stomach and intestines. It is usually strong, scattered, and hard to locate.

abdominal regions, nine parts of the belly, made by four imaginary lines, in a tic-tac-toe pattern. The **epigastric region** is in the upper middle part of the abdomen, just below the breastbone. The **hypochondriac region** is the part of the upper belly on both sides and beneath the lower ribs. The **inguinal region** is the part of the groin surrounding the inguinal canal. The **lateral region** is the part of the abdomen on both sides of the navel. The **pubic region** is in the lowest part of the intestinal area and below the navel. The **umbilical region** is the part of the abdomen around the navel (umbilicus).

abdominal surgery, any operation on the belly, usually done with general anesthesia. Before surgery, blood and urine tests are done. Often an enema is given. The skin is shaved and cleaned. A drug is often given at bedtime to aid sleep. Eating and drinking are not allowed after midnight before surgery. Shortly before surgery a calming drug is usually given, along with a drug to reduce saliva and respiratory secretions. After surgery the patient is checked to be sure all intravenous (IV) tubes and catheters are working. The dressing is checked for bleeding or drainage. The patient is turned from side to side and is helped to cough and breathe deeply. Drugs are given as needed for pain. Some kinds of abdominal surgery are **appendectomy, cholecystectomy, colostomy, gastrectomy, herniorrhaphy, laparotomy.**

abducens nerve /abdoo'sənz/, the sixth cranial nerve, which starts in the brain and goes to the muscle that turns the eye out.

abduction boots, a set of casts for the legs, with a bar joining the casts at ankle level to keep the toes pointed out. This prevents the end of the thigh bone (femur) from moving inside the hip socket. These casts are often used after hip surgery to allow the bone to heal.

abductor, a muscle that allows a body part to move away from the middle of the body, or to move one part away from another. For example, the triceps muscle that straightens the arm is an abductor muscle. Compare **adductor.**

Abernethy's sarcoma, a tumor made up of fat cells that is usually a cancer and occurs on the trunk.

aberrant /aber'ənt/, **1.** not found in the usual or expected course, such as a blood vessel that appears in an unusual place. **2.** describing an abnormal individual.

aberration, **1.** any change from the normal course or condition. **2.** abnormal growth. **3.** a thought or belief lacking reason. **4.** change in the number or structure of genes. **5.** bad image caused by unequal bending of light rays through a lens.

ability, being able to act in a certain way because of having the right skills and mental or physical fitness.

abiotrophy /ab'ē·ot'rəfē/, an early loss of energy or the breakdown of certain parts of the body, usually because of a lack of certain foods. –**abiotrophic,** adj.

abirritant /abir'ətənt/, a drug or substance that relieves irritation.

ablation, the act of cutting off any part of the body, or removal of a growth or damaged tissue.

abnormal behavior, acts that turn aside from normal. These may range from short-term inability to deal with a stress to total withdrawal from the realities of everyday life. See also **behavior disorder.**

abnormal psychology, the study of mental and emotional problems, including neuroses and psychoses. It also includes normal things that are not fully understood, as dreams and other states of consciousness.

aboiement /ä'bô·ämäN'/, uncontrolled animal-like sounds, such as barking. Aboiement may be a symptom of Gilles de Tourette's syndrome.

abort, **1.** to birth a fetus before it can survive or to end a pregnancy before the fetus is able to live. See also **abortion, miscarriage. 2.** to end anything in the early stages, as to stop the course of a disease, to stop growth, or to halt a project.

abortifacient /əbôr'tifā'shənt/, a drug or substance that causes abortion.

abortion, a spontaneous or deliberate ending of pregnancy before the fetus can be expected to live. The end of a pregnancy before the twentieth week is called an **embryonic abortion**. With a **fetal abortion,** the pregnancy ends after the twentieth week but before the fetus is able to live outside of the uterus. The intentional ending of a pregnancy before the fetus has developed enough to live if born is called an **induced abortion.** Twenty to 50% of pregnancies are ended deliberately, at the request of the mother or for medical reasons. Ending of a pregnancy by a trained person under proper conditions is safe. Unskilled abortions can be extremely hazardous because of the danger of infection and damage to the uterus. A **criminal abortion** is the intentional ending of pregnancy under any condition not allowed by law. Infection and excessive bleeding after criminal abortion have been leading causes of maternal death. An **elective abortion** refers to ending a pregnancy by choice of the pregnant woman and performed at her request. A **therapeutic abortion** refers to the ending of pregnancy as thought necessary by a physician.

A **complete abortion** is one in which the fetus or embryo is entirely removed. Because nothing remains in the uterus, a D and C (dilatation and curettage) is not necessary. **Incomplete abortion** refers to an end of pregnancy in which the products of conception are not entirely expelled or removed. It often causes bleeding that may require surgery and blood transfusion. Infection is also a frequent side effect of incomplete abortion. With **habitual abortion,** there is abrupt ending of three pregnancies in a row before week 20. Habitual abortion can result from long-term infection, abnormal fetus, mother's hormone problems, or womb problems. An **infected abortion** is an end of a pregnancy in which the products of conception have become infected. Fever is present and antibiotic therapy and emptying of the uterus is required. A **septic abortion** is one that is needed when the womb becomes infected and threatens the life of the mother. It may happen by itself or it may be done by a doctor. A **missed abortion** is a condition in which a dead embryo or fetus is not released from the uterus for 2 or more months. The uterus becomes smaller and symptoms of pregnancy slow down. Infection and disorders of the clotting of the mother's blood may follow. The fetus and placenta may decay. Less commonly, the fetus becomes hardened calcium and the placenta is absorbed by the uterus. A **tubal abortion** is a condition in which an embryo implants outside of the uterus in the fallopian tube. Tubal abortion may have no symptoms but often results in rupture of the tube, with internal bleeding that causes severe pain. The products of conception may absorb again, but, rarely, the products reimplant on the lining of the abdominal cavity (peritoneum) and continue growing to become an abdominal pregnancy. See also **dilatation and curettage, miscarriage, vacuum aspiration.**

abortion-on-demand, the right of a pregnant woman to have an abortion done at her request.

abortus, a fetus weighing less than 600 g (about 1⅓ pounds) at time of abortion.

abrasion, a scraping or rubbing away of a surface. It may be the result of injury, such as a skinned knee. Compare **laceration.**

abreaction, an emotional release from recalling a painful past event. See also **catharsis.**

abruptio placentae, parting of the placenta from the uterus before birth. It occurs about once in 200 births. Because it often results in severe bleeding, it is serious. If it is not at the end of the pregnancy, the mother rests in bed and is watched carefully. If the pregnancy is close to the end (usually 7 months or more) the baby is often delivered by cesarean section. Compare **placenta previa.**

abscess, a hole filled with pus and surrounded by red, swollen tissue. It forms as a result of a local infection. Healing usually occurs after it drains or is opened. A **cold abscess** is an infection that does not show the usual signs of heat, redness, and swelling.

absorbed dose, the energy imparted to matter by ionizing radiation per unit mass of irradiated material at the place of interest. The unit of absorbed dose is the rad.

absorbifacient /-fā′shənt/, anything that aids absorption.

absorption, **1.** taking one substance into another, as dissolving a gas in a liquid or removing a liquid with a sponge. **2.** substances passing into tissues, as digested food being absorbed into intestinal walls. **3.** taking up of substances through the mucous membranes or skin. **4.** the absorbing of energy rays, such as sunlight, by living or nonliving matter.

absorption rate constant, a value that describes how much drug is taken up by the body in a set amount of time.

abstinence, choosing to avoid some thing or activity, as no food during a religious day.

abulia /əbōō′lyə/, a loss of the ability to act on one's free will or to make decisions.

abuse, **1.** wrong use of equipment, a substance (as a drug), or a service either on purpose or not. See also **drug abuse. 2.** to attack or injure, as in **child abuse.**

abutment, a tooth, root, or implant to support dentures or a bridge.

a.c., abbreviation for *ante cibum,* a Latin phrase meaning before meals.

acalculia /a′kalkōō′lyə/, the inability to solve simple mathematic problems.

acampsia /əkamp′sē·ə/, a defect in which a joint becomes rigid. See also **ankylosis.**

acanthocyte /əkan′thəsīt′/, an abnormal red blood cell with spurlike projections giving it a thorny look. **Acanthocytosis** refers to the presence of acanthocytes in the blood.

acanthoma /ak′ənthō′mə/, any harmless or malignant tumor of the skin.

acanthosis /ak′ənthō′sis-/, a thickening of the skin, as in eczema and psoriasis. With **acanthosis nigricans,** there are dark colored, wartlike areas in the armpit or other body folds like the genital area.

acarbia /akär′bē·ə/, a decrease in the bicarbonate level in the blood.

acariasis /ak′ərī′əsis/, any disease caused by an acarid mite. Several types can infect humans. See also **chigger, scabies.**

acceptable daily intake (ADI), the most of anything that can be safely taken. Taking more than the ADI may cause problems.

acceptor, a person who receives living tissue from another person or organism, such as a blood transfusion. Compare **donor.**

accessory, a structure that serves one of the main systems of the body. For example, the hair, the nails, and the sweat glands are accessories of the skin.

accessory muscle, a muscle that is an exact copy of another. It is usually noticed as a swelling under the skin. Treatment is not necessary if it does not interfere with normal function.

accessory nerve, either of a pair of nerves in the head needed for speech, to swallow, and for certain movements of the head and shoulders. Each nerve has a cranial and a spinal part, connects with certain nerves in the neck, and connects to the brain. Also called **eleventh cranial nerve.**

acclimate /əklī′mit, ak′limāt/, to adjust to a different climate, especially to changes in altitude and weather.

accommodation (A, acc, Acc), the state of adapting to something, such as the ongoing process of a person to adjust to his or her surroundings, both physically and mentally. **Visual accommodation** refers to the way the eye is able to change its focus while seeing things either close up or far away. As the person grows older, the lens of the eye gets harder, and there may be a loss of the ability to focus on nearby things.

accommodation reflex, a change by the eyes for close vision. It includes the pupils getting smaller, the eyes moving together, and focusing. Also called **ciliary reflex.** See also **light reflex.**

accretio cordis /əkrē′shē·ō/, a state in which there is scarlike tissue of the sac (pericardium) covering the heart that has grown to a structure around the heart.

accretion /əkrē'shən/, **1.** growth or increase by adding to something. **2.** the growing together of parts that are normally separated. **3.** the gathering of foreign material, especially within a hole.

Accurbrun, a trademark for a drug to treat bronchial asthma (theophylline).

Accutane, a trademark for a drug to treat acne (isotretinoin).

acebutolol, a drug given for high blood pressure, chest pain (angina), and irregular heart beats. This drug is not given to patients with asthma, heart failure, or blood vessel disease. Side effects include slow heart beat, gas, leg pains, nausea, headache, skin rashes, and dizziness. Also called **butanamide.**

acetabulum /as'ətab'yələm/, *pl.* **acetabula,** the large, cup-shaped, hip socket holding the ball-shaped head of the thigh bone (femur).

acetaldehyde, a colorless liquid with a strong odor. In the body, acetaldehyde is made in the liver. It is also made commercially to make various aromas and flavors. Exposure to high levels of this liquid can cause headache, eye injury, runny nose, and lung problems.

acetaminophen /əset'əmin'əfin/, a pain relieving and fever reducing drug used in many over-the-counter drugs. Known allergy to this drug prohibits its use. Side effects include severe allergy and anemia. Overdose can result in fatal liver failure.

acetanilide, a pain relieving drug that reduces fever and joint swelling in arthritis. Because acetanilide can cause defective red blood cells, it has been replaced by acetaminophen in most cases.

acetazolamide, a drug used for treating fluid buildup (edema), pressure buildup in the eye (glaucoma), and epilepsy.

Acetest, a trademark for tablets used to test urine for abnormal amounts of acetone. Patients with diabetes mellitus can have high levels of this substance in the urine. This test allows patients to check their acetone level at home.

acetoacetic acid /as'ətō·əsē'tik/, a colorless compound that is in normal urine in small amounts and in large amounts in the urine of patients with diabetes mellitus, especially in an acid buildup (ketoacidosis).

acetohexamide, a drug taken by mouth to treat diabetes mellitus when insulin is not required.

acetone /as'ətōn/, a colorless, sweet-smelling liquid found in small amounts in normal urine and in larger amounts in the urine of patients with diabetes.

acetylcholine /as'ətilkō'lēn/, a substance in the body that allows messages to travel from one nerve to another. For example, a person who decides to pick up a pen can act on the thought only when the hand receives the message from the brain. This process in normal persons occurs in a fraction of a second.

acetylcholine chloride, a liquid that causes the pupil of the eye to get smaller during eye surgery. It also reverses the effects of other eye drugs. There are no known reasons not to use the liquid as prescribed. It may cause dry mouth and stomach cramps. Some solutions may cause the lens of the eye to become cloudy.

acetylcholinesterase /-es'tərās/, an enzyme that stops acetylcholine. It reduces or prevents the movement of nerve signals.

acetylsalicylic acid /as'ətilsal'əsil'ik/. See **aspirin.**

achalasia /ak'əlā'zhə/, the inability of a muscle to relax.

Achard-Thiers syndrome /äshär'-tērz'/, a disorder seen in women after menopause who have diabetes. It causes growth of body hair in a male pattern. See also **hirsutism.**

ache, a pain that is steady and dull. An ache may be local, as a stomach ache, headache, or bone ache. It may be general, as the ache of the flu. See also **pain.**

achievement test, a standard test that measures a person's knowledge in many fields of study. The score from an achievement test, divided by the person's actual age and multiplied by 100, is called an **achievement quotient (AQ).**

Achilles tendon /əkil'ēz/, the tendon of the calf muscles. It is the thickest and strongest tendon in the body. It begins near the middle of the back of the leg and connects to the heel bone. Also called **calcaneal tendon.**

Achilles-tendon reflex. See **deep tendon reflex.**

achlorhydria /ā'klôrhī'drē·ə/, a state in which hydrochloric acid is missing from the gastric juice in the stomach. Digestion of protein, such as in meat, is hard for patients with this problem, but otherwise digestion is close to normal.

acholia /əkō'lyə/, **1.** the absence or decrease of bile fluids. **2.** anything that stops the flow of bile from the liver into the small intestine.

acholuria, the lack of bile colors in the urine, indicating a possible liver problem.

achondroplasia /ākon'drōplā'zhə/, an inherited problem with the growth of cartilage in the long bones and skull. The bones fuse too soon. Growth stops and dwarfism results. The most common type of dwarf (achondroplastic) has short limbs, a normal-sized trunk, large head with a sunken nose and small face, stubby hands, and a sway back. Usually these people have normal intelligence.

Achromycin V, a trademark for an antibiotic (tetracycline hydrochloride).

achylia /əkī′lyə/, a lack or not enough of certain chemicals (hydrochloric acid and pepsinogen) needed for digesting food in the stomach.

achylous /əkī′ləs/, **1.** describing a lack of gastric or other digestive juices. **2.** referring to a lack of chyle, a milky fluid made in the intestines during digestion.

acid, 1. a substance that turns blue litmus paper red, has a sour taste, and reacts with bases to form salts. See also **alkali. 2.** *slang.* LSD. See **lysergide.**

acid-base balance, a normal condition in which the body makes acids and bases at the same rate they are removed. See also **acid, base.**

acid-base metabolism, the acts that maintain the balance of acids and bases in the body. When this balance is upset, either too much acid is present (acidosis) or the opposite (alkalosis). Acidosis may be caused by diarrhea, vomiting, kidney disease (uremia), uncontrolled diabetes mellitus, and some drugs. Alkalosis may be caused by too much of an alkaline drug (antacids), vomiting, and some drugs (diuretics) that increase urine production. See also **acidosis, alkalosis, metabolism.**

acid bath, a bath taken in water with a mineral acid. It helps reduce excess sweating.

acid dust, highly acid bits of dust that collect in the air. This is the reason for much of the smog over towns and cities. High levels can be dangerous for patients with lung problems. See also **acid rain.**

acidophilic adenoma /as′idōfil′ik/, a tumor of the pituitary. These can cause the pituitary to make too much growth hormone, causing abnormal growth (gigantism or acromegaly).

acidosis, an abnormal increase in hydrogen in the body from too much acid or the loss of base. The many forms of acidosis are named for the cause. For example, **lactic acidosis** describes a buildup of lactic acid in the blood that causes oxygen starvation in tissues. It may occur after vigorous exercise, or from liver impairment, respiratory failure, tumors, or heart and blood vessel diseases. **Metabolic acidosis** results when excess acid is added to the body fluids or bicarbonate is lost from them. In starvation and in uncontrolled diabetes mellitus, sugar (glucose) is not present or is not available to burn for body fuel. The blood plasma bicarbonate of the body is used up in neutralizing substances (ketones) that result from the breakdown of body fat used for energy in the lack of glucose. Metabolic acidosis also occurs when carbohydrates are burned without enough oxygen, as in heart failure or shock. Excess blood potassium is often seen with the condition. **Renal tubular acidosis** results when the kidney fails to get rid of hydrogen or is unable to use a salt (bicarbonate) properly and to put acid in the urine. Long-term disease can cause excess blood calcium and kidney stones. Depending on the treatment and the amount of kidney damage, the outlook for recovery is often good. Some common signs and symptoms, especially in children, may be loss of appetite, vomiting, constipation, slowed growth, having to urinate often, and rickets. In children and adults it can also cause urinary tract infections. Treatment includes giving sodium bicarbonate tablets, potassium, vitamin D, and antibiotics. Surgery may be needed to remove kidney stones. **Respiratory acidosis** is an abnormal condition with high blood levels of carbon dioxide. A lowered breathing rate slows the release of carbon dioxide, which then joins with water and makes large amounts of an acid (carbonic acid). This causes more acid in the blood. Many disorders can cause it, such as a block in an airway, a muscle disease, chest injuries, pneumonia, and fluid in the lungs. It may also be caused by narcotics, sleeping pills, tranquilizers, or anesthetics, which hold down breathing reflexes. Some common symptoms are headache, breathing difficulty, tremors, rapid heart beat, and high blood pressure. Failed treatment can lead to coma and death. Any block in an airway must be taken out at once. Treatment may include oxygen and drugs. Compare **alkalosis.**

acid-perfusion test, a test of the response of the esophagus to acid. Sensitivity to acid may be caused by stomach acid moving into the esophagus (reflux esophagitis).

acid phosphatase, an enzyme found in the kidneys, blood serum, semen, and prostate. It is higher in serum of patients with cancer of the prostate and in injury victims. See also **alkaline phosphatase.**

acid poisoning, a condition caused by swallowing a toxic acid, such as hydrochloric, nitric, phosphoric, or sulfuric acids. Emergency treatment includes giving large amounts of water or milk to weaken the acid. Vomiting should not be brought on. The victim must be taken quickly to the hospital. Compare **alkali poisoning.**

acid rain, rain with high acid content caused by air pollution from industry, motor vehicles, and other sources. Acid rain is blamed for many health problems, fish kills, and the ruin of timber.

Acidulin, a trademark for a drug used to add hydrochloric acid to the stomach (glutamic acid hydrochloride).

acinus /as′inəs/, *pl.* **acini, 1.** any small saclike structure, as one found in a gland. Also called **alveolus. 2.** a part of the lung.

acmesthesia /ak′misthē′zhə/, the feeling of a pinprick or a sharp point touching the skin.

acne /ak′nē/, a breakout of pimples. It usually occurs in or near the oil glands on the face, neck, shoulders, and upper back. Its cause is not known but involves bacteria that bother the skin. **Acne artificialis** is caused by an external irritation such as tar. It can also be caused by swallowing some irritating substance. **Acne vulgaris** is a common form of acne seen in teenagers and young adults. It is probably caused by male sex hormones working on the oil glands. Bacteria, which live around the hair root, become more active and pimples are formed. **Chronic acne vulgaris** often makes severe scars. Treatment for the various forms of acne may include antibiotics, topical vitamin A, benzyl benzoate, and dermabrasion.

acneform drug eruption, an acnelike skin response to a drug.

acne rosacea. See **rosacea.**

acoria /akôr′ē·ə/, a state of always being hungry even when the desire for food is small.

acousma /əkooz′mə/, hearing strange sounds which are not there.

acoustic, referring to sound or hearing.

acoustic nerve, a pair of nerves in the skull important to hearing. The nerves connect the inner ears with three areas in the brain. Also called **eighth cranial nerve.**

acoustic trauma, a loss of hearing. This can be caused by loud noise over a long time. A sudden loss of hearing may be caused by an explosion, a blow to the head, or other accident. Hearing loss may be for a short time or permanent, partial or total. See also **deafness.**

acquired, referring to a feature, state, or disease that happens after birth. It is not inherited but is a response to the environment. Compare **congenital, familial, hereditary.**

acquired immune deficiency syndrome (AIDS) /ādz/, a disease of the system that fights infection. The problem is found mostly in gay men and intravenous (IV) drug users. AIDS can also occur in women who have sex with bisexual men and in children whose parents have the disease. The cause is thought to be a virus called HTLV-3. This virus is thought to spread through exchange of body fluids, as in sex. The first symptoms are extreme fatigue, fever, night sweats, chills, swollen lymph glands, swollen spleen, loss of appetite with weight loss, severe diarrhea, and depression. As the disease goes on, the patient may become weaker because of many infections. A form of pneumonia (*Pneumocystis carinii*) often occurs, as does inflammation of the cover of the spine (meningitis) or of the brain (encephalitis). Most patients get cancer, especially Kaposi's sarcoma, Burkitt's lymphoma, and non-Hodgkin's lymphoma. Treatment is mainly with chemotherapy. Drugs have been used, with little success. The death rate is 90% for patients who have had the disease more than 2 years.

acrid, sharp, bitter, and unpleasant to the smell or taste.

acrochordon /ak′rōkôr′don/, a harmless skin tag growing on the eyelids or neck or in the armpit or groin.

acrocyanosis /-sīnō′sis/, a problem of the hands and feet, more often the hands. The symptoms are a blue color,

coldness, and sweating of the hands and feet. It is caused by a spasm of the blood vessels and is usually started by cold or by mental stress. Also called **Raynaud's sign.**

acrodermatitis, any breaking out of the skin of the hands and feet caused by a parasitic mite.

acrodermatitis enteropathica, a rare, long-term disease of infants. The symptoms are blisters on the skin and mucous membranes, hair loss, diarrhea, and failure to thrive. It may cause death if not treated.

acrodynia /-din′ē·ə/, a disease in infants and young children. The signs are itching, swelling from water, reddish skin rash on the arms, legs, and face, sweating, stomach upsets, problems with light, crabby times, or no energy. Also called ,**pink disease.**

acromegalic eunuchoidism /-məgal′ik/, a problem in men with a disease that makes the bones in the arms and legs get larger. The signs are wasting of the genitals and breast growth. It is caused by a benign tumor (adenoma) in the pituitary.

acromegaly /-meg′əlē/, a long-term problem in which bones of the face, jaw, arms, and legs get larger. It occurs in middle-aged patients. It is caused by too much growth hormone. Treatment is by x-rays to shrink the pituitary gland or removal of part of it. See also **gigantism, growth hormone.**

acromioclavicular joint /-mī′əkləvik′yələr/, the hinge between the collarbone and shoulder blade.

acromion /əkrō′mē·ən/, the outer part of the shoulder blade. It forms the highest point of the shoulder and connects with the collarbone.

acroparesthesia /-per′isthē′zhə/, very sensitive arms or legs. It is often caused by pressure or irritation of the nerves. The signs are tingling, numbness, and stiffness in the fingers, hands, and forearms.

acrophobia, a fear of high places that does not make sense and causes one to be very nervous. See also **phobia.**

ACTH. See **adrenocorticotropic hormone.**

Acthar, a trademark for a drug used to treat arthritis and allergies (corticotropin).

Actidil, a trademark for a drug used to treat allergies (triprolidine hydrochloride).

Actifed, a trademark for a drug used to treat allergies and hay fever (pseudoephedrine hydrochloride and triprolidine hydrochloride).

actin, a protein found in muscles that helps them tighten and relax.

acting out, showing mental pain in acts that are usually slightly crazy and uptight. Acting out may be destructive or harmful. See also **transference.**

actinomycosis /ak′tinōmīkō′sis/, a long-term problem that causes deep, lumpy holes with a thin, grainy pus. It is

A–B

seen most often in patients who live in the country. It is caused by a germ (*Actinomyces israelii*) that normally lives in the bowel and mouth.

activated charcoal, a general-purpose antidote used to treat poisoning and to control intestinal gas. There are no known serious side effects or other reasons for not using it, but activated charcoal does not work for poisoning caused by a strong acid or base or by cyanide.

activated partial thromboplastin time (APTT), a timed blood test for the speed of clotting. This test is used to learn about clotting problems.

activator, 1. a substance, force, or device that prompts activity of something. **2.** a device worn in the mouth that works on the muscles around the mouth.

active specific immunotherapy, a treatment for cancer in which the patient is injected with irradiated tumor cells. The injected cells promote the making of antibodies that kill the tumor cells.

activities of daily living (ADL), normal, everyday actions, as eating, dressing, washing, or brushing the teeth. Accidents or illnesses may make it hard to do these.

activity, the word used to describe the rate at which the particular material is decaying. It is generally expressed in terms of the average number of nuclear disintegrations per second. Since this number is generally large, it is given in units of curies or fractions thereof. See also **curie.**

activity intolerance, a condition of general weakness, sitting much of the time, oxygen imbalance, or bed rest. The patient may have weakness, fast heart rate, blood pressure changes, and shortness of breath when activity is tried.

actual charge, the amount charged by a medical person for a service. This may not be the same as that paid by an insurance plan.

acuity /əkyōo'itē/, the clearness or sharpness of one of the senses, as visual acuity.

acupressure, a therapy of putting pressure on set points of the body. It is used to relieve pain or control a body function.

acupuncture, a therapy for relieving pain or changing a function of the body. Thin needles are put into the skin at set places along a series of lines called meridians. Sometimes the needles are twirled, given a slight electric charge, or warmed.

acupuncture point, a point on the skin along the meridians, or lines, of the body.

acute, 1. beginning quickly and intense or sharp, then slowing after a short time. **2.** sharp or severe. Compare **chronic.**

acute care, treatment for a serious illness, for an accident, or after surgery. It is usually given in a hospital by trained persons. It may also involve intensive care. This kind of care is usually for only a short time. Compare **chronic care.**

acute health hazard, marked by a single dose or exposure generally having a sudden onset for a course of time (e.g., acute toxicity, acute exposure).

acute lymphocytic leukemia (ALL). See **leukemia.**

acute myelocytic leukemia (AML). See **leukemia.**

acyclovir, an antiviral drug used to treat herpes, including genital herpes (acycloguanosine). It is an ointment for treating herpes of the eye (herpes simplex keratitis) and other types of herpes. Acyclovir does not work on other viral infections. Known allergy to this drug prohibits its use. The ointment may cause itching. The form taken by mouth may cause too much sweating, headache, and nausea.

adactyly /ādak'tilē/, a birth defect in which one or more fingers or toes are missing.

Adam's apple, *informal.* the bulge at the front of the neck made by the thyroid cartilage of the voice box. Also called **laryngeal prominence.**

Adams-Stokes syndrome. See **heart block.**

adaptation, a change or response to stress of any kind.

addiction, a great need for something. Stopping is very hard and there is usually a severe response. Compare **habituation.**

Addison's disease, a life-threatening disease caused by partial or complete failure of the adrenal gland. This gland makes many hormones that control many body functions. Symptoms are weakness, darkening of the skin, lack of appetite, loss of water, weight loss, and stomach and intestine problems. Other symptoms are anxiety, depression, and sensitivity to cold. The onset is usually gradual, over a period of weeks or months. Causes include autoimmune diseases, infection, tumor, or bleeding in the adrenal gland. Treatment includes replacing the natural hormones with glucocorticoid and mineralocorticoid drugs, drinking more fluids, control of salt and potassium, and a diet high in carbohydrate and protein.

adduction, movement of a limb toward the body. Compare **abduction.**

adductor, a muscle that acts to draw a part toward the midline of the body. The **adductor brevis** is a triangular muscle in the thigh. It acts to pull and turn the thigh to the center of the body and to bend the leg. The **adductor longus** is the top-most of the three adductor muscles of the thigh. It flexes the thigh. The **adductor magnus** is the long, heavy, triangular muscle of the middle of the thigh. It turns the thigh to the center of the body and bends it on the hip. The lower section straightens the thigh and turns it to the side. Compare **abductor, tensor.**

adenectomy /ad'ənek'təmē/, the removal by surgery of any gland.

adenitis /ad′ənī′tis/, an inflammation of a lymph gland. Serious adenitis in the neck causes a sore throat and stiff neck. It can look like mumps. In the belly, the disorder is often painful and may cause symptoms like appendicitis.

adenoacanthoma /ad′ənō-ak′anthō′mə/, a tumor that may be cancerous or harmless, made from gland tissue.

adenocarcinoma, any one of a large group of cancerous tumors of the glands. The types of tumors are named for the tissue. For example, **acinic cell adenocarcinoma,** an uncommon cancer, usually grows in the salivary glands. **Adenocarcinoma in situ** refers to a growth of abnormal gland tissue that may become cancerous. It is most common in the lining of the uterus (endometrium) and in the large intestine. **Follicular adenocarcinoma** is a cancer that usually comes from the thyroid gland. It has a tendency to spread to the lungs and bones. **Papillary adenocarcinoma** is a cancer with small bumps (papillae) of connective tissue with blood vessels that reach into organ spaces (follicles), glands, or cysts. The tumor is most common in the ovaries and thyroid gland.

adenocyst /ad′ənōsist′/, a harmless tumor in which the cells form glandlike lumps (cysts).

adenocystic carcinoma, a cancerous tumor that occurs most often in the salivary glands, breast, and mucous glands of the upper and lower breathing tract.

adenofibroma /-fībrō′mə/, a tumor of the connective tissues that contains glandlike parts.

adenoid /ad′ənoid/, one of two masses of spongy lymph tissue (pharyngeal tonsil) on the back wall of the throat, behind the nasal space. During childhood these masses often swell with infected material and block air passing from the nose to the throat, preventing the child from breathing through the nose.

adenoidal speech, a muted, nasal way of speaking caused by large adenoids. This usually occurs in children. It is fixed by removal.

adenoidectomy /-ek′-/, removal of the adenoids. Surgery is done because the adenoids are large, cause blockage, or are infected. Normal adenoids may be removed with the tonsils. Before surgery blood tests are done to check blood clotting. A sickle cell test is done for black patients. A general anesthesia is used in children, but local anesthesia may be used in adults. See also **tonsillectomy.**

adenoma /ad′ənō′mə/, a tumor that grows from gland tissue or shows glandlike structure. This may cause a gland to secrete a great deal. An example is a **chromophobic adenoma,** a tumor of the pituitary gland. Diabetes insipidus and other conditions caused by lack of one or more pituitary hormones are linked to this tumor. A disorder in which two or more glands grow tumors is called **adenomatosis.** The most common glands in which this occurs are the thyroid, adrenals, and pituitary.

adenomyoma /-mī·ō′mə/, a tumor of the lining (endometrium) of the womb. It usually causes menstrual cramps (dysmenorrhea).

adenomyosis /-mī·ō′-/, **1.** a condition with harmless tumors made of gland tissue and muscle cells. **2.** a cancerous state of tumors in the wall of the womb or the ducts from the ovary to the womb (oviducts).

adenopathy /ad′ənop′əthē/, a growth of any gland, especially a lymph gland. **–adenopathic,** *adj.*

adenosarcoma, a cancerous glandlike tumor of the soft tissues of the body.

adenovirus, a virus that causes problems with upper lung infection, or stomach and intestine infection.

adermia /ədur′mē·ə/, defect in or lack of skin. This state may be a birth defect or it may be acquired.

adhesion, a band of scar tissue that binds two surfaces normally apart from each other. This occurs most commonly in the belly after surgery, inflammation, or injury. More surgery may be needed to pull apart the tissues.

Adie's syndrome, a disorder of the eyes in which one pupil reacts much more slowly to light or focusing than the other (tonic pupil). There are also slowed or no tendon reflexes, in particular the ankle and knee-jerk reflexes.

adiphenine hydrochloride, a drug that relaxes smooth muscles, which are in most organs. It is used for treating spasms of the intestines and urinary tract. Side effects include widening of the pupils and dry mouth.

adipocele /ad′ipōsel′/, a loop of an organ or tissue through an opening and holding fat or fatty tissue. Also called **lipocele.**

adiponecrosis /-nikrō′-/, breaking down of fatty tissue in the body. **–adiponecrotic,** *adj.*

adiponecrosis subcutanea neonatorum, skin of newborns with patchy spots of hard fatty tissue and bluish-red bruises. It is often a result of delivery, and it clears up in a few days.

adipose /ad′ipōs/, fatty. Adipose tissue is made of fat cells arranged in lobes. See also **fat, fatty acid, lipoma.**

adipose tumor. See **lipoma.**

adipsia /ədip′sē·ə/, lack of thirst.

adjunctive psychotherapy, a form of therapy that works on improving a person's outlook without trying to solve basic emotional problems. Some kinds are **occupational therapy, physical therapy, recreational therapy.**

adjunct to anesthesia, any drug given before or during surgery that aids the patient's comfort and safety. Drugs may be given before surgery to calm the patient, reduce mouth watering and secretions of the lungs, and prevent slowed heart beat. During surgery hypnotic and pain-killing drugs are given to help the effects of other drugs. Drugs are given to relax the muscles during surgery. Drugs that excite the nerves (analeptics) are given after surgery to

A–E

reverse the effects of the anesthetic. Carbon dioxide and oxygen are given to maintain normal breathing.

adjustment reaction, a sudden, short-term response to great stress in people who have no mental illness. It may occur at any age and can be mild or severe. Symptoms include worry, withdrawal, depression, brooding, temper outbursts, crying spells, acting out to get attention, bed wetting, loss of appetite, aches, pains, and muscle spasms. See also **neurotic disorder.**

adjuvant therapy /ad′jəvənt/, the treatment of a disease with substances that help the action of drugs. The term is used to describe drugs that help the body produce antibodies.

adnexa, *sing.* **adnexus,** tissue or structures in the body that are next to or near another structure. The ovaries and the uterine tubes are adnexa of the uterus, for example.

adnexitis, an inflammation of the adnexal organs of the uterus, such as the ovaries or the fallopian tubes.

adolescence, the time in growth between the onset of sexual maturity (puberty) and adulthood. It usually begins between 11 and 13 years of age, when breast growth, beard growth, pubic hair growth, and other related changes occur (secondary sex characteristics). It spans the teen years, and ends at 18 to 20 years of age when the person has a fully developed adult body. During this time the person (adolescent) undergoes great physical, psychologic, emotional, and personality changes. See also **puberty.**

adrenal cortical carcinoma /ədrē′nəl/, a cancerous tumor of the adrenal cortex. Such tumors vary in size, occur at any age, and are more common in females than in males. The cancer often spreads to the lungs, liver, and other organs. See also **adrenogenital syndrome, Cushing's syndrome.**

adrenal crisis, a sudden, life-threatening lack of a hormone (glucocorticoid) made by the adrenal cortex. There is a drop in fluids, such as blood, urine, and saliva, and high potassium levels in the blood (hyperkalemia). The patient seems to be in shock or coma with a low blood pressure and loss of pulses. The patient may have Addison's disease. An intravenous (IV) solution of sodium chloride with the hormone glucocorticoid is given right away. Drugs may be needed to correct the low blood pressure. After the first crucial hours the patient is treated for Addison's disease and the steroid is given at lower doses. The reason for the adrenal crisis is not known. Infection and a failure to increase the steroid dose is a common cause of crisis in patients who have Addison's disease.

adrenalectomy /-ek′-/, removal of one or both adrenal glands, or part of the gland. This lowers the excess secretion of adrenal hormones when there is an adrenal tumor or a cancer of the breast or prostate. Steroids are given by mouth for a few days after surgery. When both glands are taken out, the steroids are given for life. Stress and fatigue must be avoided. See also **Addison's disease, Cushing's syndrome.**

adrenal gland, the organ that sits on top of each kidney. The gland has two parts: the cortex and the medulla. The **adrenal cortex** is the outer part of the gland. It is divided into three parts. The **zona glomerulosa** is the outer portion of the adrenal cortex. The middle part (**zona fasciculata**) acts together with the innermost part (**zona reticularis**) in making male sex hormones (androgens) and some female sex hormones (estrogen and progesterone). They also produce hormones (aldosterone and hydrocortisone) that help in the body's water balance. The inner part of the gland is the **adrenal medulla**. It makes epinephrine (adrenaline) and norepinephrine. These regulate blood pressure and heart rate.

Adrenalin, a trademark for a drug used to treat severe allerges, spasms of the large air channels of the lungs (bronchial spasms), and a clogged nose and throat (epinephrine).

adrenaline /ədren′əlin/. See **epinephrine.**

adrenalize /ədrē′nəlīz/, to stimulate or excite.

adrenergic /ad′rinur′jik/, referring to nerves that release epinephrine or epinephrine-like substances. Compare **cholinergic.** See also **sympathomimetic.**

adrenergic blocking agent. See **antiadrenergic.**

adrenergic drug. See **sympathomimetic.**

adrenocorticotropic hormone (ACTH), a hormone made by the pituitary gland. It stimulates the growth of the adrenal gland cortex and its secretion of corticosteroids. ACTH secretion is controlled by the hypothalamus gland. ACTH increases when a patient has stress, fever, sudden low blood sugar, and major surgery. Commercially made ACTH is used to treat rheumatoid arthritis, severe allergy, skin diseases, and many other disorders. Also called **corticotropin.**

adult day care center, a place for the supervised care of older adults. These centers provide services as meals and company during set day hours. The people go to their homes each night.

adulteration, a lowering of quality and purity of any substance, process, or act.

adult respiratory distress syndrome (ARDS), an emergency caused by failure of the lungs to work. This may follow heart and lung bypass surgery, severe infection, blood transfusions, too much oxygen, injury, pneumonia, or other lung infections. It may also occur in Guillain-Barré syndrome, muscular dystrophy, myasthenia gravis, emphysema, asthma, or polio. Symptoms include shortness of breath, falling blood pressure, and a blue skin color (cyanosis) from lack of oxygen. Tests of the blood show low amounts of oxygen and more carbon dioxide in the blood. The changes that occur within the lungs may include damage to the very small blood vessels, bleeding, and swelling. Treatment includes mechanical assistance with breathing. Oxygen, mist, and respiratory therapy are also used.

adventitious, referring to a state that is brought on by accident or to a random action.

adventitious bursa, a defect of the liquid sacs in a joint that is due to rubbing or pressure.

adverse drug effect, a harmful side effect of a drug given in normal amounts.

adynamia /ad′īnā′mē·ə/, physical and mental fatigue caused by a disease.

adynamia episodica hereditaria, a rare inherited defect seen in infants. The patient may suffer from attacks of muscle weakness and be unable to move. The drug acetazolamide is often given to prevent the attacks.

aerate /er′āt/, to add air, carbon dioxide, or oxygen to a substance.

aerial torch, an ignition device suspended under a helicopter, capable of dispensing ignited fuel to the ground for assistance in burnout or backfiring.

aerobe /er′ōb/, a tiny organism that needs oxygen to live and grow. Compare **anaerobe.**

aerobic exercise, any physical exercise that makes the heart and lungs work harder to meet the muscles' need for oxygen. The exercise causes harder breathing than light exercise and improves the heart and lungs. Running, bicycling, swimming, and cross-country skiing are types of aerobic exercise. Also called **aerobics.** See also **exercise.**

aerodontalgia /er′ōdontal′jə/, a pain in the teeth caused by air trapped in the teeth when the air pressure changes, as may occur at high altitudes.

aerophagia /er′ōfā′jə/, swallowing air, often leading to belching, stomach upset, and gas.

aerosinusitis, soreness, inflammation, or bleeding of the sinuses. It is caused when air expands in the sinuses. This occurs when air pressure goes down. Also called **barosinusitis.**

aerosol, **1.** small particles in a gas or air. **2.** a gas under pressure that contains a drug which is breathed in. Drugs for asthma attacks and problems in the canals of the nose are often given in aerosols.

Aerosporin, a trademark for an antibiotic used to treat meningitis, liver infection, blood poisoning due to bacteria (septicemia), and infections of the ear, lungs, urinary tract, and joints (polymyxin B sulfate).

aerotitis media, soreness or bleeding in the middle ear. It is caused by a difference between the air pressure in the middle ear and the air outside. This can occur with quick changes in altitude, in diving, or in pressure chambers.

Symptoms are pain, ringing in the ear (tinnitus), trouble hearing, and dizziness (vertigo). Also called **barotitis media.**

affect, the way in which a person's feelings are shown. **–affective,** *adj.*

afferent /af′ərənt/, moving toward the center of an organ or system. This usually refers to blood vessels, lymph channels, and nerves. Compare **efferent.**

afibrinogenemia /əfī′brinōjənē′mē·ə/, a rare blood disorder known by a low or absent clotting factor in the blood (fibrinogen).

aflatoxins, a group of cancer-causing, poisonous factors made by *Aspergillus flavus* food molds. These poisons cause liver death (necrosis) and liver cancer in test animals. Aflatoxins are thought to be the cause of the high rate of liver cancer in people in regions of Africa and Asia who may eat moldy grains, peanuts, or other *Aspergillus* infected foods. See also **aspergillosis.**

African sleeping sickness. See **trypanosomiasis.**

Afrin, a trademark for a drug that clears the nose and decreases stuffiness for easy breathing (oxymetazoline hydrochloride).

afterbirth, the material expelled from the womb after a baby is born.

aftercare, health care after release from a hospital. A patient may need care for a health problem that no longer requires hospital care.

afterload, the pressure against which the left lower chamber of the heart (ventricle) must eject the blood during a beat. The presssure is made by the amount of blood that is already flowing and the vessel walls themselves. About 90% of the oxygen needed by the heart is used in the afterload effort.

afterpains, cramps that often occur in the first days after giving birth.

agammaglobulinemia /əgam′əglob′yəlinē′mē·ə/, a rare defect in which there is not enough gamma globulin in the blood. This increases the chances of infection. The disorder may be temporary. inborn, or acquired. When present at birth, it is called **Bruton's agammaglobulinemia.**

agency representative, an individual assigned to an incident from an assisting or cooperating agency who has been delegated full authority to make decisions on all matters affecting that agency's participation at the incident. Agency representatives report to the incident liaison officer.

agenesia corticalis /ā′jənē′zhə/, the failure of some of the brain cells to grow in the embryo. It causes loss of motor function in the brain of the infant (infantile cerebral paralysis), and severe mental retardation.

agenesis /ājen′əsis/, **1.** birth without an organ or part. **2.** the state of being unable to reproduce (sterility) or maintain an erection (impotence). Also called **agenesia.** Compare **dysgenesis.** –**agenic,** *adj.*

agenetic fracture /ā′jənet′ik/, a bone break caused by faulty bone growth.

ageniocephaly /ājen′ē·ōsef′əlē/, faulty skull growth in which the brain, skull, and sense organs are normal but the lower jaw is malformed.

agenitalism /ājen′itəlizm/, the absence of the ovaries or testicles or problems of function. It is caused by lack of sex hormones.

agenosomia /ājen′əsō′mē·ə/, a birth defect in which the genitals are defective or missing, and the intestines stick out through the abdominal wall.

Agent Orange, a U.S. military code name for a mixture of two chemicals, 2,4-D and 2,4,5-T, used to kill crops in Southeast Asia during the war in Vietnam. The chemical mix contained the highly poisonous chemical dioxin. This chemical causes cancer and birth defects in animals and chloracne and slight or severe long-term scarring (porphyria cutanea tarda) in humans. See also **dioxin.**

agglutinin /əgloo′tinin/, a kind of defender cell (antibody) that interacts with foreign invaders (antigens) by agglutination. **Cold agglutinin** refers to a substance that causes red blood cells to clump at temperatures below 39°F (4° C). It may also break down the red blood cells. This does not occur when the body is at its normal temperature.

aggression, physical, verbal, or symbolic act or attitude that is carried out with force and assertion of the self. **Destructive aggression** is an act of hostility that is not needed for self-protection. It is directed toward an object or person. **Inward aggression** is destructive behavior against oneself.

aggressive personality, type of person who is quick to anger, has tantrums, and is destructive or violent when frustrated.

aging, the process of growing old, caused in part by a failure of body cells to work normally or to make new cells to replace those that are dead or defective. Normal cells may be lost through infection, poor nutrition, contact with health hazards, or gene problems. The **developmental theory of aging** refers to the idea that characteristics developed early in life tend to last into the later years. The **immunologic theory of aging** is the belief that normal cells are not recognized as such by the body's immune system, thereby triggering immune reactions within the person's own body. See also **assessment of the aging patient, senile.**

agitated, being in a state of physical and mental excitement known by restless actions that have no purpose.

agitophasia /-fā′zhə/, too rapid speech in which words, sounds, or parts of words are left out, slurred, or distorted. Also called **agitolalia.**

agnosia /agnō′zhə/, total or partial loss of the ability to know familiar objects or persons, due to brain damage. The state may affect any of the senses and is therefore noted as hearing (auditory), sight (visual), smell (olfactory), taste (gustatory), or touch (tactile) agnosia. **Body-image agnosia** is an inability to recognize and identify the parts of one's own body. It is diagnosed when a person is unable to perform a task such as touching the right ear with the left thumb.

agonal respiration /ag′ənəl/, a type of breathing pattern of gasping, followed by no breathing. It often means the onset of lung failure.

agonist /ag′ənist/, **1.** a contracting muscle that is opposed by another muscle (an antagonist). **2.** a drug or other substance that causes a response that can be known in advance.

agoraphobia /ag′ərə-/, mental defect in which the patient is afraid to be alone in an open, crowded, or public place, as a field, tunnel, bridge, busy street, or store, where escape may be hard or help may not be at hand. The disorder can sometimes be treated with success through psychiatric help.

agranulocytosis /əgran′yəlōsītō′-/, a sudden condition of the blood. There is a severe decrease in the number of a type of white blood cells (granulocyte). This results in fever, severe fatigue, and bleeding sores of the rectum, mouth, and vagina. It can occur as a side effect to a drug or be the result of radiation therapy.

agraphia /əgraf′ē·ə/, a nerve defect in which the person can no longer write. This can be caused by injury to the language center in the brain.

agrypnotic /ag′ripnot′ik/, a drug or other substance that prevents sleep.

AIDS. See **acquired immune deficiency syndrome.**

air, the clear gas with no odor that surrounds the earth. It is made of 78% nitrogen, 21% oxygen, almost 1% argon, small amounts of carbon dioxide, hydrogen, and ozone, traces of helium, krypton, neon, and xenon, and amounts of water vapor that vary.

air cylinder, a metal tank in which is carried an SCBAs supply of compressed breathing air.

air purifier, an air-purification system for compressed breathing air.

airplane splint, a method used to prevent a broken arm from moving while it heals. The splint holds the arm up at shoulder level, with the elbow bent.

air tanker, any fixed-wing aircraft certified by the FAA as being capable of transporting and delivering fire-retardant solutions.

airway, any tube that allows air to move into and out of the lungs. Examples are tubes on an anesthesia machine, a tube used for mouth-to-mouth resuscitation, and the nose, mouth, and throat.

airway obstruction, anything that blocks the windpipe and will not let oxygen enter or be absorbed by the lungs. Causes include choking, croup, goiter, tumor, and other severe lung disorders. If the blockage is minor, the patient is able to breathe, but not normally. If the blockage is severe, the patient may grasp the neck, gasp, become blue (cyanotic), and faint. Severe airway obstruction is a life-threatening emergency. Food, mucus, or a foreign object may be removed by hand, by suction, or with the Heimlich maneuver. Blockage of the airway due to swelling or allergies may be treated with drugs to open the passages, by inserting a tube to open the airway, and by giving oxygen. Inserting a tube through a cut in the throat (tracheotomy) may be needed if the blockage cannot be cleared within a few minutes. See also **aspiration, cardiopulmonary resuscitation, Heimlich maneuver.**

akinesia /ā′kinē′zhə/, an abnormal state of physical and mental inactivity or inability to move the muscles.

Akineton, a trademark for a drug (biperiden hydrochloride or biperiden lactate) used to treat a nervous system disorder (parkinsonism).

ala /ā′lə/, *pl.* **alae,** any winglike structure.

alanine (Ala) /al′ənin/, an amino acid found in many proteins in the body. It is broken down by the liver. See also **amino acid, protein.**

alanine aminotransferase (ALT), an enzyme normally present in the clear liquid part of the blood (serum) and tissues of the body, specially the tissues of the liver. The level may grow in patients with severe liver damage. Also called **glutamic-pyruvic transaminase.**

Al-Anon, a worldwide group. They give help and guidance to people who have alcoholics in their lives (families, friends, coworkers). See also **Alcoholics Anonymous.**

alar ligament /ā′lər/, one of a pair of ligaments that joins the cervical vertebra (axis) to the occipital bone at the base of the skull and limits turning of the head.

alarm reaction, the first stage of adapting. One uses the many defenses of the body or the mind to cope with a stress. See also **stress.**

Alateen, a worldwide group. They give help and guidance to the children of alcoholics. See also **Alcoholics Anonymous.**

albinism /al′binizm/, a birth defect marked by partial or total lack of pigment in the body. Total albinos have pale skin that does not tan, white hair, pink eyes, and other eye problems. Compare **piebald, vitiligo.**

Albright's syndrome, a state in which parts of the bone act like tumors, brown spots form on the skin, and hormones do not work right. It causes very early puberty in girls but not in boys.

albumin /albyoo′min/, a protein found in almost all animal tissues and in many plant tissues. Amounts and types of albumin in urine, blood, and other body tissues form the basis of many laboratory tests.

albumin A, a blood serum substance that gathers in cancer cells but does not circulate in cancer patients.

albumin (human), a substance that expands the volume of blood and is used for treating hypoproteinemia, hyperbilirubinemia, and hypovolemic shock. Severe iron-poor blood (anemia) or heart failure prohibits its use. Side effects include chills, low blood pressure, fever, and itching.

albuterol, a drug used to treat spasms in the windpipe in patients with obstructive airway disease. Known allergy to this drug prohibits its use. Side effects include rapid heart beat, inability to sleep (insomnia), dizziness, and high blood pressure.

Alcaine, a trademark for a local numbing drug (proparacaine).

Alcock's canal, a canal formed by the muscles in the pelvis (obturator internus muscle and the obturator fascia). The nerve and vessels effecting the outer sex organs pass through the canal. Also called **pudendal canal.**

alcohol, **1.** (*USP*) a liquid that contains between 92.3% and 93.8% ethyl alcohol. It is used as a skin cleaner and solvent. **2.** a clear, colorless liquid that is made by brewing sugar with yeast. Examples are beer and whiskey. **3.** a compound derived from a hydrocarbon.

alcohol bath, a way to lower a high body temperature. Alcohol is mixed with an equal amount of warm water. The patient is sponged on the arms and legs, then on the trunk. A hot-water bottle can be placed at the feet and a cold cloth on the head to speed up heat loss, to make the patient feel better, and to reduce the heat of the blood flowing to the brain.

Alcoholics Anonymous (AA), a worldwide nonprofit group, founded in 1935, whose members are alcoholics who no longer drink. The purpose of AA is to help others stop drinking and stay sober.

alcoholism, the extreme dependence on alcohol that is marked by bad behavior. It is a long-term illness that starts slowly and may occur at any age. The most frequent medical problems are mental changes and breakdown (cirrhosis) of the liver. The problems are worse when not enough food has been eaten. Patients may suffer from belly problems (gastritis), nerve damage, hearing things that are not there, and heart problems. **Alcoholic-nutritional cerebellar degeneration** is a sudden loss of ability to move the legs together, as seen in poorly nourished alcoholics. The patient walks, if at all, with the legs far apart. An **alcoholic psychosis** is any severe mental disorder, such as delirium tremens, or Korsakoff's psychosis, that is caused by brain damage from too much alcohol. **Alcohol withdrawal syndrome** refers to the symptoms that come with suddenly not drinking alcohol. These may include trembling muscles, seeing and hearing things that are not there, nervous system problems, and seizures. Caution must be used in giving drugs to the patient, because side effects with alcohol are common. Chronic alcoholism is a condition that results from the regular use of alcohol in extreme amounts. This disease involves complex cultural, social, and physical factors. Withdrawal from alcohol should be done in a hospital because withdrawal symptoms can be severe. These may include trembling muscles, weakness, sweating, and delirium. Death can also result. The treatment of alcoholism consists of mental therapy (such as in Alcoholics Anonymous), electroshock treatments, or drugs, as disulfiram, that cause one to not want any alcohol. See also **delirium tremens.**

alcohol poisoning, poisoning caused by drinking alcohol, as ethyl, isopropyl, or methyl. Ethyl alcohol (grain alcohol) is in whiskies, brandy, gin, and other drinks. In most cases, it is lethal only if large amounts are drunk in a short time. Isopropyl alcohol, found in cosmetics and solvents, is more poisonous, and drinking 8 ounces may cause breathing or heart failure. Methyl alcohol (wood alcohol) is very poisonous. It may cause nausea, vomiting, belly pain, and blindness. Death may come after drinking only 2 ounces. Treatment includes pumping the belly, giving baking soda and sugar through the veins, and, if necessary, blood dialysis (hemodialysis).

Aldactazide, a trademark for a drug that causes one to empty the bladder. It has two diuretics (hydrochlorothiazide and spironolactone). It is used for treating high blood pressure and to reduce fluids.

Aldactone, a trademark for a diuretic (spironolactone).

aldolase /al'dəlās/, an enzyme in muscle tissue that is necessary for storing energy in the cells.

Aldomet, a trademark for a drug used for treating high blood pressure (methyldopa).

Aldoril, a trademark for a drug that is used to treat too much fluid in the body (diuretichydroclorothiazide) and high blood pressure (antihypertensive-methyldopa).

aldosterone /al'dōstərōn', aldos'tərōn/, a steroid hormone made by the adrenal cortex that controls sodium and potassium in the blood. See also **adrenal gland.**

aldosteronism /al'dōstərō'nizm/, a state in which too much aldosterone is made. This can occur from a disease of the adrenal cortex or a response caused by another disorder, such as liver disease, burns, or other kinds of stress. Too much aldosterone causes the body to keep salt and get rid of potassium. Symptoms include increased blood pressure, weakness, muscle contractions (tetany), numbness

(paresthesias), kidney disease (nephropathy), and heart failure. Also called **hyperaldosteronism.**

aldosteronoma /al'dōstir'ənō'mə/, an aldosterone-secreting tumor (adenoma) of the adrenal cortex that causes the body to retain salt, increased blood volume, and high blood pressure.

aleukemic leukemia /ālookē'-/, a type of leukemia in which the white blood cell (leukocyte) count is normal and few abnormal leukocytes are found in the blood. Also called **subleukemic leukemia.** See also **leukemia.**

aleukia /āloo'kē-ə/, a marked decrease or total lack of white blood cells or blood platelets.

alexia /ələk'sē-ə/, a nervous system defect, in which the person cannot understand written words. Compare **dyslexia.** –**alexic,** adj.

algologist, /algol'-/, **1.** a person who studies or treats pain. **2.** also called **phycologist.** A person who studies water plants (algae).

alienation, the act or feeling of being separated from others or isolated. See also **depersonalization disorder.**

alimentary canal. See **digestive system.**

alkali /al'kəlī/, a compound with the chemical qualities of a base. Alkalis join with fatty acids to make soaps, turn red litmus paper blue, and enter into chemical reactions. See also **acid, base.** –**alkaline,** adj.; **alkalinity,** n.

alkali burn. See **burn.**

alkaline-ash /al'kəlin/, substance in the urine that has a pH higher than 7.

alkaline-ash producing foods, foods that are eaten to make an alkaline pH in the urine, reducing the chance of stones (calculi) forming in the urinary tract. Some of the foods that result in alkaline ash are milk, cream, buttermilk, fruit (except prunes, plums, and cranberries), vegetables (except corn and lentils), almonds, chestnuts, coconuts, and olives.

alkaline bath, a bath in which sodium bicarbonate is mixed in the water. This is used for skin problems.

alkaline phosphatase, an enzyme in bone, the kidneys, the intestine, blood plasma, and teeth. It may be present in the blood serum in high levels in some diseases of the bone or liver, and in some other illnesses.

alkali poisoning, a poisoning caused by swallowing an alkaline agent, as ammonia, lye, and some soap powders. Emergency treatment includes giving large amounts of water or milk to water down the alkali. The patient must not vomit, and mild acids should not be given. The patient is taken without delay to the hospital to watch for any damage to the esophagus, and for flushing out the stomach. Compare **acid poisoning.**

alkaloid, any of a large group of organic compounds made by plants or made synthetically. Examples include many drugs, as atropine, caffeine, cocaine, morphine, nicotine, and quinine. The term also may be applied to some synthetic chemicals, as procaine.

alkalosis, a disorder of body fluids and tissues in which there is too much alkali. **Hypochloremic alkalosis** is an increase in the body's alkalinity resulting from increased blood bicarbonate and loss of chloride from the body. **Hypokalemic alkalosis** results from the buildup of alkalinity or the loss of acid from the body associated with a low level of potassium in the blood. **Metabolic alkalosis** occurs with great loss of acid in the body or by increased levels of base bicarbonate. The acid loss may be caused by heavy vomiting, not enough replacement of minerals, or too many adrenal hormones. The condition may also be caused by using too much baking soda (bicarbonate of soda) and other antacids during the treatment of peptic ulcers. Symptoms include breathing difficulty, headache, drowsiness, irritability, nausea, vomiting, and rapid heart beat. Severe, untreated metabolic alkalosis can lead to coma and death. **Respiratory alkalosis** occurs with low blood levels of carbon dioxide and large amounts of alkali in the blood. Causes include asthma, pneumonia, aspirin poisoning, anxiety, fever, blood poisoning, and liver failure. Deep and rapid breathing at rates as high as 40 breaths per minute is a major sign. Other symptoms are light-headedness, dizziness, numbness or spasms of the hands and the feet, muscle weakness, and an irregular heart beat. Treatment includes removing the cause. Severe cases, as those caused by excess anxiety, may be treated by having the patient breathe into a paper bag and breathe in exhaled carbon dioxide to make up for the loss. Sedatives may also be given to slow the breathing rate. Treatment of alkalosis restores the normal acid-base balance. Compare **acidosis.**

Alkeran, a trademark for a drug used to treat cancer (melphalan).

alkylating agent /al'kilā'ting/, a drug that causes a chemical process to disrupt cell division, especially in fast-growing tissue. Such drugs are very useful in the treatment of cancer. The types of alkylating agents used in medicine are the alkyl sulfonates, the ethylenimines, the nitrogen mustards, the nitrosoureas, and the triagenes. The most widely used agent is cyclophosphamide.

Allen test, a method to test the function of the artery on the thumb side of the wrist (radial artery). A catheter is put in the artery. The patient then makes a fist while a nurse presses the middle (ulnar) artery of the wrist. This causes the hand to become pale. Pressure is continued while the fist is opened. If the flow of blood through the radial artery is good, the hand should flush and get its color back.

allergen /al'ərjən/, a foreign substance that can cause an allergic response in the body but is only harmful to some people. Some common allergens (also called antigens) are pollen, animal dander, house dust, feathers, and varied foods. About one of every six Americans is allergic to one or more allergens. Normal people are immune to allergens, but in others the immune system may be too sensitive to foreign substances and even to substances made by the body. The body normally protects itself against allergens by the complex chemical workings of the immune system. –**allergenic,** *adj.* See also **allergy, allergy testing, antigen.**

allergy, a reaction to generally harmless substances. Allergies are labeled according to how the body's cells react to the substance (allergen). Allergies are also divided into those that cause responses right away and those that cause delayed responses. Those allergic reactions which occur right away release substances into the blood flow, such as histamine. Delayed allergic reactions may take many days to show up. Some common symptoms of allergy are lung congestion, allergic eye inflammation, fluid buildup, fever, itching, and vomiting. Severe allergic reactions can cause shock and death. A **food allergy** results from a specific food substance. Symptoms can include runny nose, asthma, hives, itching, headache, nausea, vomiting, diarrhea, stomach pains, constipation, and skin rashes. Allergic substances in foods are mostly proteins. The most common foods causing allergic reactions are wheat, milk, eggs, fish and other seafoods, chocolate, corn, nuts, and strawberries. A **gastrointestinal allergy** is a digestive system allergy to certain foods or drugs. It differs from food allergy, which can affect organ systems other than the digestive system. Symptoms include itching and swelling of the mouth and oral passages, nausea, vomiting, diarrhea, severe abdominal pain, and, if severe, allergic shock. In childhood, gastrointestinal allergy is most often caused by cow's milk. **Physical allergy** refers to an allergic response to conditions such as cold, heat, light, or injury. Symptoms are itching, hives, and swelling beneath the skin (angioedema). The cause may be some cosmetics or drugs. Treatment for any allergy includes identifying and removing the allergen. When allergic reactions are life-threatening, steroids may be given in the vein. For milder diseases, as hay fever, antihistamines are usually given. Building up a patient's resistance to an allergen by injecting larger and larger amounts over a period of time (called desensitization) may also be done. See also **allergy testing.**

allergy testing, any one of the many tests used to find the allergens that cause the allergy. Such tests are helpful to know which treatment will stop allergies or reduce their severity. Skin tests are used most often for allergy testing. A **conjunctival test** identifies allergens by placing a small amount of a suspected substance in the eye. If the patient is allergic to the substance, the eye waters and turns red in 5 to 15 minutes. An **intradermal test** is done by injecting the skin with extracts of the suspected allergens at timed intervals. A control injection without the allergen is also given. The test is positive if, in 15 to 30 minutes, the injection of extract produces a wheal surrounded by redness and the control injection causes no symptoms. A gradual method of injections is done to prevent a systemic reaction. This is more of a risk with intradermal testing than with other kinds of allergy testing, but it tends to be more accurate than a scratch test. A **scratch test** is done by placing a small amount of liquid containing a suspected substance on a lightly scratched area of the skin. If a bump on the skin forms within 15 minutes, the patient is allergic to that substance.

A **passive transfer test** is a skin test in which an allergic reaction in one person is given to a person who does not have that allergy. It is done to help find out what substance (allergen) is causing the allergy. A small amount of the patient's blood serum is injected beneath the skin at several places on the person who is not allergic, usually a relative. After 24 to 48 hours, suspected allergens are put on these places on the nonallergic person. An allergic reaction on the skin shows that an allergen is indeed the cause. The test is only done when skin testing cannot be done directly on the allergic person. A **patch test** is usually done to locate substances that cause a skin condition (contact dermatitis). The substance, as food, pollen, or animal fur, is stuck to a patch that is placed on the patient's skin. Another patch, with nothing on it, is a control. After a time, usually 24 to 48 hours, both patches are removed. If the skin under the suspect patch is red and swollen and the control area is not, the test is said to be positive, and the person is likely allergic to that substance. A **use test** is a way to find offending allergens in foods, cosmetics, or fabrics by cutting out and adding specific items of the life-style of the patient. Allergic reactions to the use test may be right away or spread over a long time. Some patients having the test become frustrated and discouraged, needing encouragement to keep looking for the sources of their allergies by this method.

allocated resources, resources dispatched to an incident that have not yet checked in with the incident communications center.

allogenic, 1. referring to a being or cell that is from the same species but looks distinct due to different genes. **2.** referring to tissues that are transplanted from the same species but have distinct genes.

allopathic physician, a doctor who treats disease and injury with active treatments, as medicine and surgery. The treatment is meant to have the opposite effect from that which is caused by the disease or injury. Almost all doctors

in the United States are allopathic. Compare **chiropractic, homeopathy.**

allopathy /əlop′əthē/, a system of treatment in which a disease is treated by creating a state in which it cannot thrive. For example, an antibiotic that kills a certain germ is given for an infection.

allopurinol, a drug used to prevent gout attacks and kidney stones caused by uric acid. It is not prescribed for children (except those with too much uric acid in the blood from cancer), for nursing mothers, or for patients with a sudden, short-term attack of gout. Known allergy to this drug prohibits its use. Side effects include blood defects, rashes, and other allergies. Stomach upset and problems with vision also may occur.

alloxan /al′oksən/, a substance that is found in the intestine in diarrhea. Because it can kill the cells of the pancreas that secrete insulin, alloxan may cause diabetes.

aloe /al′ō/, the juice of the varied species of *Aloe* plants. Once used to empty the bowels, the practice has been stopped because it often causes severe cramps. The most common use of aloe today is for mild skin burns and rash.

alopecia /al′əpē′shə/, partial or complete loss of hair that results from aging, hormone defects, drug allergy, anticancer treatment, or skin disease. See also **baldness.**

alpha (α), the first letter of the Greek alphabet, often used in chemistry to denote one type of a chemical compound from others.

Alphalin, a trademark for vitamin A. This vitamin is given to aid normal growth and health, especially of the eyes and skin, and to prevent night blindness.

alpha particle or alpha radiation, alpha particles are ejected spontaneously from the nuclei of some radioactive elements. The alpha particle is identical to a helium-4 nucleus ($^4_2$He), which has an atomic mass number of 4 and an electrostatic charge of +2. It has low penetrating power and short range. The most energetic alpha particle will generally fail to penetrate the skin. The major hazard occurs when matter containing alpha-emitting nuclides is introduced into the body. Symbol: α.

alpha receptor, the nerve cells to which certain hormones of the adrenal gland (norepinephrine) and certain drugs attach. When attached in this way, the receptors cause the blood vessel to get smaller, the pupils of the eye to get bigger, and some skin muscles to contract. Compare **beta receptor.**

alpha state, a waking state that is relaxed, and peaceful. It can be known by the alpha rhythm of the brain waves. In the alpha state there are tranquil feelings and a lack of tension. Biofeedback training and meditation techniques are ways of reaching the state. See also **brain waves.**

alpha-tocopherol. See **vitamin E.**

alphavirus, any of a group of very small viruses made of a single molecule. Many alphaviruses live in the cells of insects and are given to humans through insect bites.

alpha wave. See **brain waves.**

altered state of consciousness (ASC), any state of awareness that differs from the normal aware state. Altered states of consciousness have been achieved by persons using techniques such as deep breathing, whirling, and chanting. Western science now knows that such techniques can affect the chemistry of the body and help to bring on the desired state. Most people are able to enter altered states of consciousness. These states can be used to improve health and help fight disease.

alt.h., abbreviation for the Latin prescription term *alternis horis,* meaning every other hour.

altitude sickness, a sickness linked with the low oxygen in the air at high altitudes. The sickness is often brought on by mountain climbing or travel in unpressurized aircraft. Persons with altitude sickness may feel dizzy, crabby, breathless or blissful, or have a headache. Older people and those with lung or heart disorders may suffer breathing problems, heart failure, or fainting, needing emergency treatment. See also **polycythemia.**

alum, a substance that causes the skin cells to contract (astringent). It is used mainly in lotions and douches.

alum bath, a bath taken in water and alum, used mainly for skin defects.

aluminum (Al), a widely used metal and the third most abundant of all the elements. It is found in many antacids, antiseptics, astringents, and styptics. Aluminum salts, as aluminum hydroxychloride, can cause allergies in some people. Aluminum hydroxychloride is the most often used agent in antiperspirants.

Alupent, a trademark for a drug (metaproterenol sulfate) used to treat breathing disorders, such as asthma, bronchitis, and emphysema.

alveolar cell carcinoma /alvē′ələr/, a cancerous tumor of the lung. This form of lung cancer is less common than others. It is known by a bad cough and a large amount of spit.

alveolar process, the part of the jaw that forms the curve (dental arch) shaped by the grouping of a normal set of teeth. It serves as a bony structure to hold the teeth.

alveolectomy /-ek′-/, removal of part of the jaw to take out a tooth, change the line of the jaw after tooth removal, or prepare the mouth for false teeth.

alveolitis /al′vē·əlī′-/, an inflammation of the tiny air sacs in the lungs. See also **hypersensitivity pneumonitis.**

alveolus /alvē′ələs/, *pl.* **alveoli,** a small saclike structure. For example, a **dental alveolus** is a tooth socket in either of the jaws. **Pulmonary alveolus** refers to one of the tiny air sacs in the lungs. This is where carbon dioxide leaves the blood and oxygen is taken on by the blood. **–alveolar,** *adj.*

alymphocytosis /əlim′fəsītō′-/, an abnormal decrease in the number of white cells (lymphocytes) in the blood.

Alzheimer's disease /älts′hīmərz, ôls′-/, a form of brain disease. It can lead to confusion, memory loss, restlessness, problems with perception, speech trouble, trouble moving, and fearing things that are not there. The patient may become too excited, refuse food, and lose bowel or bladder control. The disease often starts in late middle life with slight defects in memory and behavior. Alzheimer's disease occurs as often in men as it does in women. The exact cause is not known, but breakdown of the cells of the brain occurs. There is no treatment, but good nutrition may slow the progress of the disease, which lasts about 7 years in most people who have it. Also called **senile dementia-Alzheimer type (SDAT).**

amalgam /əmal′gəm/, a mixture or combination, such as in dentistry, the substances used to fill cavities, often a mix of silver and another substance.

Amanita /-ī′tə/, a genus of mushrooms. Some species, as *Amanita phalloides,* are poisonous if eaten, causing images to appear that are not real, stomach upset, and pain. Liver, kidney, and nervous system damage can result.

amantadine hydrochloride, a drug used to prevent and treat the flu virus A_2, and for relief of symptoms of Parkinson's disease. It is used with caution in patients with heart failure and during pregnancy and breast feeding. Known allergy to this drug prohibits its use. Side effects include confusion, mood changes, and skin blotches. Nervousness, blurred sight, and slurred speech also may occur.

amasesis /am′əsē′-/, a defect in which the person is not able to chew food. This may be caused by failure of the chewing muscles to work, crowded teeth, poorly fitted false teeth, or a mental problem.

amaurosis /am′ôrō′-/, blindness caused by something outside the eye itself. For example, amaurosis can be caused by a disease of the optic nerve or brain, diabetes, kidney disease, or poisoning from alcoholism.

Ambenyl, a trademark for a drug used to treat coughs from colds or allergies (codeine sulfate, bromodiphenhydramine hydrochloride and diphenhydramine hydrochloride, potassium guaiacolsulfonate).

ambient air standard /am′bē·ənt/, the highest amount allowed of any air pollutant, such as lead, nitrogen dioxide, sodium hydroxide, or sulfuric dioxide. Federal authorities in the United States have said that the air in some cities is dangerous to breathe. Research has shown a strong link between many diseases and poisonous chemicals. Little is known about the exact effects and movement of air pollutants.

ambivalence /ambiv′ələns/, **1.** a state in which a person has conflicting feelings, attitudes, drives, or desires, as love and hate, tenderness and cruelty, pleasure and pain. To some degree, ambivalence is normal. **2.** the state of being uncertain or unable to choose between opposites.

amblyopia /am′blē·ō′pē·ə/, reduced vision in an eye that appears to be normal.

Ambu-bag, a trademark for a breathing bag used to aid patients' breathing in an emergency.

ambulance, an emergency vehicle used to take patients to a hospital or other treatment center in cases of accident, injury, or severe illness.

ambulatory, able to walk; referring to a patient who is not confined to bed.

ambulatory care, health services given to those who come to a hospital or other health care center and who leave after treatment on the same day.

ambulatory surgery center, a health care center that deals with relatively minor surgeries, which do not need overnight hospitalization. For example, cataract repair, hernia repair, and some knee surgeries are types of surgery done in these centers.

amcinonide, a steroid ointment and cream used to treat skin inflammations. Viral and fungal diseases of the skin, blood flow problems, or known allergy to steroids prohibits its use. Side effects include skin allergies that may occur from long-term use or from covering the area with dressings.

ameba /əmē′bə/, pl. **amebae** /-bē/, a microscopic, single-celled organism. Several species may live in humans, including *Entamoeba coli* and *E. histolytica*. Also spelled **amoeba.** **See also amebiasis. –amebic,** adj.

amebiasis /am′ēbī′əsis/, an infection of the intestine or liver by an ameba, often *Entamoeba histolytica*.

amebic dysentery. See **dysentery.**

ameloblastoma /-blastō′mə/, a highly destructive, cancerous, fast-growing tumor of the jaw.

amelogenesis /-jen′əsis/, the forming of the enamel of the teeth. **–amelogenic,** adj.

amelogenesis imperfecta, an inherited defect in which the teeth are yellow or brown in color where the dentin under the enamel is showing. Also called **hereditary brown enamel.**

amenorrhea /ā′menôrē′ə/, the absence of the monthly flow of blood and discharge of mucous tissues from the uterus through the vagina (menstruation).

American Medical Association (AMA), a society made up of licensed doctors in the United States. The AMA keeps lists of all qualified doctors (including those who are not members) in the United States, and publishes many journals.

American Nurses' Association (ANA), the society of registered nurses in the United States. The ANA publishes the *American Nurse* and *The American Journal of Nursing*.

American Psychiatric Association (APA), a society of psychiatrists. It publishes the *Diagnostic and Statistical Manual of Mental Disorders*.

American Red Cross, a national organization that seeks to help people with many health, safety, and disaster relief programs. It is connected with the International Committee of the Red Cross. The Red Cross was begun at the Geneva Convention of 1864. The American Red Cross has more than 130 million members in about 3100 chapters. It depends largely on volunteers to make the programs work. They collect and give more blood than any other agency in the United States. American Red Cross nursing and health programs have courses at home on being a parent, care before and after birth, and first aid. The mark for the American Red Cross is a red cross on a field of white.

Ameslan /am′islan/, abbreviation for American Sign Language, a way of talking with the deaf. Words and letters are made with the hands and fingers.

Ames test, a way of testing if something causes cancer. Also called **mutagenicity test.**

ametropia /am′itrō′pē·ə/, an eye problem. The image seen is wrong because of the way light is bent when it enters the eye. Astigmatism, farsightedness (hyperopia), and nearsightedness (myopia) are types of ametropia. **–ametropic,** adj.

Amicar, a trademark for a drug used to treat bleeding that may happen after surgery or in severe illness (aminocaproic acid).

amide-compound local anesthetic, a compound that causes a loss of feeling in an area. Some kinds are **bupivacaine, dibucaine, etiodocaine, lidocaine, mepivacaine, prilocaine.**

amikacin sulfate, an antibiotic used to treat various severe infections.

Amikin, a trademark for an antibiotic (amikacin sulfate).

amiloride hydrochloride, a drug used to treat heart failure or high blood pressure. It is often given with water pills (diuretic). It must not be used with potassium-conserving drugs. Too much potassium in the blood, poor kidney function, or known allergy to this drug prohibits its use. Side effects include headache, diarrhea, vomiting, too much calcium in the blood, brain disease, impotence, muscle cramps, and irregular heart beats.

amine pump /am′in/, *informal*. a system in some nerve endings that absorbs epinephrine, a chemical of the nervous system. Bad reactions to some drugs, as antidepressants, block this. This causes a large amount of another chemical, norepinephrine, in heart tissue, resulting in heart rhythm disorders. See also **monoamine oxidase inhibitor.**

amino acid /am′inō, əmē′nō/, an organic compound necessary for forming peptides, a piece of protein, and proteins. Digestion releases the individual amino acids from food. Over 100 are found in nature, but only 22 occur in animals. An **essential amino acid** is an organic compound that is not produced in the body but is essential for health in adults and growth in infants and children. Essential amino acids must be obtained from the diet. Adults require isoleucine, leucine, lysine, methionine, phenylalanine, threonine, tryptophan, and valine. Infants need these eight amino acids, plus arginine and histidine. Cysteine and tyrosine are considered semiessential.

aminoaciduria /-as′ido͞or′ē·ə/, the abnormal presence of amino acids in the urine. It usually indicates an inborn chemical defect, as in cystinuria.

aminocaproic acid /-kəprō′ik/, a drug given to stop bleeding. Active blood clotting within blood vessels prohibits its use. Side affects include blood clots and low blood pressure. A man may be unable to ejaculate. Nasal congestion, diarrhea, and allergic reactions may occur.

aminophylline /-fil′in/, a drug used in treating asthma, emphysema, and bronchitis. Known allergies to this or a similar drug prohibits its use. It is used with caution in patients who have peptic ulcer and those in whom heart stimulation would be harmful. Side effects include stomach and intestinal upsets, uneven or rapid heart beat, and nervousness.

aminotransferase, an enzyme that helps move an amino group from one chemical compound to another. Aspartate amino transferase (AST) is present in blood and many tissues, especially the heart and liver. It is given off by cells that have been damaged. Also called **transaminase.**

amitriptyline, a drug used to treat depression.

ammonia, a pungent colorless gas made of nitrogen and hydrogen. It is used as a stimulant, a detergent, and an emulsifier.

amnesia, a loss of memory caused by brain damage or by severe emotional stress. **Anterograde amnesia** is the loss of memory of the events that occur after an injury. **Retrograde amnesia** is the loss of memory for events occurring before a set time in a patient's life, often before the event that caused the amnesia. The condition may result from disease, brain injury, or an emotional injury.

amniocentesis /am′nē·ōsente′-/, removing a small amount of the fluid (amniotic) that is in the womb during pregnancy. It is usually done between the sixteenth and twentieth weeks. Testing the fluid can check for fetal abnormalities, such as Down's syndrome, spina bifida, and Tay-Sachs disease. The sex of the fetus can also be learned. Later in pregnancy it may be done to learn the age of the fetus. The woman must sign an informed consent form. This form explains the procedure and possible adverse effects. Using ultrasound scanning, the position of the fetus and the location of the placenta can be learned. The skin on the woman's belly is cleaned. A local anesthetic is given. A needle attached to a syringe is put into a part of the womb where there is the least chance of touching the placenta or the fetus. Less than 1 ounce of fluid is removed. In testing for birth defects, 3 or more weeks are usually needed before a diagnosis can be made. This waiting period can be stressful. The woman is warned to report any signs of infection or labor. Problems are rare. Miscarriage occurs in approximately 1% of the women. Putting a hole in the placenta or in a blood vessel of the umbilical cord may cause bleeding and blood disease of the fetus. This could be fatal.

amnion. See **amniotic sac.**

amniotic fluid /am′nē-ot′ik/, a liquid made by the amnion and the fetus. It usually totals about 1500 ml (a little over 1½ quarts) at 9 months. It surrounds the fetus during pregnancy, providing it with protection. It is swallowed, processed, and excreted as fetal urine at a rate of 50 ml (more than 2 ounces) every hour. Amniotic fluid is clear, though cells and fat give it a cloudy look.

amniotic sac, a thin-walled bag that contains the fetus and fluid during pregnancy. The wall of the sac extends from the edge of the placenta and surrounds the fetus. There are two layers of membranes forming the sac. The **amnion** is the inner layer. It contains the amniotic fluid. The **chorion** is the outermost of the two layers of membrane. This membrane at first contains fluid and loose pieces of tissue. As pregnancy proceeds, the amnion grows into the chorionic space. The chorion continues to expand around the fetus as it grows. In this way the amniotic sac protects the fetus and separates it from the wall of the uterus. Also called **bag of waters.**

amobarbital, a barbiturate given to relieve nervousness and to help one sleep. It is also given to prevent tremors.

amoxapine, a drug used to treat depression.

amoxicillin, a type of penicillin taken by mouth. It is used to treat different infections. Known allergy to any penicillin prohibits its use. Side effects include allergic reactions, nausea, and diarrhea.

Amoxil, a trademark for an antibiotic (amoxicillin).

amphetamines, a group of drugs that work on the nervous system. These drugs are abused by some people. Abuse causes the user to act driven, feel fearful, hear and see things that are not there, and consider suicide. They have street names, such as **pep pills,** and **speed.** See also **drug abuse.**

amphetamine sulfate, a drug that works on the nervous system. It is used to treat an inability to stay awake (narcolepsy) or to pay attention. Drug abuse, high blood pressure, glaucoma, overactive thyroid, hardening of the arteries, heart disease, use of monoamine oxidase drugs, or known allergy to this drug prohibits its use. Side effects include nervousness, high blood pressure, heart problems, nausea, loss of appetite, and drug dependence.

amphotericin B /am'fəter'əsin/, a drug used to treat fungus infections. Known allergy to this drug prohibits its use. Side effects include blood clots, blood defects, kidney problems, nausea, and fever. When used on the skin, allergic reactions can occur.

ampicillin /am'pəsil'in/, a penicillin used to treat many infections caused by a broad range of organisms.

ampule /am'pyool/, a small, sterile glass or plastic container. It holds a dose of a drug to be given in the vein or in the muscle.

ampulla /ampul'ə, -pool'ə/, a rounded, saclike opening of a duct, canal, or tube, as the tear duct, fallopian tube, or rectum.

amputation, the removal of a part of the body, often a leg, arm, finger, or toe. Amputations are done in cases of severe infections or gangrene, to remove cancerous tumors, and in severe injury. **Closed amputation** is a removal of a limb in which flaps of muscle and skin are used to make a cover over the end of the bone. It is done only when no infection is present. **Congenital amputation** is the absence of a limb or part at birth. It is due to a defect in development. **Open amputation** refers to the removal of parts of the body in which a straight cut is made without skin flaps. Open amputation is done if an infection is likely or present. The cut is left open to drain away fluids, and the skin is pulled back to keep the section from closing. Drug treatment for infection is used. Surgery is later done to close the cut when the infection is gone. **Primary amputation** is removal of a body part after severe injury, when the patient has gotten over shock, and before infection has set in. **Secondary amputation** refers to surgery done after an infection with pus has begun after an injury. A place is left open for drainage, and antibiotics are given.

amputee, a patient who has had one or more arms or legs removed.

amygdalin /əmig'dəlin/, a chemical that is found in bitter almonds and apricot pits. It is thought by some to be a potential cure for cancer. It is sold under the trademark of Laetrile. Also called **vitamin B₁₇.**

amylene hydrate, a clear liquid that smells like camphor. It can be mixed with alcohol, chloroform, ether, or glycerin and is used as a solvent and as a calming drug (sedative).

amyl nitrite /am'il/, a drug that opens up blood vessels. It is used to relieve smothering chest pain (angina pectoris). Known allergy to this drug or to other nitrites prohibits its use. Side effects include low blood pressure, allergies, nausea, headache, and dizziness.

amylo-, amyl-, a combining form referring to starch.

amyotonia /ā'mī·ətō'nē·ə/, a defect of the muscles. The muscles lose tone, become weak, and waste. It is usually due to disease of the nerves that supply the muscles (motor neurons).

amyotrophic lateral sclerosis (ALS) /-trof'ik/, a disease of the nerves that supply the muscles (motor neurons). Symptoms are wasting of the muscles of the hands, forearms, and legs. It can spread to most of the body. It results from a breaking down of the nerves that supply the muscles where they begin, in the brain and spinal cord. ALS usually starts in middle age and quickly gets worse, causing death within 2 to 5 years. There is no known treatment. Also called **Lou Gehrig's disease.**

Amytal, a trademark for a depressant used to cause sleep (amobarbital).

anabolic steroid /an'əbol'ik/, any of many drug compounds that are taken from a male hormone (testosterone), or prepared synthetically. Anabolic steroids aid body growth, counter the effects of a female hormone (estrogen), and cause physical features to become more male. They are also used to treat severe anemias, leukemia, and breast cancer.

anabolism /ənab'əlizm/, any process that produces energy in which simple substances are converted into more complex matter. It is a process that occurs in living matter. Compare **catabolism.** –**anabolic,** *adj.*

anaclitic depression /-klit'ik/, a disorder in infants that occurs after sudden separation from the mother figure. Symptoms include tension, fear, withdrawal, constant crying, refusal to eat, and sleep problems. Stupor sets in, which can lead to severe damage to the infant's physical, social, and mental growth. If the mother figure returns or is replaced in 1 to 3 months, the infant recovers quickly with no long-term effects.

anadipsia /-dip'sē·ə/, extreme thirst. It often occurs in the manic phase of manic-depressive psychosis.

Anadrol-50, a trademark for hormones that is used as an anabolic steroid (oxymetholone).

anaerobe /aner'ōb/, a microorganism that grows and lives without oxygen.

anaerobic exercise, a type of exercise that does not need extra oxygen. The exercise uses up the food stored in the muscles quickly, often within 3 or 4 minutes. Lactic acid builds up in the tissues, which makes muscles feel sore. Examples of anaerobic exercise are weight lifting, wrestling, and sprinting. Compare **aerobic exercise.** See also **exercise.**

anaerobic infection, an infection caused by an anaerobic organism. It usually occurs in deep puncture wounds. Tissue that has little oxygen because of injury, cell death, or too many bacteria may also be infected with anaerobes.

anal canal, the end of the intestinal tract, about 4 cm (about 1½ inches) long, that ends at the anus.

anal crypt, the place in the wall of the rectum that holds networks of veins. This place can become sore and swollen, which is then called hemorrhoids. An **anal fistula** is an open sore on the skin surface near the anus, usually as a result of an infection of the anal crypt.

analeptic. See **central nervous system stimulant.**

analgesia, pain relief that does not cause the patient to fall asleep.

analgesic /an′əljē′zik/, a drug that relieves pain. There are two kinds. One causes a stupor and is habit-forming (narcotic). The other lacks these side effects. Narcotics are usually given for severe pain. See also **pain intervention.**

analgesic cocktail, *informal.* a tailored mix of drugs used for pain relief in certain diseases. For example, cancer patients may be given a mix of alcohol and morphine. See also **lytic cocktail.**

analog /an′əlog/, **1.** something that is similar in appearance or function to another object. However, the source or final product differ. For example, the eye of a fly and the eye of a human are analogs. **2.** a drug or other compound that acts like another substance but has different effects. Compare **homolog.**

anal stage, the period in development between 1 and 3 years of age, when bowel functions and the sensations of the anus are the major source of physical pleasure.

analysis, 1. the act of breaking down substances into their parts. It is done so that the nature and qualities of these parts may be understood. **Qualitative analysis** is naming the elements in a substance; **quantitative analysis** is the measurement of each element in a substance. **2.** *informal.* psychoanalysis. **–analytic,** *adj.* **analyze,** *v.*

analyst, 1. a psychoanalyst. **2.** a person who analyzes the chemical, physical, or other properties of a substance.

anaphylactic shock /-fəlak′-/, a severe and sometimes fatal allergic response to a foreign substance (allergen), as a drug, vaccine, certain food, insect venom, or chemical. It can occur within seconds from the time of contact with the substance. It is commonly marked by trouble in breathing and extremely low blood pressure. The more quickly any reaction occurs in a person after contact, the more severe the shock is likely to be. Anaphylactic shock can occur within seconds or minutes after contact with an allergen.

The first symptoms are intense worry, weakness, sweating, and shortness of breath. Other symptoms may include falling blood pressure, shock, uneven heart beat, wheezing, trouble in swallowing, nausea, and diarrhea. The person should be rushed to an emergency care center. A shot is given in the muscle or vein to treat the shock.

anaphylaxis /-fəlak′sis/, a severe allergic response to a foreign substance (antigen) that the patient has had contact with before. The response may be skin redness and swelling, itching, and water build-up. In severe cases there may be extremely low blood pressure, spasm of the lungs, and shock. The severity of symptoms depends on the amount of the foreign substance and how it got into the body. Anaphylaxis can be caused by insect stings; fluids that contain iodide for x-ray testing which are given in the vein; aspirin; and antitoxins from animal serum. Substances used to test and treat patients with allergies can cause this response. Allergy to penicillin is a common cause. **Aggregate anaphylaxis** refers to a severe allergy from an injection of a foreign substance (antigen). **Antiserum anaphylaxis** is an extreme allergic reaction in a person normally without allergies. It can occur after an injection of serum from a person with that allergy. **Cutaneous anaphylaxis** refers to a strong skin reaction of allergy. It shows as a raised, red area (wheal and flare) that is caused by a foreign material (antigen) injected into the skin. **Indirect anaphylaxis** is a strong reaction to a person's own antigen that occurs because the antigen has been altered in some way. **Inverse anaphylaxis** is a strong allergic reaction caused by an antibody rather than an antigen. **–anaphylactic, anaphylactoid,** *adj.*

anaplasia /-plā′zhə/, a breakdown in the structure of cells and in their relation to each other. Anaplasia occurs in cancer. Compare **metastasis.** **–anaplastic,** *adj.*

anasarca, general, massive fluid build up (edema). Anasarca is often seen in kidney disease when fluid retention is a problem that goes on for a long period of time. See also **edema.**

anastomosis /ənas′tōmō-/, joining two parts, such as blood vessels, to allow flow from one to the other. See also **aneurysm, bypass.**

anatomic curve, a normal curve of the segments of the spinal column. When looking at the spine from the side, the neck (cervical) curve is seen to go inward, as does the lower (lumbar) curve. The upper back (thoracic) curve shows an outward curve.

anatomy, 1. the study of structures and organs of the body. In **applied anatomy,** body structures in relation to disease are studied. **Comparative anatomy** relates the various stages of growth in different animals. For example, the adult stage in some animals may resemble the youth stage in others. **Cross-sectional anatomy** studies the relation of the structures of the body to each other. This involves examining cross sections of the tissue or organ. **Descriptive anatomy** is the study of the form and structure of various systems of the body, as the digestive system and the nervous system. **Gross anatomy** means the study of the organs or parts of the body large enough to be seen with the naked eye. **2.** the structure of an organism. Compare **physiology.**

Anavar, a trademark for a hormone (androgen) used as a growth promoting (anabolic) drug (oxandrolone).

anconeus, a muscle of the forearm. It works to straighten the forearm.

ancrod, the poison of the Malayan pit viper, a snake. It prevents clotting of the blood. It is used to treat certain clotting defects.

ancylostomiasis /an'silōstōmī'əsis/. See **hookworm infection.**

Andersen's disease. See **glycogen storage disease.**

andro-, andr-, a combining form referring to man or to the male.

androgen /an'drəjen/, any steroid hormone that increases growth of male physical qualities.

androgynous /androj'ənəs/, having some qualities of both sexes. Social role, behavior, personality, and appearance are not due to the physical sex of the person. −**androgyny,** n.

androsterone /andos'tərōn/, one of the male sex hormones (androgens). It is seldom used in therapy. See also **testosterone.**

anecdotal, referring to medical knowledge based on observations and not yet confirmed by scientific studies.

Anectine, a trademark for a muscle relaxant used with anesthesia (succinylcholine chloride).

anemia, a decrease in red cells in the blood. The ability to carry oxygen is reduced. Anemia is noted by the hemoglobin content of the red cells and by red cell size. Depending on its severity, anemia may cause one or more symptoms. These include fatigue, difficult breathing during activity, dizziness, headache, insomnia, and pale skin and mucous membranes. Loss of hunger, unsettled stomach, irregular heart beats and murmurs also occur. Blood tests are done to find the type of anemia and the cause. With **aplastic anemia,** the bone marrow can no longer make blood cells. This may be caused by cancer of the bone marrow, or by contact with poisonous chemicals, radiation, or antibiotics or other drugs. **Hemolytic anemia** is a disorder involving the premature destruction of red blood cells. Anemia may be slight or absent if the bone marrow is able to increase production of red blood cells. The condition may occur with some infectious diseases, with certain inherited red cell disorders, or as a response to drugs or other poisonous agents. **Hypochromic anemia** refers to any of a large

group of anemias marked by decreased hemoglobin in the red blood cells. **Hypoplastic anemia** refers to a broad class of anemias marked by low production of red blood cells. **Leukoerythroblastic anemia** is an abnormal condition in which there are large numbers of immature white and red blood cells. Some anemias of this kind result from a tumor in bone marrow. **Microcytic anemia** features abnormally small red blood cells. It is usually linked to long-term blood loss or a disease of poor nutrition, such as iron deficiency anemia. **Myelophthisic anemia** results from a defect of the red blood cell forming tissues of the bone marrow. **Anemia of pregnancy** results from a decrease of red cells in the blood. The cause may be a problem in the making of red cells (erythrocytes), a loss of red blood cells through bleeding, or a lack of iron, folic acid, or vitamin B_{12}. This type of anemia is common in about one half of all pregnancies. The treatment of anemia depends on the cause. Severe anemia may call for blood transfusion. Treatment also includes giving vitamins to replace what the blood lacks, as iron for iron deficiency anemia. See also **nutritional anemia, sickle cell anemia, antianemic.**

anencephaly /an'ənsef'əlē/, a birth defect in which there is no brain or spinal cord, the skull does not close, and the spinal canal remains a groove.

anergy, 1. lack of activity. **2.** an immune defect in which the body does not fight off foreign substances well enough. This state may be seen in advanced tuberculosis and other serious infections, in AIDS, and in some cancers. −**anergic,** adj.

anesthesia, the lack of normal sensation, especially awareness of pain. It is brought on by an anesthetic drug or by hypnosis. It can also occur with damage to nerve tissue. Anesthesia for medical purposes may be used on the skin (topical) or in part or all of the body. See also **general anesthesia, local anesthesia, obstetric anesthesia, regional anesthesia, topical anesthesia.**

anesthesia dolorosa, a bad pain in an anesthetized area.

anesthesia patients, classification of, the system by which the American Society of Anesthesiologists lists anesthesia patients in five categories. Class I includes patients who are generally healthy, without serious physical or mental problems. For these patients anesthesia is needed only for a local problem, as a hernia or fibroid uterus. Class II includes patients who have mild to moderate health problems, as anemia, mild diabetes, high blood pressure, too much fat, or long-term bronchitis. Class III includes patients who have severe health problems or disease, as severe diabetes. Class IV includes patients who have a life-threatening problem, as kidney disease. Class V includes patients who have little chance of survival, as a person in shock with a massive lung clot (pulmonary

22

embolus). The letter E is added to the roman numeral to indicate an emergency.

anesthesiologist /an′əsthē′zē·ol′-/, a doctor trained to give anesthetics and to support lungs, heart, and blood flow systems during surgery. A person who gives anesthesia may also be called an **anesthetist.**

anesthesiology, the branch of medicine that deals with the control of sensations of pain and with giving drugs to relieve pain during surgery.

aneurysm /an′yŏŏrizm/, a bulging of the wall of a blood vessel, usually caused by hardening of the arteries (atherosclerosis) and high blood pressure (hypertension). It is sometimes caused by injury, infection, or an inherited weakness in the vessel wall. A sign of an arterial aneurysm is a pulsating swelling. It makes a blowing murmur that can be heard with a stethoscope. Aneurysms are most dangerous in the large artery (aorta) of the heart. An **aortic aneurysm** can result from deposits of cholesterol (atherosclerosis), often in the abdominal section of the aorta. This may get in the way of the urinary tract, spine, or other structure, and cause pain. In many cases the first sign is life-threatening bleeding that occurs from rupture of the lesion. Aortic aneurysms may also occur from high blood pressure or syphilis. A **dissecting aneurysm** is one with a tear in one of the layers of the artery wall, most often in the aorta. Men between 40 and 60 years of age with high blood pressure are most likely to have dissecting aortic aneurysms. Symptoms include severe pain that may mimic a heart attack, lack of pulse in the neck or arm, and sometimes heart failure. A **ventricular aneurysm** is one that occurs in the wall of the left ventricle of the heart, most often after a heart attack (myocardial infarction). Scar tissue may be formed as a result of inflammation caused by the infarction. This tissue weakens a layer of the heart wall (myocardium), allowing it to bulge outward when the ventricle contracts.

Intracranial aneurysm refers to any aneurysm of the cerebral arteries in the brain. Rupture results in mortality approaching 50%. There is high risk of recurrence in survivors. **Cerebral aneurysm** also refers to one in the brain (cerebrum). It is commonly the result of inborn weakness of the artery wall, but may be caused by infection, tumors, hardening of the arteries, and injury. Depending on the size and location of a cerebral aneurysm, symptoms may be headache, drowsiness, confusion, dizziness, weakness, and pain of the face. Ringing in the ears, vision problems, stiff neck, and partial paralysis also occur. Because about half of all cerebral aneurysms break, the patient is closely watched for signs of bleeding. If surgery is needed for an aneurysm in the brain, it usually involves opening the skull (craniotomy) and clamping the aneurysm off from the flow of blood.

angiitis /an′jē·ī′-/, an inflamed state of a blood or lymph vessel.

angina /anjī′nə, an′jinə/, a symptom of some diseases that is known by a feeling of choking, suffocation, or crushing pressure and pain. **Angina dyspeptica** is a painful state caused by gas swelling of the stomach. It has the same symptoms as angina pectoris. **Angina epiglottidea** refers to pain caused when the top of the windpipe (epiglottis) becomes inflamed. **Angina pectoris** is a cramping pain in the chest. It is caused most often by a shortage of oxygen to the heart (myocardial anoxia). It is often linked with hardening of the arteries (atherosclerosis) of the heart. The pain usually travels down the inside of the left arm. It often occurs with a feeling of suffocation and impending death. Attacks of angina pectoris are often related to exertion, emotional stress, and contact with intense cold. The pain may be relieved by rest and drugs, as nitroglycerin. **Angina decubitus** is a type of angina pectoris that occurs when the patient is lying down. **Prinzmetal's angina** is a form of heart disease in which the attacks occur during rest rather than from activity. With **streptococcal angina,** feelings of choking, lack of air, and pain occur as the result of a streptococcal infection. See also **Ludwig's angina.**

angioblastoma /an′jē·ōblastō′mə/, a tumor of blood vessels in the brain.

angiocardiogram /-kär′dē·ō·gram/, an x-ray film (radiograph) of the heart and the vessels of the heart. A fluid with a dye that can be seen on x-ray films is put into a vein that goes directly to the heart. X-rays films are taken as the fluid passes through the heart and its vessels.

angiogenesis /-jen′əsis/, the ability to grow blood vessels. It is a common feature of cancerous tissue.

angiography /an′jē·og′rəfē/, the x-ray study of the inside of the heart and blood vessels, or other areas. It is done after a dye is injected. It is used to test for heart attacks (myocardial infarction), blocked vessels (vascular occlusion), hardened deposits in the arteries, stroke, high blood pressure, kidney tumors, lung clots, and lung vessel problems. **Cerebral angiography** refers to an x-ray test for seeing the blood vessels of the brain. **Renal angiography** is an x-ray test of the kidney blood vessel (renal artery) and related blood vessels. –**angiographic,** *adj.*

angiokeratoma /-ker′ətō′mə/, a horny tumor on the skin. It appears as clumps of swollen blood vessels, clusters of warts, and thickened skin, especially in the scrotum and the fingers and toes.

angiolipoma /-lipō′mə/, a harmless tumor that has blood vessels and tissue.

angioma /an′jē·ō′mə/, any harmless tumor made up mainly of blood vessels (hemangioma) or lymph vessels (lymphangioma). Most angiomas are present at birth.

angiomatosis /-mətō′-/,   a state in which the patient has many blood vessel tumors (angiomas).

angiomyoma /-mī·ō′mə/,   a tumor made of blood vessels and muscle tissue.

angiomyosarcoma /-mī-ō′mə/,   a tumor made of blood vessels, muscles, and connective tissue.

angiosarcoma,   a rare, cancerous tumor made of tissue that grows around blood vessels. This condition occurs most often in older patients. It is also linked to contact with vinyl chloride and arsenic. Compare **angioma.**

angiospasm /an′jē·ōspazm′/,   a sudden, short-term spasm of a blood vessel. Also called **vasospasm.** See also **vasoconstriction.**

angiotensin /-ten′-/,   a substance in the blood that causes blood vessels to tighten. This raises blood pressure. It causes the hormone aldosterone to be released from the adrenal cortex.

angle,   the geometric relationships between the surfaces of the body.

angular movement,   one of the four basic kinds of movement by the joints of the body. For example, the angle between the forearm and upper arm gets smaller when the arm is bent and gets larger when the arm is extended. Compare **circumduction, gliding, rotation.**

angulated fracture,   a break in which the fragments of bone are angled.

Anhydron,   a trademark for a drug used to treat high blood pressure (cyclothiazide).

aniline /an′ilēn/,   an oily, colorless, poisonous liquid with a strong odor and burning taste. It is used in making some dyes. Workers who come in contact with aniline are at risk of getting blood diseases.

anima /an′imə/,   **1.** the soul or life. **2.** the active substance in a drug. **3.** a person's true, inner being, as distinct from outward personality (persona). **4.** the female part of the male persona.

animus /an′iməs/,   **1.** the active or rational soul; the active agent of life. **2.** the male part of the female persona. **3.** a deep resentment that is under control but may break out under stress.

aniseikonia /an′īsīkō′nē·ə/,   a defect in which each eye sees the same image differently in size or shape.

anisocytosis /anī′sōsītō′-/,   a defect of the blood in which the red blood cells differ in size.

anisopoikilocytosis /-poi′kilōsītō′-/,   a defect of the blood. The red blood cells differ in size and shape.

anisotropine,   a drug used for treating peptic ulcer. Glaucoma, a blocked urinary system or digestive tract, heart defects, severe inflammation of the large intestine (ulcerative colitis), or a nerve disorder (myasthenia gravis) prohibits its use. Side effects include blurred vision, rapid heart beat, dilation of the pupils and other eye problems,

impotence, confusion, trouble in urinating, constipation, allergies, and itching.

ankle,   **1.** the joint of the three bones of the foot at the leg (tibia, talus, fibula). **2.** the part of the leg where it joins the foot.

ankle bandage,   a figure-of-eight bandage that is looped under the sole of the foot and around the ankle. The heel may be covered or left bare, although it is better to cover it.

ankle bone   the second largest bone of the ankle. It is made up of a body, neck, and head. Also called **talus.**

ankylosing spondylitis /ang′kilō′sing/,   a long-term disease with inflammation of unknown cause. It first affects the spine and nearby structures. It often progresses to a joining together (ankylosis) of the bones of the spinal column.

ankylosis /ang′kilō′-/,   "freezing" of a joint, often in a position that is not normal. It is due to destruction of cartilage and bone, as occurs in rheumatoid arthritis.

anodyne /an′ədīn/,   a drug that relieves or lessens pain. Compare **analgesic.**

anomaly /ənom′əlē/,   **1.** change from what is regarded as normal. **2.** inherited problem with growth of a structure, as the lack of a limb or the presence of an extra finger.   – **anomalous,** *adj.*

anoplasty /ā′nōplas′tē/,   an operation to restore function of the anus.

anorectic /an′ôrek′-/,   referring to appetite loss, such as caused by a drug.

anorexia /an′ôrek′sē·ə/,   a loss of appetite that results in the patient not being able to eat. The state may be caused by unpleasant food, illness, or surroundings. It may also have a mental cause. **Anorexia nervosa** is a disorder in which there is a long-term refusal to eat. It causes wasting, lack of menstrual cycles, a mental problem with body image, and a fear of becoming fat. The state is seen mainly in teenage girls. It is often linked with mental stress or conflict, as worry, anger, and fear. This stress may be due to a big change in the patient's life. Treatment consists of improving health, followed by therapy to get over the emotional conflicts.   –**anorexic,** *adj.*

anosmia /anoz′mē·ə/,   loss or damage of the sense of smell. This is often a short-term state caused by a head cold or lung infection. Blocked nasal passages keeps odors from getting to the place that senses smells (olfactory region). The loss can become permanent when any part of the olfactory nerve is destroyed. Also called **olfactory anesthesia.** Compare **hyperosmia.**

anosognosia /an′əsognō′zhə/,   a condition in which the patient is not able to tell when there has been an injury to the body. It may be caused by an injury in the brain.

anovulation /an'ovyəlā'shən/, failure of the ovaries to produce, mature, or release eggs. Anovulation may be a side effect of drugs given for other defects.

anoxia /anok'sē·ə/, a lack of oxygen. Anoxia may occur in a small space or affect the whole body. It can be the result of poor supply of oxygen to the lungs. It can also occur when the blood is not able to carry oxygen to the tissues, or the tissues are not able to absorb the oxygen from the blood. **Anemic anoxia** refers to a state in which there is lack of oxygen in body tissues. The cause is a decrease in the number of red blood cells. A condition in which too little oxygen reaches the brain is called **cerebral anoxia.** This state, which is caused by failure of circulation, can exist for no more than 4 to 6 minutes before permanent brain damage occurs. **Stagnant anoxia** is a condition in which there is not enough blood flowing through the body. This state is linked with shock, a failure of heart contactions (cardiac standstill), and blood clots.

ANSI, American National Standards Institute.

Antabuse, a trademark for a drug used to treat alcohol abuse (disulfiram).

antacid /antas'id/, **1.** opposing acidity. **2.** a drug or substance in the diet that buffers, makes neutral, or absorbs hydrochloric acid in the stomach. Antacids that contain aluminum and calcium may cause constipation; those with magnesium have a laxative effect.

antagonist /antag'ənist/, anything, such as a drug or muscle, that has an opposite action or competes for the same thing. An **associated antagonist** is one of a pair of muscles or group of muscles that pull in opposite directions. Their combined action results in moving a part in one direction. A **direct antagonist** is one of a pair of muscles that pull in opposite directions. Their combined action keeps the part from moving. Antagonist also refers to a tooth in the upper jaw that comes in contact during chewing or biting with a tooth in the lower jaw. See also **narcotic antagonist.**

antecubital /an'təkyoo'bitəl/, at the bend of the elbow on the inside of the arm.

anteflexion, a position of an organ in which it is tilted forward, folded over on itself. This is not a normal state.

antegonial notch, a depression or low place that is present at the corner of the lower jaw.

Antepar, a trademark for a drug used to treat infection from worms (piperazine citrate).

antepartal care, care of a pregnant woman throughout the maternity cycle. See also **intrapartal care, postpartal care.**

anterior (A), the front of a structure or a part facing toward the front. Compare **posterior.**

anterior cardiac vein, one of many small blood vessels that return blood to the heart when the blood is out of oxygen.

anterior cutaneous nerve, one of a pair of branches of the network of nerves near the top of the spine (cervical plexus). It arises from the second and the third nerves in the neck, and branches to the skin of the neck and upper chest.

anterior longitudinal ligament, the broad, strong ligament attached to the front surfaces of the backbones (vertebrae). It goes from the skull to the lower back.

anterior mediastinal node, a lymph node in one of the three groups of chest (thoracic) nodes of the lymph system. This node drains lymph from nodes of the thymus, heart area, and breastbone (sternum).

anterior tibial artery, one of the two branches of the major leg (popliteal) artery. The anterior tibial artery starts in back of the knee, splits into six branches, and supplies the muscles of the leg and foot.

anterior tibial node, one of the small lymph glands of the leg.

anteroposterior /an'tərō-/, from the front to the back of the body. The term is often used to describe the direction of an x-ray beam.

anthracosis /an'thrəkō'-/, a long-term lung disease of coal miners. It is caused by coal dust in the lungs. It forms black lumps on the bronchioles that lead to emphysema. Cigarette smoking worsens the condition. There is no real treatment. The progress of the disease may be halted by staying away from coal dust. Also called **black lung.**

anthralin, a drug that is put on the skin. It is used to treat psoriasis and long-term inflammation of the skin. Kidney disease or known allergy to this drug prohibits its use. It is not put on broken skin or near the eyes. Side effects include kidney failure.

anthrax /an'thraks/, a disease that affects mostly farm animals (cattle, goats, pigs, sheep, and horses). Humans most often get it through a break in the skin when in direct contact with infected animals and their hides. The type that infects the skin begins with a reddish-brown sore that breaks open and then forms a dark scab. Symptoms that follow include internal bleeding, muscle pain, headache, fever, nausea, and vomiting. Anthrax of the lungs (**woolsorter's disease**) occurs from breathing in the germs. It is so named because it is a work hazard to those who handle sheep's wool. Early symptoms look like influenza. However, the patient soon develops high fever, breathing distress, and a blood disease with bluish skin (cyanosis). If the disease is not treated at this point, it often leads to death. Treatment for both forms is penicillin G or tetracycline. A vaccine is available for people for whom anthrax is a work hazard.

anthropometry /an'thrəpom'ətrē/, the science of measuring the human body for height, weight, and size of different parts. This includes measuring skinfolds. Also called **anthropometric measurement.**

antiadrenergic /an'ti·ad'rənur'jik/, **1.** referring to blocking signals sent by the nerves that release the chemical norepinephrine. These nerves, called "adrenergic nerves," have two types of receivers called "alpha" and "beta." **2.** an antiadrenergic drug. These are drugs that block the response to norepinephrine by alpha-adrenergic receptors. They cause blood flow to increase and blood pressure to decrease. Drugs that block beta-adrenergic receptors slow the heart beat. Also called **sympatholytic.** Compare **adrenergic.**

antianemic /-ənē'mik/, referring to a drug, substance or method that corrects or prevents a shortage of red blood cells (anemia). Whole blood transfusions are given to treat anemia from sudden blood loss. Packed red cells are usually given when the shortage is due to constant blood loss. Transfusions of parts of the blood are used to treat aplastic anemia. See also **anemia.**

antiantibody, an antibody formed by the blood to fight off a foreign antibody that can cause an allergic response. See also **antibody, immune gamma globulin.**

antiarrhythmic, referring to a treatment or drug that prevents, relieves, or corrects a heart rhythm problem. A device that gives an electric shock is often used to restore a normal rhythm in patients with rapid, uneven heart beats. A pacemaker can be surgically placed in a patient with a very slow heart rate or other heart beat problems. The electrode tube (catheter) of an external pacemaker may be threaded through a vein to the heart in cases of complete heart block. Drugs may be given to restore normal heart rate. See also **arrhythmia.**

antibacterial, referring to a substance or drug that kills bacteria or prevents their growth.

antibiotic, referring to the ability to kill or prevent the growth of a living organism. Antibiotics are also called antibacterial or antimicrobial drugs. They can be made from cultures of microorganisms. They can also be made artificially. Side effects to antibiotics include rash, fever, spasm of the bronchial tubes, inflamed blood vessels, kidney and ear problems, stomach upset, vomiting, fatigue, and lack of sleep. They are used to treat infections.

antibiotic sensitivity tests, a method to find out what antibiotic will work to get rid of a certain bacteria. After the organism has been found in a sample of mucus, blood, or other body tissue, it is grown in the laboratory.

antibody (Ab), a molecule made by lymph tissue. It defends the body against bacteria, viruses, or other foreign bodies (antigens). Each antibody reacts to a certain foreign body. Antibodies are also called immunoglobulins.

anticholinergic, 1. referring to a blocking of certain receivers on the nerve. This causes the body to stay in a "fight or flight" state, with high blood pressure, rapid breathing, and dry mouth. **2.** an anticholinergic drug that lessens muscle spasms in the bladder, lung, and intestine. It also relaxes the iris muscles of the eye, decreases substances released by the stomach, lung, and mouth, decreases sweating, and speeds up the heart. Many anticholinergic drugs reduce symptoms like those in Parkinson's disease. Compare **cholinergic.**

anticholinesterase, a drug that stops the action of a chemical that sends nerve signals (acetylcholine). Anticholinesterase drugs are used to treat a disorder of sudden, local muscle fatigue (myasthenia gravis).

anticoagulant, referring to a substance or drug that prevents or delays blood clots (coagulation).

anticonvulsant, referring to a drug or treatment that prevents seizures, such as in epilepsy, or makes them less severe. Many of these drugs may cause birth defects when given to pregnant women.

antidepressant, referring to a drug or a treatment that prevents or relieves depression. See also **antipsychotic.**

antidiuretic, referring to a drug or substance that keeps the body from making urine. –**antidiuresis,** n.

antidiuretic hormone (ADH), a hormone made in the hypothalamus of the brain and stored in the pituitary gland. It decreases the making of urine by causing water to be absorbed in the kidneys. ADH is released when the blood volume falls, when a large amount of salt shows up in blood, or when pain, stress, or some drugs are present. Nicotine and large doses of certain drugs cause ADH to be released. Alcohol slows the making of the hormone. Artificial ADH is used to treat a type of diabetes. Also called **vasopressin.**

antidote /an'tidōt/, a drug or other substance that stops the action of a poison. An antidote may coat the stomach. This keeps the poison from being absorbed. It may also work to oppose the action of the poison, as a relaxing drug given to a patient who has taken a large amount of a stimulant. **Chemical antidote** refers to any substance that reacts with a poison to form a compound that is harmless or less harmful. There are few true antidotes. Treatment of poisoning depends largely on destroying the toxic agent before it can be absorbed by the body.

antiembolism hose, elastic stockings worn to prevent blood clots (emboli). They help the return flow of blood to the heart. This keeps the blood from pooling in the veins.

antiemetic, referring to a drug or treatment that prevents or relieves nausea and vomiting.

antifogging chemical, a chemical that keeps fog (condensation) from forming on the inside of a facepiece lens.

antifungal, referring to a substance that kills or controls fungi.

antigen /an'tijən/, a substance foreign to the body, often a protein. It causes the body to form an antibody that responds only to that antigen. Antigens can cause allergic reactions in some people. See also **allergen.**

antigen-antibody reaction, a process of the immune system in which certain white blood cells (lymphocytes) respond to a foreign body (antigen) by making antibodies. The antigens are made harmless when they are bound to these antibodies.

antiglobulin, an antibody against a certain type of human protein (globulin). It can occur normally or be made in laboratory animals. Antiglobulins are used to find antibodies, as in blood typing.

antiglobulin test, a test to find antibodies that damage red blood cells as a result of disease. It is used to check for a number of blood defects. Also called **Coombs' test.**

antihemophilic factor (AHF), blood clotting factor VIII, a substance that stops bleeding. It is used to treat a lack of factor VIII (hemophilia A). Hepatitis can occur if the blood plasma used to treat the patient is infected. Allergic reactions may also occur.

antihistamine /-his'təmin/, a substance that reduces the effects of histamine, a chemical made by the body. Although histamine has a normal role in the body, it can also cause the symptoms in allergic reactions. Many antihistamine drugs can be bought over the counter to treat allergies, such as hay fever and itching. Antihistamines should not be overused or left in reach of children who could swallow them. Misuse of these drugs can cause death. Side effects of prescribed use can include fatique, nausea, constipation, and dryness of the throat and breathing tract.

antihypertensive, referring to a drug or treatment that reduces high blood pressure. Some drugs that increase urine-making (diuretics) lower the blood pressure by decreasing blood volume.

antiinflammatory, referring to a drug or treatment that reduces heat, redness, swelling, and pain (inflammation) in a body area.

antilipidemic /-lip'idem'-ik/, referring to a diet or drug that reduces the amount of fats (lipids) in the blood. Antilipidemics are prescribed to reduce the risk of disease of the blood vessels and heart muscle. Fat collects in the vessel or heart that has cholesterol in it. A low-fat diet is thought to help to prevent heart disease, in the view of many heart specialists. A number of drugs are used to reduce fats in the bloodstream. Side effects of these drugs may include gallstones, uneven heart beat, blood clots, and the loss of vitamins. See also **hyperlipidemia.**

Antilirium, a trademark for a drug that is used to reverse the effects of anesthesia (physostigmine salicylate).

antilymphocyte serum (ALS). See **antiserum.**

antimalarial /-məler'ē·əl/, referring to a drug that kills or stops the growth of malaria organisms (plasmodia). Antimalarial also refers to a way to kill mosquitos that carry the disease, as spraying insecticides or draining swamps. See also **malaria.**

antimetabolite, a drug or substance that closely resembles another that is required by the body for normal functioning. Its effect comes from its interference with the needed substance. Antimetabolites are used as anticancer drugs.

antimicrobial, referring to a substance that kills microorganisms, such as bacteria, or stops their growth.

Antiminth, a trademark for a drug used to treat infection from worms (pyrantel pamoate).

antimitochondrial antibody /-mī'təkon'drē·əl/, an antibody that acts against structures in the body's cells (mitochondria) that make the cell's energy. These antibodies are not normally present in the blood of healthy people. Low levels may occur in long-term hepatitis and liver disease caused by drugs. High levels are found in severe liver disease.

antimony /an'təmōnē/, a chemical element that occurs in nature. Antimony compounds are used to treat parasite infections. It is also used to bring on vomiting in cases of poisoning. Antimony is common in many substances used in medicine and industry.

antimony poisoning, poisoning caused by swallowing or breathing antimony or antimony compounds. The symptoms are vomiting, sweating, diarrhea, and a metallic taste in the mouth. Irritation of the skin or mucous membrane may result from contact. Severe poisoning will look like arsenic poisoning. Dimercaprol is used to treat antimony poisoning.

antimutagen /-myoo'təjən/, any substance or method that lowers the rate of changes in cell structure (mutation). An antimutagen may also protect cells against agents that cause cell mutations. **–antimutagenic,** *adj.*

antineoplastic, a drug that controls or kills cancer cells.

antineoplastic antibiotic, a drug made from a microorganism or by artificial means. It is used to treat cancer. Antineoplastic antibiotics slow down bone marrow function and often cause nausea and vomiting. Some types also cause hair loss.

antineoplastic hormone, a chemical made by the body or by artificial means. It is used to control the growth of some cancers. Hormones are used with other methods to treat cancer of the prostate, and breast cancer.

antiparasitic, referring to a drug or treatment that kills parasites or stops their growth.

antiparkinsonian, referring to a drug or treatment used to treat a nervous system defect (parkinsonism). The drugs are of two kinds. One kind makes up for the lack of a chemical (dopamine) in the brain. Another kind balances the effects of too much of another chemical (acetylcholine) in the brain. Levodopa is a substance that converts to dopamine (hydrochloride) in the brain. It is given to patients to reduce the stiffness, slowness, drooling, and lack of balance that is typical of the disease. The drug does not stop the course of the disease. Other drugs may help to relieve tremors and rigidity and make movement easier.

antipruritic, referring to a drug or treatment that helps relieve or prevent itching. Anesthetics that are put on the skin, corticosteroids, and antihistamines are used as antipruritic agents.

antipsychotic, referring to a drug or treatment that lessens the symptoms of a severe mental illness (psychosis).

antipyretic, referring to a drug or treatment that reduces fever. The most widely used drugs are acetaminophen, aspirin, and other salicylates. A lukewarm alcohol sponge or tub bath may decrease a high fever. A cooling blanket is sometimes used for patients with a prolonged, high fever.

antiseptic, a substance or treatment used to stop the growth of microorganisms.

antiserum, a fluid (serum) in the blood of an animal or human that contains antibodies against a certain disease. Antiserum is normally used to transfer temporary (passive) immunity.

antisocial personality disorder, repeated behavior patterns that lack morals and ethics. These patterns bring a person into conflict with society. A person with this defect may be aggressive, impulsive, irresponsible, hostile, and immature and show poor judgment.

antistreptolysin-O test (ASOT, ASLT), a test to find and measure antibodies in the blood to streptolysin-O. This is a poison that is made by certain types of the bacteria streptococci. The test is often used to help diagnose rheumatic fever. High levels may mean the patient has had a recent infection.

antithyroid drug, any one of many drugs that can lower the level of thyroid hormones. These drugs are often used to treat an overactive thyroid (hyperthyroidism). The main antithyroid drugs are thioamides. These drugs should not be taken during pregnancy. They can cause low levels of thyroid hormones (hypothyroidism) and goiter in the baby. Mothers who breast-feed their children should not take these drugs.

antitoxin. See **antiserum.**

antitussive /-tus′iv/, any of a large group of drugs that act on the nervous system to reduce the action of the cough reflex. These drugs should not be used with a cough that produces sputum because the cough reflex is needed to clear released fluids. Antitussives may be either habit-forming (narcotic) or not habit-forming (nonnarcotic). Codeine and hydrocodone are narcotic antitussives. Dextromethorphan is not habit-forming. Antitussives are often in a syrup with a substance to help bring up the mucus (expectorant), and alcohol. They may also be given in a capsule with an antihistamine and a mild painkiller.

antivenin. See **antiserum.**

Antivert, a trademark for an antihistamine drug (meclizine hydrochloride).

antiviral, destructive to viruses.

antivitamin, a substance that stops the action of a vitamin.

Anturane, a trademark for a drug used to treat gout (sulfinpyrazone).

anuria /ənoŏr′ē·ə/, the state of being unable to urinate, the failure to produce urine, or urinating less than about 3½ ounces a day. Anuria may be caused by kidney failure, a severe decline in blood pressure, or blockage of the urinary tract. A fast decline in urinary output occurs in sudden kidney failure. Also called **anuresis** /an′-yoŏrē′-/.

anus /ā′nəs/, the opening at the end of the anal canal.

anxiety, a feeling of worry, upset, uncertainty, and fear that comes from thinking about some threat or danger. Anxiety is often mental, rather than a response to real events. The cause of the problem is complex and may involve a mental conflict about values and goals of life. It can also be due to a change in health, income, role, home life, or friendships.

anxiety attack, a sudden response of intense anxiety and panic. Symptoms often include fast heart beat, shortness of breath, dizziness, faintness, sweating, paleness, stomach upset, and a vague feeling of doom. Attacks often occur suddenly, and last from a few seconds to 1 hour or longer. They may come many times a day or once a month. Treatment may include giving drugs and psychotherapy to understand the stresses.

anxiety neurosis, a mental conflict or problem in which anxiety lasts for a long time. The person may feel tense, worried, afraid, unable to make a decision, and restless. In more severe cases, there may be hostility towards others. In extreme cases, the mental upset may lead to physical problems, as tremors, muscle tension, rapid heart beat, breathing problems, high blood pressure, and sweating. Others are nausea, vomiting, diarrhea, lack of sleep, and changes in appetite. Treatment may include drugs and psychotherapy.

aorta /ā·ôr′tə/, the main artery of the heart. It starts at the opening of the heart's lower left chamber (ventricle). The **abdominal aorta,** one of the four parts of the aorta, passes through the belly. It supplies blood to many different parts of the body, such as the testicles, ovaries, kidneys, stomach, and the legs. The **ascending aorta** branches into the right and left coronary arteries. It continues as the **arch of the aorta.** From the aortic arch, the **descending aorta** leads to the trunk of the body and supplies blood to many areas, including the throat, ribs, and stomach. The **thoracic aorta,** the large, upper portion of the descending aorta, divides into seven branches. It supplies many parts of the body, as the heart, ribs, chest muscles, and stomach.

aortic arch syndrome, a blockage of the part of the aorta that forms an arch. Conditions as atherosclerosis, inflamed arteries (arteritis), and syphilis may cause the problem. Symptoms include fainting, short-term blindness, loss of use of part of the body, and memory loss.

aortic body reflex, a normal chemical reaction in the body. It is caused by a decrease in oxygen in the blood. This causes faster breathing to build up oxygen supplies. See also **carotid body reflex.**

aortic regurgitation, the reverse flow of blood from the aorta back into the left lower heart chamber (ventricle). Also called **aortic insufficiency.**

aortic stenosis. See stenosis.

aortic valve. See **heart valve.**

aortitis /ā′ôrtī′-/, an inflammation of the aorta. It can occur in syphilis and sometimes in rheumatic fever.

aortography /a′ôrtog′rəfē/, a method to diagnose heart diseases. The aorta and its branches are injected with a fluid that will show on x-ray films.

aortopulmonary fenestration, a birth defect in which there is an opening between the ascending aorta and the main artery to the lungs (pulmonary artery). This allows blood with oxygen and blood without oxygen to mix. As a result, there is less oxygen available to the body.

apathy /ap′əthē/, a lack of emotion; a lack of care for things that are normally exciting or moving. The state is often seen in patients with certain types of mental illness, as schizophrenia.

apatite /ap′ətīt/, a mineral made of calcium and phosphate that is found in the bones and teeth.

Apert's syndrome, a rare defect in which the head and face are deformed and the fingers and toes are fused together.

aperture /ap′ərchər/, an opening in an object or structure, such as the **aperture of larynx,** the opening between the two sections of the windpipe (pharynx and larynx).

apex /ā′peks/, *pl.* **apices** /ā′pisēz/, the top, the end, or the tip of a structure, such as the **apex cordis,** the pointed lower border of the heart, or the **apex pulmonis,** the rounded upper border of each lung.

apex beat, a pulsation of the left lower chamber (ventricle) of the heart. It can sometimes be seen on the skin of the chest.

Apgar score /ap′gär/, a test to determine a newborn baby's physical health. It is done 1 minute and 5 minutes after birth. Scoring is based on a rating of five factors that refer to how well the infant is able to adjust to life outside the womb. A doctor, Virginia Apgar, MD, created the system to tell quickly which infants require treatment right away or transfer to an intensive care nursery. The infant's heart rate, breathing, muscle tone, reflexes, and color are scored from a low value of 0 to a normal value of 2. The five scores are combined, and the totals at 1 minute and 5 minutes are written. For example, Apgar 9/10 is a score of 9 at 1 minute and 10 at 5 minutes. A low 1-minute score requires on-the-spot treatment, oxygen is given, the nose and throat are cleared of mucus, and the infant may be transferred to an intensive care nursery. A baby with a low score after 5 minutes needs expert care. This may include assisted breathing, putting in a catheter, heart massage, or drugs. A score of 0 to 3 is given to infants with severe distress, a score of 4 to 7 means moderate distress, and a score of 7 to 10 is normal. About 50% of infants with 5-minute scores of 0 to 1 die, and infants that survive have three times as many defects at 1 year of age as at birth.

aphagia /əfā′jə/, loss of the ability to swallow, either from disease or mental causes. See also **dysphagia.**

aphakia /əfā′kē·ə/, a state in which part or all of the lens of the eye is missing, usually from removal, as in the treatment of cataracts.

aphasia /əfā′zhə/, a nerve defect in which there are problems with speaking or speech is lost. There are many forms and degrees of aphasia. Aphasia may result from a severe head injury, lack of oxygen, or stroke. It is sometimes short-term, as when a swelling in the brain goes down and language returns. **Anomia** is a form of aphasia in which the patient cannot name objects. It is caused by an injury to a part of the brain. With **conduction aphasia,** the patient has problems in self-expression. Words can be understood, but the patient may mix words similar in sound or meaning. He or she cannot repeat things, spell, or read aloud. The patient is alert and aware of the problem. A common cause is a blood clot in part of the middle brain artery. **Motor aphasia** is the inability to say remembered words because of a lesion in the brain. It involves brain tissue known as Broca's motor speech area in the left side of the brain in right-handed patients. Most commonly, the cause is a stroke. The patient knows what to say but cannot make the mouth movements for the words. With **receptive aphasia,** the patient may see or hear words but does not understand what they mean. Treatment includes constant hard work and practice by the patient to help restore normal speaking ability.

apheresis. See **leukapheresis, plasmapheresis, platelet-pheresis.**

A–E

aphonia /əfō′nē·ə/, a defect in which the patient is not able to make normal speech sounds.

-aphrodisia, a combining form meaning a state of sexual arousal.

apical odontoid ligament, a ligament that connects the spine to the skull.

aplasia /əplā′zhə/, a failure of normal development of an organ or tissue.

apnea /apnē′ə, ap′nē·ə/, an absence of automatic breathing. **Cardiac apnea** is an abnormal, short-term absence of breathing, as in Cheynes-Stokes respiration. The apnea alternates with periods of deep, rapid breathing. **Deglutition apnea** is the normal absence of breathing during swallowing. **Periodic apnea of the newborn** is a normal condition in the full-term newborn. Rapid breathing is followed by a brief period in which breathing stops. It most often occurs with rapid eye movement (REM) sleep. Apnea in the newborn not linked to REM sleep may be a sign of brain bleeding, seizures, or other disorders. **Primary apnea** refers to a total lack of breathing. It may come after a blow to the head and is common right after birth in the newborn baby who may not breathe until the carbon dioxide in the blood reaches a certain level. Within seconds the baby usually begins breathing, becomes pinker, moves the arms and legs, and cries. **Secondary apnea** is an abnormal condition in which breathing has stopped and will not start again. Artificial breathing is needed at once. Secondary apnea may be caused by any event that does not allow oxygen to be absorbed into the blood. **Reflex apnea** is caused by irritating, harmful vapors or gases.

apneustic breathing /apnoo′stik/, a pattern of breathing in which the person breathes in for a long time and then fails to breathe out. The rate of apneustic breathing is usually around 1.5 cycles per minute. See also **respiratory rate.**

apocrine gland /ap′əkrīn/, one of the large, deep glands that are in the armpit, anal, genital, and breast areas of the body. The apocrine glands become active only after puberty, and they release sweat that has a strong, easy-to-identify odor.

aponeurosis /ap′ōnŏŏrō′-/, pl. **aponeuroses,** a strong sheet of fiberlike tissue that attaches muscles to bone (tendon) or holds muscles together (fascia).

apophyseal fracture /-fiz′ē·əl/, a break that separates an outgrowth (apophysis) of a bone from the main bone tissue at a point where a tendon attaches.

apophysis /əpof′i·sis/, the part near the end of a long bone that is enlarged and somewhat uneven. This is the growth portion of a bone. **Apophysitis** refers to a state in which the outgrowth becomes inflamed.

A-post, first roof pillar from the windshield of a vehicle.

apothecaries' measure /əpoth′əker′ēz/, a system of liquid measurements. It was first based on the minim, equal to one drop of water. It has now been set at 0.06 ml. The measures are 60 minims equal 1 fluid dram, 8 fluid drams equal 1 fluid ounce, 16 fluid ounces equal 1 pint, 2 pints equal 1 quart, 4 quarts equal 1 gallon. See also **metric system.**

apothecaries' weight, a system of weights. The system was based on the weight of a plump grain of wheat. It is now set at 65 mg. The weights are 20 grains equal 1 scruple, 3 scruples equal 1 dram, 8 drams equal 1 ounce, 12 ounces equal 1 pound. Compare **avoirdupois weight.**

appendage, an extra piece that is attached to a part or organ. Also called **appendix.**

appendectomy /-dek′-/, removal of the appendix through a cut in the right lower part of the belly. It is done in acute appendicitis to take out a swollen appendix before it breaks open. Unless the appendix has burst and infection has set in, care of the patient is routine. If the appendix has burst, a drain may be left in and drugs are given. The pain may be severe. Fluids through the vein, sedatives, and painkillers are given. See also **abdominal surgery, peritonitis.**

Apgar scoring system for infant evaluation at birth

	0	1	2
Heart rate	Absent	Slow (below 100 beats/minute)	Over 100 beats/minute
Respiratory effort	Absent	Slow or irregular	Good crying
Muscle tone	Limp	Some flexion of extremities	Active motion
Response to catheter in nostril (tested after oropharynx is clear)	No response	Grimace	Cough or sneeze
Color	Blue or pale	Body pink, extremities blue	Completely pink

appendicitis, inflammation of the appendix, usually severe, which if not dealt with leads to a break and infection (peritonitis). The most common symptom, called **Aaron's sign,** is constant pain in the right lower part of the belly. To help the pain, the patient keeps the knees bent. Symptoms include vomiting, a low-grade fever of 99° to 102° F, tenderness, a rigid belly, and few or no bowel sounds. The problem is caused by a blockage at the opening of the appendix, disease of the bowel wall, an adhesion, or a parasite. Treatment involves taking out the appendix within 24 to 48 hours of the first symptoms. Delay usually results in rupture of the appendix, and infection from feces can then spread throughout the belly. The fever rises when infection begins. The patient may have sudden relief from pain followed by more, widespread pain. Appendicitis occurs most often in young adults and more often in males. With **chronic appendicitis,** previous inflammation has caused thickening or scarring of the appendix. See also **peritonitis.**

appendix, *pl.* **appendices,** a wormlike, blunt tube closed at one end extending from the large intestine. Its length varies from 3 to 6 inches, and its diameter is about 1/3 inch. Also called **vermiform appendix.**

appliance, something made for a set purpose, as a dental device.

apraxia /əprak′sē·ə/, loss of the ability to do simple or routine acts. This involves the nervous system and occurs in many forms.

Apresoline Hydrochloride, a trademark for a drug used to treat high blood pressure (hydralazine hydrochloride).

aprosody /āpros′ədē/, a speech defect. There are no normal changes in pitch, sound, and rhythm.

aptitude, a natural talent to learn or know a skill.

aptitude test, any standard test to check a person's ability to learn certain skills.

AquaMephyton, a trademark for vitamin K. It is used to treat blood clotting and other blood problems (phytonadione).

aqueous /ā′kwē·əs, ak′-/, **1.** watery or waterlike, such as the **aqueous humor,** the clear fluid that moves in the eyeball. **2.** a drug made with water.

arachidonic acid. See **fatty acid.**

arachnoid /ərak′noid/, a weblike structure, such as the **arachnoid membrane,** one of the three thin membranes covering the brain and the spinal cord.

Aramine, a trademark for a drug used for severe, life-threatening high blood pressure (metaraminol bitartrate).

Aran-Duchenne muscular atrophy /aran′-dōōshen′/, a form of breakdown of the nerves in the muscles (amyotrophic lateral sclerosis). It affects the hands, arms, shoulders, and legs in the beginning. It later spreads throughout the body. Also called **progressive spinal muscular atrophy.**

arbovirus, any one of more than 300 viruses carried by insects. These viruses cause infections. The infections have symptoms of two or more of the following: fever, rash, brain inflammation, and bleeding into the internal organs or skin. There are vaccines that prevent infection from some arboviruses.

arch bar, any one of many types of wires, bars, or splints that are shaped like the arch of the teeth. They are used to treat broken jaws and to make injured teeth stable.

archetype /är′kətīp/, **1.** an original model or pattern from which something is made. **2.** (in Jungian psychology) an idea or way of thinking that is inherited from the experiences of the human race. It is believed present in the unconscious of a person in the form of drives or moods.

area, a space that contains a specific structure of the body or within which certain functions take place. For example, the aortic area is the space around the large heart artery.

areflexia /ā′rēflek′sē·ə/, a condition of the nervous system in which the reflexes are missing.

arenavirus, a genus of viruses usually carried to humans by mouth or skin contact with the waste matter of wild rodents.

areola /erē′ōlə/, *pl.* **areolae,** **1.** a small space or a cavity within a tissue. **2.** a circular area of a different color surrounding a feature. For example, the **areola mammae** is the colored, circular area around the nipple of each breast. A second ring, called a **secondary areola,** appearing around the areola of the breast during pregnancy, is darker in color than the areola before pregnancy. **3.** the part of the iris around the pupil.

areolar gland /erē′olər/, one of the large oil glands in the areolae around the nipples on the breasts of women. The areolar glands give off an oily fluid that protects the nipple during nursing. They have bundles of muscles that cause the nipples to become erect when aroused.

Arfonad, a trademark for a drug used to control high blood pressure (trimethaphan camsylate).

argentaffin cell /-taf′in/, a cell that gives off serotonin. Serotonin is a chemical that narrows blood vessels. These cells occur in most parts of the stomach and intestines.

argentaffinoma /-taf′inō′mə/, a small yellow, cancerous tumor growing from argentaffin cells in the stomach and intestines.

arginine (Arg) /är′jinin/, an amino acid made by the digestion of proteins. It can also be made artificially. Some compounds made from arginine are used to treat excess ammonia in the blood caused by of liver disease.

argininemia /-ē′mē·ə/, an inherited disorder with an increased amount of arginine in the blood from a lack of an enzyme (arginase).

Argyll-Robertson pupil, a pupil of the eye that narrows when focused for near vision but not in response to light. It is most often seen with syphilis that affects the nervous system.

ariboflavinosis /ārī′bōflā′vinō′-/, a condition caused by lack of vitamin B_2 in the diet. Symptoms include sores at the corners of the mouth, on the lips, and around the nose and eyes. Other symptoms are scaling of the skin (seborrheic dermatitis) and many vision disorders. See also **riboflavin.**

Aristocort, a trademark for a steroid drug (triamcinolone). The tablets, syrup, and injections are used for severe allergies, rheumatic diseases, and other severe diseases. The cream and ointment are used for skin inflammations.

Arlidin, a trademark for a drug that widens blood vessels. It is used for diseases of the circulation (nylidrin hydrochloride).

arm, 1. the part of the upper limb of the body between shoulder and elbow. The bone of the arm is the humerus. The muscles of the arm are the coracobrachialis, biceps brachii, brachialis, and triceps brachii. The nerves are the ulnar nerve and the radial nerve. Blood is supplied by many arteries, as the brachial artery and the radial collateral artery. **2.** *nontechnical.* the arm and the forearm.

arm bone. See **humerus.**

arm cylinder cast, a cast made of plaster of paris or fiberglass used to keep the arm rigid from the wrist to above the elbow. It is most often applied to aid the healing of a dislocated elbow or to correct a defect of the elbow.

armpit. See **axilla.**

arrest, to inhibit, restrain, or stop. For example, to arrest the course of a disease. **Development arrest** is fetal growth that stops. See also **cardiac arrest.**

arrhenoblastoma /arē′nōblastō′mə/, a tumor of the ovary that releases male sex hormone. This causes a woman to develop male characteristics, as deep voice and body hair.

arrhythmia /ərith′mē·ə/, any change in the normal pattern of the heart beat. Causes include a defect in the pacemaker function, failure of electrical conduction, and increased energy need, as in exercise or fever. A heart beat that is abnormal in timing or origin of signal with respect to the normal rhythm of the heart is called an **extrasystole. Aberrant ventricular conduction (AVC)** refers to the brief abnormal electric signal of the heart found with some types of irregular heart beats. This can be caused by scar tissue or by an overdose of digitalis, a drug given for heart failure. An **accelerated idiojunctional rhythm** refers to a heart rhythm that is faster than the normal rate. If the heart is otherwise normal, this condition is not a problem. An **accelerated idioventricular rhythm (AIVR)** is a condition in which the heart beats faster than the normal rate but slower than 100 beats per minute (50 to 100 per minute). **Atrial flutter** refers to rapid, regular contractions of the upper heart chambers (atria), about 300 beats per minute. The lower chambers of the heart (ventricles) cannot respond to this. They contract at a lower rate, usually about 150 beats per minute. A **premature contraction** is a drawing together of a heart chamber before it would normally occur. This often means the heart muscle is unsteady and may lead to poor heart function. Arrhythmias are controlled by a number of drugs, as beta-blockers and calcium blockers. See also **bradycardia, fibrillation, heart block, tachycardia.** Also called **cardiac arrhythmia.** Compare **dysrhythmia.**

arsenic (As) /är′sənik/, an element that occurs throughout the earth's crust. This element has been used for centuries as a drug and as a poison. It continues to have limited use in some drugs used to treat tropical disease (trypanosomiasis). The introduction of drugs without arsenic that have less dangerous side effects has greatly reduced its use. Many compounds with arsenic are used as dyes, pesticides, herbicides, and feed additives for poultry and livestock. Federal laws on arsenic levels in food and industry have greatly lessened the number of arsenic poisonings. –**arsenic** /ärsen′ik/, **arsenical,** *adj.*

arsenical stomatitis, a mouth condition linked to arsenic poisoning. The symptoms are dry, red, and painful mucous membrane in the mouth, ulcers, bleeding gums, and loose teeth. See also **stomatitis.**

arsenic poisoning, poisoning caused by eating or breathing arsenic. Small amounts absorbed over a period of time may result in long-term poisoning. Nausea, headache, coloring and scaling of the skin, thickened skin, loss of desire for food, and white lines across the fingernails are symptoms of long-term poisoning. Consuming large amounts of arsenic results in severe stomach and intestine pain, diarrhea, vomiting, and swelling of the feet and hands. Kidney failure and shock may occur. Death may result. Diagnosis is confirmed when arsenic is found in the urine, hair, or fingernails. Treatment includes flushing the stomach with water and giving the drug dimercaprol. Fluids given in the veins and other treatment as needed for anemia, kidney failure, or shock, are also helpful.

Artane, a trademark for a drug used to treat parkinsonism (trihexyphenidyl hydrochloride).

arterial insufficiency. See **vascular insufficiency.**

arteriogram /ärtir′ē·ə gram′/, an x-ray film of an artery that has been injected with a dye. See also **angiography.**

arteriole /ärtir′ē·ōl/, any of the tiny vessels of the arterial circulation. Blood from the heart is pumped through the arteries to the arterioles, which form part of the capillaries.

The blood flows from the capillaries into the veins and returns to the heart. The wall of the arterioles narrows and widens in response to chemicals made by nerves, playing an important role in control of blood pressure. See also **artery.**

arteriosclerosis /ärtir′ē·əsklerō′-/, a common disorder of the arteries. There is thickening, loss of elasticity, and hardening of the walls from calcium. This results in less blood supply, especially to the brain and legs. The condition often develops with aging. Other causes include high blood pressure, kidney disease, diabetes, and excess fats (lipids) in the blood. Symptoms include leg cramps when walking (intermittent claudication), changes in skin temperature and color, altered pulses, headache, dizziness, and memory defects. See also **atherosclerosis.**

arteriovenous angioma of the brain /-vē′nəs/, an inborn tumor. It is made up of a tangle of arteries and veins, and areas of hardened brain tissue. The tumor may grow deeply into the brain, causing seizures and paralysis. See also **angioma.**

arteriovenous fistula, an abnormal link between an artery and vein. It can occur from a birth defect, injury, infection, bulge in an artery wall (aneurysm), or cancer. An arteriovenous fistula is often made by surgery. It gives access to the bloodstream of patients receiving dialysis.

arteritis /är′tərī′-/, inflammation of the walls of one or more arteries. It may occur as a disease in itself. It also may go together with another disorder, as rheumatoid arthritis and rheumatic fever.

artery, any one of the large blood vessels carrying blood with oxygen from the heart to the rest of the body. The artery is a hollow tube enclosed by three layers of tissue: the inner layer (tunica intima), the middle layer (tunica media), which makes up most of the arterial wall, and the outer layer (tunica adventitia). The middle layer is almost entirely muscular. The thickness of the outer layer changes with the location of the artery. Larger arteries have a thick inner layer. In older patients the layer may have deposits of cholesterol and calcium salts or other deposits. Most of the arteries in the body are about ³/₁₆ inch (4 mm) in diameter. The muscle walls of arteries move blood with oxygen from the heart to structures throughout the body. Nerves that supply the arteries direct the flow of blood.

arthralgia /ärthral′jə/, any pain that affects a joint. – **arthralgic,** *adj.*

arthritis, any inflammation of the joints. **Acute pyogenic arthritis** is a bacterial infection of one or more joints. It occurs most often in children and is caused by injury. Symptoms include pain and swelling in the joint, muscle spasms, chills, fever, and sweating. Treatment is mainly with antibiotics, although in some cases the fluid in the joint is removed. **Septic arthritis** may be caused by the spread of bacteria through the bloodstream from an infection elsewhere in the body or by infection of a joint during injury or surgery. The joint is stiff, painful, tender, warm, and swollen. Physical therapy as the joint heals helps to restore it to full motion. See also **osteoarthritis, rheumatoid arthritis.**

arthrocentesis /är′thrōsentē′-/, puncturing a joint with a needle and withdrawing fluid (synovial fluid) from the joint. This is done to get samples of the fluid for diagnosis.

arthrodesis /ärthrod′əsis/, fixing a joint by uniting the bones through surgery to relieve pain or give support.

arthrogryposis multiplex congenita /-gripō′-/, stiffness of one or more joints that is present at birth.

arthropathy /ärthrop′əthē/, any disease or abnormal condition affecting a joint.

arthroplasty /är′thrəplas′tē/, surgery for a painful, broken-down joint. Arthroplasty gives movement to a joint in joint disease (osteoarthritis and rheumatoid arthritis). It can correct an inborn defect.

arthropod /-pod/, a member of the Arthropoda, a large major group of animal life that includes crabs and lobsters, mites, ticks, spiders, and insects. Arthropods generally have a jointed shell (exoskeleton) and paired, jointed legs. They bite, sting, and cause allergic reactions. They carry viruses and other disease-causing organisms.

arthroscopy /ärthros′kəpē/, examination of the interior of a joint, usually in knee problems. A specially designed microscope-like device (endoscope) is put through a small cut. Arthroscopy permits removal of cartilage or fluid (synovial) from the joint, and the diagnosis of a torn meniscus.

Arthus reaction, a rare, severe, direct allergic reaction to injection of a foreign substance (allergen). The allergen is usually not harmful. However, in some individuals it causes a reaction. A sudden red, painful swelling with bleeding and tissue death occurs at the site of injection.

articular capsule, an envelope of tissue that surrounds a joint. See also **fibrous capsule.**

articular disk, the platelike end of some bones in movable joints. It can be closely linked to surrounding muscles or with cartilage.

articular fracture, a broken bone involving the articular surfaces of a joint.

artifact, anything irrelevant or unwanted, as a substance, structure, or piece of information. In x-ray films electronic signals may appear as an artifact on an image, thereby confusing the results of any examination.

artificial fever. See **fever therapy.**

artificial heart, a mechanical device of molded polyurethane. It is made up of two chambers implanted in the body and powered by an air compressor outside the body. The first artificial heart for humans was implanted in December 1982. The mechanical heart was attached to the upper chambers (atria) and major blood vessels of the patient's normal heart with Dacron fittings.

artificial insemination, putting semen into the vagina or uterus by mechanical means rather than by sexual intercourse. This is planned along with the expected time of the discharge of the egg (ovum) from the ovary. Thus fertilization can occur. **Artificial insemination donor (AID)** refers to semen given by an unknown donor. It is used mainly in cases where the husband is sterile. When semen is given by the husband, it is called **artificial insemination husband (AIH)**. It is used mainly in cases of impotency or when the husband is incapable of sexual intercourse because of some physical disability.

artificial kidney, a device used to rid the blood of substances that should be released in urine. It usually is made up of a set of tubes for passing the blood between the patient and a dialysis machine. Also called **kidney machine.** See also **dialysis.**

artificial limb. See **prosthesis.**

artificial lung, an airtight breathing machine consisting of a metal tank that encloses the entire body, except for the head. It is used for long-term therapy. It provides artificial breathing by contracting and expanding the walls of the chest. Also called **iron lung, respirator.**

artificial pacemaker. See **pacemaker.**

artificial respiration, the process of continuing breathing by the hands and mouth of another person or mechanical means when normal breathing has stopped. Breathing may stop because of swelling, an object stuck in the throat, mucus, nerve disorders, and severe asthma. Other causes are exhaustion, drug overdose, or injury to the chest wall. Before trying to give artificial respiration, the airway is checked. Any obstruction is removed. See also **cardiopulmonary resuscitation (CPR).**

aryl hydrocarbon hydroxylase (AHH), an enzyme that changes cancer-causing chemicals in tobacco smoke and in polluted air into active cancer-causing agents within the lungs.

asbestosis, a life-long lung disease caused by breathing asbestos fibers. It results in lung disorders, as pleural fibrosis, with shortness of breath. Asbestos miners and workers are most often affected. The disease sometimes occurs in other people who have been exposed to asbestos building materials. See also **pulmonary disease.**

ascariasis /as'kərī'əsis/, an infection caused by a parasitic worm, *Ascaris lumbricoides*. The eggs are passed in human feces. The infection is carried on to others through hands, water, or food.

ascending pharyngeal artery, one of the smallest arteries that branch from the outer carotid artery, deep in the neck. It takes blood to many organs and muscles of the head.

ascites /əsī'tēz/, an abnormal pooling of fluid in the abdominal cavity containing large amounts of protein and other cells. See also **paracentesis.** –**ascitic,** *adj.*

ascorbemia /as'kôrbē'mē·ə/, the presence of vitamin C (ascorbic acid) in the blood in larger than normal amounts. It usually means an excess in the diet.

ascorbic acid. See **vitamin C.**

ascorburia /-ōōr'ē·ə/, ascorbic acid in the urine in larger amounts than normal.

Asellacrin, a trademark for a drug used to stimulate growth in children who have some types of dwarfism (somatotropin).

Asendin, a trademark for a drug used to relieve depression (amoxapine).

asepsis /āsep'-/, the absence of germs. **Medical asepsis** is the removal of disease organisms or infected material. **Surgical asepsis** is protection against infection before, during, or after surgery by using sterile technique. –**aseptic,** *adj.*

Asepto syringe, a trademark for a blunt-tipped syringe fitted with a bulb at the top. It is used mainly for flushing out wounds.

asexual /āsek'shoo·əl/, **1.** referring to an organism that has no sexual organs. **2.** referring to a process that is not sexual. –**asexuality,** *n.*

asexual dwarf, an adult dwarf whose sex organs are not well developed.

asexualization /āsek'shoo·əlīzā'shən/, the process of making one unable to reproduce. This may be by castration, vasectomy, taking the ovaries away, tying the tubes, or other means.

Asherman syndrome, lack of menstruation (amenorrhea) in a woman with normal hormones.

asparagine (Asn) /asper'əjin/, an amino acid found in many proteins in the body. It acts as a drug that promotes the release of urine. See also **amino acid.**

aspartame, a white, almost odorless crystalline powder with an intensely sweet taste. It is used as an artificial sweetener. It is about 180 times as sweet as the same amount of sugar. Aspartame tends to lose its sweetness in the presence of heat and moisture.

aspartate aminotransferase (AST) /aspär'tāt/, an enzyme normally present in blood serum and in the heart and liver. AST is released into the blood after injury and as a result of heart attack and liver damage.

aspartic acid (Asp), an amino acid in sugar cane, beet molasses, and the breakdown products of many proteins. Aspartic acid is used in dietary supplements and in drugs that kill funguses and germs. See also **amino acid.**

aspergillosis /as′pərjilō′-/, an infection caused by the fungus *Aspergillus*. It usually affects the ear but is capable of infecting any organ. Relatively uncommon, it typically occurs in a patient already weakened by another disorder.

asphyxia /asfik′sē·ə/, severe oxygen lack. It leads to blood with low oxygen content, loss of consciousness, and, if not corrected, death. Some of the more common causes of asphyxia are drowning, electric shock, breathing vomit, and an object stuck in the breathing tract. Breathing toxic gas or smoke and poisoning are other causes. Artificial respiration and oxygen are promptly given to avoid damage to the brain. See also **artificial respiration.** – **asphyxiate,** *v.,* **asphyxiated,** *adj.*

aspiration, 1. the act of taking a breath, inhaling. 2. the act of withdrawing fluid, as mucus or blood, from the body by a suction device. 3. the act of taking foreign material or vomit into the lungs. –**aspirate,** *n.*

aspiration pneumonia. See **pneumonia.**

aspirator, any instrument that takes a substance away from body cavities by suction, as a bulb syringe, pump, or hypodermic needle.

aspirin, a drug used to reduce fever and to relieve pain and inflammation. Bleeding disorders, peptic ulcer, pregnancy, the use of anticlotting drugs, or known allergy prohibits its use. Side effects include stomach and intestine problems (ulcers, bleeding), and ringing in the ears. Use of large doses over a long time can cause blood clotting defects and liver and kidney damage. Reye's syndrome in children may be caused by aspirin. Some asthmalike and other allergic reactions are occasionally seen.

aspirin poisoning. See **salicylate poisoning.**

assertive training, a method used in behavior therapy to help people become more self-confident in their relationships. It teaches direct, honest statement of feelings and beliefs.

assessment, 1. an evaluation of a condition. 2. an examiner's evaluation of the disease or condition based on the patient's report of the symptoms and the examiner's findings. It includes data gotten through laboratory tests, physical examination, and medical history.

assessment of the aging patient, an evaluation of the changes brought about by advancing years in an elderly patient. In many cases, changes considered normal in elderly patients are actually diseases that may respond to treatment.

assigned resources, resources checked in and assigned work tasks on an incident.

assimilation, 1. the process of incorporating nutrition into living tissue. 2. the incorporation of new experiences into a person's consciousness.

assisting agency, an agency directly contributing suppression, rescue, support, or service resources to another agency.

association, 1. a connection, union, joining, or combination of things. 2. connecting feelings, emotions, sensations, or thoughts with particular persons, things, or ideas.

astereognosis /əstir′ē·ognō′-/, a nervous system disorder. It is marked by an inability to recognize objects by touch.

asthenia /asthē′nē·ə/, the lack or loss of strength or energy; weakness.

asthenic habitus. See **somatotype.**

asthenic personality, a personality with low energy, lack of enthusiasm, and oversensitivity to physical and emotional strain.

asthenopia, /as′thənō′pe·ə/, a condition in which the eyes tire easily because of weakness of the eye muscles. Symptoms include pain in or around the eyes, headache, dimness of vision, dizziness, and slight nausea.

asthma /az′mə/, a lung disorder with attacks of breathing difficulty. The attacks can range from occasional periods of wheezing, mild coughing, and slight breathlessness to severe attacks that can lead to airway obstruction and total inability to breathe. Asthmatic attacks are caused by a narrowing of the airways. This results from muscle spasm in the lungs, inflammation and swelling of the bronchial tubes, or excess mucus. The episodes may be started in various ways. **Allergic asthma** occurs from breathing in an airborne substance (allergen). Antibodies form in the cells of the lung sacs to fight the allergen. The histamine then released causes the bronchial muscles to contract, which leads to the coughing and wheezing of asthma. Treatments are more effective for pollen sensitivity than for house dust, animal hair, molds, and insects. Often, a daily pattern of histamine release is seen, causing many degrees of attacks at different times of the day. **Intrinsic asthma** is a nonseasonal, nonallergic form of asthma usually starting later in life than allergic asthma. It tends to be chronic and long-lasting rather than episodic. The trigger factors include breathing irritating pollutants, as dust particles, smoke, aerosols, strong cooking odors, paint fumes, and other volatile substances. An example is **grinder's asthma,** caused by breathing in fine particles put out during industrial grinding processes. Persons who work with soaps, Western red cedar, cotton, flax, hemp, grain, flour, and stone are subject to **occupational asthma.** Bronchospasm may also occur in cold, damp weather, after sudden breathing of cold, dry air, and after exercise or violent coughing or laughing. Breathing infections, as the common cold, and mental factors, as anxiety, may also cause attacks.

An acute, severe, and long-lasting asthma attack is called **status asthmaticus.** A lack of oxygen in the blood, blue skin, and unconsciousness may follow. This is a medical emergency. Treatment includes the giving of certain drugs and the use of artificial breathing methods. A bronchodilator may be given by aerosol inhalation from a ventilator. An asthmatic attack needs direct relief with drugs that widen the bronchi and remove excess mucus. The major drugs used to relieve bronchospasm are the beta-adrenergic agents, the methylxanthines, steroids, expectorants, and sedatives. Antibiotics are used when infection is the cause of an attack.

Treatment includes getting rid of the cause if possible.

astigmatism /əstig′mətizəm/, an abnormal condition of the eye in which the curve of the cornea is unequal. As a result, light rays cannot be focused clearly. Vision is blurred. The eyes tire easily. The condition usually can be corrected with contact lenses or with eyeglasses.

astringent /əstrin′jənt/, a substance that causes tissues to contract. It is usually used on the skin. Alum and tannic acid are common astringents.

astringent bath, a bath in which an astringent is added to the water.

astroblastoma /as′trōblastō′mə/, a cancerous tumor of the brain and spinal cord. Cells of an astroblastoma lie around blood vessels or, in some cases, around connective tissue.

astrocytoma /-sītō′mə/, a tumor of the brain. There is slow growth, lump (cyst) formation, and invasion of surrounding structures.

asymmetrical, referring to parts of the body that are unequal in size or shape, or that are different in arrangement. Compare **symmetrical.**

asynclitism /āsing′klitizm/, during labor, a presentation of the top of the baby's head that is not in proper alignment with the mother's pelvis for birth. In normal labor, the baby's head is usually out of correct position at some time, especially during early labor.

asynergy /āsin′ərjē/, faulty coordination among groups of organs or muscles that normally function well together.

asyntaxia /ā′sintak′sē·ə/, any interference with the proper order of growth of the fetus during development. This results in one or more birth defects. See also **birth defect.**

asystole /āsis′tōlē/. See **cardiac arrest.**

Atabrine Hydrochloride, a trademark for a drug used to treat malaria (quinacrine hydrochloride).

Atarax, a trademark for a drug used to treat distress and itching from allergies (hydroxyzine hydrochloride).

atavism /at′əvizm/, traits or characteristics in a person that are more like those of a grandparent or earlier ancestor

than like the parents. This data may offer hints of genetic or family health factors to a physician.

ataxia /ətak′sē·ə/, a blocked ability to coordinate movements. A staggering walk and poor balance may be caused by damage to the spinal cord or brain. This can be the result of birth trauma, inborn disorder, infection, tumor, poison, or head injury.

ataxic breathing, a disorder of breathing linked to an injury in the brain. Symptoms include poorly coordinated breathing movements.

atelectasis /at′ilek′təsis/, an abnormal condition with the collapse of lung tissue. This prevents the exchange of carbon dioxide and oxygen by the blood. Symptoms include difficulty in breathing, reduced breath sounds, and fever. Loss of lung tissue may also cause increased heart rate and higher blood pressure. The condition may be caused by a block in the major airways, pressure on the lung from fluid or air in the area around the lungs (pleural space), or by pressure from a tumor outside the lung.

atenolol, a drug used to treat high blood pressure. Abnormally slow heart beat or heart failure prohibits its use. Side effects include slow heart beat, dizziness, and nausea.

atheroma /ath′ərō′mə/, an abnormal mass of fat, as in an oil gland cyst or in deposits in an artery wall.

atherosclerosis /ath′ərōsklərō′-/, a common disorder of the arteries. Yellowish plaques of cholesterol, fats, and other remains are deposited in the walls of large and medium-sized arteries. The vessel walls become thick and hardened. The vessel narrows. This lessens circulation to organs and other areas normally supplied by the artery. These plaques (atheromas) are major causes of heart disease, chest pain (angina pectoris), heart attacks, and other disorders of the circulation. How atherosclerosis develops is not clear. It may begin with injury to the artery or with an increase of muscle in vessel walls. Excess saturated fats in the diet, faulty carbohydrate processing, or a genetic defect may be other causes. Atherosclerosis usually occurs with aging. It is often linked to overweight, high blood pressure, and diabetes. See also **arteriosclerosis.**

athetosis /ath′ətō′-/, a condition of the nerves supplying the muscles. Symptoms include slow, twisting, continuous, and involuntary movement of the arms and legs.

athiaminosis /əthī′əminō′-/, a condition resulting from lack of thiamine (vitamin B₁) in the diet.

athlete's foot, a long-term fungal infection of the foot. It occurs especially on the skin between the toes and on the soles. It is common worldwide. Adults are most susceptible. Drying the feet well after bathing and applying powder between the toes help prevent it.

athlete's heart, the typical, normal but large heart of an athlete trained for endurance. The condition has slow heart beats, an increased pumping capacity, and greater than average ability to carry oxygen to muscles. Also called **athletic heart syndrome (AHS).**

athletic habitus. See **somatotype.**

Ativan, a trademark for a drug used in tablet form to treat anxiety. Injections are given before surgery to deepen the anesthesia (lorazepam).

atlantooccipital joint /-oksip′itəl/, one of a pair of joints formed where the atlas of the vertebral column meets the occipital bone of the skull.

atlas. See **vertebra.**

atmosphere, 1. the natural air, composed of about 20% oxygen, 78% nitrogen, and 2% carbon dioxide and other gases, that covers the surface of the earth. **2.** an envelope of gas, which may not be identical to the natural atmosphere, in chemical components.

atmospheric pressure, the pressure of the weight of the atmosphere. The atmospheric pressure at sea level is about 14.7 pounds per square inch. With increasing altitude the pressure becomes less. At 30,000 feet, the air pressure is 4.3 pounds per square inch. Also called **barometric pressure.**

atom, the smallest particle of an element that retains all the chemical characteristics of the element. It consists of a central core called the nucleus, which contains protons and neutrons, and electrons, which revolve in orbits around the nucleus.

atomic energy, energy released in nuclear reactions. Of particular interest is the energy released when a neutron initiates the splitting of an atom's nucleus into smaller pieces (fission) or when two nuclei are joined together under millions of degrees of heat (fusion). "Atomic energy" is really a popular misnomer. It is more correctly called nuclear energy.

atomizer, a device for spraying a liquid as a fine mist or vapor.

atonic /ətonˈik/, **1.** weak, or lacking normal tone, as a muscle that is soft. **2.** lacking vigor, as an atonic ulcer, which heals slowly.

atopic /ātopˈik/, referring to an inborn tendency to develop immediate allergic reactions, as asthma, allergic skin disease, or hay fever. Atopic reactions are caused by an antibody in the skin and sometimes the bloodstream.

atopic dermatitis, an intensely itching inflammation of the skin on the face, knees, and elbows of allergy-prone patients. It is most common in infants.

atresia /ətrēˈzhə/, the absence of a normal body opening, duct, or canal, as the anus, vagina, or ear canal.

atrial fibrillation /āˈtrē·əl/. See **fibrillation.**

atrioventricular (AV) block /āˈtrēōventrikˈyələr/. See **heart block.**

atrioventricular (AV) node, an area of specialized heart muscle that receives the electric impulse of the heart from the sinoatrial (SA) node. The impulse then travels to the atrioventricular bundle of His, which carries it to the ventricles. The AV node is located in the wall (septum) of the right atrium.

atrioventricular septum, a small portion of wall that separates the upper heart chambers (atria) from the lower heart chambers (ventricles) of the heart.

atrioventricular valve, a valve in the heart through which blood flows from the upper heart chambers (atria) to the lower heart chambers (ventricles). The valve between the left atrium and left ventricle is called the mitral valve. The right valve is called the tricuspid valve. Also called **cuspid valve.**

at risk, able to be hurt by a particular disease or injury. The risk may be environmental or physical. An example of an environmental risk is exposure to toxic wastes. An example of a physical risk is a genetic tendency to develop a disease.

atrium /āˈtrē·əm/, pl. **atria,** a chamber or cavity, such as the nasal cavity. The **atrium of the heart** is one of the two upper chambers of the heart. Blood lacking oxygen returns from the body to the right atrium. The left atrium receives blood with oxygen from the veins in the lungs. Blood is emptied into the lower heart chambers (ventricles) from the atria.

atrophic fracture /ātrofˈik/, a spontaneous fracture caused by wasting away (atrophy). This sometimes occurs in elderly patients.

atrophy /atˈrəfē/, a wasting or loss of size of a part of the body because of disease or other influences. A muscle may atrophy because of lack of physical exercise. Nervous system or muscle disease are other causes. Cells of the brain and nervous system may atrophy in old age because of restricted blood flow to those areas.

atropine sulfate /atˈrəpin/, a drug used to treat spasms of the stomach and intestines, inflammation of the eye, irregular heart beats, nerve disorders (parkinsonism), some kinds of poisoning, and with anesthesia. Blockage of the digestive tract, glaucoma, hepatitis, kidney disease, or known allergy to this or similar drugs prohibits its use. Side effects include rapid heart beat, chest pain, dry mouth, nausea, diarrhea or constipation, skin rash, blurred vision, and eye pain.

attachment, 1. the state or quality of being attached. **2.** a mode of behavior in which one person relates in a dependent manner to another; a feeling of affection or loyalty that binds one person to another. See also **bonding.**

attending physician, the physician who is responsible for a particular patient.

attention deficit disorder, a condition of learning and behavior problems affecting children, adolescents, and, rarely, adults. It may result from genetic factors, chemical imbalance, or injury or disease at or after birth. Also called **hyperactivity, minimal brain dysfunction.** See also **learning disability.**

attenuation, the process of reduction, as the weakening of a disease organism.

Attenuvax, a trademark for a vaccine against measles virus.

attraction, a tendency of the teeth or other jaw structures to grow above their normal position.

attrition, the process of wearing away or wearing down by friction.

audiometer /ô′dē·om′ətər/, an electric device for testing the hearing and for measuring the conduction of sound through bone and air. Earphones are placed over the ears. The ear not being tested gets a masking noise from the machine. The ear being tested is aroused by a series of tones, from very low to very high frequencies at various decibels. The patient signals when a tone is heard. The results are noted on a chart (**audiogram**).

audiometry /ô′dē·om′ətrē/, testing the sense of hearing. **Pure tone** audiometry determines the patient's ability to hear frequencies, usually ranging from 125 to 8000 hertz (Hz). It can determine if a hearing loss is caused by a middle-ear problem or by one in the inner ear or the auditory nerve. In this test the patient sits in a soundproof booth. The operator slowly increases the decibel level. The patient signals when sounds are first heard through the earphones.

auditory ossicles /ô′ditôr′ē/, the small bones in the middle ear (incus, malleus, and stapes) that connect with each other and the ear drum (tympanic membrane). Sound waves are carried through these bones as the tympanic membrane vibrates.

auditory system assessment, an evaluation of the patient's ears and hearing.

auditory tube. See **eustachian tube.**

Auer rod /ou′ər/, abnormal, needle-shaped or round bodies in the white blood cells of a patient with leukemia.

aura /ôr′ə/, *pl.* **aurae** /ôr′ē/, a sensation of light or warmth that may be noted before an attack of migraine headache or an epileptic seizure.

aural /ôr′əl/, referring to the ear or hearing. **−aurally,** *adv.*

Aureomycin, a trademark for a tetracycline antibiotic (chlortetracycline hydrochloride).

auricle /ôr′ikəl/, **1.** the external ear. Also called **pinna. 2.** the left or right upper heart chamber (atrium), so named because of its earlike shape.

auricularis /ôr′ikyələr′is/, referring to the ear, such as one of three outer muscles of the ear.

auriculin /ôrik′yəlin/, a hormonelike substance made in the upper chambers (atria) of the heart. It promotes the release of urine.

aurothioglucose /ôr′ōthī′ōgloo′kōs/, gold used to treat adult and juvenile rheumatoid arthritis. Uncontrolled diabetes, kidney or liver disease, high blood pressure, heart failure, pregnancy, or known allergy to this drug prohibits its use. Side effects include kidney damage, allergic reactions, and ulcers of the mucous membranes.

auscultation /ôs′kəltā′shən/, the act of listening for sounds within the body to evaluate the condition of the heart, lungs, intestines, or other organs or to hear the fetal heart beat. The listening may be done with the ear alone, but usually a stethoscope is used. During auscultation of the chest, the patient usually sits upright and breathes slowly and deeply through the mouth. The heart and stomach may be auscultated with the patient lying down or sitting upright.

Australian lift, a type of shoulder lift used to move patients who are unable to sit upright by themselves.

autism /ô′tizm/, a disorder with extreme withdrawal into fantasy.

autoantibody, an antibody that reacts against the patient's own body. Normally antibodies attack foreign invaders (antigens). Several processes may lead to the making of autoantibodies. For example, antibodies made against some streptococcal bacteria during infection may react with heart tissue. This causes rheumatic heart disease. Another way is that normal body proteins may be changed to antigens by chemicals, infection, or drugs.

autoantigen /-an′tijən/, a normal body substance that causes an abnormal production of autoantibody. This results in a reaction of the body against tissues in the body. See also **autoantibody.**

autodiploid /-dip′loid/, referring to a person, organism, or cell containing two genetically identical or nearly identical chromosome sets.

autoeroticism /-irot′isizm/, **1.** sensual, usually sexual, satisfaction of the self. It is usually done through stimulating one's own body without another person. Satisfaction comes from stroking, masturbation, fantasy, or other oral, anal, or visual sources. **2.** (in Freudian psychoanalytic theory) an early phase of sexual development. It occurs in the oral and the anal stages.

autoerythrocyte sensitization /-ərith′rəsīt/, an unusual disorder with painful bleeding under the skin on the front areas of the arms and legs. The cause is allergy to the patient's own red blood cells.

autogenous /ôtoj′ənəs/, **1.** self-creating. **2.** originating from within the organism, as a poison or vaccine.

autograft. See **transplant.**

autoimmune disease, one of a large group of diseases marked by a change of the immune system of the body. Normally, the immune system controls the body's defenses against infection. Sometimes these defenses are turned against the body itself. This leads to chronic and often deadly diseases. The cause of autoimmune disease is not known.

autoimmunity. See **immunity.**

automatism /ôtom′ətizm/, **1.** involuntary function of an organ system. It can be independent of outer stimulation, as beating of the heart, or dependent on outer stimulation but not consciously controlled, as the dilation of the pupil of the eye. **2.** mechanical, repetitive, and undirected behavior that is not consciously controlled, as in brain disorder (psychomotor epilepsy), hysteric states, and sleepwalking.

autonomic, **1.** having the ability to function independently without outside influence. **2.** referring to the autonomic nervous system.

autonomic drug, any of a large group of drugs that copy or change the function of the autonomic nervous system.

autonomic nervous system, the part of the nervous system that regulates vital functions of the body that are not consciously controlled (involuntary). It includes the activity of the heart, the smooth muscles (such as digestive muscles), and the glands. It has two divisions: the **sympathetic nervous system** speeds up heart rate, narrows blood vessels, and raises blood pressure; the **parasympathetic nervous system** slows heart rate, increases intestinal and gland activity, and relaxes ringlike muscles which close passages (sphincters). See also **peripheral nervous system.**

autonomic reflex, any of a large number of normal reflexes that regulate the functions of the body's organs. Autonomic reflexes control activities such as blood pressure, heart rate, intestinal activity, sweating, and urination.

autonomy /ôton′əmē/, the quality of having the ability to live independently. –**autonomous,** *adj.*

autoplastic maneuver, a process that is part of adaptation, involving an adjustment within the self. The opposite, **alloplastic maneuver,** involves a change in the external environment.

autopsy /ô′topsē/, an examination after death that is done to determine the cause of death.

autosomal /-sō′məl/, **1.** referring to or characteristic of a non-sex-determining chromosome (autosome). **2.** referring to any condition carried by an autosome.

autosomal recessive inheritance, a pattern of inheritance in which a non-dominant (recessive) gene on a non-sex-determining chromosome (autosome) results in a person being either a carrier of a trait or being affected.

autosome /ô′təsōm/, any chromosome that is not a sex chromosome and appears as an identical (homologous) pair.

autosplenectomy /-splinek′-/, a continuous shrinking of the spleen. It may occur in sickle-cell anemia. The spleen is replaced by fiberlike tissue and becomes nonfunctional.

autosuggestion, an idea, thought, attitude, or belief suggested to oneself, often as a formula or chant, as a means of controlling one's behavior.

auxanology /ôks′ənol′-/, the scientific study of growth and development.

available resources, resources assigned to an incident and available for an assignment.

avascular /āvas′kyələr/, referring to an area not receiving a sufficient supply of blood. The reduced flow may be the result of blockage by a blood clot. It may also be from stopping the blood flow during surgery or when controlling bleeding.

Aventyl Hydrochloride, a trademark for a drug used to relieve depression (nortriptyline hydrochloride).

aversion therapy, a form of behavior therapy in which punishment or an unpleasant or painful stimulation are used to stop undesirable behavior. Electric shock and drugs that cause nausea are examples of aversion therapy. Conditions such as drug abuse, alcoholism, gambling, overeating, smoking, and various sexual abnormalities are treated.

avidin, a protein in raw egg white that reacts with a B complex vitamin (biotin).

avitaminosis /āvī′-/, a lack of one or more essential vitamins. It may result from lack of vitamins in the diet or inability to use the vitamins because of disease. Also called **hypovitaminosis.**

AV nicking, a blood vessel abnormality on the retina of the eye. The vein appears ''nicked'' because of narrowing or spasm. It is a sign of high blood pressure, hardening of the arteries (arteriosclerosis), and other disorders of the blood vessels.

avoidance, a conscious or unconscious defense mechanism, physical or psychologic in nature. A person tries to escape from something unpleasant. See also **conflict.**

avoirdupois weight /av′ərdəpoiz′/, the English system of weights in which there are 7000 grains, 256 drams, or 16 ounces to 1 pound. One ounce in this system equals 28.35 grams. 1 pound equals 453.59 grams. See also **metric system.**

avulsion /əvul′zhən/, the separation, by tearing, of any part of a structure.

avulsion fracture, a bone fracture caused when a ligament or tendon forcibly pulls a piece of bone away.

axial, referring to or situated on the center (axis) of a structure or part of the body.

axial gradient, the variation in the chemical processes (metabolic rate) in different parts of the body.

axilla /aksil′ə/, *pl.* **axillae,** a pyramid-shaped space forming the underside of the shoulder between the upper part of the arm and the side of the chest. Also called **armpit.**

axillary artery /ak′sələr′ē/, the artery that supplies each arm. Called the subclavian artery at the collar bone, it becomes the axillary at the shoulder. Where it crosses the bicep it becomes the brachial artery.

axillary nerve, the nerve that runs through the armpit (axilla), winds around the bone in the upper arm (humerus), and supplies part of the shoulder muscles (deltoid) and the shoulder joint.

axillary node, one of the lymph glands of the armpit (axilla) that help to fight infections in the chest, armpit, neck, and arm. They also drain lymph from those areas. See also **lymphatic system, lymph node.**

axillary vein, one of a pair of veins of the arm that begins at the top of the arm near the bicep and becomes the subclavian vein near the collarbone. It receives oxygen-poor blood from certain veins.

axis, *pl.* **axes** /ak′sēz/, an imaginary line that passes through the center of the body, or a part of the body. See also **vertebra.**

axis artery, one of a pair of extensions of the subclavian arteries. It runs into the upper arm and continues into the forearm as the palmar interosseous artery.

axon, the cylinderlike extension of a nerve (neuron) cell that conducts electric impulses (synapses) away from the neuron. Compare **dendrite.**

axon flare, widening of the blood vessels, reddening, and increased sensitivity of skin surrounding an injured area. It is caused by nerve damage. Histamine or a histaminelike substance is released and the rash of hives occurs.

azathioprine, an immunosuppressive drug used to prevent organ rejection after an organ transplant. It is also used to treat systemic inflammatory diseases.

Azlin, a trademark for an antibiotic (azlocillin).

azlocillin sodium, a penicillin antibiotic used to treat various infections. Allergy to any of the penicillins prohibits its use. Side effects include allergic reactions, seizures, pain, blood disorders, and kidney and liver problems.

azoospermia /āzō′əspur′mē·ə/, lack of sperm in the semen. It may be caused by dysfunction of the testicles, blockage of the tubes in which sperm is stored (epididymis), or vasectomy. Infertility but not impotence is linked to with azoospermia.

azotemia /āz′ōtē′mē·ə/, excess amounts of nitrogen compounds in the blood. This poisonous condition is caused by failure of the kidneys to remove urea from the blood. See also **uremia.** –**azotemic,** *adj.*

azygous /az′igəs/, occurring as a single being or part, as any unpaired physical structure (for example, the mouth).

azygous vein, one of the seven veins of the chest.

B

Ba, symbol for **barium.**

babesiosis /bəbē′sē·ō′-/, an infection caused by the protozoa *Babesia,* which enters the body through the bite of ticks. Symptoms include headache, fever, nausea and vomiting, aching, and blood disorders.

Babinski's reflex /bəbin′skēz/, extending the big toe upward and fanning the other toes when the sole of the foot is stroked. The reflex is normal in newborn infants. It is abnormal in children and adults, in whom it may indicate a brain injury. Also called **Babinski's sign.** Compare **Chaddock's sign.**

baby, **1.** an infant or young child, especially one who is not yet able to walk or talk. **2.** to treat gently or with special care.

Baby Jane Doe regulations, rules established in 1984 by the United States Health and Human Services Department. State governments are required to investigate complaints about parental decisions involving the treatment of handicapped infants. The rules also allowed the federal government to have access to children's medical records. Hospitals are required to post notices urging doctors and nurses to report any suspected cases of infants denied proper medical care. Also called **Baby Doe rules.**

baby talk, **1.** the speech patterns and sounds of young children learning to talk. It features mispronounced words, repetition, and speech changes, as lisping or stuttering. **2.** the manner of speech that imitates young children learning to talk. It is often used by adults in addressing children or pets. **3.** the speech patterns that occur in some mental disorders, especially schizophrenia.

bacampicillin hydrochloride, a penicillin used to treat respiratory tract, urinary tract, skin, and gonococcal infections. Known sensitivity to this drug or other penicillins prohibits its use. Side effects include allergic reactions, gastritis, enterocolitis, and transient blood disorders.

Bacillaceae /-lā′si·ē/, a family of *Schizomycetes* bacteria of the order *Eubacteriales,* consisting of rod-shaped cells. These bacteria commonly appear in soil. Some are parasitic on insects and animals and can cause disease. The family includes the genus *Bacillus,* which needs air (aerobic), and the genus *Clostridium,* which can live without air (anaerobic).

bacille Calmette-Guérin (BCG) /kälmet′gāraN′/, a weakened strain of tubercle bacilli, used in many countries as a vaccine against tuberculosis.

bacitracin /-trā′sin/, an antibacterial used to treat some skin infections. Known allergy to this drug prohibits its use. Side effects include kidney damage and skin rash.

back, the back part of the trunk between the neck and the pelvis. The back is divided by a furrow created by the spine. The skeletal portion of the back includes the chest (thoracic) and lower (lumbar) backbones (vertebrae) and both shoulder blades (scapulas).

backache, pain in the spine or muscles of the back. Causes may include muscle strain or other muscular disorders, pressure on the root of a nerve, or a ruptured vertebral disk. Treatment may include heat, ultrasound, and devices to provide support, bed rest, surgery, pain relievers, and muscle relaxers.

backdraft, an "explosion" or rapid burning of heated gases resulting from the introduction of oxygen when air is admitted to a building that is heavily charged with smoke from a fire that has depleted the oxygen content of the building.

background radiation, naturally occurring radiation given off by materials in the soil, ground waters, and building material. Radioactive substances in the body, especially potassium 40 (^{40}K), and cosmic rays from outer space also give off background radiation. The average person is exposed each year to 44 millirad (mrad) of cosmic radiation, 44 mrad from the environment, and 18 mrad from naturally occurring internal radioactive sources.

backpack, the assembly that holds the air cylinder and has straps to secure the SCBA to the wearer.

back pressure, pressure that builds in a blood vessel or a cavity as fluid accumulates. The pressure increases and extends backward if the normal passageway for the fluid is not opened.

baclofen, a muscle relaxant used to treat spasticity in multiple sclerosis. Known allergy to this drug prohibits its use. Side effects include confusion, low blood pressure, shortness of breath, impotence, nausea, and temporary drowsiness.

bacteremia /-tirē′mē·ə/, the presence of bacteria in the blood. Bacteremia is diagnosed by growing organisms from a blood sample. Treatment is antibiotics. Compare **blood poisoning.**

bacteria /baktir′ē·ə/, *sing.* **bacterium,** the one-celled microorganisms of the class Schizomycetes. Some are round (cocci), rod-shaped (bacilli), spiral (spirochetes), or comma-shaped (vibrios). The nature, severity, and outcome of any infection caused by a bacterium depend on the species.

bactericidal /-sī′dəl/, destructive to bacteria. Compare **bacteriostatic.**

bacteriology, the scientific study of bacteria.

bacteriolysin /-lī′sin/, an antibody that breaks down a particular species of bacteria. See also **antibody.**

bacteriophage /baktir′ē·əfāj′/, any virus that causes bacteria to disintegrate. **Bacteriophage typing** is the process of identifying a species of bacteria according to the type of virus that attacks it.

bacteriostatic, tending to restrain the development of bacteria. Compare **bacteriocidal.**

bacteriuria /-ēyo͝or′ē·ə/, the presence of bacteria in the urine. More than 100,000 bacteria per ml of urine usually means a urinary tract infection is present. See also **urinary tract infection.**

Bacteroides /-oi′dēz/, a genus of bacilli that can live without air (anaerobic). They are normally found in the large intestine, mouth, genital tract, and upper respiratory system. Severe infection may result when a break occurs in the mucous membranes and the bacillus enters the circulation.

Bactrim, a trademark for a drug containing two antibacterials (sulfamethoxazole and trimethoprim).

bag, a flexible pouch designed to contain gas, fluid, or semisolid material, as crushed ice. Several types of bags are used to widen the anus, vagina, or other body openings. See also **bagging.**

bagging, *informal.* artificial respiration performed with a respirator bag, as an Ambu-bag. The bag is squeezed to force air into the patient's lungs as the mask is held over the mouth. During surgery, the anesthetist may also use this technique to correct the breathing pattern of an unconscious patient.

bag of waters. See **amniotic sac.**

Bainbridge reflex, a heart reflex with an increased pulse rate, resulting from stimulation of the wall of the left upper heart chamber (atrium). It may be produced by large amounts of intravenous fluids.

balance, 1. an instrument for weighing. **2.** a normal state of physical equilibrium. **3.** a state of mental or emotional equilibrium.

balanced diet, a diet containing all of the essential nutrients in adequate amounts needed by the body for growth, energy, repair, and maintenance of normal health.

balanic /bəlan′ik/, referring to the penis or the clitoris.

balanitis, inflammation of the penis.

balanoplasty /bal′ənō-/, an operation involving plastic surgery of the penis.

balanoposthitis /-posthī′-/, a generalized inflammation of the penis and foreskin. The symptoms are soreness, irritation, and discharge, occurring as a complication of bacterial or fungal infection. The cause is often a common venereal disease, in which case it is treated with antibiotics. Circumcision may be considered in severe cases.

balantidiasis /bal′əntidī′əsis/, an infection caused by swallowing the cysts of the protozoan *Balantidium coli.* It is transmitted from hogs. Infection with *B. coli* usually causes diarrhea. The protozoan may invade the intestinal wall and produce ulcers or abcesses.

baldness, absence of hair, especially from the scalp. See also **alopecia.**

BAL in Oil, a trademark for a drug used to treat poisoning with arsenic, gold, mercury, and lead (dimercaprol).

ball-and-socket joint, a synovial joint in which the round head of one bone is held in the cuplike cavity of another bone. This allows a limb to move in many directions. The hip and shoulder joints are ball-and-socket joints. See also **joint.**

ballismus, an abnormal condition characterized by violently flinging the arms about and, occasionally, the head. The cause is a brain injury.

ballistocardiogram /-kär′-/, a recording of the vibrations of the body that are caused by the beating of the heart. When the blood is pumped into the large heart artery (aorta) and the pulmonary arteries, it causes a vibration beginning at the head and traveling to the feet. The patient is placed on a special table, a ballistocardiograph, that is so delicately balanced that vibrations of the body can be recorded by a machine attached to the table. It is used to determine how elastic the aorta is and the amount of blood the heart is able to handle.

ballottement /bä′lôtmäN′, bəlot′mənt/, a technique of feeling (palpating) an organ or structure by bouncing it gently and feeling it rebound. In late pregnancy, a fetal head that can be ballotted is said to be **floating** or **unengaged.** This is in contrast to a fixed or an engaged head which cannot be easily dislodged from the pelvis.

ball-valve action, the opening and closing of a hole by a buoyant, ball-shaped mass that acts as a valve. Some kinds of objects that may act in this manner are kidney stones, gallstones, and blood clots.

balneotherapy /bal′nē·ō-/, use of baths in the treatment of many diseases and conditions. **Balneology** is a field of medicine that deals with the healing characteristics of various mineral waters, especially in baths.

bamboo spine, the typically rigid spine of advanced ankylosing spondylitis. Also called **poker spine.**

band, 1. a bundle of fibers that encircles a structure or binds one part of the body to another. **2.** a strip of metal that fits around a tooth and serves as an attachment for orthodontic appliances.

bandage, a strip of cloth that is wound around a part of the body in a variety of ways. It is used to hold a dressing, put pressure over a compress, or immobilize a limb or other part of the body.

bandage shears, scissors used to cut through bandages. The blades of most bandage shears are angled, and the lower blade has a rounded blunt tip to avoid harming the skin when the scissors are inserted under the bandage.

bank blood, preserved blood collected from donors in pints (500 ml) and refrigerated for future use. Bank blood is used after it is matched to the recipient's blood. See also **blood bank.**

Banthine, a trademark for a drug used to treat peptic ulcer and irritable bowels (methantheline bromide).

Banti's syndrome /ban'tēz/, a serious disorder involving several organ systems. The blood vessels that lie between the intestines and the liver are blocked, leading to congestion of the veins, an enlarged spleen, stomach and intestinal tract bleeding, cirrhosis of the liver, and destruction of red and white blood cells. Early symptoms are weakness, fatigue, and anemia. The spleen is sometimes removed, and a passage between the portal vein and the vena cava (portacaval shunt) is created to improve circulation to the liver.

barbiturate /bärbich'oorāt/, a class of drugs that act as sedatives or induces sleep. These drugs depress the respiratory rate, blood pressure, temperature, and nervous system. They are addictive.

barbiturism /bärbich'ər-/, **1.** sudden or long-term poisoning by any of the barbiturates. Excessive amounts of these drugs may be fatal or may produce physical and psychologic changes, as depressed respiration, lack of oxygen, disorientation, and coma. **2.** addiction to a barbiturate.

Bard-Pic syndrome, a condition of jaundice, enlarged gallbladder, and growing worse with advanced pancreatic cancer.

Bard's sign, the increased movements of the eyeball in uncontrolled rapid eye movement (nystagmus) when the patient tries to follow a target moved from side to side.

bariatrics /ber'ē·at'riks/, the field of medicine that focuses on the treatment and control of obesity and diseases associated with obesity.

barium (Ba) /ber'-/, a pale yellow, metallic element classified with the alkaline earths. Fine, milky barium sulfate is given to patients before x-ray films are taken of the digestive tract.

barium enema, an enema of barium sulfate given before x-ray films are taken of the lower intestinal tract. The x-rays cannot pass through the barium, so abnormalities can be seen on the x-ray film. This is used for diagnosing obstruction, tumors, or disorders as ulcerative colitis. The patient takes only liquids the night before and has no breakfast before the examination. After the x-ray films are taken, the barium is removed by a cleansing enema. Also called **contrast enema.**

barium meal, swallowing barium sulfate before x-ray films are taken of the esophagus, stomach, and intestinal tract. It is used to diagnose conditions as inability to eat (dysphagia), peptic ulcer, and other disorders. The movement of the barium through the stomach and intestinal tract is followed by fluoroscopy, x-ray films, or both. Before the test, the patient receives nothing by mouth for at least 8 hours. Also called **barium swallow.**

Barlow's syndrome, an abnormal heart condition with the sound of a murmur and a click. These symptoms are associated with back flow of blood caused by prolapse of the mitral valve located between the upper and lower heart chambers.

baroreceptor /-risep'-/, one of the pressure-sensitive nerve endings in the walls of the upper chambers (atria) of the heart and in some large blood vessels. Baroreceptors stimulate reflex mechanisms that allow the body to adapt to changes in blood pressure by dilating or constricting the blood vessels.

barotrauma /-trô'mə/, physical injury that occurs from exposure to increased environmental pressure. For example, rupture of the lungs or sinuses may occur among deep-sea divers.

barrel chest, a large, rounded chest, considered normal in some stocky people and others who live in high-altitude areas. They develop larger lung capacities. Barrel chest, however, may also be a sign of emphysema.

Barrett's syndrome, an ulcerlike area in the esophagus. Not cancer, it is caused most often by long-term irritation of the esophagus from digestive juices flowing back into the esophagus. Treatment is similar to that for heartburn.

barrier, 1. a wall or other obstacle that can block the passage of substances. Barrier methods of contraception, as the condom or diaphragm, prevent sperm from entering the uterus. Membranes of the body act as screenlike barriers to permit water or certain other molecules to move from one side to the other, while preventing the passage of other substances. **2.** something nonphysical that obstructs, as barriers to communication.

barrier nursing, nursing care of a patient in isolation to prevent the spread of infection. Gown, mask, and gloves are worn by anyone entering the room. The number of staff and visitors are limited. Contaminated substances are handled according to strict guidelines.

Bartholin's gland, one of two small glands located on the wall near the opening of the vagina. These glands help lubricate the vagina. **Bartholinitis** is an inflammation of one or both Bartholin's glands, caused by bacterial infection.

Barton's fracture, a fracture of the forearm involving the bone on the thumb side of the arm (radius) near the wrist. A dislocated wrist often goes along with the broken bone.

Bartter's syndrome, a rare hereditary disorder with kidney enlargement and overactive adrenal glands.

basal /bā′səl/, referring to the fundamental or the basic. For example, "basal metabolic rate" means the lowest rate at which chemical activity (metabolism) occurs in the body.

basal acid output (BAO), the minimum amount of digestive juice produced in a given period of time. This measurement is used in the diagnosis of various diseases of the stomach and intestines.

basal body temperature. See **body temperature.**

basal body temperature method of family planning. See **natural family planning method.**

basal bone, 1. the bone of the upper and lower jaw, which provides support for artificial dentures. **2.** the fixed bone structure that limits the movement of teeth.

basal cell, any one of the cells in the base layer of epithelium. Epithelium is the lining of the internal and external surfaces of the body, including organs, blood vessels, and skin (epidermis).

basal cell carcinoma, a slow-growing cancer on the face that begins as a small bump and enlarges to the side. It develops a central crater that erodes, crusts, and bleeds.

basal ganglia, the islands of gray matter within the lobes of the brain (cerebrum). They are involved in posture and coordination.

basal membrane, a sheet of tissue that lies just under the pigmented layer of the retina in the eye.

basal metabolism, the amount of energy needed to maintain essential body functions, as respiration, circulation, temperature, intestinal activity, and muscle tone.

basaloid carcinoma, a rare, malignant tumor of the anal canal. These tumors contain areas that resemble basal cell carcinoma of the skin. The tumor may spread to the skin of the genital area.

basal temperature. See **basal body temperature.**

base, 1. a chemical compound that combines with an acid to form a salt. Compare **alkali. 2.** the major ingredient of a compounded material, particularly one that is used as a drug. Petroleum jelly is frequently used as a base for ointments.

baseline fetal heart rate, the fetal heart rate pattern during labor between contractions of the uterus. An electronic fetal monitor is used to detect very fast or slow rates (less than 120 or more than 160 per minute). An abnormal rate can mean the baby's oxygen supply is interrupted.

baseplate, a temporary form that represents the base of a denture.

bas-fond /bäfôN′/, the bottom or base of any structure, especially the urinary bladder.

basic health services, the minimum amount of health care considered necessary to maintain health and protection from disease.

basilar artery, the artery at the base of the skull that is formed by the junction of the two vertebral arteries. It supplies blood to the internal ear and parts of the brain.

basilar artery insufficiency syndrome, a lack of blood flow through the basilar artery. The cause can be a blockage. Symptoms include dizziness, blindness, numbness, depression, speech problems, difficult swallowing, and weakness on one side of the body.

basilar plexus, the network of veins between the layers of the membrane that protects the brain (dura mater) over the base of the skull.

basilic vein /bəsil′ik/, one of the four veins of the arm near the surface. It runs along the inside of the forearm.

basiloma, a cancer composed of basal cells. **Basiloma terebrans** is a basal cell cancer that invades surrounding tissue.

basioccipital /-oksip′-/, referring to the base of the back of the skull (occipital bone).

basophilic adenoma, a tumor of the pituitary gland. Cushing's syndrome is often caused by a basophilic adenoma. See also **adenoma.**

basophilic leukemia, a cancer of blood-forming tissues, characterized by large numbers of immature basophils. See also **leukemia.**

basophilic stippling, the abnormal presence of spotted basophils in the red blood cells. Stippling is characteristic of lead poisoning. See also **lead poisoning.**

basosquamous cell carcinoma /-skwā′-/, a malignant skin tumor composed of basal and squamous cells.

Bassen-Kornzweig syndrome. See **hypolipoproteinemia.**

bath, a cleansing routine performed daily by or for almost all hospitalized patients. A daily bath helps prevent infection, preserves the unbroken condition of the skin, stimulates circulation, promotes oxygen intake, maintains muscle tone and joint mobility, and provides comfort. A **cold bath** has a water temperature of about 50° F (10° C) to 65° F (18° C). Cold baths are used mainly to reduce body temperature.

bathesthesia /bath′əsthē′zhə/, a sensitivity of internal parts of the body. It is associated with organs or structures beneath the surface, as muscles and joints.

bathycardia /bath′ə-/, an unusually low position of the heart in the chest. It usually does not cause any problems with functioning.

battered woman syndrome (BWS), repeated episodes of physical assault on a woman by the man with whom she lives, often resulting in serious physical and emotional damage to the woman. Such violence tends to follow a pattern, such as verbal abuse on almost any subject— housekeeping, money, or childrearing. Often the violent episodes become more frequent and severe over time. Studies show that the longer the woman stays in the relationship the more likely she is to be seriously injured. The use of alcohol increases the severity of the assault; a man who usually shoves or slaps his partner is more likely to punch or kick her if he is drunk. Other drugs do not have this effect; the man is more likely to be abusive as the drug is wearing off. Battering occurs in cycles of violence. Verbal abuse, insults, and criticism increase, and shoves or slaps begin. As the tension mounts, the woman becomes unable to calm the man, and she may argue or defend herself. The man uses this to justify his anger and assaults her, often saying that he is ''teaching her a lesson.'' Apology and remorse on the part of the man may occur, with promises of change, until tension builds again. The battered woman syndrome occurs at all social and economic levels. Men who grew up in homes in which the father abused the mother are more likely to beat their wives than are men who lived in nonviolent homes. Aggressive behavior is a normal part of male socialization in most cultures; physical aggression may be condoned as a means of resolving a conflict. The battered woman syndrome is better recognized now than a decade ago, and there are agencies to assist and protect the woman. In many communities the police have programs to remove the man and to refer the woman to help.

Battey bacillus, any of a group of mycobacteria that cause a long-term lung disease resembling tuberculosis. These organisms are resistant to most of the common antibiotic drugs. Surgical removal of involved lung tissue may be necessary and may improve the outcome in serious cases.

Battle's sign, a small area of bleeding under the skin behind the ear. It may indicate a fracture of a bone of the lower skull.

Baudelocque's method /bôdloks′/, turning the baby from a face-first position to a crown-first position just before delivery.

B cell, a type of white blood cell (lymphocyte) that comes from the bone marrow. It is one of the two lymphocytes that play a major role in the body's immune response. Compare **T cell.** See also **plasma cell.**

BCG vaccine, an immunizing vaccine (**bacille Calmette-Guérin**) against tuberculosis. It is not given after vaccination for smallpox, or to patients with a positive tuberculin reaction or a burn. Side effects include severe allergic reactions and rarely the development of tuberculosis. Pain, inflammation, and lumps may develop at the site of injection.

B complex vitamins, a large group of water-soluble substances that includes **vitamin B$_1$ (thiamine), vitamin B$_2$ (riboflavin), vitamin B$_3$ (niacin), vitamin B$_6$ (pyridoxine), vitamin B$_{12}$ (cyanocobalamin), biotin, choline, carnitine, folic acid, inositol,** and **para-aminobenzoic acid.** The B complex vitamins are essential in breaking down carbohydrates into glucose to provide energy, and for breaking down fats and proteins. They are also needed for normal functioning of the nervous system, for maintenance of muscle tone in the stomach and intestinal tract, and for the health of skin, hair, eyes, mouth, and liver. They are found in brewer's yeast, liver, whole-grain cereals, nuts, eggs, meats, fish, and vegetables and are produced by the intestinal bacteria. Maintaining milk-free diets or taking antibiotics may destroy these bacteria. Symptoms of vitamin B deficiency include nervousness, depression, insomnia, nerve problems, anemia, hair loss, acne or other skin disorders, and excessive cholesterol in the blood. See also specific vitamins.

Beck operation, a type of surgery that provides additional circulation to the heart. It is performed when the vessels of the heart are diseased and supply inadequate amounts of blood to the heart.

Beck's triad, a combination of three symptoms that show compression of the heart: high pressure in the veins, low pressure in the arteries, and a small, quiet heart.

Beckwith's syndrome, a hereditary disorder in infants of low blood sugar (hypoglycemia) and overproduction of insulin.

beclomethasone dipropionate, a type of steroid (glucocorticoid) used in an inhaler in the treatment of bronchial asthma. Severe asthma attack or known allergy to this drug prohibits its use. Side effects include symptoms of adrenal insufficiency, hoarseness, sore throat, and fungal infections of the throat.

bed, a supporting tissue, as the nail beds of specialized skin over which the fingernails and the toenails move as they grow.

bedbug, a bloodsucking arthropod of the species *Cimex* that feeds on humans and other animals. The bedbug can be removed after covering it with petrolatum. The bite causes itching, pain, and redness. See also **petrolatum.**

bedsore, an inflamed ulcer (decubitus) on the skin over a bony part of the body. It results from prolonged pressure on the part.

bee sting, an injury caused by the venom of bees, usually accompanied by pain and swelling. The stinger of the honeybee usually remains implanted and should be removed carefully. Pain may be relieved by applying an ice pack or a paste of sodium bicarbonate and water. Allergic individuals are encouraged to carry emergency kits with them when the possibility of bee sting exists.

behavior, **1.** the manner in which a person acts or performs. **2.** any or all of the activities of a person, including physical and mental activity.

behavior disorder, any of a group of antisocial behavior patterns occurring mainly in children and adolescents. The behavior disorders include overaggressiveness, overactivity, destructiveness, cruelty, truancy, lying, disobedience, perverse sexual activity, criminality, alcoholism, and drug addiction. The most common reason for such behavior is hostility. It is started by a disturbed relationship between the child and the parents, an unstable home situation, and, in some cases, organic brain dysfunction. See also **antisocial personality disorder.**

behaviorism, a school of psychology founded by John B. Watson that studies and interprets behavior by observing people's responses to things. Behaviorism is not concerned with consciousness, mental states, or ideas and emotions.

behavior therapy, a kind of psychotherapy that attempts to modify patterns of behavior by substituting a new response to a given stimulus. Some "quit smoking" programs use this technique successfully. Also called **behavior modification.** See also **biofeedback.**

bel, a unit that expresses intensity of sound. An increase of 1 bel approximately doubles the intensity or loudness of most sounds.

belladonna, the dried leaves, roots, and flowering or fruiting tops of *Atropa belladonna,* a common perennial called deadly nightshade. It contains hyoscyamine, which is a source of atropine.

Bell's law, an axiom stating that the nerves at the internal part of the spinal cord control the muscles and those at the outer part control the senses.

Bell's palsy, a paralysis of the facial nerve. It is caused by injury to the nerve, compression of the nerve by a tumor, or, possibly, an unknown infection.

belly. See **abdomen.**

belly button. See **navel.**

belonephobia /bel'ənə-/, an abnormal fear of sharp-pointed objects, especially needles and pins.

Benadon, a trademark for vitamin B$_6$.

Benadryl, a trademark for an antihistamine used to treat allergic reactions (diphenhydramine hydrochloride).

bending fracture, a fracture indirectly caused by bending an extremity, as the foot or the big toe.

bendroflumethiazide, a diuretic and antihypertensive drug used to treat high blood pressure and water retention. Kidney dysfunction or known allergy to this or other similar drugs prohibits its use. Side effects include loss of potassium, high blood sugar, excess uric acid in the blood, and various allergic reactions.

Benedict's qualitative test, a test for sugar in the urine.

Benemid, a trademark for a drug used to treat gout (probenecid).

benign /bənīn'/, not harmful; describing a condition or disorder that is not a threat to health. Compare **malignant.**

benign neoplasm. See **neoplasm.**

benign prostatic hypertrophy, enlargement of the prostate gland, common among men after 50 years of age. The condition is not malignant or inflammatory. It may lead to blockage of the urethra and interfere with the flow of urine. This can increase frequency of urination, the need to urinate during the night, pain, and urinary tract infections. Treatment consists of regular sexual release, hot baths, massage of the prostate, avoiding alcohol and drinking excessive fluids, and urinating as soon as the urge occurs. Surgery is sometimes necessary. Compare **prostatitis.**

Bennett's fracture, a fracture of the hand that runs through the base of the thumb and into the wrist. Bennett's fracture may be caused by the thumb being forced backwards or by being dislocated.

Benoxl, a trademark for an antiseptic used on the skin to treat acne (benzoyl peroxide).

bent fracture, a fracture caused by the bone being forcibly bent. The actual fracture may be some distance from the area that was bent.

bentonite, aluminum silicate (colloidal, hydrated). When added to water, it swells to approximately 12 times its dry size. It is used as a bulk laxative and as a base for skin care preparations.

Bentyl, a trademark for a drug used to treat intestinal irritability and spasms (dicyclomine hydrochloride).

benzalkonium chloride, a disinfectant and fungicide prepared in water. It comes in various strengths.

Benzedrex, a trademark for a drug used to treat low blood pressure (propylhexedrine).

benzene poisoning, poisoning caused by swallowing benzene, inhaling benzene fumes, or exposure to benzene-related products, as toluene or xylene. Symptoms include nausea, headache, dizziness, and incoordination. In severe cases, respiratory failure or extremely rapid heart beat may cause death. Long-term exposure may result in aplastic anemia or a form of leukemia. Benzene poisoning by inhalation is treated with breathing assistance and oxygen. Poisoning from swallowing benzene is treated by flushing the stomach with water. See also **nitrobenzene poisoning.**

benzethonium chloride, a disinfectant for the skin and for treating some infections of the eye, nose, and throat. It is also used as a preservative in some drugs.

benzocaine, an anesthetic for the skin used in many over-the-counter compounds for itching and pain. Although not poisonous, some people become sensitive to it from too much use. Use of benzocaine may cause a blood disorder (methemoglobinemia) in infants and small children.

benzodiazepine derivative /ben′zōdī·az′əpin/, one of a group of drugs used to relieve anxiety or insomnia, including tranquilizers and hypnotics. Tolerance and physical dependence occur with prolonged high doses. Withdrawal symptoms, including seizures and serious psychosis, may occur if the drug is abruptly stopped. Side effects include drowsiness, muscle incoordination, and increased aggression and hostility. However, these reactions are not commonly seen in patients who take only the usual recommended dose.

benzoic acid /-zō′ik/, a substance usually used with salicylic acid as an ointment for treating athlete's foot and ringworm of the scalp. Mild irritation may occur at the site of application.

benzonatate, a drug used to suppress coughing. It is not a narcotic. Known allergy to this drug prohibits its use. Side effects include convulsions, vertigo, headache, constipation, and allergic reactions.

benzoyl peroxide, an antibacterial drying agent used to treat acne. Known allergy to this drug prohibits its use. It is not used in the eye, on inflamed skin, or on mucous membranes. Side effects include excess drying of the skin and allergic contact dermatitis.

benzphetamine hydrochloride, a drug that causes loss of appetite and is used to treat obesity. Arteriosclerosis, cardiovascular disease, high blood pressure, glaucoma, overactive thyroid gland, or known allergy to this or other similar drugs prohibits its use. Side effects include restlessness, insomnia, rapid heart beat, increased blood pressure, and dry mouth.

benzthiazide, a drug used to treat high blood pressure and water retention.

benztropine mesylate, a drug used to treat parkinsonism. It is used in combination with other drugs, as levodopa. Known allergy to this drug prohibits its use. It is not given to children under 3 years of age. Side effects include

blurred vision, dry mouth, nausea and vomiting, constipation, depression, and skin rash.

benzyl alcohol, a clear, colorless, oily liquid, derived from certain balsams. It is used as an anesthetic on the skin and to prevent bacteria from growing in solutions for injection.

benzyl benzoate, a clear, oily liquid with a pleasant, aromatic odor. It is used to destroy lice and scabies, as a solvent, and as a flavor for gum.

beriberi, a disease of the nerves of the arms and legs caused by a deficiency of thiamine. It is usually caused by a diet limited to polished white rice and is common in eastern and southern Asia. Rare cases in the United States are linked with stressful conditions, as underactive thyroid gland, infections, pregnancy, breast feeding, and alcoholism. Symptoms include fatigue, diarrhea, appetite and weight loss, disturbed nerve function causing paralysis and wasting of limbs, water retention, and heart failure. See also **thiamine.**

Berlock dermatitis, a skin disorder caused by a reaction to oil of bergamot (psoralens), which is commonly used in perfumes, colognes, and pomades. Dark patches and sores appear on the skin. This condition affects mostly women and children and may result from using products that contain psoralens and exposure to ultraviolet light. The level of ultraviolet radiation reaching the earth on a sunny day is enough to cause the condition to appear.

Bernard-Soulier syndrome /-soōlyā′-/, a blood-clotting disorder caused by lack of an essential glycoprotein in the platelets.

berylliosis /bəril′ē·ō′-/, poisoning that results from inhaling dusts or vapors that contain beryllium, a steel-gray light-weight metallic element.

bestiality, 1. conduct or behavior with beastlike appetites or instincts. 2. sexual relations between a human being and an animal. 3. sodomy.

beta (β), the second letter of the Greek alphabet, used as a combining form with chemical names to distinguish one of two or more forms or to show the position of substituted atoms in certain compounds. Compare **alpha.**

beta-adrenergic blocking agent. See **antiadrenergic.**

beta-adrenergic stimulating agent. See **adrenergic.**

beta-carotene, an ultraviolet screening agent used to reduce sensitivity to the sun. It is used with caution in patients with impaired kidney or liver function. Known allergy to this drug prohibits its use. Side effects include slight yellowing of skin and diarrhea.

beta cells, 1. cells in the pancreas that produce insulin. The insulin production by the beta cells tends to speed up the movement of glucose, amino acids, and fatty acids out of the blood and into the cells. 2. cells in the pituitary gland.

Betadine, a trademark for an antiinfective that is used on the skin (povidone-iodine).

Betalin S, a trademark for vitamin B_1 (thiamine hydrochloride).

betamethasone, a steroid (glucocorticoid) available as an oral drug or as a lotion, cream, or ointment. The skin preparations are used to treat skin inflammation, as dermatitis. The oral form is given for severe allergy and a variety of serious diseases. Systemic fungal infections, viral and fungal infections of the skin, impaired circulation, or known allergy to this drug prohibits its use. Side effects linked to long-term use of the drug include stomach and intestinal, hormone, nerve, and fluid and electrolyte disturbances.

beta particle or **beta ray,** a small particle ejected spontaneously from a nucleus of a radioactive element. It has the mass of the electron and a charge of minus 1 or plus 1. It has a medium or intermediate penetrating power; its range in air is from a few inches to several feet. The most energetic beta particles will penetrate the skin and a fraction of an inch of tissue. The damage is manifested primarily as skin burns. Symbol: β^- or β^+.

beta receptor, any one of the adrenergic receptors of the nervous system that responds to an adrenal gland hormone, epinephrine. Activation causes various reactions, as relaxation of the bronchial muscles, and an increase in the speed and force of the heart beat.

betatron, a machine that produces high-energy electrons for x-ray treatment.

beta wave. See **brain waves.**

bethanechol chloride, a drug used to treat retaining of urine and to increase intestinal action. Uncertain bladder strength, blockage in the digestive or urinary tract, overactive thyroid gland, peptic ulcer, asthma, heart and blood vessel disease, epilepsy, Parkinson's disease, low blood pressure, pregnancy, or known allergy to this drug prohibits its use. Side effects include flushing, headache, digestive distress, diarrhea, excess saliva, sweating, and low blood pressure.

bezoar /bē′zôr/, a hard ball of hair and vegetable fiber that may develop within the intestines of humans but usually is found in the stomachs of cud-chewing animals, such as cattle or sheep.

bicarbonate of soda. See **sodium bicarbonate.**

bicarbonate precursor, an injection of sodium lactate used to treat acidosis (metabolic). It is changed by the body to sodium bicarbonate.

biceps brachii, the long muscle that stretches over the bone of the upper arm (humerus). It flexes the arm and the forearm. Also called **biceps.**

biceps femoris. See **hamstring muscle.**

biconcave, curved in (concave) on both sides, a term usually applied to a lens.

biconvex, bulging out (convex) on both sides, a term usually applied to a lens.

bicornate uterus /bīkôr′nāt/, an abnormal uterus that may be either a single or a double organ with two branches. It is associated with a high incidence of premature labor, miscarriage, and infertility.

bicuspid /bīkus′pid/, **1.** having two cusps or points. **2.** one of the two teeth between the molars and canines of the upper and lower jaw.

b.i.d., (in prescriptions) abbreviation for *bis in die,* a Latin phrase meaning twice a day. A drug prescribed this way should be taken 12 hours apart, for example at 7 AM and 7 PM.

bidactyly /bīdak′tilē/, an abnormal condition in which the second, third, and fourth fingers on the same hand are missing.

biduotertian fever. See **malaria.**

bifocal, referring to an eyeglass lens that has two areas, one for near vision and the other for distant vision.

bifurcation, a splitting into two branches, as the windpipe (trachea), which branches into the two bronchi of the lungs just below the collarbone.

bigeminy /bījem′inē/, **1.** an association in pairs. **2.** an irregular heart beat characterized by two beats in rapid succession followed by a pause. –**bigeminal,** *adj.*

bilateral, 1. having two sides, or layers. **2.** occurring or appearing on two sides. A patient with bilateral hearing loss may have partial or total deafness in both ears.

bile, a bitter, yellow-green secretion of the liver. Bile is stored in the gallbladder and is released when fat enters the first part of the small intestine (duodenum). Bile emulsifies these fats, preparing them for further digestion and absorption in the small intestine. Also called **gall.**

bile ducts, any of several passageways that convey bile from the liver to the small intestine. Also called **biliary ducts.**

bile solubility test, a test used to determine whether an infection is caused by pneumococci or streptococci.

biliary /bil′ē·er′ē/, referring to bile or to the gallbladder and its ducts, which transport bile to the duodenum. These are often called the **biliary tract** or the **biliary system.**

biliary atresia, an inborn absence or poor development of one or more of the biliary structures. It causes jaundice and early liver damage. See also **biliary cirrhosis.**

biliary calculus. See **gallstone.**

biliary cirrhosis, an inflammatory condition in which the flow of bile through the liver is obstructed. With **primary biliary cirrhosis,** there is abdominal pain, jaundice, and enlargement of the liver and spleen. Other symptoms are general itching, weight loss, and diarrhea with pale, bulky stools. Blood coagulation defects may also occur with pinpoint bleeding in the skin, and nose bleeds. Broken bones

A–E

and collapsed back bones may occur from a lack of absorbed vitamin D and calcium. See also **cirrhoses.**

biliary duct.   See **bile ducts.**

biliary fistula,   an abnormal passage from the gallbladder, a bile duct, or the liver to an internal organ or to the surface of the body. A biliary fistula may open into the large intestine, duodenum, liver duct, or abdominal cavity.

biliary obstruction,   blockage of the common or cystic bile duct, usually caused by one or more gallstones. Stones, consisting chiefly of cholesterol, bile pigment, and calcium, may form in the gallbladder and liver duct in persons of either sex at any age but are more common in middle-aged women. This interferes with bile drainage and produces an inflammatory reaction. Symptoms of biliary obstruction include severe pain near the breastbone that may radiate to the back and shoulder, nausea, vomiting, and profuse sweating. The dehydrated patient may have chills, fever, jaundice, clay-colored stools, dark, concentrated urine, and an electrolyte imbalance. There may also be a tendency to bleed because the absence of bile prevents the synthesis and absorption of vitamin K, which is necessary for clotting. Uncommon causes of biliary obstruction include cysts or inflammation of the common bile duct, pancreatic and duodenal tumors, Crohn's disease, pancreatitis, and roundworm infection. Removal of the gallbladder (cholecystectomy) is the usual treatment, but, in most cases, surgery is delayed until the patient's condition is stabilized and any clotting problems (caused by vitamin K malabsorption) are corrected. If surgery is not done, the person must stay on a low-fat diet and report any recurrence of symptoms.

biliary tract cancer,   an uncommon malignant tumor in a bile duct, occurring slightly more often in men than in women. Symptoms include progressive jaundice, itching, weight loss, and, in the later stages, severe pain. X-ray studies are done to determine the site of the tumor.

bilious /bil′yəs/,   referring to bile, such as an excessive secretion of bile, or a disorder affecting the bile.

bilirubin /-roo′-/,   the orange-yellow pigment in bile, formed mainly by the breakdown of hemoglobin in red blood cells. Bilirubin normally travels in the bloodstream to the liver, where it is changed to a water-soluble form and excreted into the bile. In a healthy person, most of the bilirubin produced daily is excreted from the body in the stool. The yellow skin of jaundice is caused by bilirubin in the blood and in the tissues of the skin. See also **jaundice.**

biliuria /-yŏŏr′ē·ə/,   the presence of bile in the urine.

Billings method,   a method of estimating ovulation time by changes in the mucus of the cervix that occur during the menstrual cycle.

Billroth's operation,   the surgical removal of the area (pylorus) where the stomach joins the beginning of the small intestine (duodenum). The duodenum is attached to the stomach. This surgery is performed for stomach cancer. It may also refer to the surgical removal of the pylorus and duodenum. The cut end of the stomach is joined to the small intestine.

Biltricide,   a trademark for a drug used to rid the body of Schistosoma flukes (praziquantel).

bimaxillary /bīmak′siler′ē/,   referring to the right and left upper jaw (maxilla).

bilobate /bīlō′bāt/,   having two lobes.

bimanual,   referring to the functioning of both hands.

binary fission,   direct division of a cell or nucleus into two equal parts. It is the common form of asexual reproduction of bacteria, protozoa, and other lower forms of life.

bind,   **1.** to bandage or wrap in a band. **2.** to join together with a band. **3.** to combine or unite molecules.

binocular,   **1.** referring to both eyes, especially regarding vision. **2.** a microscope, telescope, or field glass that can accommodate viewing by both eyes.

binocular fixation,   the process of having both eyes directed at the same object at the same time. This is essential to having good depth perception.

binocular vision,   the use of both eyes together so that the images seen by each eye are combined to appear as a single image. Compare **diplopia.**

bioavailability,   the amount of drug or other substance that is active in the tissues.

biochemistry,   the chemistry of living organisms and life processes.

bioelectricity,   electric current that is produced by living tissues, as nerves, brain, heart, and muscles. The electric impulses of human tissues are recorded by electrocardiograph, electroencephalograph, and similar sensitive devices.

bioenergetics,   a system of exercises based on the concept that healing is increased by bringing into harmony the patient's body rhythms and the natural environment.

bioequivalent,   referring to a drug that has the same effect on the body as another drug, usually one nearly identical in its chemical structure.

biofeedback,   a method used in learning to alter certain functions of the body, as blood pressure, muscle tension, and brain wave activity, through relaxation. A device may be used to allow the patient to monitor this information. Some conditions, as high blood pressure, insomnia, and migraine headache, may be treated this way.

bioflavonoid /-flā′-/,   a term for any of a group of substances found in many fruits and essential for the absorption and processing of vitamin C (ascorbic acid). Also called **vitamin P.** See also **vitamin C.**

biogenic /-jen'ik/, **1.** produced by the action of a living organism, as fermentation. **2.** essential to life and the maintenance of health, as food, water, proper rest.

biogenic amine, one of a large group of naturally occurring compounds, most of which transmit nerve impulses. The most dominant, norepinephrine, is involved in functions as emotional reactions, memory, sleep, and arousal from sleep. Acetylcholine and dopamine are other biogenic amines.

biologic, any substance made from living organisms or the products of living organisms that is used as diagnosis, prevention, or treatment of disease. Kinds of biologics are **antigens, antitoxins, serums, vaccines.**

biological half-life, the time required for the body to eliminate one half of an internally deposited radioactive substance by normal processes of elimination. This time is the same for both stable and radioactive isotopes of a particular element.

biology, the scientific study of plants and animals.

biomechanics, the study of mechanical laws and their application to living organisms, especially the human body and its movement.

biomedical engineering, a system of techniques in which knowledge of biologic processes is applied to solve practical medical problems.

bionics /bī·on'iks/, the science of applying electronic principles and devices, as computers and solid-state miniaturized circuitry, to medical problems. Artificial pacemakers used to correct abnormal heart rhythms are an example. –**bionic,** *adj.*

biopsy /bī'əpsē/, a small piece of living tissue or its removal from an organ or other part of the body for microscopic examination to establish a diagnosis or follow the course of a disease. An aspiration biopsy is made with a fine needle attached to a syringe. A cone biopsy means surgical removal of a cone-shaped piece from the cervix to help make a diagnosis. This is most often used to test for cancer. A needle biopsy is made by putting a hollow needle through the skin on the surface of an organ or tumor and turning it within the cell layers. A punch biopsy refers to the removal of a sample of tissue (usually bone marrow) by means of an instrument with punch action. Tissue removal done by scraping the surface of a sore or tumor is called a surface biopsy. This method is used mainly to detect cancer of the cervix.

biorhythm, any cyclic, biologic event, as the sleep cycle, the menstrual cycle, or the respiratory cycle. –**biorhythmic,** *adj.*

biostatistics. See **vital statistics.**

biosynthesis /-sin'thəsis/, any of thousands of chemical reactions continually occurring throughout the body. In biosynthesis, molecules form more complex biomolecules, especially carbohydrates, fats, proteins, nucleotides, and nucleic acids.

biotechnology, the study of the relationships between humans or other living organisms and machinery. An example is the health effects of word processor equipment on office workers.

biotin /bī'ətin/, a colorless, crystalline, water-soluble B complex vitamin that helps produce fatty acids. It also helps the body use protein, folic acid, pantothenic acid, and vitamin B_{12}. Rich sources are egg yolk, beef liver, kidney, unpolished rice, brewer's yeast, peanuts, cauliflower, and mushrooms.

biotransformation, the chemical changes a substance undergoes in the body, as by the action of enzymes. See also **metabolism.**

Biot's respiration /bē·ōz'/, an abnormal breathing pattern that occurs with brain disorders, as meningitis or pressure on the brain. Symptoms are irregular breathing with periods of not breathing. The breathing may be slow and deep or rapid and shallow and is often accompanied by sighing.

biperiden, a drug used to treat Parkinson's disease and drug-caused disorders of movement and coordination (extrapyramidal symptoms). Glaucoma, asthma, blockage of the digestive or urinary tract, or known allergy to this drug prohibits its use. Side effects include blurred vision, nervous system problems, rapid heart beat, dry mouth, reduced sweating, and allergic reactions.

bipolar /bīpō'lər/, **1.** having two poles, as in certain types of electrotherapy using opposite poles (positive and negative). **2.** referring to a nerve cell that has electric signals traveling both to and away from the center (afferent and efferent).

bipolar disorder, a mental disorder with periods of mania and depression. The manic phase shows excess emotional displays, excitement, overactivity, excess joy, a high degree of energy, inability to concentrate, and reduced need for sleep, often coupled with unrealistic ideas about one's worth. In the depressive phase, apathy and underactivity are seen along with feelings of excess sadness, loneliness, guilt, and lowered sense of one's worth. Most people with this disorder respond well to the drug lithium.

bipolar lead, two electrodes for heart test (electrocardiogram) that are placed on different parts of the body.

birth, event of being born, the coming of a new person out of its mother into the world. Kinds of birth are **breech birth, live birth, stillbirth.**

birth canal, *informal.* the passage that extends from the opening in the pelvis to the vaginal opening, through which an infant passes during birth.

birth control. See **contraception.**

birth defect, any abnormality present at birth, mainly a structural one. Also called a **congenital anomaly,** it may be inherited, obtained during pregnancy, or inflicted during childbirth. A **developmental anomaly** refers to any birth defect that results when the normal growth of the fetus is disturbed. Such defects can occur at any stage of development. They vary greatly in type and severity and may be caused by a number of things. These include chromosome abnormalities, drugs, diseases of the mother (such as measles), and environmental factors.

birth injury, damage to a baby while being born. Also called **birth trauma.**

birthmark. See **nevus.**

birth rate, the number of births during a given period in relation to the total population of a certain area. The birth rate is usually counted as the number of births per 1000 of population. A **crude birth rate** is the number of births per 1000 people in a population during 1 year. The ratio of total births to the total female population of childbearing age, between 15 and 45 years of age is called the **true birth rate.**

birth weight, the weight of a baby when born, usually about 3500 g (7.5 lbs). In the United States, 97% of newborns weigh between 2500 g (5.5 lbs) and 4500 g (10 lbs). Babies who are full term but weigh less than 2500 g are called **small for gestational age.** This is smaller than 90% of all babies born. Factors linked with smallness other than heredity include any disorder causing short stature, as dwarfism, malnutrition in the womb, and some infections, as rubella virus. Other causes linked with the smallness of an infant include cigarette smoking by the mother during pregnancy, and addiction to alcohol or heroin. Babies who weigh more than 4500 g are called **large for gestational age,** whether delivered prematurely, at term, or later than term. Diabetes mellitus in the mother is a cause of rapid fetal growth. These infants are generally obese, with very pink skin and red, shiny cheeks. They are often listless and limp, feed poorly, have breathing problems, and have low blood sugar (hypoglycemia) within the first few hours.

bisacodyl /bisak'ōdil/, a laxative given for constipation, to empty the bowel before or after surgery, or before x-ray studies are done. Stomach and bowel pain, nausea, vomiting, open hemorrhoids, or known allergy to this drug prohibits its use. Side effects include cramping, stomach and bowel pain, and diarrhea.

bisexual, 1. having sex organs of both sexes (hermaphroditic). **2.** having physical or psychologic features of both sexes. **3.** engaging in both heterosexual and homosexual activity.

bismuth (Bi) /biz'məth/, a reddish metal element. It is combined with other elements, as oxygen, to make salts used in making many drugs.

bismuth stomatitis, an abnormal mouth condition caused by using bismuth compounds over long periods. A blue-black line shows on the gum next to the teeth, or there may be darkening of the inside cheek in the mouth. Other symptoms are a sore tongue, metal taste, and a sense of burning in the mouth. See also **stomatitis.**

bite, 1. the act of cutting, tearing, holding, or gripping with the teeth. **2.** a record of the bite or relationship of the teeth to each other. An **open bite** is a condition in which the lower front teeth do not touch the upper front teeth when the jaws are closed. **Overbite** refers to the up and down (vertical) overlapping of lower teeth by upper teeth. A **closed bite** is an abnormal overbite.

bitegage, a dental device that helps gain proper bite of the teeth in the upper and lower jaw.

biteplane, a removable dental device for covering the biting surfaces of the teeth to prevent them from touching.

biteplate, a device used in dentistry for diagnosis or treatment. It is made of wire and plastic, worn in the palate, and may also be used to correct problems of the jaw joint.

biting in childhood, a natural behavior and reflex in infants. It begins at about 5 to 6 months of age in response to solid foods in the diet and the beginning of teething.

biuret test /bī'yŏŏrət/, a method for finding urea and other proteins in blood. In an alkaline solution, copper sulfate reacts with proteins to produce a purple color, which is called the biuret reaction.

blackhead, a buildup of skin cells and oil in the pouch (follicle) from which a hair grows. It is dark because of the effect of oxygen on the skin oil, not because of dirt. Also called **comedo.**

black lung. See **anthracosis.**

blackout, *informal.* a temporary loss of vision or consciousness resulting from lack of oxygen to the brain.

blackwater fever. See **malaria.**

black widow spider, a poisonous spider (arachnid) found in many parts of the world. The poison injected with its bite causes sweating, stomach cramps, nausea, headaches, and many degrees of dizziness. Small children, old people, or those with heart conditions are most severely affected.

black widow spider antivenin, a vaccinating drug used to treat a black widow spider bite. Known allergy to this drug or to horse serum prohibits its use. Side effects include allergic reactions.

bladder, 1. a sac that holds fluids. **2.** the urinary bladder.

bladder cancer, the most common cancer of the urinary tract. Cancer of the bladder is more than twice as common in men than in women, and is more common in urban than in rural areas. Early symptoms of a bladder cancer include bloody urine, frequent or painful urination, and the growth of lumps (cystitis). The risk for developing bladder cancer is increased with cigarette smoking and exposure to cancer-causing agents (carcinogens), as aniline dyes, aromatic hydrocarbons, or benzidine. Other risk factors are long-term urinary tract infections, kidney stone disease, and infection with the fluke that causes schistosomiasis. See also **cystectomy.**

bladder stone. See **urinary calculus.**

Blalock-Taussig procedure /blā'loktô'sig/, joining two arteries by surgery as a temporary way to correct an inborn heart defect (tetralogy of Fallot). The artery above the collarbone (subclavian) is joined end-to-end with the artery that carries blood to the lungs. This moves blood from the circulation to the lungs. Permanent correction is done later in early childhood.

blanch, 1. causing to become white or pale. **2.** becoming white or pale, as from narrowing of the blood vessels that happens with fear or anger.

bland, mild or having a soothing effect.

bland diet, a nonirritating diet. It is often given to treat many different stomach and bowel diseases, and after stomach or bowel surgery. The diet may include eggs, meat, poultry, fish, and enriched fine cereals; milk is usually important. A bland diet may be planned that includes or excludes any specific foods. Spicy or highly seasoned foods, carbonated beverages, raw fruits and vegetables, and rich desserts are avoided.

blanket bath, wrapping the patient in a wet pack and then in blankets.

blast cell, any immature cell, as a red blood cell (erythroblast), a white blood cell (lymphoblast), or a nerve cell (neuroblast).

blastema /blastē'mə/, **1.** any mass of living protoplasm able to grow and separate. **2.** in certain animals, a group of cells able to grow back a lost or damaged part or to make a complete organism in asexual reproduction.

blastid, the site in the fertilized egg (ovum) where the nucleus forms.

blastin, any substance that gives food to or helps the growth or reproduction of cells.

blastocyte /blas'təsīt/, a very early embryonic cell before any cell layer has formed.

blastogenesis /-jen'əsis/, **1.** nonsexual reproduction by budding. **2.** the theory that hereditary traits are carried by the first cell of an organism (germ plasm). **3.** the development of the embryo during the separation and formation of the germ layers. **–blastogenetic,** *adj.*

blastoma /blastō'mə/, a tumor of embryonic tissue that develops from the early substance (blastema) of an organ or tissue. The development of many tumors of embryonic tissue is **blastomatosis.**

blastomycosis /-mīkō'sis/, an infectious disease caused by a fungus, *Blastomyces dermatitidis.* It usually affects only the skin but may invade the lungs, kidneys, nervous system, and bones. The disease is most common in young men living in the southeastern United States. Skin infections often begin as small bumps on exposed areas where there has been a cut, bruise, or other injury. These bumps spread into surrounding areas. When the lungs are involved, symptoms include cough, shortness of breath, chest pain, chills, and a fever with heavy sweating.

blastula /blas'tyələ/, an early stage of the process in which a fertilized egg develops into an embryo. The blastula is the form in which the embryo becomes planted in the wall of the uterus. Also called **blastosphere.**

bleb, a gathering of fluid under the skin, forming bumps that are smaller than normal blisters.

bleed, 1. to lose blood from the blood vessels. The blood may flow out through a natural opening, or a break in the skin, or it may flow into a space, an organ, or the spaces between the tissues. **2.** to cause blood to flow from a vein or an artery.

bleeder, 1. *informal.* a patient who has a blood clotting disease (hemophilia) or any other vessel or blood condition linked to a tendency to bleed. **2.** *informal.* a bleeding blood vessel, especially one cut during surgery.

bleeding time, the time needed for blood to stop flowing from a tiny wound. A test of bleeding time is the Ivy method, in which a blood pressure cuff on the upper arm is inflated and a small wound is made with a scalpel on the inner surface of the arm. Normal Ivy bleeding time is from 2 to 6 minutes.

Blenoxane, a trademark for an anticancer drug (bleomycin sulfate).

bleomycin sulfate, an anticancer antibiotic used to treat many cancers. Allergy to this drug prohibits its use. Side effects include lung problems (pneumonitis, pulmonary fibrosis), high fever, and collapse of the circulation. Rashes and skin reactions commonly occur.

blepharitis /blef'ərī'tis/, an inflammatory, often contagious condition of the eyelash and oil glands of the eyelids. It features swelling, redness, and crusts of dried mucus on the lids.

blepharoatheroma /blef'ərō·ath'ərō'mə/, a tumor of the eyelid.

blepharoplegia /-plē'jə/, paralysis of the eyelid.

blepharospasm /blef'ərospazm'/, a spasm of the eyelid.

blighted ovum, a fertilized egg (ovum) that fails to develop. On x-ray films or ultrasound it appears to be a fluid-filled lump (cyst) attached to the wall of the uterus. Many miscarriages in the first 3 months of pregnancy are actually a blighted ovum being released.

A–B

blind loop, a part of the intestine that is blocked off from the rest of the intestines so that nothing can pass through it. Blind loops are sometimes created surgically during bowel operations.

blindness, being unable to see. **Cortical blindness** results from injury to the visual center brain cortex.

blind spot, 1. a small, normal gap in sight caused when an image is focused on the optic disc of the retina. **2.** an abnormal gap in sight caused by an injury of the retina or other part of the eye. It is often sensed as light spots or flashes.

blister, a thin, rounded swelling of the skin that contains fluid. It is caused by irritation or burns. Also called **vesicle** or **bulla.**

bloat, a swelling or filling with gas, as when the stomach is distended from swallowing air or from intestinal gas.

Blocadren, a trademark for a drug used to treat high blood pressure (timolol maleate).

blocking, 1. preventing the sending of an electric signal impulse of the nervous system. For example, spinal anesthesia blocks the nerve signals to part of the body. **2.** interrupting some of the body's processes, as with some drugs. **3.** being unable to remember an event.

blood, the liquid pumped by the heart through all of the arteries, veins, and capillaries. It is made up of a clear yellow fluid, called plasma, and many cells called the formed elements. The formed elements include red blood cells (erythrocytes), white blood cells (leukocytes), and platelets. The erythrocytes move oxygen and food to the cells and remove carbon dioxide and other wastes from the cells. The leukocytes defend the body against foreign invaders. The platelets function in blood clotting. Hormones and proteins are also contained in the blood. The normal adult has about 1 ounce of blood per pound of body weight (70 ml/kg for men and 65 ml/kg for women).

blood bank, an organization that collects, processes, and stores blood to be used for transfusions and other purposes. Blood banks routinely examine blood for **hepatitis B surface antigen (HBsAG).** It is found in the blood of a patient who has serum hepatitis or who is a carrier for that virus. The purpose is to avoid passing on the infection to a patient receiving a transfusion.

blood-brain barrier (BBB), a feature of the brain thought to be made up of walls of small vessels (capillaries) that surround the membranes. The blood-brain barrier normally prevents many chemicals and disease-causing organisms in the blood from entering the nervous system.

blood buffers. See **buffer.**

blood cell, any one of the many cells (formed elements) of the blood, including red cells (erythrocytes), white cells (leukocytes), and platelets. Together they normally make up about 50% of the total volume of the blood. See also **erythrocyte, leukocyte, platelet.**

blood clot, a semisolid, gelatin-like mass that results from the clotting process of blood. It is mostly made up of red cells, white cells, and platelets mixed in a protein (fibrin) grouping. Compare **embolus, thrombus.**

blood clotting, changing blood from a liquid to a semisolid gel. The process usually starts with tissue damage and exposure of the blood to air. Within seconds of injury to the vessel wall, platelets clump at the site. A chain reaction of clotting factors (prothrombin, thrombin, and fibrinogen) produces a substance called fibrin. Fibrin forms a mesh over the wound in which the blood cells are kept rigid. Clotting can also occur in abnormal conditions within the blood vessel, forming an embolus or thrombus. Also called **blood coagulation.**

blood count, a measure of the number of cells found in the blood. A **complete blood count (CBC)** is the number of red and white blood cells per cubic millimeter of blood. All patients admitted to the hospital receive a complete blood count. It is one of the most valuable diagnostic tests. The count can be done by staining a smear of blood on a slide and counting the types of cells under a microscope. Most laboratories use an electronic counter. In a **red blood cell count (RBC),** only the red blood cells (erythrocytes) are measured in a sample of whole blood. In a **differential white blood cell count,** the number of different types of white blood cells (leukocytes) are measured in a small blood sample. The different kinds of white cells are reported as percentages of the total examined. A **hematocrit** is a measure of the number of red cells found in the blood, stated as a percentage of the total blood volume. The normal range is between 43% and 49% in men, and between 37% and 43% in women.

blood donor, anyone who donates blood to a blood bank or to another person. A **universal donor** is a person with blood of type O, Rh factor negative. Such blood may be used for emergency transfusion with little risk of incompatibility.

blood doping, a new technique that has been used by some athletes to increase their performance and endurance. It consists of giving a blood transfusion to add red blood cells to increase the oxygen-carrying ability of the blood. It is illegal in most competitions. Also called **blood boosting, blood packing.**

blood dyscrasia, a condition in which any of the blood elements are abnormal, as in leukemia or hemophilia.

blood gas, gas dissolved in the liquid part of the blood. Blood gases include oxygen, carbon dioxide, and nitrogen. This is measured to see whether oxygen intake and distribution is normal and whether the acid-base status (pH) is adequate. The oxygen content of blood becomes less in disorders such as obstructive lung disease, chest deformities, and some muscle diseases. Overweight has the same effect. Carbon dioxide content is increased in disorders such as shortness of breath (emphysema) and severe vomiting. It is decreased in starvation and acute kidney failure.

blood-gas determination, an analysis of the acid-base balance (pH) of the blood. This includes measuring the amount and pressure of oxygen, carbon dioxide, and hydrogen in the blood. Blood-gas determination is important for evaluating heart failure, bleeding, kidney failure, drug overdose, shock, uncontrolled diabetes, or any other condition of severe stress. See also **acid-base balance.**

blood group, the labeling of blood based on the presence or lack of specific chemical substances on the surface of the red cell. There are several different grouping systems. **ABO blood groups** refers to the main system for labeling blood based on properties of the red blood cell. The four blood types in this group are A, B, AB, and O.

blood plasma. See **plasma.**

blood poisoning, an infection of the whole body (septicemia) caused by germs that spread from an infected part of the body through the bloodstream. It is treated with antibiotic drugs. Usually septicemia causes fever, chill, prostration, pain, headache, nausea, or diarrhea. **Toxemia** refers to the presence of poisons (toxins) from bacteria in the bloodstream.

blood pressure (BP), the stress placed on the walls of the arteries, the veins, and the heart chambers by the flow of blood. The amount of arterial pressure is the product of how much blood the heart pumps and the resistance in the blood vessels. Stress, high blood volume, low blood volume, and many drugs may alter the arterial pressure. Blood pressure is most often measured by using a device with a blood pressure cuff (sphygmomanometer) and a stethoscope.

blood pump, 1. a pump for controlling the flow of blood into a blood vessel during a transfusion. 2. the part of a heart-lung machine that pumps the blood through the machine to put oxygen into it and then through the circulation system of the body.

blood serum. See **serum.**

blood substitute, a substance used to replace circulating blood or to increase its volume. For example, plasma, human serum albumin, and white cells (leukocytes) are often given in place of whole blood transfusions in the treatment of many disorders.

blood sugar, 1. one of a group of closely related substances, as glucose, fructose, and galactose, that are normally in the blood and are needed to process food. 2. the amount of glucose in the blood. Also called **blood glucose.** See also **hyperglycemia, hypoglycemia.**

Classification of blood pressure*

Diastolic blood pressure (mm Hg)	Category
<85	Normal blood pressure
85 to 89	High normal blood pressure
90 to 104	Mild hypertension
105 to 114	Moderate hypertension
≥115	Severe hypertension

Systolic blood pressure (mm Hg) when DBP <90 mm Hg	Category
<140	Normal blood pressure
140 to 159	Borderline isolated systolic hypertension
≥160	Isolated systolic hypertension

*A classification of borderline isolated systolic hypertension (SBP 140 to 159 mm Hg) or isolated systolic hypertension (SBP ≥ 160 mm Hg) takes precedence over a classification of high normal blood pressure (DBP 85 to 89 mm Hg) when both occur in the same individual. A classification of high normal blood pressure (DBP 85 to 89 mm Hg) takes precedence over a classification of normal blood pressure (SBP <140 mm Hg) when both occur in the same person.

From The 1984 Report of the Joint National Committee on Detection, Evaluation, and Treatment of High Blood Pressure, U.S. Dept. of Health and Human Services, Public Health Service, NIH Publication No. 84-1088, Bethesda, MD, June 1984, National Institutes of Health.

blood test, 1. any test that finds out something about the traits or properties of the blood. 2. *informal.* a test for syphilis.

blood transfusion, giving whole blood or a part, as red cells, to replace blood lost through injury, surgery, or disease. A needle is placed into a vein, usually in the arm, and a tube is connected to allow the blood to drip in slowly. Whole blood may be given to a patient by transfusion directly from a donor, but more often the donor's blood is collected and stored by a blood bank. Blood must be checked, typed, and cross matched carefully. A healthy donor's blood group and specific chemical substances must match those of the patient.

blood typing, noting the specific chemical substances (antigens) on the surface of the red blood cell. This process is used to determine a person's blood group. It is the first step in testing donor's and patient's blood to be used in transfusion and is followed by cross matching. See also **blood group.**

blood urea nitrogen (BUN), the amount of nitrogen in the blood in the form of urea. It is a waste product of normal body functions. BUN is a rough sign of kidney function. It is high in kidney failure, shock, stomach and bowel bleeding, diabetes mellitus, and some tumors. BUN levels are lowered in liver disease, bad dietary situations, and normal pregnancy.

levels are lowered in liver disease, bad dietary situations, and normal pregnancy.

blood vessel, any one of the group of tubes that carries blood. Kinds of blood vessels are **arteries, arterioles, capillaries, veins, venules.**

bloody show. See **vaginal bleeding.**

Bloom's syndrome, a genetic disease occurring mainly in Ashkenazi Jews and carried as a recessive trait. It features slowed growth, large blood vessels on the face and arms, sensitivity to sunlight, and a risk of leukemia.

blow-out fracture, a broken bone beneath the eyeball caused by a blow that suddenly increases the pressure within the eye.

blue baby, an infant born with bluish skin (cyanosis) caused by an inborn heart problem or incomplete expansion of the lungs. Tetralogy of Fallot is the most common inborn cyanotic heart defect. These defects are diagnosed by certain tests (cardiac catheterization, angiography, or echocardiography) and are corrected surgically, usually in early childhood. See also **congenital heart disease.**

blue nevus, a steel-blue skin lump (nodule) with a diameter between 2 and 7 mm (less than ⅓ inch). It is found on the face or arms, grows very slowly, and lasts throughout life. Those on the buttocks or near the tailbone occasionally become cancerous. Any sudden change in the size demands a physician's attention and tissue tests. Compare **melanoma.**

blue spot, **1.** any of the small grayish-blue spots (macula cerulea) that may appear near the armpits or around the groin of individuals infested with body or pubic lice. **2.** any of the dark blue or mulberry-colored round or oval spots (Mongolian spots) that may appear as a temporary birth defect on the tailbone.

blush, a brief reddening of the face and neck, commonly the result of the widening of small blood vessels. Blushing is a response to heat or sudden emotion.

BMR, abbreviation for **basal metabolic rate.**

board certified, referring to a physician who has passed an examination given by a medical specialty board and has been certified as a specialist in a particular field of medicine.

board of health, a board generally concerned with noting the health needs of the people and bringing projects and resources together to meet these needs. The functions, powers, and duties of boards of health vary with their location.

Boas' test, a test for hydrochloric acid in the contents of the stomach. Also called **resorcinol test.**

body, **1.** the whole structure of an individual including the organs. **2.** the largest or the main part of any organ.

body fluid, a liquid contained in the three fluid spaces of the body: the blood plasma, the fluid between the cells (interstitial), and the cell fluid within the cells. Blood plasma and interstitial fluid make up the extracellular fluid. The cell fluid is the intracellular fluid.

body image, a person's own concept of physical appearance. The mental picture, which may be realistic or unrealistic, is created from self-observation, the reactions of others, and the interaction of attitudes, emotions, memories, fantasies, and experiences.

body jacket, a cast that covers the body but does not cover the neck or arms and legs. It is used to treat a crooked spine (scoliosis) and for keeping the patient rigid after spinal surgery.

body language, a set of nonspeaking signals that can express many physical, mental, and emotional states. These include body movements, postures, gestures, expressions, and what one wears.

body movement, motion of all or part of the body, especially at a joint. Some kinds of body movements are **abduction, adduction, extension, flexion, rotation.**

body odor, a smell linked to stale sweat. Fresh sweat is odorless, but after exposure to the air and bacteria on the surface of the skin, chemical changes occur to make the odor. Body odors also can be the result of discharges from many skin conditions, including cancer, fungus, hemorrhoids, leukemia, and ulcers.

body position, posture of the body. The **anatomic position** is one in which a person stands erect, facing directly forward, feet pointed forward and slightly apart, arms hanging down at the sides with palms facing forward. This is the standard neutral position referred to in medical texts. It is used to describe sites or motions of parts of the body. **Decerebrate posture** is usually seen in patients who are in a coma. The arms are extended and turned toward the body and the legs are extended with the feet flexed downward. **Decubitus** refers to a reclining or flat position, such as lying on one side. In the **knee-chest (genupectoral) position,** the person kneels so that the weight of the body is supported by the knees and chest. The belly is raised, the head is turned to one side and the arms are bent so that the upper part of the body can be supported in part by the elbows. The **lithotomy position** is one used on an examining table. The patient lies on the back with the hips and knees fully flexed. For Ob-Gyn procedures, the buttocks are at the edge of the table and the feet are held in stirrups. **Trendelenburg's position** is one in which the head is low and the body and legs are on an upward angle. It is sometimes used in pelvic surgery to move the stomach and intestinal organs upward, out of the pelvis. See also **prone, supine.**

body-righting reflex, any one of the nerve and muscle responses to restore the body to its normal upright position when it has been displaced. The righting reflexes involve

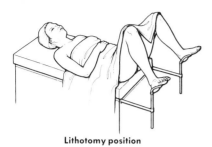

Lithotomy position

complex mechanisms linked to the structures of the internal ear. Also involved in the righting mechanism are the many nerves to the inner ear, to muscles and tendons, and to the eyes. Interruption of the nerve signals linked to body-righting reflexes may disturb the sense of balance and cause nausea and vomiting.

body temperature, the level of heat made by the body. Variations in body temperature are major signs of disease and other defects. Heat is created in the body through processing (metabolism) of food. Heat is lost from the body surface through radiation, convection, and evaporation of sweat. Heat production and loss are regulated by the hypothalamus and brain stem. Fever is usually caused by increased heat production. However, some abnormal conditions, as congestive heart failure, cause slight fevers because the heat-loss function is damaged. Diseases of the hypothalamus may cause below normal body temperatures. **Basal body temperature** is the temperature of the body taken in the morning, by mouth or in the rectum, after at least 8 hours of sleep. It is taken before doing anything else, including getting out of bed, moving around, talking, eating, or drinking. Normal adult body temperature, as measured by mouth, is 98.6° F. Mouth temperatures ranging from 96.5° F to 99° F are consistent with good health, depending on the physical activity and the normal body temperature for that person. When the temperature is taken under the armpit, it is usually 1° F lower than the mouth temperature. Rectal temperatures may be 0.5° to 1.0° F higher than mouth readings. Body temperature appears to vary 1° to 2° F throughout the day, with lows recorded early in the morning and peaks between 6 PM and 10 PM. See also **fever.**

boil, a pus-making skin infection in a gland or hair gland (follicle). It features pain, redness, and swelling. The center of the swollen area forms a core of matter from tissue death. To prevent spread of infection, it is important to avoid irritating or squeezing the sore. Treatment includes antibiotics, local moist heat, and draining. Also called **furuncle.**

boiling point, the temperature at which a substance passes from a liquid to a gas at a particular air pressure. For example, water boils at 212 degrees Fahrenheit at sea level.

bolus /bō′ləs/, **1.** a chewed, round lump of food ready to be swallowed. **2.** a large round mass of a drug for swallowing that is usually soft and not prepackaged. **3.** a dose of a drug or a drug injected all at once into the vein.

bonding, the attachment process that occurs between an infant and the parents, especially the mother. These ties of affection later influence the physical and mental growth of the child. Bonding often starts at birth when the nude infant is placed on the mother's stomach so that the parents and child can see and touch one another and begin to interact. The newborn is alert for about 30 minutes to 1 hour after birth and cries, sucks, clings, grasps, and follows with the eyes, which in turn begins the parenting instincts. Especially important in starting bonding is eye-to-eye contact, holding the infant, soothing talk, and other behavior that creates emotional ties. New concepts in birth procedures help to build stronger parent-infant relationships, such as the trend toward more natural childbirth, allowing the father to help in the birth, and involving parents in the care of premature and ill newborns. Certain behaviors are common for each parent during the early bonding process. Mothers are usually more concerned with touching and holding the infant. Fathers are more intent on eye contact with the child.

bone, 1. the dense, hard, and slightly stretchy connective tissue that makes up the 206 bones of the human skeleton. It is made up of dense bone tissue (osseous) surrounding spongy tissue that contains many blood vessels and nerves. Covering the bone is a membrane called the periosteum. Long bones contain yellow marrow in the long spaces and red marrow in the ends near the joints. Red marrow also fills the spaces of the flat and the short bones, the backbones (vertebrae), the skull, the breastbone (sternum), and the ribs. Blood cells are made in active red marrow. **2.** any single element of the skeleton, as a rib, the sternum, or the femur. See also **connective tissue.**

bone cancer, a skeletal cancer occurring as the first tumor in an area of rapid growth or as a spreading tumor from cancer elsewhere in the body. First bone tumors are rare. The risk peaks during adolescence, then decreases, and rises again after 35 years of age. Paget's disease, overactive parathyroid gland, long-term bone infection (osteomyelitis), areas where the blood supply is cut off, and a thickening at a bone fracture increase the risk of bone tumors. Most bone cancers are spreading tumors found in the spine, pelvis, or other areas. Bone cancers develop rapidly but are often difficult to detect; pain that increases at night may be the only symptom. The most common bone cancers are osteosarcomas, chrondrosarcomas, fibrosarcomas, and

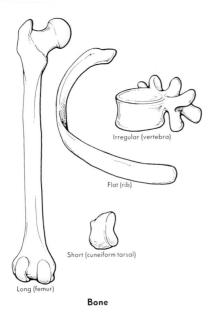

Irregular (vertebra)

Flat (rib)

Short (cuneiform tarsal)

Long (femur)

Bone

Ewing's sarcoma. Treatment includes surgery, x-ray therapy, and chemotherapy. The use of interferon and other forms of immune therapy has been experimental.

bone marrow, soft tissue filling the spaces in the spongy part of bone shafts. Its main function is to make the blood cells. Fatty, **yellow marrow** is found in the compact bone of most adult long bones, as in the arms and legs. **Red marrow** is found in many bones of infants and children and in the smaller bones, as the sternum, ribs, and backbones of adults. Red blood cells are made in red marrow.

Bonine, a trademark for a drug used to treat nausea from motion sickness (meclizine hydrochloride).

booster injection, giving an antigen, as a vaccine or toxoid, usually in a smaller amount than the original vaccination. A booster is given to keep the immune response at the correct level.

booster pump, a pump used to increase the pressure of compressed air.

borax bath, a bath in which borax and glycerin are added to the water.

borborygmus /bôr'bərig'məs/, *pl.* **borborygmi,** a stomach and bowel sound caused by overactive intestine movement (peristalsis). Borborygmi are rumbling and gurgling noises. Although increased intestinal movement may be noted in cases of gastroenteritis and diarrhea, true borborygmi are more intense and periodic. Borborygmi along with vomiting, bloating, and cramps may mean a blockage of the small intestine.

boric acid, a white, odorless powder or crystal-like substance used as a buffer. It is sometimes used in weak solution as an eye wash.

born out of asepsis (BOA), referring to a newborn infant that was not delivered in a disinfected birthing unit. A BOA infant may have been born on the way to the hospital, in the hospital on the way to the delivery room, or in a labor room. The usual steps in caring for a newborn are carried out. In many hospitals BOA infants are placed in a special nursery, isolated from other infants to prevent contagion should the BOA baby be infected. Daily care for the newborn BOA is the same as that given to other newborns, but the baby is also watched for signs of infection.

boron (B), a nonmetal element, similar to aluminum. It is the main part of boric acid.

Boston exanthem, an epidemic disease caused by a virus. Symptoms are a scattered, pale red rash on the face, chest, and back, sometimes with small ulcers on the tonsils and soft palate. The lymph glands usually do not swell, and the rash disappears by itself in 2 or 3 weeks. It needs no treatment.

bottle feeding, feeding an infant or young child from a bottle with a rubber nipple on the end. It is sometimes called artificial feeding because it is a substitute for or an addition to breast feeding. The formula contains protein, fats, carbohydrates, vitamins, and minerals in amounts similar to those in breast milk. Bottle feeding is used as a substitute for breast feeding when the mother is unable or chooses not to breast-feed. It can also be a supplement to breast feeding. Bottle feeding is urged if the mother has a contagious disease or a serious long-term disease, or has recently had surgery. Severe breast infection (mastitis), drug addiction, or use of drugs that are released in the breast milk usually means bottle feeding.

botulism /boch'əlizm/, an often fatal form of food poisoning caused by a poison (endotoxin) made by rod-shaped germs (*Clostridium botulinum*). Most botulism occurs after eating improperly canned or cooked foods. In rare cases, the toxin may come into the human body through a wound infected by the organism. Botulism differs from most other types of food poisoning in that it develops without stomach upset. Nausea and vomiting occur in less than one half of the cases. Symptoms may not occur from 18 hours up to 1 week after the infected food has been eaten. Botulism features a period of weakness followed by sight problems, as double vision, difficulty in focusing the eyes, and sensitivity to light. Muscles may become weak, and the person often develops difficulty in swallowing. Hospitalization is necessary, and antitoxins are given. About two thirds of the cases of botulism are fatal, usually as a result of late diagnosis and lung problems. For those who survive, recovery is slow. **Infant botulism** is a condition of poisoning that occurs in children less than 6 months of age. It is marked by severe loss of tone in all muscles, constipation, lethargy, and feeding difficulties, and it may lead to inability to breathe. Treatment includes fluids, electrolytes, and nutrition. Help in breathing may also be necessary.

Bouchard's node /booshärz´/, a swelling of a knuckle. It usually occurs in wasting diseases of the joints, as osteoarthritis. Compare **Heberden node.**

bougie /boo´zhē, boozhē´/, a thin cylinder made of rubber or other flexible material. It is put into canals of the body to widen, examine, or measure them.

boutonneuse fever /boo´tənooz´/, an infectious disease carried to humans through the bite of a tick. The disease begins with a sore at the site of the bite. A fever lasting from a few days to 2 weeks and a red rash that spreads over the body including the palms and soles develop. It is common in parts of Europe, Asia, Africa, and the Middle East. See also **Rocky Mountain spotted fever.**

bowel. See **intestine.**

bowel training, a method of creating regular bowel movements by reflex conditioning. It is used to treat undesired defecation, constipation, long-term diarrhea, and other bowel problems.

bowleg, a deformity in which one or both legs are bent out at the knee. Also called **genu varum.**

boxer's fracture, a break of one or more of the bones in the hands (metacarpals). It usually involves the base of the fourth or fifth finger and is caused by punching a hard object.

B-post, second roof pillar from a vehicle's windshield.

brace, a device, sometimes jointed, to support and hold any movable part of the body in the correct position. It allows that part of the body to function, as a leg brace that permits walking and standing. Compare **splint.**

brachial /brā´kē·əl/, referring to the arm.

brachial artery, the main artery of the upper arm. It ends just below the inside bend of the elbow where it branches into the radial artery and the ulnar artery.

brachialis /brā´kē·a´lis/, a muscle of the upper arm that extends from the shoulder to below the inside of the elbow. It lies under the biceps and flexes the forearm.

brachial plexus, a group of nerves that branch from the upper spine and neck. The brachial plexus supplies the muscles and skin of the chest, shoulders, and arms.

brachiocephalic /brāk´ē·ōsəfal´ik/, relating to the arm and head.

brachioradialis /-rā´dē·a´lis/, the muscle just under the skin on the thumb (radial) side of the forearm. It flexes the forearm.

brachycephaly /brak´ēsef´əlē/, a birth defect of the skull in which premature closing of the soft spot (coronal suture)

results in excess growth of the head from side to side, giving it a short, broad appearance.

brachytherapy, the use of radioactive materials in the treatment of cancer by placing the radioactive sources in direct contact with the tissues to be treated.

Bradford frame, a rectangular frame made of pipes with straps of canvas attached to support a patient lying on the back or the face. The straps can be removed to permit the patient to urinate or defecate while remaining rigid.

Bradley method, a method of preparing for childbirth developed by Robert Bradley, MD. It includes education about the physical nature of childbirth, exercise and diet during pregnancy, and ways of breathing for control and comfort during labor and birth. The father is involved in the classes and is the mother's ''coach'' during labor. Also called **husband-coached childbirth.** Compare **Lamaze method, Read method.** See also **natural childbirth.**

bradycardia /brad´ēkär´dē·ə/, an abnormal condition in which the heart contracts steadily but at a rate of less than 60 beats a minute. The heart normally slows during sleep, and, in some physically fit people, the pulse may be quite slow. Bradycardia may be a symptom of a brain tumor, digitalis overdose, or an abnormal response of the vagus nerve (vagotonia). There may be dizziness, chest pain, fainting, and collapse of the circulation. Treatment may include giving atropine, implanting a pacemaker, or reducing the digitalis dose.

bradycardia-tachycardia syndrome, a heart disorder with a heart rate that shifts from very slow to very fast rhythms.

bradykinesia /-kinē´zhə/, an abnormal condition that features slowness of all voluntary movement and speech. This may be caused by parkinsonism, other nerve disorders, and some tranquilizers.

bradykinin, a chemical made by the body that widens the blood vessels.

bradypnea /-pnē´ə/. See **respiratory rate.**

Braille /brāl/, a system of printing for the blind. It is made up of patterns of raised dots or points that can be read by touch.

brain, the portion of the brain and spinal cord (central nervous system) contained within the skull. It is made up of the cerebrum, cerebellum, and brainstem (pons, medulla, and mesencephalon). The **cerebrum** is the largest and uppermost section of the brain, divided by a deep groove at the top into the left and the right halves of the brain. **Cerebral hemisphere** refers to one of the halves of the cerebrum. The two cerebral hemispheres are connected at the bottom by the corpus callosum. Each cerebral hemisphere is made up of the large outer **cerebral cortex** layer (the ''gray matter'' of the brain), the underlying white substance, the internal basal ganglia, and certain other structures. The internal structures of the hemispheres join with the brainstem through the cerebral stalks. Prominent grooves further subdivide each hemisphere into four major lobes. The **frontal lobe** is the largest of the brain. The **occipital lobe** lies under the occipital bone of the skull. The **parietal lobe** rests on the side of the skull next to the parietal bone. The **temporal lobe** is the outer lower region of the brain. The **cerebellum** is the part of the brain located at the base of the skull behind the brainstem. It consists of two cerebellar lobes, one on each side, and a middle section called the vermis. Three pairs of stalks link it with the brainstem. **Cerebellar cortex** refers to the outer layer of gray matter of the cerebellum. It covers the white substance in the core. The **brainstem** is the part of the brain that includes the medulla oblongata, the pons, and the mesencephalon. It has motor, sense and reflex functions and contains the spinal tracts. The 12 pairs of nerves from the brain to the rest of the body branch off the brainstem. The **medulla oblongata** continues as the bulblike part of the spinal cord just above the opening into the skull (foramen magnum). It contains mostly white substance with some gray substance. The medulla contains the heart, blood vessel, and breathing centers of the brain. Thus, any injury or disease in this area is often fatal. The **mesencephalon,** also called midbrain, is mostly made up of white matter with some gray matter. A red nucleus is in the mesencephalon. It contains the ends of nerve fibers from the other parts of the brain. Deep inside the mesencephalon are nuclei of several skull nerves. The mesencephalon also contains nerve nuclei for certain hearing and seeing reflexes. The **pons** is a mass of nerve cells on the surface of the brainstem. It has nuclei of various nerves, including the facial and the trigeminal nerves.

Special cells in the brain's mass of complex, soft, gray or white tissue bring together and control the functions of the central nervous system. The cerebrum has sensory and motor functions, and functions linked to integration of many mental activities. The cerebral cortex has cells that integrate higher mental functions, general movement, stomach functions, and behavioral reactions. Research has described more than 200 different areas and 47 separate functions of the cerebral cortex. The left cerebral hemisphere is dominant in right-handed people, and those who are left-handed have dominant right hemispheres. The motor speech area is better developed in the left hemisphere of right-handed persons, for example. Its destruction causes loss of speech (aphasia) or other speech defects. Stimulation of the frontal area affects circulation, breathing, widening of the pupils, and other activity. The cerebrum makes a variety of electrical waves that can be recorded (electroencephalogram). Some of the other processes that are controlled by the cerebrum are memory,

speech, writing, and emotional response. The frontal lobe influences personality and is linked to the higher mental activities, as planning and judgment. Damage to the parietal lobe causes disorders of speaking (aphasia) and sight. The parietal lobe also helps to tell the sizes, shapes, and textures of objects. The center for smell is located within the temporal lobe of the brain. It also has some association areas for memory and learning, and a region where thoughts are selected. **Association area** refers to any part of the main portion of the brain (cerebrum) involved in integrating sensory information, such as vision. The cerebellum is concerned with coordinating voluntary muscular activity, as walking, and maintaining equilibrium.

brain concussion, a violent jarring or shaking injury to the brain. After a mild concussion there may be a brief loss of consciousness with a headache on awakening. Sometimes no loss of consciousness occurs. Severe concussion may cause lengthy unconsciousness and disruption of certain vital functions of the brainstem, as breathing. Because concussions can be fatal, medical attention should be sought if any of the following symptoms develop even 4 weeks after a head injury: unequally widened pupils, severe headache, confusion, loss of memory, continual drowsiness, personality changes, speech difficulties, paralysis, or loss of coordination.

brain death, an irreversible form of unconsciousness. A complete loss of brain function occurs while the heart continues to beat. The legal definition of this condition varies from state to state. The usual medical definition of brain death includes the lack of reflexes, movements, and breathing. The pupils are widened and fixed. Because cold exposure (hypothermia), anesthesia, poisoning, or drug overdose may cause a state that resembles brain death, a diagnosis of brain death requires that the electric activity of the brain is proved to be absent. This is proven by doing two brain tests (electroencephalograms) 12 to 24 hours apart. Also called **irreversible coma.** Compare **coma, sleep, stupor.**

brain electric activity map (BEAM), a map of the brain created by a computer that is able to respond to the brain's electric signals by a flash of light. An abnormal pattern of disordered or blocked signals may indicate a tumor or other problem. See also **brain waves.**

brain fever, *informal.* any inflammation of the brain or lining of the brain (meninges). See also **encephalitis.**

brain scan, a painless diagnostic test to identify injury, tumors, or areas where the blood supply is blocked. Radioisotopes are injected into a vein, which circulate to the brain where they gather in abnormal tissue. The radioisotopes are traced and photographed by a scanner (scintillator) to find the size and place of the abnormality. See also **radioisotope scan.**

brainstem. See **brain.**

brain tumor, a tumor of the brain that usually does not spread beyond the brain and spinal cord. Brain tumors cause high rates of illness and death, but many are successfully treated. Brain tumors in children are usually the result of a defect during fetal growth. In adults 20% to 40% of cancers in the brain are spread from cancers in the breast, lung, stomach, intestines, kidney, or any site of a cancerous skin tumor. The cause of first brain tumors is not known, but the risk is greater for people exposed to vinyl chloride, for the brothers and sisters of cancer patients, and for patients with kidney transplants who are treated with immune supressing drugs. Symptoms of a brain tumor include headache, nausea, vomiting, swelling of the optic disc in the eye, weakness, and confusion. Many other signs also occur, as loss of sight in the eye on the side of the tumor. Treatment for brain tumors includes surgery and x-ray therapy. A normally protective feature of the brain (blood-brain barrier) prevents many anticancer drugs from being effective for brain tumors.

brain waves, the repeating changes, or rhythms, in the electrical activity of the brain. There are four types of brain waves. These can be recorded on a machine that graphs brain impulses (electroencephalograph). They can be used to diagnose brain problems or to identify changed states of consciousness. They can also show brain death. **Alpha waves** are the ''relaxed waves'' of the brain and are the main waves recorded. Blinking the eyes affects the patterns of the alpha waves. **Beta waves** are the ''busy waves'' of the brain, when a person is awake and alert with eyes open. **Delta waves** are the slowest of the brain waves. They are ''deep-sleep waves'' linked with a dreamless sleep from which a person is not easy to awaken. **Theta waves** are the ''drowsy waves'' of the temporal lobes of the brain, when a person is awake but relaxed and sleepy.

bran bath, a bath in which bran has been boiled in the water. Bran baths are used to relieve skin irritation.

branch, that organizational level having functional/geographic responsibility for major segments of incident operations. The branch level is organizationally between section and division/group.

branched chain ketoaciduria. See **maple syrup urine disease.**

branchial fistula /brang′kē·əl/, an inborn, abnormal passage from the throat to the outside surface of the neck. Also called **cervical fistula.**

Braxton Hicks contraction. See **false labor.**

Brazelton assessment, a system for assessing the behavior of newborns with a series of 27 reaction tests. The tests check response to solid objects, to a pinprick, to light, and to the sound of a rattle or bell.

breakthrough bleeding. See **vaginal bleeding.**

breast, the front part of the surface of the chest. See also **mammary gland.**

breast cancer, a malignant tumor of breast tissue, the most common cancer in women in the United States. The rate increases between 30 to 50 years of age and reaches a second peak at 65 years of age. Risk factors include a family history of breast cancer, no children, exposure to radiation, young age when menstruation began, late menopause, being overweight, diabetes, high blood pressure, long-term cystic disease of the breast, and, possibly, hormone therapy after menopause. Women who are over 40 years of age when they bear their first child or with cancer in other areas also have a greater risk of getting breast cancer. First symptoms include a small painless lump, thick or dimpled skin, or nipple withdrawal. As the tumor grows, there may be a nipple discharge, pain, ulcers, and swollen lymph glands under the arms. The diagnosis is made by a careful physical examination, a breast scan (mammography), and examination of tumor cells. Tumors are more common in the left than in the right breast and in the upper and outer parts of the breast. Spreading through the lymph system to lymph nodes under the arm (axillary) and to bone, lung, brain, and liver is common. Surgical treatment may be a radical, modified radical, or removal of the breast (mastectomy), with the removal of axillary nodes. X-ray therapy, chemotherapy, or both are usually given after surgery. The ovaries, adrenal glands, or the pituitary gland may also be removed. Androgen or antiestrogen drugs may be given to prevent the return of the cancer. Breast cancer seldom occurs in men, but those with Klinefelter's syndrome are at 60 times greater risk. See also **mastectomy.**

breast examination, a process in which the breasts and the surrounding structures are inspected for changes that could indicate cancer. The breasts are examined with the woman sitting with her arms at her sides, sitting with her arms over her head, back straight, then leaning forward, and sitting upright while contracting the pectoral muscles. The breasts are checked for identical shape and size and for surface changes, including moles or colored areas, dimpling, swelling, nipple withdrawal, unusual vein patterns showing through the skin, lumps, sores, or abnormal hair growth. The lymph nodes under the arms and around the collarbones are checked for swelling. With the woman lying on her back, each breast is shifted, and the gland area in each is felt with the flat of the fingers in circles working from the outer edges toward the nipples. The areolar areas, the nipples, and the area extending toward the armpit are then felt. The breast examination done thoroughly is a valuable means of finding women who need further examination by tests, as xeroradiography, mammography, biopsy, or thermoradiography.

breast feeding, 1. suckling or nursing, giving a baby milk from the breast. Breast feeding causes the uterus to return to its nonpregnant size. **2.** taking milk from the breast.

breast milk, human milk, the ideal food for most babies. It is easily digested, clean and warm, passes some immunities from the mother, and helps the emotional bonding between mother and baby. Infants fed breast milk are less likely to become overweight or to develop a poor bite.

breast milk jaundice, liver disease (jaundice) and excessive bile coloring (bilirubin) in breast-fed infants that occur in the first weeks of life. It is caused by a substance in the mother's milk that makes the infant unable to process and release bilirubin. The infant seems normal and healthy, but the skin and the whites of the eyes are yellowish. Breast feeding may be stopped until there is a decrease of bilirubin to normal levels, usually a period of 1 to 3 days. During this time, the infant is bottle-fed.

breast pump, a device for taking milk from the breast.

breathing. See **respiration.**

breathing air, compressed air that contains no more contaminants than are allowed by standards.

breathing tube, a device put into the windpipe (trachea) through the mouth or nose to create an open airway for good breathing during breathing assistance.

breathlessness. See **dyspnea.**

breath sound, the sound of air passing in and out of the breathing system as heard with a stethoscope. Decreased breath sounds may mean a blocked airway, collapsed lung, a lung disease (emphysema), or other long-term blocking lung disease. An **amphoric** breath sound is an abnormal, hollow blowing sound caused by a hollow place opening into the bronchus, or by air in the chest (pneumothorax). A **bronchial** breath sound is heard over the lungs and caused by pneumonia or pressure. There are loud, high-pitched sounds of equal length. A **tracheal** breath sound refers to a normal breath sound heard in the windpipe. Breathing in and out are equally loud. A **vesicular** breath sound is a normal sound of rustling or swishing heard with a stethoscope over the lung. There is a higher pitch when breathing in which fades rapidly while breathing out.

breech birth, birth in which the baby comes out feet, knees, or buttocks first. Breech birth is often dangerous. The body may come out easily, but the head may become trapped by an incompletely widened cervix because babies' heads are usually larger in diameter than their bodies. A **complete breech** is a position of the fetus in the womb in which the buttocks and feet are toward the birth canal. The posture of the fetus is the same as in a normal head-first position, but upside down. A **footling breech**

refers to a position in which one or both feet are folded under the buttocks. One folded foot coming out is a single footling breech, both feet a double footling breech. **Frank breech** means the buttocks of the baby are at the mother's pelvic opening. The legs are straight up in front of the body, and the feet are at the shoulders. Babies born in this position tend to hold their feet near their heads for some days after birth.

breech extraction, a birth method in which a baby being born feet or buttocks first is grabbed before any part of the trunk is born and delivered by guiding and pulling. With **assisted breech,** the baby is permitted to be born spontaneously as far as its navel. The infant is then helped the rest of the way by the physician or midwife.

bregma /breg′mə/, the joining of the frontal and roof (parietal) bones on the top of the skull. –**bregmatic,** *adj.*

Brenner tumor, a noncancerous tumor of the ovary that is made up of skin (epithelial) cells covered by fiberlike connective tissue.

Brethine, a trademark for a bronchodilator drug used to treat asthma, bronchitis, and emphysema (terbutaline sulfate).

bretylium tosylate, a drug used to treat life-threatening irregular heart beats (ventricular arrhythmias). Known allergy to this drug prohibits its use. Side effects include low blood pressure, nausea and vomiting, chest pain (angina), and nasal stuffiness.

Bretylol, a trademark for a drug used to treat severe heart beat irregularities (bretylium tosylate).

Brevital Sodium, a trademark for a barbiturate used for anesthesia (methohexital sodium).

brewer's yeast, a preparation containing the dried cells of a yeast, used as a diet additive. It is one of the best sources of the B complex vitamins and of many minerals and amino acids.

Bricanyl, a trademark for a bronchodilator drug used to treat asthma, bronchitis, and emphysema (terbutaline sulfate).

bridging, positioning a patient so that bony areas of the body are free of pressure on the mattress by using pads, bolsters, or pillows.

brim, the edge of the upper pact on the inside of the pelvis (pelvic inlet). See also **pelvis.**

Brissaud's dwarf /brisōz′/, a person affected with a severe form of underactive thyroid (myxedema) in infancy that results in short height.

British Medical Association (BMA), a professional organization of physicians in the United Kingdom.

brittle bones. See **osteogenesis imperfecta.**

broad beta disease, a hereditary disorder (a type of hyperlipoproteinemia) in which a fatty substance, lipoprotein, gathers in the blood. The condition features yellowish lumps (xanthomas) on the elbows and knees, disease of the blood vessels, and high blood cholesterol levels. Patients with this disease are at risk of having early heart disease. See also **hyperlipoproteinemia.**

broad ligament, a folded sheet of membrane in the abdomen (peritoneum) that is draped over the uterine tubes, the uterus, and the ovaries.

Broca's area /brō′kəz/, the part of the brain that is involved in speech making. It is located on the front part of the brain.

Brodie's abscess, a type of bone infection (osteomyelitis) caused by a staphylococcal infection. It usually occurs near a joint in the growth zone (metaphysis) of a long bone of a child. See also **osteomyelitis.**

Brodmann's areas, the many local areas of the brain. They are linked to specific brain functions. Compare **motor area.** See also **brain.**

bromhidrosis /brō′midrō′sis/, an abnormal condition in which the sweat has an unpleasant odor. The odor is usually caused by the breakdown of sweat by bacteria on the skin.

bromide /brō′mīd/, a compound of bromine, a toxic, red-brown, liquid element. Once widely used as sleeping pills, bromides are now seldom used for that purpose because they may cause serious side effects. Long-term use of these products may cause a toxic condition (brominism) with symptoms of an acnelike skin disorder, headache, loss of sexual interest, drowsiness, and weakness.

bromocriptine, a drug used to treat female infertility, Parkinson's disease, and the making of too much of the hormone prolactin. Allergy to any ergot alkaloid prohibits its use. Side effects include irregular heart rate, low blood pressure, slow heart beat, hallucinations, fainting, nausea, difficulty walking, shortness of breath, swallowing difficulty, weakness, and confusion.

brompheniramine, an antihistamine used to treat many allergic reactions, including nasal congestion, skin reactions, and itching.

bronchial hyperreactivity /brong′kē·əl/, an abnormal breathing condition with spasms of the bronchus. It is a reflex response to histamine or a cholinergic drug. This is a feature of asthma and is used to tell the difference between asthma and heart disease.

bronchial tree, a complex of the bronchi and the bronchial tubes. The bronchi branch from the windpipe (trachea), and the bronchial tubes branch from the bronchi. The right bronchus is wider and shorter than the left bronchus. The right bronchus branches into three bronchi, one passing to each of the lobes that make up the right lung. The left bronchus is smaller in diameter but about twice as long as the right bronchus and branches into the bronchi for the upper and the lower lobes of the left lung.

bronchiectasis /brong′kē·ek′təsis/, an abnormal condition of the bronchial tree. There is irreversible widening and destruction of the bronchial walls. It usually results from bronchial infection or blockage by a tumor or a foreign body, but sometimes is a birth defect. Symptoms include a constant cough with excess, blood-stained sputum, a long-term sinus infection, clubbing of the fingers, and continual moist-sounding breathing.

bronchiole /brong′kē·ōl/, a small airway of the breathing system from the bronchi to the lobes of the lung. The bronchioles allow the exchange of air and waste gases between the alveolar ducts and the bronchi. —**bronchiolar,** *adj.*

bronchiolitis, a viral infection of the lower breathing tract that occurs mainly in infants under 18 months of age. The condition typically begins with watery nasal discharge and, often, mild fever. Rapid breathing and a fast heart rate, cough, wheezing, and fever develop. The chest may appear barrel-shaped, and breathing becomes more shallow. Treatment includes humidity and oxygen in a mist tent, vaporizer, or Croupette; giving fluids, usually through a vein; suctioning the airways to remove fluids; and rest. An airway tube is sometimes inserted. The infection typically runs its course in 7 to 10 days, with good recovery. A major problem is bacterial infection, most commonly following long-term use of a mist tent.

bronchitis /brong·kī′tis/, inflammation of the mucous membranes of the air passages (bronchi) beyond the windpipe that lead to the lungs. **Acute bronchitis** features a cough that releases sputum, fever, mucus-secreting structures growing larger, and back pain. Caused by the spread of viral infections to the bronchi, it often occurs with childhood infections, as measles, whooping cough, diphtheria, and typhoid fever. Treatment includes bed rest, aspirin, cough drugs, and antibiotics. With **chronic bronchitis** there is an excess release of mucus in the bronchi with a cough that releases sputum for at least 3 months in at least 2 years. The disease is noted for frequent pus-forming infections of the lungs. Difficult breathing results from narrow airways and often brings lung failure. Sharp attacks of breathing distress with blue skin from lack of oxygen can result. Patients who suffer from these symptoms are called ''blue bloaters.'' A risk to develop a heart disease (cor pulmonale) or heart failure is a common result. Factors that may cause chronic bronchitis include cigarette smoking, air pollution, long-term infections, and abnormal growth of the bronchi. Treatment includes antibiotics during the acute attack of symptoms, and drugs that open the airways (bronchodilators). Heart failure is managed by restricting salt in the diet, diuretics, and sometimes digitalis. Patients with chronic bronchitis should be vaccinated against influenza and lung infections.

bronchodilator /-dī′lātər/,   a drug that relaxes contractions of the bronchioles to improve breathing. Bronchodilators are given for asthma, bronchiectasis, bronchitis, and emphysema. Commonly used bronchodilators include steroids, ephedrine, isoproterenol hydrochloride, theophylline, and many related combinations of these drugs. The steroids beclomethasone dipropionate and triamcinolone can be used in aerosol form.

bronchogenic carcinoma /-jen′ik/,   a common form of lung cancer that starts in the bronchi. Usually linked to cigarette smoking, it may cause coughing and wheezing, weakness, chest tightness, and aching joints. In the late stages, symptoms are bloody sputum, clubbing of the fingers, weight loss, and fluid around the lungs. Diagnosis is made by a wide range of tests. Surgery is the most effective treatment, but about 50% of cases are too advanced and not helped by surgery when first seen. Other treatment includes x-ray therapy and chemotherapy.

bronchography /brongkog′rəfē/,   an x-ray examination of the bronchi after they have been coated with a radiopaque substance.

bronchopneumonia,   an inflammation of the lungs and bronchioles. Symptoms include chills, fever, fast pulse and breathing, cough with bloody sputum, severe chest pain, and bloated stomach. The disease usually results from the spread of bacterial infection from the upper breathing tract to the lower breathing tract. Bronchopneumonia may also occur in viral and rickettsial infections. The most common cause in infants is a respiratory virus. Treatment includes an antibiotic, oxygen therapy, measures to keep the bronchi clear of fluids, and pain relievers. See also **pneumonia.**

bronchopulmonary /-pul′məner′ē/,   referring to the bronchi and the lungs.

bronchoscopy /brongkos′kəpē/,   an examination of the bronchial tree. A narrow, flexible tube (bronchoscope) is used. It contains fibers that carry light down the tube and project a large image up the tube to the viewer. Bronchoscopy is done after the patient fasts and is given a relaxing drug and a local anesthesia. The purpose can be to suction, to get a tissue or fluid sample for examination, to remove foreign bodies, and to diagnose diseases.

bronchospasm /brong′kōspazm′/,   an abnormal contraction of the bronchi, resulting in narrowing and blockage of the airway. A cough with wheezing is the usual symptom. Bronchospasm is the main feature of asthma and bronchitis.

bronchus /brong′kəs/, *pl.* **bronchi,**   any one of several large air passages in the lungs through which breathed in air and breathed out waste gases pass. Each bronchus has a wall made up of three layers. The outer layer is made of dense fiber strengthened with cartilage. The middle layer is a grouping of smooth muscle. The inner layer is made up of mucous membrane with hairlike structures (cilia). **Primary bronchus** refers to one of the two main air passages that branch from the wind pipe (trachea) and take air to the lungs. A hook-shaped ridge (carina) at the bottom of the trachea separates the two primary bronchi. It is located to the left of the middle line so that the right primary bronchus is a more direct continuation of the trachea than the left. As a result, foreign objects that come into the trachea usually drop into the right bronchus rather than the left.

Bronkephrine,   a trademark for a bronchodilator drug injected into the muscle. It is used to treat asthma, emphysema, and bronchitis (ethylnorepinephrine hydrochloride).

Bronkodyl,   a trademark for a bronchodilator drug used to treat asthma, bronchitis, and emphysema (theophylline).

Bronkosol,   a trademark for a bronchodilator drug used to treat asthma, bronchitis, and emphysema (isoetharine hydrochloride).

brown fat,   a type of fat in newborn infants that is rarely found in adults. Brown fat is a unique source of heat energy for the infant because it makes more heat than ordinary fat.

Brown-Séquard syndrome /-sākär′/,   a serious nerve disorder resulting from pressure of one side of the spinal cord at about the level of the bottom of the shoulder blades. The disorder includes spastic paralysis on the injured side of the body, loss of a sense of posture, and loss of the senses of pain and heat on the other side of the body.

brown spider,   a poisonous spider, also known as the brown recluse or violin spider, found in both North and South America. The poison from its bite usually creates a blister surrounded by white and red circles. This so-called ''bull's eye'' appearance is helpful in telling it apart from other spider bites. The wound usually turns into an open sore and can become infected. Pain, nausea, fever, and chills are common, but the reaction usually goes away by itself. Steroids are sometimes given, and cleaning and applying antibiotics to the area will prevent infection. Although painful, the bite is not always a danger to adults. However, small children should get medical attention to avoid possible serious reactions.

brucellosis /broo̅′səlō′sis/,   a disease caused by any of several species of *Brucella* bacteria. Mainly a disease of livestock, humans usually get it by drinking infected milk or milk products or through a break in the skin. The symptoms are fever, chills, sweating, and weakness. The fever often comes in waves, rising in the evening and lowering during the day, occurring at times separated by periods of no symptoms. Although brucellosis itself is rarely fatal, treatment is important because serious problems, as pneumonia, meningitis, and encephalitis, can develop. **Abor-**

tus fever is a form of brucellosis with similar routes of infection and of symptoms.

Brudzinski's sign /broŏodzin′skēz/, an involuntary flexing of the arm, hip, and knee when the neck is passively flexed. This is seen in patients with meningitis.

bruise, darkening of an area of the skin or mucous membrane caused by blood leaking into the tissues under the skin. Also called **ecchymosis,** it occurs as a result of damage to the blood vessels or by brittle vessel walls. A **contusion** is a bruising injury that does not break the skin. It is caused by a blow and features swelling and pain. Treatment is applying cold.

bruit /broo′ē/, an abnormal sound heard by the physician while listening to an organ or gland, as the liver or thyroid. The specific character of the bruit, where it is, and when it occurs in a cycle of other sounds are all important in diagnosis.

Brushfield's spots, pinpoint, white or light yellow spots on the iris of a child with Down's syndrome. Occasionally, they are seen in normal infants, but their lack may help to rule out Down's syndrome.

bruxism /bruk′sizm/, the continuous, unconscious grinding of the teeth. This occurs especially during sleep, or during waking hours to release tension in periods of high stress.

bubble oxygenator, a heart-lung device that puts oxygen in the blood while it is outside the patient's body.

bubo /byoo′bō/, pl. **buboes,** a very swollen lymph node usually in the armpit or groin. Buboes are linked to diseases such as chancroid, bubonic plague, and syphilis. Treatment includes antibiotics, using moist heat, and sometimes opening and drainage.

bubonic plague /byoobon′ik/. See **plague.**

buccal /buk′əl/, referring to the inside of the cheek, or the gum or side of a tooth next to the cheek.

buccal flange, the part of a denture that fits next to the cheek in the mouth.

buccinator /buk′sinā′tər/, the main muscle of the cheek, one of the 12 muscles of the mouth. It puts pressure on the cheek, acting as an important muscle of chewing by holding food under the teeth.

buccopharyngeal /buk′ōfərin′jē·əl/, referring to the cheek and the throat (pharynx) or to the mouth and the pharynx.

bucket-handle tear, a tear in the knee cartilage (meniscus) that occurs lengthwise. It is a common injury in athletes and active young people. The usual cause is twisting the knee. Symptoms are pain when squatting or twisting, some swelling, and tenderness. Often the knee pops or it may lock suddenly. These tears may heal over time if the knee is supported and protected, but sometimes surgery is needed.

bucking, informal. **1.** gagging on an airway tube. **2.** unconsciously fighting back the air pushed into the lungs by a respirator.

Budd-Chiari syndrome /-kē·är′ē/, a disorder of liver circulation. Blockage of the veins leads to a swollen liver, fluid filling the abdomen (ascites), and excess growth of more blood vessels. There is severe high blood pressure within the liver vessels.

Buerger's disease, a condition in which the veins close, usually in a leg or a foot. The small and medium-sized arteries are inflamed and clotted. Early signs of the condition are burning, numbness, and tingling of the foot or leg. Dead tissue (gangrene) may develop as the disease progresses. Pulsation in the limb below the damaged blood vessels is often absent. The goal of therapy is to avoid all factors that lessen the blood supply to the extremity, as cigarette smoking, and to use all means possible to increase the supply. Also called **thromboangiitis obliterans.**

buffer, a substance or group of substances that controls the hydrogen levels in a solution. Buffer systems in the body keep the acid-base balance (pH) of the blood and the proper pH in kidney tubules. **Blood buffers** are made mostly of dissolved carbon dioxide and bicarbonate.

bulbar paralysis /bul′bər/, a wasting nerve condition with continually worsening paralysis of the lips, tongue, mouth, throat, and vocal cords.

bulimia /byoolē′mē·ə/, an unsatisfied desire for food, often resulting in periods of continuous eating. This is followed by periods of depression and self-denial, and, in some cases, forced vomiting. –**bulemic,** n., adj.

bulk. See **dietary fiber.**

bulk packaging, bulk packaging has an internal volume greater than 119 gallons (450 L) for liquids, a capacity greater than 882 pounds (400 kg) for solids, or a water capacity greater than 1000 pounds (453.6 kg) for gases. They can be an integral part of a transport vehicle (e.g., tank cars and barges), packaging placed on or in a transport vehicle (e.g., portable tanks, intermodal portable tanks, ton containers), or fixed or processing containers.

bulla /bul′ə/, pl. **bullae,** a thin-walled blister of the skin or mucous membranes containing clear fluid. Compare **vesicle.** –**bullous,** adj.

bullous myringitis /bul′əs/, a condition of inflammation in the ear with fluid-filled sores on the eardrum (tympanic membrane) and severe pain. The condition often occurs with bacterial ear infection (otitis media). Treatment includes antibiotics, pain relievers, and surgical draining of the sores. See also **otitis media.**

bumetanide, a diuretic used to treat excess fluid pooling caused by heart, liver, or kidney disease. Kidney shutdown, electrolyte loss, or known allergy to this drug prohibits its use. Side effects include loss of potassium in the blood, and excess uric acid in the blood.

Bumex, a trademark for a diuretic drug used to treat congestive heart failure and in liver and kidney disease (bumetanide).

Buminate, a trademark for a drug that expands the blood volume (human albumin).

BUN, abbreviation for **blood urea nitrogen.**

bundle branch block. See **heart block.**

bundle of His /his/, a band of fibers in the heart through which the electric signal is carried from the atrioventricular node to the lower chambers (ventricles). Also called **atrioventricular bundle, His bundle.**

bunion /bun'yən/, an abnormal swelling of the joint at the base of the big toe. It is caused by inflammation of the bursa, usually as a result of long-term irritation and pressure from poorly fitted shoes.

bupivacaine hydrochloride /byo͞opiv'əkān/, a local anesthetic used in various nerve blocks. Known allergy to this or similar drugs prohibits its use. Side effects include central nervous system disturbances, low blood pressure, breathing difficulties, heart attack, and allergic reactions.

burn, any injury caused by heat, electricity, chemicals, radiation, or gases. Burns are rated according to how many layers of skin are damaged. Partial-thickness burns may be first or second degree. First degree burns involve only the top skin layer (epidermis). Second degree burns involve the epidermis and second layer of skin (corium), whereas full-thickness or third degree burns involve all skin layers. Second degree burns covering more than 30% of the body and third degree burns on the face and arms and legs, or more than 10% of the body surface, are critical. In the first 48 hours of a severe burn, fluid from the vessels, salt (sodium chloride), and protein pass into the burned area causing swelling, blisters, low blood pressure, and very low urine output. This is followed by a shift of fluid in the opposite direction resulting in excess urine, high blood volume, and low blood electrolytes. Other problems in serious burns include collapse of the circulation, kidney damage, shutdown of the stomach and bowel system, infections, pneumonia, and shock.

A **chemical burn** refers to tissue damage caused by exposure to a strong acid or alkali. The damage to the body caused by an **acid burn** depends on the kind of acid and the length of time and amount of tissue exposed. Emergency treatment includes washing the area with large amounts of water. With an **alkali burn,** tissue damage is caused by an alkaline compound, as lye. Treatment includes flushing with water to wash off the chemical. Then vinegar or another mildly acidic substance mixed with water is put on the burn to make neutral any alkali that is left and to lessen the pain. The patient should be taken to a hospital if the damage is severe. Breathing a hot gas or burning particles, as may occur in a fire or explosion, causes a **respiratory burn,** with tissue damage in the breathing system. The person often must have oxygen treatment and go to the hospital at once. Exposure to extreme heat will cause a **thermal burn,** which is usually tissue injury of the skin.

The treatment of burns includes pain relief, stopping infection, keeping fluids and electrolytes balanced, and good diet. Often a urinary tube (catheter) and a tube through the nose to the stomach are inserted. Treatment of the burn may be by either a closed or open method. In the open method the injured area is cleaned and exposed to air. In the closed method, a cream, ointment, or solution is placed on the burn, and the wound is covered with a dressing. A temporary skin graft may be used to prevent loss of fluid and reduce the risk of infection. Newly developed artificial skin holds great promise for treating severe burns. If fluids by mouth are allowed, juices and carbonated drinks are given. Fluid intake and output are measured hourly. Blood transfusions, steroid therapy, and drugs to reduce fever may be ordered, but aspirin is not given. Excess chilling and exposure to upper lung infections and wound infections are carefully avoided. Burned arms and legs are raised, and cramps are prevented by using firm supports to keep affected areas in line. The patient may grasp a ball when the back of the hand is burned. After the first important period, a high-calorie, high-protein, high-potassium diet is given in many small meals. Vitamins may be needed. Recovery may take a long time. A large amount of plastic surgery and repeated skin grafts may be needed to restore function and the physical appearance of burn patients.

burn center, a health care center that is set up to care for patients who have been badly burned.

burnout, a popular term for a loss of mental or physical energy following a period of long-term, continuous job-related stress. There may also be physical illness.

Burow's solution, a liquid that contains aluminum sulfate, acetic acid, solid calcium carbonate, and water. It is used as a skin cream and antiseptic for many skin disorders. Also called **aluminum acetate solution.**

bursa /bur'sə/, *pl.* **bursae,** one of the many closed sacs in the connecting tissue between the muscles, tendons, ligaments, and bones. Lined with a membrane that releases fluid (synovial), the bursa acts as a small cushion. This makes the gliding of muscles and tendons over bones easier. An example is the **bursa of Achilles** that separates the tendon of Achilles and the heel.

bursitis /bərsī'tis/, an inflammation of the bursa, the connective tissue structure surrounding a joint. Bursitis may

65

be caused by arthritis, infection, injury, or excess activity. The main symptom is severe pain in the joint, particularly on movement. Treatment for the pain is usually an injection of a steroid into the bursa. Other treatments are pain relievers, antiinflammatory drugs, cold packs, and keeping the area rigid.

bursting fracture, any broken bone that scatters bone fragments, usually at or near the end of a bone.

busulfan, a drug used to treat long-term myelocytic leukemia. Radiation, low white cells or platelets in the blood, anticancer drugs, or known allergy to this drug prohibits its use. Side effects include lung problems, blood abnormalities, and severe nausea and diarrhea. It often causes menstrual periods to stop.

butabarbital sodium, a sleeping pill used to relieve anxiety, nervous tension, and lack of sleep (insomnia). Porphyrin disturbances, seizure disorders, or known allergy to this drug prohibits its use. Side effects include liver disease (jaundice), skin rash, and excitement.

Butazolidin, a trademark for a drug used to treat gout, rheumatoid arthritis, osteoarthritis, and bursitis (phenylbutazone).

Butesin Picrate, a trademark for an anesthetic ointment for burns (butamben picrate).

Butisol Sodium, a trademark for a drug used to cause sleep (butabarbital sodium).

butorphanol tartrate, a narcotic given before and during surgery. It is used for moderate to severe pain after surgery. Overdose may result when butorphanol is used with other narcotic drugs.

butterfly bandage, a narrow adhesive strip with winglike ends used to close and hold the edges of a surface wound. It is used instead of stitches in certain cases.

butterfly fracture, a bone break in which two cracks form a triangle.

butterfly rash, a scaling rash of both cheeks joined by a narrow band of rash across the nose. It is seen in lupus erythematosus, rosacea, and seborrheic dermatitis.

buttocks, the large fleshy knobs at the lower back of the body made up of fat and the gluteal muscles. Also called **nates.**

buttonhole fracture, any broken bone caused by a bullet.

butyl alcohol /byoo′til/, a clear, poisonous liquid used as a solvent. Also called **butanol.**

butyr-, a combining form referring to butter.

bypass, any one of many types of surgery to move the flow of blood or other fluids from their normal courses. A bypass may be either temporary or permanent. Bypass surgery is often done to treat heart, stomach, and bowel disorders. An example is a **cardiopulmonary bypass.** This is a technique used in heart surgery in which blood is sent through plastic tubes from the heart and lungs. A pump adds oxygen to the blood and returns it to the patient's blood system. An **internal mammary artery bypass** refers to surgery to clear a coronary artery blockage. A **partial bypass** is a system in which a person's heart keeps a part of the blood flow while the rest of the flow depends on a pump. See also **coronary bypass.**

byssinosis /bis′inō′sis/, a job-related lung disease that is an allergic reaction to dust or fungus in cotton, flax, and hemp fibers. Symptoms are shortness of breath, cough, and wheezing. The disease is curable in the early stages. Exposure for several years results in long-term airway blockage, bronchitis, and emphysema, leading to lung failure.

C

C, 1. symbol for **carbon.** 2. abbreviation for **Celsius.**

Ca, symbol for **calcium.**

cabinet bath, a heated bath in which the patient is placed in a cabinet from the neck down. Also called **box bath.**

Cabot's splint, a metal support splint worn behind the thigh and leg.

cachet /käshā′/, any wafer-shaped, flat capsule that holds a dose of a bitter tasting drug. It is swallowed whole.

cachexia /kəkek′sē·ə/, general ill health and faulty diet. It is usually linked to a wasting disease, as tuberculosis or cancer.

cachinnation /kak′ənā′shən/, excess laughter for no reason, often part of the behavior in schizophrenia.

cacodemonomania /kak′ədē′mənō-/, a confused state in which a person claims to be possessed by the devil or an evil spirit.

cadaver, a dead body used for study.

cadmium (Cd), a bluish-white metal element. Once used in drugs, cadmium has since been replaced by less poisonous drugs. It is used in engraving, printing, and photography. Breathing the fumes during metal-plating processes can cause poisoning. A lung disease (**cadmiosis**) is caused by breathing in cadmium dust. Acid foods (as tomatoes and lemonade) that are prepared and stored in cadmium-lined containers can also cause poisoning.

cadmium poisoning, the effects of swallowing cadmium, eating foods stored in cadmium cans, or breathing cadmium fumes from welding, smelting, or other industrial processes. Symptoms from breathing fumes include vomiting, difficulty in breathing, headache, and exhaustion. Cadmium causes severe stomach and bowel symptoms 30 minutes to 3 hours after swallowing. Treatment for poisoning includes fluids through the veins, special drugs, and oxygen.

caduceus /kədoo′sē·əs/, the wand of the god Hermes or Mercury, shown as a staff with two serpents coiled around it. The caduceus is a medical symbol and the official symbol of the U.S. Army Medical Corps.

café-au-lait spot /kaf′ā·ōlā′/, a pale tan patch of skin. It occurs in a type of bone disease (Albright's syndrome), but these spots can also occur normally. Many café-au-lait spots may develop with a tumorlike growth all over the body (neurofibromatosis).

cafe coronary, a popular term for choking on a piece of food that gets stuck in the windpipe. Because the patient is suddenly unable to talk or breathe and collapses while eating, it is often mistaken for a heart attack. Death or brain damage can result within a few minutes if emergency treatment is not given immediately to remove the food blockage. The Heimlich maneuver is a simple and effective treatment if the person hasn't collapsed. See also **cardiopulmonary resuscitation, Heimlich maneuver.**

Cafergot, a trademark for a drug that contains caffeine and ergotamine. It is used to treat migraine headaches.

caffeine /kafēn′, kaf′ē·in/, a substance found in coffee, tea, cola, and other plant products. It is used as a stimulant and given to treat migraine headaches. Patients with heart disease and peptic ulcer must use it with caution. Known allergy prohibits its use. Side effects include rapid heart beat, excess urination, stomach and bowel distress, restlessness, and lack of sleep.

caffeinism, a poisoning condition caused by the long-term use of excess amounts of caffeine in beverages or other products. Symptoms include restlessness, anxiety, general depression, rapid heart beat, tremors, nausea, high urine output, and lack of sleep. A fatal dose is estimated to be 10 g (equal to 100 cups of coffee) for a healthy adult. See also **xanthine derivative.**

cal., abbreviation for **small calorie** (or **gram calorie**). See also **calorie.**

Cal., abbreviation for **large calorie** (or **kilocalorie, kilogram calorie**). See also **calorie.**

Caladryl, a trademark for a lotion that contains a protectant (calamine) and an antihistamine (diphenhydramine hydrochloride). It is used to relieve minor skin irritations and itching.

calamine /kal′əmīn/, a pink powder containing zinc oxide and a small amount of ferric oxide. It is used to protect and dry the skin.

Calan, a trademark for a drug (verapamil) used to treat chest pain (angina pectoris).

calcaneal spur /kal′kā′nē·əl/, a painful, bony growth on the lower surface of the heel bone (calcaneus). The spur is usually caused by long-term pressure on the heel.

calcaneus /kal′kā′nē·əs/, the heel bone. The largest of several bones that forms the ankle.

calcar /kal′kär/, *pl.* **calcaria,** a spur or spurlike structure that occurs normally on many bones of the human skeleton.

calcemia, an excess level of calcium in the blood.

calcifediol /kal′səfē′dē·ôl/, a form of Vitamin D used to treat bone disease and lack of blood calcium caused by long-term kidney failure. Calcifediol should not be given to patients with excess blood calcium, vitamin D overdose, or known allergy to this drug. Side effects include kidney poisoning, soft tissue hardening, stomach and bowel problems, brain disturbances, or excess blood levels of calcium.

calciferol /kalsif′ərôl/, a crystal-like form of vitamin D_2. It occurs naturally in milk and fish liver oils. It is used in the diet to prevent and treat rickets, osteomalacia, and other disorders with low blood calcium. Also called **ergocalciferol.**

calcific aortic disease, abnormal deposits of calcium in the large artery of the heart (aorta).

calcification, the gathering of calcium deposits in body tissues. Normally, about 99% of all the calcium in the human body is deposited in the bones and teeth. The remaining 1% is dissolved in body fluids, as the blood. Disorders that cause deposits in arteries, kidneys, lungs, and other soft tissues usually are related to parathyroid hormone activity and vitamin D levels.

Calcimar, a trademark for a thyroid hormone used to treat Paget's disease of bone and excess blood calcium (calcitonin).

calcinosis /kal′sənō′-/, an abnormal condition with deposits of calcium in the skin and muscles. The disease usually occurs in children.

calcitonin /-tō′nin/, a hormone made in the thyroid gland. It controls the levels of calcium and phosphorus in the blood and acts to prevent the loss of calcium from the bones.

calcitriol /kalsit′rē·ôl/, a hormone related to vitamin D_3, made in the kidney. It increases the absorption of calcium and phosphorus in the bowels. It is used to prevent calcium loss in patients undergoing kidney dialysis. Calcitriol should not be given to patients with high blood levels of calcium, vitamin D poisoning, or an allergy to the drug. Side effects include kidney poisoning, soft tissue hardening, and stomach, bowel, and nervous system problems.

calcium (Ca), an alkaline earth metal element. It is the most common mineral and the fifth most common element in the human body, found mainly in the bones and teeth.

The body needs calcium to carry nerve signals, to contract muscles, to clot blood, to help heart functions, and to work with enzymes. Calcium is absorbed mainly by the small intestine. The adult human body contains about 2.5 pounds of calcium. Only about one third of the calcium taken in by humans is absorbed. The **calcium balance** is the relation between the amount of calcium absorbed by the body and the amount lost each day in urine, feces, and sweat. Excess calcium in the body can cause stones (calculi) in the kidney. Too little calcium can cause rickets in children and fragile bones (osteoporosis), especially in older women.

calcium channel blocker, a drug that prevents calcium from entering smooth muscle cells. This causes the smooth muscles to relax and reduces muscle spasms. Calcium channel blockers are used mainly to treat heart diseases with spasms in the artery of the heart (angina pectoris). Also called **calcium antagonist, calcium blocker.**

calcium carbonate, a white chalklike powder that occurs naturally in bones and shells. It is used in certain antacids. Calcium carbonate antacids are effective for short-term relief but are not suggested for constant use. They can cause excess alkali buildup (alkalosis) or kidney damage.

calcium chloride, a white crystal-like powder or granules usually made into a solution. It is used to replace calcium in the blood, to control the acid-base balance, and to treat muscle spasms from lack of calcium (hypocalcemic tetany). Kidney problems, irregular heart beat, excess calcium in the body, or known allergy to this drug prohibits its use. Side effects include excess calcium blood levels, nausea, vomiting, widening of the blood vessels, and heart disorders.

calcium lactate, a calcium replacer used to treat a lack of calcium, particularly in cases of muscle spasm (tetany) resulting in difficult breathing. It is given by mouth.

calcium EDTA, calcium disodium edetate, used to treat metal poisoning.

calcium gluconate, a calcium salt used to treat a lack of calcium and as an antidote for fluoride or oxalic acid poisoning. It may be given in the vein or by mouth.

calcium-phosphorus ratio, the proportion of calcium to phosphorus suggested for the daily diet to keep a desired calcium balance.

calcium pyrophosphate dihydrate disease (CPPD), a disorder with calcium deposits in the joints. The symptoms look like arthritis or gout.

calculus /kal′kyələs/, *pl.* **calculi,** an abnormal stone formed in tissues when mineral salts clump together. Calculi may form anywhere in the body. The most common places are the kidneys, the gallbladder, and the joints.

Calderol, a trademark for a drug used to treat bone disease and lack of blood calcium (calcifediol).

calefacient /kal′əfā′shənt/, **1.** making or tending to make anything warm or hot. **2.** an agent that gives off a sense of warmth when used, as a hot-water bottle or a hot compress.

calf, *pl.* **calves,** the fleshy mass at the back of the leg below the knee. It is made up mainly of the gastrocnemius and soleus muscles.

calf bone. See **fibula.**

calibration, determining accuracy of a measuring instrument and ascertaining necessary correction factors.

caligo /kəlī′gō/, dim sight, usually caused by cataracts, a cloudy cornea, or failure of the pupil to widen properly.

calipers, an instrument with two hinged jaws used to measure the thickness or diameter of an object. In obstetrics calipers are used to measure a woman's pelvis.

calisthenics /kal′isthen′-/, exercising the many muscles of the body according to certain routines. They may be done with or without equipment, as dumbbells. The goal of calisthenics is to keep physical health while increasing muscle strength.

callus, **1.** a common, usually painless thickening of the skin at locations of pressure or friction. **2.** a bony deposit formed around the broken ends of a broken bone during healing. The bone callus is replaced by normal hard bone as the bone heals.

calomel /kal′əmel/, a white odorless powder that darkens when exposed to light. It is sometimes used in ointments or dusting powders. Because it irritates the bowel, calomel was once used as a laxative.

calor /kā′lər/, heat in the body. Examples are heat caused by inflammation or from the normal processes of the body.

caloric /kəlôr′ik/, referring to heat or calories.

caloric balance, the proportion of the number of calories taken in food and beverages to the number of calories used during work and exercise.

caloric test, a test used to see if the inner ear is diseased or normal. The test involves flushing the ear with warm and cool water. Also called **Barany's test.**

calorie, **1.** also called **gram calorie, small calorie (cal.).** The amount of heat needed to raise 1 g of water 1°C at 1 atmosphere pressure. **2.** also called **great calorie, kilocalorie, kilogram calorie, large calorie (Cal.).** A quantity of heat needed to raise the temperature of 1 kg of water 1°C at 1 air pressure. The kilocalorie unit is used by food experts when referring to the fuel or energy value of many foods. **–caloric,** *adj.*

calorimetry /kal′ərim′ətrē/, the method of measuring heat loss or energy loss. Human body heat can be measured by putting the person in a tank of water and noting the temperature change in the water. This change is caused by the body heat. Human calorie use can also be measured in terms of the amount of oxygen breathed in and the amount of carbon dioxide breathed out during a given time.

calusterone /kəloo′stərōn/, a male sex hormone that slows or prevents the growth of cancer cells. It is used to treat breast cancer in women. Heart and kidney disease, high blood levels of calcium, or known allergy to the drug prohibits its use. It is not given to pregnant or nursing women. Side effects include excess fluid and excess blood calcium levels, enlargement of the clitoris, increased body hair growth, acne, hair loss, and changes in red blood cells.

Calvé-Perthes disease. See **Perthes' disease.**

calyx /kā′liks/, a cup-shaped structure of the body. An example is the kidney (renal) calyx which collects urine and directs it into a tube (ureter) that carries the urine to the bladder.

camp, a geographical site, within the general incident area, separate from the base, equipped and staffed to provide food, water, and sanitary services to incident personnel.

camphor, a clear or white crystal-like substance with a strong odor and taste. It is used as a mild irritant and antiseptic in lotions and soaps.

camptodactyly /kamp′tədak′tilē/, an abnormal condition in which one or more fingers become permanently bent.

camptomelia /-mē′lyə/, an inherited defect in which one or more limbs are bent. This causes a permanent curve of the arm or leg.

canal, **1.** any narrow tube or channel through an organ or between structures. An example is the **adductor canal,** a channel for vessels and nerves in the thigh muscle. The **canal of Schlemm** is a tiny vein at the corner of the eye that drains the water in the eye (aqueous humor) and funnels it into the bloodstream. A blockage of the canal can result in glaucoma. **2.** (in dentistry) the root and tissue canals in the teeth.

cancellous /kan′sələs/, referring to the spongy, inner part of many bones, mainly bones that have marrow.

cancer (CA), a general term for a malignant tumor or for forms of new tissue cells that lack a controlled growth pattern. Cancer cells usually invade and destroy normal tissue cells. A cancer tends to spread to other parts of the body by releasing cells into the lymph or bloodstream. In this way cancer cells can be carried to a place in the body that may be far from the first tumor. The first site of cancer is sometimes called a primary cancer. The tumor which grows as a result of the cancer spreading is called a secondary cancer. A secondary cancer often is noticed before the primary cancer can be found. There are more than 150 different kinds of cancer and many different causes, including viruses, too much exposure to sunlight or x-rays, cigarette smoking, and chemicals in the environment. The most common sites for the growth of cancers are the lung, breast, colon, uterus, mouth, and bone marrow. Many cancers are curable if found in the early stage. Warning signs for cancer may be a change in bowel or bladder habits, a nonhealing sore, unusual bleeding or discharge, a thickening or lump in the breast or elsewhere, indigestion or difficulty in swallowing, an obvious change in a wart or mole, or a nagging cough or continuing hoarseness. Treatments include surgery, radiation treatment, and chemotherapy.

cancericidal /-isī′dəl/, referring to a drug or treatment that destroys cancer cells.

cancer of the small intestine, a cancer of the upper, middle, or lower portion (duodenum, jejunum, or ileum) of the small intestine. The type of tumor may differ from site to site. Adenocarcinomas are found in the upper or middle portion. They form lumplike, ''napkin ring'' growths. Lymphomas are found in the lower portion. They can harm bowel function by attacking the nerves and prevent the small intestine from taking in nutrients. Less common tumors of the small intestine are carcinoids and sarcomas. Cancer of the small intestine occurs more often in men than in women.

cancer staging, a way to describe a cancer, its extent, and how far it has spread, in order to plan treatment and predict outcome.

cancer tests, certain tests always done by doctors to find early signs of cancer. They include:

1. Guaiac test for bowel cancer, which uses a stool sample from the patient. The sample is looked at for traces of blood.

2. Rectal exam, done by a doctor with a gloved finger to detect tumors in men or women and prostate cancers in men.

3. Sigmoidoscopy exam of the bowels with a lighted instrument.

4. Pelvic exam for women, done by a doctor using a gloved finger to check the female reproductive organs.

5. Pap test, done at the same time as the pelvic exam, in which cells are scraped from the surface of the cervix and looked at under a microscope.

6. Breast exam for women, for changes such as a lump or thickening of tissue. A breast exam may include an x-ray film of the breast (mammography) to find tumors before they can be felt.

cancriform /kang′krifôrm/, referring to a tumor that looks like a cancer.

cancroid, 1. resembling a cancer. 2. a mild skin cancer.

cancrum oris, a cankerlike sore of the mouth. It can begin as a small sore of the gum and spread to the mouth and face.

Candida albicans /kan′didə al′bəkanz/, a tiny, common, yeastlike fungus normally found in the mouth, digestive tract, vagina, and on the skin of healthy persons. In some situations, it may cause long-term infections of the skin, nails, scalp, mucous membranes, genitals, or internal organs. See also **candidiasis.**

candidiasis /kan′didī′əsis/, any infection caused by a species of the *Candida* genus of yeastlike fungi. Many common diseases, as diaper rash, thrush, vaginitis, and dermatitis, are caused by *Candida* infestations. A warm, moist environment will aid the growth of the fungus. Some drugs destroy helpful bacteria as well as harmful ones and allow the fungus to grow. Gentian violet is a drug used on the skin. Antifungal drugs, as candicidin, clotrimazole, or nystatin may be used for some infections. **Chronic mucocutaneous candidiasis** is a rare form of the infection. There are sores on the skin, viral infections, and repeated lung infections. It usually occurs during the first year of life but can develop as late as the 20s, and is linked to an inherited defect of the body's immune system. Other prob-

Cancer's seven warning signals

Adults	Children
Change in bowel or bladder habit	Marked change in bowel or bladder habits; nausea and vomiting for no apparent cause
Unusual bleeding or discharge	Bloody discharge of any sort: blood in urine, spontaneous nosebleed or other type homorrhage, failure to stop bleeding in the usual time
Thickening or lump in breast or elsewhere	Swellings, lumps, or masses anywhere in the body
Obvious change in wart or mole	Any change in the size or appearance of outward growths, such as moles or birthmarks
Nagging cough or hoarseness	Unexplained stumbling in a child
A sore that does not heal	A generally run-down condition
Indigestion or difficulty in swallowing	Pains or the persistent crying of a baby or child, for which no reason can be found

From American Cancer Society: cancer facts and figures (1982), New York, 1982, American Cancer Society.

lems linked to the disease include diabetes, Addison's disease, thyroid deficiency, and pernicious anemia. Some patients also develop disfigurements and hormone imbalances. These hormone disorders can result in low blood levels of calcium, abnormal liver function, high blood sugar, iron deficiency, and abnormal vitamin B_{12} absorption. Chronic mucocutaneous candidiasis does not react to agents that kill fungus being placed on the skin. Most success in treating severe cases has been with an antibiotic that kills fungus (amphotericin B) given in the vein. Plastic surgery may also be part of the treatment to correct disfigurements caused by the disease. Hormone disorders linked to the disease must be treated separately. Treatment may also include extra iron to correct the anemia.

canine tooth, any one of the four teeth, two in each jaw, found on either side of the four front teeth (incisors) in the human. Canine teeth are larger and stronger than the front teeth and have deeper roots. The first set of canine teeth show around 18 months after birth. They are replaced by adult canines at 11 or 12 years of age. Canines in the upper jaw are also called **eyeteeth.**

canker, a sore, found mostly in the mouth. Causes include a food allergy, herpes infection, and emotional stress. See also **gingivitis, stomatitis.**

cannabis /kan′əbis/, American or Indian hemp (*Cannabis sativa*) used as a source of marijuana, hashish, and other mind-altering drugs. The dried flower tops of this annual contain the chemical tetrahydrocannabinols (THC). All parts of the plant have some mind-altering chemicals, but the highest amounts are in the flowers. Cannabis and its products are classified as controlled substances by the U.S. government. Cannibis is sometimes approved for cancer patients to relieve the nausea caused by chemotherapy. It is also given to patients with an increase of pressure within the eye (glaucoma) to reduce that pressure.

cannula /kan′yələ/, *pl.* **cannulas, cannulae,** a flexible tube containing a pointed metal rod (trocar) that can be put in the body, such as in a vein or the bladder. When the rod is removed, fluid can drain through the tube.

cantharis /kan′thəris/, *pl.* **cantharides** /kanther′idēz/, the dried insects *Cantharis vesicatoria,* which contain an irritating chemical once thought to stimulate sex. Also called **Spanish fly.**

canthus /kan′thəs/, *pl.* **canthi,** each corner of the eye; the angle at which the upper and lower eyelid meet on either side of the eye.

Cantil, a trademark for an antispasm drug used to treat peptic ulcers (mepenzolate bromide).

Capastat, a trademark for an antibiotic drug used to treat tuberculosis (capreomycin).

capeline bandage /kap′əlin/, a caplike bandage used for protecting the head, shoulder, or a stump of a limb.

capillary /kap′iler′ē/, any of the tiny blood vessels in the system that link the arteries and the veins. The size of a capillary may be 0.008 mm, so tiny that red blood cells must pass through one at a time. Through their walls, blood and tissue cells exchange various substances. The blood gives oxygen and nutrients to the cells and collects waste from the cells.

capillary fracture, any thin hairlike break.

capitate bone, a large bone in the center of the wrist.

capitulum /kəpich′ələm/, *pl.* **capitula,** a small, rounded high place on a bone where it joins another bone. The capitula of the wrist and ankle can be seen as bulges under the skin.

capotement /käpōtmäN′/, a splashing sound made by the stomach.

capsule, 1. a small, oval-shaped, gelatin container that holds a powdered or liquid drug. It is taken by mouth. Liquid drugs are usually packaged in soft gelatin capsules that are sealed to prevent leakage. Powdered drugs may be packaged in hard capsules. A capsule is coated with a substance to keep from dissolving in the stomach when the drug must be absorbed in the lower tract. Compare **tablet. 2.** a membrane or other body structure that covers an organ or part, as the capsule of the adrenal gland or the capsule of a joint.

capsulectomy /-ek′-/, the surgical removal of a capsule, usually the capsule of a joint or the capsule of the lens of the eye.

caput /kā′pət, kap′ət/, the head or the enlarged portion of an organ or part. The term is used with another word naming the organ part, as **caput costae,** for head of a rib, or **caput epididymidis,** the head of the epididymis, which is the long tube in the testicles through which sperm travel.

caput succedaneum. See **molding.**

caramiphen edisylate, a drug used to treat coughs. Known allergy to this drug prohibits its use. Side effects include dizziness, stomach upset, nausea, and lack of sleep.

carbachol, a drug used to treat pressure within the eye (glaucoma). It is also used in eye surgery, and to reverse other drugs used for the eyes, as atropine. Carbachol is not given to patients with inflammation of the iris, or known allergy to this drug. Side effects include eye spasm and blood in the eyelids (conjunctival hyperemia).

carbamazepine /kär′bəmaz′əpin/, a painkilling and muscle-relaxing drug used to treat a face nerve disorder (trigeminal neuralgia) and some kinds of seizures. It should not be used with monoamine oxidase inhibitors or by anyone with blood problems or known allergy to this or similar drugs. Side effects include life-threatening blood problems, loss of sleep, dizziness, loss of balance, and nausea.

carbamide peroxide, a growth-stopping drug used to treat canker sores and other minor inflammations of the gums and mouth, and to soften impacted earwax. Punctured eardrum prohibits its use in the ears. A side effect is local irritation.

carbenicillin disodium, a penicillin antibiotic used to treat some infections in burns, wounds, and the urinary tract. Known allergy to penicillin prevents its use. The drug should be used carefully by persons with allergies or kidney problems, or by persons on a low-salt diet. The high salt content may disturb fluid and mineral balances in patients with heart, liver, or kidney problems. Convulsions, bleeding, and blood and nerve problems can result.

carbidopa, a drug used in combination with levodopa to treat Parkinson's disease. Carbidopa allows smaller doses of levodopa to be given, with fewer side effects. Pressure within the eye (glaucoma), high blood pressure, the use of a monoamine oxidase inhibitor, or known allergy to this drug prohibits its use. Side effects include stomach bleeding, uneven heartbeat, slowed muscle movements, depression, and blurred vision.

carbinoxamine maleate, a drug used to treat many allergies, including sneezing, skin reactions, and itching. Asthma or allergy to this drug prevents its use. It is not given to newborn infants or nursing mothers. Side effects include rapid heart beat, lack of sleep, skin rash, and dry mouth.

Carbocaine Hydrochloride, a trademark for a local pain-killer (mepivacaine hydrochloride).

carbohydrate, a large group of sugars, starches, celluloses, and gums that all contain carbon, hydrogen, and oxygen in similar proportions. Carbohydrates are the main source of energy for all body functions and are needed to process other nutrients. They are formed by all green plants, which use the sun to combine carbon dioxide and water into simple sugar molecules. They can also be made in the body. Lack of carbohydrates can result in fatigue, depression, breakdown of body protein, and mineral imbalance.

carbohydrate loading, a diet practice of some endurance athletes. A low-carbohydrate diet is eaten for many days. Then for many days just before competing, a diet very high in carbohydrates is eaten. The theory is that the muscles will be overfull with energy for the event.

carbolated camphor, a germ-preventing wound dressing made of 1.5 parts camphor and 1.0 parts each of alcohol and carbolic acid.

carbol-fuchsin paint, a substance used to treat fungus infections on the skin. It is made of boric acid, carbolic acid, resorcinol, fuchsin, acetone, and alcohol in water.

carbolic acid, a germ-preventing and germ-killing compound made from coal tar. While fairly safe in very weak solutions of about 1% for cleaning small wounds or to relieve itching, carbolic acid is a strong poison. It can be absorbed through the skin, and destroy the tissue. If swallowed, it depresses the nerves and causes the lungs and blood flow to stop working. It will cause death unless emergency treatment is given promptly. Because carbolic acid has no color, it often contains a dye to warn against mistaken use. Also called **phenol.**

carbon (C), a nonmetallic chemical element. Carbon occurs throughout nature as a part of all living tissue and is essential to the chemistry of the body. It occurs in a vast number of carbon compounds, such as in diamonds, coal, charcoal, coke, and carbon dioxide. Carbon dioxide is important in the acid-base balance of the body and in controlling breathing. Carbon monoxide can be deadly if breathed in. Dusts with carbon in them can cause many on-the-job lung diseases, such as coal worker's pneumoconiosis, black lung disease, and byssinosis.

carbon dioxide (CO_2), a clear, odorless gas. It is found in nature, but it is also made in diverse ways. Plants and animals make carbon dioxide in breathing. Although it is mostly not poisonous, carbon dioxide can cause suffocation. The acid-base balance of the body is affected by the level of carbon dioxide in the blood and other tissues. Solid carbon dioxide (dry ice) is made by compressing carbon-dioxide gas at very cold temperatures. It is sometimes used to treat warts, lupus, or moles.

carbon monoxide, a clear, odorless, poisonous gas made when carbon or other fuel is burned, as in gasoline engines. Poisoning occurs when carbon monoxide gas has been breathed and absorbed by the blood. **Carboxyhemoglobin** is a compound produced when carbon monoxide links with red blood cells. It blocks the sites on the cells that carry oxygen. This limits the ability of the blood to transport oxygen. Oxygen in the blood decreases and, when the decrease is too much, suffocation and death result. A sign of carbon monoxide poisoning in a person is a cherry-pink skin color. In a small enclosed space, death can occur within minutes unless emergency treatment is given. This includes removing the person from the source right away and giving oxygen.

carbon tetrachloride, a clear, poisonous liquid that quickly changes to vapor. It is used as a solvent in dry-cleaning fluids, and in fire extinguishers. Accidentally swallowing the liquid or breathing the fumes results in headaches, nausea, depression, stomach pain, and convulsions. In poisoning by fumes, artificial respiration and oxygen may be needed. In poisoning by swallowing, the usual treatment is pumping the stomach. Carbon tetrachloride is very poisonous to the kidneys and liver, and can cause permanent damage.

carboprost tromethamine, a male hormone used to induce abortion during the second 3 months of pregnancy. The drug should not be given to patients with severe pelvic inflammation and known allergy to this drug. It is used with caution in many disorders. Side effects include fever, vomiting, and diarrhea.

carbuncle /kär′bungkəl/, a group of staphylococcal sores in which pus is present in deep, connected pockets under the skin. Common sites for carbuncles are the back of the neck and the buttocks. Treatment includes antibiotics, hot compresses, and drainage. **Carbunculosis** refers to the presence of a group of carbuncles. The infecting bacteria invade the skin through hair follicles. The problem can occur with diabetes mellitus.

carcinectomy /kär′sinek′-/, the removal of a cancerous tumor.

carcinoembryonic antigen (CEA) /kär′sinō·em′brē·on′ik/, a substance that is sometimes measured in searching for tumors. It is found in very small amounts in normal adult tissues. In patients with cancers of the colon, bladder, breast, and pancreas, the levels are higher. CEA is thought to be released into the bloodstream by tumors. However, finding CEA is not thought to be proof of cancer.

carcinogen /kärsin′əjən, kär′sinəjən/, a substance that can cause the growth of cancer. An **environmental carcinogen** is any of many natural or manufactured substances that can cause cancer. These substances may be chemical agents, physical agents, or certain hormones and viruses. They include arsenic, asbestos, uranium, vinyl chloride, radiation, ultraviolet rays, x-rays, and various things derived from coal tar. **Carcinogenic** refers to the ability to cause cancer.

carcinolysis /kär′sinol′isis/, the killing of cancer cells, as by chemotherapy.

carcinoma /kär′sinō′mə/, any cancerous tumor that starts with the cells (epithelial) that cover inner and outer body surfaces. Carcinomas invade nearby tissue and spread to far regions of the body. It occurs most often in the skin, large intestine, lungs, stomach, prostate gland, cervix, and breast. The tumor is usually a firm, uneven, knotty mass, with a well-defined edge in some places.

carcinoma en cuirasse /äN kēräs′/, a rare cancer that occurs along with advanced breast cancer. It is known by progressive growth of fibers in the tissues. It causes the skin of the chest, neck, back, and sometimes the stomach to become rigid.

carcinoma in situ, a precancerous tumor that has not invaded the nearby tissues, but looks like it is invasive

cancer. Such tumors are often seen on the cervix. They also occur in the anus, lung tissue, mucous membranes in the mouth, throat, eye, lip, penis, wall of the uterus, vagina, and skin growths in the aged (senile keratosis). Cervical carcinoma in situ is treated with success in various ways. These can include cryosurgery, electrocautery, and hysterectomy.

carcinosarcoma /-särkō′mə/, a cancerous tumor made of two kinds of cancer cells that are called carcinoma and sarcoma. Tumors of this type may occur in the throat, thyroid gland, and uterus.

carcinosis /kär′sinō′-/, the growth of many cancers throughout the body.

carcinostatic /-stat′ik/, referring to the slowing or halting of the growth of a cancer.

cardiac, 1. referring to the heart. 2. referring to a person with heart disease. 3. referring to the part of the stomach that is joined by the esophagus.

cardiac arrest, a sudden stopping of heart output. The blood stops flowing, and delivery of oxygen does not get to vital tissues. Carbon dioxide builds up in the tissues, and cell functions fail. Cardiac arrest usually occurs with fibrillation, in which electric activity persists, but contraction stops. Cardiac arrest may also occur with **asystole.** Also called **cardiac standstill,** this is the absence of a heart beat. Cardiotoxic asystole is a brief period of cardiac arrest. It is caused by speeding up of the heart rate. Heart and lung revival is needed right away to prevent permanent heart, lung, kidney, and brain damage. Cardiopulmonary resuscitation, cardiac massage, or a defibrillator may be used to start heart contractions.

cardiac atrophy, a breaking down of the heart muscle.

cardiac catheterization, a test in which a long fine tube (catheter) is passed into the heart through a large blood vessel in an arm or a leg. The blood pressures in the heart chambers (atria and ventricles) and nearby blood vessels are measured during catheterization. A catheter nearly 4 feet long is passed through a cut into the vein. It is then passed into either the right upper chamber (atrium), the left lower chamber (ventricle) of the heart, or other parts to be studied. The catheter is guided by the doctor who watches its course on a fluoroscope. X-ray films may also be taken. An electrocardiogram monitors the heart during the procedure. As the catheter tip passes through the chambers and vessels of the heart, the pressure of the flow of blood is watched. Samples of the blood are taken for testing. An antibiotic may be given the day before to reduce the risk of infection. After the test the patient may run a fever for a few hours, and there may be pain at the site of the incision. Many conditions may be identified and assessed by using cardiac catheterization. These include hereditary heart disease, narrowing of the heart valves, and valve failure.

Among the risks of the test are infection, uneven heart beat, and inflammation of a vein.

cardiac conduction defect, any impairment in the electric signals that control the pumping of the heart. Defects may occur in special fibers of the heart. See also **fibrillation, heart block.**

cardiac cycle, the cycle of the heart from the start of one beat until the start of the next. The cycle begins with the electrical signal from special heart fibers (the sinoatrial node). The signal travels the pathways that run through the heart muscle. This causes the heart chambers to contract, first the atria and then the ventricles. The cycle ends when the heart fibers become charged for the next contraction. The whole cycle lasts about 0.8 seconds.

cardiac hypertrophy, an enlargement of the heart.

cardiac impulse, the movement of the chest caused by the beating of the heart. It is easy to feel and easy to record.

cardiac massage. See **heart massage.**

cardiac monitoring, an electronic process that provides continuous reading of the heart on an oscilloscope. Each contraction of the heart chambers is indicated by either a flashing light or a sound. The equipment also has an alarm system that is triggered by heart beats above or below normal rates. See also **electrocardiograph.**

cardiac murmur. See **heart murmur.**

cardiac output, a measure of the amount of blood put out by the heart in a given space of time. A normal heart in a resting adult puts out from about 2.5 to 4 quarts (2.5 to 4.0 liters) of blood per minute. An output at rest of less than 2.5 liters usually indicates that something is wrong with the heart. Cardiac output is measured in many ways. One way is to measure the amount of oxygen in blood samples taken from a patient whose breathing has been measured for oxygen.

cardiac pacemaker. See **pacemaker.**

cardiac plexus, a set of nerves near the arch of the main trunk where the system of arteries begins (aorta). It has nerve fibers that both speed up the heart rate (sympathetic fibers) and slow the heart rate (parasympathetic fibers). Both types of nerves follow along with the arteries of the heart. They go into the heart, and end in the fibers which control electrical signals of the heart.

cardiac reserve, the potential of the heart to increase output and blood pressure above its normal level in response to needs of the body.

cardiac sphincter, a ring of muscle fibers where the gullet (esophagus) joins the stomach. Its function is to keep the stomach contents from backing up into the gullet. **Cardiochalasia** is a state in which the muscle is relaxed. This allows the stomach contents to back up.

cardiac stimulant, any drug that increases heart action. Drugs such as digitalis increase the force of contractions and slow the heart rate. This allows more time for the heart to relax and become filled with blood between beats.

cardiac tamponade, squeezing of the heart caused by blood or fluid collecting in the sac around the heart. This can result when a blood vessel in the heart breaks or by a wound to the heart. Signs of cardiac tamponade may include neck veins that stand out, low blood pressure, decreased heart sounds, fast breathing, and weak or absent pulses. The person can be anxious and restless, tending to sit upright or lean forward. The skin may be pale or blue. See also **tamponade.**

cardiac valve. See **heart valve.**

cardialgia /kär′dē·al′jə/, any pain in the region of the heart. The term is used even if the heart is not directly involved. Also called **cardiodynia.**

cardiectomy /-ek′-/, removing the area of the stomach where it joins the gullet (esophagus).

Cardilate, a trademark for a drug used to treat smothering chest pain which is called angina pectoris (erythrityl tetranitrate).

cardinal, referring to the main feature of an organ or its function.

cardinal position of gaze, one of the positions to which the normal eye may be turned. Each position depends on certain eye muscles and nerve fibers. The positions include to the left, to the right, up, up and to the right, up and to the left, down, down and to the right, and down and to the left.

cardiocele /kär′dē·əsēl′/, an event in which the heart pushes through the muscle that holds it in place above the stomach (diaphragm), or through a nearby wound.

cardiogenic shock. See **shock.**

cardiogram. See **electrocardiogram.**

cardiologist /-ol′-/, a doctor who finds and treats heart problems.

cardiolysis /-ol′isis/, a procedure to separate scar tissue (adhesions) that constrict the heart. Part of the ribs and breastbone are cut out. The sac around the heart is cut from the membrane on the inside of the breastbone.

cardiomegaly /-meg′əlē/, enlargement of the heart caused most often by high blood pressure within the heart. It can also occur with various heart defects. In athletes an enlarged heart is normal.

cardiomyopathy /-mī·op′əthē/, any disease that affects the heart muscle. **Secondary cardiomyopathy** refers to a problem that is linked to another form of heart disease or illness, as high blood pressure.

cardioneurosis, a state of mental upset that occurs with heart symptoms, such as chest pains or fluttering heart beat. It may be set off by a heart condition or the fear of heart disease (cardiophobia).

cardiopericarditis /-per′ikärdī′-/, inflammation of the heart and the sac around the heart (pericardium).

cardioplegia /-plē′jə/, paralysis of the heart, which may be caused by drugs, low body heat, or electrical excitement used in order to operate on the heart.

cardiopulmonary /-pul′məner′ē/, referring to the heart and the lungs.

cardiopulmonary resuscitation (CPR), a basic emergency method of life saving. Artificial respiration and heart massage is used to restart the heart and lungs. CPR is done for cardiac arrest, electric shock, and drowning. It is vital that blood flow and breathing be kept up until trained help arrives. Permanent damage to the brain can occur if oxygen flow is not restored within about 4 minutes. Chest compression presses the heart between the lower breastbone and the spine. During pressure, blood is forced into moving through the blood vessels. Blood refills the heart when the pressure is released. Mouth-to-mouth breathing is used at the same time to put oxygen in the blood that is pumped through the body by heart massage. The American Heart Association, the American Red Cross, and other places offer CPR courses all over the United States. It is best if the rescue is handled by persons trained in CPR. Equipment is not needed. CPR can be done by one or two persons. CPR involves three actions: opening the airway, restoring breathing, and restoring blood flow. For an adult, CPR is done in the following way:

1) The patient is quickly placed on a hard flat surface, as a board or the floor.

2) Look at the patient closely. If unresponsive, the patient is tapped on the shoulder. The rescuer asks loudly, "Can you hear me? Are you all right?" If there is no response, assume the patient is not conscious.

3) Open the airway to the lungs. If the patient is lying face up, the tongue will drop back in the throat, blocking the airway. This can be fixed by tilting the head. To do this, place one hand beneath the patient's neck and the other on the patient's forehead and lift up. This extends the neck and lifts the tongue from the back of the throat. However, if there is any sign of a neck injury, the method is different. Otherwise, the head is held, either tilted back or with jaw lifted, throughout the procedure.

4) The rescuer should assess the need for artificial respiration by looking, listening, and feeling for signs of breathing. Regular mouth-to-mouth artificial respiration should start quickly if there are none.

5) To begin artificial respiration, pinch the patient's nostrils closed. The rescuer's mouth should be put tightly around the mouth of the patient. Four quick breaths, each of increasing strength and size, are forced into the patient's

lungs. The rescuer's mouth is removed between each breath, and the patient is allowed to exhale without help. The cycle is repeated every 5 seconds as long as the patient does not start breathing. If the chest does not expand, move the head and try again. If this does not work, the airway is blocked. If the airway seems to be blocked, or the chest does not rise, use the Heimlich maneuver or look in the patient's mouth for a foreign object.

6) Take the patient's pulse at the neck artery for 5 seconds and check for signs of heart stoppage right after the first four breaths are given. Absent or weak pulse at that time means that chest compression is needed.

7) To start compression, take a position facing the side of the patient. To find the right place to put the hands, uncover the patient's chest and find the lower end of the breastbone. Place the heel of one hand just above the tip of the breastbone. With the fingers pointing upward and away from the ribs, the other hand is placed on top of the first and the fingers are interlocked. With arms straight, the rescuer rocks back and forth from the hips, using enough downward pressure with the forward swing of the body to push down the adult patient's breast bone from 1½ to 2 inches. The fingers should be held so that they do not touch the ribs. (It is important to avoid hurting the victim.) After each compression, a rest is allowed for a time equal to the time of compression, but the hands must not be moved from their place on the chest. The cycle is repeated using a rate of 15 chest compressions to 2 breaths. A rate of about 60 compressions a minute should be maintained. The right rhythm may be found by counting "one and two and three," up to 15. If there are two persons, CPR is done with one person giving compressions and the other giving breaths, at a 5-to-1 ratio at a rate of 60 compressions a minute. Check results by feeling for the pulse in the neck and by watching for "pinking" of the skin, eye signs, and a return of breathing. If the person doing compressions gets tired, a switch may be made by changing the counting rhythm to "switch-one thousand, two-one thousand," up to "five-one thousand." At the end of that cycle, the person giving compressions moves to the patient's head and checks the pulse. The person at the head, after giving a breath, moves to the patient's side, and checks the pulse for 5 seconds. If the pulse is absent or weak, the person says, "No pulse. Continue CPR."

For children 8 years of age and older, the technique is like that for adults. Younger children and infants need special treatment. CPR is an emergency treatment used until medical help is available. Once started, it is kept up until one of the following occurs: breathing and blood flow are restored; someone else takes over; a doctor takes charge of the patient; the patient is handed over to the care of a hospital; or the rescuer is not able to continue. Even if CPR is begun as soon as possible and all steps are done correctly, there are some cases, as with severe emphysema or crushing chest injuries, in which it will not work. Even when done correctly, CPR may cause rib fractures in some patients. Other problems include fracture of the breastbone, and liver or lung injuries. There is less danger of problems when technique is correct.

cardiospasm /kär′dē·əspazm′/, a failure of the muscle at the end of the gullet (esophagus) to relax. This makes it hard to swallow and vomit. It sometimes requires surgery to correct the defect.

cardiotachometer /-təkom′ətər/, a device that watches and records the heartbeat over a long time.

cardiotomy /-ot′-/, **1.** an operation in which the heart is cut into. **2.** an operation in which the heart or gullet end of the stomach is cut.

cardiotonic /-ton′ik/, a substance that makes the heart work better. Examples include drugs such as digitalis, digitoxin, and digoxin. They increase the force of contractions and slow the heart beat.

cardiotoxic, referring to a substance that has a poisonous or harmful effect on the heart.

cardiovascular /-vas′kyələr/, referring to the heart and blood vessels.

cardiovascular assessment, a way to assess the state, function, and defects of the heart and blood flow. The patient's history of heart and blood flow problems is noted, including the onset, quality, length of time, and place of any pain. Also noted are weakness, fatigue, shortness of breath, fever, coughing, wheezing, and uneven heart beat. Questions are asked about fainting, stomach upset, swelling of the feet and hands, bluish skin, changes in sight, and whether the hands and feet ever feel numb or cold. The patient's appearance, color, posture, the rate and rhythm of the pulses, and the neck veins are observed. The blood pressure, temperature, and rate and type of breaths are checked. The sounds the heart and breath make are checked. The color and condition of the skin is noted. The patient's level of awareness, reflexes, and responses to pain are noted. High blood pressure, weight, diabetes, and any lung and kidney problems are noted. Past heart surgery and illness are discussed. A number of tests are done on the blood itself as it relates to heart disease. A graph of the electrical signals of the heart may also be done (electrocardiogram). A thorough test of the heart and blood flow is an important part of a complete physical. It is vital to the care of a patient who has cardiovascular disease.

cardiovascular disease, any one of many defects that may cause problems with the heart and blood vessels. In the United States cardiovascular disease is the main cause of death. It accounts for more than 50% of all deaths from disease every year. More than a quarter of a million persons under 65 years of age in the United States die each year from this disorder.

cardiovascular system, the network of structures, which include the heart and the blood vessels, that pump and carry the blood through the body. The system has thousands of miles of blood vessels (arteries, veins, and capillaries). Many controls in the system send the blood to the places where it is most needed and at the proper rate. The arteries deliver nutrients to the fluids that surround the cells, and the veins take away waste products from the cells. The cardiovascular system works closely with the lungs and related structures (respiratory system) to transport oxygen from the lungs to the tissues and carry carbon dioxide to the lungs to be exhaled. Special nerves control the heart rate and blood pressure so that constant changes are made to deal with the needs of the body. Many conditions, as diet, exercise, and stress, affect the cardiovascular system.

cardioversion /-vur′zhən/, a method to restore the heart's normal rhythm in treating severe arrhythmias. An electric shock is given through two metal paddles placed on the patient's chest. One of the metal paddles, covered with a thick layer of special paste, is placed below the heart on the left side of the chest. The other paddle is placed over the upper right chest. The device is first set at a low level of voltage. If the normal rhythm of the heart does not resume, higher shocks can be given. A sedative is given before cardioversion. A constant graph of the heart's electric impulses is made. The person must sign an informed consent before treatment can start. Cardioversion will usually work to restore the heart's normal rhythm.

carditis /kärdī′-/, an inflammation of the muscles of the heart. It usually results from infection. Chest pain, uneven heartbeats, failure of the blood system, and damage to the heart may occur.

caries /ker′ēz/, decay, breaking down, and destruction of a bone or tooth. See also **dental caries, nursing-bottle caries, radiation caries.**

carisoprodol, a drug used to relieve muscle spasm. Porphyria or known allergy to this or similar drugs prohibits its use. Side effects include loss of sense of balance, fatigue, weakness, problems with eyesight, confusion, and allergic reactions.

carminative /kärmin′ətiv/, a substance that relieves bloating due to gas and painful spasms, especially after meals. Oils of anise, mints, and wintergreen were once used as carminatives but are rarely used in modern medicine except as flavorings.

carmustine /kärmus′tin/, an anticancer drug used alone or with other chemotherapeutic drugs. Carmustine is used to treat brain tumors, multiple myeloma, Hodgkin's disease, and non-Hodgkin's lymphomas. Also called **BCNU.**

carotene /ker′ətin/, a red or orange compound found in carrots, sweet potatoes, milk fat, egg yolk, and leafy vegetables. Carotene is changed to vitamin A in the body. A body that cannot make use of carotene may become lacking in vitamin A. See also **vitamin A.**

carotenemia /-ē′mē·ə/, the presence of too much carotene in the blood. This results in yellow appearance of the blood and skin.

carotenoid /kərot′ənoid/, any of a group of red, yellow, or orange pigments that are found in foods, as carrots, sweet potatoes, and leafy green vegetables. They can also be found in some animal tissue. Many of these substances, such as carotene, are needed to make vitamin A in the body.

carotid artery /kərot′id/, one of the major blood vessels bringing blood to the head and neck. The **common carotid artery** begins at the large artery of the heart (aorta) on the left side and at the innominate artery on the right side. About an inch above the collar bone, it forms two branches. The **external carotid** supplies the face, scalp, and most of the neck and throat tissues. The **internal carotid** supplies the brain, ears, and eyes. The carotid artery pulse can be felt just below the jaw bone.

carotid body reflex, a normal chemical reflex that begins when there is decreased oxygen in the blood or increased carbon dioxide. The carotid body is a small structure that contains nerve tissue at the branch of the carotid arteries. It controls the oxygen content of the blood by sending nerve signals to the brain's breathing center. The center sends back nerve signals that increase the breathing rate.

carotid body tumor, a benign round, firm growth that occurs at the branch of the common carotid artery. The tumor usually has no symptoms, but it sometimes causes dizziness, nausea, and vomiting, especially if it blocks the flow of blood. It may be removed in some cases.

carotid plexus, a network of nerves around the carotid artery and its branches.

carotid sinus, a bulge of the artery wall at the branch of the common carotid artery. It holds nerve ends that respond to changes in blood pressure.

carotid sinus reflex, the decrease in the heart rate as a normal response to pressure on the carotid artery where it branches.

carotid sinus syndrome, a short-term fainting spell that is sometimes seen with convulsions. It is caused by the strength of the carotid sinus reflex.

carotodynia /kərot′ōdin′ē·ə/, a soreness along the length of the common carotid artery.

carpal /kär′pəl/, referring to the wrist (carpus).

carpal tunnel syndrome, a common, painful defect of the wrist and hand. It occurs in the carpal tunnel, a channel in the wrist for the middle nerve (median nerve) and the tendons of the hand. The middle nerve serves the palm and the thumb side of the hand. Pressure on the nerve causes weakness, pain when the thumb is bent toward the palm, and burning, tingling, or aching that may spread to the forearm and the shoulder. The disorder is seen more often in women, especially in pregnant and in menopausal women. Symptoms may result from a blow, swelling, a tumor, rheumatoid arthritis, or a small carpal tunnel that squeezes the nerve. Weakness and wasting of muscles may occur from lack of use. Treatment includes drugs given by injection or an operation to relieve nerve pressure.

carpus. See **wrist.**

carrier, 1. a person or animal who carries and spreads disease, as typhoid fever, to others but who does not become ill. 2. one who carries a gene that has no effect unless it is combined with the gene of another person (recessive gene).

cartilage, a tissue that connects and supports. It is made of cells and fibers, found mostly in the joints, the chest, and stiff tubes of all sorts, as the voicebox (larynx), windpipe (trachea), nose, and ear.

caruncle /kär′ungkəl/, a small piece of flesh that bulges out. An example is the tissue that remains when the membrane (hymen) that covers the vagina is broken after birth. Also called **hymenal tag,** it disappears without treatment.

cascade system, three or more large air cylinders, each usually with a capacity of 300 cubic feet (8490 L), from which SCBA cylinders are recharged.

cascara sagrada /kasker′ə səgrä′də/, a drug made from the bark of a tree (*Rhamnus purshianus*). It is used to treat constipation.

caseation /kā′sē·ā′shən/, a form of tissue death in which the area looks like crumbly cheese. It is common in tuberculosis.

cast, 1. a stiff, solid dressing of plaster of paris or other material. It is formed around a limb or other body part to keep it from moving while it heals. A cast is used in treatment of bone breaks or dislocations, for positioning the part after surgery, and to correct deformities. A **bivalve cast** is one that is cut in half to watch for pressure under the cast, especially with a patient who has little or no feeling in the area. If dangerous pressure areas are found, ''windows'' are often cut out of the cast over the pressure areas to correct the problem. A **long-arm cast** covers the arm from the hand to the upper arm. A **short-arm cast** is used to keep the hand or wrist from moving. A **long-leg cast** covers the leg from the toes to the upper thigh. A **short-leg cast** covers the leg from the knee to the toes. The person can walk, wearing the leg casts, when weight-bearing on the foot is allowed, with the addition of a rubber walker. **2.** a mold of a part or all of a patient's teeth and inner jaw for fitting dental work. **3.** a small structure made when mineral or other substances collect on the walls of kidneys, bronchia, or other organs. Casts often show up in urine or blood collected for laboratory tests.

castor oil, an oil from the castor bean seed. It is used as a laxative for constipation and for cleansing the bowel before examination. Symptoms of appendicitis, blocked or torn bowels, and tightly-packed feces prohibit its use. It is not to be used during menstruation or pregnancy. Side effects include rectal bleeding, laxative dependence, nausea, cramps, and dizziness.

castration, the removal of one or both testicles or ovaries. It is usually done to reduce hormone production that may cause the growth of cancer cells in women with breast cancer or in men with cancer of the prostate. The removal of both ovaries or testicles (gonads) causes the person to become sterile.

catabasis /kətab′əsis/, the phase in which a disease declines and health begins to return.

catabiosis /kət′əbī·ō′-/, the normal aging of cells.

catabolism /kətab′əlizm/, a complex, chemical process of the body in which energy is released for use in work, energy storage, or heat production. The energy is released in the cells by breaking down complex substances into simple compounds. Compare **anabolism.** −**catabolic,** adj.

catalase /kat′əlās/, an enzyme, found in most living cells. It speeds up (catalyzes) the breakdown of hydrogen peroxide to water and oxygen.

catalepsy /kat′əlep′sē/, an abnormal condition with a trancelike level of awareness and rigid muscles. It occurs in hypnosis and in some physical and mental defects, as schizophrenia, epilepsy, and hysteria.

catalyst /kat′əlist/, a substance that speeds up the rate of a chemical reaction without being changed by the process. See also **enzyme.**

cataplexy /kat′əplek′sē/, a state in which sudden muscle weakness and loss of muscle tone occurs. It is caused by emotions, as anger, fear, or surprise. It is linked with narcolepsy, a desire to sleep that cannot be controlled. −**cataplectic,** adj.

Catapres, a trademark for a drug used to treat high blood pressure (clonidine hydrochloride).

cataract, a condition in which the eye lens loses its clearness. A gray-white film can be seen in the lens, behind the pupil. Most cataracts are caused by a loss of function in the lens tissue, most often after 50 years of age. Injury, as a puncture wound, may result in cataracts. Contact with poisons, as dinitrophenol or naphthalene, may cause cataracts.

catastrophic reaction, the confused response to a bad shock or a sudden threatening state. This reaction often occurs in the victims of car crashes and disasters.

catatonia /-tō′nē·ə/, a state of not being able to move due to a problem in the nerves of the muscles, which become very stiff. −**catatonic,** adj.

catecholamine /-kəlam′in/, any of a group of chemicals made by the body that work as important nerve transmitters. The main catecholamines made by the body are dopamine, epinephrine (also called adrenaline), and norepinephrine. Norepinephrine and epinephrine are made by the adrenal glands. Dopamine is found mainly in certain types of nerve tissue in the brain. The main job of catecholamines is to prepare the body to act, which includes increasing the blood pressure, heart beat, and breathing. At the same time other processes shut down, as digestion. Catecholamines are also made as drugs and are used to raise blood pressure and excite the heart in emergencies.

cat-eye syndrome, a rare, inherited disorder in which the pupils of the eye look like the narrow pupils of a cat. A closed anus, heart defects, and severe mental retardation may also be present.

catharsis /kəthär′-/, **1.** a cleaning out. **2.** the process of bringing memories of events that were not pleasant to the surface of thought. The technique of free association may be used with hypnosis and hypnotic drugs.

cathartic /kəthär′-/, referring to a substance that aids bowel movement by exciting intestinal waves (peristalsis), increasing the bulk of feces, making the feces soft, or adding fluid to the wall of the intestines. The term *cathartic* implies a fluid bowel movement; this is in contrast to *laxative,* which implies a soft, formed stool. See also **laxative.**

catheter /kath′ətər/, a hollow, flexible tube that can be put into a vessel or space in the body to take out or to add fluids. Most catheters are made of soft plastic or rubber and may be used for treatment or tests. Kinds include: an **acorn-tipped catheter,** a tube with an acorn-shaped tip, often used in urology; an **angiocatheter,** a tube put into a blood vessel to take blood or give fluids; and a **balloon-tip catheter,** which has an inflatable sac around one end. After the catheter is inserted, the sac is inflated with air or sterile water. The inflated sac secures the catheter in the correct position. An **indwelling catheter** is any catheter designed to be left in place for a prolonged period. A **self-retaining catheter** is an indwelling urinary catheter that has two channels. One channel allows urine to drain from the bladder into a collecting bag. The other channel has a system to hold the catheter in place. A **two-way catheter** has two tubes within it, one for injection of drugs or fluids and the other for taking out fluid or specimens.

C–D

catheterization, putting a tube (catheter) into a body cavity or organ to add or take out fluid. The most common practice is putting a catheter into the bladder through the urethra to empty it before surgery. It is also done when a sterile urine sample is needed or if voluntary urination is not possible. In **hepatic vein catheterization,** the tube is inserted through a vein in the arm and passed through the heart and down into a liver vein. The purpose is to record vein pressure within the liver. In **laryngeal catheterization,** a tube is put into the voicebox (larynx) to remove secretions or introduce gases. **Umbilical catheterization** refers to a procedure in which a catheter is passed through an umbilical artery to give a newborn fluids or to take blood samples. The tube may also go into the umbilical vein for a transfusion or for giving emergency amounts of

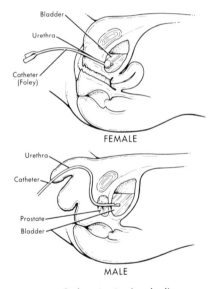

Catheterization (urethral)

drugs or fluids. See also **cardiac catheterization.**

cathexis /kəthek′sis/, to attach importance and feeling to a set idea, person, or object.

CAT scan. See **computerized tomography.**

cat-scratch fever, a disease that may be caused by a virus. It results from the scratch or bite of a cat that looks healthy. The first signs are inflammation and bumps filled with pus near the scratch. Lymph nodes in the neck, head, groin, or armpits swell 2 weeks later. The symptoms can last for months.

cauda equina /kô′də/, the nerve roots that come out from the end of the spinal cord and go down the spinal canal through the lower part of the spine and tailbone (coccyx).

caudal anesthesia. See **local anesthesia.**

caudate /kô′dāt/, having a tail.

caudate process, a small, raised tissue that comes out of the lower part of the tail end of the liver.

caul, the intact bag of waters (amniotic sac) that surrounds a baby at birth. The sac usually breaks open during the course of labor or birth. When it remains whole it must be torn or cut to allow the baby to breathe. In the past, pieces of the caul were sold to sailors as a good luck charm that would protect from death by drowning.

cauliflower ear, a thick, deformed ear caused by being hit many times, as suffered by boxers.

caumesthesia /kô′məsthē′zhə/, a problem in which a patient has low body heat but feels a sense of intense heat.

causalgia /kôzal′jə/, a feeling of severe burning pain, sometimes with local redness of the skin. It is caused by damage to a sensory nerve.

cause, anything that has an effect.

caustic, any substance that destroys living tissue, or causes burning or scarring, as silver nitrate, nitric acid, or sulfuric acid.

cautery /kô′tərē/, a device or substance that scars and burns the skin or other tissues. With **actual cautery,** heat is applied to destroy tissue. A **cautery knife** is an electric knife that cuts tissue and seals it with heat so it will not bleed. The breakdown or burning of living tissue by a caustic chemical, as potassium hydroxide, is **chemocautery.** It is done to remove severely infected or damaged tissue so that healthy tissue can grow. Placing a needle that is heated by electric current on tissue is **electrocautery.** This destroys the tissue. The method is often used to remove warts or polyps. **Thermocautery** also uses a hot needle or loop wire in the destruction of tissue.

cavernous sinus /kav′ərnəs/, one of a pair of unevenly shaped channels for blood vessels between the bone of the skull and the membrane covering the skull (dura mater). It is one of the five sinuses in the lower front portion of the skull that drain the blood from the skull membrane into the large vein in the neck (jugular vein).

cavernous sinus syndrome, a disorder with swelling of the membrane that lines the eye (conjunctiva), the upper eyelid, and the root of the nose. There is deadening of the nerves that serve the eye. It is caused by a blood clot in a blood vessel of the cavernous sinus. Called **cavernous sinus thrombosis,** the blood clot is usually the result of infections near the eye or nose. The infection may spread to the fluid of the brain and spinal cord (cerebrospinal fluid), and to the membranes that cover the brain and spinal cord (meninges). Treatment is with antibiotics and, sometimes, with drugs that slow the clotting action of the blood.

cavitation, the making of hollow spaces in the body, as those made in the lung by tuberculosis.

cavity, a hollow space in a larger structure, as the space which holds the lower organs of the body (peritoneal cavity), or the mouth (oral cavity). A space in a tooth formed by decay of the tooth (caries) is also called a cavity. An **access cavity** is a hole made in a tooth for cleaning, shaping, and filling the pulp space.

cavity classification, the listing of tooth decay (cavities) that refers to the tooth surfaces on which they occur, as labial, buccal, or occlusal; type of surface, as pitted or smooth. A cavity may be classified in one of six groups. Class 1: cavities linked to structural tooth defects, as pits and fissures. Class 2: cavities in the sides of premolars and molars. Class 3: cavities in the sides of the canines and incisors that do not interfere with the edge of the tooth. Class 4: cavities in the sides of canines and molars that require restoring the edge of the tooth. Class 5: cavities, except pit cavities, near the gum. Class 6: cavities on the edges and cusp tips of the teeth.

cecal /sē′kəl/, **1.** referring to the top part of the large intestine (cecum). **2.** referring to a blind spot in the field of vision.

Ceclor, a trademark for an antibiotic drug (cefaclor).

cecum /sē′kəm/, the first part of the large intestine.

Cedilanid-D, a trademark for a drug that makes the heart pump harder. (deslanoside).

CeeNU, a trademark for an anticancer drug (lomustine).

cefaclor, an antibiotic (cephalosporin) used to treat infections. Allergy to any cephalosporin drug prohibits its use. Persons who are allergic to penicillin need caution. Side effects include allergies, diarrhea, nausea, and vomiting.

cefadroxil monohydrate, an antibiotic (cephalosporin) used to treat infections. Allergy to any cephalosporin drug prohibits its use. Persons who are allergic to penicillin need caution. Side effects include allergies, diarrhea, nausea, and vomiting.

Cefadyl, a trademark for an antibiotic (cephapirin).

cefamandole nafate, an antibiotic (cephalosporin) used to treat infections. Allergy to any cephalosporin drug prohibits its use. Persons who are allergic to penicillin need caution. Side effects include allergies, blood clots in the legs (phlebitis), and pain when given in the muscle.

cefazolin sodium, an antibiotic (cepalosporin) used to treat a number of infections. Allergy to any cephalosporin drug prohibits its use. Persons who are allergic to penicillin need caution. Side effects include pain at the site where it is given, and allergies.

Cefizox, a trademark for a cephalosporin antibiotic (ceftizoxime).

Cefobid, a trademark for a cephalosporin antibiotic (cefoperazone).

cefoperazone sodium, an antibiotic (cephalosporin) used to treat lung infections, bowel, skin, and female reproductive tract infections and blood poisoning caused by bacteria. Allergy to any cephalosporin drug prohibits its use. Side effects include itching, rash, blood defects, and skin reactions to the shot.

cefotaxime sodium, an antibiotic (cephalosporin) used to treat infections of the lungs, genitals, urinary tract, bowels, skin, bones and joints, and central nervous system and blood poisoning caused by bacteria. Allergy to any cephalosporin drug prohibits its use. Side effects include itching, bowel trouble, fungal infections, and skin reactions to the shot.

cefoxitin sodium, an antibiotic (cephalosporin) used to treat bacterial infections. Allergy to any cephalosporin drug prohibits its use. Persons who are allergic to penicillin need caution. Side effects include allergies, blood clots in the legs (phlebitis), and muscle pain where the shot is given.

ceftizoxime sodium, an antibiotic (cephalosporin) used to treat infections. Allergy to any cephalosporin drug prohibits its use. Persons who are allergic to penicillin need caution. Side effects include allergies, blood disorders, and pain at the place where the shot is given.

cefuroxime sodium, an antibiotic (cephalosporin) used to treat lung, urinary tract, and skin infections, blood poisoning caused by bacteria, meningitis, and gonorrhea, and to prevent infections after surgery. Allergy to any cephalosporin drug prohibits its use. Side effects include itching, rash, and blood defects.

Celestone, a trademark for a drug used to treat severe disorders, as lung disease, leukemia, allergies, rheumatic disease, and eye disease (betamethasone).

celiac artery /sē′lē·ak/, a thick branch of the blood vessel that serves the belly (abdominal aorta). It starts below the muscle that holds the lungs above the stomach (diaphragm). The celiac artery divides into three arteries that serve the stomach, the liver, and the spleen.

celiac disease, a defect in the chemistry of food breakdown that is present from birth. A person with this defect cannot digest the gluten of some grain foods. The disease affects adults and young children, who may suffer from a swollen belly, vomiting, diarrhea, muscle wasting, and extreme fatigue. See also **malabsorption syndrome, sprue.**

celiocolpotomy /sē′lē·ōkəlpot′-/, a cut into the belly region through the vagina.

cell, the basic unit of all living tissue. The **cell body** is the part of a cell that contains the nucleus and cytoplasm around it. The cell body does the work that keeps the cell alive. Within the **nucleus,** the controlling part of the cell, are the nucleolus (containing RNA) and chromatin granules (containing protein and DNA) that grow into chromosomes, which determine hereditary traits. Some cells lack a nucleus when they are mature, as red blood cells. The **cytoplasm** is all of the substance of a cell other than the nucleus. Bits of substance in the cytoplasm, the organelles, are a network of membrane-enclosed tiny tubes (endoplasmic reticulum), ribosomes, the Golgi complex, mitochondria, lysosomes, and the centrosome. The thin and fragile outer wall of a cell is called the **cell membrane.** The membrane takes care of the exchange of materials between the cell's cytoplasm and the area around it.

cell death,   **1.** the death of a cell. **2.** the point in the process of dying at which the cells of the body no longer perform their work.

cell division.   See **meiosis, mitosis.**

cellulitis,   an infection of the skin that usually stays in one place, as the lower leg. Symptoms include heat over the area, redness, pain, and swelling, and occasionally fever, chills, and headache. Abscess and tissue destruction usually follow if antibiotics are not taken.

cellulose /sel′yəlōs/,   a colorless, transparent solid carbohydrate that is the main part of the cell walls of plants. It is nondigestible by humans. However, it provides the bulk needed for proper functioning of the stomach and intestines. See also **dietary fiber.**

cell wall,   the structure that covers and protects the cell membrane of some kinds of cells, as certain bacteria and all plant cells.

Celontin,   a trademark for a drug used to prevent convulsions (methsuximide).

Celsius (C) /sel′sē·əs/,   a temperature scale in which 0° is the freezing point of water and 100° is the boiling point of water at sea level. Also called **centigrade.** Compare **Fahrenheit.**

cement,   **1.** a sticky, gluelike substance that helps neighboring tissue cells stay together. **2.** any of a variety of dental materials used to fill cavities or to hold bridgework or other dental prostheses in place. **3.** a material used to position an artificial joint in adjacent bone.

cementoma,   a pooling of cementum at the tip of a tooth. It may be caused by injury.

cementopathia /sim′əntop′əthē/,   an abnormal condition of the teeth caused by dead cementum. Cementopathia contributes to the inflammation (periodontitis) and breakdown (periodontosis) of the tissues that support the teeth.

cementum,   the bonelike connective tissue that covers the roots of the teeth and helps to support them.

cenesthesia /sē′nəsthē′zhə/,   the general sense of existing, based on all the various stimuli and reactions throughout the body at any specific moment.

censor,   a form of mentally holding back thoughts and only letting them rise to consciousness if they are heavily masked.

center,   **1.** the middle point of the body. **2.** a group of nerve cells with a common function, as the center in the brain that controls the heart beat.

Centers for Disease Control (CDC),   an agency of the United States government that offers facilities and services for the investigation, identification, prevention, and control of disease. The CDC's interests include environmental health, smoking, hunger, poisoning, and problems of health in the workplace.

centigrade.   See **Celsius.**

centimeter (cm) /sen′timē′tər/,   a metric unit of measurement. It is equal to one hundredth of a meter, or 0.3937 inches.

centimeter-gram-second system (CGS, cgs),   an internationally accepted scientific system of expressing length, mass, and time in basic units of centimeters, grams, and seconds. The CGS system is slowly being replaced by the International System of Units based on the meter, kilogram, and second.

centipede bite,   a wound produced by the poison claws and the jaws of a centipede, a wormlike insect with many pairs of legs. The bite of a few species, particularly in the southern United States, may cause painful swelling, fever, headache, vomiting, and dizziness.

central nervous system (CNS),   one of the two main divisions of the nervous system of the body. It is made up of the brain and the spinal cord. The central nervous system carries impulses to and from the peripheral nervous system. It is the main network of coordination and control for the entire body. The brain controls many functions and sensations, such as sleep, sexual activity, muscle movement, hunger, thirst, memory, and the emotions. The spinal cord contains various types of nerve fibers from the brain and acts as a switching and relay terminal for the peripheral nervous system. The 12 pairs of cranial nerves emerge directly from the brain. The nerves of the peripheral system leave the spinal cord separately between the vertebrae of the backbone. However, they unite to form 31 pairs of spinal nerves containing sensory fibers and motor fibers. Sensory nerves carry impulses to the spinal cord and brain. Motor nerves carry impulses (or "commands") from the central nervous system to the muscles and glands. The brain contains more than 10 billion nerve cells. Billions of other cells help form the soft, jellylike substance of the brain. Flowing through many cavities of the central nervous system is the fluid of the brain and spine. This fluid helps to protect the central nervous system from injury. It affects the rate of breathing through cells that measure its content of carbon dioxide. The brain and the spinal cord are made up of gray matter and white matter. The gray matter has mainly nerve cells and linked filaments. The white matter is made up of bundles of mainly insulated (myelinated) nerve fibers. The central nervous system grows from the neural tube of the embryo, which first appears in the third week of pregnancy. The cavity of the neural tube is kept after birth in the spaces (ventricles) of the brain and in the central canal of the spinal cord. Compare **peripheral nervous system.** See also **brain, spinal cord.**

central nervous system depressant,   any drug that lowers activity of the central nervous system (CNS), such as alcohol, barbiturates, and sleeping pills. Depressants, especially the tranquilizers, are the most widely given drugs throughout the world. These drugs work by decreasing the flow of nerve impulses. Alcohol affects the CNS more than any other part of the body. All depressants can be abused. Constant use of these drugs can make a condition in which the person's body needs the drugs to feel normal. This dependence leads to compulsive drug use. Sudden withdrawal of CNS depressants that have been used in high doses for prolonged periods can be fatal. Withdrawal treatment commonly involves substituting pentobarbital, then gradually reducing the dosage over a 10-day to 3-week period.

central nervous system stimulant,   a substance that speeds up the activity of the central nervous system (CNS). CNS stimulants work by increasing the rate of nerve impulses or by blocking substances that would calm the nervous system. Many natural and artificial chemicals stimulate the CNS. Only a few are used in therapy. Caffeine, a potent CNS stimulant, is used to help restore mental alertness and overcome depressed breathing. It may cause nausea, nervousness, ringing in the ears, tremor, abnormal heart beats, increased urination, and visual disturbances. Amphetamines have been used to treat long-term drowsiness and overweight. However, amphetamines have a high potential for abuse. They may cause dizziness, restlessness, rapid heart beat, high blood pressure, headache, mouth dryness, an unpleasant taste, digestive disorders, and hives. Amphetamines are sometimes given for overactivity, as in attention deficit disorder, because some stimulants have a calming effect on patients. Some are used to stimulate the breathing center and to restore consciousness after anesthesia or for overdose of depressants. Also called **analeptic.**

central nervous system tumor.   See **brain tumor, spinal cord tumor.**

central scotoma,   an area of blindness or lowered vision involving the central area of the retina.

central venous pressure (CVP) monitor,   a device for measuring and recording the blood pressure inside a large vein by means of a catheter and a pressure gauge.

central venous return,   the blood from the body's veins that flows into the right upper chamber (atrium) of the heart through the major vein in the trunk (vena cava).

central vision,   vision that results from images falling on the center of the retina.

Centrax,   a trademark for a drug that relieves anxiety (prazepam).

centrifugal /sentrif′yəgəl/,   referring to a force that is directed outward, away from a central point or axis. See also **centripetal.**

centrifuge /sen′trifyŏŏj/,   a device for separating substances in a liquid by spinning the mixture at high speeds. The heavier substances move to one part of the container, leaving the lighter ones in another. Blood is centrifuged, for example, for transfusions of plasma.

centriole /sen′trē·ōl′/,   an organ within a cell usually as a part of the center of a cell (centrosome). Often occurring in pairs, centrioles are linked to cell division. The precise function of centrioles is still unclear.

centripetal /sentrip′ətəl/,   **1.** referring to a direction, as a sensory nerve impulse traveling toward the brain. **2.** the direction of a force pulling an object toward the center or an axis of rotation, as opposed to a centrifugal force.

centromere /sen′trəmir/,   a specialized region of the chromosome. It joins 2 chromosome halves (chromatids) to each other and attaches to the spindle fiber in cell reproduction. During cell division the centromeres split lengthwise, half going to each of the new daughter chromosomes.

centrosome /-sōm/   a region present in animal cells and in some plants. It is located near the nucleus and is involved in cell division.

centrosphere /-sfir/,   a condensed area of cytoplasm surrounding the centrioles in the centrosome of a cell.

cephalalgia /sef′əlal′je/,   headache, often combined with another word to describe the type of headache, as histamine cephalalgia. See also **headache.**

cephalexin,   an antibiotic (cephalosporin) used to treat some infections. Known allergy to any cephalosporins prohibits its use. Persons who are allergic to penicillin need caution. Side effects include nausea, diarrhea, and allergic reactions.

cephalhematoma /sef′əlhē′mətō′mə/,   swelling caused by the pooling of blood under the scalp. It may begin to form in the scalp of a baby during labor and slowly become larger in the first few days after birth. It is usually a result of injury, often from forceps. Compare **molding.**

cephalic /səfal′ik/,   referring to the head.

cephalic presentation, a classification of a baby's position during labor in which the head is at the narrow lower end of the uterus (cervix). Cephalic presentation is usually further qualified by the part of the head presenting, as the back (occiput) or front (bregma).

cephalic vein, one of the four superficial veins of the arm. It begins in the network of veins in the hand and winds upward to end at a vein near the shoulder.

cephalometry /sef'əlom'ətrē/, the scientific measurement of the head. It may be done in dentistry to decide orthodontic methods for straightening the teeth.

cephalopelvic disproportion (CPD) /sef'əlōpel'vik/, a condition in which a baby's head is too large or a mother's birth canal too small to allow normal labor or birth. In **relative CPD,** the size of the baby's head may be normal but larger than average, or the size of the mother's birth canal may be normal but smaller than average, or both. Relative CPD is often overcome by shaping of the head, the forces of labor, or the use of forceps to effect childbirth. In **absolute CPD,** the baby's head is definitely large or the mother's birth canal is very small. This makes vaginal birth impossible. See also **pelvimetry.**

cephalosporin /-spôr'in/, an antibiotic originally derived from the fungus *Cephalosporium acremonium.* Cephalosporins are similar in chemical structure to penicillins.

cephalothin sodium, an antibiotic (cephalosporin) used to treat many infections. Allergy to any cephalosporin drugs prohibits its use. Persons who are allergic to penicillin need caution. Side effects include pain at the site of injection and allergic reactions.

cephapirin, an antibiotic used to treat infections, including blood poisoning (septicemia), heart infection (endocarditis), bone infection (osteomyelitis), and infections of the breathing tract, urinary tract, and skin. Known sensitivity to cephalosporin antibiotics prohibits its use. Side effects include anemia and other blood disorders and allergic reactions.

cephradine, an antibiotic (cephalosporin) used to treat some bacterial infections. Allergy to any cephalosporin drugs prohibits its use. Persons who are allergic to penicillin need caution. Nausea, diarrhea, and allergic reactions may occur.

cercaria /sərker'ē·ə/, *pl.* **cercariae,** a tiny, wormlike form of the class Trematoda. It develops in a freshwater snail. Cercariae enter the body of a human, usually by direct invasion through the skin, or through a cut or other break in the skin. They form cysts and end their growth in many organs of the body. Each species tends to go to a particular organ, as *Fasciola hepatica,* which becomes a liver fluke. See also **fluke, schistosomiasis.**

cerclage /serkläzh'/, **1.** a way in which the ends of a fractured bone or the chips of a broken kneecap are bound together with a wire loop or a metal band. This holds the bone parts in position until the break is healed. **2.** a way in which a silicone band is put around the white of the eye (sclera) to restore contact between the retina and the blood vessel layer (choroid) when the retina is detached. **3.** an obstetric method in which stitches (suture) are used to hold the lower end of the uterus (cervix) closed to prevent miscarriage. The band is usually released when the pregnancy is at full term. This allows labor to begin.

cerebellar /ser'əbel'ər/, referring to a part of the brain (cerebellum).

cerebellum /ser'əbel'əm/. See **brain.**

cerebral /ser'əbrəl, sərē'brəl/, referring to a part of the brain (cerebrum).

cerebral cortex. See **brain.**

cerebral dominance, the role of each of the two halves of the cerebrum (cerebral hemispheres) in the integration and control of different functions. The left hemisphere houses the logical, reasoning activities and controls reading, writing, speech, and analytic activities. The right hemisphere concerns imagination, intuitions, creativity, spatial skills, art, and left-hand control. In 90% of the population, the left cerebral hemisphere dominates the ability to speak, write, and understand spoken and written words. In the other 10% of the population, either the right hemisphere or both hemispheres dominates. The right cerebral hemisphere also dominates the integration of certain sounds other than speaking, such as the sounds of coughing, laughter, crying, and melodies. The right cerebral hemisphere perceives touch stimuli and visual relationships better than the left cerebral hemisphere.

cerebral hemisphere. See **brain.**

cerebral hemorrhage, bleeding from a blood vessel in the brain. Cerebral hemorrhages are classified by location, the kind of vessel involved, and the cause. Each type has its own symptoms, some of which include headache, partial paralysis, loss of consciousness, nausea, vomiting, and seizures. They are caused by the breaking of a hardened artery as a result of high blood pressure. Other causes of rupture include inborn ballooning of brain arteries (aneurysm) and head injury. Bleeding may lead to destruction of brain tissue. Extensive bleeding leads usually to death. Blood may be found in the spinal fluid. Surgery is often necessary to stop the bleeding in order to prevent death. The person is kept without movement. The neck is held straight to allow adequate blood flow to and from the head. Physical therapy and speech therapy may be needed during recovery. Depending on the extent and the location of the damaged tissue, effects may include loss of speech or understanding speech (aphasia), diminished mental function, or loss of the function of one of the special senses.

cerebral palsy, a motor nerve disorder caused by a permanent brain defect or an injury at birth or soon after. Symptoms depend on the area of the brain involved and the extent of damage. Milder cases have spastic paralysis of the legs or both limbs on one side and normal intelligence. More severe cases have widespread loss of normal muscle control, seizures, numbness, mental retardation, blocked speech, vision, and hearing. The disorder is usually linked to too early or abnormal birth and lack of oxygen during birth, causing damage to the nervous system. Abnormalities in breathing, sucking, and swallowing are often visible soon after birth. The stiff, awkward movements of the infant's limbs may be overlooked for several months. Walking is usually delayed, and when tried, the walk has a scissorslike quality. The arms may be affected only slightly but the fingers are often spastic. Some reflexes are too strong. There may be slurred speech, and delay in acquiring bowel and bladder control. There also may be slow movements of the face and hands. Identifying the disorder early is important. Treatment may include braces, correcting deformities by surgery, speech therapy, and drugs that relax the muscles and prevent convulsions. Many patients can lead near normal lives with the proper therapy. Even the severely affected can benefit from training and learn self-care activities, as washing, dressing, and feeding.

cerebrocerebellar atrophy /ser'əbrōser'əbel'ər/, a breakdown of a part of the brain (cerebellum) caused by some nutritional diseases.

cerebroma /ser'əbrō'mə/, any unusual mass of brain tissue.

cerebroretinal angiomatosis /-ret'ənəl/, a hereditary disease of small tumorlike growths in the retina of the eye and part of the brain (cerebellum). Similar growths on the spinal cord, pancreas, kidneys, and other organs are also common. Seizures and mental retardation may be present.

cerebroside /ser'əbrōsīd'/, any of a group of fatty carbohydrates found in the brain and other parts of the nervous system.

cerebrospinal /-spī'nəl/, referring to the brain and the spinal cord.

cerebrospinal fluid (CSF), the fluid that flows through and protects the brain and the spinal canal. It has small amounts of proteins, glucose, and electrolytes. Changes in the carbon dioxide content of CSF affect the breathing center in the brain, helping to control breathing. A brain tumor may stop the flow of the fluid. This results in a form of water on the brain (hydrocephalus). Other blockages of the flow of cerebrospinal fluid may occur, as those caused by blood clots. Examination of CSF is important in diagnosing diseases of the central nervous system. See also **lumbar puncture.**

cerebrovascular /-vas'kyələr/, referring to the blood vessels and blood supply of the brain.

cerebrovascular accident (CVA). See **stroke.**

cerebrum /ser'əbrəm, sərē'brəm/. See **brain.**

cerium (Ce), a gray rare earth element. A compound of cerium (cerium oxalate) is used as a sedative, to relieve nausea, and to control coughing.

ceroid /sir'oid/, a golden, waxy pigment appearing in the stomach and intestines, the nervous system, and the muscles. It is sometimes found in the livers of people with cirrhosis.

certified milk, raw milk that is handled in accordance with state health laws. The milk must be made by disease-free cows, which are regularly inspected by a veterinarian. The cows are milked by sterilized equipment in hygienic surroundings. The milk must have less than a certain low bacterial count. The milk must not be older than 36 hours when delivered.

certify, 1. to guarantee that certain requirements have been met based on expert knowledge of significant facts. **2.** to claim, by a legal process, that someone is insane. **3.** to claim the fact of someone's death in writing, usually on a form as required by local authority.

Cerubidine, a trademark for an anticancer drug (daunorubicin hydrochloride).

cerumen /siroo'mən/, a yellowish or brownish waxy substance. It is made by tiny glands (ceruminous) in the ear canal that release the waxy matter instead of watery sweat. Also called **earwax.**

ceruminosis /siroo'minō'-/, excess buildup of earwax in the outer ear canal. It can cause discomfort, hearing loss, and irritation leading to an ear infection. Removal of excess cerumen is done by inserting a wax softening agent. This is followed by carefully flushing the ear with an ear syringe.

cervical /sur'vikəl/, referring to the neck or a necklike structure, as the narrow lower end of the uterus (cervix).

cervical cancer, a malignant tumor of the uterine cervix. It can be detected in the early, curable stage by the Papanicolaou (Pap) test. The growth of cervical cancer is linked to sexual activity at an early age, having many sexual partners, genital herpesvirus infections, and multiple pregnancies. Poor obstetric and gynecologic care are other factors. Early cervical tumor growth is usually without symptoms. There may be a watery vaginal release or some spotting of blood. Advanced tumors may cause a dark, foul-smelling vaginal release, leakage from bladder or rectal canals (fistulas), weight loss, and back and leg pains. Pap smears of cervical cells are very important in screening. Diagnosis may require a biopsy. Cervical cancer invades the tissues of nearby organs. It may spread cancer cells through lymph channels to distant sites, including the lungs, bone, liver, or brain. Treatment depends on the kind and the extent of the cancer. It also depends on the woman's age and general health. Also considered are her wishes about keeping her reproductive function. Invasive tumors are treated with x-ray therapy or surgery (hysterectomy).

cervical cap, a birth control device. It is a small rubber cup that fits over the narrow lower end (cervix) of the uterus. It prevents sperm from entering the cervix. Some experts claim it is as effective as the diaphragm. It may be more comfortable than the diaphragm. It can be left safely on the cervix for days or weeks and remain effective. Accurate initial fitting by a trained person is needed. Practice by the user may be required to put the cap into proper position. The cap has become a popular contraceptive in Europe.

cervical disk syndrome, a spinal disorder in which nerves (cervical) around the neck and shoulders are squeezed or irritated. The cause may be herniated disks, degenerative disk disease, or neck injuries, especially those that overextend the vertebrae. Fluid usually pools around the injured area. Pain, the most common symptom, usually centers around the neck. It may also radiate down the arm to the fingers. See also **herniated disk.**

cervical erosion, a condition in which the lining (epithelium) of the narrow lower end of the uterus (cervix) is eroded as a result of infection or injury, as during childbirth. Treatment includes tissue destruction (cauterization) and douches.

cervical fistula, an abnormal passage from the narrow lower end of the uterus (cervix) to the vagina or bladder. The cause may be cancer, x-ray therapy, surgical injury, or injury during childbirth. A cervical fistula connecting with the bladder permits leakage of urine. When surgical repair is not possible, sitz baths, use of a deodorizing douche or powder, and protective pants may be advised.

cervical plexus, the network of nerves formed by divisions of the first four cervical nerves in the neck.

cervical polyp, an outgrowth of tissue on the wall of the passageway (cervical canal) through the uterine cervix. It is usually attached to the wall by a slender skin flap. Often there are no symptoms. However, polyps may cause bleeding, especially from contact during intercourse. Polyps are most common in women over 40 years of age. The cause is not known. A polyp is removed during surgery by turning the polyp on its stalk while pulling gently until it tears off. Little bleeding and prompt healing usually follow.

cervical smear, a small amount of the secretions and cells scraped from the narrow lower end of the uterus (cervix) with a sterile device. For a Pap smear, it is taken from the tissues of the uterine cervix and from the vaginal walls. The specimen is spread on a glass slide. It is then sent to a laboratory for microscopic examination.

cervical vertebra. See **vertebra.**

cervicitis /sur'visī'-/, sudden or long-term inflammation of the narrow lower end of the uterus (cervix). **Acute cervicitis** is an infection with redness, swelling, and bleeding of the cervix. Symptoms may include a foul-smelling discharge from the vagina, pelvic pressure or pain, slight bleeding with intercourse, and itching or burning of the outer genitals. The main causes are *Trichomonas vaginalis, Candida albicans,* and *Haemophilus vaginalis.* Specific antibiotics may be effective. Acute cervicitis tends to be a returning problem because of reexposure to the germ, ineffective treatment, multiple sexual partners, or poor general health. **Chronic cervicitis** is a persistent inflammation of the cervix. It usually occurs among women in their reproductive years. Symptoms are like those of the acute form. The cervix is congested and swollen. Cysts are often present. There may be old cuts from childbirth. A Pap smear is taken before treatment is started. Antibiotics are seldom effective. The symptoms of mild chronic cervicitis may lessen with creams or suppositories. The most effective treatments are hot or cold cautery to remove the diseased tissue. See also Candida albicans, **cautery, cervical cancer, cervical polyp.**

cervix /sur'viks/, the part of the uterus that protrudes into the cavity of the vagina. The cervix is divided into two parts: the portion above the vagina (supravaginal) and the vaginal portion. The outside of the supravaginal part is next to the bladder. They are separated by a band of tissue. The vaginal part of the cervix projects into the vagina. It has the **cervical canal,** the opening within the cervix. The canal is a passageway through which the menstrual flow escapes. It is completely widened during labor. The infant passes through this canal when childbirth is done vaginally. Many diagnostic and therapeutic procedures need widening of the canal, including obtaining samples of the uterine lining (endometrial biopsy), scraping of the surface (D&C), or putting in radium to treat cancer. Sperm must travel upward through the canal to reach the uterus and fallopian tubes. The mucus that is released by cervical glands changes in appearance and consistency through the menstrual cycle. The mucous membrane lining of the cervix is broken by many ridges, lumps, and cavities.

cesarean section /səser'ē·ən/, a surgical procedure in which the abdomen and uterus are cut open for childbirth. It is done when abnormal conditions exist that are judged likely to make vaginal birth dangerous for mother or child. About 15% of births in the United States are by cesarean section. The operation is performed less frequently in other countries. The maternal death rate is 0.1% to 0.2%. Reasons for the operation include severe bleeding from placenta abnormalities (placenta previa or abruptio placenta), severe toxemia (preeclampsia), fetal distress (such as from the umbilical cord around the neck), a baby too large to fit through the pelvis, a breech or transverse (sideways) presentation, and very difficult labor. A previous birth by cesarean section is no longer considered a good reason for doing it again in future births. Cesarean birth is less cause for injury to babies than a difficult forceps delivery. The cut in the skin of the abdomen may be horizontal or vertical. **Classical cesarean section** refers to a vertical cut, running from below the navel to above the pubic bone. For many doctors this is the fastest method of cesarean delivery and often used in emergencies. **Low cervical cesarean section** refers to a sideways (horizontal) cut in the thin lower part of the uterus. This bleeds less during surgery and heals with a stronger scar. A **bladder flap** is a fold of stomach lining (peritoneum) that is cut open during a low cesarean section (a ''bikini cesarean''). It allows the bladder to be separated from the uterus so that the cut can be made low on the uterus. An **extraperitoneal cesarean section** is a method for delivering a baby through a cut in the lower part of the uterus without entering the peritoneal cavity. This is done to avoid spreading infection from the uterus into the peritoneal cavity. It is somewhat slower to perform than other cesarean operations.

cesium 137, a radioactive material used in x-ray therapy to treat various cancers.

cestode infection. See **tapeworm infection.**

Cetacaine, a trademark for an anesthetic available as a spray, ointment, gel, or liquid. It is used to relieve pain of mucous membranes.

cetyl alcohol /sē′til/, a fatty alcohol. It is used as an emulsifier and stiffening agent in creams and ointments.

cetylpyridinium chloride, an antiinfection substance used as a skin cleanser to prevent infection of the skin or mucous membranes. Known allergy to this drug prohibits its use. The surface of the skin must be clean and well rinsed before use.

Ce-Vi-Sol, a trademark for a vitamin C (ascorbic acid) supplement.

CFM, cubic feet per minute.

CGA, Compressed Gas Association.

Chaddock reflex, an abnormal reflex induced by firmly stroking the skin of the forearm on the side opposite the thumb. This causes the wrist to flex and the fingers to spread like a fan. This reflex occurs on the affected side in partial paralysis.

Chaddock's sign, a variation of the Babinski reflex. It is induced by firmly stroking the side of the foot. This causes the great toe to extend and the other toes to fan. It is seen in disease of an area of the brain (pyramidal tract).

Chadwick's sign, the bluish color of the vulva and vagina that develops after the sixth week of pregnancy as a normal result of congestion of the blood vessels. It is an early sign of pregnancy.

chafe, an irritation of the skin by friction, as when rough material rubs against an unprotected area of the body.

Chagres fever /chag′ris/, an arbovirus infection carried to humans through the bite of a sandfly. Symptoms include fever, headache, and muscle pains of the chest or stomach. Also called **Panama fever.**

chain, 1. a length of units linked together, as a polypeptide chain of amino acids. 2. a group of individual bacteria linked together, as streptococci formed by a chain of cocci. 3. the relationship of some body structures, as the chain of small bones in the middle ear. Each bone moves in order in response to vibration of the eardrum, thus carrying the sound to the inner ear.

chain reaction, 1. a chemical reaction that makes a compound needed for the reaction to continue. 2. an atomic reaction that continues itself by continuing the splitting of nuclei and the release of atomic particles, which cause more nuclear splitting.

chalasia /kəlā′zhə/, the abnormal relaxation of a muscle (cardiac sphincter) at the junction of the esophagus with the stomach. This results in the stomach contents backing up into the esophagus. Infants with this disorder vomit after every feeding. Most grow out of it by about 6 months of age. See also **reflux.**

chalazion /kəlā′zē·on/, a small swelling of the eyelid. It results from obstruction of the glands in the eyelid. It often requires surgery for correction. See also **sty.**

chalkitis /kalkī′-/, an inflammation of the eyes. It is caused by rubbing the eyes with the hands after touching or handling brass. Also called **brassy eye.**

chamber, a hollow but not always empty space or cavity in an organ. An example is the upper and lower (atrial and ventricular) chambers of the heart.

chancre /shang′kər/, 1. a skin sore, usually from syphilis (venereal sore). It begins as a small lump and grows into a red, bloodless, painless ulcer with a scooped-out appearance. It heals without treatment, but is highly contagious. It leaves no scar. 2. an ulcerated area of the skin that marks the point of infection of a nonsyphilitic disease, as tuberculosis.

chancroid /shang′kroid/, a highly contagious, sexually carried disease caused by infection with *Haemophilus ducreyi.* It usually begins as a pimple on the skin of the external genitals. The chancroid grows and ulcerates. If untreated, the infection spreads, causing swollen lymph glands in the groin. A skin test is used to diagnose this condition. Sulfonamide drugs are given to treat chancroid. Because the ulcer looks like syphilis and other venereal infections, the diagnosis must be made before treatment in order to avoid obscuring other infections.

change of life, *informal.* the end of the female reproductive period. See also **menopause.**

channel, a passageway or groove that passes fluid, as the central channels that connect the small arterial branches (arterioles) with the small veins (venules).

chapped, referring to skin that is roughened, cracked, or reddened by exposure to cold or excess evaporation of sweat. Stinging or burning sensations are often felt with chapped skin. Treatment includes avoiding frequent washing, replacing ordinary soaps and detergents with super-fatted soaps, and applying softening drugs (emollients).

character, the group of traits and behavioral tendencies that enable a person to react in a relatively consistent way. Character, as contrasted with personality, implies choice and morality.

character disorder, a persistent, habitual, badly adaptive, and socially unacceptable pattern of behavior and emotional response. See also **antisocial personality disorder.**

Charcot-Marie-Tooth atrophy /shärkō′-mərē′-/, a hereditary disorder with breakdown of the nerves and muscles of the lower legs. This results in clubfoot, footdrop, and lack of muscle coordination.

Charcot's fever /shärkōz′/, a disorder with fever, yellowing of the skin (jaundice), and stomach pain on the right upper side linked to inflammation of the bile ducts. It is caused by a gallstone becoming lodged in the bile ducts.

charging station, container in which SCBA cylinders rest while being charged. Usually shielded to prevent injury to personnel if the cylinder ruptures.

charley horse, a painful condition of muscles in the back of the thigh (quadricep or hamstring). There is soreness and stiffness. It is the result of a strain, tear, or bruise of the muscle. Compare **cramp.**

chart, *informal.* a patient record.

chauffeur's fracture, any fracture of the wrist, caused by a twisting or a snapping type injury.

check-in, locations where assigned resources check in at an incident. The locations are: incident command post (resources unit), incident base, camps, staging areas, helibases, division supervisors (for direct line assignments). Check in at one location only, and complete ICS form 211.

check-up, a thorough study of the health of an individual.

Chediak-Higashi syndrome /ched′ēak·higä′shē/, an inherited disorder with partial absence of skin color (albinism), abnormal white blood cells, nervous system problems, returning infections, and early death.

cheek, a fleshy rise, especially the fleshy parts on both sides of the face between the eye and the jaw and the ear and the nose and mouth. Also called **bucca.**

cheilitis /kīlī′-/, inflammation and cracking of the lips. There are several forms including those caused by excessive exposure to sunlight, allergic sensitivity to cosmetics, and vitamin lack. Compare **cheilosis.**

cheilocarcinoma /kī′lōkär′sinō′mə/, a cancerous tumor of the lip.

cheiloplasty /kī′ləplas′tē/, correction by surgery of a defect of the lip.

cheilorrhaphy /kīlôr′əfē/, a surgical procedure that stitches the lip, as in the repair of a cleft lip or a cut lip.

cheilosis /kīlō′-/, a disorder of the lips and mouth. It features scales and cracks resulting from a lack of riboflavin (vitamin B_2) in the diet.

cheiromegaly /kī′rōmeg′əlē/, extremely large hands. –**cheiromegalic,** *adj.*

cheiroplasty /kī′rəplas′tē/, an operation involving plastic surgery of the hand.

chelation /kēlā′shən/, a chemical reaction in which a metal combines with another chemical to form a ring-shaped molecular complex. The process is used in chemotherapy for metal poisoning.

chemical, a substance made up of elements that can react with other substances; a substance produced by or used in chemical processes.

chemical abstract service (CAS) number, often used by state and local right-to-know regulations for tracking chemicals in the work place and the community. It is sometimes referred to as a chemical's ''social security number.''

chemical action, any process in which natural elements and compounds react with each other to produce a chemical change or a different compound. For example, hydrogen and oxygen combine to produce water.

chemical burn. See **burn.**

chemical equivalent, a drug with similar amounts of the same ingredients as another drug.

chemical gastritis, an inflammation of the stomach. It is caused by swallowing a chemical compound. The amount of damage depends on the substance. **Corrosive gastritis** is a severe condition caused by swallowing an acid, alkali, or other substance that eats away the lining of the stomach. **Erosive gastritis** is a condition in which a wearing away of areas in the mucous membrane lining the stomach has occured. Symptoms include nausea, loss of appetite, pain, and stomach bleeding. Correct treatment for gastritis depends on what was swallowed and how long it remained in the stomach. Treatment for erosion includes removing the irritating substance. Washing out the stomach (gastric lavage) is often advisable. However, neither lavage nor drugs to cause vomiting are given in cases involving the most corrosive poisons. See also **acid poisoning, alkali poisoning, gastritis.**

chemical name, the name of a drug by its chemical structure.

chemical stress, the result of a chemical reaction of two or more materials. Examples include corrosive materials attacking a metal, the pressure or heat generated by the decomposition or polymerization of a substance, or any variety of corrosive actions.

chemistry, the science dealing with the elements, their compounds, and the chemical structure and interactions of matter. **Applied chemistry** refers to the practical use of the study of chemical elements and compounds.

chemonucleolysis /kē'mōnoō'klēol'isis, kem'ō-/, a method of dissolving the cartilage between the vertebrae of the spine (intervertebral disk) by injecting a substance, such as chymopapain. It is done mainly to treat a herniated disk.

chemoreceptor, a sensory nerve cell that is activated by chemicals. An example is the chemoreceptor in the main artery (carotid) in the neck. It is sensitive to carbon dioxide in the blood, which signals the breathing center in the brain to increase or decrease breathing. The activity or reflex triggered by the stimulation of chemoreceptors is called **chemoreflex.**

chemosis /kimō'-/, an abnormal swelling of the mucous membrane covering the eyeball and lining the eyelids. It is usually the result of injury or infection. A blockage of normal lymph flow may be the cause of chemosis. Also called **conjunctival edema.**

chemosurgery, the destruction of cancerous, infected, or dead (gangrenous) tissue by applying chemicals. The technique is used to remove skin cancers.

chemotherapy, the treatment of disease with chemicals or drugs. The term is most often used in treating cancer. The drugs interfere with DNA synthesis by the tumor. Thus they kill off new cells as the tumor grows. However, normal body cells are destroyed as well. The drugs are given for short periods of time, followed by a rest to allow the body to recover. Side effects of chemotherapy include hair loss, nausea and vomiting, diarrhea, skin rash, mouth ulcers, severe anemia, and extreme weakness. There are four basic classes of anticancer drugs: alkylating agents, antimetabolites, antibiotics, and alkaloids. The drugs are most often used in combination. Chemotherapy is often started after surgery or radiation treatments. Chemotherapy has been very successful in some types of cancer.

chenodeoxycholic acid, an acid found in bile. It is given to dissolve gallstones. See also **ursodeoxycholic acid.**

cherry-red spot, an abnormal red area with white tissue around it on the retina of the eye. It is linked to retinal artery disorders. It sometimes appears in people with Tay-Sachs disease. Also called **Tay's spot.**

cherubism /cher'əbizm/, a hereditary disorder with swelling at the angles of the lower jaws, especially in children.

In some cases of cherubism, the entire jaw swells and the eyes turn up. This promotes the cherubic facial appearance.

chest. See **thorax.**

chest pain, a physical complaint that may be a symptom of heart or lung disease. Chest pain may also be caused by muscle or skeletal problems, digestive disorders, or other problems. Over 90% of severe chest pain is caused by coronary heart disease, compression of a spinal nerve, or a psychological disturbance. Because of its link to life-threatening heart disease, chest pain causes extreme anxiety. This tends to mask other symptoms that would aid in diagnosis and treatment. The quality of the pain (dull, sharp, or crushing) is important to the doctor's diagnosis. The site of the pain (in the center or side of the chest) must be located, including the spread of pain to other parts of the body. Also important are how long the pain has gone on, how it has developed, and whether it has occurred in the past. Factors must be identified that worsen or relieve the pain, as physical efforts, emotional distress, or deep breathing. Some conditions that can cause chest pain include rib fractures, swelling of the rib cartilage, muscle strain, inflammation of the esophagus, and peptic ulcers.

Cheyne-Stokes respiration (CSR) /chān'-/, an abnormal pattern of breathing. There are periods of breathlessness and deep, fast breathing. The breathing cycle begins with slow, shallow breaths that increase to abnormal depth and speed. Breathing slowly becomes shallower, climaxing in a 10- to 20-second period without breathing before the cycle is repeated. Each cycle may last from 45 seconds to three minutes. The cause of Cheyne-Stokes respiration is a complex change in the functioning of the breathing center in the brain. This pattern of breathing may occur in a patient who has taken a drug overdose. It occurs more often during sleep.

Chiari-Frommel syndrome /kē·är'ē-/, a hormonal disorder that occurs after a pregnancy in which weaning the baby does not spontaneously end milk production. It may go together with lack of menstruation. Treatment includes hormone therapy and investigation to determine if a pituitary tumor exists.

chickenpox, a highly contagious disease caused by a herpes virus, varicella zoster virus (VZV). It occurs mainly in young children and is usually benign. It features many itching, blisterlike eruptions on the skin. The fluid and scabs from the blisters are infectious until entirely dry. The disease may also be spread by droplets from the breathing tract of infected persons, usually in the early stages of the disease. The incubation period averages 2 to 3 weeks. A slight fever, mild headache, and loss of appetite occurs about 24 to 36 hours before the rash begins. The early period is usually mild in children, but may be severe in adults. The rash begins as flat red spots and develops in a day or two to raised bumps. These become blisters surrounding a reddened base and containing clear fluid. Within 24 to 48 hours the blisters turn cloudy. They are easily broken, and become encrusted. They erupt in crops so that all three stages are present at the same time. They appear first on the back and chest, and then spread to the face, neck, and limbs. They occur only rarely on the soles and palms. In severe cases, blisters in the throat may cause breathing difficulty and pain with swallowing. Fever, swollen lymph glands, and extreme irritability from itching are other symptoms. The symptoms last from a few days to 2 weeks. Treatment includes bed rest, drugs to reduce fever, antihistamines, and wet compresses. Calamine lotion may be used to relieve itching. Infected blisters may be treated with antibiotics. People who are susceptible and at risk for severe disease when exposed to the infection may be protected with immune globulin. Babies born to women who develop chickenpox within 5 days of birth may get a severe case of the disease. One attack of the disease gives permanent immunity. However, herpes zoster virus (HZV), like all herpes viruses, lies dormant in certain sensory nerve roots following a main infection. The virus is sometimes reactivated later in life (usually after age 50), with the eruption following the path of a nerve on the trunk, face, or limbs. Common complications are secondary bacterial infections, as abscesses, pneumonia, and blood poisoning. Less common complications are inflammation of the brain (encephalitis), Reye's syndrome, blood disorders, and liver disease (hepatitis). Also called **varicella.**

chigger, the larva of *Trombicula* mites found in tall grass and weeds. It sticks to the skin, causing irritation and severe itching.

chilblain /chil′blān/, redness and swelling of the skin caused by excess exposure to cold. Burning, itching, blistering, and ulceration may occur. Treatment includes protection against cold and injury, gentle warming, and avoiding tobacco. Also called **pernio.** Compare **frostbite.**

child, **1.** a person between the time of birth and adolescence. **2.** an unborn (fetus) or recently born (neonate or infant) human being. **3.** an offspring or descendant.

child abuse, the physical, sexual, or emotional mistreatment of a child. It often results in permanent physical or mental injury or, sometimes, death. Child abuse occurs mostly with children less than 3 years of age. Factors that contribute to child abuse include a stressful environment, as poor economic conditions, lack of physical and emotional support within the family, and any major life change or crisis, especially those arising from marital strife. Parents that abuse their children often have unsatisfied needs and difficulty in forming healthy relationships. Unrealistic

expectations of the child and a lack of nuturing experience also often occur. Many of those parents were neglected or abused in their own childhoods. Obvious physical marks on a child's body, as burns, welts, or bruises, and signs of emotional distress, including symptoms of failure to thrive, are common signs of neglect or abuse.

child bearing period, the reproductive period in a woman's life, from puberty to menopause. It is the time during which she is physically able to become pregnant.

childbirth. See **birth.**

childbirth center, a health facility where prenatal care and childbirth services are available to women who are healthy and have normal, uncomplicated pregnancies. The health care team includes nurse-midwives, obstetricians, jediatricians, and other health professionals.

child development, the various stages of physical, social, and psychological growth that occur from birth to adulthood.

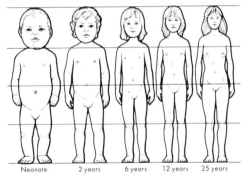

Child development and proportion

childhood, the period in human development that extends from birth until the beginning of puberty.

child welfare, any service sponsored by the community or special organizations that provide for the physical, social, or psychologic care of children in need.

chill, **1.** the sensation of cold from exposure to a cold environment. **2.** an attack of shivering with paleness and a feeling of coldness. Often it occurs at the beginning of an infection and goes together with a fast rise in body temperature.

Chinese restaurant syndrome, a reaction that occurs soon after eating food with the flavor additive monosodium glutamate. Symptoms include tingling and burning sensations of the skin, facial pressure, headache, and chest pain.

chip, a relatively small piece of a bone or tooth.

chip fracture, any small fracture that detaches from the bone. It usually involves a bone near a joint.

chiropodist /kirop′ədist, shir-/, a health professional trained to diagnose and treat diseases and disorders of the feet. Also called **podiatrist.**

chiropody /kirop′ədē, shir-/, the study of disorders of the feet and the practice of treating these disorders.

chiropractic /kī′rōprak′-/, a system of treatment that involves manipulation of the spinal column. It is based on the theory that the state of a person's health is determined by the condition of the musculoskeletal and nervous systems. Some practitioners take x-rays for diagnosis. Chiropractic therapy does not use drugs or surgery.

chisel fracture, any fracture in which a bone fragment becomes detached from the head of the radius in the forearm.

Chlamydia /kləmid′ē·ə/, a genus of microorganisms that live as parasites within the cell. They are classified as specialized bacteria. Two species of *Chlamydia* cause diseases in humans. *Chlamydia trachomatis* are organisms that live in the membrane lining the eye (conjunctiva) and the lining of the urine passage (urethra) and lower end of the uterus (cervix). They cause inflammation of the conjunctiva (inclusion conjunctivitis), venereal disease (lymphogranuloma venereum), and eye disease (trachoma). It is one of the most common sexually transmitted diseases in North America, and often causes sterility. *Chlamydia psittaci* are organisms that infect birds. They cause a type of pneumonia in humans. See also **psittacosis.**

chloasma /klō·az′mə/, tan or brown coloring, particularly of the forehead, cheeks, and nose. The condition is commonly linked to pregnancy and the use of birth control pills. Also called **mask of pregnancy.**

chloracne /klôrak′nē/, a skin condition caused by contact with chlorinated chemical compounds, as cutting oils, paints, varnishes, and dioxin. Symptoms are blackheads and pimples, usually on the face, arms, neck, and any other exposed areas.

chloral hydrate, a sedative and sleep inducer. It is used to relieve the inability to sleep (insomnia), anxiety, or tension. Liver or kidney disorders or known allergy to this drug prohibits its use. Side effects include upsets of the stomach and intestines, skin rash, excitability, and low blood pressure.

chlorambucil, an alkylating agent used to treat a variety of cancers. Severe anemia or known allergy to this drug prohibits its use. It is not given during the first three months of pregnancy or within 28 days of other chemotherapy or radiation therapy. Side effects include severe anemia, disturbance of stomach and intestines, skin rash, and liver disease.

chloramphenicol, an antibacterial and antiricksettsial drug used to treat a wide variety of serious infections. Mild or unidentified infections, pregnancy, breast feeding, or known allergy to this drug prohibits its use. Side effects include blood disorders and severe anemia.

chlorcyclizine hydrochloride, an antihistamine. It has been used for nasal congestion, sinus infection, and hayfever. As a cream, it is also used for skin conditions.

chlordiazepoxide, a minor tranquilizer used to treat anxiety, nervous tension, and alcohol withdrawal symptoms. Psychosis, eye disease (glaucoma), or known allergy to this drug prohibits its use. Side effects include withdrawal symptoms occurring on discontinuation of treatment. Drowsiness and weakness commonly occur.

chlorhexidine /klôrhek′sidin/, an antimicrobial agent. It is used as a surgical scrub, hand rinse, and antiseptic for the skin.

chloride /klôr′īd/, a chemical compound with chlorine.

chlorine (Cl) /klôr′ēn/, a yellowish-green, gaseous element of the halogen group. It has a strong, distinctive odor.

C–D

Guidelines for identifying potential child abusers

One or both parents were often abused as children.
  Studies indicate over 90% of abusive parents were abused children.
Parents tend to be lonely adults, attracted to each other as they search for loving parent figures.
Extreme personal and social isolation. These parents lack group and community integration and most often lack family support.
Unstable marital relationship. Parents lack positive feedback and support.
Low self-esteem.
Parent-child role reversal. The parents want the infant to meet their unfulfilled needs for mothering.
Unrealistic expectations of infants. Parents expect children to act older.
Parents unable to reach out and ask for help.

Special traits that make a child vulnerable to abuse
Usually young child, under 3 years of age.
Something different about child (i.e., pregnancy or delivery uncomfortable, child unwanted, premature birth).
Child is extremely irritable or cries often.
Birth order. Most often the first or last child is abused.

It is irritating to the breathing tract. It is poisonous if swallowed or inhaled. It occurs in nature chiefly as a component of sodium chloride in sea water and in salt deposits.

chloroform /klôr′əfôrm/, a nonflammable liquid. It was the first gas anesthetic to be discovered. Chloroform is a dangerous anesthetic drug, however. Delayed poisoning, even weeks after apparently complete recovery, can occur. Serious eye damage is often reported.

chloroformism /klôr′-/, the habit of inhaling chloroform for its narcotic effect.

chloroleukemia /klôr′əlo͞oke̅′me̅·ə/, a kind of myelocytic leukemia in which body fluids and organs get a green color. See also **leukemia.**

chlorolymphosarcoma /-lim′fo̅-särko̅′mə/, a greenish tumor of bone marrow (myeloid) tissue. It occurs in patients with myelocytic leukemia.

chloroma /klôro̅′mə/, a cancerous, greenish tumor. It occurs anywhere in the body in patients with myelocytic leukemia. The green pigment has no definite function. Also called **granulocytic sarcoma, green cancer.**

Chloromycetin, a trademark for an antibacterial and antirickettsial drug (chloramphenicol).

chlorophyll /klôr′əfil/, a plant pigment that absorbs light and changes it to energy. Chlorophylls a and b are found in green plants. Chlorophyll c occurs in brown algae. Chlorophyll d occurs in red algae. See also **photosynthesis.**

chloroprocaine /-pro̅′kān/, a local anesthetic with a chemical structure similar to procaine hydrochloride.

chloroquine /klôr′əkwīn′/, an antimalarial drug used to treat malaria, amebiasis, rheumatoid arthritis, some forms of skin disease (lupus erythematosus), and allergic reactions to light. Visual changes, porphyria, or known allergy to this drug prohibits its use. Side effects include disturbances of the stomach and intestines, headache, visual problems, and itching.

chlorothiazide, a diuretic and antihypertensive used to treat high blood pressure and water retention. Kidney dysfunction or known allergy to thiazide or sulfonamide drugs prohibits its use. Side effects include loss of potassium, high blood sugar, excess uric acid in the blood, and allergic reactions.

chlorotrianisene, an estrogen used to treat menopausal symptoms and prostatic cancer and to dry up breast milk after childbirth. Liver dysfunction, blood clots, unusual vaginal bleeding, known or suspected pregnancy, cancer that is stimulated by estrogen, or known allergy to this drug prohibits its use. Side effects include stomach and intestinal distress and breakthrough bleeding. In men, breast enlargement, decreased sexual interest, and impotence can occur.

chlorpheniramine maleate, an antihistamine used to treat a variety of allergic reactions, including rhinitis, skin rash, and itching. Asthma or known allergy to this drug prohibits its use. It is not given to newborn infants or nursing mothers. Side effects include skin rash, allergic reactions, and rapid heart beat.

chlorpromazine /klôrpro̅′məze̅n/, a tranquilizer and anti-nausea drug used to treat psychotic disorders, severe nausea and vomiting, and intractable hiccups.

chlorpropamide, an oral antidiabetic drug used to treat mild, stable non-insulin-dependent diabetes mellitus.

chlorprothixene, a drug used to treat psychotic disorders. Parkinson's disease, taking depressant drugs, liver or kidney failure, low blood pressure, or known allergy to this drug prohibits its use. Side effects include low blood pressure, liver toxicity, a variety of nervous system reactions, blood disorders, and allergic reactions.

chlortetracycline hydrochloride, an antibiotic used to treat many infections. Kidney or liver dysfunction, pregnancy, or known allergy to this drug or to other tetracycline drugs prohibits its use. Side effects include stomach and intestines disturbances, sensitivity to sunlight, and allergic reactions. Discoloration of teeth may occur in children exposed to this drug before 8 years of age.

chlorthalidone, a diuretic and antihypertensive. It is used to treat high blood pressure and fluid pooling. Inability to urinate or known allergy to this drug, to other thiazide drugs, or to sulfonamide drugs prohibits its use. Side effects include low calcium levels, high blood sugar, excess urea in the blood, and allergic reactions.

Chlor-Trimeton, a trademark for an antihistamine (chlorpheniramine maleate).

chlorzoxazone /klôrzok′səzo̅n/, a skeletal muscle relaxant. It is used to relieve muscle spasms. Known allergy to this drug prohibits its use. Side effects include liver disease (jaundice) and bleeding in the stomach and intestines.

choke, to interrupt breathing by compression or obstruction of the throat or windpipe.

chokes, a breathing condition that occurs in decompression sickness. Decompression sickness occurs from reduction of the surrounding pressure by deep sea diving or flying at high altitudes. Symptoms include shortness of breath, chest pain, and a cough caused by bubbles of gas in the blood vessels of the lungs. If not treated promptly by chamber recompression, death can result.

choking, the condition in which a breathing passage is blocked by constriction of the neck, an obstruction in the windpipe, or swelling of the throat. There is sudden coughing and a red face that rapidly becomes bluish from lack of oxygen. The person cannot breathe and clutches the throat. Emergency treatment requires removing an obstruction and resuscitation if necessary. See also **Heimlich maneuver.**

cholangeostomy /kōlan'jē·os'təmē/, a surgical operation to form an opening in a bile duct.

cholangiography /kōlan'jē·og'rəfē/, a special x-ray procedure for viewing the major bile ducts. A special dye is injected slowly into a vein. X-rays are taken of the region of the gallbladder. If the gallbladder has not been removed, a fatty meal may then be given and further x-rays taken to show contraction of the gallbladder.

cholangiohepatoma /kōlan'jē·ōhep'ətō'mə/, a liver cancer that has a mixture of liver cells and bile duct cells.

cholangioma /kōlan'jē·ō'mə/, a cancer of the bile ducts.

cholangitis /kō'lanjī'-/, inflammation of the bile ducts. Causes include bacterial infection, and blocking of the ducts by stones or a tumor. Symptoms include severe pain in the right upper part of the belly, yellow skin (jaundice) if an obstruction is present, and fever.

cholecalciferol. See **vitamin D₃.**

cholecystectomy /kō'lisistek'-/, the removal by surgery of the gallbladder. The bile duct is tied off. Any stones found in the bile duct are removed. A T-tube is placed in the incision temporarily to drain bile to the outside of the body. Usually after about 10 days it is removed. The most common complication is a disruption of the liver or other ducts of the biliary system. This needs surgical correction. Wound infection, bleeding, bile leakage, and jaundice may also occur.

cholecystitis /-sistī'-/, sudden or long-term inflammation of the gallbladder. **Acute cholecystitis** is usually caused by a gallstone that cannot pass through the bile duct. Pain is felt in the right upper part of the belly. Other symptoms include nausea, vomiting, belching, and intestinal gas (flatulence). **Chronic cholecystitis,** the more common type, has a slower beginning. Pain, often felt at night, may follow a fatty meal. Complications include gallstones, inflammation of the pancreas, and cancerous growth (carcinoma) of the gallbladder. Diagnosis of either form of the disorder is usually made with x-rays. Surgery is the usual treatment.

cholecystography /-sistog'rəfē/, an x-ray examination of the gallbladder. At least 12 hours before the study the patient has a fat-free meal and swallows a tablet containing iodine. The iodine material may also be injected into a vein. The iodine is released by the liver into the bile in the gallbladder. The patient then may consume a fatty meal. This stimulates the gallbladder to contract, expelling bile and the dye into the bile duct. Additional x-rays are taken about an hour later.

cholecystokinin /-sis'təkī'nin/, a hormone produced by cells of the small intestine. It stimulates contraction of the gallbladder and the release of enzymes from the pancreas.

Choledyl, a trademark for a bronchi widener (bronchodilator) used to treat asthma (oxtriphylline).

cholelithiasis /-lithī'əsis/, the presence of gallstones in the gallbladder. The condition affects about 20% of the population over age 40. It is more common in women. Many patients complain of general stomach discomfort, burping, and intolerance to certain foods. Other patients have no symptoms at all. See also **gallstone.**

cholelithotomy /-lithot'-/, a surgical operation to remove gallstones through an incision in the gallbladder.

cholera /kol'ərə/, a serious bacterial infection of the small intestine. Symptoms include severe diarrhea and vomiting, muscular cramps, and dehydration. The disease is spread by water and food that have been contaminated by feces of infected persons. The symptoms are caused by toxic substances made by the bacterium *Vibrio cholerae*. The profuse, watery diarrhea (as much as a quart or a liter an hour) depletes the body of fluids and minerals. Complications include circulatory collapse, destruction of kidney tissue, and pooling of acid (acidosis). Mortality is as high as 50% if the infection is untreated. Treatment includes antibiotics and restoring fluids and electrolytes with intravenous solutions. A cholera vaccine is available for people traveling to areas where the infection is common. Other preventive measures include drinking only boiled or bottled water and eating only cooked foods.

cholera vaccine, an agent used to immunize persons against cholera. Acute infection, use of corticosteroids, or known allergy to this drug prohibits its use. The most serious side effect is an allergic reaction.

cholestasis /-stā'-/, interruption in the flow of bile through any part of the biliary system, from liver to intestine. The cause may be within the liver (intrahepatic) or outside it (extrahepatic). Intrahepatic causes include liver disease (hepatitis), drug and alcohol use, and pregnancy. Extrahepatic causes may be an obstructing gallstone or tumor in the common bile duct or cancer of the pancreas. Symptoms of both types of cholestasis include yellowing of skin (jaundice), pale and fatty stools, dark urine, and intense itching of the skin. If liver disease is suspected, liver biopsy can confirm the suspicion, and attempts can be made to treat the underlying disorder. Extrahepatic cholestasis usually requires surgery.

cholesteatoma /kōles'tē·ətō'mə/, a cyst in the middle ear. It occurs as an inborn defect or as a complication of an ear infection (otitis media).

cholesterase /koles'tərās/, an enzyme in the blood and other areas of the body that forms cholesterol and fatty acids.

cholesterol /koles'trôl/, substance found in animal fats and oils, egg yolk, and the human body. It is most common in the blood, brain tissue, liver, kidneys, adrenal glands, and fatty covers around nerve fibers. It helps to absorb and move fatty acids. Cholesterol is necessary for the making of vitamin D on the surface of the skin. It is also needed for the making of various hormones, including the sex hormones. It sometimes hardens in the gallbladder to form gallstones. Cholesterol is found in foods from animals and is constantly made in the body, mainly in the liver and the kidneys. High amounts of cholesterol in the blood may be linked to the development of cholesterol deposits in the blood vessels (atherosclerosis).

cholesterolemia /-ē'mē·ə/, the presence of too much cholesterol in the blood.

cholesterolosis /-ō'sis/, a rare condition, found in about 5% of patients with long-term inflammation of the gallbladder (cholecystitis). It produces deposits of cholesterol in the lining of the gallbladder. Cholesterolosis is often linked to gallstones.

cholestyramine resin, a drug used to reduce too much cholesterol in the blood (hyperlipoproteinemia) and for itching resulting from partial blockage of bile. Complete blockage of bile or known allergy to this drug prevents its use. Side effects include severe constipation, stomach problems, and loss of vitamins A, D, and K.

choline /kō'lēn/, one of the B complex vitamins, essential for the use of fats in the body. It is a large part of the nerve signal carrier (acetylcholine). It stops fats from being deposited in the liver and helps the movement of fats into the cells. The richest sources of choline are liver, kidneys, brains, wheat germ, brewer's yeast, and egg yolk. Lack of choline leads to cirrhosis of the liver, resulting in bleeding stomach ulcers, damage to the kidney, high blood pressure, high blood levels of cholesterol, cholesterol deposits in blood vessels (atherosclerosis), and hardening of the arteries (arteriosclerosis). See also **inositol, lecithin.**

cholinergic /-ur'jik/, **1.** referring to nerve fibers that release a nerve signal carrier (acetylcholine) at the connections of muscles and nerves. **2.** the tendency to pass on or to be stimulated by a nerve signal carrier (acetylcholine). Compare **adrenergic, anticholinergic.**

cholinergic blocking agent, any drug that blocks the action of the nerve signal carrier (acetylcholine) and similar substances.

cholinesterase /-es'tərās/, an enzyme that causes the breakdown of the nerve signal carrier (acetylcholine).

Choloxin, a trademark for a drug used to reduce excess cholesterol in the blood (dextrothyroxine sodium).

chondrectomy /kondrek'-/, the surgical removal of cartilage.

chondroangioma /kon'drō·an'jē·ō'mə/, a harmless tumor containing blood vessels and cartilage.

chondroblastoma /-blastō'mə/, a benign tumor formed from simple cartilage cells. It develops most often in growth areas of the thigh bone (femur) and upper arm bone (humerus) in young men. Also called **Codman's tumor.**

chondrocalcinosis /-kal'sinō'-/, a type of arthritis in which calcium deposits are found in the joints of hands and feet. Chondrocalcinosis is similar to gout. It is often found in patients over 50 who have long-term joint disease (osteoarthritis) or diabetes. Also called **pseudogout.** Compare **gout.**

chondrocostal /-kos'təl/, referring to the ribs and the cartilages of the ribs.

chondrodystrophia calcificans congenita /-distrō'fē·ə kalsif'ikəns konjen'itə/, an inherited defect that affects the growth of long bones. This defect can be seen on x-ray films of newborn infants. Dwarfism, shortening of muscles, cataracts, mental retardation, and short stubby fingers develop as the infant grows into childhood.

chondrodystrophy /-dis'trəfē/, a group of illnesses in which cartilage changes to bone, especially in the long bones. Patients are dwarfed, with normal trunks and short arms and legs.

chondrofibroma /-fībrō'mə/, a fiberlike tumor containing cartilage elements.

chondroma /kondrō'mə/, a fairly common, harmless tumor of cartilage cells. These cells grow slowly inside cartilage (enchondroma) or on the surface (ecchondroma).

chondromalacia /-məlā'shə/, a softening of cartilage.

chondromyxofibroma /-mik'sōfībrō'mə/, a benign tumor that grows from connective tissues that form cartilage. The tumor is typically a firm, grayish-white, somewhat rubbery mass. These tumors tend to occur in the knee and small bones of the foot. Also called **chondromyxoid fibroma.**

chondroplasty /kon'drəplas'tē/, the surgical repair of cartilage.

chondrosarcoma /-särkō'mə/, a cancerous tumor of cartilage cells. This tumor occurs most often on long bones, the pelvis, and the shoulder. The usual tumor is a large, smooth, well-defined growth. A **central chondrosarcoma** is one that forms inside a bone.

chordae tendineae /kôr'dē tendin'i·ē/, *sing.* **chorda tendinea,** strong fibrous bands in the heart that attach the corners of the heart valves to the muscles of the lower heart chambers (ventricles). They prevent the valves from protruding into the upper heart chambers (atria) as the heart beats.

chordee /kôr′dē, -dā/, a birth defect of the genital and urinary systems. The penis curves, caused by a fiberlike band of tissue instead of normal skin along the shaft of the penis. This is often linked to a defect in the placement of the urinary opening on the penis (hypospadias). It is surgically corrected in early childhood. The surgery improves the appearance of the genitals and constructs an organ that allows the boy to urinate in a standing position. It also produces a sexually functional organ.

chordencephalon /kôrd′ənsef′əlon/, the part of the central nervous system that develops in the early weeks of pregnancy from the nerve tube. It later becomes the nerves of the spinal cord that control senses and movement.

chorditis /kôrdī′-/, inflammation of a spermatic cord or of the vocal cords.

chordoma /kôrdō′mə/, a rare, inherited tumor of the brain. It is usually found in the center of the brain. Although it grows slowly, it spreads very easily. Surgical removal is rarely possible.

chordotomy /kôrdot′-/, an operation in which parts of the spinal cord are surgically divided to relieve pain.

chorea /kôrē·ə/, a condition of uncontrolled, purposeless, rapid motions. Typical movements are bending and extending the fingers, raising and lowering the shoulders, or grimacing.

chorioadenoma /kôr′ē·ō·ad′ənō′mə/, a tumor of the outer membrane protecting the fetus (chorion).

chorioamnionitis /-am′nē·oni′-/, inflammation in the membranes protecting the fetus (amniotic sac) caused by organisms in the fluid surrounding the fetus.

choriocarcinoma /-kär′sinō′mə/, a cancer that develops from the membranes protecting the fetus, usually from a cystic mole. Less often it grows following an abortion, during a normal or tubal (ectopic) pregnancy, or from a tumor of the genitals. The tumor most often first appears in the uterus as a soft, dark red, crumbling mass. It may attack and destroy the wall of the uterus and spread through lymph or blood vessels. It then forms more tumors in the wall of the vagina, vulva, lymph nodes, lungs, liver, and brain. The urine often contains much more of the hormone chorionic gonadotropin than is usual in pregnancy. The hormone level returns to normal when the tumor is completely removed.

choriocele /kôr′ē·əsēl′/, a hernia or bulging of tissue in the back (choroid layer) of the eyeball.

chorion /kôr′ē·on/. See **amniotic sac.**

chorioretinitis /-ret′əni′-/, inflammation of the outer membrane and retina of the eye, usually as a result of infection. Symptoms are blurred vision, sensitivity to light, and distorted images.

chorioretinopathy /-ret′inop′əthē/, a disease of the eye that involves the outer membrane of the eye (choroid) and the retina. Inflammation does not occur.

choroid /kôr′oid/, a thin membrane richly supplied with blood that covers the white of the eyeball. It begins near the iris and wraps around the back of eye. The choroid supplies blood to the retina. It conducts nerves and arteries to the front of the eye.

choroidal malignant melanoma, a tumor of the membrane surrounding the eyeball (choroid) that causes the retina to separate from the eye.

choroiditis, inflammation of the outer membrane of the eye (choroid). See also **chorioretinitis.**

choroidocyclitis /-siklī′-/, an inflammation of the eye that affects the outer membrane and the process that controls focusing of the lens.

choroid plexus, any one of the tangled masses of tiny blood vessels found in several parts of the brain.

Christchurch chromosome (Ch^1), an abnormally small chromosome that is linked to long-term leukemia centered in the lymph tissues. It has also been found in patients with various other inherited defects.

chromaffin cell /krō′məfin/, any one of the special cells linked to sympathetic nerves, which are nerves that produce the "flight or fight" response. Chromaffin cells in the adrenal glands secrete hormones (epinephrine and norepinephrine) that increase heart rate, raise blood pressure, increase breathing, and slow digestion. They are most highly responsive to stress.

chromatic, 1. referring to color. 2. able to be stained by a dye. 3. referring to chromatin. Also **chromatinic.**

chromatic dispersion, the splitting of light into its wavelengths or frequencies. A prism is often used to separate and study the different colors.

chromatid /krō′mətid/, one of the two identical threadlike fibers of a chromosome. It results when the chromosome reproduces itself. The two chromatid fibers making up each chromosome are joined in the center. During cell division, it divides lengthwise to form identical chromosomes.

chromatin /krō′mətin/, the material in the center of a cell (nucleus) that forms the chromosomes. It is made up of fine, threadlike strands of DNA attached to protein. During cell division, parts of the chromatin condense and coil to form the chromosomes. **Chromatin-negative** refers to the centers of cells (nuclei) that lack sex chromatin. This is distinctive of the normal male. **Chromatin-positive** refers to the nuclei that contain sex chromatin. This is distinctive of the normal female.

chromatism, 1. an abnormal condition in which the person suffers hallucinations and sees colored lights. 2. abnormal pigmentation.

chromatopsia /-top′se̅·ə/,   **1.** a visual defect that makes colorless objects appear touched with color. **2.** a form of color blindness in which the patient may not see various colors correctly. It may be caused by a lack of one or more of the cells in the retina or from incorrect color messages being carried. See also **color blindness.**

chromesthesia /kro̅′məsthe̅′zhə/,   a condition in which the person confuses other senses, as hearing, taste, or smell, to be sensations of color.

chromhidrosis /kro̅′midro̅′-/,   a rare disorder in which the sweat glands secrete colored sweat. The sweat may be yellow, blue, green, or black and often also glows (fluoresces). A cause is regular exposure to copper, catechols, or ferrous oxide.

-chromic, -chromatic,   **1.** a combining form meaning the number of colors seen by the eye. **2.** a combining form meaning a specific color of the blood indicating the hemoglobin content. **3.** a combining form meaning the ability of bacteria and tissues to be stained. **4.** a combining form meaning a specified skin color as a symptom of disease.

chromium (Cr),   a hard, brittle, metallic element. It does not occur naturally in pure form but exists with iron and oxygen in chromite. Traces of chromium occur in plants and animals. This element may be important in human nutrition, especially in digestion of carbohydrates. Workers in chromite mines are susceptible to a long-term lung disorder (pneumoconiosis) caused by breathing chromite dust.

chromobacteriosis /kro̅′məbaktir′e̅·o̅′-/,   a rare, usually fatal infection caused by bacteria found in fresh water in tropic and subtropic regions. They enter the body through a cut in the skin. The symptoms are fever, liver abscesses, and severe exhaustion. Early diagnosis, surgical drainage of abscesses, and giving the drug chloramphenicol greatly improve the chance of survival.

chromoblastomycosis /-blas′təmiko̅′-/,   an infectious skin disease caused by a fungus. Symptoms include itching, warty bumps that develop in a cut or other break in the skin. These first appear as a small dull-red bump, slowly becoming a large ulcerlike growth. Over weeks or months, more warty growths may appear on the skin. Treatment includes surgical removal and, in some cases, applying antibiotics to the skin.

chromonema /-ne̅′mə/,   a twisted thread in a chromosome to which beadlike structures (chromomeres) attach. It forms the central part of the chromosome during cell division.

chromosomal aberration /-so̅′məl/,   any change in the normal structure or number of any of the chromosomes. This can result in birth defects ranging from mild to severe. In humans, a number of physical disabilities are linked to defects of both the non-sex chromosomes (autosomes) and the sex chromosomes. Some of these include Down's syndrome, Turner's syndrome, and Kleinfelter's syndrome.

chromosomal nomenclature,   a system used to identify the groupings of chromosomes in a person. The system features the number of chromosomes, sex, and the lack or addition of a specific chromosome or part of a chromosome. The grouping for a normal female is 46,XX, and for a normal male, 46,XY (X and Y are sex chromosomes). Any defect in the normal number or structure of the chromosomes can be indicated by this system.

chromosome /kro̅′məso̅m/,   any one of the threadlike structures in the center of a cell (nucleus) that carries genetic information. Each is made up of a double strand of twisted DNA (deoxyribonucleic acid). Along the length of each strand of DNA lie the genes, which contain the genetic material that controls the inheritance of traits. In cell division chromosomes reproduce themselves. **Daughter chromosome** refers to either of the two spiral strands (chromatids) that make up a chromosome. These separate and go to opposite ends of the cell before cell division. Each contains the complete genetic information of the original chromosome. In this way each new cell has a full set of chromosomes. Each species has a certain number of chromosomes, called a **chomosome complement**. Humans have 46 chromosomes. These include 22 pairs of nonsex chromosomes (autosomes) and one pair of sex chromosomes. Each parent contributes one sex chromosome. –**chromosomal,** *adj.*

chronic,   referring to a disease or disorder that develops slowly and persists for a long period of time. This is different from the course of an acute disease that attacks suddenly and ends quickly. The symptoms of chronic disease are usually less severe than those of the acute form of the same disease. Chronic disease can sometimes remain for the person's lifetime and result in complete or partial disability. Chronic glaucoma is an example of this type of disease. Compare **acute.**

chronic brain syndrome (CBS),   an abnormal condition that is caused by damage to the brain tissue. The symptoms are loss of memory and disorientation. It may occur in several diseases (dementia paralytica, cerebral arteriosclerosis, brain injury, and Huntington's chorea).

chronic care,   a type of medical care that concentrates on lasting care of people with long-term disorders. This care may be given either at home or in a medical facility. It includes medical treatment, as well as helping the patients to care for themselves and to eat properly. Physical therapy is also used to prevent loss of function.

chronic health hazard,   marked by a long or permanent duration, consistent or continuous (e.g., chronic toxicities are usually permanent or irreversible). Often occurs from repeated exposures over a period of time.

chronic lymphocytic leukemia (CLL). See **leukemia.**

chronic myelocytic leukemia (CML). See **leukemia.**

chronic obstructive pulmonary disease (COPD). See **pulmonary disease.**

chronologic age, the age of a person stated as the amount of time that has passed since birth. For example, the age of an infant is stated in hours, days, or months, and the age of children and adults is stated in years.

chronotropism /krənot′rəpizm/, anything that affects the rhythm of a function of the body, such as interfering with the rate of heartbeat.

chrysotherapy /kris′ō-/, the treatment of any disease with gold salts.

Churg-Strauss, an allergy in which tumorlike masses appear, usually in the lungs. This often involves the circulatory system.

Chvostek's sign /khvosh′teks/, an abnormal spasm of the face muscles when the facial nerve is lightly tapped. This spasm occurs in patients who have low blood calcium. It is a sign of a disorder of the nerves supplying the muscles (tetany).

chyle /kīl/, the cloudy liquid that results from digestion in the small intestine. Consisting mainly of fats, chyle passes through tiny fingerlike bulges (lacteals) in the small intestine. It then goes into the lymph system for transport to the blood veins.

chylothorax /kī′lōthôr′aks/, a condition in which fluid caused by digestion in the intestine (chyle) makes its way through the thoracic duct in the chest to the space around the lungs. The cause is usually an injury to the neck or a tumor that attacks the thoracic duct. Treatment is surgical repair of the duct.

chyluria /kīlŏŏr′ē·ə/, milky appearing urine caused by the presence of digestive juices (chyle) from the intestine.

chyme /kīm/, the thick and gummy contents of the stomach during digestion of food. Chyme then passes through into the beginning of the small intestine (duodenum), where further digestion takes place.

chymopapain /kī′mōpəpā′in/, an enzyme found in the tropical fruit papaya. It is used to treat ruptured or herniated vertebral disks.

chymotrypsin /-trip′sin/, an enzyme, produced by the pancreas, that speeds the breakdown of milk protein (casein) and gelatin. It is used to treat digestive problems in which the enzyme is deficient or totally gone.

chymotrypsinogen /-tripsin′əjən/, a substance that is made in the pancreas. It is turned into the digestive enzyme chymotrypsin by trypsin.

cibophobia /sē′bō-/, an abnormal aversion to food or to eating.

cicatrix /sik′ətriks, sikā′-/, scar tissue that is pale, tight, and firm. As the skin begins to heal, it becomes red and soft.

ciclopirox, an antifungal drug used to treat ringworm (tinea) and yeast (candidiasis) infections. Known allergy to this drug prohibits its use. Side effects include allergy of the skin.

cicutism /sik′yətizm/, poisoning caused by water hemlock. Symptoms include lack of oxygen which results in blue skin, widened pupils, convulsions, and coma.

cigarette drain, a drain to allow fluids to escape from a wound or surgical cut. It is made from a piece of gauze drawn into a narrow tube.

ciguatera poisoning /sē′gwəter′ə/, food poisoning that results from eating fish infected with the ciguatera poison. The poison comes from tiny creatures that the fish eat. Over 400 types of fish from the Caribbean and South Pacific are thought to carry this poison. Symptoms include vomiting, diarrhea, tingling or numbness of limbs and the skin around the mouth, itching, muscle weakness, and pain. Symptoms last 6 to 18 hours. Abnormal nerve sensations may last for months. Cold liquids feel hot to the mouth and throat. No treatment has been developed.

cilia /sil′e·ə/, *sing.* **cilium, 1.** the eyelashes. **2.** small, hairlike projections on the outer layer of some cells, helping processing by making motion in a fluid. **–ciliary,** *adj.*

ciliary body /sil′ē·er′ē/, the part of the eye that joins the iris with the blood vessel layer (choroid). Continuous with the ciliary body is the **ciliary margin,** the outer border of the iris of the eye.

ciliary gland, one of the many tiny sweat glands found in several rows on the eyelids. These glands lie near the eyelashes. Bacterial infection of one or more of the ciliary glands causes sties.

ciliary muscle, a partly clear, round band of smooth muscle fibers of the eye. These help adjust the eye to view near objects.

ciliary reflex. See **accommodation reflex.**

Ciliata /sil′ē·ā′tə/, a type of tiny primitive creature (protozoa) that has cilia through its whole life. The only important ciliate in humans is the intestinal parasite *Balantidium coli,* which causes dysentery.

ciliospinal reflex /sil′ē·ōspī′nəl/, a normal reflex caused by scratching or pinching the skin of the back of the neck. This results in widening (dilation) of the pupils. Also called **pupillary-skin reflex.**

cimetidine, a drug used to treat duodenal ulcer, pancreatitis, and too much stomach acid.

cineradiography /sin′irā′dē·og′rəfē/, the filming with a movie camera of body images that appear on a fluorescent screen. A nontoxic dye is first injected into the patient.

This is done to study the action of body structures, such as the blood vessels, for diagnostic purposes.

cingulectomy /sing′gyəlek′-/,   the surgical removal of part of the bundle of nerve fibers (cingulate gyrus) and nearby tissue in the front part of the brain.

cingulotomy /sing′gyəlot′-/,   brain surgery to relieve constant pain. The operation stops the nerves in the bundle of nerve fibers (cingulum gyrus) by applying heat or cold to the tissues.

circadian rhythm /sərkā′dē·ən, sur′kədē′ən/,   the biologic clock in humans based on a 24-hour cycle. At regular intervals each day, the body becomes hungry or tired, active or peevish. Body temperature is highest in the afternoon or evening. It drops to its lowest point from 2 A.M. to 5 A.M. Heart beat, blood pressure, breathing, urine flow, hormones, and enzymes rise and fall in a rhythmic pattern. Interference with this rhythm can cause impatience, less mental alertness, problems with sleep, stomach upsets, and rapid heart beat. Jet lag and some sleeping disorders are common causes of circadian disturbance. Some drugs affect the body more at certain times during the day than at others.

circle of Willis,   a group of arteries at the base of the brain. The circle is formed by the connections between branches of the arteries that supply the brain.

CircOlectric (COL) bed,   a trademark for a bed run by electricity that can be rotated up 210 degrees. This type of bed is used in orthopedics, for patients with severe burns, and for cardiovascular patients. The bed is made up of a round frame and two straight frames inside the circle. The patient is "sandwiched" between the straight frames during rotation.

circular bandage,   a bandage wrapped around an injured part, usually an arm or leg.

circular fold,   one of the many ring-shaped folds in the small intestine formed by mucous tissue.

circulation,   movement of a substance in a round course so that it returns to its starting point. An example is the circulation of blood through the arteries and veins.

circulation time,   the time it takes for blood to flow from one part of the body to another. A dye or radioactive substance is injected into a vein and timed to find how long it takes to return to the same point in the body. A substance such as saccharin can also be injected. Then the time it takes to travel to the tongue is noted.

circulatory failure,   an inability of the heart and blood vessel (cardiovascular) system to supply enough blood to meet the needs of the cells. One cause is an abnormal function of the heart, such as from a heart attack. Other causes are not enough blood in the body, as in severe bleeding, or from collapse of the blood vessels, such as in blood poisoning. See also **shock.**

circulatory system,   the network consisting of the heart, blood vessels, and lymph vessels through which the blood and lymph circulates. See also **cardiovascular system, lymphatic system.**

circumcision,   a surgical removal of the foreskin of the penis or, rarely, the hood of the clitoris. Circumcision is often performed on newborn boys in spite of a lack of known medical benefit. There is also a small but real risk of complications. Circumcision can be performed on adult males to treat tightness of the foreskin (phimosis) and inflammation of the penis (balanitis). Circumcision is required by the religions of about one sixth of the people of the world.

circumduction,   1. the round movement of a limb or the eye. **2.** the motion of the head of a bone in a socket, as the hip joint. Circumduction is one of the 4 basic kinds of motion of the joints of the skeleton. Compare **angular movement, gliding, rotation.** See also **joint.**

circumoral /sur′kəmôr′əl/,   referring to the part of the face around the mouth.

circum-speech,   the behaviors that are linked to conversation. They include body language, keeping of personal space between persons, handsweeps, head nods, and activity, as walking or knitting, while carrying on a conversation.

circumstantiality,   a disorder in which a person is unable to separate important from unimportant facts while describing an event. The person may include every detail, losing the train of thought. Very often the person may need to have questions repeated. It may be a sign of chronic brain dysfunction. Compare **flight of ideas.**

circus movement,   1. an abnormal involuntary rolling or somersaulting. It is caused by injured parts of the brain that control body posture. **2.** an abnormal circular walk caused by injury to the brain or other nerve centers.

cirrhosis /sirō′-/,   a long-term disease of the liver in which the liver becomes covered with fiberlike tissue. This causes the liver tissue to break down and become filled with fat. All functions of the liver then decrease, such as making of glucose and vitamin absorption. Stomach and bowel function and making of hormones are also affected. Blood flow through the liver is blocked. Symptoms include nausea, appetite loss, weight loss, light-colored stools, weakness, stomach pain, varicose veins, and noticeable veins (often on the face). Unless the cause of the disease is removed, coma, bleeding in the stomach and bowels, and kidney failure occur. Cirrhosis is most often the result of long-term alcohol abuse. It can also result from malnutrition, hepatitis, or other infection. X-ray tests, physical examination, and blood tests of liver function are done to watch the growth of the disease. Treatment includes a balanced diet rich in protein, vitamins (especially folic acid), rest, and total avoidance of alcohol. The liver is able to restore itself, unless too much tissue is destroyed, but recovery may be very slow. See also **biliary cirrhosis.** – **cirrhotic,** *adj.*

cisplatin, an anticancer drug used to treat many types of cancerous tumors, such as those of the testicles, prostate, and ovaries. Kidney failure, hearing loss, or known allergy to this drug prohibits its use. Side effects include poisoning, severe nausea, appetite loss, vomiting, and allergic reactions.

cisterna /sistur′nə/, *pl.* **cisternae,** a cavity that holds lymph or other body fluids. An example is a **cisterna subarachnoidea,** any one of many spaces in the brain that hold fluid from the brain and spine (cerebrospinal fluid).

cisternal puncture, insertion of a needle into a space containing fluids of the brain and spine (cerebellomedullary cistern) near the base of the skull. The purpose is to take out the fluid for examination.

cisvestitism /sisves′titizm/, wearing clothing correct for the sex, but not the age, occupation, or status of the wearer.

Citanest Hydrochloride, a trademark for a local anesthetic (prilocaine hydrochloride).

citric acid, a white, crystal-like organic acid which dissolves in water and alcohol. It is taken from citrus fruits, especially lemons and limes. Citric acid is used to flavor foods, carbonated drinks, and medicinal products, as laxatives. It is also used to prevent scurvy.

citrin, a crystal-like substance that is used as a source of bioflavonoid, which maintains the walls of small blood vessels.

Cl, symbol for **chlorine.**

Claforan, a trademark for an antibiotic (cefotaxime sodium).

clairvoyance /klervoi′əns/, the alleged ability to be aware of objects or events without the use of the physical senses, as sight or hearing.

clamp, an instrument with notched tips and locking handles. In surgery, clamps are most often used to control bleeding.

clang association, the mental connection between unrelated ideas that is made because the two words sound similar. This happens often during manic-depression (bipolar disorder).

clasp, **1.** a fitting that is fastened over a tooth to hold a partial denture in place. **2.** any surgical device for holding tissues together, especially bones.

clasp-knife reflex, an abnormal reflex in which a spastic arm or leg can not be moved and then suddenly jerks, like the the blade of a jackknife. It indicates damage to the brain's involuntary control system.

claudication, a pain of the legs with cramps in the calves caused by poor circulation of blood in the legs. The condition is often linked to hardening of the arteries (atherosclerosis) and may include lameness or limping. **Intermittent claudication** is a form of the disorder that occurs only at certain times, often after a period of walking. It is relieved by rest.

claustrophobia /klôs′trə-/, a great fear of being trapped in closed or narrow places. This fear is seen more often in women than in men. Sometimes it can be traced to some very frightening event involving closed spaces, usually occurring in childhood. Treatment includes finding the cause, if possible, and changing the person's behavior towards the feared situation. See also **behavior therapy.**

claustrum /klôs′trəm/, *pl.* **claustra,** **1.** a barrier, as a membrane that partly closes an opening. **2.** a thin sheet of gray matter in the brain.

clavicle /klav′ikəl/, the collarbone. It is a long, curved, horizontal bone just above the first rib, forming the front portion of the shoulder. It starts to form before any other bone in the body, but does not totally unite with the breastbone (sternum) until about the twenty-fifth year. It is shorter, thinner, less curved, and smoother in women than in men. In persons who perform regular heavy manual labor, it becomes thicker, more curved, and more ridged for muscle attachment.

clawhand, a hand seriously bent into a fixed position. Also called **main en griffe** /menäNgrēf′/.

clearance, the removal of a substance from the blood by the kidneys. Kidney function can be tested by measuring how much of a specific substance appears in the urine in a given length of time.

clear cell carcinoma. See **renal cell carcinoma.**

clear-liquid diet, a diet that supplies fluids and results in little waste. It consists mostly of dissolved sugar and flavored liquids, as ginger ale, sweetened tea or coffee, fat-free broth, plain gelatin, and strained fruit juices. The diet is usually given for a limited amount of time, as for one day after surgery.

clear text, the use of plain English in radio communications transmissions. No ten codes or agency-specific codes are used when using clear text.

cleavage, the series of repeated cell divisions of the egg (ovum) immediately after fertilization. A mass of cells is formed into an embryo capable of growth. **Determinate cleavage** refers to the cell division into sections that will each become a specific part of the embryo. Damage to any of these cells results in a malformed fetus. Cell division into identical sizes is called **equal cleavage.** With **indeterminate cleavage,** there is division into two parts that have similar developmental potential each of which, if isolated, can give rise to a complete individual embryo. **Total cleav-**

age is the first cell division of the ovum into two cells (blastomeres).

cleavage fracture, any broken bone that splits cartilage when a small piece of bone separates from a part of the upper arm bone (humerus).

cleavage line, any of a number of lines in the skin that mark the basic structural pattern and tension of the skin tissue. They are present in all areas of the body but are visible only in certain sites, as the palms of the hands and soles of the feet. In general, the lines run in the direction in which the skin is most loose.

cleft, 1. divided. **2.** a crack, most often one that begins in the embryo.

cleft foot, an abnormal condition in which the division between the third and fourth toes extends into the foot.

cleft lip, a birth defect consisting of one or more splits (fissures) in the upper lip. This results from the failure of the upper jaw and nasal area to close in the embryo. A cleft lip may sometimes be fixed with surgery during the infant's first 48 hours of life.

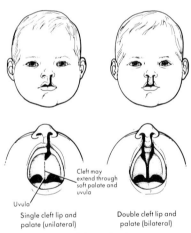

Cleft may extend through soft palate and uvula

Uvula

Single cleft lip and palate (unilateral)

Double cleft lip and palate (bilateral)

Cleft lip and palate

cleft palate, a birth defect in which there is a hole in the middle of the roof of the mouth (palate). This results from the failure of the two sides to join during the development of the embryo. The crack may be complete, going through both the hard and soft palates into the nasal area, or it may go only partly through. A cleft lip is often present as well. These two problems are the most common disorders of the skull and face. The condition affects females more than males. Surgical repair of the defect is normally not begun until the first or second year of life.

cleft uvula, birth defect in which the flap of skin hanging from the palate (uvula) is split into two halves.

clemastine, an antihistamine used to treat symptoms of allergy, as sneezing, runny nose and eyes, and itching.

Cleocin, a trademark for a substance that kills bacteria (clindamycin).

click. See **heart sound.**

climate, the average conditions of the weather in any place. Climate may be considered in the diagnosis and treatment of some illnesses, especially those affecting breathing–**climatic,** *adj.*

clindamycin hydrochloride, a drug that kills bacteria used to treat certain serious infections.

clinic, 1. a department in a hospital where persons not needing to stay in the hospital receive medical care. Formerly it was called a dispensary. **2.** a group practice of doctors, as the Mayo Clinic. **3.** a meeting place for doctors and medical students where lessons can be given at the bedside of a patient or in a similar place.

clinical, referring to direct, bedside medical care.

clinical horizon, a point in a disease at which detectable symptoms first begin to appear.

clinical laboratory, a laboratory in which tests are done to help diagnose a patient's illness. Such laboratories use material, as blood or skin samples, obtained from patients for testing. This differs from research laboratories where animal and other sources of test material are also used.

clinical research center, an organization that studies and describes medical cases. Such centers are often linked to a medical school or teaching hospital. Clinical research centers often offer free or low-cost care for patients taking part in research programs. These centers often produce important new medical information.

clinical specialist, a doctor or nurse who has advanced training in a certain field of medicine. These include nurse-midwife, pediatrician, or radiologist.

clinical trials, organized studies to provide clinical data for assessment of a treatment.

Clinitest, a trademark for tablets used to test the urine for sugar.

clinocephaly /klī'nōsef'əlē/, a birth defect in which the upper surface of the skull dips in the middle, making it saddle-shaped.

clinodactyly /-dak'tilē/, a birth defect in which one or more fingers are bent to either side.

Clinoril, a trademark for a drug to decrease inflammation (sulindac).

Clistin, a trademark for an antihistamine (carbinoxamine maleate).

clitoris /klit'əris/, the female structure that corresponds to the penis. It is a pea-shaped projection made up of nerves, blood vessels, and erect tissue. It is partially hidden by the vaginal lips (labia minora). The clitoris is very sensitive to touch and is important in the sexual excitement of the female.

cloaca /klō·ā′kə/, an opening at the end of a structure (hindgut) in an embryo that develops into the rectum, the bladder, and the genitals.

clocortolone pivalate, a corticosteroid used on the skin to treat inflammation. Viral and fungal diseases of the skin or circulation disorders prohibits its use. Systemic side effects may occur from too much use. Irritation of the skin may also occur.

Cloderm, a trademark for a steroid used to treat skin inflammation (clocortolone pivalate).

clofibrate, a drug used to treat high levels of cholesterol, triglycerides, or both in the blood.

Clomid, a trademark for a fertility drug (clomiphene citrate).

clomiphene citrate, a drug that causes ovulation. It is used mainly to treat infertility in women. Abnormal bleeding from the vagina, liver disturbance, or known allergy to this drug prohibits its use. Side effects include blurred vision, upset stomach, rashes, and stomach pain. Ovaries may become larger.

clomiphene stimulation test /klō′məfēn/, a method to study gonad function in males who show signs of abnormal sexual development. It tests for diseases of the hypothalamic or pituitary areas, and tumors of the pituitary.

clonazepam /klōnaz′əpam/, an anticonvulsant used to prevent seizures in petit mal epilepsy and other disorders involving seizures.

clone, a group of cells or organisms that have identical genes. They are a result of cell division.

clonidine hydrochloride, a drug given to help relieve high levels of anxiety (antihypertensive). It is used to reduce high blood pressure.

clonus /klō′nəs/, abnormal activity of the nerves sending signals to the muscles. In this disorder the person cannot control rapid tensing and relaxing of muscles. Compare **tonus.** –**clonic,** *adj.*

C-loop, a loop of bowel formed by surgery with a C-shape.

closed-wound suction, draining fluids, as blood and pus, from surgical wounds. Such fluids slow the healing of wounds and often cause infection. Removing these fluids helps draw healing tissues together. Closed-wound suction devices most often are made of containers attached to suction tubes and suction pumps. After flushing out the wound to remove blood clots and debris, the surgeon places a tube in the wound. It is then brought out through healthy tissue, about 2 inches from the wound. When the suction tube is in place, the wound is closed and a dressing is put on. Closed-wound suction usually continues for 2 or 3 days after sur-

gery or until the wound stops oozing fluid. Closed-wound suction is often used after chest surgery.

clostridial /klostrid′ē·əl/, referring to bacteria that form spores and need no oxygen to live. They are of the genus *Clostridium.* Gangrene, botulism, and tetanus are examples of disease caused by this kind of bacteria.

closure /klō′zhər/, the surgical closing of a wound by stitching it together. These stitches are called sutures.

clotrimazole, a drug used to treat a number of simple fungus infections. It is also used for yeast infections of the vagina. Known allergy to this drug prohibits its use. Avoid contact with eyes. Side effects include severe allergic reactions of the skin.

clotting time, the time required for blood to form a clot. It is tested by putting a small amount of blood in a glass tube. The first clot is noted and timed. This simple test has been used to diagnose hemophilias, a serious clotting disease. It will not detect mild clotting disorders. Its chief use is in watching over treatment with anticlotting drugs. Also called **coagulation time.**

cloud baby, a newborn who looks well and healthy but carries bacteria or viruses. The infant may spread these into the air when breathing. This may cause disease among other infants in the hospital nursery.

cloxacillin sodium, a drug that kills bacteria used to treat certain serious infections. It is most helpful in treating bacteria resistant to penicillin.

clubbing, an abnormal enlargement of the tips of the fingers and toes. Clubbing is most easily seen in the fingers. The fingers and toes are full, fleshy, and the skin may break away easily. Clubbing is common in patients with disorders that cause lack of oxygen, such as heart disease and long-term lung disease. It also may occur with liver, bowel, and thyroid disorders.

clubfoot, a birth deformity of the foot, sometimes resulting from crowding in the uterus. In a clubfoot the bones in the front part of the foot are misaligned. In 95% of clubfoot deformities the front half of the foot turns in and down **(equinovarus).** In the rest of the defects the front part of the foot turns out and up **(calcaneovalgus** or **calcaneovarus).**

cluster breathing, a breathing pattern in which fast breathing is followed by a period of not breathing. This is linked to a tumor or disease in the brainstem.

cluster headache. See **headache.**

cluttering, a speech defect in which words are rapid, confused, nervous, and uneven. Letters or syllables may be reversed or left out. The condition is often linked to other language disorders, as problems in learning to speak, read, and spell. It is also seen in some personality and behavior problems.

CNS, abbreviation for **central nervous system.**

CO₂, symbol for **carbon dioxide.**

coagulase /kō·ag′yəlās/, an enzyme produced by bacteria, particularly *Staphylococcus aureus*. It helps to form blood clots.

coagulation /kō·ag′yəlā′shən/, clotting; the process of turning a liquid into a solid, especially the blood. See also **blood clotting.**

coagulation factor, one of 13 elements in the blood that help to form blood clots. See also **blood clotting, factor.**

coagulopathy /-lop′əthē/, any disorder of the blood that makes it difficult for blood to coagulate.

coal tar, a substance put on the skin. It is used to treat long-term skin diseases, as eczema and psoriasis. Known allergy to this drug prohibits its use. Side effects include skin irritation and allergic reactions.

coaptation splint /kō·aptā′shən/, a small splint fitted to a broken limb to keep the fragments of bone in place. A longer splint usually covers the small one to provide for more support.

coarctation /kō·ärktā′shən/, a narrowing or contraction of the walls of a blood vessel, as the aorta.

coarctation of the aorta, a birth defect of the heart in which the major artery (aorta) is narrowed. This results in higher blood pressure on one side of the defect and lower pressure on the other side. In its most common form it causes high blood pressure in the arms and head and low blood pressure in the legs. Symptoms include dizziness, headaches, fainting, nose bleeds, and muscle cramps in the legs during exercise.

coarse, a wide range of movements, as those linked to tremors and uncontrolled movements of the muscle.

coat, 1. a membrane that covers the outside of an organ or part. 2. one of the layers of a wall of an organ or part, especially a canal or a vessel.

cobalamin /kōbôl′əmin/, a common term for part of the vitamin B₁₂ complex. See also **cyanocobalamin.**

cobalt (Co), a metallic element that is found in certain minerals. Cobalt is a part of vitamin B₁₂, and is found in most foods. It is easily absorbed by the stomach and intestines. The amount the body needs is not known. Lack of enough cobalt in humans does not seem to occur. Giving a form of cobalt seems to help some patients with anemia. A radioactive form, **cobalt 60 (⁶⁰Co),** is the source most often used in x-ray treatment for cancer.

coca, a species of South American shrub that is native to Bolivia and Peru. It is also grown in Indonesia. It is a natural source of cocaine.

cocaine hydrochloride, a white crystal-like powder used as a local anesthetic. It was taken from coca leaves, but now a synthetic form can be made. It is commonly used to examine and treat the eye, ear, nose, and throat. The drug slows bleeding. Long or frequent use may damage the mucous membranes. Too much stimulation of the central nervous system may result from use with some drugs. Cocaine is not given to patients with severe heart disease, thyroid disease, or low blood pressure. Side effects include excitement, mental depression, tremors, dizziness, nausea, vomiting, high blood pressure, stomach cramps, chills, fever, coma, or death from lung failure. Cocaine is a narcotic (Schedule II) drug under the Controlled Substances Act.

cocarcinogen /kō′kärsin′əjən/, a substance that becomes cancerous only when combined with another substance.

coccidioidomycosis /koksid′ē·oi′dōmīkō′-/, an infectious disease caused by breathing in spores of the fungus *Coccidioides immitis*. These spores are carried on dust particles in the wind. The disease occurs in hot, dry regions of the southwest United States. Early symptoms resemble the common cold or influenza. Later new problems develop which last for weeks to years. These include low fever, appetite and weight loss, bluish skin, and breathing difficulty. Also found are blood in the spit, skin sores, and arthritic pain in the bones and joints.

coccidiosis /kok′sidē·ō′-/, a parasitic disease found in tropical and subtropical regions. It is caused by swallowing eggs of a tiny organism (*Isospora belli* or *I. hominis*). Symptoms include fever, malaise, stomach pain, and watery diarrhea. The infection usually lasts 1 to 2 weeks, and health returns. No specific treatment has been found.

coccus /kok′əs/, *pl.* **cocci** /kok′sī/, a bacterium that is round, spheric, or oval. **–coccal,** *adj.*

coccygeus /koksij′ē·əs/, one of the muscles in the floor of the pelvis. It is a band of muscle and fibers. This band stretches across the pelvic cavity like a hammock.

coccygodynia /kok′sigōdin′ē·ə/, a pain in the tailbone area of the body.

coccyx /kok′siks/. See **vertebra.**

cochlea /kok′lē·ə/, a small bone of the inner ear that is the organ of hearing. It is coiled 2½ times into the shape of a snail shell. This bone has many small holes through which passes the nerve carrying signals from the ear to the brain (acoustic nerve). The cochlea connects with the organs of the acoustic nerve. **–cochlear** /kok′lē·ər/, *adj.*

Coco-Quinine, a trademark for a drug used to treat malaria (quinine sulfate).

code, 1. a system of signals for passing on information, as a genetic code. 2. *informal,* a signal used to call a specially trained and equipped team in a hospital. This is done without alarming patients or visitors. The **code team** is prepared to revive patients suffering from sudden heart and lung failure.

codeine, a narcotic used to relieve mild pain, to treat diarrhea, and to stop coughing. Known allergy to this drug prohibits its use. Side effects include constipation, nausea, drowsiness, and allergic reactions. High doses can affect breathing and circulation. The drug can be addictive.

cod-liver oil, a pale-yellow, fatty oil from the fresh livers of codfish. It may also come from other related species. It is a rich source of vitamins A and D and is useful for treating a lack of those vitamins. It is also used to treat abnormal absorption of calcium and phosphorus.

coelom /sē′ləm/, the body cavity of the developing embryo.

coelosomy /sē′ləsō′mē/, a birth defect in which the stomach and bowels protrude from the body cavity.

coenzyme /kō·en′zīm/, a substance that combines with other substances to form a complete enzyme. Coenzymes include some of the vitamins, as B_1 and B_2.

coffee, the seeds of *Coffea arabica, C. liberica,* and *C. robusta* trees. These trees grow in almost all tropical areas. Coffee beans contain caffeine and are used to make a stimulating drink. Coffee has been used to treat headache, long-term asthma, and drug poisoning.

coffee-ground vomitus, vomit that looks dark brown, like coffee grounds. It is made up of gastric juices and old blood. This is a symptom of slow bleeding in the stomach and upper bowels. Compare **hematemesis.**

Cogentin, a trademark for a drug used to treat Parkinson's disease (benztropine mesylate).

cognition, the mental process of knowing, thinking, learning, and judging.

cognitive development, the process by which an infant gains knowledge and the ability to think, learn, and reason.

cognitive dissonance, a state of mental stress. This comes from learning new information that conflicts with old ideas or knowledge.

cognitive therapy, various ways of treating mental and emotional disorders. These include behavior therapy, existential therapy, Gestalt therapy, and transactional analysis.

cogwheel rigidity, an abnormal stiffness in muscle tissue. There are jerky movements when the muscle is made to stretch.

coherence, 1. the property of sticking together, as the molecules of a substance. 2. the logical pattern of speech and thought of a normal, stable person.

cohort, a group of people who share a characteristic, as age or sex.

coiled tubular gland, a gland that has a coiled, tube-shaped part that releases fluid, such as the sweat glands.

coitus /kō′itəs/, the sexual union of two people of opposite sex. The penis is inserted into the vagina, usually resulting in orgasm. Also called **sexual intercourse.** – **coital,** *adj.*

coitus interruptus. See **withdrawal method.**

Colace, a trademark for a stool softener (docusate sodium sulfosuccinate).

colchicine /kol′chəsēn/, a drug used to treat gout and to prevent gouty arthritis attacks. Ulcer, ulcerative colitis, or known allergy to this drug prohibits its use. It is not given to elderly, weakened patients or persons with long-term kidney, liver, heart, or stomach and intestine disease. Side effects include severe stomach and bowel pain, diarrhea with blood, severe anemia, nerve disorders, liver failure, and hair loss.

cold, 1. the absence of heat. 2. a contagious viral infection (**common cold**) of the upper respiratory tract. Symptoms include stuffy nose, watery eyes, low fever, and aching. It is treated with rest, aspirin, decongestants, and drinking a lot of fluids.

cold-blooded, referring to animals not able to control body heat, as fishes, reptiles, and amphibians. Compare **warm-blooded.**

cold caloric irrigation, a procedure for testing brainstem function. It is done by pouring a cold salt solution into the ear canal with the head at a 30° angle. This causes jerky but regular eye movements in a normal patient. Absence of the reaction may be a sign of a disease of the brainstem. See also **caloric test.**

cold injury, any of several abnormal conditions caused by exposure to cold temperatures. These conditions are often serious. See also **chilblain, frostbite, hypothermia, immersion foot.**

cold-pressor test, a test for the tendency to develop high blood pressure (essential hypertension). One hand of the person is placed in ice water for about 60 seconds. A large rise in the blood pressure or a delay in the return of normal pressure when the hand is taken from the water is watched for. If either takes place, it is believed that the person may develop hypertension.

cold sore. See **herpes simplex.**

cold zone area, safe haven for those agencies directly involved in a hazardous materials operation. Includes the incident commander, command post, representatives from appropriate agencies, and usually the media.

colectomy /kəlek′-/, surgical removal of part or all of the large intestine (colon). This is done to treat cancer of the colon or severe long-term ulcerative colitis. See also **abdominal surgery.**

Colestid, a trademark for a drug used to lower cholesterol in the blood (colestipol hydrochloride).

colestipol hydrochloride, a drug that reduces high blood levels of cholesterol. It is used to treat high cholesterol and

xanthoma. A blocked gallbladder or known allergy to this drug prohibits its use. Side effects include skin rash, constipation, and lack of vitamins A, D, and K.

colic /kol′ik/,   sharp pain resulting from twisting, blockage, or muscle spasm of a hollow or tubelike organ. These can include a ureter or the intestines. A **baby's colic** is a painful condition common in infants under the age of three months. Causes include swallowed air, too much gas in the intestines, and allergy to the baby's formula. Treatment may include switching formulas, helping the infant to bring up gas, and a medication prescribed by the doctor.

coliform /kol′ifôrm/,   referring to the bacteria that live in the intestines of humans and other animals.

colistimethate sodium,   a drug that fights bacteria. It is used to treat some stomach and bowel infections and skin infections.

colistin sulfate,   a drug used to treat infections of the outer ear, and infection of the stomach and bowels caused by *Escherichia coli.* Known allergy to this drug prohibits its use. Side effects include breathing arrest, kidney poisoning, and nerve and muscle disorders.

colitis /kōlī′-/,   a general term for inflammation of the large intestine. This can refer to the disorder called **irritable bowel syndrome.** It can also mean one of the more serious long-term inflammatory bowel diseases (**Crohn's disease, ulcerative colitis**). Because persons with colitis may be irritated by different foods, a diet is created for each patient. Treatment depends on the specific disorder. See also **Crohn's disease, irritable bowel syndrome, ulcerative colitis.** –**colitic,** *adj.*

collagen /kol′əjən/,   a protein consisting of bundles of tiny fibers. Collagen forms connective tissue. These include the white inelastic fibers of the tendons, the ligaments, the bones, and the cartilage. –**collagenous** /kəlaj′ənəs/, *adj.*

collagenase ointment,   a drug used to treat bed sores, burns, and other skin disorders.

collagen disease,   any one of many disorders marked by inflammation and breakdown of fiber in connective tissue. Some collagen diseases are rheumatic fever, arteritis, and ankylosing spondylitis.

collagenoblast /kəlaj′ənōblast′/,   a cell that forms collagen. It can also change into cartilage and bone tissue.

collagenous fiber /kəlaj′əns/,   the tough, white fibers that make up much of the connective tissue of the body. These fibers contain collagen. They are often arranged in bundles which strengthen the tissues in which they are found.

collagen vascular disease,   any of a group of disorders in which inflammation occurs in small blood vessels and connective tissue. The cause of most of these diseases is unknown. Heredity, deficiencies, environment, infections, and allergies may be involved. Common features of most

of these diseases include arthritis, skin sores, and eye inflammations. Further features are infection of the membrane around the lungs (pleuritis), of the heart (myocarditis), and of the kidneys (nephritis). Diseases included in this category are rheumatic fever, rheumatoid arthritis, scleroderma, and systemic lupus erythematosus.

collapse,   1. *informal.* a state of extreme depression or of total exhaustion caused by physical or emotional problems. **2.** an abnormal condition marked by shock. **3.** the abnormal sagging of an organ.

collar,   any structure that circles another, usually around its neck. The periosteal bone collars that form around the ends of young bones are an example.

collarbone.   See **clavicle.**

collateral,   1. secondary   or   accessory. **2.** a   small branch, as any one of the arterioles in the body.

collector,   a device for collecting fluids from the bronchi of the lungs and the esophagus for laboratory examination.

Colles' fascia /kol′ēz/,   a strong, smooth sheet of tissue with stretchy fibers that fills a groove between the scrotum and the thigh in a man or between the labia and the thigh in a woman.

Colles' fracture,   a break of one of the bones in the forearm (radius). It occurs 1 inch above the wrist and causes a hand position bent to the back and side.

colliquation /kol′ikwā′shən/,   the breakdown of a tissue of the body into liquid. It is normally linked to dead tissue.

collodion baby,   a newborn baby whose skin is covered with a scaly, dry membrane.

colloid /kol′oid/,   **1.** referring to a state of matter in which large molecules remain suspended in a liquid or other material. They neither mix in nor settle to the bottom. **2.** a gelatinlike substance in the body that resembles glue. Compare **solution, suspension.**

colloid bath,   a bath in water that contains substances as bran, gelatin, or starch. Colloid baths are often used to relieve irritation and inflammation of the skin.

colloid osmotic pressure,   an abnormal condition of the kidney. It is caused by the pressure of large particles that will not pass through a membrane. Also called **oncotic pressure.**

coloboma /kol′əbō′mə/,   a birth defect in which a cleft extends along the edge of the eyeball. This affects the iris, ciliary body, or the blood vessel layer (choroid).

colon /kō′lən/,   the part of the large intestine that extends to the rectum. The **ascending colon** extends upward from the first part of the colon (cecum) in the lower right side of the stomach to where the colon turns. The **transverse colon** goes from the end of the ascending colon at the liver on the right side across the middle intestinal area to the beginning of the **descending colon** at the spleen on the left side. From there the colon descends to the **sigmoid colon,** which extends to the beginning of the rectum. The colon takes the contents of the small intestine, moving them to the rectum by contracting. Much water is added to the foodstuff by the stomach and small intestine during digestion. The colon absorbs most of this water through the walls. This firms the feces as they move into the rectum.

colonic fistula /kōlon′ik/, an abnormal passage from the colon to the surface of the body or to another organ or structure. Long-term inflammation of the intestines may cause a passage (fistula) between two loops of bowel. An opening from the colon to the surface of the skin may be made surgically after a part of the bowel is removed. This surgery is common when a cancerous section or badly infected sore in the bowel is removed. See also **colostomy.**

colony, **1.** a mass of microorganisms that grows from a single cell. This mass is grown in a special substance called a culture. **2.** a mass of cells in a culture.

Colorado tick fever, a virus infection that is carried to humans by the bite of a tick. It is most common in the spring and summer months throughout the Rocky Mountains, especially in Colorado. Symptoms occur in two phases between which there are no symptoms. They include chills, fever, headache, pain in the eyes, legs, and back, and sensitivity to light. Painkillers can be given for headache and other pains. Compare **Rocky Mountain spotted fever.**

color blindness, the inability to clearly tell one color from another. In most cases it is not a blindness but a weakness in seeing colors distinctly.

color dysnomia, an inability to name colors, even though the person can match and tell them apart. It may be caused by damaged speech centers in the brain.

colorectal cancer /kō′lərek′-/, a malignant tumor of the large intestine. Symptoms include dark sticky stools containing blood and a change in bowel habits. Cancer of the large bowel often occurs after the age of 50. It is slightly more frequent in women than in men and almost as common as lung cancer in the United States. A diet high in carbohydrates and beef and low in roughage may be a factor.

colorimetry /kol′ərim′ətrē/, **1.** measurement of the intensity of color in a fluid or substance. **2.** measurement of color in the blood to determine the content of hemoglobin.

color index (C.I.), the ratio between the amount of hemoglobin and the number of red blood cells in sample of blood.

color vision, the perception of color. Color is seen as the cones in the retina react to changing intensities of red, green, and blue light. See also **color blindness.**

colostomy /kəlos′-/, an opening made by surgery for feces to pass through the abdominal wall. The colon is cut and brought to the surface of the skin. Colostomies are performed for cancer of the colon and noncancerous tumors that block the bowel. They may also be done in the case of severe wounds to the stomach and bowels. A colostomy may be "single-barreled" with one opening or "double-barreled" with two loops opening onto the skin. The latter is done when the lower bowel is completely blocked or in paralyzed people to help daily care.

colostrum /kəlos′trəm/, the fluid released by the breast during pregnancy before milk production (lactation) begins. Colostrum is a thin, yellow fluid that contains white blood cells, water, protein, fat, and carbohydrate.

colpectomy /kolpek′-/, the surgical removal of the vagina.

colporrhaphy /kolpôr′əfē/, stitching of the vagina, usually to narrow the vagina.

colpotomy /kolpot′-/, any surgical cut into the wall of the vagina.

Coly-Mycin M, a trademark for a drug that fights bacteria (colistimethate sodium).

coma, a state of deep unconsciousness. Symptoms include the absence of eye movements and response to pain and sounds. The person cannot be awakened. Coma may result from injury, brain tumor, serious infectious disease with brain inflammation, or blood vessel disease. It may also result from poisoning, diabetic acidosis, or intoxication. See also **hepatic coma.**

combat fatigue. See **stress reaction.**

Combid, a trademark for a drug used to treat peptic ulcers, irritable bowel syndrome, and diarrhea (isopropamide iodide and prochlorperazine).

combined system disease, a disorder of the nervous system caused by a lack of vitamin B_{12}. The disorder causes anemia and breakdown of the spinal cord and the nerves. There is also difficulty in walking, feeling of vibration in the legs, and a loss of sense of body position.

comedo /kom′idō, kəmē′dō/. See **blackhead.**

comedocarcinoma /-kär′sinō′mə/, a cancer of the milk ducts of the breast. Since the growth is confined in the milk ducts, the complete cure after surgery is better than for most other types of breast cancer.

comfort measure, any action taken to increase comfort of the patient. Examples might be a back rub, a change in position, or warming a stethoscope or a bedpan before use.

command, the act of directing, ordering, and/or controlling resources by virtue of explicit legal, agency, or delegated authority.

command staff, those individuals assigned to assist the incident commander and his section officers by gathering and managing information and coordinating communications. They may be fire fighters, EMTs, line officers, or any other knowledgeable individuals on the scene.

comminuted fracture, a fracture in which there are several breaks in the bone. This creates many bone fragments.

commissurotomy /kom'ishŏŏrot'-/, surgically dividing a fiberlike band or ring connecting parts of a body structure. This is often done to separate the thickened flaps of a narrowed mitral valve in the heart.

commitment, **1.** the placement of a patient in a hospital or other facility designed to deal with the patient's special needs. **2.** the legal act of admitting a mentally ill patient to an institution for psychiatric treatment. The process usually involves court action. This act is based on medical evidence that the person is mentally ill. **3.** a pledge or promise to do something in the future. It often refers to fulfilling an agreement. It is widely used in some forms of psychotherapy or marriage counseling.

common bile duct, the duct formed by the joining of the gallbladder (cystic) duct and liver (hepatic) duct.

common carotid artery. See **carotid artery.**

common cold. See **cold.**

common hepatic artery, an artery that branches off the aorta as it goes through the area of the stomach. Its five branches supply blood to the stomach, small intestines, and liver.

common iliac artery, a division of the abdominal aorta that divides into external and internal iliac arteries. These supply blood to the pelvis and legs.

communicable disease, any disease carried from one person or animal to another by direct or indirect contact. Direct contact includes touching any discharge from the body, as saliva. Indirect might include contact through something else, as drinking glasses, toys, water, or insects. To control a communicable disease, it is important to identify the organism causing the disease and prevent its spread. The infected person must be treated, and others must be protected from contact with the organism. Many communicable diseases, by law, must be reported to the local health department. Also called **contagious disease.**

communication, transferring a message, especially from one person to another. Communication may be verbal or nonverbal. It may occur directly, as in a conversation or by a gesture. It also may occur indirectly, spanning space and time, as in writing and reading.

communication, impaired verbal. See **speech dysfunction.**

comm. unit (communications unit), a vehicle (trailer or mobile van) used to provide the major part of an incident communications center.

community health nursing, a field of nursing that blends patient health care and public health nursing. A community health nurse seeks to prevent, as well as cure, disease. This field is also concerned with rehabilitation.

community medicine, a branch of medicine concerned with the health of the members of a community or region.

community mental health center (CMHC), a community-based center that provides complete mental health care. This includes outpatient and inpatient care.

companionship, placing a staff member or another patient with a disturbed patient. This is to provide support and to protect patients from hurting themselves or others.

company, any piece of equipment having a full complement of personnel.

compartment syndrome, a condition caused by inward pressure of an artery reducing blood supply. It can result in a permanent contraction of the hand or foot. This may also cause a break in the hand or foot with or without a fracture. See also **contracture.**

compatibility, **1.** the ability to live together in harmony. **2.** the orderly, efficient mixing of elements from one system with those of another. **3.** the ability of several drugs to work together without harming the patient. **4.** the degree to which the body's defense system will accept foreign matter, as blood or organs. Usually, perfect compatibility exists only between identical twins.

Compazine, a trademark for a drug used to treat nausea and psychosis (prochlorperazine).

Compensated heart failure. See **heart failure.**

compensating curve, the curve of alignment of the biting surfaces of the teeth. It is used to ensure that the molar teeth meet properly. It also provides balancing contacts on dentures.

compensation, **1.** correction of a defect or loss of the body by the increased output of another part. **2.** the process of keeping enough blood flow in spite of heart or circulatory problems. Failure of the heart to pump enough blood indicates a diseased heart muscle. **3.** a complex defense mechanism to avoid a feeling of inferiority. This can be achieved by putting forth great effort to overcome a handicap. Another way is to scorn the lack of quality.

compensation neurosis, an unconscious process by which one keeps the symptoms of an injury or disease. This is done in order to receive other gains. Compare **malingering.**

competence, the ability of any part of the body to do what is required of it.

complaint, *informal.* any illness, problem, or symptom identified by the patient. A **chief complaint** is a statement made by a patient describing his or her most important symptoms of illness or dysfunction. It is often the reason that the person seeks health care.

complement, complex proteins in the blood that bind with substances that defend the body (antibodies) against foreign invaders (antigens). Complement is involved in reactions such as severe allergic reaction (anaphylaxis). A deficiency or defect of any of the parts of a complement can occur. Patients with complement abnormalities are more likely to get infections and collagen vascular diseases. It is difficult and often expensive to diagnose.

complete blood count (CBC). See **blood count.**

complex, **1.** a group of chemical molecules that are related in structure or function. **2.** a combination of symptoms of disease that forms a syndrome. **3.** a group of linked ideas with strong emotional overtones. These ideas affect a patient's attitudes.

compliance, fulfillment by the patient of the treatment prescribed.

component therapy, transfusion in which only certain parts (components) of blood are given. In this way it is possible to transfer more of the blood component than would be found in whole blood.

compound, **1.** a substance made up of two or more elements that cannot be separated. **2.** any substance made up of two or more ingredients. **3.** to make a substance by combining ingredients, as a drug. **4.** referring to an injury marked by several factors.

compound tubuloalveolar gland, a gland with more than one duct for fluids, as a salivary gland.

comprehensive care. See **holistic health care.**

Comprehensive Environment Response, Compensation, and Liability (CERCLA), also known as "superfund." It addresses hazardous substance releases into the environment and the clean-up of inactive hazardous waste disposal sites. It requires that those individuals responsible for the release of hazardous materials above certain levels (reportable quantities) notify the National Response Center.

compress, a soft pad, usually made of cloth. It is used to apply heat, cold, or drugs to the surface of a body. A compress also may be placed over a wound to help stop bleeding. Compare **dressing.**

compression, the act of applying pressure to an area of the body. A tumor or bleeding may cause compression of brain tissue, for example.

compression fracture, a bone break, most often found in a short bone. It breaks apart bone tissue and collapses the bone. The bones of the spine (vertebrae) are often sites of compression fractures.

compromised host, a patient who is not able to resist infection. This may be due to defective immune system or severe anemia. A severe disease or condition, as cancer or general poor health may also be involved.

compulsion, an irresistible, impulse to perform an irrational act. The impulse is usually the result of an obsession. See also **obsession.** –**compulsive,** *adj.*

compulsive personality disorder, a condition in which a compulsive need interferes with everyday work and normal behavior. The disorder features excessive devotion to order, rules, and detail and clinging to a system of behavior. The person cannot make decisions when faced with unexpected situations.

compulsive ritual, a series of acts a person feels must be carried out. This is done even though the behavior is known to be useless and inappropriate. Failure to complete the acts results in extreme anxiety. See also **obsessive-compulsive neurosis.**

computerized tomography (CT), a method for examining structures inside the body. It produces a highly accurate picture that shows relationships of structures to each other. The examination is painless and requires no special preparation. Tumors, blood clots, bone displacement, and gathering of fluid can be detected. This method can be used on the brain, chest, stomach, and pelvis. Also called **computerized axial tomography (CAT).**

conation, the mental process marked by desire, impulse, voluntary action, and striving. Compare **cognition.** –**conative,** *adj.*

concentric fibroma, a fiberlike tumor surrounding the uterus.

concept, an abstract idea or thought that begins and is held in the mind. –**conceptual,** *adj.*

conception, **1.** the beginning of pregnancy. This is usually taken to be the instant that a sperm enters an egg (ovum). **2.** the act or process of fertilization. **3.** the process of creating an idea. **4.** the idea created.

conceptional age, the number of weeks since conception of an embryo. Because the exact time of conception is difficult to know, conceptional age is said to be two weeks less than the pregnancy (gestational) age.

conceptus, the result of conception. It includes the fertilized egg and its enclosing membranes. See also **embryo, fetus.**

concordance, the appearance of one or more traits in both members of a pair of twins. Compare **discordance.** –**concordant,** *adj.*

concussion, a violent jar or shock, as caused by a blow or explosion. See also **brain concussion.**

condition, **1.** a state of being. It refers to physical and mental health or well-being. **2.** to train the body or mind.

This is done through certain exercises and repeated exposure to a state or thing.

conditioned reflex. See **reflex action.**

conditioned response, an automatic reaction to a stimulus that has been learned through training. Such responses can be physical or psychologic, conscious or unconscious. They are caused by exposure to the stimulus or event. This is done over and over until the response is automatic. A **conditioned avoidance response** is learned in order to avoid an unpleasant stimulus. A **conditioned escape response** is learned in order to stop or to escape from an unpleasant stimulus. Compare **unconditioned response.**

conditioning, a form of learning in which a response to a stimulus is developed. **Avoidance conditioning** establishes certain patterns of behavior to avoid unpleasant or painful stimulation. With **classical conditioning,** an object or event that used to hold no special meaning now causes a predictable response. **Operant conditioning** refers to a way of learning used in treatment to change the way a person thinks or does things (behavior therapy). The person is rewarded for the right response and punished for the wrong response.

condom, a soft, flexible sheath used to prevent conception during sexual intercourse. It is placed over the penis and stops semen from entering the vagina. Condoms are also used to avoid transmitting infection. They are made of plastic, rubber, or skin. Also called **prophylactic,** *(informal)* **rubber.**

conduction, **1.** a process in which heat is carried from one substance to another. **2.** the process by which a nerve signal is carried.

condylar fracture /kon′dilər/, any break of the round end of a hinge joint. This type of break most often occurs at the elbow or knee. A small bone fragment that includes the condyle often breaks off.

condyle /kon′dil/, a rounded, knucklelike bump at the end of a bone. Muscles attach to this bump and join the bone to nearby bones.

condyloid joint, a joint in which a condyle fits into an oval cavity, as the wrist joint. See also **joint.**

condyloma /-ō′mə/, a wartlike growth on the anus, vulva, or penis. One form (**condyloma latum**) is a flat, moist growth found in the groove between the thighs or on the penis. It appears in secondary syphilis. See also **venereal wart.**

cone, a cell that receives light in the retina of the eye and causes a person to see colors. There are three kinds of retinal cones, one for each of the colors blue, green, and red. Other colors are seen by combining these three colors.

confabulation, the invention of events, often told in a detailed and convincing way. This is done in order to fill in and cover up gaps in the memory. It occurs mainly as a way of defense. It is quite common in alcoholics and persons with head injuries or lead poisoning. Also called **fabrication.**

confinement, **1.** a state of being held in a specific place. This is done in order to obstruct or reduce activity. **2.** the final phase of pregnancy during which labor and childbirth occur.

conflict, a painful mental state caused by opposing thoughts, ideas, goals, or desires. This state is made worse by not being able to resolve the conflicts. This kind of stress is found to some degree in every person. **Approach-approach conflict** refers to a conflict caused by the need to choose between two or more things that are wanted. **Approach-avoidance conflict** is caused by something that is both wanted and not wanted. **Avoidance-avoidance conflict** results from the confrontation of two or more events that are equally undesirable. An **intrapsychic conflict** is an emotional conflict within oneself.

confusion, a mental state in which a patient is unsure of time, place, or person. This causes a lack of orderly thought. The person is also not able to make decisions. It often indicates an organic mental disorder. It may, however, appear with severe emotional stress. –**confusional,** *adj.*

congener /kon′jənər/, one of two or more things that are similar in structure, function, or origin. Examples are muscles that function the same way, or drugs that are similar in effect.

congenital /kənjen′ətəl/, present at birth, as a congenital defect.

congenital anomaly. See **birth defect.**

congenital dislocation of the hip, a birth defect in which the top of the thigh bone (femur) does not fit into the hip socket, because of a very shallow hip socket. Treatment consists of keeping the thigh angled to the side. This causes the top of the femur to press into the center of the socket, deepening it.

congenital heart disease, any defect of the heart or great vessels existing from birth. Congenital heart disease is a major cause of newborn problems. The basic symptoms are slow growth, frequent lung infections, rapid breathing and heart beat, bluish skin, and heart murmurs.

congenital nonspherocytic hemolytic anemia, a large group of blood disorders caused by similar inherited diseases. Most are linked to a condition in which hemoglobin, which carries oxygen, is separated from the red blood cell too soon. See also **anemia, sickle cell anemia.**

congenital pulmonary arteriovenous fistula, a direct passage (fistula) between the arteries and veins of the lung. This condition is present at birth. It permits blood that contains no oxygen to enter the circulation. There may be several fistulas in any part of the lung. Surgery may be used to correct the defect.

congestion, abnormal collection of fluid in an organ or body area. The fluid is often blood, but it may be bile or mucus.

congestive heart failure. See **heart failure.**

conjugated estrogen. See **estrogen.**

conjunctiva /kon′jungktī′və/, two membranes in the eye. The **palpebral conjunctiva** lines the inner surface of the eyelids. It is thick, dull, and supplied with blood vessels. The **bulbar conjunctiva** covers the front part of the white of the eye (sclera). It is thin and transparent.

conjunctival reflex, a way of protecting the eye. The eyelids close whenever the front of the white of the eye is touched. Compare **corneal reflex.**

conjunctivitis /kənjungk′tivī′tis/, inflammation of the lining (conjunctiva) of the eye and eyelids. This is caused by infection, allergy, or outside factors. Red eyes, a thick discharge, and sticky eyelids in the morning are the symptoms. Treatment depends on the cause. It may include antibiotics. Symptoms include itching and discharge.

connecting fibrocartilage, a disk of fiberlike cartilage between many joints. It is common between joints with little movement, as the spinal vertebrae. Each disk is made of rings of fiberlike tissue separated by cartilage. The disk swells outward if it is pressed by the vertebrae on either side. See also **intervertebral disk.**

connective tissue, tissue that supports and joins other body tissue and parts. It also carries materials for processing, nutrition, and waste release. Various kinds of cells are found in this tissue, as plasma cells and white blood cells. See also **bone, cartilage.**

consanguinity /kon′sang·gwin′itē/, a hereditary or ''blood'' relationship between persons. These persons share a common parent or ancestor.

conscience, the moral sense of what is right and wrong. This includes the ability to judge one's own actions.

conscious, 1. able to respond to outside stimuli including awareness of being awake, alert, or awareness of one's surroundings. **2.** that part of mental functioning that is aware of thoughts, ideas, and emotions.

consolidation, 1. combining of separate parts into a single whole. **2.** the process of becoming solid. This is seen in pneumonia when the lungs become firm and will not stretch.

constipation, problems in passing stools. Among the physical causes are too little food and bulk, too little physical activity, a side effect of drugs, overuse of laxatives and enemas, stomach and bowel blockage, tumors, nerve or muscle damage, weak intestinal muscles, pain, lack of privacy, and pregnancy. Symptoms are reduced times of defecation, a hard, formed stool, straining at stool, reduced

bowel sounds, a feeling of stomach or rectal fullness or pressure, and nausea. Stomach and bowel pain, loss of appetite, back pain, and headache may also occur.

constriction ring, a band of muscle in the uterus that contracts around part of the fetus during labor. This often follows early breakage of the membranes around the fetus. This can interfere with labor.

contact, 1. transfer of an infectious organism from one person to another. This can be done by direct or indirect contact, as touching food or clothes. **2.** the touching or bringing together of two surfaces, as those of upper and lower teeth.

contact dermatitis, skin rash resulting from exposure to either an irritating or allergic substance. An irritant, such as detergent or acid, causes a sore much like a burn. Treatment is to flush the area quickly with water. With an allergic substance, the reaction is delayed. Symptoms are inflammation, blisters, and large amounts of fluid in the body tissues. Poison ivy is a common example of this type. Treatment includes steroid creams and soothing or drying lotions. The irritating or allergic substance should be avoided. See also **dermatitis.**

contact lens, a small, curved plastic lens shaped to fit the patient's eye. It is used to correct poor vision. Contact lenses float on the film of tears over the cornea. They must be handled with great care to avoid damage to the eyes. Various types of contact lenses include hard lenses, soft lenses, extended-wear lenses, and tinted lenses.

contagious, communicable, as a disease that is carried by direct or indirect contact. –**contagion,** *n.*

container, the portion of a shipping package that physically houses the radioactive material.

contamination or radioactive contamination, deposition of radioactive material in any place where it is not desired, particularly where its presence may be harmful.

contingency (emergency) planning, a comprehensive and coordinated response to the plant or community hazardous materials problem. It builds upon hazard analysis and recognizes that no single public or private sector agency is capable of managing the hazardous materials problem alone.

continuous positive airway pressure (CPAP), breathing assisted by an outside flow of air. The air flows steadily throughout the breathing cycle. This is done for patients who are not able to keep enough oxygen in the blood without help. CPAP may be given through a tube inserted into the throat (endotracheal tube) or tube in the nose. It may also be given by way of a hood over the patient's head. Respiratory distress syndrome in the newborn is often treated with CPAP. Also called **continuous positive pressure breathing.**

contraception, a technique for preventing pregnancy. This may be done with a drug, device, or by blocking a process of reproduction. Contraception permits sexual union without resulting in pregnancy. Kinds of contraception are **cervical cap, condom, contraceptive diaphragm, intrauterine device, natural family planning method, oral contraceptive, spermatocide, sterilization.** Also called **birth control, conception control, family planning.**

contraceptive diaphragm, a birth control device made up of a thin rubber disk fastened to a flexible ring. It is inserted in the vagina together with jelly or cream that kills sperm. The diaphragm covers the cervix so that sperm cannot enter the uterus. This prevents pregnancy. About five to 10 unplanned pregnancies occur in 100 women using the method properly. The main advantages are that it has no side effects and that it needs to be used only during intercourse. There are reported disadvantages. These include claims that it is messy, it is uncomfortable for some people, and insertion may interfere with making love. The diaphragm must be left in place for at least 6 to 8 hours after intercourse. It must also be used for every act of intercourse. A **coil-spring diaphragm** has a flexible rim that is coiled and round. This kind is used by a woman whose vaginal muscles offer good support, and whose uterus is not tipped back or forward. It is also used with a normal size vagina with an abnormally deep arch behind the pubic bone. A **flat-spring diaphragm** has a rim that is thin and flat. It is given to a woman whose vaginal muscles give good support and whose uterus is in the normal position. An **arcing-spring contraceptive diaphragm** has a flexible metal spring that forms the rim. It is a combination of the flexible coil spring and the flat band spring. This kind of diaphragm is given for a patient whose vagina muscles are relaxed and will not afford strong support. This is a common problem in patients whose bladder or rectum pushes through the vagina (cystocele and rectocele), or whose uterus has sagged into the vagina (uterine prolapse). The arcing spring may offer better protection than the coil or flat spring. It is stronger and better able to hold the diaphragm in place. A **contraceptive diaphragm fitting** is done in a doctor's office or clinic. Proper fitting takes into account the size and shape of the vagina, the position of the uterus, and the muscle support in the vagina. When the correct size has been found, the woman is taught to insert it herself. A new fitting is necessary if the woman gains or loses more than 20 pounds or if she has an abortion or a vaginal delivery.

Contraceptives in common use and their modes of action

Contraceptive	Mode of action	Involvement time
Natural family planning		
Rhythm/calendar	Couple cooperation: abstinence during fertile periods	Mathematic formula calculated once every month
BBT	Couple cooperation: abstinence during fertile periods	Ovulation determined from daily record of BBT
Cervical mucus	Couple cooperation: abstinence during fertile periods	Ovulation determined from daily record of cervical mucus characteristics
Symptothermal	Couple cooperation: abstinence during fertile periods	Combination of BBT, cervical mucus observation, and record of secondary symptoms by couple
Oral contraceptives	Suppress ovulation by inhibiting hypothalamus and pituitary	Ingestion of OC at same time each day; physical examination by physician every 6 mo
IUDs (unmedicated) (now rarely used)	Prevent implantation within uterus	Inserted into uterus by trained person; placement checked often; IUD changed every 2-3 yr, prn
Mechanical barriers		
Diaphragms	Prevent sperm migration into uterus	Inserted into vagina over cervix before intercourse
Condoms	Prevent sperm migration into uterus	Applied to penis before intercourse
Chemical barriers: foams, gels, suppositories*	Destroy sperm or make them immobile within vaginal vault	Inserted into vagina before each intercourse; applied with diaphragm or condom
Fertility awareness	Family planning method combined with a barrier method of contraception	
Vaginal sponge	Releases spermicide Blocks cervical opening Absorbs semen	Inserted into upper vagina before intercourse; can be left in place to provide protection for 24 hr

*Chemicals may be combined with other forms of contraception to enhance their effectiveness (e.g., Cu-7 IUD; spermicide with diaphragm or condom).

contraceptive effectiveness, the success of a method of contraception in preventing pregnancy. It is best expressed as the number of pregnancies per 100 women per year. A contraceptive method that results in a pregnancy rate of less than 10 pregnancies per 100 women per year is considered effective.

contractility, the ability of the heart to contract when properly stimulated.

contraction, 1. a reduction in size, especially of muscle fibers. 2. an abnormal shrinkage. 3. a rhythmic tightening of the muscles in the upper part of the uterus during labor. Contractions are mild in early labor. They become quite strong late in labor, occurring as often as every 2 minutes and lasting more than a minute. Contractions make the uterus smaller and squeeze the fetus through the birth canal. 4. abnormal smallness of the birth canal. This can cause difficult labor (dystocia). See also **clinical pelvimetry, dystocia, x-ray.**

contracture, an abnormal condition of a joint. The joint is bent and will not move. This is usually a permanent condition. Contractures are caused by shortening and wasting away of muscle fibers or by loss of the normal stretchiness of the skin. Extensive scar tissue over a joint can cause contracture.

contraindication, a factor that prohibits a certain treatment for a specific patient due to some condition of the patient. For example, pregnancy is a contraindication for giving the antibiotic drug tetracycline.

contralateral, affecting the opposite side of the body.

contrast medium, a dye injected into the body that illuminates inner structures that are hard to see on x-ray films.

controlled area, an area in which entry and activities are controlled to ensure radiation protection and prevent the spread of contamination.

controlled ventilation, the use of a breathing machine to replace natural breathing by the patient.

contusion. See **bruise.**

convalescence, the period of recovery after an illness, injury, or surgery.

convalescent home. See **extended care facility.**

conversion, 1. changing from one form to another. 2. correcting the position of a fetus during labor. This is most often done when the infant's face or brow is against the cervix. The doctor moves the baby so that the head is against the cervix.

conversion disorder, a kind of hysterical neurosis. Emotional conflicts are repressed and changed into symptoms of illness. However, the symptoms have no physical cause. Common symptoms are blindness, loss of feeling, increased sensitivity, or involuntary muscle movements (as tics or tremors). More severe symptoms are paralysis, loss of voice, hallucinations, trance and rigidness (catalepsy), choking, and breathing difficulties. The person who has conversion disorder firmly believes the physical condition exists.

convulsion, a sudden, violent uncontrollable contraction of a group of muscles. Convulsions may occur in episodes, as in epilepsy. They also may occur once, such as after a brain concussion.

Cooley's anemia. See **thalassemia.**

cooling, reducing body temperature. This is done by applying a cooling blanket, cold moist dressings, ice packs, or an alcohol bath. Below normal body temperature may be produced in a patient before some kinds of surgery. This reduces the rate of the body functions. Very high fevers of any cause may be treated with cooling techniques.

coordination, the process of systematically analyzing a situation, developing relevant information, and informing appropriate *command* authority (for its decision) of viable alternatives for selection of the most effective combination of available resources to meet specific objectives. The coordination process (which can be either introagency or interagency) does not in and of itself involve command dispatch actions. However, personnel responsible for coordination *may* perform such command or dispatch functions within limits as established by specific agency delegations, procedures, and legal authority.

cooperating agency, an agency supplying assistance other than direct suppression, rescue, support, or service functions to the incident control effort (e.g., Red Cross, law enforcement agency, telephone company).

coping, a process by which a person deals with stress, solves problems, and makes decisions. The stress can be either physical or mental. Coping is done through the use of both conscious and unconscious tools. A problem in coping with crisis situations features a failure to meet one's basic needs or change in ability to take part in society. Other symptoms may be destructive behavior, a change in ways of communicating, and too many accidents and illnesses. There may be a lack of emotional support for a patient from a family member or friend. The cause is often feelings of grief, anxiety, guilt, hostility, or despair by the significant person. There may also be a marked distortion of reality in regard to the patient's health problem. This makes it hard for the patient to cope with a current health problem.

copper (Cu), a soft metallic element essential to good health. Copper deficiency in the body is rare. Little is needed daily, and it is easily obtained from a number of foods. Too much copper in the body can result from some diseases.

coprolalia /kop'rəlā'lyə/, the excessive use of obscene words.

coproporphyria /-pôrfir'ē·ə/, a rare hereditary disorder in which large amounts of nitrogen substances (porphyrins) are released in the feces. Attacks may be caused by certain drugs, as barbiturates and steroids. These attacks are marked by stomach and nervous system disorders. Patients are often helped by a high-carbohydrate diet.

cor, 1. the heart. 2. relating to the heart.

coracoid process /kôr'əkoid/, the thick, curved part of the upper edge of the shoulder blade (scapula). The pectoralis minor muscle stretches between this process and the ribs.

Coramine, a trademark for a stimulant (nikethamide). This drug is used to treat breathing and nervous system problems and circulatory failure.

cord, any long, rounded, flexible structure. The body contains many cords, as the vocal, spinal, nerve, and umbilical cords. Cords serve many purposes, depending on location and need. –**cordal,** *adj.*

corditis /kôrdī'-/, an inflammation of the sperm cord with pain in the testicles. It is often caused by an infection in the urethra or by a tumor. Other causes are a collection of fluid in the testicles (hydrocele) and varicose veins in the scrotum (varicocele). Injury to the groin often causes a blood clot in the cord.

Cordran, a trademark for a drug to treat itching and skin inflammation (flurandrenolide).

Corgard, a trademark for a drug used to treat high blood pressure and angina (nadolol).

Cori's disease. See **glycogen storage disease.**

corium /kôr'ē·əm/, the layer of skin, just below the outer layer (epidermis). It contains blood and lymph vessels, nerves and nerve endings, glands, and hair follicles.

corkscrew esophagus, a disorder of the throat (esophagus). Normal contractions are replaced by spastic movements. They may occur when swallowing or for no reason. They may also be caused by swallowing stomach acid backing up into the esophagus. Symptoms include difficulty in swallowing, weight loss, and severe pain over the upper chest. Treatment includes drugs to fight the contractions, avoidance of cold fluids, or surgical correction.

corn, a cone-shaped horny mass of thickened skin on the toes. Corns result from long-term friction and pressure. The conical shape of the corn presses down on the skin beneath, making it thin and tender. There are two types of corns. The hard corn is most often found on the outside of the little toe or the upper surfaces of the other toes. The soft corn is found between the toes and kept soft by moisture.

Treatment includes relief from the pressure and surgical or chemical removal.

cornea /kôr'nē·ə/, the transparent front part of the eye. It is dense and even in thickness. It projects like a dome beyond the white of the eye (sclera). The amount of curve varies in different persons. It can also change in one person since the cornea tends to flatten with age.

corneal grafting /kôr'nē·əl/, transplanting corneal tissue from one human eye to another. It is done to improve vision in persons with scars or warps of the cornea or when an ulcer in the cornea is removed. See also **transplant.**

corneal reflex, a way of protecting the eye in which the eyelids close when the cornea is touched. People who wear contact lenses may have a weak or no corneal reflex. Compare **conjunctival reflex.**

cornification, thickening of the skin by a buildup of dead cells.

corn pad, a device that helps relieve the pressure and pain of a corn. It transfers the pressure to surrounding areas. Corn pads are made of flexible fabric and shaped in a number of ways.

corona /kərō'nə/, 1. a crown. 2. a crownlike bulge, such as a place on a bone that sticks out.

coronal suture, the joining line (suture) between the bones of the skull that crosses the top of the skull from temple to temple.

coronary /kôr'əner'ē/, 1. referring to circling structures, as the coronary arteries; referring to the heart. 2. a nontechnical term for a heart attack.

coronary arteriovenous fistula, a birth defect that affects the heart. There is a abnormal passage (fistula) between a coronary artery and the right upper or lower chamber, or the major vein returning to the heart (vena cava). In simple cases there may be no ill effects. A severe case may result in growth failure, lack of tolerance for exercise, difficult breathing, and anginal pain. A loud continuous heart murmur is also a symptom. Treatment is with surgery.

coronary artery, one of a pair of arteries that branch from a part of the main artery (ascending aorta) of the body. The **right coronary artery** passes along the right side of the heart and divides into branches that supply both lower chambers (ventricles) and the right upper chamber (atrium). The **left coronary artery** supplys both ventricles and the left atrium of the heart.

coronary artery disease, any abnormal condition that may affect the arteries of the heart. This refers especially to those that reduce the flow of oxygen and nutrients to the heart muscle. The most common kind of coronary artery disease is coronary atherosclerosis. This is a form of hardening of the arteries (arteriosclerosis) in which fat (cholesterol) is deposited in the artery walls. This can lead to blood clots and heart attack. The disease affects more men than women. It also occurs more often in whites and the middle-aged or elderly. More younger women today are affected than in the past. This is possibly due to the effects of increased cigarette smoking, stressful office jobs, and the use of birth control pills. The disease occurs most often in people with regular diets high in calories, fat (especially saturated fat), cholesterol, and refined carbohydrates. Cigarette smokers are two to six times more likely to develop this disease or to die from it than nonsmokers. High blood pressure is also a common related cause in atherosclerosis. Other risk factors include heavy alcohol use, obesity, lack of exercise, shortage of vitamins C and E, living in large urban areas, heredity, climate, and viruses. Angina pectoris is the classic symptom of coronary artery disease. It results from blockage of an artery, causing lack of oxygen in part of the heart. Angina is a crushing pain under the breastbone that travels to the left arm, neck, jaw, and shoulder blade. It often follows physical exercise, emotional excitement, or exposure to cold. Diagnosis of coronary artery disease is usually based on patient history, an electrocardiogram (ECG) during angina, exercise tests, and x-ray test (angiography) of the heart. Treatment of coronary artery disease commonly includes giving of nitrate drugs, such as nitroglycerin, or propranolol. Bypass surgery may use vein grafts to bypass the diseased arteries. Another type of surgery is angioplasty, which opens the blocked arteries. High blood pressure may be controlled with diuretics or other drugs.

coronary autoregulation, the widening of an artery of the heart. This happens in response to lack of oxygen to the heart muscle.

coronary bypass, open-heart surgery to relieve a blocked heart artery. An artificial tube or part of a blood vessel is attached to the diseased coronary artery. It is then connected to the aorta, bypassing the damaged artery. The operation improves the blood supply to the heart muscle, eases the work of the heart, and helps anginal pain. Two or three grafts are most often done when several areas are blocked. See also **bypass.** (Illustration on page 154.)

coronary care unit (CCU), a specially equipped hospital area. It is designed to treat patients with sudden, dangerous heart conditions. Such units contain equipment to revive and watch patients. The staff is trained in heart emergencies. See also **intensive care unit.**

coronary occlusion, a blockage of any one of the heart arteries. The most common cause is buildup of fat deposits in the arteries (atherosclerosis), sometimes with blood clots (thrombosis). These deposits narrow the channel, reduce the blood flow, and lead to heart attacks. In certain heart diseases spasms of an artery can narrow the opening and block blood flow. This causes symptoms of a heart attack, as crushing pain under the breastbone that spreads

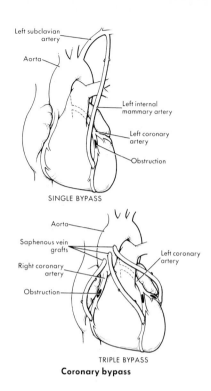

SINGLE BYPASS

TRIPLE BYPASS

Coronary bypass

to the arms, jaw, and neck. Occlusions that lead to heart attack are common. Delayed treatment often results in death. Almost half of the deaths caused by heart attacks occur before the person gets to the hospital, often within 1 hour of the beginning of symptoms. Occlusions often lead to irregular heart beats. Some types also cause fainting. Treatment includes drugs to correct irregular heart beat, nitroglycerin to relieve pain, oxygen, and bed rest. A temporary pacemaker may also be implanted. See also **coronary artery disease.**

coronary sinus, the wide channel, in the left upper heart chamber (atrium). It is about 1 inch long.

coronary thrombosis. See **thrombosis.**

coronary vein, one of the veins of the heart. It takes blood from the capillaries of the heart to the right upper heart chamber (atrium).

coronavirus /kôr′ənə-/, a member of a group of viruses. Several types can cause severe breathing illnesses.

coroner /kôr′ənər/, a public official who looks into the causes and events of a death, especially one resulting from unnatural causes. Also called **medical examiner.**

cor pulmonale /kôr pŏŏl′mənā′lē/, an abnormal condition of the heart with increase in size of the right lower chamber (ventricle). This results from high blood pressure (hypertension) of the lung circulation. Long-term cor pulmonale enlarges the right ventricle because it cannot adjust to a rise in pressure as easily as the left ventricle. In some patients, however, the disease also increases the size of the left ventricle. Some diseases linked to cor pulmonale are cystic fibrosis, myasthenia gravis, heart disease, and inflammation of the lung arteries (pulmonary arteritis). Chronic obstructive pulmonary disease and emphysema are others. Cor pulmonale accounts for about 25% of all types of heart failure. The disease affects middle-aged and elderly men more than women. It may occur in children. Some of the early signs of cor pulmonale include constant cough, difficulty breathing, fatigue, and weakness. As the disease grows worse, breathing difficulty may become more severe. Signs of this condition include water retention, swollen neck veins, and rapid heart beat. A weak pulse and low blood pressure may result from decreased heart function. Treatment tries to increase oxygen, increase exercise tolerance, and correct the defect if possible. The outcome is usually poor, however. This is because cor pulmonale is most often the result of an incurable disease, chronic obstructive pulmonary disease. Treatment includes bed rest, digitalis, drugs to fight lung infection, oxygen, low-salt diet, a small amount of fluids, diuretics, and anticlotting drugs.

corpus cavernosum,   a type of spongy tissue in the penis or clitoris. The tissue becomes filled with blood during sexual excitement.

corpuscle /kôr′pəsəl/,   **1.** any cell of the body. **2.** a red or white blood cell.

corpus luteum,   a mound of yellow tissue that forms in the ovary. It occurs in the wall of the ovary where an egg (ovum) has just been released. Its purpose is to release hormones to help prepare the body for pregnancy. If the egg is impregnated, it grows larger and lasts for several months. If the egg is not impregnated, it shrinks and is shed during menstruation.

corrosive,   **1.** eating away a substance or tissue, especially by chemical action. **2.** a substance that eats away a substance or tissue.   **–corrode,** *v.,* **corrosion,** *n.*

corrosivity hazards,   a material that causes visible destruction of, or irreversible alterations to, living tissue by chemical action at the point of contact.

corrugator supercilii,   one of the three muscles of the eyelid. It draws the eyebrow downward and inward, as in a frown.

Cortef,   a trademark for a glucocorticoid cream used to treat itching of the vaginal area and rectum (cortisol).

Cortef Fluid,   a trademark for a steroid used to treat allergies and inflammation (cortisol cypionate).

cortex /kôr′teks/,   *pl.* **cortices** /kôr′tisēz/,   the outer layer of a body organ or other structure.

cortical fracture,   any break that involves the outer layer (cortex) of the bone.

corticosteroid /kôr′tikōstir′oid/,   any one of the hormones made in the outer layer of the adrenal gland (adrenal cortex). They influence or control key functions of the body, as making carbohydrates and proteins, working of the heart and lung systems, and functions of the muscles, kidneys, and other organs. The release of these hormones increases during stress, especially in anxiety and injury. Too much of these hormones in the body is linked with various disorders, as Cushing's syndrome.

corticotropin.   See **adrenocorticotropic hormone.**

cortisol /kôr′-/,   a steroid hormone found naturally in the body. It is made in synthetic form to treat inflammation. Also called **hydrocortisone.**

cortisone /kôr′-/,   a steroid hormone made in the liver. It is made artificially and is used to treat inflammation.

Corti's organ,   a small, spiral structure inside the organ of hearing (cochlea) in the inner ear. It contains hair cells that touch the acoustic nerve, sending sound waves to the brain.

Cortisporin,   a trademark for a drug used in the eyes for infection and inflammation.

Corynebacterium /kôr′inē-/,   a group of rod-shaped, curved organisms. The most common disease-causing types are *Corynebacterium acnes,* found in acne sores, and *C. diphtheriae,* the cause of diphtheria.

Cosmegen,   a trademark for an anticancer drug (dactinomycin).

cosmetic surgery,   repair of skin or tissues, usually around the face and neck. It is generally done to correct a defect, remove a scar or birthmark, or correct the effects of aging on the skin. The surgery is usually done with a local anesthetic. **Rhinoplasty** is a method in which the structure of the nose is changed. It is most often done for cosmetic reasons. Bone or cartilage may be removed, tissue taken from another part of the body, or artificial material planted to change the shape. After surgery, any breathing difficulty is reported at once and the patient is kept with the head and knees raised. Edema and discoloration around the eyes is expected to last for several days. See also **plastic surgery.**

cosmic rays,   high-energy particulate and electromagnetic radiations that originate outside the earth's atmosphere.

costal,   **1.** referring to a rib. **2.** located near a rib or on a side close to a rib.

costochondral /kos′təkon′drəl/,   referring to a rib and its cartilage.

costovertebral,   referring to a rib and the spinal column.

Cotazym,   a trademark for a drug that replaces enzymes in the pancreas (pancrelipase).

cotyledon /kot'ilē'dən/, one of the segments on the surface of the placenta that attaches to the uterus. A normal placenta may have 15 to 20 cotyledons.

cough, a sudden, forceful release of air from the lungs. Coughing clears the lungs and throat of irritants and fluid. It also prevents breathing foreign matter into the lungs. It is a common symptom of diseases of the chest and throat. Tuberculosis, lung cancer, and bronchitis can cause long-term coughing. Ear infection, congestive heart failure, and heart valve disease may be linked with severe coughing. A **productive cough** usually forces sputum from the breathing tract, clearing the air passages and allowing oxygen to reach the air sacs (alveoli). Coughing is brought on by irritation of the breathing tract. Inhaling deeply and then contracting the diaphragm and muscles between the ribs and exhaling with force helps patients with breathing tract infections bring on productive coughing. Drugs that turn mucus into liquid (mucolytic agents) in the breathing tract help bring it up so it can be forced out more easily. Other drugs, as atropine, reduce the amount of mucus.

cough fracture, any break of a rib, caused by violent coughing. This most often happens to the fifth or seventh rib.

Coumadin, a trademark for an anticlotting drug (warfarin sodium, also called coumarin).

coumarin /kōō'mərin/, an anticlotting drug used to prevent and treat various kinds of blood clots (thrombosis and embolism). A serious side effect can be bleeding in the body (hemorrhage). It should not be used when this is a risk. Also called warfarin sodium.

countertraction, a force that pulls against traction, as the force of body weight. Countertraction is begun slowly by changing the position of a patient and by adding or by removing weights from weight hangers.

coup /kōō/, any blow to the body. It is most often used with a French word indicating a type of blow or wound. **Coup de sabre** /dəsäb'r(ə)/ means a wound similar to a sword cut. A **coup de soleil** /dəsōlā'ē/ is a sunstroke. **Coup sur coup** /sYrkōō'/ refers to giving a drug in small amounts over a short period of time rather than in one large dose. **Contre coup** /kôNtrəkōō'/ means an injury most often linked to a blow to the skull. The force of the blow carries through the skull to the other side of the head where the bruise or break appears.

coupling, the act of coming together, joining, or pairing.

Courvoisier's law /kōōrvō·äzē·āz'/, the rule that the gallbladder is smaller than usual if a gallstone blocks the common bile duct. However, the gallbladder is enlarged if the common bile duct is blocked by something else, as cancer of the pancreas.

Couvelaire uterus /kōōvəler'/, a bleeding condition of the uterus. It may occur after sudden tearing loose of the placenta (abruptio placenta). The uterus turns purple and does not contract well. See also **abruptio placenta.**

Cowper's gland /kou'pərz/, either of two pea-sized glands found at the end of the urine canal (urethral sphincter) of the male. They consist of several lobes with ducts that join and form a single duct.

cowpox, a mild infectious disease marked by a rash with pus-filled blisters. It is a disease of cattle caused by a virus that may be given to humans by direct contact. It may also be given by deliberate injection as cowpox infection usually makes a person immune to smallpox. Also called **vaccinia.** See **also smallpox.**

coxa magna, an abnormal widening of the head and neck of the thigh bone (femur).

coxa valga, a hip defect in which the thigh bone (femur) angles out to the side of the body.

coxa vara, a hip defect in which the thigh bone (femur) angles toward the center of the body. Also called **coxa adducta, coxa flexa.**

coxsackievirus /koksak'ē-/, any of 30 different viruses that infect the intestines (enterovirus). These cause a number of symptoms and affect mostly children during warm weather. These infections are linked to many diseases. These include hand, foot, and mouth disease, infection of the heart, infection of the membrane around the brain, and several diseases linked to skin eruptions. Treatment is relief of symptoms. See also **viral infection.**

CPR, abbreviation for **cardiopulmonary resuscitation.**

crab louse, a type of body louse. It infests the hairs of the genital area and is often carried between persons by sexual contact. Also called *Pediculus pubis (informal)* **crab.** See also **pediculosis.**

cradle cap. See **seborrheic dermatitis.**

cramp, 1. a spastic and often painful contraction of one or more muscles. 2. a pain similar to a muscle cramp. See also **charley horse, dysmenorrhea, heat cramp, writer's cramp, wryneck.**

cranial nerves /krā'nē·əl/, the 12 pairs of nerves emerging from the cranial cavity through openings in the skull. They are referred to by Roman numerals and named as follows: (I) olfactory, sense of smell; (II) optic, sight; (III) oculomotor, eye muscles; (IV) trochlear, eye muscles; (V) trigeminal, jaws, chewing; (VI) abducens, eye muscles; (VII) facial, taste; (VIII) acoustic, hearing; (IX) glossopharyngeal, throat, swallowing; (X) vagal, heart, lungs, digestion; (XI) accessory, upper spine; (XII) hypoglossal, tongue, speaking.

craniopharyngeal /-fərin'jē·əl/, referring to the skull and the throat.

craniopharyngioma /-fərin'jē·ō'mə/, a tumor of the pituitary gland. It appears most often in children and adolescents. The tumor is solid and may expand into the brain, where it often becomes calcified. It may result in water on the brain (hydrocephalus) and disrupt control of the nervous system. Increased pressure in the brain, severe headaches, vomiting, stunted growth, defective vision, and genitals that do not develop are often linked to the tumor in children. Appearance of the tumor after puberty often results in absence of menstruation in women, and in men loss of sexual interest.

craniostenosis /-stənō'-/, a birth defect of the skull. It results from premature closing of the borders (sutures) between the skull bones. The extent of the defect depends on which sutures close and when the closure occurred. Impaired brain growth may or may not be involved. Surgery is necessary to relieve pressure on the brain when several sutures are fused. Surgery may also be done to improve appearance.

craniotomy /krā'nē·ot'-/, any surgical opening into the skull. It may be done to relieve pressure in the brain, to control bleeding, or to remove a tumor. A curved cut is made in the skin, holes are drilled in a circle, and the flap of bone is removed.

cranium /krā'nē·əm/, the bony skull that holds the brain. It is made up of eight bones: frontal, occipital, sphenoid, and ethmoid bones, and paired temporal and parietal bones. –**cranial,** *adj.*

cravat bandage /krəvat'/, a triangular bandage, folded lengthwise. It may be used to control bleeding or to tie splints in place.

crease, a wrinkle formed by a folding back of tissue, as on the palm of the hand.

creatine /krē'ətēn/, an important nitrogen compound made in the body. It combines with phosphorus to form high-energy phosphate.

creatinine /krē·at'inēn/, a substance formed from the making of creatine. It is common in blood, urine, and muscle tissue.

Crede's prophylaxis, a 1% silver nitrate solution dropped into the eyes of newborn infants. This is done to prevent gonorrhea infection of the eyes, which can result in blindness. State laws requiring this have greatly reduced blindness.

creeping eruption, a skin disorder with irregular, wandering red lines. These are made by burrowing larvae of hookworms and some roundworms. The worms make their way into the body when people walk barefoot where these parasites are known to be common. Treatment includes giving antiparasite drugs. In some cases the worms are surgically removed from the skin. Also called **larva migrans.**

cremaster /krimas'tər/, a thin muscle layer covering the spermatic cord through which sperm travels. The function of the cremaster is to pull the testicles up toward the body in response to cold or stimulation of nerves.

cremasteric reflex. See **superficial reflex.**

crepitus /krep'itəs/, **1.** the noisy release of gas from the intestine through the anus. **2.** a sound heard in gas gangrene or the rubbing together of bone fragments in damaged joints.

cresol /krē'sol/, a liquid obtained from coal tar. It is used as an antiseptic and disinfectant and is poisonous.

cretinism /krē'tənizm/, a condition marked by severe lack of thyroid function during infancy. It is often linked to other hormone defects. **Familial cretinism** is a genetic disorder. Signs of cretinism include dwarfism, mental deficiency, puffy facial features, a large tongue, navel hernia, and lack of muscle coordination.

crib death. See **sudden infant death syndrome.**

cricoid /krī'koid/, **1.** having a ring shape. **2.** a ring-shaped cartilage in the voicebox (larynx). It moves as the pitch of the voice raises or lowers.

cricopharyngeal /krī'kōfərin'jē·əl/, referring to the cricoid cartilage and the upper part of the esophagus (pharynx).

cricothyrotomy /-thīrot'-/, an emergency surgical cut into the larynx to open the throat in a choking person. A small vertical cut is made just below the Adam's apple and above the cricoid cartilage. The wound is then spread open with an object as a retractor. A tube is usually inserted through the opening. Compare **tracheostomy.**

Crigler-Najjar syndrome /-naj'är/, a hereditary defect in which an enzyme (glucuronyl transferase) is deficient or absent. The condition features yellow skin (jaundice) and severe disorders of the central nervous system.

crisis, 1. a turning point for better or worse during a life. A crisis is most often noted by a marked change in the strength of symptoms. **2.** events that strongly affect the emotional state of a person, as death or divorce.

crisis intervention, help given to solve a mental problem. The goal is to restore the patient to the level of coping that existed before the crisis. A **crisis intervention unit** is a group trained in emergency treatment and in methods for giving mental help to a patient during a period of crisis, as suicide attempts or drug abuse. Such groups are found in community hospitals, in health care centers, or as special units, as suicide prevention centers, and are open 24 hours a day.

crisis theory, a way of defining and explaining the events that occur when a person faces a problem that appears to have no solution.

crista supraventricularis /kris'təsoo'prəventrik'yəler'is/, the muscle ridge on the inside wall of the right lower chamber (ventricle) of the heart.

critical care. See **intensive care.**

critical organs, tissues that are the most reactive to radiation, as the sex glands, lymph organs, and intestine. The skin, cornea and lens of the eye, mouth, esophagus, vagina, and cervix are the next most reactive organs to radiation.

Crohn's disease, a long-term bowel disease with inflammation. The cause is unknown. It most often affects the lower part of the small intestine (ileum), the main part of the large intestine (colon), or both structures.

cromolyn sodium, a drug used to prevent bronchial asthma. The drug has no effect after an attack has started. Known allergy to this drug prohibits its use. Side effects include lung spasms, wheezing, a stuffy nose, throat irritation, and other allergic reactions.

Cronkhite-Canada syndrome, an abnormal inherited condition of growths (polyps) in the intestines with skin defects, as nail wasting, hair loss, and excess amounts of skin color. In some patients, there may also be faulty intestine activity and a lack of blood calcium, potassium, and magnesium.

cross-bite tooth, any of the back teeth that allow the cusps of the upper teeth to fit in the central grooves of the lower teeth.

crossed reflex, any nerve reflex in which stimulating one side of the body causes a response on the other side.

cross-eye. See **strabismus.**

crossmatching of blood, a means used by blood banks to find out whether donated blood can be used by a patient. This is done after the samples have been matched for major blood type, as A, B, AB, and O. Serum from the donor's blood is mixed with red cells from the patient's blood, and cells from the donor are mixed with serum from the patient. If clumping (agglutination) occurs, a foreign (antigenic) substance is present and the bloods are not usable. If no agglutination occurs, the donor's blood may safely be given to the patient. See also **blood group.**

croup /kroop/, a virus infection of the upper and lower breathing tract that occurs mostly in infants and young children. Croup occurs after another upper breathing tract infection. Symptoms include hoarseness, fever, a distinct "barking" cough, and many degrees of breathing distress from blockage of the windpipe. Infection is carried by airborne particles or by contact with infected fluids. The acute stage starts rapidly, most often occurs at night, and may be triggered by exposure to cold air. Treatment includes bed rest, drinking a lot of fluids, and relieving airway blockage, as with vaporizers. Children with mild infections are treated at home. It may be necessary to put children in the hospital who have high fevers, breathing distress, and bluish or pale skin. A tube in the throat to open the airway may be necessary. The infection may spread to other areas of the breathing tract, causing problems, as bronchiolitis, pneumonia, and ear infections. In most children the condition is mild and runs its course in 3 to 7 days.

Croupette, a trademark for a device that gives cool humidity with oxygen or compressed air. It is used for children from 1 month to 10 years of age. The Croupette is made up of a machine that lets out a fine spray with attached tubing that connects to a canopy. It is often used to treat croup, bronchiolitis, cystic fibrosis, asthma, laryngitis, dehydration after surgery, and extremely high fever.

crown, 1. the upper part of an organ or structure, as the top of the head. 2. the upper part of a human tooth that is covered by enamel. An **artificial crown** is a dental device (prosthesis) that restores part or all of the crown of a natural tooth.

crowning, the phase at the end of labor in which the baby's head is seen at the opening of the vagina. The labia are stretched around the head during crowning just before birth. See also **labor.**

cruciate ligament of the atlas /kroo'shē·ăt/, a crosslike ligament that attaches the top spinal bone (atlas) to the base of the skull above and connecting to the second spinal bone (axis) below.

crush syndrome, 1. a severe, near fatal condition caused by a major crushing injury. It occurs when there is destruction of muscle and bone tissue, severe bleeding, and fluid loss. These injuries cause shock, bloody urine, kidney failure, and coma. Treatment includes giving fluids and electrolytes in the vein, antibiotics, pain relievers, and oxygen. Intensive care with close watching of all vital functions is often needed. 2. a severe problem caused by heroin overdose. It is marked by coma, water buildup, blockage of the blood system, and lymph channel blockage.

crust, a solid, hard outer layer formed by the drying of body fluids; a scab. Crusts are common in skin conditions, as eczema, impetigo, seborrhea, and during the healing of burns and sores.

Crutchfield tongs, a device put into the skull to hold the head and neck straight. The device is used in patients with broken necks. The tongs are placed into small bur holes drilled in each side of the skull. The surrounding skin is stretched and covered with a dressing. A rope attached to the tongs is set up with a pulley, and weights are hung at the other end. A patient's body may be kept straight by Crutchfield tongs for weeks before surgery is done.

cry, 1. a sudden, loud, willful or automatic sound in response to pain, fear, or a startle reflex. 2. weeping, because of pain or as a response to depression or grief.

cryoanesthesia /krī'ō-/, freezing a part to deaden nerve feelings to pain during brief minor surgery.

cryocautery /-kô'tərē/, applying any substance, as solid carbon dioxide, that destroys tissue by freezing. Also called **cold cautery.**

cryogen /krī'əjən/, a chemical that causes freezing. It is used to destroy diseased tissue without injury to nearby structures. An example is carbon dioxide. –**cryogenic,** *adj.*

cryoglobulinemia /-glob'yəlinē'mē·ə/, an abnormal condition in which an abnormal plasma protein (cryoglobulin) is in the blood. The disorder occurs in a cancer (multiple myeloma) and fluid buildup (angioneurotic edema).

cryonics /krī·on'-/, the ways in which cold is applied for many treatments, as brief local anesthesia.

cryosurgery /krī-ō-/, use of subfreezing temperature to destroy tissue. Cryosurgery is used to destroy nerve cells in the thalamus to treat Parkinson's disease, to destroy the pituitary gland to halt some kinds of spreading cancer, and to treat many cancers and skin disorders. The process is also used to heal the edges of a detached retina in the eye and to remove cataracts.

cryotherapy /krī-ō-/, a treatment using cold to destroy cells. Skin tags, warts, and actinic keratosis are some of the common skin disorders treated by cryotherapy.

crypt, a blind pit or tube on a surface. An example is any of the small pits in the iris of the eye along its outside margin, called **crypt of Fuchs.** See also **anal crypt.**

cryptitis /kriptī'-/, inflammation of a crypt, most often an anal crypt. Symptoms include pain, itching, and spasm of the sphincter.

cryptococcosis /krip'təkokō'-/, an infection caused by a fungus, *Cryptococcus neoformans.* It spreads through the lungs to the brain, skin, bones, and urinary tract. In North America it is most likely to affect middle-aged men in the southeastern states. Tumors filled with a jellylike material grow in organs and under the skin. Symptoms include coughing or breathing problems, headache, blurred sight, and difficulty in speaking.

Cryptomenorrhea /-men'ôrē'ə/, an abnormal condition in which the products of menstruation stay in the vagina because of a closed hymen. The disorder can also be caused by a blockage in the cervical canal that holds the products in the uterus. The symptoms are signs of menstruation with very little or no flow and sometimes severe pain. If the flow is completely blocked, menstrual flow may back up into the pelvic space causing severe infection (peritonitis), pain, scar tissue, and tissue shedding (endometriosis).

cryptophthalmos /-fthal'məs/, a defect of a fetus with complete joining of the eyelids, most often found with defects in form or lacking eyes.

cryptorchidism /kriptôr'kidizm/. See **undescended testis.**

crystal, a solid inorganic substance with the atoms or molecules in a regular, repeating three-dimension pattern. The exact pattern marks the shape of the crystal. –**crystalline,** *adj.*

crystalline lens /kris'təlin, -līn/, a clear structure of the eye that is in a capsule. It is located between the iris and the fluid in the eyeball (vitreous humor). The lens is a biconvex structure with the back surface more convex than the front. It is attached to the ciliary body and retina by ligaments that adjust the shape of the lens. This allows the lens to keep an object focused on the retina. For distant sight the lens thins, and for near sight it thickens. See also **eye.**

Crystodigin, a trademark for a drug used to strengthen a weak heart muscle and correct irregular heart beats (digitoxin).

cuboid bone, the foot (tarsal) bone on the outside of the foot next to the heel bone.

cul-de-sac /kYdesok', kul'dəsak/, a blind pouch.

Cullen's sign, the appearance of faint, irregularly formed patches when bleeding under the skin occurs around the navel. The discolored skin is blue-black and becomes greenish-brown or yellow. Cullen's sign may appear with pancreatitis, severe bleeding in the upper bowels, and a ruptured ectopic pregnancy.

culture-bound, referring to a health belief that is specific to a culture, as belief in certain kinds of prayer or the "evil eye."

culture procedure, any of several ways for growing colonies of microorganisms in a laboratory. Cultures are grown to note an organism and to find out which antibiotics are effective in fighting infections.

culture shock, the mental effect of a drastic culture change in the life of a person. There may be feelings of helplessness, discomfort, and confusion when trying to adapt to a different culture with unfamiliar practices, values, and beliefs.

cumulative, increasing by steps with an eventual total that may go past the expected result.

cumulative action, 1. the increased action of a treatment or drug when given repeatedly, as the cumulative action of a regular exercise program. **2.** the increased effect of a drug when repeated doses build up in the body.

cumulative dose, the total dose that builds up from repeated exposure to radiation or a radioactive drug.

cuneiform /kyo͞onē'əfôrm/, (of bone and cartilage) wedge-shaped.

cup arthroplasty of the hip joint, surgery to replace the head of the thigh bone (femur) with a metal or plastic mold to relieve pain and increase motion in arthritis or to correct a deformity. See also **arthroplasty, hip replacement.**

Cuprimine, a trademark for a drug used to treat rheumatoid arthritis, kidney stones, and poisoning by heavy metals (D-penicillamine).

curare /kyŏŏrä′rē/, a substance taken from tropical plants of the genus *Stryknos*. It is a very strong muscle relaxer. Large doses can cause complete paralysis, but use is most often short-term with drugs or with general anesthesia. See also **tubocurarine chloride.**

cure, **1.** restoring the health of a patient with a disease or other disorder. **2.** the favorable result of treating a disease or other disorder. **3.** a course of treatment, a drug, or another method used to treat a medical problem.

curettage /kyŏŏr′ətäzh′/, scraping material from the wall of a body cavity or other surface. It is done to remove tumors or abnormal tissue, or to get tissue for tests. It may be done with a blunt or a sharp knife (curet) or by suction.

curie, defined as the quantity of any radioactive nuclide such that 37 billion (3.7×10^{10}) disintegrations occur per second. Abbreviation: Ci. Also see **millicurie** and **microcurie.**

current, **1.** a flowing or streaming movement. **2.** a flow of electrons along a conductor in a closed circuit; an electric current. **3.** certain electric activity in the body, such as that of the heart, allowing blood to flow, or a current that passes to and through a muscle.

curve of Carus, the normal axis of the opening at the base of the pelvis.

Cushing's disease, a disorder resulting from the high release of ACTH (adrenocorticotropic hormone) by the pituitary gland. The cause is often a tumor on the pituitary gland. Symptoms include fat pads on the chest, upper back, and face; water buildup; high blood sugar; round "moon" face; muscle weakness; purplish streaks on the skin; infection; fragile bones; acne; and heavy growth of hair on the face. The high blood sugar most often does not respond to treatment, and diabetes mellitus may become a long-term condition. Treatment includes removal of the tumor by surgery or shrinking the tumor by x-ray treatments. Also called **hyperadrenalism.** Compare **Cushing's syndrome.**

Cushing's syndrome, a disorder resulting from excess ACTH (adrenocorticotropic hormone) made by the pituitary gland. It occurs when large doses of steroid drugs are given over a period of several weeks or longer. Symptoms include high blood sugar levels, overweight, a round "moon" face, a pad of fat on the chest and stomach, lowered sex hormone levels, muscle wasting, water buildup, low potassium levels, and some emotional change. The skin may be highly colored and fragile; minor infections may become severe and long-lasting. Children with the disorder may stop growing. Lowering or changing the drug may relieve the symptoms. Also called **hyperadrenocorticism.** Compare **Cushing's disease.**

cusp, **1.** a sharp or rounded projection that rises from the chewing surface of a tooth. The **anterior determinants of cusp** are the shapes of the front teeth that decide the "hills and valleys" of the back teeth. They are important in restoring the back teeth. **2.** any one of the small flaps on the valves of the heart.

custodial care, nonmedical care given on a long-term basis, most often for invalids and patients with long-term diseases.

cutaneous /kyŏŏtā′nē·əs/, referring to the skin.

cutaneous horn, a hard, skin-colored bulge of the skin, most often on the head or face. It may be a forerunner of cancer and is usually removed.

cutaneous papilloma. See **skin tag.**

cutdown, cutting into a vein to insert a tube (catheter). It is done when a vein cannot be entered with a needle. It is also done for nutrition (hyperalimentation) therapy when highly packed solutions are needed. After the catheter is removed, the cut is stitched shut, and a sterile dressing is applied. See also **hyperalimentation, venipuncture.**

cuticle /kyŏŏ′tikəl/, **1.** skin. **2.** the sheath of a hair sac (follicle). **3.** the thin edge of thick skin at the base of a nail.

cyanide poisoning /sī′ənīd/, poisoning from swallowing or breathing in cyanide. It may be in substances such as bitter almond oil, wild cherry syrup, prussic acid, hydrocyanic acid, or potassium or sodium cyanide. Symptoms include rapid heart beat, tiredness, seizures, and headache. Cyanide poisoning can result in death within 1 to 15 minutes. Treatment includes flushing the stomach out, giving amyl-nitrite, oxygen, and sodium thiosulfate.

cyanocobalamin /sī′ənōkōbal′əmin/, a red, crystal-like substance that can be dissolved in water. It is also known as **vitamin B_{12}.** It is used by the body in processing protein, fats, and carbohydrates, normal blood making, and nerve function. A lack of cyanocobalamin results in pernicious anemia and brain damage.

cyanosis /sī′ənō′-/, bluish discoloration of the skin and mucous membranes from lack of oxygen. The cause can be hemoglobin without oxygen in the blood or a defect in the hemoglobin molecule. **–cyanotic,** *adj.*

cyclacillin, a penicillin antibiotic used to treat bacteria infections. Known allergy to the penicillin drugs prohibits its use. Side effects include allergic reactions, severe diarrhea, nausea, and skin rash.

Cyclaine, a trademark for a local anesthetic (hexylcaine hydrochloride).

cyclamate /sī'kləmāt/, an artificial sweetener with no food value. It was taken from the market in the United States because it caused cancer in laboratory animals.

cyclandelate, a drug that widens the blood vessels. It is used to treat blockage of blood flow or blood vessel spasm. Pregnancy or known allergy to this drug prohibits its use. Side effects include rapid heart beat, stomach upset, and flushing.

Cyclapen-W, a trademark for a penicillin antibiotic (cyclacillin).

cyclencephaly /sīk'lənsef'əlē/, a birth defect marked by the fusion of the two parts of the brain (cerebral hemispheres).

cyclitis /sīklī'-/, inflammation of the focusing part of the eye (ciliary body). Cyclitis causes redness of the white (sclera) next to the cornea of the eye.

cyclizine hydrochloride, an antihistamine used to treat or prevent motion sickness. Asthma or known allergy to this drug prohibits its use. It is not given to newborn infants or nursing mothers. Side effects include skin rash, allergic reactions, rapid heart beat, drowsiness, and dry mouth.

cyclobenzaprine hydrochloride, a muscle-relaxing drug used to treat muscle spasm.

Cyclocort, a trademark for a steroid drug used to treat itching and inflammation of the skin (amcinonide).

Cyclogyl, a trademark for a solution dropped into the eyes to widen and paralyze the eyes (cyclopentolate hydrochloride).

cyclomethycaine sulfate, a local anesthetic used on mucous membranes before tests are done on the area.

Cyclopar, a trademark for an antibiotic (tetracycline).

cyclophosphamide, a drug used to treat many cancers and to prevent rejection in organ transplants.

cycloplegic /sī'kləplē'jik/, **1.** referring to a drug or treatment that causes paralysis of the muscles of the eye that focus the lens (ciliary muscles). **2.** one of a group of drugs used to paralyze the ciliary muscles of the eye for tests or surgery.

cyclopropane /-prō'pān/, a highly flammable and explosive anesthetic gas now used for anesthesia only when other anesthetic drugs prohibit their use in a specific patient.

cycloserine /-ser'ēn/, an antibiotic used to treat active tuberculosis of the lungs and other parts of the body. Seizures, depression, severe anxiety, psychosis, severe kidney disease, excess use of alcohol, or known allergy to this drug prohibits its use. Side effects include tremor, drowsiness, seizures and mental changes.

Cyclospasmol, a trademark for a drug that widens blood vessels. It is used to treat hardening of the arteries, thrombophlebitis, night leg cramps, and Raynaud's phenomenon (cyclandelate).

cyclosporine, a drug that slows down the immune system. It is used in transplant surgery to prevent rejection.

cyclothymic disorder /-thī'mik/. See **bipolar disorder.**

Cylert, a trademark for a drug used to treat overactive children (pemoline).

cyproheptadine hydrochloride, an antihistamine used to treat many allergic reactions, including stuffy nose, skin rash, and itching.

cyst, a closed sac in or under the skin lined with skin tissue and containing fluid or semisolid material, as a **sebaceous cyst.**

cystadenoma /sis'tadinō'mə/, **1.** a benign skin tumor (adenoma) linked to a tumor with cysts (cystoma). **2.** an adenoma with many cysts. The cysts may contain blood, clear fluid, or thick, sticky fluid.

cystectomy /sistek'təmē/, a kind of surgery in which all or a part of the bladder is removed. This is most often done for cancer of the bladder.

cysteine (Cys) /sis'tēn/, an amino acid found in many proteins in the body, including keratin. It is an important source of sulfur for many body actions.

cystic carcinoma, a cancer with cysts or cystlike spaces. Tumors of this kind occur in the breast and ovary.

cysticercosis /sis'tisərkō'-/, an infection by the larval stage of the pork tapeworm (*Taenia solium)* or the beef tapeworm (*T. saginata).* See also **tapeworm infection.**

cystic fibroma, a fiberlike tumor in which saclike (cystic) breakdown has occurred.

cystic fibrosis, an inherited disorder of the glands that secrete through ducts (exocrine glands). It causes the glands to make very thick releases of mucus. The glands most affected are those in the pancreas, the breathing system, and the sweat glands. Cystic fibrosis is often diagnosed in infancy or early childhood. It occurs mainly in whites. The earliest symptom is often a blockage of the small bowel by thick stool that appears in newborns (meconium ileus). Other early signs are a long-term cough, many foul-smelling stools, and constant upper lung infections. Diagnosis is made by the sweat test, which shows high levels of both sodium and chloride. Because there is no known cure, treatment is directed at preventing lung infections, which are the most common cause of death.

cystic tumor, a tumor with spaces or sacs with a semisolid or a liquid material.

cystine /sis'tin/, an amino acid found in many proteins in the body, including keratin and insulin.

cystinosis /-ō'sis/, an inborn disease with amino acid (cystine) deposits in the liver, spleen, bone marrow, and cornea in the eye. Other symptoms include sugar and proteins in the urine, rickets, kidney defects, and slowed growth. Also called **cystine storage disease.**

cystinuria /-ŏŏr′ē·ə/, **1.** high amounts of an amino acid (cystine) in the urine. **2.** an inherited defect of the kidney filtering tubes, marked by excess urinary release of cystine and many other amino acids. In high amounts, cystine forms kidney or bladder stones.

cystitis /sistī′-/, an inflammation of the urinary bladder and ureters. Symptoms include bloody urine, pain, and the need to urinate often. It may be caused by a bacteria infection, stone, or tumor.

cystocele /sis′təsēl/, sagging of the urinary bladder through the wall of the vagina. A large cystocele may cause voiding difficulty or incontinence, urinary tract infection, and painful sexual union. Compare **rectocele.**

cystogram /-gram′/, a series of x-ray films of the bladder and ureters.

cystometry /sistom′ətrē/, the study of bladder function by use of a **cystometer,** an instrument that measures ability in relation to changing pressure.

cystoscopy /sistos′kəpē/, the examination of the urinary tract with a special device (cystoscope) placed in the urethra. Before the test, the patient either is given a tranquilizer or is put to sleep. For the test, the bladder is filled with air or water and the cystoscope is put into place. In addition to testing, cystoscopy is used for taking samples of tumors or other growths and for removing growths (polyps).

Cystospaz, a trademark for an antispasm drug used to treat urinary tract disorders (hyoscyamine).

Cytadren, a trademark for a drug used to slow down adrenal gland action in some patients with Cushing's syndrome (aminoglutethimide).

cytarabine, an anticancer drug used to treat myelocytic leukemia, lymphocytic leukemia, and erythroleukemia. Known allergy to this drug prohibits its use. Side effects include severe anemia, inflammation of the mouth and blood vessels, liver damage, and fever.

cytocide /sī′təsīd/, any substance that destroys cells. –**cytocidal,** adj.

cytoctony /sītok′tənē/, destroying of cells, as killing cells in culture by viruses.

cytogene /sī′təjēn/, a particle in the cytoplasm of a cell that reproduces itself and can carry inherited data. –**cytogenic,** adj.

cytogenesis /sī′təjen′əsis/, the beginning, growth, and dividing of cells. –**cytogenetic, cytogenic,** adj.

cytogenetics /-jənet′-/, the branch of genetics that studies the cell parts that concern heredity, mainly the chromosomes.

cytogenic gland /-jen′ik/, a gland that releases living cells, as the testicles and ovaries.

cytology /sītol′-/, the study of cells, their growth, beginnings, structure, action, and diseases.

cytolysis /sītol′isis/, the destruction of a living cell, mainly by breaking down the outer membrane. –**cytolytic,** adj.

cytomegalic inclusion disease (CID) /-məgal′ik/, an infection caused by a virus (cytomegalovirus) related to the herpes viruses. It is mainly an acquired disease of infants before birth. It results in a very small head, slowed growth, liver and spleen defects, hemolytic anemia, and broken long bones.

cytomegalovirus (CMV) /-meg′əlō-/, a member of a group of large herpes-type viruses that can cause many diseases. It causes serious illness in newborns and in patients being treated with drugs that slow down the immune system, as after an organ transplant.

cytomegalovirus (CMV) disease, a virus infection caused by a virus (cytomegalovirus). Symptoms include fatigue, fever, swollen lymph glands, pneumonia, and liver and spleen defects. Another infection with many bacteria and fungi often occurs as a result of slowing down the immune response, a common effect of herpesviruses.

Cytomel, a trademark for a thyroid hormone drug used to treat an underactive thyroid gland (liothyronine sodium).

cytometry /sītom′ətrē/, counting and measuring cells, as blood cells. –**cytometric,** adj.

cytomorphosis /-môrfō′-/, the many changes that occur in a cell during the course of its life cycle, from the first stage until death.

cyton /sī′tən/, the cell body of a nerve, or the part of a nerve with the nucleus and its surrounding cytoplasm. Also called **cytone** /sī′tōn/.

cytophoresis /-fôr′əsis/, a process of removing red or white blood cells or platelets from patients with certain blood disorders.

cytoplasm. See **cell.**

Cytosar-U, a trademark for an anticancer drug (cytarabine).

cytosine /sī′təsin/, a substance that is an important part of DNA and RNA. It occurs in small amounts in most cells.

cytotoxic drug, any drug that blocks the growth of cells in the body. These drugs are able to destroy abnormal cells while saving as many normal cells as possible. They are commonly used in cancer treatments. Cytotoxic drugs can themselves cause cancer, so they are used only for a short time.

cytotoxin, a substance that has a harmful effect on some cells. A substance that defends the body against foreign bodies (antibody) may act as a cytotoxin. –**cytotoxic,** adj.

Cytoxan, a trademark for an anticancer drug (cyclophosphamide).

D

D & C, abbreviation for **dilatation and curettage.**

dacarbazine, a drug used to treat cancerous melanoma, sarcoma, and Hodgkin's disease. Known allergy to this drug prohibits its use. Side effects include severe anemia, intestinal symptoms, kidney and liver failure, hair loss, and fever.

Dacriose, a trademark for a solution for rinsing the eyes.

dacryocyst /dak'rē·əsist'/, a tear sac at the inner corner of the eye. It is a normal feature.

dacryocystitis /dak'rē·ōsistī'-/, an infection of the tear sac. It is caused by blockage of the duct that drains into the nose (nasolacrimal duct). Symptoms include tearing and discharge from the eye.

dacryostenosis /-stəno'-/, an abnormal narrowing of the duct that drains into the nose (nasolacrimal duct). This occurs either as a birth defect or as a result of infection or injury.

dactinomycin, an antibiotic used as an anticancer drug. Herpes zoster infection or known allergy to this drug prohibits its use. Side effects include severe anemia, severe intestinal problems, inflammation of the rectum, hair loss, and ulcers of the mouth.

dactyl /dak'təl/, a digit (finger or toe).

Dakin's solution, a solution for killing bacteria (antiseptic).

Dalmane, a trademark for a drug that produces sleep or has a calming effect (flurazepam hydrochloride).

damp, a harmful gas found in caves and mines. **Black damp** or **choke damp** is caused by coal seams soaking up the oxygen in the tunnels. **Fire damp** is made up of explosive gases. **White damp** is another name for carbon monoxide.

danazol, a drug that stops the output of some pituitary hormones. It is used to treat endometriosis. Genital bleeding, heart, liver, or kidney malfunction, or known allergy to this drug prohibits its use. It is not used in pregnancy or during nursing. Side effects include muscle spasms, nausea, weight gain, acne, water retention, oily skin, and voice changes and other masculinizing effects.

dander, dry scales shed from the skin or hair of animals or the feathers of birds. Dander may cause an allergic reaction in some persons.

dandruff, scaly material shed from the scalp. It is made up of dead skin. Treatment with a dandruff (keratolytic) shampoo is often given to soften and remove the scales. See also **seborrheic dermatitis.**

Danocrine, a trademark for a drug that suppresses the action of the pituitary gland (danazol).

danthron, a laxative used to treat constipation. It is also used to empty the bowels before x-ray tests or surgery. Abdominal pain, nausea, or vomiting prohibits its use.

Dantrium, a trademark for a drug that relaxes muscles and is used in anesthesia (dantrolene sodium).

dantrolene sodium, a drug that relaxes muscles. It is used to treat muscle spasms resulting from injury to the spinal cord or brain. It is not used for spasm from rheumatic disorders. Liver malfunction or allergy to this drug prohibits its use. Side effects include possible liver poisoning, confusion, drowsiness, diarrhea, dizziness, fatigue, and muscle weakness.

dapsone (DADPS), a drug used to treat leprosy. Pregnancy or known allergy to this drug prohibits its use. Side effects include red blood cell disorders, episodes of active disease, nervous system disorders, nausea, loss of appetite, and skin rash.

Daraprim, a trademark for a drug used to treat malaria (pyrimethamine).

Darbid, a trademark for a drug used to treat peptic ulcers (isopropamide iodide).

Daricon, a trademark for a drug used to treat peptic ulcers (oxyphencyclimine hydrochloride).

dark-adapted eye, an eye in which the pupil has widened, making it more sensitive to dim light.

Darvon, a trademark for a drug that relieves pain (propoxyphene hydrochloride).

Darvon Compound, a trademark for a combination drug containing a pain reliever (propoxyphene hydrochloride) and APC (aspirin, phenacetin, and caffeine).

daunorubicin hydrochloride, an antibiotic used to treat cancer, such as leukemia and tumors of the nervous system. Severe anemia caused by drugs or known allergy to this drug prohibits its use. Side effects include severe anemia, heart poisoning, intestinal disorders, inflammation of the mouth, and hair loss.

day blindness, an abnormal visual condition (hemeralopia) in which bright light causes blurring of vision. It is an unpleasant side effect of certain drugs used to prevent convulsions, such as in treating children affected with petit mal epilepsy.

day health care services, centers that provide health services to adult patients who are mobile but do not require constant hospital care.

day hospital, a psychiatric center that offers a program during the day for patients released from hospitals.

D.D.S., abbreviation for *Doctor of Dental Surgery*.

DDT (dichlorodiphenyltrichloroethane), a substance once used worldwide as a major insecticide, most often in agriculture. It does not break down naturally in the environment. In recent years, its use has been restricted because DDT is a danger to the environment.

DDT poisoning. See **insecticide poisoning.**

deaf-mute, a person who is unable to hear or speak.

deafness, a condition of partial or complete loss of hearing. In assessing deafness, the patient's ears are examined to determine the cause of the hearing loss. **Conductive hearing loss** is a condition in which sound does not travel well to the sound organs of the inner ear. The volume of sound is less, but the sound remains clear. If volume is raised, hearing is normal.

death, the absence of life. **Apparent death** is the end of life as indicated by the absence of heartbeat or breathing. **Legal death** is the total absence of activity in the brain, heart, and lungs, as observed and declared by a physician. See also **stages of dying.**

debility, feebleness, weakness, or loss of strength. See also **asthenia.**

debride /dibrēd′/, to remove dirt, and damaged tissue from a wound or a burn. This prevents infection and aids healing. In treating a wound, this is the first step in cleaning it. −**debridement,** *n.*

Debrox, a trademark for drops that soften ear wax and aid its removal (carbamide peroxide).

Decadron, a trademark for a steroid drug used to treat inflammation (dexamethasone).

Deca-Durabolin, a trademark for a male hormone used to build tissue after severe injuries and to control the spread of breast cancer and bone weakness (nandrolone decanoate).

decalcification, loss of calcium salts from the teeth and bones. It is caused by malnutrition, failure of the body to absorb nutrients (malabsorption), or other factors. It may result, especially in older people, from a diet that lacks enough calcium. Malabsorption of calcium may be caused

by a lack of vitamin D, by a lack of stomach acids, and other disorders.

decay, radioactive, the decrease in activity of any radioactive material with the passage of time as a result of the spontaneous disintegration of the material.

decibel (db), a unit of measure of the intensity of sound. A decibel is one tenth of a bel; an increase of 1 bel is approximately double the loudness of a sound.

Declomycin, a trademark for a drug that kills bacteria (demeclocycline hydrochloride).

decompensation, the failure of a system, as cardiac decompensation in heart failure.

decomposition, the breakdown of a substance into simpler chemical forms.

decompression sickness, a painful, sometimes deadly condition caused by nitrogen bubbles forming in the body tissue. It is most often found in deep-sea divers, caisson workers, and aviators. It is caused by moving too quickly from areas of higher atmospheric pressures to lower pressures, as divers coming up from the bottom of the ocean too fast. Disorientation, severe pain, and fainting result. Treatment includes returning the person to an environment of higher pressure and reducing the pressure to allow the body time to adjust (decompression). Also called **bends.**

decongestant, referring to a drug, substance or procedure that reduces congestion or swelling, especially of the nasal passages.

decontamination procedure, the process of making personnel, equipment, and supplies safe by the elimination of harmful substances.

deep palmar arch, the end of the radial artery in the lower arm. It joins the end of the ulnar artery, which also travels down the lower arm, in the palm of the hand.

deep tendon reflex (DTR), a quick contraction of a muscle when its tendon is sharply tapped by a finger or rubber hammer. Absence of the reflex may be caused by damage to the muscle, the nerve, nerve roots, or the spinal cord. A violent reflex may be caused by disease of the nervous system or by overactive thyroid gland. The **Achilles-tendon reflex** is the response of the tendon at the back of the ankle causing the foot to move up. This does not happen in patients with nerve damage in the legs. Patients with an underactive thyroid often have a slow reflex. A very quick reflex may be caused by an overactive thyroid or by a disease of the brain. The **biceps reflex** is a contraction of a biceps muscle when the tendon is tapped. A **brachioradialis reflex** is caused by striking the side of the forearm near the head of the radius. It features normal slight elbow flexion and forearm rotation outward. The **patellar** or **knee-jerk reflex** occurs with a sharp tap on the tendon just below the kneecap (patella). The normal response is a quick upward jerk of the leg at the knee. The reflex is stronger in disease of the nervous system. A **triceps reflex** is brought on by tapping sharply the triceps tendon next to the elbow with the forearm in a relaxed position. The response is a clear extension of the forearm. A stronger response may occur with a spinal cord injury. **Hung-up reflex** refers to a delayed deep tendon reflex. After a stimulus is given and the reflex action takes place, there is a slow return of the limb to its neutral position. This delayed return is typical of the reflexes in patients with underactive thyroid.

deep vein, one of the many veins that accompany the arteries. The vein and artery are usually wrapped together in a sheath. Compare **superficial vein.**

defecation /def′ikā′shən/, the ridding of feces from the digestive tract through the rectum. See also **constipation, diarrhea, feces.**

defense mechanism, an unconscious reaction that offers protection from a stressful situation. Examples include conversion, denial, and dissociation. Also called **ego-defense mechanism.**

deferent duct /def′ərənt/. See **vas deferens.**

deferoxamine mesylate, a drug used to treat iron overdose. Kidney disease or inability to urinate prohibits its use. Side effects include low blood pressure, fast heart beat, urination problems, visual problems, and allergies.

defervescence /di′fərves′əns/, the dropping or ending of a fever. –**defervescent,** *adj.*

defibrillation /difī′brilā′shən, difib′-/, the process of stopping very rapid contractions of the heart (fibrillation) by delivering a direct electric shock to the patient's heart with a device called a defibrillator. Defibrillation by electric shock through the chest wall is a common emergency procedure.

deficiency disease, a condition resulting from the lack of one or more essential nutrients in the diet. It can be caused by failure of the body to absorb the nutrients from food or digestive problems. Compare **malnutrition.**

deformity, a condition of being distorted or flawed. A deformity may affect the body in general or just part of it. It may be the result of disease, injury, or birth defect.

degenerative disease /dijen′ərətiv/, any disease in which there is decay of structure or function of tissue. Some kinds of degenerative disease are **arteriosclerosis, osteoarthritis.**

degenerative joint disease. See **osteoarthritis.**

degeneration, the gradual decay of normal cells and body functions.

degradation, the physical destruction or decomposition of a clothing material as a result of exposure to chemicals, use, or ambient conditions (e.g., storage in sunlight). Degradation is noted by visible signs such as charring, shrinking or dissolving, or testing the clothing material for such

factors as weight changes, and loss of fabric tensile strength.

degree of solubility, an indication of the solubility of the material — negligible, less than 0.1%; slight, 0.1% to 1%; moderate, 1% to 10%; appreciable, greater than 10%; complete, soluble at all proportions.

dehiscence /dihis′əns/, the separation of a surgical cut (incision). Dehiscence may also refer to the splitting open of a closed wound.

dehydrated alcohol, a clear, colorless, liquid containing at least 99.5% ethyl alcohol. Also called **absolute alcohol.**

dehydration, **1.** the large loss of water from the body tissues. Dehydration may occur after fever, diarrhea, vomiting, or any condition where there is rapid loss of body fluids. It is of particular concern in infants, young children, and the elderly. An example is the drying of gum (gingival) tissue, often the result of breathing through the mouth. This lowers the resistance of the gum tissue to infection. **2.** completely removing water from a substance.

déjà vu /dāzhävY′, -vē′, -voo′/, The feeling that one has lived an event or been in a place before. It is normal in everyone, but occurs more often in some emotional and physical disorders. Déjà vu results from an unconscious connection with the present experience.

Deladumone OB, a trademark for a combination drug containing a masculine hormone (testosterone enanthate), female hormone (estradiol valerate), and a sleep-inducing drug (chlorobutanol).

Delalutin, a trademark for a female hormone used in pregnancy to prevent miscarriage (hydroxyprogesterone caproate).

Delatestryl, a trademark for an androgen used to treat lack of enough masculine hormones in men (testosterone enanthate).

Delestrogen, a trademark for an estrogen (estradiol valerate).

delirium /dilir′ē·əm/, a serious mental disorder. It features confusion, speech disorders, anxiety, excitement, and often hallucinations. The condition is caused by an upset in brain functions that can result from many physical disorders. These include nutritional or hormone disorders, exposure to various poisons (as gas, drugs, or alcohol), stress, or high fever. **Acute delirium** refers to a mental problem that is quick, severe, and short-lived. **Exhaustion delirium** may result from long-term physical or emotional stress, fatigue, or shock. It is linked with severe metabolic or nutritional problems. **Senile delirium** is linked with very old age and marked by restlessness, insomnia, aimless wandering, and, less commonly, hallucination. **Traumatic delirium** may occur after severe head injury. There is alertness and conciousness with disorientation, talk of imagined things (confabulation), and amnesia.

delirium tremens (DTs),   a serious and sometimes fatal reaction to sudden withdrawal of alcohol in the alcoholic. The reaction may follow an alcoholic binge during which no food was eaten. It can also be triggered by a head injury, infection, or withdrawal of alcohol after extended drinking. Symptoms include loss of appetite, difficulty in sleeping, excitement, mental confusion, and hallucinations. There may also be body tremors, fever, fast heart rate, sweat, and chest pain. The episode generally lasts from 3 to 6 days and is a medical emergency. A deep sleep often follows. Sedatives and tranquilizers are useful for calming the patient.

delivery,   the birth of a child.

delivery room,   a unit of a hospital for childbirth.

Delta-Cortef,   a trademark for a steroid drug (prednisolone).

delta-9-tetrahydrocannabinol (THC),   the active ingredient of marijuana (cannibas). It has been used to treat some cases of nausea and vomiting caused by cancer chemotherapy. See also **cannabis.**

delta wave,   in study of the heart (cardiology), a part of the tracing of a heartbeat on an electrocardiogram. See also **brain waves.**

deltoid muscle,   a large, thick muscle that covers the shoulder joint. It bends, extends, rotates, and moves the arm away from the body. The deltoid attaches to the collarbone, several points of the shoulder blade, and the upper arm bone (humerus).

delusion,   a belief or perception held to be true by a person even though it is illogical and wrong. Kinds of delusion include the **delusion of being controlled,** the false belief that one's feelings, thoughts, and acts are controlled by something else; the **delusion of grandeur,** a wild exaggeration of one's importance, wealth, power, or talents; and the **delusion of persecution,** an extreme belief that one is being mistreated and harassed by unknown enemies. Delusions are seen in various forms of schizophrenia. Compare **illusion.**

demand apparatus,   breathing apparatus with a regulator that supplies air to the face piece only when the wearer inhales or when the bypass valve has been opened; hence, ''demand.''

demand valve,   the valve that lets breathing air pass to the wearer when the wearer inhales.

Demazin,   a trademark for a respiratory, combination drug containing a stimulant (phenylephrine hydrochloride) and an antihistamine (chlorpheniramine maleate).

demecarium bromide,   a drug used to treat a type of disorder in the eye (open-angle glaucoma). Eye inflammation, some types of glaucoma, asthma, peptic ulcer, epi-

lepsy, recent heart attack, or known allergy to this drug prohibits its use. Side effects include slow heart beat, diarrhea, eye irritation, low blood pressure, and headaches.

demeclocycline hydrochloride,   an antibiotic used to treat a number of infections and often given when penicillin cannot be used. Kidney or liver disorders, pregnancy, or known allergy to this drug prohibits its use. It is not given to young children. Side effects include blood disorders, intestinal problems, sensitivity to light, and allergy.

dementia /dimen'shə/,   a disorder in which mental functions break down. It grows worse with time. It features personality change, confusion, and lack of energy. Thinking, reason, memory, and judgment are affected. The cause is usually brain disease. **Secondary dementia** results from another form of insanity that the patient has at the same time. **Multiinfarct dementia** is caused by a blood vessel disease. Symptoms include emotional upsets and defects in memory. There also may be nervous system defects, as walking abnormalities, mild paralysis, and numbness in the arms and legs. The condition is more likely to affect men than women. It may be caused by a stroke. **Toxic dementia** results from excess use of or exposure to a poisonous substance. See also **Alzheimer's disease, Pick's disease.**

Demerol,   a trademark for a narcotic drug that relieves pain (meperidine).

Demerol Hydrochloride,   a trademark for a narcotic drug that relives pain (meperidine hydrochloride).

demineralization,   a decrease in the amount of minerals or salts in tissues. This occurs in certain diseases.

Demser,   a trademark for a drug that reduces high blood pressure (metyrosine).

Demulen 1/50-28,   a trademark for a birth control pill. It contains an estrogen (ethinyl estradiol) and a progestin (ethynodiol diacetate).

denatured alcohol,   ethyl alcohol made unfit for drinking. This is done by adding several poisonous chemicals.

dendrite /den'drīt/,   a structure that extends from the cell body of a nerve (neuron). It receives signals that are sent on to the cell body. Compare **axon.**

dengue fever /deng'gē, den'gā/,   a serious virus infection given to humans by a mosquito. It occurs in tropical and subtropical regions. Symptoms include fever, a bright-red rash, and severe head, back, and muscle pain.

denial,   **1.** refusal of something requested or needed. It often results in physical or emotional deficiency. **2.** an unconscious defense mechanism. Thoughts and feelings that cause emotional conflict are avoided. It often involves failure to admit what is true or real.

dens, *pl.* **dentes** /den'tēz/,   a tooth or toothlike structure. See also **dentition, tooth.**

dental anomaly, a defect in which one or more teeth are not normal in form or position.

dental arch, the curve formed by the grouping of a normal set of teeth. See also **alveolar process.**

dental caries, holes made in tooth enamel, often called "cavities" or "tooth decay."

dental hygienist, a person trained to provide minor dental services. These services include cleaning the teeth, taking x-ray films, and applying drugs when needed.

dental plaque, a film made up of mucin secreted by the salivary glands and that clings to the teeth. Microorganisms are also a part of plaque. It often causes tooth decay and infections of the gums. Also called **bacterial plaque.**

dental sealants, plastic films that are applied to the chewing surfaces of teeth. These are used to cover the pits and to seal grooves where food becomes trapped.

dentate fracture /den′dāt/, any break that causes jagged bone ends that fit together like the teeth of gears.

dentifrice /den′tifris/, a substance used with a toothbrush for cleaning and polishing the teeth. It may also contain drugs to prevent tooth decay. This substance is commonly called tooth paste.

dentin /den′tin/, the chief material of teeth. It surrounds the inner part of the tooth (pulp) and is covered by the enamel. It is harder and denser than bone.

dentist, a person who is educated and licensed to practice dentistry.

dentistry, practice of preventing and treating diseases and disorders of the teeth and gums. This includes repairing teeth and replacing missing teeth. It also includes detecting signs of diseases, as tumors, that would require treatment by a doctor. There are dental specialties, each needing extra training.

dentofacial anomaly /-fā′shəl/, a defect of the mouth structure in form, function, or position.

dentogingival junction /-jinjī′vəl/, the place of meeting between the surface of the teeth and the gum (gingiva).

denture /den′chər/, an artificial tooth or a set of teeth that are not permanently fastened in the mouth.

Denver Articulation Screening Examination (DASE), a test to judge the ability to speak clearly. It is given to children between 2½ and 6 years of age.

Denver Developmental Screening Test (DDST), a test to judge the development in children from 1 month to 6 years of age. The child's level of motor, social, and language skills is compared with the average performance of other children.

deoxyribonucleic acid (DNA) /dē·ok′sirī′bōnōōklē′ik/, a large nucleic acid molecule, found mainly in the chromosomes of the nucleus of a cell. It is the carrier of genetic information. Also called **desoxyribonucleic acid.** See also **nucleic acid, ribonucleic acid.**

Depakene, a trademark for a drug used to treat convulsions (valproic acid).

dependence, the state of being addicted to drugs or alcohol. As time passes, more and more of the substance is needed to prevent withdrawal symptoms.

dependent, relying on someone or something for help, support, and other need. For example, a child is dependent on a parent.

dependent personality, behavior in which there is an extreme need for attention, acceptance, and approval from other people.

depersonalization disorder, an emotional disorder in which there is a loss of the feeling of personal identity (depersonalization). Everything becomes dreamlike. The body may not feel like one's own, and important events may be watched with detachment. It is common in some forms of schizophrenia and in severe depression.

depilation /dep′ilā′shən/, the removal of hair from the body. It may be temporary, as in shaving, or permanent, as by electrolysis, which destroys the hair root.

depilatory /dipil′ətôr′ē/, referring to a substance or method that removes hair.

depot, **1.** any area of the body in which drugs or other substances, as fat, are stored until needed. **2.** a drug that is injected in the body and absorbed over a period of time into the blood.

depressant, a drug that tends to decrease the activity of a part of the body, as a heart depressant.

depressed fracture, any break of the skull in which pieces of bone are below the surface of the skull.

depression, **1.** a depressed area or hollow; downward movement. **2.** a decrease of body activity. **3.** an emotional state in which there are extreme feelings of sadness, dejection, lack of worth, and emptiness. The obvious signs range from a slight lack of motivation and failure to concentrate to severe changes of body functions. The cause of depression can be hereditary, drug-related, lack of balance of hormones, or diet. Depression can also result from diseases such as nervous system disorders, infection, or cancer. See also **bipolar disorder.** –**depressive,** *adj.*

depressor, any drug that reduces activity when applied to nerves and muscles. See also **depressant.**

depressor septi, one of the three muscles of the nose. It serves to narrow the nostril.

deprivation, the loss of something considered valuable or necessary. It may be taken away or access may be denied. In experimental psychology, human subjects may be deprived of something in order to study their reactions.

depth perception. See **perception.**

derivative, anything that is obtained from another substance. For example, penicillin is derived from a fungus.

dermatitis /dur′mətī′-/, an inflammation of the skin. It is marked by redness, pain, or itching. The condition may be long-term or sudden. Treatment depends on the cause.

dermatofibroma /dur′mətō·fībrō′mə/, a bump on the skin. It is painless, round, firm, and gray or red. It is most commonly found on the arms and legs and needs no treatment.

dermatoglyphics /-glif′-/, the study of the skin ridge patterns on fingers, toes, palms of hands, and soles of feet. These patterns are often called prints, as fingerprints. The patterns are used for identification. They can also help diagnose some chromosome defects.

dermatology /dur′mətol′-/, the study of the skin. This includes the diagnosis and treatment of skin disorders by a **dermatologist,** a doctor specializing in the skin.

Dermatophagoides farinae /-fəgoi′dēz/, a common household dust mite. It causes allergic reactions in sensitive persons. Bug killers and vacuum cleaning can help to control them. The mites thrive on skin, hair, pet foods, carpets, and bedding, as well as house dust.

dermatophytid /-fī′tid, dur′mətof′itid/, an allergic skin reaction. It is marked by small blisters and is linked to fungal infections.

dermatosis /dur′mətō′-/, any disorder of the skin that does not cause inflammation. An example is **dermatosis papulosa nigra,** a common abnormal skin condition in blacks. It features many noncancerous, tiny, dark bumps on the cheeks. Compare **dermatitis.**

dermoid cyst, a tumor with a fiberlike wall. It is filled with fatty material and cartilage. More than 10% of all tumors on the ovary are dermoid cysts. They are most often noncancerous.

DES, abbreviation for **diethylstilbestrol.**

Desenex, a trademark for a drug used on the skin for the treatment of athletes's foot (undecylenic acid and zinc undecylenate).

desensitize, 1. to make a person not react to any of the various foreign substances (antigens) that might cause an allergy. **2.** to help an emotionally disturbed person become free of phobias and neuroses by talking about the fears and events that cause the problems. **3.** in dentistry, to reduce the pain in the teeth caused by irritating substances and temperature changes.

deserpidine, a drug used to treat mild high blood pressure and anxiety. Depression, ulcers, or known allergy to this drug prohibits its use. It can react with other drugs to increase high blood pressure. Side effects include possible severe mental depression, dizziness, blurred vision, and fainting when a person stands up.

Desferal Mesylate, a trademark for a drug used to treat too much iron in the body (deferoxamine mesylate).

desiccant /des′ikənt/, any drug or way that causes a substance to dry up. Also called **exsiccant.**

desipramine hydrochloride, drug used to treat mental depression.

deslanoside, a drug used to treat heart failure and certain forms of irregular heart beats. Irregular heart contractions, fast heart beat, or known allergy to this drug prohibits its use. Side effects include irregular heart beat.

desmoid tumor /dez′moid/, a cancerous tumor of the muscle that may occur in the head, neck, upper arm, stomach, or legs.

desmopressin acetate, a drug that slows down urine making in the kidneys. It is used to treat diabetes. Known allergy to this drug prohibits its use. Side effects include a lack of salt with extreme fluid buildup in the body, headache, and cramps.

desmosis /dezmō′-/, any disease of the connective tissue.

desonide, a drug put on the skin to reduce inflammation. Viral or fungal diseases of the skin, poor circulation, or known allergy to this drug prohibits its use. Side effects include streaks in the skin, loss of skin color, and skin irritation. They occur most often after long use.

desoximetasone, a drug put on the skin to reduce inflammation. Viral and fungal diseases of the skin, poor circulation, or known allergy to this drug prohibits its use. The wound should not be sealed from the air with a bandage. Side effects include streaks in the skin, loss of skin color, and skin irritation. They occur most often after long use.

Desoxyn, a trademark for a drug that stimulates the central nervous system on the body as a whole (methamphetamine hydrochloride).

desquamation /des′kwəmā′shən/, a normal process in which the top layer of the skin comes off in tiny flakes. Some conditions, injuries, and drugs speed up desquamation. Also called **exfoliation.**

Desyrel, a trademark for a drug used to treat depression (trazodone).

detached retina. See **retinal detachment.**

detergent, a cleaning agent.

detonation, an explosive chemical reaction with a release rate less than .01 second. This gives responders NO time to react. Examples include military munitions, dynamite, and organic peroxides.

detoxification, removal of the poison from a substance or speeding up its removal from the body.

detoxification service, a hospital service that treats the effect of chemical poisons, as alcohol or drugs. Detoxification is the first step in helping people overcome their dependence (addiction) on these substances.

C–D

deutoplasm /do͞o′təplazm/, the parts of the yolk that store nutrition. Also called **deuteroplasm.**

development, 1. the gradual process of change from a simple to a more complex level. The ability of humans to adapt to surroundings and to function in society is gained through growth and learning. **2.** the series of events that occur in an organism from the time the egg is fertilized to the adult stage. –**developmental,** *adj.*

developmental age (DA), a way to express a child's progress. It is stated in age and is determined by accepted measurements. The child is judged by body size, social and psychologic abilities, and motor skills. Mental and aptitude tests are also given.

developmental disability (DD), a disorder that starts developing before 18 years of age. Most disorders of this type last the person's lifetime, but many can be treated.

developmental model, a guide that outlines four stages of a patient's therapy for mental problems. In the first stage the patient starts to recognize the problem with the help of the therapist. In the second stage a sense of closeness to the therapist develops. This allows them to work well together. In the third stage the patient assumes some control of the meetings and grows more independent. During the last stage the patient is independent and no longer needs the therapist.

deviate /dē′vē·it/, a person or an event that varies from the normal standard.

deviated septum, a condition in which the center section (septum) of the nose shifts to one side. It affects many adults. The septum often shifts to the left during normal growth. This shift may be increased by a blow to the nose or by other problems. A severe shift of the septum may block the nasal passages and cause infection, sinusitis, shortness of breath, headache, or frequent nosebleeds.

device, an item other than a drug that is used to aid healing. Devices include splints, crutches, artificial heart valves, pacemakers, wheelchairs, hearing aids, and eye glasses.

dexamethasone, a drug used to treat numerous disorders with inflammation.

dexchlorpheniramine maleate, a drug used to treat a number of allergic reactions. These include runny nose, skin rash, and severe itching.

Dexedrine, a trademark for a drug that stimulates the central nervous system (dextroamphetamine sulfate).

dextran, a form of liquid sugar (glucose) given in the vein to treat shock from blood loss.

dextromethorphan hydrobromide, a drug used to help stop coughing. Known allergy to this drug prohibits its use. Side effects include breathing difficulty caused by large doses.

dextrose /dek′strōs/, a liquid sugar solution (glucose) given in the vein to treat low blood sugar.

D.H.E.-45, a trademark for a drug used to treat migraine and certain other forms of headache (dihydroergotamine mesylate).

dhobie itch /dō′bē/, a skin infection caused by laundry marking fluids.

diabetes /dī′əbē′tēz/, a condition in which there is too much excretion of urine. It can be caused by a lack of the hormone (called antidiuretic or ADH) that limits the amount of urine made, as in **diabetes insipidus.** It can also result from a high blood sugar level, as in **diabetes mellitus.** See these entries.

diabetes insipidus /insip′idəs/, a type of diabetes with symptoms of extreme thirst and heavy urination. It is usually caused by a lack of ADH (antidiuretic hormone) that limits urine production. It may also be caused by a failure of the kidneys to respond to ADH (**nephrogenic diabetes insipidus**). The condition may be inborn, result from a kidney disorder, or have an unknown cause. The disorder may begin quite suddenly, and the urine output may be as much as 2½ gallons in 24 hours. The patient seldom suffers from any other problems except the constant need to drink. If enough fluids are not taken, the person can become severely dehydrated. In mild cases, no treatment is necessary. Drugs may be given to help the kidneys respond to ADH and to reduce the amount of urine.

diabetes mellitus (DM) /məlī′təs/, a complex disorder that is mainly caused by the failure of the pancreas to release enough insulin into the body. It may also be caused by a defect in the parts of cells that accept the insulin. The disease tends to run in families. Symptoms include the need to urinate often, increased thirst, weight loss, and increased appetite. The levels of sugar in the blood and urine will be high. The eyes, kidneys, nervous system, and skin may be affected. Infections are common, and hardening of the arteries often develops. There are four main types of diabetes mellitus. Type I is also called **insulin-dependent diabetes.** This is the more serious form of the disease. Type I diabetes most often develops during childhood, although young adults also can develop this form. Symptoms include loss of weight, weakness, and marked irritability. The onset is usually rapid, but about one third of the patients have a remission within 3 months. This stage may continue for years, but diabetes can progress quickly to a state of total dependence on insulin. This type of diabetes tends to be unstable and hard to control. Coma from not enough insulin (ketoacidosis) is a constant danger. Type II is also called **non-insulin-dependent diabetes.** The disease usually begins after 40 years of age, but can occur at any age. The patients are not dependent on injections of insulin, although they may use insulin for correction of symptoms, as excess sugar in the blood (hyperglycemia). Type II often develops in overweight adults, and the condition may be improved by weight loss. Type III, or **gestational diabetes,** occurs in some women during pregnancy. It disappears after childbirth, but many women later develop Type II diabetes. Type IV includes other types of diabetes linked to disease of the pancreas, hormonal changes, side effects of drugs, or genetic defects.

diabetic /-bet′ik/, **1.** referring to diabetes. **2.** a person who has diabetes mellitus.

diabetic retinopathy, a disorder of broken blood vessels in the retina of the eye.

Diabinese, a trademark for a drug used to treat diabetes (chlorpropamide).

diacondylar fracture /dī′əkon′dilər/, any break that runs across the top of a rounded bone projection (condyle).

diagnosis /dī′əgnō′-/, pl. **diagnoses,** identification of a disease or condition. Physical signs, symptoms, history, laboratory tests, and procedures are used. A **clinical diagnosis** is one based on the facts learned from the medical history and physical examination alone, without use of laboratory tests or x-ray films. **Differential diagnosis** is the process of telling the difference between two or more similar diseases. This is done by comparing their signs and symptoms.

diagnostician /dī·əgnostish′ən/, a person skilled and trained in making diagnoses.

Dialose plus, a trademark for a drug containing a stool softener (docusate potassium) and a laxative (casanthranol).

dialysate /dī·al′isāt/. See **dialysis.**

dialysis /dī·al′isis/, a method for removing unwanted elements from the blood. It is used in treating kidney failure and other poisonous conditions. This is done by passing the blood through a membrane that filters out the unwanted elements. A tube (catheter) is put in place and connected to tubing that allows flow in and out of the body. There are two ways in which dialysis is done. With **hemodialysis,** the patient's blood is run from the body through a machine (**dialyzer**) containing the filtering membrane. A constant flow of blood passes on one side of the membrane. On the other side flows a cleansing solution (**dialysate**) that attracts the waste products through the membrane. The purified blood is then returned to the patient's blood vessels. The procedure takes from 3 to 8 hours and may be needed daily in serious situations or two or three times a week in long-term kidney failure. With **peritoneal dialysis,** the membrane lining the abdominal wall (peritoneum) is used as the filtering membrane. This form of dialysis may be done nightly for very ill children while they sleep and may also be done at home. The kind of cleansing fluid (dialysate) used also differs because it can be put directly into the peritoneal space. The fluid is first warmed to body temperature, and drugs used to stop blood clotting, antibiotics, or other additives may be given. Drugs may be given for pain. There are three phases in each cycle. During the

Classification of diabetes mellitus and descriptive characteristics for each type

Class	Clinical and associated factors and former terminology
Type I: insulin-dependent diabetes mellitus (IDDM)	Patients dependent on insulin to prevent ketosis; onset usually in youth but may occur in adults; associated with certain HLA types, islet cell antibodies are frequently present; formerly called juvenile-onset diabetes, ketosis-prone diabetes, brittle diabetes
Type II: noninsulin-dependent diabetes mellitus (NIDDM)	Patients not dependent on insulin to preserve life, although they may be treated with insulin (even if treated with insulin, they are still classified as NIDDM); ketosis resistant except in very special circumstances such as presence of infection; not HLA related; onset usually after 40 years of age but may occur in youth; serum insulin levels may be depressed, normal, or elevated; 60% to 90% of diabetics in this class are obese; formerly called maturity-onset diabetes, adult-onset diabetes, ketosis-resistant diabetes, and stable diabetes; class may be subdivided into two classes: (1) obese type II, and (2) nonobese type II
Type III: gestational diabetes mellitus (GDM)	Glucose intolerance occurs during pregnancy; group does not include known diabetics who become pregnant; after delivery, glucose intolerance may remain but not be serious enough to be treated or the patient may have characteristics of type I or type II diabetes, or glucose intolerance may disappear; patient is reclassified after delivery; formerly called gestational diabetes
Type IV: other types, includes diabetes mellitus associated with pancreatic disease, other hormonal abnormalities, drugs	Patients in this class must have diabetes mellitus and one of the other diseases, syndromes, or casual factors; formerly called secondary diabetes

first phase (inflow), the dialysate is sent into the peritoneal space. During the second phase (equilibration), the dialysate stays in the space. The needed substances pass to the blood. Waste products pass from the blood vessels through the peritoneum into the dialysate. During the third phase (outflow), the dialysate drains from the peritoneal space by gravity. Problems may occur, including puncturing (perforation) the bowel, infections, and bruises. Bruises often develop because the tissues are irritated by the catheter.

dialysis disequilibrium syndrome, a disorder caused by a rapid change in body fluid that sometimes occurs in dialysis. The condition may feature brain or nervous system disorders, irregular heart beat, and fluid in the lungs.

dialyzer. See **dialysis.**

Diamox, a trademark for a drug (acetazolamide), used with other drugs in treating certain seizure disorders and to reduce eye pressure in glaucoma.

diapedesis /dī′əpədē′-/, the passage of red or white blood cells through the walls of blood vessels. This occurs without damage to the vessels.

diaphoresis /dī′əfôrē′-/, profuse sweating that occurs with a fever, physical exertion, exposure to heat, or stress. Sweating is controlled by the nervous system and is mainly a way to control body temperature. However, the sweat glands on the palms and soles respond to motional conditions.

diaphragm /dī′əfram/, a dome-shaped muscle that separates the chest cavity from the abdominal cavity. This muscle has holes through which pass the large artery (aorta), esophagus, and large vein (vena cava). The diaphragm aids breathing by moving up and down. When breathing in, it moves down and increases the space in the chest. When breathing out, it moves up, decreasing the volume. See also **contraceptive diaphragm.**

diaphragmatic hernia. See **hernia.**

diaphysis /dī·af′isis/, the shaft of a long bone. It consists of a tube of bone enclosing the bone marrow.

Diapid, a trademark for a pituitary hormone (lypressin). It is in the form of a nasal spray and is used to treat excessive urination and other problems in diabetes insipidus.

diarrhea /dī′ərē′ə/, the frequent passage of loose, watery stools. It is usually the result of increased activity of the large intestine (colon). The stool may also contain mucus, pus, blood, or large amounts of fat. The condition may be caused by stress and anxiety, diet, the side effects of drugs, inflammation, irritation, or faulty absorption of the bowel, or the effects of poison, infectious waste material, or radiation. Diarrhea may be accompanied by vomiting and various other symptoms. The symptoms include stomach and bowel pain, cramping, increased bowel sounds, loose or liquid stools, and often a change in the color of the feces. Diarrhea is usually a symptom of some other disorder. It is

common symptom in some types of flu, food poisoning, and after eating foods that are highly spiced. It is also a symptom of more severe diseases. These include various disorders, as tumors of the intestines, malabsorption syndrome, or milk intolerance. In addition, patients may complain of stomach cramps and weakness. Untreated, diarrhea may lead to dehydration.

diastasis /dī·as′tə-/, the separation of two body parts that normally are joined together, as the separation of parts of a bone.

diastole /dī·as′təlē/, **1.** the period of time between contractions of the heart. During this state blood enters the relaxed chambers of the heart to be pumped throughout the body. Compare **systole.** See also **blood pressure.** –**diastolic** /dī′əstol′ik/, *adj.*

diastolic blood pressure. See **blood pressure.**

diastrophic dwarf /dī′əstrof′ik/, a person in whom short height is caused by any disorder of bone and cartilage. It is linked to various deformities of the bones and joints. The condition may be inherited.

diathermy /dī′əthur′mē/, the production of heat in body tissues with high-frequency electric currents. The currents are not intense enough to destroy tissues or to damage function. Diathermy is used to treat arthritis, bursitis, fractures, gynecologic diseases, and inflammation of the sinuses.

diathesis /dī·ath′əsis, dī′athē′-/, *pl.* **diatheses,** an inherited condition of the body which makes it more susceptible to certain diseases or disorders than is normal.

diazepam /dī·az′əpam/, a sedative and tranquilizer used to treat anxiety, nervous tension, muscle spasm, and convulsions.

diazoxide, a drug used to reduce very high blood pressure in emergencies. It may also be used in some cases to treat low blood sugar.

Dibenzyline, a trademark for a drug used to improve circulation of the arms and legs in certain conditions (phenoxybenzamine hydrochloride).

dicalcium phosphate and calcium gluconate with vitamin D, a source of calcium and phosphorus used to treat low levels of calcium, especially in pregnancy and nursing. Poor thyroid function or known allergy to any of the ingredients of this drug prohibits its use. There are no known side effects.

Dick test, a skin test for determining the lack of ability to resist scarlet fever. A small dose of the scarlet fever bacteria is injected under the skin. A small area of redness indicates that the person is not immune. Larger doses may then be given to create immunity.

dicloxacillin sodium, a drug used to treat staph infections.

dicumarol, a drug that prevents blood from clotting. It is used to prevent and treat blood clots.

dicyclomine hydrochloride, a drug used to treat ulcers.

Didrex, a trademark for a drug that decreases the appetite (benzphetamine hydrochloride).

Didronel, a trademark for a drug that regulates calcium in the body (etidronate disodium).

diencephalon /dī'ensef'əlon/, the middle part of the brain

dienestrol /dī'ines'trôl/, an estrogen used to treat a wasting away of the vulva. Pregnancy, cancer of the breast, inflammation of a vein, vaginal bleeding, or known allergy to this drug prohibits its use. Side effects include risk of cancer, inflammation of a vein, tumor of the liver, blood clots, and gallbladder disease.

diet, 1. food and drink judged by nutritional value, composition, and effects on health. 2. food and drink restricted in type and amount for treatment or other purposes. 3. the usual amount of food and drink consumed. Compare **nutrition.** –**dietetic,** *adj.*

dietary fiber, a term for substances found in plants that the body does not digest. Fiber promotes healthy intestinal action and prevents constipation. It may also help protect against cancer of the large intestine (colon). Major sources of dietary fiber are vegetables, fruits, and whole grains. Also called **bulk, roughage.**

dietetic food /dī'ətet'ik/, 1. a specially made low-calorie food. It often contains artificial sweeteners. 2. a food prepared for any special need or restriction of the diet, as food without salt or meals with no meat.

dietetics, the study of foods and their nutrients and how they relate to both health and disease.

diethylpropion hydrochloride, a drug that curbs the appetite. It is used to treat obesity.

diethylstilbestrol (DES), a hormone which is made to be similar to estrogen. Also called **stilbestrol.**

diethylstilbestrol diphosphate, an anticancer drug used to treat cancer of the prostate that cannot be treated by surgery. Inflammation of a vein, blood clot disorders, liver disorders, or stroke prohibits its use. Side effects include vein inflammation, blood clots in the lungs or brain, jaundice, mental depression, severe skin rashes, changes in sexual interest, and dizziness.

dietitian, a person who has completed a special training in nutritional care of groups and persons.

Dietl's crisis /dē'təlz/, a sudden, very severe pain in the kidney. It is caused by rapidly drinking very large amounts of liquid, or by blockage in the tube that carries urine from the kidneys to the bladder.

differentiation, 1. a process in development in which simple cells or tissues change to take on specific physical forms, functions, and chemical properties. 2. taking on functions and forms different from those of the original. 3. telling apart one thing or disease from another, as in differential diagnosis.

diffuse, widely spread, as through a fluid.

diflorasone diacetate, a drug placed on the skin to reduce inflammation. Virus and fungus diseases of the skin, poor circulation, or known allergy to this drug or to other steroids prohibits its use. Side effects include streaks, loss of color, or irritation of the skin.

diflunisal, a drug that relieves mild pain and inflammation in the skeletal muscles. Allergy to aspirin and similar drugs or known allergy to this drug prohibits its use. Side effects include intestinal pain, diarrhea, ulcer, loss of appetite, and water retention.

digastricus /dīgas'trikəs/, one of the lower jaw muscles. It acts to open the jaw and to move the bone (hyoid) under the tongue.

DiGeorge's syndrome, an inherited disorder marked by severe losses in the immune system and structural defects. The defects include notched low-set ears, small mouth, downward slanting eyes, set far apart, and heart defects. There may also be a lack of the thymus and parathyroid glands. Death, often from infection, usually occurs before two years of age. Also called **thymic parathyroid aplasia.**

digest, 1. to soften by heat and moisture. 2. to convert food into a form that can be absorbed by the body. This is done by chewing the food, adding water, and the action of stomach and intestinal fluids.

digestion, the changing of food into substances able to be absorbed by the body. This takes place in the stomach and intestines. –**digestive,** *adj.*

digestive gland, any of the many structures that releases substances that break down food so that it can be absorbed by the body. Some kinds of digestive glands are the salivary glands, gastric glands in the stomach, intestinal glands, liver, and pancreas.

digestive system, the organs, structures, and glands of the digestive tube of the body through which food passes. The digestive system includes the mouth, throat, stomach, and small and large intestines. The digestive tube is a muscular tube, about 30 feet (9 meters) long, which extends from the mouth to the anus.

digital, referring to a digit, that is, a finger or toe.

digitalis /dij'ital'is/, a drug that stimulates the heart. It is used to treat heart failure and certain forms of irregular heart beats.

digitalis therapy, giving the drug digitalis to a person with a heart disorder. Digitalis increases the force of heart contractions and produces a slower and more regular heart rate. Digitalis therapy can also reduce blood pressure, improve circulation, reduce water retention, and stop extremely rapid heart beat. Digitalis is given with extreme care, in the exact dosage, and at the exact times prescribed. The pulse is checked for a full minute before the drug is taken.

digitate /dij′itāt/, having fingers or fingerlike projections. See also **digital.**

digitoxin, a drug that stimulates the heart. It is used to treat heart failure and certain forms of irregular heart beats.

digoxin, a drug that stimulates the heart. It is used to treat heart failure and certain forms of irregular heart beats.

dihydroergotamine mesylate, a drug used to treat migraine headaches and other forms of headache. Heart disease, high blood pressure, liver or kidney disorders, blood poisoning, pregnancy, or known allergy to this drug prohibits its use. Side effects include gangrene, nausea, vomiting, diarrhea, headache, weakness, visual disturbances, and irregular heart beats.

dihydrotachysterol /dīhī′drōtəkis′tərôl/, a form of vitamin D. It is used to treat calcium deficiency resulting from an underactive parathyroid gland. Low calcium levels linked to kidney malfunction, kidney insufficiency, or known allergy to this drug or to vitamin D prohibits its use. Caution is advised for nursing mothers. Side effects include an excess increase of calcium, hardening of soft tissues, and heart or kidney failure.

diking, application of a barrier that prevents passage of a hazardous material to an area where it will produce more harm.

Dilantin, a trademark for a drug used to prevent convulsions (phenytoin).

dilatation /dil′ətā′shən/, normal increase in the size of a body opening, blood vessel, or tube. An example is the widening of the pupil of the eye in dim light. Also called dilation. –**dilatate, dilate** /dī′lāt/, v.

dilatation and curettage (D & C), widening of the opening to the uterus (cervix) and scraping the lining (endometrium) of the uterus. A D & C is done to diagnose diseases of the uterus, to correct heavy vaginal bleeding, or to empty the uterus of substances from conception (as after a miscarriage or in an abortion). **Fractional dilatation and curettage** is a way in which each section of the uterus is examined and scraped to get samples from all parts of the uterus. It is often done in the diagnosis of cancer of the uterus. See also **abortion.**

dilatator pupillae, a muscle that contracts the iris of the eye and widens the pupil.

Dilaudid Hydrochloride, a trademark for a drug that relieves pain (hydromorphone hydrochloride).

Dilor, a trademark for a drug that widens the openings of the air passages to the lungs (dyphylline).

diltiazem, a drug used to treat pain in the chest caused by physical exertion. Irregular heart beats, heart block, or low blood pressure prohibits its use. Side effects include water retention, irregular heart beats, very slow heart beats, low blood pressure, fainting, rash, headache, and dizziness.

dilution, making a less concentrated solution from a solution of greater concentration.

dimenhydrinate, a drug used to treat nausea and motion sickness. Asthma or known allergy to this drug prohibits its use. It is not given to newborn infants or nursing mothers. Side effects include skin rash, allergic reactions, and very rapid heart beats. Drowsiness and dry mouth are common.

dimercaprol /dī′mərkap′rôl/, a drug used to treat Wilson's disease. It is also used to treat severe arsenic, mercury, or gold poisoning. Liver or kidney disorders, poisoning with certain metals, or known allergy to this drug prohibits its use. Side effects include kidney damage, high levels of acid in the blood, convulsions, and abnormal heart functions.

Dimetane, a trademark for an antihistamine drug (brompheniramine maleate).

dimethyl sulfoxide (DMSO), a drug used to treat inflammation of the bladder. It also has been used on the skin to relieve sports injuries. Known allergy to this drug prohibits its use. Side effects include intestinal disturbances, sensitive eyes in light, disturbance of color vision, and headache. A garliclike body odor and taste in the mouth may occur. When applied to the skin, it can cause skin irritations.

dioxin /dī′ok′sin/, an ingredient in a certain herbicide used widely throughout the world to help control plant growth. Because of its high level of poison, it is no longer made in the United States. Dioxin was an ingredient of Agent Orange sprayed by the U.S. military aircraft over areas of Southeast Asia from 1965 to 1970 to kill concealing trees and shrubs. No safe exposure levels have been found. It has been strongly linked to many cancers and is very harmful to all living things.

dioxybenzone, a sunscreen used to prevent sunburn. Known allergy to this drug prohibits its use. It should not come into contact with the eyes. The only known side effect is skin rash.

diphenhydramine hydrochloride, a drug used to treat motion sickness and a number of allergic reactions, including runny nose, skin rash, and itching.

diphenidol, a drug used to treat vertigo and to control nausea and vomiting. Absence of urination or known allergy to this drug prohibits its use. Side effects include low blood pressure, hallucinations, and mental confusion.

diphenoxylate hydrochloride, a drug used to treat diarrhea and cramps of the intestines. Liver disease, diarrhea from antibiotics, or known allergy to this drug prohibits its use. It is not given to children under 2 years of age. Side effects include stomach pain, intestinal blockage, skin rash, and nausea.

diphenylpyraline hydrochloride, a drug used to treat a number of allergic reactions, including runny nose, skin rash, and itching. Asthma or known allergy to this drug prohibits its use. It is not given to newborn infants or nursing mothers. Side effects include skin rash, allergic reactions, and fast heart beats.

diphtheria /difthir′ē·ə, dipthir′ē·ə/, a serious, contagious disease. It produces a poison throughout the body and a false membrane lining of the throat. The poison is very harmful to the tissues of the heart and central nervous system. The thick membrane lining the throat may interfere with eating, drinking, and breathing. The membrane may also occur in other body tissues. Lymph glands in the neck swell. If not treated, the disease is often fatal, causing heart and kidney failure. Patients are usually put in the hospital in isolated rooms. Immunization against diphtheria is available to all children in the United States. It is usually given early in infancy. See also **Schick test.**

diphtheria and tetanus toxoids (DT), a drug used for immunizing persons against diphtheria and tetanus.

diphtheria, tetanus toxoids, and pertussis vaccine (DTP), a drug used for immunizing children under 6 years of age against the diseases diphtheria, tetanus, and pertussis (whooping cough).

diplegia /dīplē′jə/, paralysis affecting the same parts on both sides of the body.

diploë /dip′lō·ē/, the spongy tissue between the skull bones.

diplopia /diplō′pē·ə/, double vision. It may be caused by defective eye muscles or it may result from a disorder of the nerves that signal the muscles. A temporary diplopia is usually not serious and is common after a mild brain concussion. Also called **ambiopia, double vision.** Compare **binocular vision.**

dipsomania /dip′sō-/, an uncontrollable craving for alcoholic beverages.

dipyridamole, a drug that increases blood flow to the heart. It is used for the long-term treatment of chest pain. The drug should be used with caution in patients with low blood pressure and those taking drugs that decrease blood clotting. Side effects include headache, dizziness, rash, nausea, and flushing.

direct contact, mutual touching of two persons or organisms. Many communicable diseases may be spread by the direct contact between an infected and a healthy person.

direct fracture, any bone break that occurs exactly at a point of injury.

disability, the loss or damage of physical or mental fitness. Compare **handicap.**

disaccharide /dīsak′ərid/, a sugar made up of two simple sugars, as lactose and sucrose.

disc. See **disk.**

discharge, **1.** to release a substance or object. **2.** to release a burst of energy from or through a nerve. **3.** to release an electric charge. **4.** a release of emotions. **5.** to release a patient from a hospital.

discharge summary, a report prepared by a physician at the end of a patient's hospital stay or series of treatments. The summary outlines the patient's problem and the diagnosis. It then lists the treatment given and the patient's response to it. It ends with suggestions for the patient after discharge.

disease, **1.** a condition of abnormal function involving any structure, part, or system of an organism. **2.** a specific illness or disorder marked by a specific set of signs and symptoms. It may stem from heredity, infection, diet, or environment. An **acute disease** is one with symptoms that are usually severe but last only a short time. The patient gets better, moves into a long-term phase, or dies. A **chonic disease** is one that persists over a long period of time, but is often less severe than an acute disease. **Functional disease** has two meanings. It may refer to a disease that affects function or performance rather than body tissue. It may also be a condition with symptoms of a physical disease or disorder although careful examination fails to show any sign of physical problems. The symptoms of a functional disorder are as real as those of a physical disease. Headache, lack of sexual function (impotence), certain heart problems, and constipation may be symptoms of functional disease. An **intercurrent disease** is one that develops in and may alter the course of another disease.

disease prevention, procedures to protect people from health threats and their harmful results.

disengagement, **1.** moving the part of the baby lowest in the pelvis in order to aid childbirth. **2.** the detachment of oneself from other persons or responsibilities.

dishpan fracture, a break that causes a hollow or depression in the skull.

disinfectant, a chemical that can destroy bacteria.

disk, **1.** also spelled **disc.** A flat, round, platelike structure, as a joint (articular) disk or an optic disc. **2.** a term for the cartilage between the backbones. Also called **discus.**

dislocation, the displacement of any part of the body from its normal position. This applies most often to a bone moved from its normal position with a joint. See also **subluxation.** –**dislocate,** *v.*

disopyramide phosphate, a drug used to treat irregular or very rapid heart beats.

C–D

disorientation, a state of mental confusion as to place, time, or personal identity.

dispatch, the implementation of a *command* decision to move a resource or resources from one place to another.

dispatch center, a facility from which resources are directly assigned to an incident.

dispersing agent, a chemical used to distribute the ingredients throughout the product, as in lotions with both oil and water.

displaced fracture, a bone break in which two ends of the bone are separated from each other. The ends of broken bones often pierce through the skin.

displacement, 1. the state of being moved from the normal position. 2. an unconscious defense mechanism to avoid emotional conflict. Emotions or ideas are transferred from one object or person to another that is less threatening.

disseminated intravascular coagulation (DIC), a severe disorder that results from too much of the body's clotting substance being made in response to disease or injury. DIC can be caused by blood poisoning (septicemia), severe low blood pressure, poisonous snake bites, cancer, childbirth emergencies, severe injury, or extensive surgery and bleeding.

dissemination, a phase of cancer in which cells spread (metastasize) to other parts of the body.

dissociation, 1. the act of separating into parts or sections. 2. an unconscious defense mechanism by which an idea or emotion is separated from the consciousness. In this way it loses emotional significance.

dissociative disorder, a type of hysterical neurosis. Emotional conflicts are denied to the point that a split in the personality occurs. This causes a confusion in identity. Symptoms include amnesia, sleep walking, flight from reality, dream state, or multiple personality. The disorder is caused by failure to cope with severe stress or conflict. It most often occurs suddenly, after a shocking situation. Compare **conversion disorder.**

distal /dis′tal/, away from or being the farthest from a point of origin, such a central point of the body. For example, the distal phalanx is the bone at the tip of the finger. Compare **proximal.**

distance regulation, behavior that is related to the control of personal space. Most humans need a certain space between themselves and others. This space offers security, but does not create a sense of isolation. The amount of social distance varies with different persons and in different cultures.

distension, the state of being expanded or swollen.

distraction techniques, ways to prevent or lessen the feeling of pain. They focus attention on feelings unrelated to the pain.

disulfiram, a drug used to discourage the drinking of alcohol. It is used to treat long-term alcoholism. It causes severe stomach cramping, severe perspiration, and nausea if alcohol is drunk.

disuse phenomena, the physical and mental changes that result from not using part of the body. Patients who are treated for broken bones and other orthopedic disorders must often be confined to beds and immobilized in traction for long periods. Such patients often lack communication with others. They lose motivation and abilities from lack of practice.

Ditropan, a trademark for a drug that relieves spasms (oxybutynin chloride).

Diucardin, a trademark for a drug that lowers blood pressure and stimulates urine release (hydroflumethiazide).

Diupres, a trademark for a drug that stimulates urine release (chlorothiazide) and lowers blood pressure (reserpine).

diuresis /dī′yo͞orē′-/, increased formation and release of urine. Diuresis occurs in conditions such as diabetes mellitus and diabetes insipidus. It is normal in the first 48 hours after childbirth. Coffee, tea, certain foods, diuretic drugs, and some steroids cause diuresis. In **osmotic diuresis,** urine release is caused by certain substances in tubes of the kidney, as urea or glucose, that cannot be absorbed.

diuretic /dī′yo͞oret′ik/, a drug or other substance that promotes the formation and release of urine. Diuretics are given to lessen the volume of fluid in the treatment of many disorders, as high blood pressure, congestive heart failure, and water retention. Allergy to sulfur drugs prohibits use of this class of drug. Several side effects are common to all diuretics, including a decrease of fluid volume and electrolyte imbalance.

Diuril, a trademark for a drug that stimulates urine release (chlorothiazide).

diurnal /dī′ur′nəl/, occurring during the day. Compare **nocturnal.**

diurnal variation, the range of the release rate of a substance, as urine, being collected for laboratory analysis over a 24-hour period.

diversion, controlled movement of a hazardous material to an area where it will produce less harm.

diverticulitis /dī′vərtik′yəlī′tis/, inflammation of one or more pouches (diverticula) in the wall of the large intestine (colon). It is caused by fecal matter seeping through the thin-walled diverticula. Inflammation and abcesses form in the tissues surrounding the colon. The opening of the colon narrows and may become blocked. During an attack of diverticulitis, the patient will experience crampy pain, often in the lower abdomen, and fever. Mild and moderate attacks are treated with bedrest and antibiotics. Severe attacks require surgery. An opening between colon and body surface is created (colostomy) to rest the bowel for about 6 months. See also **colostomy.**

diverticulosis /-lō′sis/, a pouchlike bulging through the muscular layer of the large intestine (colon) without inflammation. This occurs most often in the sigmoid colon, which is above the rectum. Diverticulosis affects mainly people over age 50. Most patients with this condition have few symptoms except for occasional bleeding from the rectum, gas, and vague stomach distress. Barium enemas and examination with a device called a proctoscope are used to make the diagnosis. Diverticulosis may lead to diverticulitis. Treatment is to add roughage to the diet, rest, a heating pad to relieve discomfort, and sometimes medication to relieve the pain.

diverticulum /dī′vərtik′yələm/, *pl.* **diverticula,** a pouchlike bulging through the muscular wall of a tubular organ. A diverticulum may occur in the stomach, in the small intestine, or, most commonly, in the colon.

division, **a,** the separation of something into two or more parts. A kind of division is **cell division. b,** that organizational level having responsibility for operations within a defined geographic area or with functional responsibility. The division level is organizationally between the strike team and the branch. See also **group.**

dizygotic /dī′zīgot′ik/, referring to twins from two fertilized eggs. Compare **monozygotic.** See also **twin.**

dizziness. See **vertigo.**

DNA, abbreviation for **deoxyribonucleic acid.**

dobutamine hydrochloride, a drug used to increase heart output in long-term congestive heart failure. It is also used in heart surgery. Narrowing of the large artery of the heart (aorta) or known allergy to this drug prohibits its use. It is not recommended for use in pregnancy. Side effects include too rapid heart beats (tachycardia), high blood pressure, irregular heart beats (arrythmias), chest pain, nausea, vomiting, and headache.

Dobutrex, a trademark for a drug used to increase heart output (dobutamine hydrochloride).

Doctor of Medicine, Doctor of Osteopathy. See **physician.**

docusate /dok′yəsāt/, a stool softener. It is used to relieve constipation. Symptoms of appendicitis, use of mineral oil at the same time, or known allergy to the drug prohibits its use. No serious side effects are known.

Doederlein's bacillus, a bacterium present in normal vaginal discharge.

Dolene, a trademark for a painkiller (propoxyphene hydrochloride).

doll's-eye reflex, a normal response in newborns to keep the eyes stationary as the head is moved to the right or left. The reflex disappears as ability to focus the eyes develops.

Dolobid, a trademark for a drug that reduces inflammation (diflunisal).

Dolophine Hydrochloride, a trademark for a narcotic painkiller (methadone hydrochloride).

dome fracture, any bone break of the hip socket which the thigh bone fits into (acetabulum).

dominance, a basic genetic principle stating that not all genes operate with equal strength. If two genes produce a different trait, as eye color, the gene that is expressed is dominant.

dominant gene. See **gene.**

Donath-Landsteiner syndrome, a rare blood disorder. It features separation of hemoglobin from the red cells (hemolysis) minutes or hours after exposure to cold. Symptoms include dark urine, severe pain in the back and legs, headache, vomiting, and diarrhea. When the condition occurs with syphilis, treatment with pencillin may cure the disorder.

Donnatal, a trademark for a drug (phenobarbital) with a calming effect and three nerve blockers (hyoscyamine sulfate, atropine sulfate, and hyoscine hydrobromide). It is used to decrease the activity of the intestinal tract and relieve diarrhea.

donor, a human or other organism that gives living tissue to be used in another body, for example, blood for transfusion or a kidney for transplantation. See also **blood donor, transplant.**

dopamine hydrochloride /dō′pəmin/, a drug used to treat shock, low blood pressure, and low heart output.

Dopar, a trademark for a drug used to treat Parkinson's disease (levodopa).

dope, *slang.* morphine, heroin, marijuana, or another illegal substance.

Doppler scanning. See **ultrasound imaging.**

Dopram, a trademark for a drug that stimulates the breathing tract (doxapram hydrochloride).

Doriden, a trademark for a drug that induces sleep (glutethimide).

dorsal /dôr′səl/, referring to the back or posterior. Compare **ventral.** –**dorsum,** *n.*

dorsal digital vein, one of the veins along the sides of the fingers. The veins from both sides of the fingers unite to form three dorsal metacarpal veins, which end in a dorsal vein network on the back of the hand.

dorsal interventricular artery, the branch of the right coronary artery. It branches to supply both lower heart chambers (ventricles).

dorsalis pedis artery /dôrsā′lis pē′dis/, the continuation of the anterior tibial artery of the lower leg. It starts at the ankle joint, divides into five branches, and supplies various muscles of the foot and toes.

dorsal scapular nerve, one of a pair of nerve branches above the collarbone. It supplies the muscles of the shoulder blade (rhomboideus major and the rhomboideus minor) and sends a branch of nerves to the levator muscle in the neck.

dorsiflect /dôr'siflekt/, to bend or flex backward, as in the upward bending of the fingers, wrist, foot, or toes.

dorsiflexor /-flek'sər/, a muscle causing backward flexion of a part of the body, as the hand or foot.

dosage, the size, frequency, and number of doses of a drug to be given to a patient.

dose, the amount of a drug or other substance to be given at one time. **Effective dose** refers to the amount of a drug that may be expected to have a specific effect. With the **limited fluctuation method of dosing,** the dose is not allowed to rise or fall beyond certain maximum and minimum limits. A **maintenance dose** is the amount of drug needed to keep a desired amount of the drug in the tissues. A part of a drug is lost through the body's normal processes, as excretion. With the **peak method of dosing,** a drug dose is given so that a certain maximum level is reached to cause a desired effect, as lowering the blood pressure. See also **pediatric dose.**

dose, radiation, an accumulated quantity of ionizing radiation. It is a measure of the energy absorbed per gram of absorbing material. The unit of absorbed dose is the rad. The term ''dose'' is often used in the sense of the exposure, expressed in ''roentgens,'' which is a measure of the total amount of ionization that the quantity of radiation could produce in air. The absorbed dose in tissue is about 1 rad when the exposure in air is 1 roentgen.

dose equivalent, a quantity used in radiation protection. It expresses all radiations on a common scale for evaluating and comparing the effects of radiation in man. It is defined as the product of the absorbed dose in rads and certain modifying factors. The unit of dose equivalent is the rem. For the most common forms of radiation (X, gamma, and beta), the dose equivalent in rems is numerically equal to the absorbed dose in rads.

dose rate, the amount of radiation absorbed in a certain amount of time.

dose threshold, the minimum amount of absorbed radiation that produces an effect.

dose to skin, the amount of absorbed radiation at the center of the irradiation field on the skin.

dosimeter /dōsim'ətər/, an instrument to detect and measure total radiation exposure.

DOT hazard class, the designation for hazardous material as found in the Department of Transportation regulations, CFR part 49.

double-blind study, an experiment made to test the effect of a treatment or drug. Groups of experimental and control subjects are used in which neither the subjects nor the investigators know the identity of the treatment being given to any group. In a double-blind test of a new drug, the drug may be identified to the investigators only by a code.

double fracture, a fracture that has breaks or cracks in two places in a bone, resulting in more than two bone segments.

Down's syndrome, a disorder present at birth that features mental retardation and many physical defects. It is more frequent in infants born to women over 35 years of age. The incidence is as high as 1 in 80 for offspring of women older than 40 years. Infants with the disorder are small with weak muscles. They have a small head with a flat back skull, a mongoloid slant to the eyes, depressed nose bridge, low-set ears, and a large, protruding tongue that is furrowed and lacks the central groove. The hands are short and broad with a single crease across the palm (called a simian crease). Other abnormalities include bowel defects, inborn heart disease, long-term breathing infections, vision problems, and susceptibility to acute leukemia. The most significant feature of the disorder is mental retardation, which varies considerably, although the average IQ is in the range of 50 to 60. Also called **mongolism.**

Downey cells, white blood cells (lymphocytes) identified in patients with infectious mononucleosis.

doxapram hydrochloride, a breathing stimulant. It is given to improve breathing after anesthesia, in drug overdose, and for long-term disease linked to an acute condition of excess carbon dioxide in the blood (hypercapnia). Seizure disorder, lung disease, coronary artery disease, high blood pressure, or known allergy to this drug prohibits its use. Side effects include convulsions, spasms of the bronchial tubes, heart symptoms, and vein inflammation (phlebitis).

doxepin hydrochloride, an antidepressant drug used to treat depression.

doxorubicin hydrochloride, an antibiotic drug used to treat several forms of cancer.

doxycycline, an antibacterial used to treat some infections. Kidney or liver problems or known allergy to this drug or to other tetracyclines prohibits its use. It is not given during pregnancy or to children under 8 years of age. Side effects include intestinal disturbances, excess reaction to sunlight (phototoxicity), potentially serious new infections, and allergic reactions. Tooth color may be harmed in children exposed to the drug before birth or under 8 years of age.

doxylamine succinate, an antihistamine. It is used to treat acute allergic symptoms. Known allergy to this drug prohibits its use. It is not recommended for use during pregnancy or nursing. It is not given to children under 6 years of age. Side effects include poor muscle coordination (ataxia), fast heart beat (tachycardia), anemia, and decrease in blood platelets.

dozer company, any dozer with a miminum complement of two persons.

DPT vaccine, abbreviation for **diphtheria, tetanus toxoids, and pertussis vaccine.**

dracunculiasis /drakun′kyəlī′əsis/, a parasitic infection. It is caused by the worm (nematode) *Dracunculus medinensis.*

drainage, the removal of fluids from a body cavity, wound, or other source of discharge by one or more methods. **Closed drainage** involves attaching a tube to the area to remove fluid to an airtight container, preventing contaminants from entering the wound or cavity. In **open drainage** the discharge passes through an open-ended tube into a container. **Suction drainage** uses a pump to assist in removing fluid. With **tidal drainage,** a body area is washed out by alternately flooding and then emptying it with the aid of gravity. This method may be used in treating a urinary bladder disorder. The use of body position to drain fluids released from the breathing tubes (bronchi) and lungs into the throat is called **postural drainage.** Coughing usually gets rid of these fluids from the throat. Positions are chosen that help drainage. Pillows and other devices are used to support or raise parts of the body. The patient begins with the body straight out and level, and the head is slowly lowered. Breathing in through the nose and breathing out through the mouth is best. Tapping and shaking the body over the affected area of the lungs helps to loosen the fluids. The patient is then helped to a position to cough and breathe deeply. Outcome of this method depends on using positions that allow drainage by gravity, and breathing well and deeply.

drainage tube, a heavy-gauge tube (catheter) used to remove air or a fluid from a cavity or wound in the body. The tube may be attached to a suction device or it may simply allow flow by gravity into a container.

Draize test, a controversial method of testing the toxicity of drugs and other products to be used by humans. A small amount of the substance is placed in the eyes of rabbits. A substance that irritates the rabbit's eyes is considered a measure of the possible effect the product could have on similar human tissues.

dram, a unit of mass equivalent to an apothecaries' measure of 60 grains or ⅛ ounce and to 1/16 ounce or 27.34 grains avoirdupois.

Dramamine, a trademark for an antihistamine. It is used to prevent nausea and motion sickness (dimenhydrinate).

drape, a sheet of fabric or paper for covering all or a part of a person's body during a physical examination or treatment. It is usually the size of a small bed.

drawing, *informal.* a vague sensation of muscle tension.

dream, **1.** ideas, thoughts, emotions, or images that pass through the mind during the rapid eye movement stage of sleep. **2.** a creation of the imagination during wakefulness. **3.** the expression of thoughts, emotions, memories, or impulses repressed from the consciousness.

dream analysis, a process of gaining access to the unconscious mind by examining the content of dreams. It is usually done through the method of free association.

dream state, a condition of altered consciousness in which a person does not recognize the environment and reacts in a manner not like his or her usual behavior, as by flight or an act of violence. The state is seen in epilepsy and certain neuroses. See also **automatism, fugue.**

dressing, a clean or sterile covering applied directly to wounded or diseased tissue. The uses are varied. An **absorbent dressing** is placed on a wound or cut to absorb fluid or other drainage. An **antiseptic dressing** is treated with a germ or bacteria-killing drug to prevent or treat infection. A **dry dressing** has no medication. It is applied to prevent contamination or injury or to absorb releases. A **fixed dressing** is usually made of gauze with a hardening agent, as plaster of paris or starch. It supports or keeps rigid a part of the body. An **occlusive dressing** prevents air and germs from reaching a wound. It stores moisture, heat, body fluids, and drugs. A **pressure dressing** is put on firmly, most often on a wound to stop loss of blood. A **wet dressing** is used to treat some skin diseases. As the moisture evaporates, it cools and dries the skin, softens dried blood and sera, and stimulates drainage. Drugs may be added if necessary.

Dressler's syndrome, a disorder that may occur several days after severe heart attack. It results from the response of the body's immune system to a damaged heart. Symptoms include fever, fluid in the lungs, joint pain, and inflammation of the sac around the heart and the membrane around the lungs.

drift, a change that occurs in a strain of virus so that variations appear periodically with alterations in the virus' qualities.

drip, the process of a liquid or moisture forming and falling in drops. It is used in health care to put a liquid continuously into the body, as into the stomach or a vein. One device used for putting specific volumes of solutions into a vein is called a **drip system.** Another is called a **nasal drip,** a method of giving liquid to a dehydrated infant by a tube placed through the nose and into the esophagus. See also **postnasal drip.**

Drisdol, a trademark for vitamin D₂ (ergocalciferol).

Drolban, a trademark for a synthetic drug that stimulates male characteristics, used in cancer therapy (dromostanolone propionate).

droperidol, a drug with a calming, sleep-inducing effect. It is used to decrease anxiety and pain before anesthesia (fentanyl).

drop foot, a condition in which the foot is flexed down and cannot voluntarily be flexed up. It is usually caused by nerve damage.

droplet infection, an infection caused by inhaling germs that are in particles of liquid sneezed or coughed by an infected person or animal.

drowning, suffocation from being submerged in a liquid. **Near drowning** is a state in which a person has survived conditions that usually cause drowning. Cardiopulmonary resuscitation (CPR) is done at once, followed by hospitalization. The return of consciousness does not necessarily mean the patient will recover. Strong, close treatment may be needed for several days.

drug, 1. any substance taken by mouth, injected into a muscle, the skin, a blood vessel, or a cavity of the body, or applied to the skin to treat or prevent a disease. **2.** *informal.* a narcotic substance.

drug abuse, the use of a drug for a nontherapeutic effect. Some of the most commonly abused drugs are alcohol, amphetamines, barbiturates, cocaine, methaqualone, and opium alkaloids. Drug abuse may lead to organ damage, addiction, and disturbed patterns of behavior. Some illegal drugs have no known therapeutic effect in humans. See also **drug addiction.**

drug action, the means by which a drug has a desired effect. Drugs are usually classified by their actions. For example, a vasodilator, which is prescribed to decrease the blood pressure, acts by widening the blood vessels.

drug addiction, a condition marked by an overwhelming desire to continue taking a drug because it produces a desired effect, usually an altered mental activity, attitude, or outlook. Addiction goes along with a tendency to increase the dose, a psychological or physical dependence, and harmful effects for the person and society. A newborn infant of an addicted mother can show withdrawal symptoms, usually within the first 24 hours of life. Most commonly these are caused by maternal dependence on heroin, methadone, diazepam, phenobarbital, or alcohol. Typical symptoms include tremors, breathing distress, excessive sweating, high temperature, vomiting, diarrhea, and excess water loss. The infants cry shrilly, often sneeze, frantically suck their fists but feed poorly. They often yawn but have trouble falling asleep. They are usually pale, and are often born with nose and knee abrasions. They are subject to convulsions. These infants need special treatment including protection from stimulation. See also **alcoholism, drug abuse.**

drug allergy, allergy to a drug shown by reactions ranging from a mild rash to severe allergic reaction and shock. The seriousness of the reaction depends on the person, the drug, and the dose. Allergic responses may be caused by any drug. A **drug eruption** is any skin reaction or rash caused by a drug.

drug dependence, a psychologic craving for or a physical dependence on a drug. It results from habituation, abuse, or addiction. See also **drug abuse, drug addiction.**

drug dispensing, the preparation, packaging, labeling, record keeping, and transfer of a prescription drug to a patient or to one who is responsible for giving the drug.

drug-drug interaction, a change of the effect of a drug when given with another drug. The effect may be an increase or a decrease in the action of either drug. The effect may also be a side effect that is not normally linked to either drug. See also **side effect.**

dry skin, skin lacking moisture or oil. It features a pattern of fine lines, scaling, and itching. Causes include too frequent bathing, low humidity, and low oil production in aging skin. Treatment includes bathing less often, increased humidity, bath oils, drugs that soften the skin such as lanolin and glycerine, and water absorbing ointments. Also called **xerosis** /zērō′-/.

DTIC-Dome, a trademark for a drug used to treat cancer (dacarbazine).

DTs, abbreviation for **delirium tremens.**

Duchenne's muscular dystrophy /dooshenz′/. See **muscular dystrophy.**

duct, a narrow tubelike structure, especially one through which material is released.

duct carcinoma, a cancer developed from the lining of ducts, especially in the breast or pancreas.

ductless gland, a gland lacking a duct. Endocrine glands, which release hormones directly into blood or lymph, are ductless glands.

Dulcolax, a trademark for a laxative (bisacodyl).

dumping syndrome, a disorder with profuse sweating, nausea, dizziness, and weakness. It is experienced by patients who have had part of their stomachs removed (gastrectomy). Symptoms are felt soon after eating, when the contents of the stomach empty too rapidly into the first part of the small intestine (duodenum). A high-protein, high-calorie diet, with small frequent meals should prevent discomfort and ensure good nutrition. See also **gastrectomy.**

duodenal /doo′ədē′nəl/, referring to the first part of the small intestine (duodenum).

duodenal ulcer. See **peptic ulcer.**

duodenoscope /dōō′ədē′nəskōp′/, an instrument, usually fiberoptic, for the visual examination of the duodenum.

duodenum /dōō′ədē′nəm, dōō·od′ənəm/, *pl.* **duodena, duodenums,** the shortest, widest, portion of the small intestine that joins the stomach at the pyloric valve. It is about 10 inches (25 cm) long. It is divided into superior, descending, horizontal, and ascending portions. Compare **jejunum, ileum.**

Durabolin, a trademark for a steroid used to build up tissues damaged from severe disease or injury (nandrolone phenpropionate).

dura mater /dōōr′ə mā′tər, dyōō′rə/, the fiberlike, outermost of the three membranes surrounding the brain and spinal cord. The **dura mater encephali** covers the brain. The **dura mater spinalis** covers the cord. See also **meninges.**

Duranest, a trademark for a drug used to produce local anesthesia (etidocaine hydrochloride).

dust, any fine, particulate, dry matter. **Inorganic dust** refers to dry, finely powdered particles of an inorganic substance. especially dust. When inhaled, it can cause abnormal conditions of the lungs. **Organic dust** is dried bits of matter from plants, animals, fungi, or germs that are fine enough to be carried by the wind. Many kinds of this dust cause different types of breathing problems.

Duverney's fracture /dōōvərnāz′/, fracture of the pelvic bone (ilium) just below the spine.

dwarf, an abnormally short person, especially one whose bodily parts are not proportional. See also specific entry.

dwarfism, the abnormal underdevelopment of the body. It features extreme shortness. The condition is linked to numerous other defects and sometimes includes varying degrees of mental retardation. Dwarfism has numerous causes, including genetic defects, hormone lack involving either the pituitary or thyroid glands, chronic diseases (as rickets, kidney failure, and intestinal malabsorption defects), and psychosocial stress (as the maternal deprivation syndrome).

Dyazide, a trademark for a drug containing two drugs that stimulate urine release (triamterene and hydrochlorothiazide).

Dyclone, a trademark for a drug used to produce local anesthesia (dyclonine hydrochloride).

dyclonine hydrochloride, a local anesthetic drug that also destroys bacteria and fungus. It is used for mouth pain, severe itching, insect bites, and minor skin burns and injuries.

dye, 1. to apply coloring matter to a substance. **2.** a chemical compound that colors a substance to which it is applied. Various dyes are used as to color drugs, to stain tissues, as therapeutic agents, and in tests.

Dymelor, a trademark for a drug used to treat diabetes (acetohexamide).

dynamometer /dī′nəmom′ətər/, a device for measuring the amount of energy used in the contraction of a muscle or a group of muscles. For example, a squeeze dynamometer measures the force of the hand when squeezing the device.

Dynapen, a trademark for an antibacterial drug used to treat infections (dicloxacillin sodium).

dyphylline, a drug that relaxes the bronchial muscle of the airway. It is used to treat acute bronchial asthma, bronchitis, and emphysema. It is used carefully in patients with ulcer or heart disease. Known allergy to this or to other xanthines prohibits its use. Side effects include digestive distress, dizziness, too rapid heart beat, and headache.

Dyrenium, a trademark for a drug that stimulates urine release (triamterene).

dysadrenia /dis′adrē′nē·ə/, abnormal adrenal gland function. It features decreased or increased production of gland hormones.

dyscholia /-kō′lyə/, any abnormal condition of the bile, either regarding the amount released or the condition of the contents.

dyscrasia /-krā′zhə/, an abnormal blood or bone marrow condition, as leukemia, aplastic anemia, or Rh incompatibility.

dyscrasic fracture, any broken bone caused by the weakening of a specific bone as a result of a debilitating disease.

dysentery /dis′inter′ē/, an inflammation of the intestine, especially of the large intestine (colon). It may be caused by chemical irritants, bacteria, protozoa, or parasites. The symptoms are frequent and bloody stools, stomach pain, and straining. Dysentery is common when sanitary living conditions, clean food, and safe water are not available. **Amebic dysentery** is an inflammation of the intestine caused by *Entamoeba histolytica.*

dysfunctional, unable to function normally, as a body organ or system. –**dysfunction,** *n.*

dysfunctional uterine bleeding (DUB), a disorder of bleeding from the uterus caused by hormone imbalance rather than a disease.

dysgenesis /-jen′əsis/, **1.** defective formation of an organ or part, primarily during early fetal development. **2.** loss of the ability to reproduce.

dysgenitalism /-jen′ətəlizm/, any condition involving the abnormal growth of the genital organs.

dysgerminoma /dis′jərminō′mə/, a rare cancerous tumor of the ovary that is found in young women.

dysgraphia /-graf′ē·ə/, a blockage of the ability to write, caused by a disease process.

dyskinesia /dis′kinē′zhə/,   impaired ability to make voluntary movements.   **−dyskinetic** /-et′ik/, *adj.*

dyslexia /-lek′sē·ə/,   a blockage of the ability to read, as a result of a variety of disorders. Some are linked to the central nervous system. Dyslexic persons often reverse letters and words. They cannot determine the order of letters in written words. They also have difficulty determining left from right.   **−dyslexic,** *adj.*

dysmaturity,   1. the failure of an organism to develop or mature in structure or function. **2.** a fetus or newborn who is abnormally small or large for the length of pregnancy (age of gestation). See also **birth weight.**

dysmelia /-mē′lyə/,   a birth defect marked by missing or shortened arms and legs. This is linked to abnormalities of the spine in some individuals. See also **phocomelia.**

dysmenorrhea /dis′menôrē′ə/,   pain linked to menstruation.

dysmorphophobia /dis′môrfō-/,   **1.** a delusion of body image. **2.** the morbid fear of deformity or of becoming deformed.

dysostosis /dis′ostō′-/,   an abnormal condition with defective bone formation (ossification), especially in fetal cartilages.

dyspareunia /dis′pəroo͞′nē·ə/,   an abnormal condition of women in which sexual intercourse is painful. The pain may result from abnormal conditions of the genitals, a psychologic reaction to sexual union, rape, or incomplete sexual arousal. See also **vaginismus.**

dyspepsia /-pep′sē·ə/,   a vague feeling of discomfort under the breastbone after eating. There is an uncomfortable feeling of fullness, heartburn, bloating, and nausea. Dyspepsia is not a distinct condition, but it may be a symptom of an underlying disorder, such as peptic ulcer, gallbladder disease, or long-term inflammation of the appendix (appendicitis). **Cholelithic dyspepsia** refers to sudden attacks of indigestion linked to the dysfunction of the gallbladder. **Fermentative dyspepsia** is impaired digestion linked to the fermenting of digested food. **Functional dyspepsia** results from a smooth muscle or nervous system problem. **Gastric dyspepsia** is another term for pain or discomfort in the stomach. Faulty digestion that is linked to a disease or a change in an organ other than an organ of digestion is called **reflex dyspepsia.**

dysphagia /-fā′jə/,   difficulty in swallowing, commonly linked to blockage or motor disorders of the esophagus. Patients with blockages as esophageal tumor or lower esophageal ring are unable to swallow solids but can tolerate liquids. Patients with motor disorders, as muscle problems related to esophagus (achalasia), are unable to swallow solids or liquids.

dysphasia /-fā′zhə/,   difficulty in speaking, not as severe as aphasia. It usually results from an injury to the speech area of the brain. Symptoms include lack of coordination in speaking and getting words out of order. It may follow a stroke or brain tumor. It may occur with other language disorders, such as inability to write (dysgraphia).

dyspnea /-pnē′ə/,   a shortness of breath or a difficulty in breathing. It may be caused by some heart conditions, strenuous exercise, or anxiety. **Cardiac dyspnea** is linked with the first stages of heart failure. It happens when the heart is unable to keep up with the increased oxygen needs during exercise. **Nocturnal paroxysmal dyspnea** occurs with sudden attacks of shortness of breath, heavy sweating, rapid heartbeat, and wheezing which awaken the patient from sleep. The attacks may be caused by nightmares, noises, or coughing. It is usually linked to heart failure or fluid in the lungs, and is relieved by getting up and opening a window.

dyspraxia /-prak′sē·ə/,   a partial loss of the ability to perform skilled, coordinated movements. See also **apraxia.**

dysprosium (Dy),   a rare earth metallic element. Radioactive isotopes of dysprosium are used in studies of the bones and joints.

dysproteinemia /-prō′tēnē′mē·ə/,   an abnormality of the protein content of the blood.

dysreflexia /dis′riflek′sē·ə/,   a nerve or muscle condition with abnormal reflexes.

dysrhythmia /-rith′mē·ə/,   any abnormality in a normal rhythmic pattern. This especially refers to irregularity in the brain waves or pattern of speech. Compare **arrhythmia.**

dyssebacea /dis′ibā′shē·ə/,   a skin condition marked by red, scaly, greasy patches on the nose, eyelids, scrotum, and lips. It results from a lack of vitamin B_2. It is commonly seen in persons with long-term alcoholism, liver disease, and protein malnutrition. Also called *(informal)* **shark skin.**

dystocia /-tō′shə/,   a difficult labor. It may be caused by an blockage or narrowing of the birth passage or an abnormal size, shape, or position of the fetus.

dystrophy /dis′trəfē/,   any abnormal condition caused by defective nutrition. The term is often applied to a change in muscles that does not involve the nervous system, as fatty breakdown linked to increased muscle size but decreased strength. See also **muscular dystrophy.**

dysuria /-yoŏr′ē·ə/,   painful urination. It usually results from a bacterial infection or blockage in the urinary tract. Dysuria is a symptom of such conditions as inflammation of the urine bladder (cyctitis), the urethra (urethritis), or the prostate (prostatitis), tumors, and some gynecologic disorders. Compare **hematuria, pyuria.**

E

ear, the organ of hearing. The ear has three parts: the inner, middle, and outer ear. The outer ear is both the skin-covered cartilage (**auricle**) that sticks out on either side of the head, and the tube (**external auditory canal**) that leads from the outside of the head to the middle ear. The two parts of the outer ear focus sound waves on the eardrum, between the outer and middle ear. Also called the **tympanic membrane**, the eardrum carries sound vibrations to the inner ear by means of the bones of the middle ear. The **middle ear** is the space between the eardrum and the inner ear. It is filled with air carried from the back of the throat by the auditory (eustachian) tube. It holds three small bones called the hammer (malleus), anvil (incus), and stirrup (stapes). These bones pick up the vibrations caused by sound waves hitting the eardrum. The bones pass the vibrations on to the inner ear. The **inner ear** (labyrinth) is filled with fluid, and holds two organs. One of the organs gives a sense of balance (vestibular apparatus), the other picks up the sound vibrations from the inner ear fluid and carries them to the nerve endings that sense sounds.

earache, a pain in the ear that may be sharp, dull, burning, on and off, or constant. The cause does not have to be a disease of the ear, because infections and other disorders of the nose, mouth, throat, and jaw joint can cause pain to be felt in the ear. See also **otitis externa, otitis media.**

eardrops, a liquid drug for treating various conditions of the ear, including inflammation or infection or hardened wax.

earwax. See **cerumen.**

eccentric implantation, rooting of the fertilized egg in a fold of the wall of the womb (uterus). The fold then closes off from the main cavity.

eccentricity, behavior that is seen as odd or peculiar for a given culture or community, although not unusual enough to be considered dangerous or insane.

ecchondroma /ek′əndrō′mə/, a harmless tumor that grows on the surface of a cartilage or under bone covering (periosteum).

ecchymosis /ek′imō′-/. See **bruise.**

eccrine /ek′rin/, referring to fluid released through a duct to the surface of the skin. See also **exocrine.**

eccrine gland, one of two kinds of sweat glands in the skin. These glands are unbranched, coiled, and tubelike. They are placed throughout the skin covering of the body. They cool the body by evaporation of the fluid (sweat) they release, which is clear, has a faint odor, and contains water, sodium chloride, and traces of albumin, urea, and other compounds. Compare **apocrine gland.**

ECG, **1.** abbreviation for **electrocardiogram. 2.** abbreviation for **electrocardiograph.**

echo beat, a heartbeat that is restarted when an electric impulse returns to one of the chambers of the heart.

echocardiography /ek′ōkär′dē·og′rəfē/, a method of diagnosis that studies the structure and motion of the heart. Sound waves (ultrasonic) directed through the heart are reflected backward, or echoed, when they pass from one type of tissue to another, such as from heart muscle to blood. This test can find tumors in the upper chambers, and fluid in the sac around the heart. It can spot problems with the movement of the valve (mitral) between the upper and lower chambers on the left side of the heart. Also called **ultrasonic cardiography.**

echoencephalography /-ensef′əlog′rəfē/, the use of sound waves (ultrasonic) to study the brain. The method is useful for showing widening of the hollows (ventricles) and a shift of the tissues between the hollows caused by a growing tumor. See also **ultrasound imaging.**

echolalia /-lā′lyə/, the automatic and meaningless repeating of another's words or phrases, especially as seen in schizophrenia.

echoradiography /-rā′dē·og′rəfē/, a method of diagnosis using ultrasonography and various devices for visualizing inner parts of the body.

echothiophate iodide, a drug used to treat open-angle glaucoma and some forms of crossed eyes. Persons with eye inflammation, most types of angle-closure glaucoma, or known allergy to this drug should not take it. Side effects include retinal detachment, lens thickening, and other eye problems.

echovirus, a virus linked to many infections but not identified as a cause of any disease. There are many echoviruses, and most are harmless.

eclampsia /iklamp'sē·ə/, the gravest form of poisoning of pregnancy, marked by grand mal convulsion, coma, high blood pressure, water retention, and protein in the urine. Symptoms of convulsions coming on include anxiety, pain under the breastbone, headache, blurred vision, extremely high blood pressure, and overactive reflexes. Convulsions may be prevented by bed rest and by a calming drug. Treatment of a convulsion includes keeping the airway open, protection against injury, and drugs to stop the convulsion and lower the blood pressure. Convulsions rarely happen after the child has been born. Eclampsia occurs in 0.2% of pregnancies, and the cause is not known.

Eclipse, a trademark for a drug containing an ultraviolet sunscreen for use on the skin (padimate).

econazole, a drug that destroys fungus. It is used to treat ringworm, candidiasis, and other fungus infections. Patients who are allergic to this drug should not use it. Side effects include skin irritation and allergy.

Econochlor, a trademark for a drug that destroys bacteria and rickettsia (chloramphenicol).

Econopred, a trademark for a steroid drug (prednisolone acetate).

ectoderm /ek'tədurm/. See **embryonic layer.**

ectomorph /-môrf/. See **somatotype.**

ectoparasite /-per'əsīt/, an organism that lives on the outside of the body of the host, as a louse.

ectopic /ektop'ik/, **1.** referring to an object or organ located in an unusual place, away from its normal area. For example, an ectopic pregnancy is one that occurs outside the uterus. **2.** referring to an event occurring at the wrong time, such as a premature heartbeat.

ectromelia /-mē'lyə/, a birth defect marked by the lack or faulty growth of the long bones of one or more of the arms or legs.

eczema /ek'simə/, inflammation of the outer layer of skin from unknown cause. In the early stage it may be itchy and red, have small blisters, and be swollen and weeping. Later it becomes crusted, scaly, and thickened. Eczema is not a distinct disease but a symptom. See also **dermatitis.**

eczema herpeticum, a skin disease with pus-filled blisters. It is caused by herpes simplex virus or vaccinia virus infection of a rash already present. Hospitalization is advised because this disease can be fatal. Also called **Kaposi's varicelliform eruption.**

Edecrin, a trademark for a diuretic (ethacrynic acid).

edema /idē'mə/, the abnormal pooling of fluid in tissues. Many conditions can cause edema. Among therm are congestive heart failure, kidney failure, cirrhosis, overactive adrenal glands, draining wounds, excessive bleeding, malnutrition, allergic reactions, and blockage of blood or lymph vessels. One form, **angioedema,** affects the face, neck, lips, throat, hands, feet, genitals, or abdominal

organs. It may be caused by a food or drug allergy, infection, or mental stress, or it can be inherited. **Sequestered edema** refers to fluid collected in the tissues surrounding a surgical wound. Treatment of edema is directed at correcting the basic cause. Some drugs may be given to promote the removal of sodium and water. When a limb has edema because blood is pooling in a vein, raising the limb and wrapping it with an elastic stocking or sleeve helps the fluid move back into the vein and return to the heart.

edetate disodium, a drug used to treat a serious condition resulting from excess calcium. It is also used for irregular heartbeats and heart block resulting from reaction to the drug digitalis, and for lead poisoning. Patients who have low levels of calcium, kidney disease, or known allergy to this drug should not use it. Side effects include low levels of calcium, vein inflammation linked to clotting, kidney damage, and excess bleeding linked to lowered ability of the blood to clot.

edrophonium chloride, a drug used to treat severe reactions to the drug curare, to aid in diagnosis of myasthenia gravis, and to slow rapid heartbeats. Blockage of the digestive or urinary tract, low blood pressure, slow heartbeats, or known allergy to this drug prohibits its use. Side effects include stopping of breathing, low blood pressure, slow heartbeats, spasms of the air passages.

EEG, **1.** abbreviation for **electroencephalogram. 2.** abbreviation for **electroencephalography.**

effacement, the shortening of the cervix and thinning of its walls as it is stretched and widened by the fetus during labor. See also **birth, labor.**

efferent /ef'ərənt/, directed away from a center, such as certain arteries, veins, nerves, and lymph channels. Compare **afferent.**

efferent duct, any duct through which a gland releases its fluids.

efficacy /ef'əkəsē/, the greatest ability of a drug or treatment to produce a result, regardless of dosage.

effort syndrome, an abnormal condition with chest pain, dizziness, fatigue, and rapid, uneven heartbeat. This condition is often found in soldiers in combat but occurs also in other persons. The symptoms of effort syndrome often mimic angina pectoris but are really anxiety states.

effusion, **1.** the escape of fluid from blood vessels because of a break or leaking, usually into a body hollow. The condition is usually linked with a circulatory or kidney disease. It is often an early sign of heart disease. The term may refer to an affected body area, as pleural effusion. **2.** the outward spread of a bacterial growth.

Efudex, a trademark for a drug used to treat cancer (fluorouracil).

ego /ē'gō, eg'ō/, **1.** the conscious sense of the self; those elements of a person, such as thinking and feeling, that mark the person as an individual. **2.** the part of the self that experiences and maintains conscious contact with reality and balances the drives and demands of the self with the social and physical needs of society.

ego boundary, a sense or awareness that there is a difference between the self and others. In some psychoses the person does not have an ego boundary and cannot tell the difference between his or her own personal feelings and other people's feelings.

egocentric, seeing the self as the center of all experience and having little regard for the needs, interests, ideas, and attitudes of others.

ego ideal, the image of the self that a person strives to be both consciously and unconsciously and against which he or she measures him or herself. It is usually based on a positive identification with the important and influential figures of early childhood years. See also **identification.**

egoism /ē'gō·iz'əm, eg'-/, the belief that individual self-interest is, or ought to be, the basic motive for all conscious behavior.

ego libido, focusing of the sexual interest (libido) on the self; self-love, narcissism.

egomania, an extreme, long-term focus on the self and magnified sense of one's own importance.

ego strength, the ability to keep up the ego by a group of traits that together contribute to good mental health.

egotism /ē'gətizm, eg'-/, a magnifying of the importance of the self and the contempt of others. See also **egoism.**

egress /ē'gres/, the act of coming out or moving forward.

eidetic image /īdet'ik/, an unusually vivid, elaborate, and apparently exact mental image coming from a visual experience and happening as a fantasy, dream, or memory. See also **image.**

ejaculation, the sudden release of semen from the male urethra, usually happening during intercourse, masturbation, and sleep (nocturnal emission). It is a reflex action in two phases: First, sperm fluid and releases from the prostate and bulbourethral gland are moved into the urethra; second, strong spasms (peristaltic) force ejaculation. The feeling of ejaculation is called orgasm. The fluid volume of semen released at one time, called **ejaculate,** is usually less than 0.2 ounces (2 to 5 ml). Each milliliter usually contains 50 million to 150 million sperm. **−ejaculatory** /ijak'yələtôr'ē/, *adj.*

ejaculatory duct, the passage through which semen enters the urethra.

ejection clicks. See **heart sound.**

ejection fraction (EF), the amount of blood that is released during each contraction of the lower heart chamber (ventricle) compared with the total volume of blood released by both ventricles.

Elase, a trademark for a combination drug containing enzymes (fibrinolysin and desoxyribonuclease). It is put on the skin to cure many infections.

elastic bandage, a bandage of stretchy fabric that gives support and allows movement.

elastic band fixation, a method of treating breaks of the jaw using rubber bands to join metal splints or wires that are attached to the upper and lower jaws. The rubber bands pull the jaws together and align the teeth properly while the break heels. Rubber bands are thought to be safer than rigid wires.

elasticity, the ability of tissue to regain its original shape and size after being stretched or squeezed. Muscle tissue is generally thought of as elastic, because it is able to change size and shape and return to its original state.

elastin /ilas'tin/, a protein that forms the main part of yellow elastic tissue fibers.

Elavil, a trademark for an antidepressant drug.

elbow joint, the hinged joint of the arm. The bone of the upper arm (humerus) and the two bones of the forearm (ulna and vadius) join at the elbow. The elbow joint allows the forearm to bend and extend and to roll from side to side. The elbow is a common site of injury, especially from sports.

elective, referring to a treatment that is done by choice but that is not required, as elective surgery.

electric burns, the tissue damage that results from heat of up to 5000° C given off by an electric current. The point of contact on the skin is burned, and the muscle and tissues under the skin may be hurt. If the burn is severe, failure of circulation and breathing may occur and are treated before the burn. In this case, artificial respiration and cardiac resuscitation are done as the person is taken rapidly to a medical facility.

electric shock, a damaged physical state caused by electric current passing through the body. It usually occurs from accidental contact with exposed parts of electric circuits in home appliances and power supplies. It may also result from lightning or contact with high-voltage wires. The damage electricity does in passing through the body depends on the intensity of the electric current. Alternating current (AC) and direct current (DC) cause different kinds and degrees of damage to tissues. High-frequency current (measured in Hz, or Hertz) gives off more heat than low-frequency current and can cause burns, blood clotting, and tissue death. Low-frequency current can burn tissues. Severe electric shock commonly causes unconsciousness, muscle spasms, bone breaks, and heart disorders, and stops breathing. Even small electric currents passing through the heart can cause dangerously rapid heartbeats. Treatment of severe electric shock includes cardiopulmonary resuscitation, defibrillation, and giving electrolytes in the vein to help bring vital functions back to normal levels. See also **shock.**

electric shock therapy. See **electroconvulsive therapy.**

electrocardiograph (ECG) /-kär′dē-əgraf′/, a device used to record the electric activity of the heart to detect abnormal electric impulses through the muscle. The record made, called an **electrocardiogram,** allows diagnosis of heart problems. To make an ECG recording, the patient lies quietly on a table. Electrodes, called leads, are placed on the patient's chest, usually with a gluey gel that helps send the electric impulse to the recording device. The record made varies, depending on the site of the electrode. Electrocardiography is generally performed with six leads placed over the heart and three leads placed at different points (one on each upper arm and one below a knee is common). The ECG is also used for stress tests, which require that the patient be active (usually walking or running on a treadmill) while the machine is working.

electrocautery. See **cautery.**

electroconvulsive therapy (ECT), causing a brief convulsion by passing an electric current through the brain. It is used to treat some mental disorders, especially in patients who have not been helped by drug therapy. The patient has no memory of the shock. A side effect is memory loss. Also called **electric shock therapy.**

electrocution, death caused by an electric current passing through the body. See also **electric shock.**

electrode /ilek′trōd/, **1.** a contact for bringing on or recording electric activity. **2.** a substance that conducts an electric current from the body to measuring equipment.

electrodynograph (EDG) /-din′əgraf/, an electronic device used to measure pressures made by the body as it moves, such as the foot in walking, running, or jogging.

electroencephalogram (EEG) /-ənsef′ələgram′/, a chart of·the electric impulses, called brain waves, made by the brain cells, as picked up by electrodes placed on the scalp. Changes in brain wave activity can show nervous system disorders, mental states, and level of consciousness. For example, a **flat electroencephalogram** means that no tracings were recorded during a brain wave test. It indicates a lack of brain wave activity. Flat readings are a sign of brain death except in cases of central nervous system problems. See also **brain waves.**

electroencephalography (EEG) /-ensef′əlog′rəfē/, the process of recording brain wave activity with an instrument called an **electroencephalograph.** Electrodes are attached to areas of the patient's head. The patterns of electric activity received are then recorded on a chart. During the procedure the patient remains quiet, with eyes closed, although in certain cases some activities may be done, such as breathing rapidly. The test is used to diagnose seizure disorders, brainstem disorders, tumors or clots, and

impaired consciousness. During surgery on the nervous system, the electrodes can be set directly on the brain or placed within the brain tissue to detect injury or tumors. See also **electroencephalogram.**

electrogram /ilek′trəgram/, record of electric activity of the heart as sensed by electrodes inside the heart chambers or on the surface of the heart.

electrohemodynamics (EHD) /-hē′mōdīnam′-/, a method for measuring the workings of the blood flow system of the body. This measures blood pressure in the arteries, the strength of nerve impulses, and the ability of the system to hold and direct flowing blood.

electrohydraulic heart /-hīdrôlik/, a type of artificial heart in which the lower chambers (ventricles) are driven by the alternate pumping of a fluid rather than by compressed air. See also **artificial heart.**

electrolyte /ilek′trəlīt/, an element or compound that, when melted or dissolved in water or other solvent, breaks up into ions (atoms able to carry an electric charge). Electrolyte amounts vary in blood plasma, in tissues, and in cell fluid. The body must have the correct amounts of the main electrolytes to use energy. For example, calcium (Ca^{++}) is needed to relax the heart muscles and contract the heart. Potassium (K^+) is needed to contract muscles and relax the heart. Sodium (Na^+) is needed to maintain fluid balance. Some diseases, defects, and drugs may lead to a lack of one or more electrolytes. Watching the levels of electrolytes and replacement of fluids and electrolytes are part of care in many illnesses. An **electrolyte solution** may be made to give a patient by mouth, rectally, or in the vein. The loss of potassium (K^+) from vomiting, diarrhea, or the action of some drugs (as diuretics and steroids) is corrected by giving a solution high in potassium. Other electrolyte solutions with calcium, sodium, phosphate, chloride, or magnesium may be given to treat an imbalance from disease, as long-term kidney disease or lack of insulin in diabetes (ketoacidosis).

electromagnetic radiation, a packet of emitted energy in the form of a wave resulting from changing electric or magnetic fields. Familiar electromagnetic radiations range from x-rays (and gamma rays) at short wavelengths through the ultraviolet, visible, and infrared regions to radar and radio waves of relatively long wavelength.

electromyogram /-mī′əgram/. See **electroneuromyography.**

electronarcosis, a way to reduce pain that does not use gases or drugs. The patient loses consciousness when an electric current is passed through the brain. The method is experimental.

electroneuromyography /-nyŏŏr′ōmī·og′rəfē/, a method to test and record nerve and muscle function. Electrodes are placed on the skin, or a needle electrode is put into a muscle. An electric current is passed through the electrodes to stimulate the nerves. The record made is called an **electromyogram.** The method helps with the study of nerve injury and reflex responses.

electronic fetal monitor (EFM), a device that allows the fetal heartbeat and the contractions of the uterus to be observed. When used outside the body, two belts are put around the mother's belly, one to pick up heartbeats and one to detect contractions. When done internally, the fetal heart is observed by clipping an electrode to the fetal scalp. The strength, number, and length of time of the uterine contractions are detected by a catheter inside the uterus.

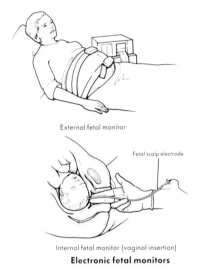

External fetal monitor

Fetal scalp electrode

Internal fetal monitor (vaginal insertion)

Electronic fetal monitors

electron microscopy, using an electron microscope, a beam of electrons is focused by a special lens onto very thin tissue or other sample. A second lens takes the image and projects it onto a screen. The image that is made is 1000 times greater than with an optical microscope.

electronystagmography /-'nīstag-mog'rəfē/, a method of testing and recording eye movements by measuring the electric impulses of the eye muscles.

electroresection /-risek'shən/, a method to remove bladder tumors. An anesthetic is given, and an electric wire is put in through the urethra.

electrosleep therapy, a method to bring about sleep, especially in mental patients. A low-level electric current is passed through the brain.

electrosurgery, surgery that is done with electric instruments. **Electrocoagulation** is a form of electrosurgery in which tissue is hardened with an electric cautery device. A high frequency current is sent through the tissue. Another method, called **electrodesiccation,** burns away tissue with

an electric spark. It is used mainly for removing small surface growths. It may also be used to remove abnormal tissue deep in the skin, in which case layers of skin are burned, then scraped away. The burning is done under local anesthesia.

eleidin /elē'idin/, a clear protein substance that looks like keratin, found in the skin, mucous membrane, and other surface tissues.

element, one of more than 100 primary, simple substances that cannot be broken down by chemical means into any other substance.

elimination diet, a way to test for food to which a person is allergic. Certain foods are left out of the diet one at a time until the symptoms go away.

elixir, a clear liquid made of water, alcohol, sweeteners, or flavors mainly in drugs that are taken by mouth.

Elixophyllin, a trademark for a muscle relaxant used to make the airway passages open wider (theophylline).

elliptocytosis /əlip'tōsītō'-/, a mild defect of the blood in which there are increased numbers of oval-shaped red blood cells (elliptocytes). Less than 15% of the red cells appear in this form in normal blood. Small increases occur in some anemias.

Elspar, a trademark for a drug used to treat cancer antineoplastic (asparaginase).

emaciation /imā'sē·ā'shən/, extreme leanness caused by disease or lack of nutrition.

embedded tooth, a tooth that has not cut through the gums. It is usually completely covered with bone. Compare **impacted tooth.**

embolectomy /em'bōlek'-/, a cut made in an artery to remove a clot (embolus). It is done as emergency treatment within 4 to 6 hours after pain has started, if possible.

embolism /em'bəlizm/, a defect in which a clot (embolus) travels through the bloodstream and becomes lodged in a blood vessel, usually in the heart, lungs, or brain. The symptoms vary with the degree of blockage that the embolism causes, the type of embolus, and the size, nature, and location of the blocked vessel. **Air embolism** refers to the presence of air in the blood that blocks the flow of blood through a vessel. Air can enter a vessel by needle, during surgery, or through a puncture wound. A **cerebral embolism** is a blood clot that stops the flow of blood through vessels of the brain. This results in lack of oxygen in cells beyond the clot. A **fat embolism** is a blob of fat blocking an artery. It may follow the breaking of a long bone or, less commonly, after injury to fat tissue or a fatty liver. This usually occurs 12 to 36 hours after the injury. Symptoms include severe chest pain, pale skin, breathing difficulty, rapid heartbeat, exhaustion, confusion, and, in some cases, coma. A **gas embolism** is caused by expanding bubbles of gases that block one or more small blood vessels,

E–F

especially in the muscles, tendons, and joints. This affects deep-sea divers who rise too quickly to the surface and is most dangerous in the central nervous system. Such embolisms are very painful. Treatment of gas embolisms involve slow decompression of gases, especially nitrogen, that are dissolved in the blood. **Pulmonary embolism** refers to a lung (pulmonary) artery blocked by foreign matter, such as fat, air, tumor tissue, or a blood clot. It may be caused by damage to blood vessel walls; total slowing of blood flow, especially when linked with childbirth; congestive heart failure; or surgery. Symptoms are like those of a heart attack or pneumonia. There may be breathing difficulty, sudden chest pain, shock, and bluish skin coloring.

embolotherapy /em'bəlō-/,   a method of blocking a blood vessel with a tube (catheter) that balloons at one end. It is used to treat bleeding ulcers within the body, and blood vessel defects. During surgery it is used to stop blood flow to a tumor.

embolus /em'bələs/,   *pl.* **emboli,**   a foreign object such as a large bubble of air or gas, a bit of tissue or tumor, or a piece of a blood clot that travels through the bloodstream until it becomes lodged in a vessel. See also **blood clot, thrombus.**

embryectomy /em'brē·ek'-/,   the removal of an embryo. It is done most often in pregnancy outside the uterus (ectopic pregnancy).

embryo /em'brē·ō/,   in humans, the stage of growth between the time the fertilized egg is implanted in the uterus, which occurs about 2 weeks after conception, until the end of the seventh or eighth week of pregnancy. The period involves early growth of the major organ systems, and of the main external features. Compare **fetus.**

embryologic development,   the stages in the growth and development of the embryo from the time of fertilization of the egg until about the eighth week of pregnancy. The stages are divided into two periods. The first is the formation of the embryo (**embryogenesis**). It occurs during the 10 days to 2 weeks after fertilization until the embryo is implanted in the wall of the uterus. The second period (**organogenesis**) involves the growth of organs and organ systems during life in the womb. This stage occurs from about the end of the second week to the eighth week of pregnancy. During this time the embryo grows and changes rapidly and is very likely to be damaged by infections, drugs, radiation, or other agents in the mother that can cause birth defects. Anything that alters the normal processes of organogenesis can stop the growth of a body part, resulting in one or more birth defects. See also **prenatal development.**

embryology /em'brē·ol'-/,   the study of the origin, growth, and function of an organism from the time it is fertilized to birth. **Descriptive embryology** is the study of the changes that occur in the fetus during pregnancy.

embryoma /em'brē·ō'mə/,   a tumor growing from embryonic cells or tissues.

embryonal carcinoma /em'brē·ənəl/,   a fast-spreading cancer that usually grows in gonads, especially the testicles. It is a firm, lumpy mass with many bleeding areas. Bodies that look like a 1- or 2-week-old embryo are sometimes seen in these tumors.

embryonic layer /em'brē·on'ik/,   one of the three layers of cells in the embryo: the endoderm, the mesoderm, and the ectoderm. From these layers, all of the structures and organs of the body grow. The **endoderm** is the first to appear. It is the innermost of the cell layers that grow from the early embryo. From the endoderm comes the lining of the upper system, stomach tract, liver, pancreas, urinary bladder and canal, thyroid, ear cavity, tonsils, and parathyroid glands. The endoderm thus lines most of the internal organs and spaces. The **ectoderm** follows in growth. It is the outer of the three main cell layers of an embryo.

embryonic rest,   a portion of embryonic tissue that stays in the adult. Such tissue may act as a sign for certain types of cancer.

embryopathy /em'brē·op'əthē/,   any defect in the embryo or fetus as a result of problem with growth. A kind of embryopathy is **rubella embryopathy.**

Emcyt,   a trademark for a drug used to treat cancer of the prostate (estramustine phosphate sodium).

emergency,   a serious situation that arises quickly and threatens the life or welfare of a person or a group of people, as a tornado or a health crisis.

emergency childbirth,   a birth that occurs accidentally in or out of the hospital, without standard procedures. It may also be called **precipitate delivery,** childbirth that occurs with such speed or in a place where the usual preparations cannot be made. Signs of childbirth about to begin include increased bloody show, strong contractions, desire to bear down or to have a bowel movement, bulging of the bag of waters, or the baby's head showing at the vaginal opening. See **childbirth.**

emergency department,   part of a health center set up to provide quick emergency care, specially for sudden acute illness or severe injury.

emergency doctrine,   a doctrine that assumes a person agrees to treatment when in immediate danger and not able to approve of the care. It assumes that they would agree if they could.

Emergency Medical Service (EMS),   a national network of services providing aid from the first response to the selected care. The staff is trained in emergency care. EMS is linked by a local and regional communications system. There is usually an emergency number.

emergency medicine, a branch of medicine dealing with the diagnosis and care of conditions coming from injury or sudden illness. The patient is stabilized. Care is then given by the person's doctor or a specialist.

emergency room (E.R., ER), a hospital area set up to receive and treat patients suffering from sudden injury or medical problems, as bleeding, poisoning, broken bones, heart attack, and breathing failure.

Emete-con, a trademark for a drug used to prevent nausea and vomiting after anesthesia (benzquinamide hydrochloride).

emetic /imet′ik/, referring to a substance that causes vomiting.

EMG syndrome, an inherited disorder with bulging eyes, enlarged tongue, and gigantism. It is often accompanied by larger organs, kidney problems, and larger cells in the adrenal gland. Also called **exophthalmos-macroglossia-gigantism syndrome.**

emissary veins /em′əser′ē/, the small vessels that connect the spaces in the membrane over the brain (dura) with the veins on the outside of the skull.

emmetropia /em′ətrō′pē·ə/, the state of normal (20/20) vision. Compare **amblyopia, hyperopia, myopia.** – **emmetropic,** adj.

emollient /imol′yənt/, a substance that softens tissue, specially the skin and mucous membranes.

emotion, the feeling part of awareness as compared with thinking. Physical changes, as illness, can come with changes in emotion, whether the feelings are conscious or not.

emotional need, a psychologic need centered on such basic feelings as love, fear, anger, sorrow, anxiety, frustration, and depression. Such needs occur in everyone and become greater during times of stress and physical and mental illness, and at various stages of life, as infancy, early childhood, and old age.

emotional response, a response to a certain feeling. It occurs with physical changes that may not be obvious. An example is crying as a response to death of a loved one.

emotional support, the sensitive, understanding approach that helps patients accept and deal with their illnesses, talk about their fears, take comfort from a caring person. It can help a patient to better care for him- or herself. It is vital to respect the patient's needs, wants, and independence. It helps to understand what the patient has gone through. See also **stages of dying.**

empathy /em′pəthē/, the ability to know and to some extent share the emotions of another and to understand the meaning of that person's behavior. –**empathize,** v.

emphysema /em′fəsē′mə/, a defect of the lung system. There are destructive changes of the pouches where air exchange occurs (alveolar walls). This causes the lungs to inflate too much, become too rigid, and handle less oxygen. Symptoms include shortness of breath, cough, blue-toned skin, troubled breathing while lying down, fast and shallow breathing, unequal chest expansion, rapid heart beat, and a fever. Anxiety, high levels of carbon dioxide, lack of sleep, confusion, weakness, appetite loss, congestive heart failure, fluid in the lungs, and lung failure are common in advanced cases. A respirator and oxygen equipment may be prescribed.

Empirin, a trademark for a combination drug that has two drugs to relieve pain and reduce fever (aspirin and phenacetin) and a drug that stimulates the nervous system (caffeine).

emprosthotonos /em′prosthot′ənəs/, a position of the body in which it is stiffly bent forward at the waist. It is the result of a long-term muscle spasm, most often seen with tetanus infection or strychnine poisoning.

empty sella syndrome, enlargement of the cavity inside the base of the skull. This cavity normally holds the pituitary gland. In this defect, the gland may be smaller than normal, or it may be absent. The cause is unknown.

empyema /em′pī·ē′mə/, pus in a body cavity, especially the space between the lung and the membrane that surrounds it (pleural space). It is caused by an infection, as pleurisy or tuberculosis.

emulsify, to mix a liquid into another liquid, making a suspension that has globules of fat. Bile is an emulsifier in the digestive tract. An **emulsion** is a mix of two liquids, made so that small droplets are formed, as oil and water.

E-Mycin, a trademark for an antibiotic (erythromycin).

enamel, a hard white substance that covers a tooth.

enanthema /en′anthē′mə/, a sore on the surface of a mucous membrane.

Enarax, a trademark for a drug that slows the rate of the secretion of stomach juices. It contains a nerve blocker (oxyphencyclimine hydrochloride) and a tranquilizer (hydroxyzine hydrochloride).

encapsulated, referring to arteries, muscles, nerves, and other body parts that are enclosed in fiber or membrane sheaths.

encephalitis /ensef′əlī′-/, pl. **encephalitides** /-tidēz/, an inflammation of the brain. The cause is usually a virus infection that comes from the bite of an infected mosquito. It may also be caused by lead or other poisoning, or bleeding. **California encephalitis** (named for California where it was first found) may occur anywhere in the United States. A viral infection carried by a mosquito, it affects mainly children in rural or suburban areas. Symptoms include a fever that may reach 104° F, headache, stomach problems, and vomiting. **St. Louis encephalitis** is carried from birds to humans by mosquito bites. It occurs most commonly in the central and southern portions of the United States. Symptoms include headache, fever, stiff neck, delirium, and convulsions. Resulting conditions may include sight and speech disorders, difficulty in walking, and personality changes. Recovery may be slow, and death may result. Compare **meningitis.**

encephalocele /ensef′·əlōsəl′/, bulging of the brain through an opening in the skull; hernia of the brain. This problem may be from a birth defect or injury.

encephalography /ensef′əlog′rəfē/, a way of making x-ray pictures of the brain spaces that contain fluid. The fluid (cerebrospinal) is taken out and replaced by a gas, as air, helium, or oxygen. This is done to outline the spaces. The method is used mainly for finding the site of cerebrospinal fluid blockage. Because the method is risky, it is used only when other methods do not provide a complete picture.

encephalomyelitis /-mī′əlī′-/. See **encephalitis.**

encephalomyocarditis /-mī′əkärdī′-/, an infection of the brain, spinal cord, and heart tissue caused by a group of viruses. Rodents are a major source of the infection. Symptoms are generally similar to those of poliomyelitis. Treatment is supportive.

encephalopathy /ensef′əlop′əthē/, any defect of the structure or function of brain tissues. It often refers to long-term defects in which there is a breakdown or death of tissue. **Acute necrotizing hemorrhagic encephalopathy** is a disorder that leads to brain tissue death. Typical signs are severe headache, fever, and vomiting. Convulsions may occur, and the patient may rapidly lose consciousness. Treatment consists of removing spinal fluid to ease pressure on the brain and giving large doses of steroids.

enchondroma /en′kondrō′mə/, a slow growing tumor of cartilage cells that begins near the ends of long bones. The growth of the tumor may cause the bone to bulge.

enchondromatosis /-tō′sis/, a disorder with too much cartilage in the flared ends of many bones. This causes thinning of the bone and the length to be affected.

encopresis /en′kōprē′-/, inability to control bowel movements. —**encopretic,** adj.

encounter group, a small group of people who meet to increase self-awareness, promote growth, and improve communication. Members focus on being aware of their feelings and on learning how to express those feelings openly, honestly, and clearly. See also **group therapy.**

encyst /ensist′/, to form a cyst or capsule. See also **cyst.** —**encysted,** adj.

endarterectomy /en′därtərek′-/, a method to remove the core (tunica intima) of an artery that has become thickened by fatty deposits (atherosclerosis).

endarteritis /en′därtərī′-/, a disease in which the inner layer of one or more arteries becomes inflamed. The arteries may become partly blocked or completely blocked.

end bud, a mass of cells that grow from the remains of the growing embryo. In humans it forms the tail end of the trunk. Also called **tail bud.**

endemic /endem′ik/, a disease or infection common to a geographic area or population. See also **epidemic, pandemic.**

endemic goiter. See **goiter.**

endocardial cushion defect /en′dōkär′dē·əl/, any heart defect that results from the failure of part of the fetal heart (endocardial cushions) to fuse and form the wall that divides the upper chambers (atrial septum). See also **congenital heart disease.**

endocardial fibroelastosis /fī′brōē′lastō′-/, a defect in which the wall of the lower left chamber (ventricle) of the heart grows too much. The tissue that lines the heart (endocardium) becomes thick and fibrous. This often makes the capacity of the heart chamber larger, but it may also make it smaller.

endocarditis /-kärdī′-/, a defect in which the lining of the heart (endocardium) and the heart valves become inflamed. **Bacterial endocarditis** in either an acute or subacute form is caused by various types of *Streptococcus* or *Staphylococcus.* Prompt treatment with antibiotics is essential to prevent destruction of the valves and heart failure. This disease affects equal numbers of men and women of all ages. It causes heart murmurs in about 30% of the cases, and tends to affect the valves on the left side of the heart. There is no successful treatment of nonbacterial thrombic endocarditis. Blood-thinning (anticoagulant) drugs may reduce the risk of arterial blood clots. If not treated, all types of endocarditis are quickly fatal. They are often treated with success using drugs or surgery.

endocardium /-kär′dē·əm/, pl. **endocardia,** the lining of the heart chambers. It contains small blood vessels and a few bundles of smooth muscle. Compare **epicardium, myocardium.**

endocervicitis /-sur′visī′-/, a defect in which the lining and glands of the uterine cervix become inflamed or swollen. See also **cervicitis.**

endocervix /-sur′viks/, the membrane lining the canal of the uterine cervix.

endocrine fracture /en′dəkrīn, -krēn/, any break in a bone that results from bone weakness because of a hormone (endocrine) disorder.

endocrine system, the network of ductless glands and other structures that secrete hormones into the bloodstream. Glands of the endocrine system include the thyroid and the parathyroid, the pituitary, the pancreas, the adrenal glands, and the gonads. The pineal gland is also thought of as a endocrine gland because it lacks ducts, although its precise function is not known. The thymus gland, once thought of as a endocrine gland, is now classed with the lymph system. Secretions from the endocrine glands affect a number of functions in the body, as metabolism and growth, secretions of other organs.

endocrinology /-krinol'-/, the study of the form and function of the endocrine system and the treatment of its problems.

endoderm /en'dədurm/. See **embryonic layer.**

endogenous /endoj'ənəs/, coming from inside the body, as a disease that is caused by failure of an organ. Compare **exogenous.** −**endogenic,** *adj.*

endolymph /en'dəlimf/, the fluid in the ducts of the inner ear. The endolymph carries sound waves to the ear drum. It helps maintain balance.

endometrial /-mē'trē·əl/, referring to the cavity or lining of the uterus.

endometrial cancer, a malignant tumor of the lining (endometrium) of the uterus. It most often occurs in the fifth or sixth decade of life. Vaginal bleeding that is not normal, especially after menopause, is the main symptom. There also may be lower belly and low back pain. Causes include a history of infertility, lack of ovulation, taking drugs with estrogen, and uterine growths. Women who have diabetes or high blood pressure or are very overweight are also at greater risk. Endometrial cancer may spread to the cervix, but rarely to the vagina. It often grows in the broad ligaments, fallopian tubes, and ovaries. The disease is often tested for with a surgical exam (D & C) of the uterus. A Pap test does not always show endometrial cancer. Treatment includes removal of the uterus (hysterectomy), removal of ovaries and fallopian tubes (salpingo-oophorectomy), and x-ray therapy. High doses of a hormone may be given for advanced cases.

endometrial hyperplasia, an overgrowth of the lining of the uterus (endometrium). The cause is a hormone problem with too much estrogen for too long and not enough progesterone.

endometrial polyp, a bulblike pouch on a stem that grows from the lining of the uterus (endometrium), and is usually harmless. Polyps are a common cause of vaginal bleeding in women during menopause.

endometriosis /-mē'trē·ō'-/, a growth of endometrial tissue outside the uterus. The most typical symptom of endometriosis is pain, especially severe menstrual cramps, pain during sex, and with bowel movements. Pain is not always present, however. Other symptoms include premenstrual vaginal bleeding, too much bleeding during menstruation, and infertility. When the disease is worse, the treatment includes hormones or surgery to reduce the size and number of deposits.

endometritis /-mitrī'-/, an inflammation of the lining (endometrium) of the uterus. It is often caused by infection. Symptoms include fever, pain in the lower belly, and discharge with a bad odor. It occurs most often after childbirth or abortion and in women using an intrauterine contraceptive device (IUD). Endometritis may cause sterility because scars form and block the fallopian tubes. See also **pelvic inflammatory disease.**

endometrium /-mē'trē·əm/, the mucous membrane lining of the uterus, consisting of three layers. The endometrium changes thickness during the menstrual cycle. Two of the layers are shed with each menstrual flow. The third layer provides the surface for the placenta to attach to during pregnancy.

endomorph /en'dəmôrf/. See **somatotype.**

endophthalmitis /endof'thalmī'-/, an inflammation of the inner eye. The eye becomes red, swollen, and painful, and sometimes fills with pus. The vision is often blurred. There may be vomiting, fever, and headache. The cause may be bacteria or a fungus, injury, allergy, drug or chemical poisoning, or blood vessel disease.

endophthalmitis phacoanaphylactica /fak'ō·an'əfilak'təkə/, a disorder in which there is an allergic response of the eye to the protein in the eye lens. It often occurs after injury to the lens or after a cataract operation. Symptoms include swelling and inflammation of the eye, severe pain, and blurred vision. The other eye may also be affected.

endorphin /endôr'fin/, a substance of the nervous system. Endorphins are composed of amino acids. They are made by the pituitary gland and act on the nervous system to reduce pain. They produce effects like that of morphine. Compare **enkephalin.**

endoscopy /endos'kəpē/, examination of the inside of organs and cavities of the body with a special device (endoscope) that has a light on its end.

endothelium /-thē'lē·əm/, the layer of cells that lines the heart, the blood and lymph vessels, and the fluid-filled cavities of the body. It is well supplied with blood and heals quickly.

endotracheal /-trā'kē·əl/, within or through the windpipe (trachea).

endotracheal intubation, inserting a large tube through the mouth or nose into the trachea (windpipe). An endotracheal tube may be used to keep an open airway or to prevent material from the stomach from getting into the lungs in the unconscious or paralyzed patient.

endoxin /endok'sin/, a hormone made in the human body that is similar to the drug digoxin. Endoxin regulates the excretion of salt.

Endrate, a trademark for a drug used to treat a serious condition resulting from too much calcium. It is also used for irregular heart beats and for lead poisoning (edetate disodium).

E−F

Enduron, a trademark for a drug that lowers blood pressure and increases urine output (methyclothiazide).

Enduronyl, a trademark for a drug that increases urine output (methyclothiazide) and a drug that lowers blood pressure (deserpidine). It is used to treat heart conditions.

enema, a method in which a fluid is flushed into the rectum for cleansing or treatment. The solution is warmed to 99.0° F (37.8° C) to 105° F (40.6° C) to avoid causing cramps. The patient should lie on the left side with knees drawn close to the chest. The tip of the catheter is then lubricated and gently inserted 3 to 4 inches (7.5 cm to 10 cm) into the rectum. The enema is given slowly to avoid sudden expansion that would cause spasm of the intestine. The tip of the catheter is taken out. The fluid is held in by the patient as long as possible before expelling the fluid.

energy, the capacity to do work or to perform vigorous activity. –**energetic,** *adj.*

enervation, 1. lack of energy; weakness. 2. removal of a complete nerve or of a section of nerve.

en face /äNfäs'/, "face-to-face"; a position in which the the mother's face and the infant's face are about 8 inches apart. Examples are when the mother holds the infant up in front of her face and when she nurses the child. Studies have shown that mothers seek eye-to-eye contact, and that they will instinctively move the baby to an en face position. Babies are best able to focus at a distance of 8 to 10 inches.

engine, any ground vehicle providing specified levels of pumping, water, and hose capacity but with less than the specified level of personnel.

engine company, any ground vehicle providing specified levels of pumping, water, hose capacity, and personnel.

engorgement, swelling or congestion of body tissues. An example is the swelling of breast tissue before the mother's milk comes in.

Enisyl, a trademark for an amino acid (lysine hydrochloride).

enkephalin /enkef'əlin/, a pain-relieving substance made in the body. It is found in the pituitary gland, brain, stomach, and bowels. Enkephalins are believed to slow nerve activity through the central nervous system, including nerve signals that indicate pain. This reduces the mental and physical sensation of pain. Compare **endorphin.**

enophthalmos /en'ofthal'məs/, a drawing back of the eyeball into the socket. It is caused by an injury or birth defect.

Enovid, a trademark for a birth control pill with the female hormones estrogen (mestranol) and progestin (norethynodrel).

enriched material, material in which the relative amount of one or more isotopes (naturally occurring) has been increased.

Ensure, a trademark for a nutritional supplement that does not contain any milk product. It does contain protein, carbohydrate, fat, vitamins, and minerals.

Entamoeba /en'təmē'bə/, a family (genus) of intestinal parasites. Several types are harmful to humans. See also **amebiasis.**

enteric coating /enter'ik/, a coating added to drugs taken by mouth that need to reach the intestines. The coating resists the effects of stomach juices, which can destroy certain drugs.

enteric infection, a disease of the intestine caused by any infection. Symptoms include diarrhea, stomach pain, nausea and vomiting, and loss of appetite. There may be a great loss of fluid from severe vomiting and diarrhea. Nothing should be taken by mouth until vomiting has ceased. At that time, a clear fluid diet may be given.

entericoid fever, a typhoidlike disease that causes fever and inflammation in the stomach and bowels. See also **typhoid fever.**

enteritis /en'tərī'-/, inflammation in the lining of the bowels, often the small intestine. Causes include bacteria, viruses, and some functional disorders. Compare **enterocolitis, gastroenteritis.**

Enterobacteriaceae /en'tərōbaktir'ē·ā'si·ē/, a family of bacteria that includes both harmless and harmful organisms. Salmonella is among the most important disease-causing types.

enterococcus /-kok'əs/, *pl.* **enterococci,** any bacteria of the *Streptococcus* family that lives in the intestinal tract.

enterocolitis /-kōlī-/, an inflammation of both the large and small intestines. See also **necrotizing enterocolitis.**

enterokinase /-kī'nās/, a substance in the intestines that helps the body absorb protein.

enterolithiasis /-lithī'əsis/, the presence of stones (enteroliths) in the intestine.

enterostomy /en'təros'təmē/, surgery to produce an artificial opening in the small intestine. A hole is made in the intestine and is connected to a hole in the skin above on the abdomen. The contents of the intestine empty through the outside opening (stoma). See also **ostomy.**

enterovirus, a virus that thrives mainly in the intestinal tract. Kinds of enteroviruses are **coxsackievirus, echovirus, poliovirus.**

Entozyme, a trademark for a combination drug containing bile salts and digestive enzymes (pancreatin and pepsin).

entrainment, a natural state in which a person will move with the rhythms of speech and movement from another person. Infants seem to move in time to the rhythms of adult speech. Entrainment is thought to be important in the developing relationship of a mother and infant.

entropion /entrō'pē·on/,   a turning inward of the edge of the eyelid toward the eye. **Cicatricial entropion** can occur in either the upper or lower eyelid as a result of scar tissue. **Spastic entropion** results from inflammation or another factor that affects tissue strength. Inflammation of the eyelid may be caused by an infection or by irritation from an inverted eyelash.

ENT specialist,   a doctor who specializes in treating the ear, nose, and throat. See also **otolaryngology.**

enucleation /ēnoo'klē·ā'shən/,   **1.** removal of an organ or tumor in one piece. **2.** removal of the eyeball. This is done in case of a cancer, severe infection, or injury, or to control pain in glaucoma.

Enuclene,   a trademark for a combination drug containing a detergent drug (tyloxapol) and a preservative (benzalkonium chloride). It is used in the treatment of eyes.

enuresis /en'yŏŏrē'-/,   inability to control the need to urinate, especially in bed at night.

environment,   all of the many factors, including physical and psychological, that affect the life of a person.

environmental health,   all of the aspects in and around a community that affect the health of the population.

environmental information,   the label of a hazardous material may provide information on both the storage and disposal of the product and the environmental or wildlife hazards that could occur. This information can be most useful when planning clean up and disposal after a fire or spill.

Enzactin,   a trademark for a drug applied to the skin to treat fungus (triacetin).

enzyme /en'zīm/,   a protein that speeds up or causes chemical reactions in living matter. Most enzymes are produced in tiny amounts and affect reactions that take place within the cells. Digestive enzymes are made in large amounts and act outside the cells in the digestive tube.

eosinophil /ē'əsin'əfil/,   a two-lobed white blood cell (leukocyte). Eosinophils make up 1% to 3% of the white blood cells of the body. They increase in number with allergy and some infections. Compare **basophil, neutrophil.**

eosinophilia /-fil'yə/,   an increase in the number of eosinophils in the blood. This occurs in allergies and many conditions with inflammation.

eosinophilic leukemia,   a cancer of white blood cells, mainly eosinophils. It resembles chronic myelocytic leukemia but is most often sudden and quick. See also **leukemia.**

EPA establishment number,   the location where a hazardous material product was manufactured. This number has little significance to emergency response personnel. When faced with an incident involving poisonous or toxic containers, obtain an uncontaminated container or label for reference whenever possible. When civilian or emergency services personnel are transported to a medical facility as a result of a suspected exposure, ensure proper identification and medical care by also forwarding an uncontaminated label or container.

EPA registration number,   required for all pesticide products marketed in the United States. It is one of three ways to positively identify a pesticide. The others are by the product name or chemical ingredient statement. The registration number will appear as a two- or three-section number. When relaying this number, be sure to include each dash. A U.S. Department of Agriculture number may appear on products registered before 1970.

ependymoblastoma /ipen'dimō'blastō'mə/,   a cancer made up of cells from the lining (ependyma) of the chambers of the brain.

ependymoma /ipen'dimō'mə/,   a tumor, usually benign, made up of cells from the lining (ependyma) of the chambers of the brain.

ephapse /ef'aps/,   a point of side-to-side contact between nerve fibers. Nerve signals may be passed through the walls of the nerves rather than through the space (synapse) between the ends of two nerves. This may be a factor in epileptic seizures. Compare **synapse.**

ephedrine /əfed'rin/,   a stimulant drug that opens the airway passages. It is used to treat asthma and bronchitis and also used as a nasal decongestant.

epicanthus /ep'ikan'thəs/,   a vertical fold of skin over the inner corner of the eye. It may be slight or marked. This is normal in Oriental people. Some infants with Down's syndrome also have the folds. Also called **epicanthal fold.**

epicardium /-kär'dē·əm/,   one of the three layers of tissue that form the wall of the heart. See also **myocardium.**

epicondylar fracture /-kon'dələr/,   any bone break that involves the knob on the end of a bone (epicondyle), as at the elbow.

epicondyle /-kon'dəl/,   a knucklelike projection at the end of a bone.

epicondylitis /-ī'tis/.   See **tennis elbow.**

epicranium /-krā'nē·əm/,   the complete scalp, including the skin, muscles, and tendon sheets.

epicranius /-krā'nē·əs/,   the muscle and tendon layer covering the top and sides of the skull from the back of the head to the eyebrows. It consists of broad, thin muscles connected by an extensive tendon sheet. Branches of the facial nerves can draw back the scalp, raise the eyebrows, and move the ears.

epidemic,   a disease that spreads rapidly through a part of the population. For example, an epidemic may affect everyone in a certain geographic area (as a military base or a town), or everyone of a certain age or sex (as the children or women of a region). Compare **endemic, pandemic.**

epidemiologist /-dem′ē·ol′-/, a physician or scientist who studies the spread, prevention, and control of disease in a community or a group of persons.

epidermis /-dur′mis/, the outer layers of the skin. It is made up of an outer, dead portion and a deeper, living portion. Epidermal cells gradually move outward to the skin surface, changing as they go, until they become flakes. Also called **cuticle.** –**epidermal, epidermoid,** *adj.*

epidermoid carcinoma, a cancer in which the cells tend to develop much like the cells of the outer layer of the skin (epidermis). They then form horny cells called prickle cells.

epididymis /-did′imis/, *pl.* **epididymides,** one of a pair of long, tightly coiled tubes that carry sperm from the testicles to the tip of the penis. An **appendix epididymidis** is a cyst sometimes found on the epididymis.

epididymitis /-did′imī′-/, inflammation of the tubes (epididymides) that carry sperm from the testicles to the tip of the penis. It may result from venereal disease, urinary tract infection, or removal of the prostate.

epididymoorchitis /-did′imō·ôrkī′-/, inflammation of the testicles and the tubes (epididymides) that carry sperm from the testicles to the tip of the penis.

epidural /-do͞or′əl/, outside the outer membrane surrounding the brain and spinal cord (dura mater).

epidural blood patch, a patch to repair a tear in the outer membrane (dura mater) around the spinal cord, as may be made by a needle during spinal anesthesia. To form a patch, a small amount of the patient's blood is injected into the area of the hole. This blood forms a clot, covering the hole.

Epifrin, a trademark for a stimulant drug (epinephrine hydrochloride).

epigastric node /-gas′trik/, a lymph node in one of the groups that serve the stomach, intestines, and pelvis. See also **lymphatic system, lymph node.**

epiglottis /-glot′is/, the cartilage-like structure that overhangs the windpipe like a lid. It prevents food from entering the windpipe by closing while swallowing.

epiglottitis /-glotī′-/, inflammation of the structure that closes the windpipe while swallowing (epiglottis). **Acute epiglottitis** is a severe form of the condition, affecting mostly children, usually between 2 and 7 years of age. Symptoms include fever, sore throat, harsh breathing sounds, croupy cough, and a red swollen epiglottis. Sudden blockage can occur and be fatal. Infection occurs from air particles or direct contact. The first signs may be followed by an inability to swallow, drooling, shortness of breath, or high-pitched breathing. Treatment includes antibiotics. The infection may spread, causing ear infections, pneumonia, and bronchitis.

epilepsy /ep′ilep′sē/, a group of nervous system disorders that feature repeated episodes of convulsive seizures, sensory disorders, abnormal behavior, and blackouts. All types of epilepsy have an uncontrolled electrical discharge from brain nerve cells. Most epilepsy is of unknown cause. It may be linked to head injury, brain infection or tumor, blood vessel disturbances, intoxication, or chemical imbalance. Seizures may occur several times a day to one every few years. They can occur during sleep or after stimulation, as a blinking light or sudden loud sound. Some people have odd visual effects (aura) before a seizure, but others have no warning symptoms. Most epileptic attacks are brief. They may affect the entire body or a small area. The muscles may contract violently or only twitch slightly. Drowsiness or confusion often follow seizures. A **focal seizure** (also called partial or Jacksonian) commonly begins as spasms in the face, hand, or foot and spreads to other muscles. Symptoms include chewing, lip-smacking, swallowing movements, and excess saliva. Seizures in the eye-turning area of the brain may begin with a forced turning of the head and eyes. A **petit mal seizure** begins with a sudden, short-term loss of consciousness. Muscles may contract in the neck, face, or arms, or muscles may lose their tone. The seizures most often occur many times a day and are most common in children and adolescents. When consciousness returns, the person may have no recall of the seizure. A **grand mal seizure** features uncontrolled muscle spasms involving the entire body, and loss of consciousness. During the fit the person may clench the teeth, bite the tongue, and lose bladder control. After the seizure passes, the person may fall into a deep sleep for an hour or more. Usually, there is no recall of the seizure on waking up. A sensory warning, or aura, usually comes before each grand mal seizure. These seizures may occur once, over a period of time, or many in a short period of time. **Motor seizure** refers to a temporary disturbance in brain function. It is caused by abnormal nerve signals that begin in a local motor nerve area of the brain. The effects depend on where the abnormal electric activity is, as chewing movements caused by excess signals in the motor area of the brain controlling the jaws. The disturbance may end in a group of reflex movements or lead to a general convulsion. A **psychomotor seizure** is a brief loss of consciousness. During the seizure the person may appear drowsy, intoxicated, or violent. Symptoms may include chest pain, shortness of breath, rapid heart beat, and abnormal sensations of smell and taste. The person may see things that are not there (hallucinate), have a sense of unreality and distorted sense of time. Most people who have epilepsy can control it with drugs and should expect to live a normal life. The person should wear a medical identification tag. The kind of epilepsy determines the drug to prevent the seizures. If the cause is a tumor or metabolic imbalance, this is corrected. During an attack the patient should be protected from injury. See also **status elepticus.**

International classification of epileptic seizures

Generalized seizures
- Tonic-clonic (grand mal)
- Absence (petit mal)
- Infantile spasms
- Other (myoclonic seizures, akinetic seizures, undetermined)

Partial seizures
- Simple partial seizures (e.g., disturbances in movement only)
- Complex partial seizures (psychomotor, other)
- Secondarily generalized seizures

From The Office of Scientific and Health reports, National Institute of Neurological and Communicative Disorders and Stroke: Epilepsy: hope through research, NIH Publication No. 81-156, Bethesda, MD, July 1981, National Institutes of Health.

epinephrine /-nef′rin/, a drug that stimulates the adrenal glands and narrows the blood vessels. It is used to treat stuffy nose. It is also used to help extreme allergic reactions and as a local anesthetic.

epiphyseal fracture /-fiz′ē·əl/, a break in the area at the end of a long bone where bone growth occurs. This results in separation of the head of the bone.

epiphysis /ipif′isis/, *pl.* **epiphyses,** the rounded head of a long bone, as in the arm or leg. During childhood it is separated from the shaft of the bone by the growth plate where bone growth occurs. When the bone stops growing, the growth plate becomes solid. Compare **diaphysis.** – **epiphyseal,** *adj.*

episcleritis /-sklerī′-/, inflammation of the outer layers of the white of the eye (sclera).

episiotomy /epē′zē·ot′əmē/, an operation to enlarge the opening of the vagina with a cut. This is done during childbirth to aid in delivery or to prevent stretching of the mother's muscles and connective tissues. Such stretching is thought to cause the bladder and uterus to relax and so decrease their ability to function. The cut is then closed after the baby is delivered.

episode, an incident that stands out from everyday life, as an episode of illness.

episodic care, a type of medical service in which care is given to a person for a certain problem. The patient does not remain for continued care. Emergency rooms provide episodic care.

epispadias /-spā′dē·as/, a birth defect in boys in which the urine canal (urethra) opens on the underside of the penis. Surgical correction is usually performed in the first few years of life.

epistaxis /-stak′sis/. See **nosebleed.**

epithalamus /-thal′əmas/, a part of the brain that passes on nerve signals for the senses and movement.

epithelioma /-thē′lē·ō′mə/, a tumor derived from the epithelium.

epithelium /-thē′lē·əm/, the covering of the organs of the body, including the lining of vessels. –**epithelial,** *adj.*

epoophorectomy /ep′ō·of′ərek′-/, surgical removal of the epoophoron.

epoophoron /ep′ō·of′əron/, a structure that lies between the ovary and the uterine tube. It is made up of a few short tubules pointing toward the ovary and, on the other end, opening into a duct.

Eprolin, a trademark for vitamin E (alpha tocopherol).

Epsom salt. See **magnesium sulfate.**

Epstein-Barr virus (EBV), the herpes virus that causes mononucleosis (''kissing disease'').

Epstein's pearls, small, white, pearl-like cysts that occur on both sides of the hard palate in newborn infants. They are normal and usually go away within a few weeks.

epulis /epyōō′lis/, any tumor or growth on the gum.

Equagesic, a trademark for a combination drug containing aspirin and a sedative (meprobamate). It is used to relieve pain accompanied by anxiety or tension.

Equanil, a trademark for a sedative drug used to treat anxiety (meprobamate).

equilibrium, 1. a state of balance caused by the equal action of opposing forces, as calcium and phosphorus in the body. **2.** a state of mental or emotional balance.

equine encephalitis /ē′kwīn, ek′wīn/. See **encephalitis.**

Erb's palsy, a kind of paralysis caused by injury to the nerves branching off the spinal cord at the base of the neck (brachial plexus). It occurs most often in infants during delivery. Symptoms include numbness in the arm, and paralysis and wasting of the muscles. The arm on the affected side hangs loosely with the elbow pointed out and the palm toward the back. Physical therapy and splinting may be needed to improve function.

erectile /irek′til/, capable of being raised to an erect position, such as the spongy tissue of the penis or clitoris. This tissue becomes erect when filled with blood. The term may also be used when referring to the ''goose bumps'' on the skin (horripilation) in response to fear, anger, or cold.

erection, the condition of hardness, swelling, and raising of the penis. This may also describe the clitoris. Erection is usually caused by sexual arousal, but it also occurs during sleep or as a result of physical stimulation. Erection begins when extra blood enters the organ and blood pressure increases. See also **ejaculation, nocturnal emission, priapism.**

ergoloid mesylates, a stimulant drug used to treat lessened mental ability of unknown cause, such as in senility (senile dementia). Psychosis or known allergy to this drug prohibits its use. Side effects include irritation to the area under the tongue, passing nausea, and stomach disorder.

Ergomar, a trademark for a drug used to treat migraine headaches (ergotamine tartrate).

ergosterol /ərgos′tərôl/, a steroid of the vitamin D group. It is found in yeast, mushrooms, ergot, and other fungi. When treated with ultraviolet light, it is changed into vitamin D_2. See also **vitamin D.**

ergot /ur′gət/, the food storage body of the fungus *Claviceps purpurea*. This fungus commonly infects rye and other cereal grasses. It contains ergot alkaloids.

ergot alkaloid, one of a large group of alkaloids found in the common fungus *Claviceps purpurea*. This fungus grows on rye and other grains throughout the mild areas of the world.

ergotamine tartrate /ərgot′əmēn/, a drug that narrows blood vessels and hastens labor. It is used to treat migraine headaches and after birth when the uterus lacks strength to contract on its own. Pregnancy, blood vessel disease, infection, or known allergy to this drug forbids its use. Side effects include vomiting, diarrhea, thirst, tingling of fingers and toes, and increased blood pressure.

ergotherapy /ur′gō-/, the use of exercise to treat disease. The therapy also includes any treatment that increases the blood supply to a diseased or injured part, such as massage or hot baths.

Ergotrate Maleate, a trademark for a drug used to contract the uterus to treat or prevent bleeding after birth or after an abortion (ergonovine maleate).

Eros, a term, used by Freud, for the instinct for survival. It includes self-preservation and survival of the species through reproduction.

erosion, the wearing away or slow and steady destroying of a tissue. Erosion may be caused by infection, injury, or other disease. It usually occurs with an ulcer. See also **necrosis.**

eroticism, 1. sexual impulse or desire. 2. the arousal or attempt to arouse sexual desire.

erucic acid /ərōō′sik/, a fatty acid that has been linked with heart disease. It is found in rapeseed oil and is used in some countries as a vegetable oil.

eructation, the act of bringing up air from the stomach with a typical sound. Also called **belching.**

eruption, the rapid growth of a skin rash, especially one caused by a virus or by a drug reaction.

erysipelas /er′isip′ələs/, a skin infection with redness, swelling, blisters, fever, pain, and swollen lymph nodes. It is caused by a species of streptococci. Treatment includes antibiotics, pain relievers, and dressings on the skin.

erysipeloid /-loid/, an infection of the hands marked by blue-red bumps or patches and, sometimes, redness. It is caught by handling meat or fish infected with *Erysipelothrix rhusiopathiae*. Also called **fish-handler's disease.**

erythema /er′ithē′mə/, inflammation of the skin or mucous membranes. It is the result of widening and clogging of capillaries near the skin surface. Examples of erythema are nervous blushes and mild sunburn.

erythema infectiosum, an acute infection, mainly of children. Symptoms include fever and a rash beginning on the cheeks and appearing later on the arms, thighs, buttocks, and trunk. As the rash spreads, earlier areas fade. Sunlight worsens the rash. It usually lasts about 10 days. Also called **fifth disease.**

erythema multiforme, an allergic condition with a rash on the skin and mucous membranes. A variety of sizes and shapes appear on the patient (multiforme) and include nodules, pimples, blisters, and bull's-eye-shaped areas.

erythema nodosum, an allergy marked by blood vessel inflammation. It causes reddened, tender bumps on both shins and sometimes on other parts of the body. Other symptoms are mild fever and pains in muscles and joints. This condition occurs with streptococcal infections, tuberculosis, sarcoidosis, drug allergy, ulcerative colitis, and pregnancy.

erythema neonatorum, a common skin condition of newborns. A pink raised rash occurs that is often covered by blisters or pustules. The rash appears within 24 to 48 hours after birth, covers the chest, stomach, back, and diaper area, and disappears after several days. Also called **toxic erythema of the newborn,** *(informal)* **flea bites.**

erythrasma /er′ithraz′mə/, a bacteria-caused skin infection of the armpit or groin regions. There are irregular, reddish-brown raised patches. It is more common in diabetics and responds quickly to the oral antibiotic erythromycin.

erythremia /-rē′mē·ə/, an abnormal increase in the number of red blood cells.

erythrityl tetranitrate, a drug that dilates the blood vessels of the heart. It is used to treat chest pain resulting from heart disease. It is used with caution when glaucoma is present. Known allergy to this drug forbids its use. Side effects include low blood pressure, allergic reactions, headache, and flushing.

erythroblastosis fetalis /irith′rəblastō′mə fētā′lis/, a type of anemia that occurs in newborns who have Rh positive blood, but whose mothers are Rh negative. The maternal-fetal blood systems mix through the placenta. The mother's blood reacts to the fetal blood as a foreign substance (antigen). Her blood forms antibodies, which kill the red blood cells (erythrocytes) in the fetus's body. This causes high levels of a bile substance (bilirubin) in the fetus, the amniotic fluid, and the placenta. See also **Rh factor.**

erythrocyte /irith′rəsīt′/, a red blood cell. It is a concave disk, microscopic in size, and contains hemoglobin. As the main element of the circulating blood, its main function is to transport oxygen, which is carried by the hemoglobin. The number of cells per cu mm of blood is usually between 4.5 and 5.5 million in men and between 4.2 and 4.8 million in women. An erythrocyte usually lives for 110 to 120 days. It is then removed from the bloodstream and broken down in the body's cells. New erythrocytes are produced in the marrow of long bones at a steady rate so that a constant level is usually maintained. With acute blood loss, anemia, or chronic lack of oxygen, erythrocyte production may increase greatly. Kinds of erythrocyte include **burr cell, discocyte, macrocyte, meniscocyte, spherocyte.** Also called **red blood cell, red cell, red corpuscle.**

erythrocyte sedimentation rate (ESR), a blood test that measures the rate at which red blood cells (erythrocytes) settle out in a tube. Blood is collected in a substance that prevents clotting. The speed with which the red cells fall to the bottom of the tube indicates an amount of inflammation in a disease. See also **inflammation.**

erythrocytosis /-ō′sis/, an abnormal rise in the number of circulating red cells. See also **polycythemia.**

erythroleukemia /-lookē′mē-ə/, a malignant blood disorder marked by a excess production of red blood cells in bone marrow. Immature red blood cells in the bone marrow have odd, lobed nuclei. There are also abnormal immature red blood cells (erythrocytes) in circulating blood. Also called **diGuglielmo's disease.**

erythromycin /-mī′sin/, an antibiotic used to treat many bacterial infections, particularly infections that cannot be treated by penicillins. Liver disease or known allergy to this drug prohibits its use. Side effects include liver disease and allergic reactions.

erythrophobia, 1. an anxiety disorder with an irrational fear of blushing or of displaying embarrassment. **2.** an unnatural fear of the color red.

erythroplasia of Queyrat /-plā′shə/, a precancerous sore on or around the tip of the penis. It is a reddish patch on the skin. It is usually surgically removed.

erythropoiesis /-pō·ē′sis/, the process of red blood cell (erythrocyte) production. The bone marrow produces cells with nuclei. These cells mature into erythrocytes without nuclei that contain hemoglobin. See also **erthrocyte, hemoglobin.**

erythropoietin (EPO) /erith′rōpō·ē′tin/, a hormone produced mainly in the kidneys. It is released into the bloodstream in response to low oxygen levels. The hormone controls the production of red blood cells (erythrocytes) and is thus able to raise the oxygen-carrying capacity of the blood. See also **erythropoiesis.**

escape beat, an automatic beat of the heart that occurs when there is a pause in the dominant heart beat cycle. Escape beats act as safety mechanisms. Anything that causes a pause in the heart cycle may allow an escape to occur.

eschar /es′kär/, a scab or dry crust resulting from a burn, infection, or skin disease.

Escherichia coli /esh′ irī′kē·ə kō′lī/, a species of bacteria of the family Enterobacteriaceae. *E. coli* normally lives in the intestines and is common in water, milk, and soil. It causes urinary tract infection and serious infection in wounds.

Esidrix, a trademark for a diuretic drug used to treat high blood pressure (hydrochlorothiazide).

Eskalith, a trademark for an antidepressant used to treat bipolar disorders (lithium carbonate).

Esmarch's bandage /es′märks/, a broad, flat, elastic bandage wrapped around an elevated arm or leg to force blood out of the limb. It is used before some operations to create a blood-free area.

esophageal cancer /ēsof′əjē′əl, es′ofā′jē·əl/, a cancer of the esophagus. It occurs three times more often in men than in women, and more often in Asia and Africa than in North America. Esophageal cancer does not often cause any symptoms in the early stages. In later stages it causes painful swallowing, appetite and weight loss, vomiting, swollen lymph nodes in the neck, and often a nagging cough. Risk factors include heavy use of alcohol, smoking, hiatus hernia, and inability to relax the muscle between the esophagus and the stomach (achalasia). Treatment includes partial or total removal and radiation. See also **esophagectomy.**

esophageal dysfunction, any disease or abnormality that interferes with normal functioning of the esophagus, such as difficult swallowing or esophagitis. The condition is one of the main symptoms of scleroderma.

esophageal varices, a network of twisted veins at the lower end of the esophagus. It is enlarged and swollen as the result of high blood pressure within the portal vein in the abdomen. These vessels often form open sores and bleed. This is often a complication of cirrhosis of the liver.

esophagectomy /ēsof′əjek′-/, an operation in which all or part of the esophagus is removed. This may be required to treat severe, recurrent, bleeding esophageal varices.

E–F

esophagitis /-jī′tis/, inflammation of the lining of the esophagus. Causes include backflow of gastric juice from the stomach, infection, and irritation from a tube inserted through the nose to the stomach. See also **reflux.**

esophagoscopy /-gos′kəpē/, examination of the esophagus with an endoscope.

esophagus /ēsof′əgəs/, the muscular canal, 9½ inches long (about 24 cm), extending from below the tongue to the stomach. It is the narrowest part of the digestive tube. It is narrowest where it begins and at the point where it passes through the diaphragm. The esophagus is made up of a fibrous coat and a muscular coat and is lined with mucous membrane. Also called **gullet.** –**esophageal,** *adj.*

esophoria /es′əfôr′ē·ə/, deviation of one eye toward the other eye when the eyes are not focused on an object. Compare **strabismus.**

esotropia /-trō′pē·ə/. See **strabismus.**

essential amino acid. See **amino acid.**

essential fatty acid. See **fatty acid.**

essential hypertension. See **hypertension.**

Estar, a trademark for a coal tar substance used to treat eczema and psoriasis.

ester /es′tər/, a class of chemical compounds formed by an alcohol bonding to one or more organic acids. Fats are esters, formed by the bonding of fatty acids with the alcohol glycerol.

esterified estrogen /ester′ifīd/, a form of natural estrogen used to treat menstrual irregularities and symptoms of menopause. It is also used as a contraceptive. Pregnancy, known or suspected breast cancer, inflammation of a vein associated with clotting, vaginal bleeding of unknown origin, or known allergy to this drug prohibits its use. Side effects include gallbladder disease, blood clots, and a possible increase in risk of cancer.

Estinyl, a trademark for an estrogen used to treat postmenopausal breast cancer, menstrual cycle irregularities, cancer of the prostate, and decreased function of sexual organs, for contraception, and to relieve menopausal symptoms (ethinyl estradiol).

Estrace, a trademark for an estrogen (estradiol).

estradiol /es′trədī′ôl/. See **estrogen.**

Estradurin, a trademark for an estrogen used to treat cancer (polyestradiol phosphate).

estramustine phosphate sodium, a drug used to treat cancer of the prostate. Clotting disorders or known allergy to this drug prohibits its use. Side effects include stroke, heart attack, inflammation of a vein linked with clotting, clots in the lungs, and heart failure.

Estratab, a trademark for an estrogen (esterified estrogens).

Estraval, a trademark for an estrogen (estradiol valerate).

estriol /es′trē·ôl/. See **estrogen.**

estrogen /es′trojən/, one of a group of hormonal steroid compounds that aid the development of female secondary sex traits (such as breast development). Human estrogen is produced in the ovaries, adrenal glands, testicles, and both the fetus and placenta. Estrogen prepares the wall of the uterus for fertilization, implantation, and nutrition of the early embryo after each menstrual period. See also **esterified estrogen, estrone, estropipate.** –**estrogenic,** *adj.*

estrone /es′trōn/, a relatively strong estrogen. It is used to treat menstrual cycle irregularities, cancer of the prostate, and blood vessel symptoms in menopause, and to prevent pregnancy. Vein inflammation linked with clotting, abnormal genital bleeding, known or suspected pregnancy, or known allergy to this drug prohibits its use. Side effects include vein inflammation, clot formation, and excess levels of calcium.

estropipate, an estrogen used to treat blood vessel symptoms of menopause, vaginitis linked with menopause, atrophy of the female genitalia, decreased function of the female sex organs, and ovarian failure. Known or suspected cancer of the breast or estrogen-dependent cancer, pregnancy, inflammation of a vein linked with clotting, clotting disorders, undiagnosed abnormal genital bleeding, or complications from previous estrogen use prohibits its use. Side effects include a possible increased risk of cancer, gallbladder disease, and clotting disorders.

ethambutol hydrochloride, an antibiotic used to treat tuberculosis. Eye nerve inflammation or known allergy to this drug prohibits its use. It is not recommended for children. Side effects include vision loss and allergic reactions.

ethaverine hydrochloride, a drug that relaxes smooth muscles to relieve spasm of the intestinal or urinary tract, spasms of the arteries, and decreased blood flow to the brain. Liver disease, heartbeat irregularities, or known allergy to this drug prohibits its use. It is used with caution in patients who have glaucoma. Side effects include low blood pressure, abdominal distress, irregular heartbeats, and headache.

ethchlorvynol, a drug with calming and sleep-inducing effects. It is used to treat insomnia.

ether /ēthər/, a liquid used as a general anesthetic. It has an irritating, strong odor and is highly flammable and explosive, and often causes nausea and vomiting after surgery.

ethinamate, a drug that produces sedation. It is used to treat insomnia. Known allergy to this drug prohibits its use. It is not recommended for pregnant women, for people under 15 years of age, or for persons with a history of drug abuse. Side effects include small hemorrhages into the skin, physical and psychologic dependence, and skin rash.

ethinyl estradiol, an estrogen used to treat postmenopausal breast cancer, menstrual cycle irregularities, cancer of the prostate, and decreased function of sexual organs, for contraception, and to relieve blood vessel symptoms of menopause. Vein inflammation with clotting, abnormal genital bleeding, known or suspected pregnancy, or known allergy to this drug prohibits its use. Side effects include vein inflammation, clot formation, and excess levels of calcium.

ethionamide, an antibacterial drug used to treat tuberculosis. Liver damage or known allergy to this drug prohibits its use. This drug should not be used in pregnancy. Side effects include skin rash, jaundice, mental depression, and intestinal problems.

ethmoid bone /eth′moid/, the very light and spongy bone at the base of the skull that forms most of the walls of the upper part of the nasal cavity.

ethoheptazine citrate, a nonnarcotic drug used to relieve mild to moderate pain. Known allergy to this drug prohibits its use. Side effects include stomach and intestine distress and dizziness.

ethopropazine hydrochloride, a drug used to treat parkinsonism and other nervous system disorders. Narrow-angle glaucoma, asthma, blockage of the genitourinary or gastrointestinal tract, severe ulcerative colitis, or known allergy to this drug or to phenothiazines prohibits its use. Side effects include blurred vision, nervous system effects, rapid heart beats, dry mouth, less sweat, and allergic reactions.

ethosuximide, a drug that controls convulsions. It is used to treat petit mal epilepsy. Known allergy to this drug prohibits its use. Side effects include blood disorders, disorders of the stomach and intestines, and systemic lupus erythematosus.

ethotoin, a drug that controls convulsions. It is used for grand mal and psychomotor seizures. Liver disease, blood disorders, or known allergy to this drug or to any hydantoin prohibits its use. It is not recommended for use during pregnancy or nursing. Side effects include blood disorders, nausea, fatigue, skin rash, and chest pain.

Ethril, a trademark for an antibacterial used to treat many bacterial infections, particularly infections that cannot be treated by penicillins (erythromycin stearate).

ethyl alcohol. See **alcohol.**

ethylene dibromide (EDB), a liquid used as an insecticide and gasoline additive. Because it has been found to be a cause of cancer in animals, the Environmental Protection Agency has limited the use of EDB on grains and fruits intended for human use.

ethylestrenol, a steroid used to help rebuild body tissue in patients with severe diseases and injuries.

ethylnorepinephrine hydrochloride, a drug that widens the airway passages. It is used to treat bronchial asthma. Known allergy to this drug or to similar drugs prohibits its use. Side effects include increased or decreased blood pressure, palpitations, and a rise in heart rate.

ethyl oxide, a colorless liquid solvent similar to diethyl ether. It is widely used in making drugs.

ethynodiol diacetate, an oral contraceptive drug (progestin).

ethynodiol diacetate and ethinyl estradiol, an oral contraceptive drug. Inflammation of a vein linked with clotting, heart disease, breast or reproductive organ cancer, or known allergy to either ingredient prohibits its use. Side effects include tumors of the uterus, gallbladder disease, clot formation, and liver disorders.

ethynodiol diacetate and mestranol, an oral contraceptive drug. Vein inflammation linked with clotting, heart disease, breast or reproductive organ cancer, or known allergy to either ingredient prohibits its use. Side effects include tumors of the uterus, gallbladder disease, clot formation, and liver disorders.

etidronate disodium, a drug that regulates the metabolism of calcium. It is used to treat Paget's disease of bone and hardening of muscle into bone, and after total hip replacement. Side effects include bone pain at sites of Paget's disease, intestinal disturbances, and elevated levels of phosphate in the blood.

etiology /ē′tē·ol′-/, the study of all factors that may be involved in the development of a disease. This includes the condition of the patient, the cause, and the way in which the patient's body is affected.

Etrafon, a trademark for a combination drug containing a tranquilizer (perphenazine) and an antidepressant (amitriptyline hydrochloride).

eucholia /yookō′lyə/, the normal state of the bile. This includes the amount produced and the condition of the contents.

euchromatin /yookrō′mətin/, that part of chromosome material that is active in gene expression during cell division. See also **chromatin.** –**euchromatic,** *adj.*

eugenics /yoogen′-/, the study of methods for controlling the traits of future human populations through selective breeding.

eukaryocyte /yooker′ē·əsīt′/, a cell with a true nucleus. These cells are found in all higher organisms and in some microorganisms.

eukaryon /yooker′ē·on/, **1.** a nucleus in a cell that is very complex, organized, and surrounded by a nuclear membrane. Eukaryons usually occur only in higher organisms.

2. an organism containing a very complex, organized nucleus surrounded by a nuclear membrane. This is typical of all organisms except bacteria, viruses, and blue-green algae.

eunuch /yōō′nək/, a male whose testicles have been destroyed or removed.

eunuchoidism /yōō′nəkoidizm/, deficiency of male hormone. The deficiency leads to sterility, abnormal tallness, small testicles, poor development of secondary sexual traits, lack of sexual desire, and impotence.

euphoretic /yōō′fəret′ik/, **1.** a substance or event tending to produce a condition of euphoria. **2.** a substance tending to produce euphoria, such as LSD, mescaline, marijuana, and other hallucinogenic drugs.

euphoria /yōōfôr′ē·ə/, **1.** a feeling of well-being or elation. **2.** a greater than normal sense of physical and emotional well-being. It is not based on reality, is out of proportion to its cause, and is inappropriate to the situation. This is commonly seen in some forms of mental disorders, and in poisonous and drug-induced states.

euploid /yōō′ploid/, **1.** referring to a person, organism, or cell with a chromosome number that is an exact multiple of the normal (haploid) number of the species. For example, diploid refers to two sets of chromosomes, triploid to having three, tetraploid to four, and polyploid to over two sets. See also **homologous chromosomes.**

Eurax, a trademark for a drug used to treat scabies (crotamiton).

eustachian tube /yōōstā′shən, -stā′kē·ən/, a tube lined with mucous membrane that joins the nose-throat cavity (nasopharynx) and the inner ear (tympanic cavity). This tube allows air pressure in the inner ear to be equalized with the outside air pressure. Also called **auditory tube.**

euthanasia /yōō′thənā′zhə/, deliberately bringing about the death of a person who is suffering from an incurable disease. Euthanasia can be performed actively, such as by giving a lethal drug, or by allowing the person to die by not giving treatment. Euthanasia is both a legal and ethical issue that has received much attention in recent years. Legally, euthanasia is murder and therefore against the law. Also called **mercy killing.**

Euthroid, a trademark for a thyroid hormone used to treat underactive thyroid (liotrix).

Eutonyl, a trademark for an antidepressant drug used to treat high blood pressure (pargyline hydrochloride).

Eutron, a trademark for a combination drug containing a diuretic (methyclothiazide) and an antidepressant (pargyline hydrochloride). It is used to release high blood pressure.

evacuate, to discharge or remove a substance from a cavity, space, organ, or tract of the body. **–evacuation,** *n.*

evaporation, the change of a substance from a solid or liquid state to a gas. See also **boiling point.** **–evaporate,** *v.*

event-related potential (ERP), a type of brain wave that is a response to a specific stimulus. See also **evoked potential.**

evisceration /ivis′ərā′shən/, **1.** the removal of the organs (viscera) from the abdominal cavity; disembowelment. **2.** the removal of the contents from an organ or an organ from its cavity. **3.** bulging of an internal organ through a wound or surgical cut, especially in the abdominal wall. **–eviscerate,** *v.*

evocator, a specific chemical or hormone that is produced by embryonic tissue. The substance stimulates the embryo to grow and change.

evoked potential (EP), a tracing of a brain wave. It is measured by electrodes on the surface of the head at various places and recorded by an electroencephalograph (EEG).

evolution, **1.** a slow, steady, orderly, continuous process of change from one condition to another. In humans, it includes all aspects of life, including physical, mental, social, cultural, and intellectual development. Evolution involves a steady movement from a simple to a more complex state. **2.** the theory of the origin and continuation of all plant and animal species, including humans. It includes their development from lower to more complex forms. This occurs by natural selection through genetic changes or inbreeding.

exacerbation /igzas′ərbā′shən/, an increase in the seriousness of a disease or disorder. It is marked by greater intensity in the symptoms.

exanthema /ig′zanthē′mə/, a skin rash that often has the specific features of an infectious disease. Chickenpox, measles, roseola infantum, or rubella usually have particular types of exanthema.

exchange transfusion in the newborn. See **erythroblastosis fetalis.**

excise /iksīz′/, to remove completely, such as surgically taking out (excising) the tonsils.

excitability, the property of a cell that allows it to react to irritation or stimulation. An example is the reaction of a nerve to stimulation.

exciting eye, the eye that is mainly affected by an injury or infection, even though both eyes are disordered. Also called **inciting eye.**

exclusive (sole) use of vehicle, transport vehicle assigned for the sole use by the shipper—loaded and unloaded by the consignee or by the consignor at its origin and destination.

excoriation /ekskôr′ē·ā′shən/,   an injury to the surface of the skin or other part of the body caused by scratching or scraping. —**excoriate,** *v.*

excreta /ekskrē′tə/,   any waste matter discharged from the body; feces or urine.

excrete /ekskrēt′/,   to remove a waste substance from the body, often through normal secretion, such as a drug excreted in urine. —**excretion,** *n.*

excretion /ekskrē′shən/,   the process of getting rid of substances by body organs or tissues. Excretion usually begins at the level of the cell where water, carbon dioxide, and other waste products of cells are emptied into the capillaries. The skin, for example, excretes dead skin cells by shedding them daily.

excretory /eks′kretôr′ē/,   relating to the process of excretion.

excretory duct,   a duct that conducts substances.

exercise,   any action or skill that exerts the muscles and is performed repeatedly in order to condition the body, improve health, or maintain fitness. Exercise can also be a type of therapy for correcting a deformity or restoring the body's functions to a state of health. **Active assisted exercise** refers to moving the body or part of the body mostly through one's own efforts. A therapist or some device, as an exercise machine, assists. **Active exercise** is repeated movement of a part of the body by contracting and relaxing the muscles. During **active resistance exercise,** the body is moved against a checking force. **Corrective exercise** is a program of physical therapy. Its purpose is to restore normal function to diseased, defective, or injured parts of the body. **Passive exercise** is repeated movement of a part of the body as a result of force or willful effort of muscles directed by a physical therapist. **Progressive resistance exercise** is a way to increase the strength of a weak or injured muscle by slowly increasing the force against which the muscle works. An example is the use of heavier and heavier weights over a period of time. **Range of motion exercise** involves movements in natural directions of the arms and legs. Such exercises are used to treat bone and joint defects, to diagnose injuries, and to improve physical al health. See also **aerobic exercise, anaerobic exercise, isometric exercise, isotonic exercise.**

exercise electrocardiogram (exercise ECG).   See **stress test.**

exfoliation,   peeling and flaking off of tissue cells. This is a normal process of the skin that occurs constantly. Exfoliation may be often seen in certain skin diseases or after a severe sunburn. See also **desquamation.**

exfoliative dermatitis,   any skin inflammation in which there is too much peeling or shedding of skin. Causes include drug reactions, scarlet fever, leukemia, and lymphoma.

exhale,   to breathe out or to let out with the breath.   – **exhalation,** *n.*

exhibitionism,   **1.** the flaunting of oneself or one's abilities in order to attract attention. **2.** a disorder occurring in men in which the act of exposing the genitals to unsuspecting females in socially unacceptable situations is the preferred means of achieving sexual satisfaction.

Exna,   a trademark for a diuretic drug used to treat high blood pressure (benzthiazide).

exocrine /ek′səkrin/,   referring to the process of releasing outwardly through a duct to the surface of an organ or tissue or into a vessel. Compare **endocrine system.** See also **eccrine.**

exocrine gland,   any of a group of glands that open on the surface of the skin, organ, or into a vessel through ducts. These glands secrete specialized substances. Examples are the sweat glands and the oil (sebaceous) glands of the skin, and the salivary glands in the mouth. Exocrine glands are also found in the kidney, digestive tract, and mammary glands. See also **apocrine gland.**

exogenous /igzoj′ənəs/,   beginning outside the body or an organ of the body or produced from external causes. For example, a disease caused by bacteria or a virus is exogenous. Compare **endogenous.** –**exogenic,** *adj.*

exophoria /ek′səfôr′ē·ə/,   deviation of one eye to the side. This occurs when the eyes are at rest. When focusing on an object, the deviation disappears. See also **strabismus.** – **exophoric,** *adj.*

exophthalmia /ek′softhal′mē·ə/,   an abnormal condition with a bulging of the eyeballs (exopthalmos). Causes include a tumor pushing the eyeballs outward, bleeding or swelling of the brain or eye, paralysis or injury to the eye muscles, blood clots in the sinuses, an overactive thyroid gland, and varicose veins in the orbit.

exophthalmic goiter.   See **Graves' disease.**

exophthalmometer /-mom′ətər/,   an instrument for measuring the distance the eye bulges forward in exophthalmia.

exophytic /-fit′ik/,   referring to the tendency to grow outward. For example, an exophytic tumor grows on the surface of an organ or structure.

exophytic carcinoma,   a skin cancer that looks like a wart.

exostosis /-stō′sis/,   an abnormal, harmless growth on the surface of a bone.

exotropia /-trō′pē·ə/.   See **strabismus.**

expectation of life,   the probable number of years a person will live after a certain age. This is determined by the death rate in a specific geographic area. It may be adjusted by the person's health, race, sex, age, or other factors. Also called **life expectancy.**

E–F

expected date of confinement (EDC), the predicted date of a pregnant woman's delivery.

expectorant, referring to a substance that aids coughing up mucus or other fluids from the lungs. Also called **mucolytic.** **–expectorate,** *v.*

expectoration, removing mucus, sputum, or fluids from the throat and lungs by coughing or spitting.

experimental medicine, a branch of medicine in which new drugs or treatments are tested for safety and effect by using animals or, in certain cases, human subjects.

expiration, **1.** breathing out. Expiration depends on the elastic qualities of lung tissue and the chest. Compare **inspiration.** **2.** termination or death. **–expire,** *v.*

expiratory reserve volume (ERV) /ekspī′rətôr′ē/, the largest amount of air that can be forced out of the lungs after a normal breath has been let out.

exposure, a quantity used to indicate the amount of ionization in air produced by x or gamma radiation. The unit is the roentgen (R). One roentgen is approximately equal to 1 rad and/or 1 rem for x and gamma radiation.

exposure hazard, hazard existing from the inhalation, ingestion, or absorption of the material involved.

expression, **1.** the indication of a physical or emotional state through facial appearance or tone of voice. **2.** the act of pressing or squeezing in order to expel something, such as expressing milk from the breast.

extended care facility, an institution devoted to providing medical, nursing, or custodial care over a long period of time. Also called **convalescent home, nursing home.**

extended family, a family group consisting of the parents, their children, the grandparents, and other family members. The extended family is the basic family group in many societies.

Extendryl, a trademark for a combination drug containing a stimulant (phenylephrine hydrochloride), an antihistamine (chlorpheniramine maleate), and a nerve blocker (methscopolamine nitrate). It is used to treat nasal congestion.

extension, a movement allowed by certain joints of the skeleton that increases the angle between two adjoining bones. For example, extending the leg increases the angle between the thigh and the calf. Compare **flexion.**

extensor, one of the muscles of the forearm or of the calf of the leg.

external, **1.** being on the outside of the body or an organ. **2.** acting from the outside. **3.** referring to the outward or visible appearance. Compare **internal.**

external conjugate, a measurement made early in pregnancy to determine the ease of childbirth. It is the distance from the dent below the lowest spine bone above the pelvis (lumbar vertebra) to the upper edge of the pubic bone.

external ear. See **ear.**

external exposure, exposure of a person by radiation originating from a radiation source outside of the body.

external jugular vein, one of a pair of large blood vessels in the neck that receive most of the blood from the surface of the skull and the deep tissues of the face. It runs down the neck and joins the subclavian vein. Compare **internal jugular vein.**

exteroceptive /eks′tərōsep′tiv/, referring to stimulation that comes from outside the body. The term also refers to the nerves that are stimulated by outside events. Compare **interoception, proprioception.**

extrabuccal feeding /eks′trəbuk′əl/, giving nutrients by means other than the mouth. Also called **extraoral feeding.** See also **intravenous feeding.**

extracapsular fracture /-kap′syələr/, any bone break that occurs near a joint but does not directly involve the joint capsule. This type of break is very common in the hip. See also **capsule.**

extracellular /-sel′yələr/, referring to outside a cell in spaces between cell layers. See also **cell, interstitial.**

extracellular fluid (ECF), the part of the body fluid outside the tissue cells. This includes fluid in the spaces of tissues (interstitial fluid) and blood plasma. The adult body contains nearly 3 gallons (11.2 liters) of interstitial fluid. This accounts for about 16% of body weight. In addition, there are about 3 quarts (2.8 liters) of plasma, which is about 4% of body weight. Plasma and interstitial fluid are very similar chemically. Together with fluid inside the cells (intracellular fluid), ECF helps control the movement of water and electrolytes throughout the body.

extracorporeal /-kôrpôr′ē·əl/, outside the body. An example is extracorporeal circulation in which venous blood is routed outside the body to a heart-lung machine and returned to the body through an artery.

extract, to remove a tooth by means of elevators, forceps, or both. **–extraction,** *n.*

extradural /-dŏŏr′əl/, outside the lining of the brain and spinal cord (dura mater).

extraocular /-ok′yələr/, outside the eye.

extraocular muscle palsy, paralysis of the eye muscles. This may affect the following muscles: the superior, inferior, medial, and lateral rectus muscles, and the superior and the inferior oblique muscles. See also **strabismus.**

extraperitoneal /-per′itōnē′əl/, occurring or located outside the peritoneal cavity. The peritoneal cavity is formed by a membrane (peritoneum) lining the abdominal and pelvic walls and covering the organs.

extrapyramidal /-piram′ədəl/, referring to the nerves and fibers that coordinate and control movement.

extrapyramidal disease, any of a large group of conditions with uncontrolled movement, changes in muscle tone, and abnormal posture. Disorders such as tardive dyskinesia, chorea, athetosis, and Parkinson's disease are extrapyramidal diseases.

extrapyramidal reaction, a response to a drug marked by symptoms of extrapyramidal disease. The reaction may persist or fade after stopping the drug.

extrapyramidal system, the part of the nervous system that controls movement. These nerves include the basal ganglia, substantia nigra, subthalamic nucleus, part of the midbrain, and the motor neurons of the spine. See also **extrapyramidal tracts.**

extrapyramidal tracts, the tracts of nerves from the brain to the spinal cord that coordinate and control movement. Within the brain, the extrapyramidal tracts are nerve relays between the many motor areas of the brain. The extrapyramidal tracts are functional rather than anatomic units. They control and coordinate posture, position, support, and locomotor mechanisms. The tracts cause contractions of muscle groups in sequence or at the same time. Compare **pyramidal tract.**

extrasystole /-sis′təlē/. See **arrhythmia.**

extrauterine /-yoo′tərin/, occurring or located outside the uterus, as an ectopic pregnancy.

extravasation /-vəsā′shən/, an escape into the tissues, usually of blood, serum, or lymph. Compare **bleeding.** See also **exudate, transudate.** –**extravasate,** v.

extroversion /-vur′zhən/, **1.** the tendency to direct one's interests and energies toward things outside the self. A person who is outgoing is called an **extrovert. 2.** the state of being mainly concerned with what is outside the self. Compare **introversion.**

extrusion reflex, a normal response in infants to force the tongue outward when the tongue is touched. The reflex begins to go away by about 3 or 4 months of age. Before it fades, food must be placed well back in the mouth to be kept in and swallowed. Constant sticking out of a large tongue may be a sign of Down's syndrome.

exudate /eks′yədāt/, fluid, cells, or other substances that have been slowly discharged through small pores or breaks in cell membranes. Perspiration, pus, and serum are sometimes called exudates.

exudative /igzoo′dətiv/, relating to the oozing of fluid and other materials from cells and tissues, usually as a result of inflammation or injury.

eye, one of a pair of organs of sight, located in bony hollows at the front of the skull. The eyes are embedded in fat and supplied by one of a pair of optic nerves from the forebrain. Structures associated with the eye are the muscles, the tough muscle covering (fascia), the eyebrow, the eyelids, the membrane lining the lids (conjunctiva), and the tear (lacrimal) gland. The eyeball has 3 layers that enclose 2 spaces separated by the lens. The smaller space in front of the lens is divided by the iris into two chambers, both filled with a liquid (aqueous humor). The back chamber is larger than the front chamber and contains the jelly-like vitreous body. The outside layer of the eye consists of the transparent cornea in the front, which makes up one fifth of the layer. The lens, which is just behind the cornea, and the cornea focus images onto the retina. The white (sclera) makes up the other five sixths of the outer layer. The middle layer is supplied with blood and consists of the choroid under the sclera, the ciliary body which focuses the lens, and the iris which controls the amount of light entering the eye. The inner layer of nervous tissue is the retina. Light waves passing through the lens strike a layer of rods and cones in the retina, creating impulses that are carried by the optic nerve to the brain.

eyebrow, 1. the arch of bone over the eye that separates the eye socket from the forehead. **2.** the arch of hairs growing along the ridge of the bony arch.

eyeground, the back (fundus) of the eye. See also **funduscopy.**

eyelash, one of many small hairs (cilia) growing in double or triple rows along the border of the eyelids.

eyelid, a movable fold of thin skin over the eye. The eyelid contains eyelashes, glands (ciliary) that produce sweat, and glands (meibomian) that produce oil along its edge. It consists of loose connecting tissue containing a thin plate of fiber tissue lined with mucous membrane. The orbicularis oculi muscle and the oculomotor nerve control the opening and closing of the eyelid.

F

Fabry's disease, a somewhat rare disease that runs in families. Certain fats are stored in many parts of the body. This causes blood vessel, urinary, and skin problems and, in some cases, muscle defects. Symptoms of the disease are water retention, high blood pressure, enlarged heart, and skin bumps. Albumin and blood cells show up in the urine.

face, 1. the front of the head from the chin to the brow. It includes the skin, muscles and structures of the forehead, eyes, nose, mouth, cheeks, and jaw. **2.** to direct the face toward something. See also **en face.** –**facial,** *adj*.

facepiece, the part of an SCBA that fits over the face and includes the head harness, facepiece lens, exhalation valve, and connection for either a regulator or a low-pressure hose.

facet, a flattened, highly polished wear pattern on a tooth.

facial artery, one of a pair of arteries that come from the external carotid arteries. They divide into four neck and five face branches, and supply the organs and tissues in the head.

facial muscle, any of many muscles of the face. The five groups of facial muscles include the muscles of the scalp, the outside muscles of the ear, the muscles of the nose, the muscles of the eyelid, and the muscles of the mouth. Also called **muscle of expression.**

facial nerve, either of a pair of mixed sense and motor nerves that come from the brainstem. Also called **seventh cranial nerve.**

facial paralysis, a loss of use of the face muscles or a loss of feeling in the face. It may be caused by disease or injury. The amount of paralysis depends on the nerves affected. See also **Bell's palsy.**

facial vein, one of a pair of veins that drain blood that has lost oxygen from the surface of the face back to the heart. Because the vein has no valves that prevent the backflow of blood, infections of the skin near the nose and mouth may spread to the brain and infect its lining (meningitis).

facies /fā′shi·ēz/, *pl*. **facies** /fā′shi·ēz/, **1.** the face. **2.** the surface of any body structure, part, or organ. **3.** the face's expression or appearance.

facitis /fasī′-/, a noncancerous growth that develops in the mouth tissues under the skin, usually in the cheek. It may be mistaken for a cancer (fibrosarcoma).

factor I. See **fibrinogen.**

factor II. See **prothrombin.**

factor III. See **thromboplastin.**

factor IV, a term for calcium as an element in the process of blood clotting.

factor V, a blood clotting factor that occurs in normal plasma but is lacking in patients with a blood clotting disease (parahemophilia). It is needed to change prothrombin rapidly to thrombin. Also called **proaccelerin.**

factor VI, a chemical agent that comes from factor V (proaccelerin), in blood clotting.

factor VII, a blood clotting factor in the blood plasma and broken down in the liver if vitamin K is present. Also called **proconvertin.**

factor VIII, a blood clotting factor in normal plasma but lacking in patients with a blood clotting disease (hemophilia A). It is made up of two separate substances. The lack of one substance results in hemophilia A, and the lack of the other results in Von Willebrand's disease. See also **antihemophilic factor.**

factor IX, a blood clotting factor in normal plasma but lacking in patients with a blood clotting disease (hemophilia B). Also called **Christmas factor.**

factor IX complex, an antibleeding drug with factors II, VII, IX, and X given to treat a blood clotting disease (hemophilia B). It is a protein that depends on vitamin K in the liver.

factor X, a blood clotting factor that occurs in normal plasma but is lacking in some defects in blood clotting. Factor X is made in the liver when vitamin K is present. Also called **Stuart-Power factor.**

factor XI, a blood clotting factor in normal plasma. A lack of it results in a blood clotting disease (hemophilia C).

factor XII, a blood clotting factor in normal plasma. Also called **activation factor.**

factor XIII, a blood clotting factor in normal plasma. It acts with calcium to make a protein (fibrin) clot. Also called **fibrinase, fibrin stabilizing factor.**

Factorate, a trademark for human antihemophilic factor VIII.

faculty, any normal function or ability of a living organism, as being able to sense and recognize sense stimulations.

fagicladosporic acid /faj'iklad'ōspôr'ik/, a poison made by a fungus *(Cladosporium epiphyllum)*. This fungus causes ''black spots'' on stored meat, a skin disease (tinea negra), and black decay of the brain.

Fahrenheit /fer'ənhīt, fär'-/, a scale for measuring temperature in which the boiling point of water is 212° and the freezing point of water is 32° at sea level. Compare **Celsius.**

failure to thrive, slowed growth of an infant from conditions that affect normal body functions, appetite, and activity. Causes include birth defects, major organ system defects, sudden illness, bad nutrition, and many psychologic or social factors, as maternal deprivation syndrome.

faint, *nontechnical.* to lose consciousness, as in a fainting attack. See also **syncope.**

faith healing, a belief that a person has the power to cause a cure or recovery from an illness or injury without using normal medical treatments. It assumes the healer has been given that power by a cosmic force.

fallopian tube /fəlō'pē·ən/, one of a pair of tubes opening at one end into the uterus and at the other end into the cavity over the ovary. Each tube is the passage through which an egg (ovum) is carried to the uterus and through which sperm move toward the ovary. The parts (fimbriae) at the open end of each tube drape in fingerlike bunches over the ovary. Also called **oviduct, uterine tube.**

fallout, the spread of radioactive waste after a nuclear explosion.

false labor, irregular tightening of the pregnant uterus that begins during the first three months of pregnancy. The contractions increase in time, length, and strength as pregnancy continues. Near the end of pregnancy, strong false labor is often hard to tell apart from the contractions of true labor. Also called **Braxton Hicks contraction.**

false negative, an incorrect result of a medical test or procedure that falsely shows the lack of a finding, condition, or disease. False negative results are more common than false positive results, because the person doing the test is more likely to fail to see a finding than to imagine seeing something that does not exist.

false positive, a test result that wrongly shows the presence of a disease or other condition.

false pregnancy. See **pseudocyesis.**

familial, referring to the presence of a disease in some families and not in others, usually but not always hereditary. Compare **acquired, congenital, hereditary.**

family, 1. a group of people related by heredity, as parents, children, and brothers and sisters. The term sometimes includes persons living in the same household or those related by marriage. **2.** a group of persons having a common last name. **3.** a category of animals or plants. Humans are members of the genus *Homo sapiens,* which is a part of the hominid family which, in turn, is a part of the primate order of mammals. See also **genetics, heredity.**

family-centered care, health care that includes the health of an entire family and actions needed to keep or improve the health of the unit and its members.

family ganging, an unethical medical practice in which the patient is urged or forced to involve the entire family in a program of health care even if the other family members do not need such care. The practice allows the health care service to get insurance payments for all family members.

family history, a necessary part of a patient's medical history in which the patient is asked about the health of the other members of the family. These questions are asked to find out about any diseases that the patient may be at a high risk of getting.

family medicine, the branch of medicine that is concerned with the diagnosis and treatment of health problems in people of either sex and any age. Physicians who practice family medicine are often called family practice physicians, family physicians, or, formerly, general practitioners.

Fanconi's anemia, a usually inborn disorder marked by anemia in childhood or early adult life, bone problems, and birth defects.

Fanconi's syndrome, a group of disorders including kidney disease and sugar and phosphates in the urine. The condition is often marked by weak bones, excess acid in the urine, and low blood potassium. One form, idiopathic Fanconi's syndrome, is inherited and usually appears in early middle age. Another is acquired and is usually the result of poisoning from many sources, including the use of outdated tetracycline.

Fansidar, a trademark for an antimalaria drug (pyrimethamine and sulfadoxine).

fantasy, 1. the completely free play of the imagination; fancy. **2.** the mental process of changing undesirable experiences into imagined events to fulfill a wish, need, or desire or to express unconscious conflicts, as a daydream.

Farber test, an examination of newborn feces (meconium) for hair and skin cells. The fetus normally swallows amniotic fluid containing these proteins that then pass through the intestines to be released, usually after birth, in the first stools. The lack of hair or skin cells is a sign of blocked intestines.

E–F

farmer's lung, a lung disorder caused by breathing dusts from moldy hay. It is a form of an allergic lung disease (pneumonitis) affecting individuals who have developed an allergy to the mold spores. Symptoms include coughing, nausea, chills, and fever.

farsightedness, an eyesight disorder caused by an error of refraction in which rays of light entering the eye are brought into focus behind the retina. Also called **hyperopia.**

fascia /fash′ē·ə/, *pl.* **fasciae,** fiberlike connective tissue of the body that may be separated from other structures, as the tendons and the ligaments. It varies in thickness and weight and in the amounts of fat, fiber, and tissue fluid it contains. –**fascial,** *adj.*

fascia bulbi, a thin membrane that surrounds the eyeball from the optic nerve to the pupil and allows the eyeball to move freely.

fascial compartment, a part of the body that is walled off by fiberlike (fascial) membranes. It usually contains a muscle or group of muscles or an organ, as the heart is contained by part of the chest cavity (mediastinum).

fasciculation /fasik′yəlā′shən/, the uncontrollable twitching of a single muscle group served by a single motor nerve fiber or filament. It may be felt and seen under the skin. It results as a side effect from many drugs. It also may be a symptom of a lack in the diet, cerebral palsy, fever, a nerve disease (neuralgia), polio, or rheumatic heart disease. See also **fibrillation.** –**fascicular,** *adj.,* **fasciculate,** *v.*

fasciculus /fəsik′yələs/, *pl.* **fasciculi,** a small bundle of muscle, tendon, or nerve fibers. The shape of fasciculi in a muscle is related to the power of the muscle and its range of motion. –**fascicular,** *adj.*

fascioliasis /fas′ē·əlī′əsis/, an infection with a liver fluke (*Fasciola hepatica*). It is marked by stomach and bowel pain, fever, yellow skin (jaundice), hives, and diarrhea. One gets it by swallowing forms of the fluke found on water plants, as raw watercress. The disease is common in many parts of the world, including southern and western United States.

fascioscapulohumeral dystrophy /-skap′yəlōhyoo′mərəl/. See **muscular dystrophy.**

Fastin, a trademark for a drug used to reduce appetite (phentermine hydrochloride).

fat, **1.** a substance made up of lipids or fatty acids and occurring in many forms ranging from oil to tallow. **2.** a type of body tissue made up of cells containing stored fat (depot fat). Stored fat is usually called white fat, which is found in large cells, or brown fat, which consists of lipid droplets. Stored fat contains more than twice as many calories per gram as sugars and is a source of quick body energy. In addition, stored fat helps protect important organs. See also **fatty acid, lipid.**

fatigue, **1.** a state of exhaustion or a loss of strength or endurance, as may follow excess physical activity. **2.** an inability of tissues to respond to stimulations that normally cause muscles to contract or other activity. Muscle cells generally need a recovery period after activity. During this time cells restore their energy supplies and release waste products. **3.** a sense of weariness or tiredness. **4.** an emotional state linked to extreme or extended exposure to psychic pressure, as in battle or combat fatigue.

fatigue fracture, any broken bone that results from excess physical activity and not from any specific injury. It commonly occurs in the foot (metatarsal) bones of runners.

fat metabolism, the process by which fats are broken down and used by the cells of the body. Before the final reactions in fat use can occur, fats must be changed into fatty acids and glycerol. The body also changes fats from fatty acids and glycerol or from compounds coming from glucose or amino acids. The body can build only saturated fatty acids. Essential unsaturated fatty acids can be had only from the diet. Certain hormones, as insulin and the glucocorticoids, control fat use.

fatty acid, any of several acids found in fats. An **essential fatty acid** is one that cannot be produced by the body but is needed for its proper growth and functioning. It must therefore be included in the diet. It forms prostaglandins, which help organ muscles contract, regulate stomach acid, lower blood pressure, and regulate body temperature. It is also necessary for the normal functioning of the reproductive system, hormone regulation, and for breaking up cholesterol deposits in the arteries. Sources include natural vegetable oils, wheat germ, seeds (pumpkin, sesame, and sunflower), poultry fat, and fish oils. Symptoms of a deficiency include brittle and dull hair, nail problems, dandruff, allergies, and dermatitis, especially eczema in infants. There are three essential fatty acids, **arachidonic acid, linoleic acid,** and **linolenic acid.** Only **linoleic acid** is actually essential because the other two can be made by the body if other essential nutrients are provided. It is found mainly in vegetable oils. **Saturated** and unsaturated fatty acids differ mainly in how fluid they are. The more saturated a fatty acid is, the more solid it is. **Polyunsaturated fatty acids** are rich in liquid vegetable oils. An unsaturated fatty acid is one that is generally found in vegetables. Saturated fatty acids are found mainly in meat. A diet high in saturated fatty acids may lead to a high level of cholesterol in the blood, and in some patients is linked to heart disease.

fatty liver, a buildup of fats in the liver. Causes include alcoholic cirrhosis, injecting drugs, and exposure to poisonous substances, as carbon tetrachloride and yellow phosphorus. Fatty liver is also seen in a nutrition disease (kwashiorkor) and is a rare problem of late pregnancy. Symptoms include loss of appetite, large liver, and stomach upset. The condition will usually disappear after the cause is corrected. See also **cirrhosis.**

fauces /fô′sēz/, the opening of the mouth into the throat.

F.D.A., abbreviation for **Food and Drug Administration.**

fear, a feeling of dread that may result from natural or inborn causes, as a sudden noise, loss of physical support, pain, or heights.

febrile /fē′bril, feb′ril/, referring to high body temperature, as a feverish reaction to an infection.

fecal fistula /fē′kəl/, an abnormal passage from the colon to the outside surface of the body. It results in a release of feces from the opening. Fistulas of this kind are usually created surgically in operations involving the removal of cancerous or severely injured bowel segments. See also **colostomy.**

fecal impaction, a buildup of hardened feces in the bowel that cannot be moved naturally. See also **constipation, obstipation.**

fecal softener, a drug that allows intestinal fluids to penetrate and soften the stool. Also called **stool softener.**

feces /fē′sēz/, mostly solid waste from the digestive tract. It is formed in the intestine and released through the rectum. Feces consist of water, food remains, bacteria, and fluids of the intestines and liver. Also called **stool.** See also **defecation.** –**fecal,** *adj.*

fecundity /fəkun′ditē/, the ability to produce offspring, especially in large numbers and rapidly; fertility. – **fecund,** *adj.*

feeding, the act or process of taking or giving food. **Forced feeding** is the giving of food by force, as nasal feeding, to persons who cannot or will not eat. See also **breast feeding, nasogastric feeding.**

fee-for-service, **1.** a charge made for a professional activity, as for a physical examination or checking a patient's blood pressure. **2.** a system for paying for professional services in which the physician is paid for the particular service rather than getting a salary.

Feldene, a trademark for an arthritis drug (piroxicam).

felon, an open sore on the finger.

Felty's syndrome, a spleen disorder occurring with adult rheumatoid arthritis. See also **hypersplenism.**

female, referring to the sex that bears children; feminine.

female reproductive system assessment, an examination of a woman's genital tract and breasts including past and present disorders. The woman's age at the beginning of menstruation, the length, spacing, and regularity of cycles, and symptoms, as pain and excess bleeding, are recorded.

The problems and outcome of any pregnancies, any abortion, or the date of menopause and linked symptoms are explored. The examination may include an examination by hand, Pap test, a base body temperature figure, tests on the vaginal discharge, tests on tissues, scraping and flushing out the uterus, and blowing material into the tubes. Laboratory studies may include levels of hormones, tests for sexually carried diseases, and thyroid function tests. The breasts are examined, and the lower abdomen is felt. The space between the navel and the vagina is checked for any mass. The groin is checked for swollen lymph glands (lymphadenopathy) or hernias. If there is a possible pregnancy, listening for fetal heart tones is done. The outer parts of the vagina are examined. Any swelling, discoloration, tumor, scar, lump (cyst), discharge, or bleeding is noted. Any fluids are examined, and a sample is taken for tests. The pelvic muscles are checked. Hernia of the bladder (cytocele) or of the rectum (rectocele), or a falling (prolapse) of the uterus may be seen when the woman is asked to bear down. The color and condition of the vaginal lining are noted. Samples for tests are taken before the Pap test. For the Pap test, scrapings and fluids are taken. The physician puts pressure to the outside of the lower abdomen in many places and directions to bring the uterus, fallopian tubes, and ovaries to where they may be felt. The size, shape, position, and other features of the organs and tissues are checked. Any discomfort is noted. Examination of the rectum is done. An inability to relax, being overweight, pelvic soreness, and heavy vaginal discharge can prevent a good examination.

feminization, **1.** the normal growth or beginning of female sex characteristics. **2.** the beginning of female sex characteristics in a male. Causes include testicle tumors, advanced alcoholism, or the use of estrogen therapy for cancer. Male breasts becoming larger may be caused by Klinefelter's syndrome and by some drugs. See also **pseudohermaphroditism, virilism.**

feminizing adrenal tumor, a tumor of the adrenal gland. Symptoms in males include breasts becoming larger and loss of ability to have sexual intercourse. The testicles often begin wasting, but the prostate and penis are usually normal in size. In women, these tumors are linked to early puberty.

Feminone, a trademark for a hormone (ethinyl estradiol).

femoral /fem′ərəl/, referring to the thigh (femur).

femoral nerve, the main nerve of the thigh.

femoral vein, a large vein in the thigh.

femur /fē′mər/, the thigh bone.

fenestra /fənes′trə/, *pl.* **fenestrae,** an opening in a bandage or cast that is often cut out to reduce pressure or to give regular skin care.

E–F

fenestration, a surgery in which an opening is made to gain access to the space within an organ or a bone. Also called **window.** –**fenestrate,** *v.*

fenfluramine hydrochloride, a drug given to decrease the appetite in patients who are overweight. Glaucoma, alcoholism, high blood pressure, or known allergy to this drug prohibits its use. Side effects include drug addiction, diarrhea, mental confusion, and depression.

fenoprofen calcium, a drug given to treat arthritis and other painful conditions. Kidney or stomach and intestine diseases or known allergy to this drug, to aspirin, or to similar drugs prohibits its use. Side effects include stomach and intestine disturbances, peptic ulcers, dizziness, skin rash, and hearing problems. The drug interacts with many other drugs.

fentanyl citrate, a painkiller used with general anesthesia. Myasthenia gravis or known allergy to this drug prohibits its use. Side effects include drug addiction, itching, and throat spasm.

Feosol, a trademark for a blood builder (ferrous sulfate).

Fergon, a trademark for a blood builder (ferrous gluconate).

Ferguson's reflex, a contraction of the uterus after the cervix is stimulated. The reflex is important in labor.

ferritin /fer'itin/, an iron compound found in the intestine, spleen, and liver. It contains over 20% iron and is essential for red blood cells.

ferrous sulfate, a blood-building drug given to treat iron deficiency anemia. Side effects include diarrhea and constipation.

fertile, 1. able to reproduce or bear offspring. **2.** able to be fertilized. **3.** fruitful; not sterile. –**fertility,** *n.*, **fertilize,** *v.*

fertile eunuch syndrome, a hormone disorder of males in which the amount of sex hormone is not enough to cause sperm to develop.

fertile period, the time in the menstrual cycle during which fertilization may occur. Sperm can live for 48 to 72 hours; the egg (ovum) lives for 24 hours. Thus, the fertile period begins 2 to 3 days before ovulation and lasts for 2 to 3 days afterward.

fertilization, the union of male and female gametes to form a zygote from which the embryo develops. The process takes place in the fallopian tube of the female when a sperm comes in contact with the egg (ovum).

Festal, a trademark for a stomach and bowel drug containing digestive enzymes and bile parts.

fetal age /fē'təl/, the age of the embryo from the time since fertilization. Also called **fertilization age.** Compare **gestational age.**

fetal circulation, the pathway of blood flow in the fetus. Blood carrying oxygen from the placenta travels through the umbilical cord to the liver. The blood then flows to the heart. It goes through a hole between the right and left chambers (atria) of the heart. Blood carrying oxygen is available for circulation through the left chamber (ventricle) to the head and upper body area. The blood returning from the head and arms enters the right chamber (ventricle) and is pumped through the lung artery and into the large heart artery (aorta) for circulation to the lower parts of the body. The blood is returned to the placenta through the umbilical cord arteries.

fetal distress, a fetus with an abnormal heart rate or rhythm. If possible, the cause is found and corrected. Cesarean section may be necessary if the cause of the problem cannot be corrected.

fetal heart rate (FHR), the number of heart beats in the fetus per minute. The FHR is affected by many factors, including fever, contractions of the uterus, and drugs.

fetal hemoglobin, hemoglobin F, the major hemoglobin present in the blood of a fetus and newborn. Hemoglobin F is present in small amounts in the blood of adults.

fetal hydantoin syndrome (FHS), a disorder with a group of birth defects caused by the mother's use of hydantoin drugs to limit epileptic seizures. Symptoms include lack of nails on the fingers or toes, mental retardation, slowed growth, and heart defects.

fetal lie, the relationship between the head-to-foot position of the fetus in the uterus and that of the mother. In a longitudinal lie, the fetus is lying vertically, or up and down in the uterus. In a transverse lie, the fetus is positioned horizontally, across the opening of the cervix, making delivery difficult.

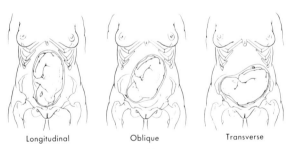

Longitudinal   Oblique   Transverse

Fetal lie

fetal position, the relationship of the body part of the fetus to the mother's pelvis. For example, if the head is directed to the back of the mother's right side, the fetal position is called **right occiput posterior.**

fetal presentation, the body part of the fetus that first appears in the pelvis at birth.

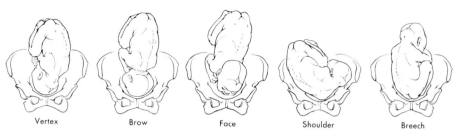

Palpation of fetal presentation

Vertex   Brow   Face   Shoulder   Breech

fetish,   1. any object or idea given unreasonable attention or worth. **2.** any inanimate object or any part of the body not of a sexual nature that arouses erotic feelings.

fetography /fētog′rəfē/,   x-ray films of the fetus in the uterus. See also **fetometry.**

fetology /fētol′-/,   the branch of medicine that is concerned with the fetus. Also called **embryatrics.**

fetometry /fētom′ətrē/,   the measurement of the size of the fetus, especially the size of the head and the body.

fetoprotein,   a substance that occurs naturally in fetuses and occasionally in adults as the result of certain diseases.

fetoscope /fē′təskōp′/,   a stethoscope for hearing the fetal heart beat through the mother's stomach. A fetoscope may also be a device like an endoscope (an instrument with a light on one end). This is used to observe the fetus through a small cut in the abdomen.

fetotoxic /fē′tōtok′sik/,   referring to anything that is poisonous to a fetus.

fetus /fē′təs/,   the human child in the uterus following the period as an embryo. The **fetal stage** is the period after the seventh week of pregnancy to birth, 38 to 42 weeks after the last menstrual period. Compare **embryo.** See also **prenatal development.**

fetus in fetu,   a birth defect in which a small, imperfectly formed twin is contained within the body of the normal twin.

fetus papyraceus,   a twin fetus that has died in the uterus and has been pressed flat against the uterine wall by the living fetus.

fever,   an abnormal temperature of the body above 98.6° F (37° C). Infection, nerve disease, cancer, anemia, and many drugs may cause fever. No single theory explains why a temperature is increased. Fever speeds up the body's chemical processes (metabolism) 7% per °C. This means more food needs to be eaten. Convulsions may occur in children whose fevers tend to rise quickly. Severe mental confusion (delirium) is seen with high fevers. It may begin quickly or gradually.

fever blister,   a cold sore caused by herpesvirus. Also called **herpes simplex.**

fever therapy,   a higher body temperature caused by artificial means. Injecting malarial parasites, a vaccine that causes fever, or applying heat to the body will produce this condition. An artificial fever may be given to a patient to stop a disease that is sensitive to higher body temperatures. Also called **artificial fever, induced fever.**

fever treatment,   the care of a patient with a high temperature. The patient is observed for rapid heart beat; a full, bounding pulse or a weak, thready pulse; rapid breathing; hot, dry skin; chills; headache; sweating; confusion; dehydration; tremors; convulsions; and coma. Treatment may include giving antibiotic, antifever, and sedative drugs. If the temperature is extremely high, an alcohol sponge bath, cooling tub bath, a cold wet sheet, or ice packs may be helpful. The patient's temperature is checked every 2 to 4 hours. The room temperature may be reduced, and air currents increased by a fan. Increased amounts of fluids are given, physical activity is reduced, and the skin is exposed to air.

fiberoptics,   a way in which an internal organ or space can be viewed, using glass or plastic fibers that reflect a magnified image.

fibril /fī′bril/,   a small threadlike structure that often is part of a cell.

fibrillation /fī′brilā′shən/,   involuntary contractions of a single muscle fiber or of an isolated group of nerve fibers. **Atrial fibrillation** is a condition of rapid, uneven contractions in the upper heart chambers (atria). This causes the lower chambers (ventricles) to beat irregularly at the rate of 130 to 150 a minute. The atria may discharge more than 350 electric impulses a minute. The lower chambers cannot contract in response to all these impulses, and the contractions become disordered. Atrial fibrillation occurs most often in heart diseases, as mitral stenosis and atrial infarction. The rapid pulsations result in a decreased amount of blood pumped to the body. The disorganized contractions of the atria can cause blood clots to form in the atria. **Ventricular fibrillation** refers to a very fast, very uneven heart beat arising from a ventricle. The condition is marked by a complete lack of a regular heart beat. Blood pressure falls to zero, resulting in unconsciousness. Death may occur within 4 minutes. Defibrillation and ventilation must be initiated immediately. See also **infarction, stenosis.**

fibrin /fī′brin/, a stringy protein that gives the semisolid character to a blood clot. Compare **fibrinogen.** See also **blood clotting.**

fibrinogen /fībrin′əjən/, a protein in the blood clotting process that is converted into protein (fibrin) by thrombin when calcium is present. Also called **factor I.** Compare **fibrin.** See also **blood clotting.**

fibrinolysin /fī′brinol′isin/, an enzyme that dissolves protein (fibrin). Also called **plasmin.**

fibrocartilage /-kär′tilij/. See **cartilage.**

fibrocystic breast disease, single or multiple lumps (cysts) in the breasts. The cysts are often harmless and fairly common, but they may be cancerous. Women with fibrocystic disease of the breast are at greater than usual risk of getting breast cancer later in life. Also called **chronic cystic mastitis.**

fibroids /fī′broidz/, an informal term for a noncancerous tumor of the smooth muscle on the uterus (leiomyoma uteri). It appears firm, round, and gray-white. Multiple tumors of this kind develop most often in the wall of the uterus.

fibroma /fībrō′mə/, a noncancerous tumor largely made up of fiberlike or fully developed connective tissue. An **ameloblastic fibroma** is a dental tumor in which there is a growth of connective and other tissues but no growth of dentin or enamel. A **fibroma cutis** occurs in the skin. An **intracanalicular fibroma** occurs in the gland lining and fibrous tissue in the breast. An **irritation fibroma** is caused by prolonged irritation, such as rubbing. It commonly develops on or near the gums. A **hard fibroma** is one in which there are few cells. A **soft fibroma** contains many cells. See also specific fibroma.

fibromyositis /-mī′əsī′-/, stiffness and joint or muscle pain, with inflammation of the muscle tissues and the fiberlike connective tissues. The condition may develop after a weather change, infection, or injury. Kinds of fibromyositis include **lumbago, torticollis.** See also **rheumatism.**

fibrosarcoma, a cancer that contains connective tissue. It develops suddenly from small bumps on the skin.

fibrosing alveolitis, a lung disorder (alveolitis) with breathlessness and air hunger, occurring in rheumatoid arthritis and other diseases. See also **alveolitis.**

fibrosis /fībrō′-/, **1.** a fiberlike connective tissue that occurs normally in the growth of scar tissue. It replaces normal tissue lost through injury or infection. **2.** the spread of fiberlike connective tissue over normal smooth muscle or other normal organ tissue. See also **cystic fibrosis.**

fibrositis /-sī′tis/, an inflammation of fiberlike connective tissue. Symptoms include pain and stiffness of the neck, shoulder, and body. Fibrositis occurs in middle age. Compare **fibromyositis, myositis.**

fibrous capsule /fī′brəs/, **1.** the layer of tissue surrounding the joint between two bones. **2.** the tough envelope of membrane surrounding some organs, as the liver.

fibrous dysplasia, a disorder in which fiberlike tissue takes the place of bone. Symptoms include a limp, pain, or a broken bone on the affected side. Girls affected may have an early start of menstruation and breast development. The involved leg may be shortened, and a deformity called "shepherd's crook" is common.

fibrous joint. See **joint.**

fibula /fib′yələ/, a bone of the lower leg, next to and smaller than the shin bone (tibia). In relation to its length, it is the most slender of the long bones. Also called **calf bone.**

field fever, a form of infection (leptospirosis) caused by a microorganism (*Leptospira grippotyphosa*). It affects mainly farm workers. Symptoms include fever, stomach and bowel pain, diarrhea, vomiting, listlessness, and eye inflammation.

figure-of-eight bandage, a bandage with successive laps crossing over and around each other like the figure eight.

filament /fil′əmənt/, a fine threadlike fiber. Filaments are found in most tissues and cells of the body and serve various functions.

filariasis /fil′ərī′əsis/, a disease caused by the presence of *Filaria* worms in the tissues of the body. After many years, the last stage occurs, called **elephantiasis,** in which an arm or leg may become greatly swollen and the skin coarse and tough.

film badge, a pack of photographic film used for approximate measurement of radiation exposure for personnel-monitoring purposes. The badge may contain two or three films of differing sensitivity, and it may contain filters that shield parts of the film from certain types of radiation for determining the types and energies of the radiations.

finger, any of the digits of the hand. The fingers are made up of a metacarpal bone and three bony hinges (phalanges). Some count the thumb as a finger, although it has one less bone. The digits of the hand are numbered 1 to 5, starting with the thumb.

Fiorinal, a trademark for a group of drugs containing a sedative-hypnotic (butalbital), an analgesic, antifever, and antiinflammatory (aspirin), an analgesic (phenacetin), and a stimulant (caffeine).

fire entry suits, suits that offer complete, effective protection for short duration entry into a total flame environment. Designed to withstand exposures to radiant heat levels as high as 2000° F. Entry suits consist of a coat, pants, and separate hood assembly. They are constructed of several layers of flame-retardant materials, with the outer layer often aluminized.

fire rescue/EMS companies,   fire, rescue, and EMS companies are those individuals who respond to the incident onboard emergency vehicles and carry out assigned tasks under the direction of the incident commander or a section officer.

first aid,   the care given to an injured or ill patient, usually where the victim was injured or became sick. It is the initial care given to the victim before medically trained people arrive or before the victim arrives at a health care center. See also **cardiopulmonary resuscitation, hemorrhage control.**

first responders,   first responders are the first trained personnel to arrive at the scene of a hazardous materials incident. Generally they will be fire fighting, law enforcement, emergency medical services (EMS), and industrial emergency brigade personnel. First responders perform these functions:

   1. Initiate the incident command system, including isolating the site and establishing a command post
   2. Initiate evacuation
   3. Recognize and identify the materials involved
   4. Notify additional resources
   5. Initiate basic hazard and risk assessment activities
   6. Select and use available personal protective equipment
   7. Perform basic containment and confinement operations (within resource and protective equipment capabilities)
   8. Implement simple decontamination activities

fish tapeworm infection.   See **tapeworm infection.**

fissile radioactive material,   material that has the capability of undergoing fission and thus requires controls to assure nuclear criticality safety during transport. Fissile materials include plutonium-238, plutonium-239, plutonium-241, uranium-233, and uranium-235.

fission /fish'ən/,   the act of splitting into parts.

fission, nuclear,   a nuclear transformation characterized by the splitting of a nucleus into at least two other nuclei and the release of a relatively large amount of energy.

fission products,   a general term for the complex mixture of substances produced as a result of nuclear fission.

fissure /fish'ər/,   **1.** a split or a groove on the surface of an organ. It often marks the division of the organ into parts, as the lobes of the lung. A fissure is usually deeper than a sulcus, but *fissure* and *sulcus* are often used as if they were the same thing. **2.** a cracklike break in the skin, as an anal fissure. Compare **sulcus.**

fissure fracture,   any broken bone in which a crack extends into the outer layer of the bone but not through the entire bone.

fistula /fis'chələ/,   an abnormal passage from an internal organ to the body surface or between two internal organs. Fistulas may occur in many sites from the mouth to the anus and may be made for treatment.

fit,   **1.** *nontechnical.* an attack or seizure. **2.** the sudden beginning of symptoms, as a fit of coughing. **3.** the manner in which one surface is placed next to another, as the fit of a denture to the gums.

fixation,   stopping at a certain stage of psychologic and sexual growth, as anal fixation.

fixative,   any substance used to bind, glue, or keep rigid.

fixed bridgework,   a dental device using artificial teeth permanently attached in the upper or the lower jaw.

fixed combination drug,   a group of mixtures with many ingredients giving specific amounts of two or more drugs at the same time.

flaccid /flak'sid/,   weak, soft, and flabby; lacking normal muscle tone, as flaccid muscles.

flaccid bladder.   See **neurogenic bladder.**

flagellant /flaj'ələnt/,   a person who gets sexual pleasure from whipping or being whipped (flagellation).

flagellate /flaj'əlāt/,   a microorganism that moves itself by waving whiplike, thready fibers (filaments), as *Trypanosoma, Leishmania, Trichomonas,* and *Giardia.* See also **protozoa.**

flagellation /flaj'əlā'shən/,   **1.** the act of whipping, beating, or flogging. **2.** a type of massage given by tapping the body with the fingers. See also **massage.**

Flagyl,   a trademark for an antiprotozoa drug (metronidazole).

flail chest,   a chest in which many broken ribs cause the chest wall to be unstable. The lung under the injured area contracts on breathing in and bulges on breathing out. The condition, if uncorrected, leads to air hunger. Symptoms include sharp pain, uneven chest expansion, shallow, rapid breathing, and reduced breath sounds. Collapsed lungs and shock may occur. Treatment includes use of a mechanical lung and traction. Chest tubes may be needed to remove air or fluid that stops the affected lung from expanding.

flammable (explosive) range,   the range of a gas or vapor concentration (percentage by volume in air) that will burn or explode if an ignition source is present. Limiting concentrations are commonly called the ''lower flammable (explosive) limit'' and the ''upper flammable (explosive) limit.'' Below the lower flammable limit, the mixture is too lean to burn; above the upper flammable limit, the mixture is too rich to burn.

E–F

flare, **1.** a red blush on the skin at the edge of a raised area from hives. **2.** the sudden worsening of a disease.

flaring of nostrils, a widening of the nostrils during breathing in, a sign of air hunger or breathing problems.

flashover, the simultaneous ignition of highly heated combustibles in an area.

flash point, the minimum temperature at which a liquid gives off enough vapors that will ignite and flash over but will not continue to burn without the addition of more heat.

flatfoot, a flat arch of the foot. Also called **pes planus.**

flatulence /flach′ələns/, an excess amount of air or gas in the stomach and intestines. It may cause the organs to bloat and in some cases mild to moderate pain.

flavoxate hydrochloride, a smooth muscle relaxing drug given for spastic conditions of the urinary tract. Stomach or bowel bleeding or blockage, urinary tract blockage, or known allergy to this drug prohibits its use. Side effects include nervousness, nausea, stomach and bowel pain, and fever.

flea bite, a small puncture wound caused by a bloodsucking flea. Fleas may carry plague, murine typhus, and tularemia.

Flexeril, a trademark for a muscle relaxing drug (cyclobenzaprine hydrochloride).

flexion /flek′shən/, a movement allowed by certain joints of the skeleton. It decreases the angle between two connecting bones, as bending the elbow. Compare **extension.**

flexor carpi radialis, a muscle of the forearm. It flexes the hand.

flexor carpi ulnaris, a muscle of the forearm. It flexes the hand.

flexor digitorum superficialis, a large muscle of the forearm.

flight into health, a reaction to an unpleasant physical sense or symptom. The person denies the reality of the symptom, insisting that nothing is wrong. See also **illness experience.**

flight of ideas, a stream of talk in which the patient switches quickly from one topic to another, each subject being hard to understand and not related to the one before it. The condition is often a symptom of sudden manic states and schizophrenia.

flight-or-fight reaction, **1.** the reaction of the body to stress. The nervous system and the adrenal gland increase the heart output and the heart beat rate, widen the pupils of the eyes, narrow the blood vessels of the skin, and cause an alert, aroused mental state. **2.** a person's reaction to stress by either fleeing from a situation or staying and trying to deal with it.

floater, one or more spots that appear to drift in front of the eye. It is made by a shadow cast on the retina from material within the eyeball. Most floaters are leftovers of blood vessels that were in the eye before birth. The cause is often injury, but sudden bleeding occurs in diabetes mellitus, high blood pressure, or brain disease. Cancer, detachment of the retina, or other eye diseases may also cause bleeding.

floating kidney, a kidney that is not securely fixed in the usual location because of a birth defect or injury. Compare **ptotic kidney.**

floating rib. See **rib.**

flocculation test /flok′yəlā′shən/, a blood test for syphilis.

flooding, a way to reduce anxiety linked to unreasonable fears (phobia). Exposure to the stimulation that causes anxiety makes a person able to resist that stimulation. Also called **implosive therapy.**

floppy infant syndrome, a general term for some childhood muscle diseases (juvenile spinal muscular atrophies).

Florinef Acetate, a trademark for a steroid hormone (fludrocortisone acetate).

Florone, a trademark for an antiinflammation drug (diflorasone diacetate).

Floropryl, a trademark for an eye ointment (isoflurophate).

flotation therapy, a way to treat and prevent bedsores. The patient's body weight is "floated" by various types of hospital equipment.

floxuridine, a drug given to treat cancers of the brain, breast, liver, and gallbladder. Infection, poor state of the diet, or known allergy to this drug prohibits its use. Side effects include bone marrow disorders, nausea, vomiting, diarrhea, and mouth inflammation.

flu, *informal.* **1.** influenza. **2.** any viral infection of the breathing or intestinal system. See also **influenza.**

flucytosine, a drug given to treat some fungus infections. Known allergy to this drug prohibits its use. Close watching is needed when used by patients with kidney disease. Side effects include stomach and bowel problems, and liver disease.

fluid, **1.** a liquid or gas that is able to flow and to adjust its shape to that of a container. **2.** a body fluid involved in moving electrolytes and other needed chemicals to, through, and from tissue cells. See also **blood, cerebrospinal fluid, lymph.**

fluke, a parasitic flatworm of the class Trematoda, some of which live in humans, infecting the liver, the lungs, and the intestines. An example is the organism that causes **schistosomiasis.** Also called **trematode.**

fluocinolone acetonide, a hormone cream given to reduce inflammation. Bad circulation, viral and fungus diseases of the skin, or known allergy to this or similar drugs prohibits its use. Side effects include various ones resulting from long-term or excess use of steroid drugs. Many allergic reactions may occur.

fluocinonide, an artificial steroid drug given to reduce inflammation. Viral and fungus diseases of the skin, tuberculosis of the skin, or known allergy to this drug prohibits its use. Side effects include other infections, skin streaks, and skin inflammation (contact dermatitis).

Fluonid, a trademark for a hormone cream (fluocinolone acetonide).

fluorescent antibody test (FA test), a test for syphilis and tuberculosis.

Fluorescent Treponemal Antibody Absorption Test (FTA-ABS test), a blood test for syphilis.

fluoridation /flôr′idā′shən/, adding fluoride, especially to a public water supply, to reduce tooth decay. See also **fluoride.**

fluoride, a form of the element fluorine (F) added to the water supply of many areas to harden the tooth enamel and decrease cavities. Excess amounts of fluoride can spot the tooth enamel.

Fluoroplex, a trademark for an anticancer drug used on the skin (fluorouracil).

fluoroscope /flo͞or′əskōp/, a device used for the immediate showing of an x-ray image. —**fluoroscopic,** adj.

fluorosis /flo͞orō′-/, excess fluorine in the body. High amounts of fluorine in drinking water causes spotting and pitting of the enamel of the teeth in children. Severe long-term fluorine poisoning will lead to bone and joint changes in adults.

fluorouracil /flo͞o′ərōyo͞or′əsil/, a drug given to treat cancer of the skin and internal organs.

fluoxymesterone, a steroid hormone used to treat breast cancer in females, and late puberty in males. Male breast or prostate cancer, liver disease, known or suspected pregnancy, or known allergy to this drug prohibits its use. Side effects include allergic shock, excess blood calcium, and liver disease (jaundice).

fluphenazine hydrochloride, a phenothiazine tranquilizer given to treat psychotic disorders.

flurandrenolide, an antiinflammation drug. Poor circulation, viral and fungus diseases of the skin, or known allergy to this drug or to steroid drugs prohibits its use. Many allergic reactions may occur.

flurazepam hydrochloride /flo͞oraz′əpam/, a tranquilizer given to treat an inability to sleep (insomnia).

flush, 1. a blush or sudden reddening of the face and neck. It may occur with a feeling of heat, as may be seen with fever, some drugs, or an overactive thyroid gland (hyperthyroidism). **2.** a sudden, rapid flow of water or other liquid.

FML, a trademark for an eye medicine (fluorometholone).

foam bath, a bath in water containing a substance that covers the surface of the liquid. Air or oxygen is used to form the foam.

focus, a specific location, as the site of an infection or the point at which a signal begins.

folic acid /fō′lik, fol′ik/, a vitamin of the B complex group able to be dissolved in water. It is needed for cell growth and reproduction. It functions with vitamins B_{12} and C in the breakdown of proteins and in the making of hemoglobin. It also increases the appetite and causes the making of hydrochloric acid in the stomach. The vitamin is stored in the liver and may be made by bacteria in the stomach and intestines. Lack of folic acid results in poor growth, gray hair, mouth and tongue inflammation, and diarrhea. Need for folic acid is increased in pregnancy, in infancy, and by stress. Rich sources include spinach and other green leafy vegetables, liver, kidneys, and whole-grain cereals.

folie /fōlē′/, a mental disorder. **Folie du doute** /dYdo͞ot′/ is one of doubting, repeating a certain act or behavior, and not being able to make a decision.

folinic acid /fōlin′ik/, an active form of folic acid used to treat some anemias (megaloblastic). Also called **leucovorin.**

follicle /fol′ikəl/, a pouchlike recessed spot, as the dental follicles that surround the teeth before they emerge or the hair follicles within the skin. —**follicular,** adj.

follicle stimulating hormone (FSH), a pituitary gland hormone that stimulates the growth and aging of follicles (graafian) that contain the ovum in the ovary. It also causes the making of sperm in the male. Also called **menotropins.**

follicular cyst /fōlik′yələr/, a lump (cyst) that comes from the tissue of a tooth bud.

folliculitis /fōlik′yəlī′-/, inflammation of hair follicles.

Follutein, a trademark for a placenta hormone (human chorionic gonadotropin).

fomentation, a treatment for pain or inflammation with a warm, moist application to the skin.

fontanel /fon′tənel′/, a space between the bones of an infant's skull covered by tough membranes. The front fontanel, roughly diamond-shaped, remains soft until about 2 years of age. The back fontanel, triangular in shape, closes about 2 months after birth. Increased brain pressure may cause a fontanel to become tense or bulge. A fontanel may be soft and sunken if the infant is dehydrated.

food, **1.** any substance, usually of plant or animal origin, made up of carbohydrates, proteins, fats, and minerals and vitamins. It is used by the body to provide energy and to cause growth, repair, and good health. **2.** nourishment in solid form, not liquid form.

Food and Drug Administration (F.D.A.), a federal agency responsible for carrying out laws covering food, drugs, and cosmetics, as protection against the sale of unsafe or dangerous substances.

food dispenser, any vehicle capable of dispensing food to incident personnel.

food exchange list, a grouping of foods in which the carbohydrate, fat, and protein values are equal for the items listed. The list is used for meal planning in many diseases. The six groups of foods included on the list are milk, vegetables, fruits, bread, meat, and fats. Starchy vegetables are listed as bread exchanges; fish and cheese are meat exchanges.

food poisoning, a condition resulting from eating food infected by poisons or by bacteria containing toxins. **Bacterial food poisoning** results from eating food contaminated by some bacteria. Symptoms of illness caused by various species of salmonella include fever, chills, nausea, vomiting, diarrhea, and general discomfort beginning 8 to 48 hours after the contaminated food is eaten and continuing for several days. Similar symptoms caused by staphylococcus appear much sooner and rarely last more than a few hours. Food poisoning caused by the organism *Clostridium botulinum* produces stomach and intestinal symptoms, disturbances of vision, weakness or paralysis of muscles, and, in severe cases, respiratory failure. An acute inflammation of the bowels may also be caused by *Clostridium perfringens*. Also called **necrotising enteritis,** this kind of food poisoning causes symptoms of strong stomach pain, bloody diarrhea, and vomiting. Some patients recover completely or survive with long-term bowel blockage. A hole in the intestine, severe lack of body fluids, poisoning of the bowel area (peritonitis), or blood poisoning may cause death. See also specific entry.

foot, the farthest part of the leg.

foot-and-mouth disease, a virus infection of animals, carried to humans by contact with infected animals or infected milk. Symptoms include headache, fever, and mouth and tongue blisters. The blisters go away in about 1 week, and total healing is complete by 2 or 3 weeks.

footdrop, an inability to flex the foot backward. It is caused by damage to a leg (peroneal) nerve. Also called **dropped foot.**

foramen /fôrā′mən/, *pl.* **foramina,** an opening (aperture) in a membrane or bone. For example, the **foramen mag-**

num is a passage in the skull (occipital) bone through which the spinal cord enters the spinal column. The **foramen ovale** is an opening in the wall between the upper chambers (atria) in the fetal heart. The foramen ovale begins to close after the newborn takes the first breath and full circulation through the lungs begins.

Forbes-Albright syndrome, a hormone disorder with lack of menstruation (amenorrhea) and with breast milk abnormalities. The cause is a tumor of the pituitary gland.

force, energy applied so that it begins motion, changes the speed or direction of motion, or changes the size or shape of an object.

forced expiratory volume (FEV), the volume of air that can be forced out in 1 second after taking a deep breath. Compare **vital capacity.**

forceps, any of a large number of surgery instruments, all of which have two handles or sides, each attached to a blade. Forceps are used to grasp, handle, press, pull, or join tissue, equipment, or supplies.

forceps delivery, a childbirth operation in which forceps are used to deliver a baby. It is done to help a difficult childbirth, to quickly deliver a baby with breathing problems, or, most often, to shorten normal labor. The forceps are put into the vagina and placed so that the baby's head is held firmly between the blades. The head is then carefully pulled from the birth passage. When the head has been delivered the forceps are removed and the delivery is completed by hand. Otherwise, cesarean section may be carried out if necessary.

forceps rotation, a childbirth operation in which forceps are used to turn a baby's head in the birth canal. It may be done to help emergency birth or as the first step in a forceps delivery.

foreign body, any object or substance found in a body organ or tissue in which it does not belong.

foreign body obstruction, a blockage caused by an object stuck in a body opening, passage, or organ. Most cases occur in children who breathe in or swallow a foreign object or put it in a body opening. In adults, pieces of hastily eaten food often stick in the throat (esophagus), causing choking and, if the airway is blocked, suffocation.

foreign medical graduate (FMG), a physician trained in and graduated from a medical school outside the United States and Canada. United States citizens graduated from medical schools outside the United States and Canada are also called FMGs.

forensic medicine /fôren′-/, a branch of medicine that deals with the legal side of health care. **Forensic psychi-**

atry also deals with legal issues, especially that of insanity for legal purposes.

foreskin, a loose fold of skin that covers the end of the penis or clitoris. Removing it is called circumcision. Also called **prepuce.**

forewaters, the amniotic fluid between the fetus and the fetal membranes.

formaldehyde /fôrmal'dəhīd/, a poisonous, colorless, foul-smelling gas that can be dissolved in water and used in that form to preserve things.

formula, a simple statement, generally using numbers and other symbols, showing the contents of a chemical compound, or a method for preparing a substance.

formulary /fôr'myələr'ē/, a list of drugs. Hospitals keep formularies that list all drugs commonly stocked in the hospital pharmacy.

fornication /fôr'nəkā'shən/, sexual intercourse between two people who are not married to each other. The specific legal definition varies from one area to another. In some, both persons are unmarried; in others, one is unmarried.

fortified milk, pasteurized milk with one or more nutrients, usually vitamin D, which has been standardized at 400 International Units per quart.

Foster bed, a special bed used in the care and treatment of severely injured patients, especially those with spinal injuries. It permits horizontal turning of the patient without moving the spine.

Fowler's position, the posture taken by the patient when the head of the bed is raised 18 or 20 inches and the patient's knees are raised. A **high-Fowler's position** places the patient in a near sitting position by raising the head of the bed at more than a 45-degree angle. In a **semi-Fowler's position,** the patient is in a leaning position, with the upper half of the body raised by elevating the head of the bed.

fractionation, the giving of a dose of radiation in smaller units over a period of time rather than in a single large dose to reduce tissue damage.

fracture, an injury to a bone in which the tissue of the bone is broken. A fracture is named by the bone involved, the part of that bone, and the nature of the break. A **complete fracture** is a bone break that completely severs the bone across its width. A **complex fracture** severely damages the soft tissue around the bone. A **fragmented fracture** results in many broken bone pieces. A **compound** or **open fracture** is a break in which the broken end or ends of the bone tear through the skin. In a **simple fracture,** the bone does not break the skin. **Multiple fracture** refers to a break in which there are several fracture lines in one bone. It can also mean the fracture of several bones at one time or from the same injury. See also specific entry.

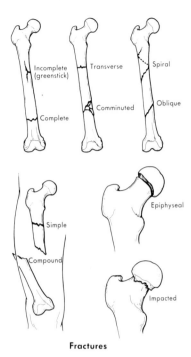

Fractures

fracture-dislocation, a broken bone involving the bony structures of any joint, with dislocation of the same joint.

fraternal twins. See **twins.**

freckle, a brown or tan spot on the skin usually caused by exposure to sunlight. There is an inherited tendency to getting freckles, often seen in persons with red hair.

free association, **1.** the automatic, unrestricted association of ideas, feelings, or mental images. **2.** automatic speaking of thoughts and emotions that enter the consciousness during psychoanalysis.

free clinic, a clinic or health program, usually located in a neighborhood, that provides health care for walk-in patients at little or no cost.

Freiberg's infarction, an abnormal condition with breakdown of bone tissue. It most commonly affects bones of the foot.

Frei test /frī/, a test for a type of cancer (lymphogranuloma venereum).

Frejka splint /frā'kə/, a device made up of a pillow that is belted between the legs of a baby born with dislocated hips. See also **congenital dislocation of the hips.**

fremitus /frem'itəs/, a trembling movement of the chest wall that can be heard or felt by an examining physician. A **bronchial fremitus** is a vibration caused by mucus rattling in a bronchus as the air passes during breathing. A **coarse fremitus** is a rough, loud vibration of the chest wall as a person breathes in and out, as with pneumonia. **Tactile fremitus** is a shaking vibration of the chest wall during breathing. It may indicate inflammation, infection, or congestion.

frenotomy /frenot′əmē/, a surgery for repairing a defective band of tissue, such as a tongue ligament to correct tongue-tie (ankyloglossia).

frequency, the number of repetitions of anything within a fixed period of time, as the number of heart beats per minute.

Freudian /froi′dē·ən/, referring to Sigmund Freud (1856–1939), his psychology ideas, and rules. These ideas stress the early years of childhood as the basis for later neurotic disorders.

friction, the act of rubbing one object against another. See also **attrition.**

friction burn, tissue injury caused by rubbing the skin. See also **abrasion.**

friction rub, a dry, grating sound heard with a stethoscope during a medical examination. It is normal when heard over the liver and spleen. A friction rub heard over the heart suggests there may be inflammation of the sac that surrounds the heart; a pleural friction rub over the lungs may be present in heart or lung disease.

Friedreich's ataxia /frēd′rīshs/. See **ataxia.**

Friedman's test, a pregnancy test. A sample of urine from a woman is injected into a mature, unmated female rabbit. If, 2 days later, the rabbit ovaries show signs of ovulation, the test indicates that the woman is pregnant.

frigid, 1. lacking warmth of feeling, emotions, or imagination; without passion or strong feeling and stiff or formal in manner. **2.** referring to a woman who has no response to sexual stimulation, or is not able to have an orgasm during sexual intercourse. Compare **impotence.** See also **orgasm.** –**frigidity,** *n.*

frôlement /frôlmäN′/, the rustling type of sound often heard in the chest in diseases of the heart sac (pericardium).

frontal lobe. See **brain.**

frontal lobe syndrome, behavior and personality changes seen following a cancer or injury of the frontal lobe of the brain. The patient may act freely, show off, and burst into a rage or become irritable. In other cases the person may become depressed, lack energy, and not care about personal appearance.

frontal sinus. See **nasal sinus.**

frostbite, the effect of extreme cold on skin and other tissues. Paleness of exposed skin surfaces, particularly the nose, ears, fingers, and toes, is the first symptom. Damage to blood vessels stops local circulation and results in oxygen starvation and tissue death. Gentle warming is first aid

treatment; rubbing the affected part is avoided. Compare **chilblain, immersion foot.**

frotteur /frôtœr′/, a person who gets sexual pleasure from rubbing against the clothing of another person (frottage).

frozen section method, a rapid way to get a tissue sample ready for a laboratory examination. The tissue is quick-frozen, and cut into thin slices. This allows the physician to examine the sample during surgery.

fructose /fruk′tōs, frook′-/, a form of sugar that is sweeter than sucrose. It is found in honey, in fruits, and combined in many carbohydrates. It is given in the veins as a food. If insulin is lacking, it is used up or changed in the body to glycogen. Also called **fruit sugar, levulose.**

fructosuria /frook′təsoor′ē·ə/, having the sugar fructose in the urine. This usually harmless condition is caused by the hereditary lack of the enzyme fructokinase, which normally helps break down fructose. One form of fructosuria is linked to symptoms of diabetes.

FUDR, a trademark for an antivirus and anticancer drug (floxuridine).

fuel tender, any vehicle capable of supplying fuel to ground or airborne equipment.

fugue /fyoog/, a mental condition with lack of memory (amnesia) and physical flight from an undesired situation. The person appears normal and acts as though aware of activities and behavior. Later, the person cannot remember the actions or behavior. The condition may last for only a few days, but may continue for several years, during which the person may start an entirely different way of life. See also **automatism.**

fulcrum /ful′krəm, fool′-/, the stable position on which a lever, such as bones of the elbow joint, turns in moving an object. Many movements of the body are lever actions using fulcrums. The muscles provide the forces that move the bones acting as levers.

fulminating /ful′minā′ting/, rapid, sudden, severe, as an infection, fever, or bleeding.

Fulvicin, a trademark for an antifungus drug (griseofulvin).

function, an act, process, or series of processes that serve a purpose.

functional disease. See **disease.**

functional residual capacity, the amount of air still in the lungs at the end of normal breathing out.

fundal height, the height of the bottom (fundus) of the uterus. It is measured in centimeters from the top of the pubic bone joint (symphysis pubis) to the top of the uterus.

fundus /fun′dəs/, the base or the deepest part of an organ; the part farthest from the mouth of an organ, as the fundus of the uterus or the fundus of an eye.

funduscopy /fundus′kəpē/, the examination of the base (fundus) of the eye by means of an ophthalmoscope.

fungal infection /fung′gəl/, any inflammation caused by a fungus. Most fungal infections are mild, but hard to cure. In older or weakened people, some may become life-threatening. Some kinds of fungal infections are aspergillosis, candidiasis, and histoplasmosis.

fungemia /funjē′mē·ə/, the presence of fungi in the blood.

fungicide /fun′jisīd/, a drug that kills fungi.

Fungizone, a trademark for an antifungus drug (amphotericin B).

fungus /fung′gəs/, *pl.* **fungi** /fun′jī/, a simple parasitic plant that lacks chlorophyll. A simple fungus reproduces by budding; many-celled fungi reproduce by making spores. Of the 100,000 known species of fungi, about 10 cause diseases in humans. See also **fungal infection.**

funiculitis /fənik′yəlī′-/, any inflammation of a cordlike structure of the body, as the spinal cord or spermatic cord.

funiculus /fənik′yələs/, a division of the white matter of the spinal cord.

Furacin, a trademark for a skin medication (nitrofurazone).

Furadantin, a trademark for an antibiotic (nitrofurantoin).

furosemide /fyərō′səmid/, a fluid-releasing drug given to treat high blood pressure, kidney failure, and fluid pooling.

Furoxone, a trademark for an antiinfection and antiprotozoa drug (furazolidone).

furuncle /fyōōr′ungkəl/. See **boil.**

furunculosis /fyōōrung′kyəlō′-/, a serious skin disease marked by boils or successive crops of boils.

fusion, 1. the act of bringing together into a single thing, as in optical fusion. 2. the act of bringing together two or more bones of a joint. 3. the surgical joining together of two or more backbones.

E–F

G

gag reflex, a normal reflex triggered by touching the soft palate or back of the throat. The response raises the palate, retracts the tongue, and contracts the throat muscles.

gait, the manner or style of walking, including rhythm and speed. A **dorsiflexor gait** is an abnormal walk caused by weakness of the dorsiflexor muscles of the ankle. There is footdrop and excess knee and hip flexion to allow the involved foot to clear during the swing phase. The sole of the foot slaps forcibly against the ground.

galactokinase deficiency /gəlak′təkī′nas/, an inherited disorder of carbohydrate processing. Dietary galactose is not used. It builds up in the blood and may cause cataracts. Food containing galactose, as milk and other milk products, must be removed from the diet.

galactorrhea /gəlak′tôrē′ə/, milk flow not related to childbirth or nursing. The condition may be a symptom of a pituitary gland tumor.

galactose /gəlak′tōs/, a simple sugar found in lactose (milk sugar), nerve cell layers, sugar beets, gums, and seaweed.

galactosemia /gəlak′təsē′mē·ə/, an inherited disease of galactose processing with a lack of an enzyme. Shortly after birth, an intolerance to milk is evident. Liver and spleen enlargement, cataracts, and mental retardation develop. Because the removal of galactose from the diet ends all symptoms except mental retardation, early diagnosis and prompt therapy are required.

Galeazzi's fracture /gal′ē·at′sēz/, a fracture of the lower arm with a separation of the joint between the lower arm bones. Also called **Dupuytren's fracture.**

Galen's bandage /gā′lənz/, a bandage for the head, made up of a strip of cloth with each end divided into three pieces.

gall /gôl/. See **bile.**

gallbladder, a pear-shaped sac near the right lobe of the liver which holds bile. During digestion of fats, it contracts, sending bile into the first portion of the small intestine (duodenum). Blocking of the bile-carrying system may lead to liver disease (jaundice) and pain. It is a common condition in overweight, middle-aged women and may require removal.

gallbladder cancer, a cancer of the bile storage sac. Symptoms include loss of appetite, nausea, vomiting, weight loss, and severe pain near the right shoulder. Tumors of the gallbladder are often connected with gallstones. They are 3 to 4 times more common in women than in men and rarely occur before the age of 40. Physical examination shows an enlarged gallbladder in about half the cases. Complete removal of the gallbladder may cure the cancer, but partial removal of the liver also may be required.

gallstone, a mineral deposit (calculus) formed in the biliary tract, consisting of bile pigments and calcium salts. Gallstones may cause right-sided pain, blockage, and inflammation of the gallbladder. Increased amounts of cholesterol in the blood (as occurs in obesity), diabetes, underactive thyroid gland, biliary stasis, and inflammation of the biliary system promote the formation of gallstones. If stones cannot pass into the small intestine, an x-ray (cholangiogram) will reveal their location, and they can be surgically removed.

gamete /gam′ēt/, **1.** a mature male or female germ cell that is able to function in fertilization and that contains the haploid number of chromosomes. **2.** the egg (ovum) or sperm (spermatozoon). See also **haploid.**

gamma-aminobutyric acid (GABA), an amino acid that carries nerve messages. It is found in the brain, heart, lungs, kidneys.

gamma-efferent fiber, any of the motor nerve fibers that carry impulses from the central nervous system to the fibers of the muscles. The gamma efferent fibers are responsible for deep tendon reflexes, spasms, and stiffness.

gamma globulin. See **immune gamma globulin.**

gamma rays or **gamma radiation,** electromagnetic radiations of high energy originating in atomic nuclei and accompanying many nuclear reactions such as fission, radioactive decay, and neutron capture. Physically, gamma rays are identical with x-rays of high energy, the only essential difference being that the x-rays do not originate from atomic nuclei but are produced in other ways, e.g., by slowing down electrons of high energy. These constitute the most penetrating type of radiation and are the major external hazard. Symbol: γ.

gamone, a chemical substance released by the egg and sperm that is thought to attract the gametes of the opposite sex to facilitate union.

Gamulin Rh, a trademark for a passive immunizing agent, Rh$_o$(D), immune human globulin.

ganglion /gang′glē·on/, *pl.* **ganglia, 1.** a knot, or knotlike mass. **2.** one of the nerve cells collected in groups outside the central nervous system. The two types of ganglia are the sensory ganglia and the autonomic ganglia.

ganglionic blocking agent, a drug used to produce controlled low blood pressure as needed in some kinds of surgery. It also may be used in emergency treatment of high blood pressure. The drugs stop response of nerves to the action of nerve impulse transmitter (acetylcholine).

ganglioside /gang′glē·əsīd′/, a fatty substance found in the brain and other nervous system tissues. Buildup of gangliosides because of a birth defect results in Sandhoff's disease or Tay-Sachs disease.

gangrene /gang′grēn/, necrosis or death of tissue, usually the result of loss of blood supply or bacterial invasion. The arms and legs are most often affected, but gangrene can occur in the intestines, gallbladder, or other organs. Gangrene may have an offensive odor, spread rapidly, and result in death in a few days. **Dry gangrene** is a problem of diabetes mellitus that has led to a thickening and hardening of the walls of the arteries (arteriosclerosis) in which the affected leg or arm becomes cold, dry, and shriveled and eventually turns black. **Moist gangrene** may follow a crushing injury or a blocking of blood flow by a clot or air bubble (embolism), tight bandages, or tourniquet. **Gas gangrene** is tissue death accompanied by gas bubbles in soft tissue after surgery or injury. It is caused by anaerobic organisms. Symptoms include pain, swelling, and tenderness of the wound area, mild fever, and rapid heart beat. The skin around the wound dies and ruptures, revealing dead muscle tissue. If untreated, gas gangrene is quickly fatal. In all types of gangrene, surgery is needed to remove the dead tissue. –**gangrenous,** *adj.*

Gantanol, a trademark for an antibiotic (sulfamethoxazole).

Gantrisin, a trademark for an antibiotic (sulfisoxazole).

Garamycin, a trademark for an antibiotic (gentamicin sulfate).

Gardner-Diamond syndrome, a disorder with large, painful, black-and-blue bruises that appear without apparent cause but often occur with emotional upsets or abnormal processing of protein.

Gardner's syndrome. See **polyposis.**

gargle, 1. to hold and move a liquid at the back of the throat by tilting the head back and forcing air through the liquid. The process cleans or medicates the mouth and throat. **2.** a solution used to rinse the mouth and throat.

gargoylism /gär′goilizm/. See **mucopolysaccharidosis.**

gas, an airlike fluid with the property of indefinite expansion. A gas has no fixed shape, and its volume is defined by temperature and pressure. Compare **liquid, solid.**

gasoline poisoning. See **petroleum distillate poisoning.**

gastrectomy /gastrek′-/, surgical removal of part or all of the stomach. It may be done to remove a peptic ulcer, to stop bleeding in an ulcer, or to remove a cancer. Usually, one half to two thirds of the stomach is removed, including the ulcer and a large area of acid-releasing mucosa. The remainder of the stomach is then joined to the middle part or the first part of the small intestine (jejunum or duodenum). If a cancer is found, the chest cavity is opened and the entire stomach is removed, along with the membrane that covers the stomach (omentum) and, usually, the spleen. The jejunum is connected to the esophagus.

gastric /gas′trik/, referring to the stomach.

gastric analysis, examination of the contents of the stomach. It is usually done to determine the quantity of acid present and the presence of blood, bile, bacteria, and abnormal cells. A sample of gastric juice and other substances is obtained via a tube passed through the nose and throat into the stomach.

gastric cancer, a cancer of the stomach. It occurs more often in men than in women and peaks at 50 to 59 years of age. Many cases show no symptoms in the early stages, and an enlarged lymph node may be the first sign of a stomach cancer. Symptoms include vague pains in the pit of the stomach (epigastrium), loss of appetite, weight loss, and unexplained iron-deficiency anemia. Treatment includes surgery (gastrectomy) with removal of involved tissues and repair of the remainder of the stomach.

gastric fistula, an abnormal passage into the stomach, usually opening on the outer surface of the abdomen. A gastric fistula may be made surgically to provide tube feeding for patients with severe disease of the esophagus.

gastric intubation. See **nasogastric intubation.**

gastric juice, digestive fluids of the gastric glands in the stomach. Excess release of gastric juice may lead to irritation of the stomach lining and to peptic ulcer.

gastric lavage. See **lavage.**

gastric motility, the movements of the stomach that aid in digestion, moving food through the stomach and into the first section of the small intestine (duodenum). Too much gastric motility causes pain that is usually treated with antispasm drugs.

gastric node, any of the lymph glands linked to an organ in the abdomen or pelvis.

gastric ulcer. See **peptic ulcer.**

G-H

gastrin /gas′trin/,   a hormone, released by the opening to the stomach (pylorus). It causes the flow of gastric juice and causes bile and pancreatic enzyme release.

gastritis /gastrī′-/,   an inflammation of the lining of the stomach. The symptoms — loss of appetite, nausea, vomiting, and discomfort after eating — usually go away after the cause has been removed. **Acute gastritis** may be caused by severe burns, major surgery, aspirin, or other drugs, by food allergens or by the presence of viral, bacterial, or chemical poisons. **Chronic gastritis** is usually a sign of underlying disease, such as peptic ulcer or stomach cancer. **Antral gastritis** refers to a defect in which the lower part (antrum) of the stomach near the opening to the duodenum (pyloris) becomes too narrow. It is not a true gastritis, but is either an ulcer or a tumor. **Atrophic gastritis** is a long-term inflammation of the stomach, with the breakdown of the mucous membranes of the stomach. This is sometimes seen in elderly patients. It is also seen in patients with severe anemia (pernicious). Atrophic gastritis may cause pain just below the breastbone. In **giant hypertrophic gastritis,** large bumpy folds of tissue cover the wall of the stomach. X-ray or endoscopic examination or surgery may be needed to identify this disease. **Hemorrhagic gastritis** is usually caused by a toxic agent, as alcohol, aspirin or other drugs, or bacterial poisons that irritate the lining of the stomach. Treatment includes drugs to shrink the blood vessels. Nausea, vomiting, and heartburn may persist after the irritant is removed. **Hypertrophic gastritis** is distinguished from other forms of gastritis by the presence of enlarged glands and lumps on the wall of the stomach. This condition often occurs with peptic ulcer, Zollinger-Ellison syndrome, or too much production of stomach fluids. **Phlegmonous gastritis** occurs as a result of an infection, peptic ulcer, cancer, surgery, or severe stress.

gastrocnemius /gas′trok·nē′mē·əs/,   a muscle in the back of the leg.

gastrocolic reflex,   a wavelike movement of the colon that often occurs when food enters the stomach. When an infant is fed, this reflex may cause a bowel movement.

gastroenteritis /-en′tərī′-/,   inflammation of the stomach and intestines that comes with many diseases. Symptoms include loss of appetite, nausea, vomiting, abdominal pain, and diarrhea. The disorder may be caused by bacterial or viral infections, chemical irritants, or other conditions, as lactose intolerance. Treatment requires bed rest, replacement of nutrients, and drugs to control vomiting and diarrhea.

gastroenterostomy /-en′təros′təmē/,   an operation to form an artificial opening between the stomach and the small intestine, usually at the middle part of the small intestine (jejunum). With part of the stomach removed, the operation is done to route food from the remainder of the stomach into the small intestine, or it is done to treat an ulcer. Compare **gastrectomy.**

gastroesophageal /-ēsof′əjē′əl/,   referring to the stomach and the esophagus.

gastrointestinal /-intes′tinəl/,   referring to the organs of the gastrointestinal tract, from mouth to anus.

gastrointestinal bleeding,   any bleeding from the stomach and intestines. Gastrointestinal bleeding is treated as a possible emergency. Vomiting of bright red blood, called **hematemesis** indicates rapid bleeding of the upper digestive tract. It is often linked to enlarged veins in the gullet or peptic ulcer. Coffee-ground-colored and textured vomit also indicates bleeding from the esophagus, stomach, or upper small intestine (duodenum). The passage of red blood through the rectum, called **hematochezia,** is usually from bleeding in the colon or rectum, but it can result from the loss of blood higher in the digestive tract. Blood passed from the stomach or small intestine generally loses its red color because of contact with enzymes. Cancer, colitis, and ulcers are among causes of hematochezia. Abnormal, black, tarry stools containing digested blood are called **melena.** This usually results from bleeding in the upper bowel or stomach. It is often a sign of peptic ulcer. See also **coffee ground vomitus.**

gastrointestinal obstruction,   any blocking of the movement of intestinal contents. Symptoms include vomiting, abdominal pain, and abdominal bloating. Loss of fluids and exhaustion may follow. Bowel sounds are softer than normal or absent. Blockage may be caused by bands of scar tissue that have developed from surgery, hernia, or tumor, or the problem may be a muscle failure. A lack of movement may follow anesthesia, abdominal surgery, or the closing of any of the arteries to the gut.

gastrointestinal system assessment,   examination of the patient's digestive system. The patient is asked if there is or has been pain or tenderness in the mouth, gums, tongue, lips, or abdomen, or instances of belching, heartburn, nausea, vomiting, constipation, diarrhea, or painful bowel movements. Changes in eating, bowel habits, the color, character, frequency of stools and urine, the use of laxatives or enemas, and swelling of the limbs are noted. The abdomen is examined for swelling, stiffness, rigidity, fluid buildup, enlarged liver, visible digestive movement, and bowel sounds. The area around the anus is inspected for its general condition, color, odor, or hemorrhoids. The family medical history, especially of stomach and bowel disease, cancer, and diabetes, is important. A complete examination will also include some laboratory tests and x-ray films.

gastroschisis /gastros′kisis/,   a birth defect of incomplete closing of the abdomen wall which causes the intestines to bulge out. Compare **omphalocele.**

gastroscopy /gastros'kəpē/, the inspection of the inside of the stomach by means of a device put in through the esophagus. See also **endoscopy.**

gastrostomy /gastros'-/, an operation to create an artificial opening into the stomach through the abdominal wall. It may be done to feed a patient with cancer of the esophagus or one who is expected to be unconscious for a long time. The front wall of the stomach is drawn forward and sewn to the abdominal wall. A tube is then inserted into an opening made in the stomach, and the opening is tightly sewn to prevent leaking of the contents of the stomach. The tube can be clamped shut, or opened to pass liquid food into the stomach. See also **colostomy, ostomy.**

gastrula /gas'troōlə/, a term used for a human embryo in an early stage of development.

gatch bed, a bed with an adjustable joint that allows the knees to bend and supports the legs.

Gaucher's disease /gōshāz'/, a disease of fat processing linked to the lack of an enzyme. It is identified by liver, spleen, lymph node, and bone marrow disorders. The death rate for this disease is high, but children with the disease who survive through their teen years may live for many years. See also **lipidosis.**

gauntlet bandage /gônt'lət/, a glovelike bandage that covers the hand and the fingers. A **demigauntlet bandage** leaves the fingers free.

gauze /gôz/, a fabric of open weave that is usually made of cotton. It is used in surgery and for bandages and dressings. **Absorbable gauze** can be taken up by the body. It is put on a wound to stop the flow of blood. **Absorbent gauze** is used for soaking up fluids. **Antiseptic gauze** is soaked in an antiseptic fluid. It is sometimes packaged in separate, sealed packets. **Aseptic gauze** refers to any gauze that is free of microorganisms. **Petrolatum gauze** is covered with white petrolatum.

gavage /gäväzh'/, the process of feeding a patient through a tube. See also **nasogastric feeding.**

gavage feeding of the newborn, a method for feeding an infant in which a tube is passed through the nose or mouth into the stomach. It is used to feed a newborn with weak sucking, uncoordinated sucking and swallowing, or difficult breathing.

gay, 1. any person who is homosexual. **2.** referring to homosexuality.

gaze palsy, a condition where the patient cannot move the eyes to all directions. It is often named for the affected direction of looking, as a right gaze palsy.

g.c., *informal.* abbreviation for **gonococcus,** the organism that causes gonorrhea.

geiger counter or **geiger-müller (GM) meter,** an instrument designed primarily for the detection of radiation or contamination. It is a very sensitive and reliable instrument, but it has a limited capacity for measuring radiation and may fail at high radiation levels.

gel, a substance that is firm even though it contains a large amount of liquid. It is used to soothe irritations, to stop oozing or bleeding, or to apply other drugs to an area to be treated.

gelatin film, an absorbable material used to control bleeding during surgery.

gelatin sponge, an absorbable material used to control bleeding in surgery and to promote healing of bed sores.

Gelusil, a trademark for a drug used to treat the stomach and bowel. It contains antigas medicine (simethicone) and antacids (aluminum and magnesium hydroxide).

gemfibrozil, a drug prescribed for excess fats in the blood.

gemmation /jemā'shən/, the way a cell reproduces by budding.

Gemonil, a trademark for an anticonvulsant drug (metharbital).

Genapax Tampon, a trademark for a tampon treated to fight infection (gentian violet).

gender, the particular sex of a person. See also **sex.**

gender identity, the sense of knowing to which sex one belongs. The process begins in infancy, continues during childhood, and is strengthened during the teenage years.

gender identity disorder, a condition marked by a long-lasting feeling of discomfort over one's sex. It usually begins in childhood with gender identity problems and may appear during the teen years or adulthood as asexuality, homosexuality, transvestism, or transsexualism.

gene /jēn/, the unit that carries physical characteristics from parent to child. The gene is thought to be a certain nucleic acid within a DNA molecule that holds a precise area on a chromosome. It also is capable of copying itself. In humans and other mammals, genes occur as pairs. They structure and regulate the way body cells and tissues develop. A **dominant gene** is one that produces a trait. A **recessive gene** carries a trait that is masked or hidden if there is a dominant gene at the same place on a matching chromosome. If genes on both chromosomes are recessive and cause the same trait, that trait is seen in the individual. A **lethal gene** produces an effect causing death of the organism at some stage of development from fertilization of the egg to adulthood. In humans, examples of diseases caused by lethal genes are Huntington's chorea and sickle cell anemia. A **mutant gene** is any that has had a change, as the loss, gain, or exchange of genetic material, which affects the normal inheritance of a trait. See also **chromosome.**

general adaptation syndrome (GAS), the defense response of the body or mind to injury or prolonged stress. It begins with a stage of shock or alarm, followed by resistance or adaptation, and ends in a state of adjustment and

G-H

healing or of exhaustion and disintegration. Also called **adaptation syndrome.** See also **stress reaction.**

general anesthesia, the total lack of sensation and consciousness as brought on by anesthetic agents. They are usually breathed-in or injected into a vein. The kind of anesthesia used and the dose and route by which it is given depend on the reason for anesthesia.

generally recognized as effective (GRAE), a standard that must be met by a drug before it can be approved by the FDA as a "new drug." To be recognized as effective, the drug must be considered safe and effective by scientific experts.

generally recognized as safe (GRAS), a classification by the Food and Drug Administration of food substances, especially colors, flavors, and other food additives, that are considered free of harmful effects when eaten by humans in small amounts.

general paresis. See **paresis.**

general practitioner (GP), a family practice doctor. See also **family medicine.**

general staff, the group of incident management personnel comprised of: incident commander, operation chief, planning chief, logistics chief, and finance chief.

generation, **1.** the act or process of producing young; procreation. **2.** the period of time between the birth of one individual or organism and the birth of its offspring.

generic /jənər′ik/, referring to the name of a kind of drug that is also the description of the drug, as penicillin or tetracycline.

generic equivalent, a drug sold under its generic name, identical in chemical composition to a drug sold under a trademark.

generic name, the official name assigned to a drug. A given drug is licensed under its generic name, and all manufacturers of the drug list it by its generic name. However, a drug is usually marketed under a trademark chosen by the manufacturer.

genesis /jen′əsis/, **1.** the origin, generation, or developmental evolution of anything. **2.** the act of producing or procreating. –**genetic,** adj.

gene splicing, the process by which a piece of DNA is attached to or inserted in a strand of DNA from another source. See also **genetic engineering.**

genetic code /jənet′ik/, information carried by the DNA molecules that decides the physical traits of an offspring, as eye color or hair color. The code fixes the pattern of amino acids that build body tissue proteins in a cell. An error in the code can result in a wrong arrangement of the amino acids in the protein, causing a birth defect.

genetic counseling, the providing of information and advice about diseases that can be inherited. Counseling may involve a child already born, a pregnancy, or a deci-

sion to end a pregnancy or to be made sterile. Special tests may be needed in genetic counseling. See also **genetic screening.**

genetic engineering, the process of making new DNA molecules. Enzymes are used to break the DNA molecule into pieces so that genes from another organism can be put into the chromosomes of another species. Through genetic engineering such human proteins as the growth hormone, insulin, and interferon have been produced in bacteria.

genetics, **1.** the science that studies the principles and mechanics of heredity, or the means by which traits are passed from parents to offspring. **Clinical genetics** is a branch of the study of genetics that looks at inherited disorders. It studies the possible genetic factors that may cause the onset of a disease. **2.** the total genetic makeup of a particular individual, family, group, or condition.

genetic screening, the study of a group for the purpose of finding an inherited disease. Genetic screening helps identify those in certain ethnic groups who have a high incidence of a particular disease, specifically sickle cell anemia in blacks and Tay-Sachs disease in Ashkenazic Jews. See also **genetic counseling.**

geniculate neuralgia /jənik′yəlāt/, a severe inflammation of the facial nerve. Symptoms include pain, loss of the sense of taste, paralysis of the face, and a decrease in saliva and tears. It sometimes follows herpes zoster infection.

geniohyoideus /jē′nē·ōhī·oi′dē·əs/, one of the muscles rising from the lower jaw. It acts to draw the hyoid bone in the neck and the tongue forward.

genitals, the reproductive organs.

genital stage, the final period in the growth of sexual emotion. It begins with the teenage years and continues through the adult years. See also **psychosexual development.**

genitourinary (GU) /jen′itōyŏŏr′iner′ē/, referring to the sexual and urinary systems of the body, either the organs or their workings, or both. Also called **urogenital.**

genome /jē′nōm/, the complete set of genes in the chromosomes of each cell of a particular individual.

genotype /jē′nōtīp′/, the complete set of genes of an organism or group, as determined by the combination and location of the genes on the chromosomes. Compare **phenotype.** –**genotypic,** adj.

gentamicin sulfate, an antibiotic given to relieve severe infections.

gentian violet /jen′shən/, A drug that attacks bacteria, fungus, and intestinal worms. It is given to treat pinworms, infections of the skin, and infections of the vagina.

genu /jē′nōō/, the knee or any angular structure in the body that is shaped like the flexed knee.

genupectoral position /-pek′tərəl/. See **body position.**

genus /jē'nəs/, *pl.* **genera** /jen'ərə/, a subdivision of a family of animals or plants. A genus usually is made up of several closely related species. The genus *Homo* has only one species, humans (Homo sapiens).

Geocillin, a trademark for an antibiotic (carbenicillin indanyl sodium).

geographic tongue, small white-to-yellow plaques that develop on the tongue. They gradually get bigger, shed cells in the center, and leave red patches surrounded by thickened white borders. The patches grow together, forming figures with curved outlines. The disease may persist for months or years. It causes a burning or itching feeling, made worse by food, and is often linked to stomach and intestine problems, especially in children.

Geopen, a trademark for an antibiotic (carbenicillin disodium).

geotrichosis /jē'ōtrikō'-/, an abnormal condition, linked with a fungus, *Geotrichum candidum,* which may cause diseases of the mouth, throat, windpipe, and intestines. Lung and windpipe problems may produce a cough with thick, bloody sputum. There may be asthmatic reactions and an intestinal disorder with stomach and bowel pain, diarrhea, and bleeding from the rectum. Geotrichosis most often occurs in people with poor disease resistance and in diabetics. Treatment includes gentian violet.

geriatrics /jer'ē·at'-/, the branch of medicine dealing with aging and the diagnosis and treatment of diseases affecting the aged.

germ, 1. any microorganism, especially one that causes disease. **2.** a unit of living matter able to develop into a self-sufficient organism, as a seed, spore, or egg. **3.** a sexual reproductive cell as a sperm or egg.

German measles. See **rubella.**

germ cell, 1. a sexual reproductive cell in any stage of development. **2.** an egg or sperm or any of their preceding forms.

germicide, a drug that kills disease causing microorganisms.

germinal stage, the space of time in which the egg becomes fertilized, undergoes cell division several times, travels to the womb, and, as a blastocyst, begins to implant itself in the lining of the womb (endometrium). The germinal stage is over at about 10 days of gestation.

germination, the first growth and development of an organism from the time of fertilization to the forming of the embryo. **–germinate,** *v.*

germ layer. See **embryonic layer.**

germ plasm, the material of the germ cells that holds the basic reproductive and hereditary codes; the sum total of the DNA in a particular cell or organism.

gerontology /jer'ontol'-/, the study of all aspects of aging, including medical, mental, and other problems met by the elderly, and their effects on both the individual and society.

gestate /jes'tāt/, **1.** to carry a growing fetus in the womb. **2.** to grow and develop slowly toward maturity, as a fetus in the womb.

gestation, the period of time from the fertilization of the egg until birth. Gestation varies with the species; in humans the average length is 266 days or approximately

G–H

Genetic diseases

Disorders of carbohydrate metabolism	Disorders of metal metabolism
Diabetes mellitus	Wilson's disease
Pentosuria	Hemochromatosis
Glycogen storage diseases	
Galactosemia	**Disorders of connective tissue, bone, and muscle**
	Familial periodic paralysis
Disorders of lipid metabolism	Muscular dystrophies
Familial lipoprotein deficiency	Mucopolysaccharidoses
Familial lecithin-cholesterol acyltranferase (L-CAT) deficiency	
Tay-Sachs disease	**Disorders of the hematopoietic system and blood**
Gaucher's disease	Sickle cell anemia
	Glucose-6-phosphate dehydrogenase deficiency
Disorders of protein metabolism	Thalassemias
Familial goiter	Hereditary spherocytosis
Phenylketonuria	
Albinism	**Disorders of exocrine glands**
Alkaptonuria	Cystic fibrosis
Tyrosinosis	
Disorders of purine and pyrimidine metabolism	
Gout	
Lesch-Nyhan syndrome	

280 days from the beginning of the last menstrual period. See also **pregnancy.**

gestational age, the age of a fetus or a newborn, usually stated in weeks dating from the first day of the mother's last menstrual period.

ghost cells, red blood cells that have lost their hemoglobin so that only the cell covering can be seen when a urine sample is examined under a microscope.

GI, abbreviation for **gastrointestinal.**

giant cell carcinoma, a cancer containing many very large primitive cells. Some lung and liver cancers contain such cells.

giant follicular lymphoma, a white blood cell disease in which many bumps change the normal structure of a lymph node. Also called **Brill-Symmer's disease.**

gibbus /gib'əs, jib'əs/, **1.** a hump, or swelling, on a body surface, usually on just one side. **2.** an abnormal curving of the spine that may happen after a back bone breaks down. It may result from a broken bone or from tuberculosis of the spine.

Gibson walking splint, a kind of leg splint that allows a patient to walk.

gigantism /jīgan'-/, an abnormal condition marked by excess height and weight. Causes include excess release of growth hormone (GH) and some genetic disorders. Gigantism with normal body proportions and normal sexual development usually comes from excess GH in early childhood. Decreased gonad function (hypogonadism), by slowing puberty and closure of the growing ends of the bones, may lead to gigantism. Excessive growth often happens in males with more than one Y chromosome, and it may occur with Klinefelter's syndrome, Marfan's syndrome, and some cases of fat disorders. See also **acromegaly.**

Gilbert's syndrome, an inherited condition with excessive bile color in the blood and liver disease (jaundice). No treatment is needed.

Gilles de la Tourette syndrome /zhēl'dəläto-oret'/, an abnormal condition of childhood, marked by face twitches, tics, and uncontrolled arm and shoulder motions. In adolescence, the condition gets worse; the child may grunt, snort, and shout without control. Obscene speech often develops. Treatment with drugs has been found to be very effective, showing an organic cause for this disorder.

Gillies' operation /gil'ēz/, an operation that reduces fractures of a skull area near the ear (zygoma and zygomatic arch) by making a cut at the hairline near the temple.

gingiva /jinjī'və/, pl. **gingivae,** the gum of the mouth, a mucous membrane and its supporting fiberlike tissue that circles the necks of teeth.

gingival hyperplasia, a disorder in which gum tissue grows too fast. It is often seen in patients treated with a drug (phenytoin) for epileptic seizures.

gingival massage, the massage of the gums to clean them, improve tissue tone and blood circulation, and harden their surface.

gingivectomy /-vek'/, removal of infected and diseased gum tissue (pyorrhea). Compare **gingivoplasty.**

gingivitis /-vī'-/, a condition in which the gums are red, swollen, and bleeding. Most gingivitis is the result of poor mouth care and the buildup of plaque on the teeth. It also may be a sign of another disorder, as diabetes mellitus, leukemia, or vitamin deficiency. It is common in pregnancy.

gingivoplasty /jin'jivəplas'tē/, the surgical shaping of the gums to maintain healthy gum tissue. Compare **gingivectomy.**

gingivostomatitis /-stō'mətī'-/, painful ulcers on the gums and mucous membranes of the mouth. It is the result of a herpesvirus infection. See also **herpes simplex.**

Giordano-Giovannetti diet /jôrdä'nōjō'vänet'ē/, a low-protein, low-fat, high-carbohydrate diet with controlled potassium and sodium intake. It is used with patients who have long-term kidney and liver failure. The foods included are eggs, small amounts of milk, low-protein bread, and some fruits and vegetables low in potassium. See also **renal diet.**

glabella /gləbəl'ə/, a flat triangular area of bone of the forehead. It is sometimes used as a baseline for head measurements.

gland, an organ of specialized cells that releases fluid and substances for use in the body. Some glands produce fluids that smooth tissues and lessen friction. Others, like the pituitary gland, produce hormones, and glands such as the spleen, thyroid, and certain lymph nodes take part in the production of blood.

glans /glanz/, pl. **glandes** /glan'dēz/, **1.** a general term for a small, round mass or body. **2.** tissue that can swell and harden, as on the ends of the clitoris and the penis.

glans of clitoris, the tissue at the end of the clitoris that can swell and harden when filled with blood. It is made up of the corpora cavernosa enclosed in a dense, fiberlike membrane. Also called **glans clitoridis.**

glans penis, the cone-shaped tip of the penis that covers the end of the corpora cavernosa penis and the corpus spongiosum like a cap. The urethral opening is normally located at the center of the tip of the glans penis. The corona glandis, the widest part of the glans penis, is around the base. A fold of dark, thin, hairless skin forms the foreskin (prepuce).

Glasgow Coma Scale, a system for describing the degree of loss of consciousness in the severely ill. It is also used to predict the length and result of coma, mostly in patients with head injuries. The system involves three responses: eye opening, verbal response, and muscle response. These responses are graded in range from mild to severe loss of consciousness. For example, the five grades of verbal response range from correctly answering the questions ''who are you? where are you? what day and month is it?'' (mild) to not responding at all to questions, or answering by making sounds that do not form words (severe).

glaucoma /glôkō′mə, gloukō′mə/, an abnormal condition of high pressure within an eye. It is caused by a blocking of the normal flow of the fluid in the space between the cornea and lens of the eye (aqueous humor). **Acute (angle-closure, closed-angle,** or **narrow-angle) glaucoma** happens if the pupil in an eye with a narrow angle between the iris and cornea opens too wide and causes the folded iris to block the flow of aqueous humor. Symptoms include extreme eye pain, blurred vision, a red eye, and an abnormally wide-open pupil. Nausea and vomiting may occur. If untreated, acute glaucoma results in complete and permanent blindness within 2 to 5 days. **Chronic (open-angle** or **wide-angle) glaucoma** is much more common, often occurring in both eyes; it develops slowly and is an inherited disease. Chronic glaucoma may show no symptoms except for gradual loss of side vision over a period of years. Sometimes headaches, blurred vision, and dull pain in the eye are present. Halos around lights and blind spots in the center of the field of vision begin to occur after the condition has developed for a while.

Glaucon, a trademark for eye drops (epinephrine hydrochloride).

gliadin /glī′ədin/, a protein that is obtained from wheat and rye.

gliding, a smooth, continuous movement, the simplest allowed by various joints of the skeleton. It is common to all movable joints and allows one surface to move smoothly over the next surface, no matter what shape.

gliding joint, a joint in which facing bones allow only gliding movements, as in the wrist and the ankle. The ligaments or other tissues around each gliding joint limit motion. An example is any one of the gliding joints between the ribs and vertebrae linked to them, called **costotransverse articulation.** This excludes the eleventh and twelfth ribs.

glioma /glī·ō′mə/, any of the largest group of cancers of the brain, made of certain nerve cells (glial cells). An example is a **ganglionic glioma,** a tumor composed of nerve cells that are nearly mature. Another, **glioblastoma**

multiforme, is a fast-growing, pulpy cancer of the brain or the spinal cord. The tumor spreads by branching out. Other kinds of gliomas are **astrocytoma, ependymoma, medulloblastoma,** and **oligodendroglioma.** Also called **gliosarcoma.**

glioneuroma /glī′ōnŏŏrō′mə/, a cancer made of nerve cells and elements of their support tissue.

globule /glob′yōol/, a small round mass.

globulin /-in/, one of a broad category of simple proteins. Compare **albumin.**

globus hystericus, a feeling of a lump in the throat that cannot be swallowed or coughed up. It often accompanies emotional conflict or acute anxiety.

glomangioma /glōman′jē·ō′mə/, a tumor that develops from a group of blood cells in the skin. Also called **angioneuroma.**

glomerular disease /glōmer′yələr/, any of a group of diseases that affect the waste product filter (glomerulus) of the kidney. There may be overgrowth, tissue death, scarring, or deposits in the kidney glomeruli.

glomerulonephritis /glōmer′yəlōnəfrī′-/, an inflammation of the waste product filter (glomerulus) of the kidney. Symptoms include blood in the urine, less urine, and build-up of fluid in the tissues. **Chronic glomerulonephritis** is a noninfectious form. Symptoms develop slowly, but the disease progresses to high blood pressure, fatigue, itching, nausea, and vomiting. This ends with kidney failure. Control of high blood pressure by salt restriction and drugs is helpful. However, transplanting a new kidney and dialysis are the only treatments in the later stages. The cause of the disease is unknown.

glomerulus /glōmer′yələs/, *pl.* **glomeruli, 1.** a tuft or cluster. **2.** a netlike structure composed of blood vessels or nerve fibers, as a kidney glomerulus.

glossitis /glosī′-/, inflammation of the tongue. Severe glossitis, with swelling and pain, may be felt as an ear disorder. It may develop during an infection or following a burn, bite, or other injury.

glossodynia /glos′adin′ē·ə/, pain in the tongue, caused by inflammation, infection, or an open sore.

glossohyal /-hī′əl/, referring to the tongue and the horseshoe-shaped bone at the base of the tongue.

glossophytia /-fit′ē·ə/, a condition of the tongue in which a black patch develops on the back. The papillae are greatly elongated and thickened like bristly hairs. The usually painless condition may be caused by heavy smoking or the use of antibiotics.

glossoplasty /glos′əplas′tē/, a plastic surgery on the tongue. It may be done to correct a birth defect, repair an injury, or restore use of the tongue following removal of a cancer.

G–H

glossopyrosis /-pīrō'-/, a burning sense in the tongue caused by inflammation or by exposure to extremely hot or spicy food.

glottis, 1. a slitlike opening between the vocal cords (plica vocalis). **2.** the voice apparatus made up of the true vocal cords and the opening between them (rima glottidis). –**glottal, glottic,** adj.

glucagon /glōō'kəgon/, a hormone, produced in the islands of Langerhans. It stimulates the changing of glycogen to glucose in the liver. Secretion of glucagon is brought on by low blood sugar and by the growth hormone.

glucagonoma syndrome /-ō'mə/, a disease linked with a tumor of the pancreas. Symptoms include excess blood sugar, mouth inflammation, anemia, weight loss, and a rash.

glucocorticoid /glōō'kōkôr'tikoid/, a hormone that aids carbohydrate processing, acts to lessen inflammation and affects many body functions. Glucocorticoids aid the release of amino acids from muscle, take fatty acids from fat stores, and increase the ability of muscles to tighten and avoid fatigue. A lack of glucocorticoids features darkening of the skin, low blood sugar, weight loss, and lack of energy. An excess is linked to damaged sugar (glucose) use by the body, thinning of the skin, poor wound healing, infection, and overweight. Glucocorticoid release is triggered by a hormone of the pituitary.

glucose /glōō'kōs/, a simple sugar found in foods, especially fruits, and a major source of energy in body fluids. Glucose, when eaten or produced by the digestion of carbohydrates, is taken into the blood from the intestines. Excess glucose in circulation is stored in the liver and muscles as glycogen and converted to glucose and released as needed. The measuring of blood glucose levels is an important test in diabetes and other disorders. See also **dextrose, glycogen.**

glucose-tolerance test, a test of the body's ability to process carbohydrates by giving a dose of glucose and then measuring the blood and urine for glucose. The test is used to help in the diagnosis of diabetes or other disorders.

glucosuria /-sōōr'ē·ə/, abnormal levels of glucose in the urine from the eating of large amounts of carbohydrate or from a kidney disease, as nephrosis, or a processing disease, as diabetes mellitus. –**glucosuric,** adj.

glue sniffing, the practice of breathing the vapors of a compound (toluene) used as a solvent in certain glues. Intoxication and dizziness result. Long-term exposure, either accidental or knowing, may damage a number of organ systems.

glutamate /glōō'təmāt/, a salt of glutamic acid.

glutamic acid (Glu) /glōōtam'ik/, an amino acid occurring widely in a number of proteins.

glutamic acid hydrochloride, a drug given for low stomach acid. This drug should not be taken by patients with excess stomach acid, peptic ulcer, or a known allergy to the drug. Side effects include loose stools and acidosis.

glutamine (Gln), an amino acid found in many proteins in the body. It works in many reactions and helps remove ammonia from the body.

gluteal tuberosity, a ridge on the surface of the thigh bone to which is attached the gluteus maximus muscle.

gluten /glōō'tən/, a protein in wheat and other grains. It can be taken from flour by washing out the starch. It is used as an adhesive agent, and makes dough tough and elastic. Some persons cannot properly digest the gluten of some grains. See also **celiac disease.**

glutethimide, a drug that is given to soothe and quiet a patient. It is used to treat anxiety and insomnia.

glycerin, a sweet, colorless, oily fluid that is used in drug preparations. Glycerin is used as a moistener for chapped skin, as an ingredient of suppositories for constipation, and as a sweetener for drugs.

glycerol /glis'ərôl/, an alcohol that is contained in fats.

glycine (Gly) /glī'sin/, an amino acid found in many animal and plant proteins.

glycogen /glī'kəjən/, the major carbohydrate stored in animal cells. It is made from glucose and stored chiefly in the liver and, to some extent, in muscles. Glycogen is changed to glucose and released into circulation as needed by the body for energy. See also **glucose.**

glycogen storage disease, any of a group of inherited disorders of glycogen processing. Glycogen is a type of sugar needed for energy. An enzyme lack causes glycogen to be stored in too large amounts in various parts of the body.

glycolic acid, a substance in bile that aids in digestion and absorption of fats.

glycolipid, a compound made of a fat (lipid) and a carbohydrate found mostly in the tissue of the nerves.

glycoside /-sīd/, any of several carbohydrates that yield a sugar and a nonsugar when broken down. The plant *Digitalis purpurea* yields a glycoside used to treat heart disease.

glycosuria /-sōōr'ē·ə/, abnormal presence of a sugar, especially glucose, in the urine. It is usually linked with diabetes mellitus. –**glycosuric,** adj.

glycosuric acid, a compound that is made by the body as it processes tyrosine. It is found in the urine of people who have alkaptonuria.

gm, abbreviation for **gram.** Preferred is the abbreviation g.

gnathion /nā'thē·on/, the lowest point in the lower border of the lower jaw. It is a common reference point in the diagnosis and orthodontic treatment of poor bite (malocclusion).

goblet cell, one of the many special cells that release mucus and form glands of the lining of the stomach, the intestine, and parts of the respiratory tract.

goiter, an overgrown thyroid gland, usually seen as a swelling in the neck. The swelling may be linked disordered thyroid function. A goiter may be cystlike or fiberlike; it may surround a large blood vessel, or a part of the swollen gland may sit beneath the sternum or in the chest hollow. Normally the thyroid gland is located behind the Adam's apple. See also **Graves' disease.** –**goitrous,** *adj.*

gold (Au), a yellowish, soft metallic element.

gold compound, a drug containing gold salts. It is usually given with other drugs to treat rheumatoid arthritis. Gold can be poisonous and is used only under the care of a specialist in gold therapy (chrysotherapy).

gold inlay, a tooth repair made of gold alloy that is melted and formed to fit a hole in the crown of a tooth.

Golgi apparatus /gôl′jē/, one of many small structures found in the cytoplasm of most cells. It is linked to the forming of carbohydrate units of various substances. Also called **Golgi body.**

Golgi-Mazzoni corpuscles, a number of thin capsules that circle the nerve endings in the tissue under the skin layers of the fingers. They are special sensory end organs.

gomphosis /gomfō′-/, *pl.* **gomphoses,** a fiberlike joint formed by the insertion of a cone-shape into a socket. An example is the root of a tooth in a hollow (alveolus) of a jaw bone.

gonad /gō′nad/, a gland that releases gametes, as an ovary or a testis. –**gonadal,** *adj.*

gonadotropin /gon′ədōtrop′in/, a hormone that causes the testes and the ovaries to act.

gonioscope /gō′nē-əskōp′/, an eye instrument used to examine the angle of the anterior chamber of the eye.

gonococcus /gon′əkok′əs/, *pl.* **gonococci** /-kok′sī/, a bacterium of the species *Neisseria gonorrhoeae,* the cause of gonorrhea.

gonorrhea /gon′ərē′ə/, a common sexually carried disease. It most often affects the sex organs, bladder, and kidneys, and sometimes the throat, eye, or rectum. It is passed by contact with an infected person or by contact with body fluids containing *Neisseria gonorrhoeae.* Symptoms include difficult urinating, greenish-yellow pus flow from the urethra or vagina, and itching, burning, or pain around the vagina or urethra. The lower abdomen may be tense and very tender. As the infection spreads, which is more common in women than in men, nausea, vomiting, fever, and rapid heart beat may occur. Inflammation of the ovaries, fallopian tubes, or lining of the abdominal wall can develop. Inflammation of the tissues around the liver may cause pain in the upper right area of the abdomen. If the disease affects the eyes (**gonorrheal conjunctivitis**), there can be scars and blindness. There may be bloodstream infection, tender sores on the skin of the hands and feet, and inflammation of the tendons of the wrists, knees, and ankles. **Gonococcal pyomyositis** is an unusual form of gonorrhea. There is an acute inflammation of a muscle, a sore with pus (abscess), and pain. Gonorrhea is diagnosed by a microscopic study of a specimen of fluid. Penicillin or other drugs are used in treatment. The patient is tested 1 or 2 weeks later to make sure the drug was effective. The infected person's sexual contacts should be treated, and great care must be taken to prevent spread of the disease. The use of condoms during sexual intercourse offers protection against future infection.

good samaritan laws, series of laws written to protect emergency care personnel. These laws require a standard of care to be provided in good faith, to the level of training, and to the best of ability.

Goodell's sign, softening of the narrow opening of the womb (cervix), usually a sign of pregnancy.

Goodpasture's syndrome, a chronic disorder usually linked to an inflammation of the kidneys. Symptoms include coughing of blood, breathing difficulty, anemia, and kidney failure. Treatment may require a kidney transplant.

gooseflesh. See **pilomotor reflex.**

Gordon reflex, an abnormal change in the Babinski reflex. It is made by compressing the calf muscles. It results in stretching of the great toe and fanning of the other toes. The reflex is evidence of disease of the central nervous system. See also **Babinski's reflex.**

Gosselin's fracture /gôslaNz′/, a V-shaped break in the shinbone (tibia) that extends to the ankle.

gout, a disease of uric acid processing. It increases production or interferes with the passing of uric acid. Excess uric acid is converted to sodium urate crystals that settle into joints and other tissues. Men are more often affected than women. The great toe is a common site for the buildup of urate crystals. The condition can result in painful swelling of a joint, along with chills and fever. The disease is crippling and, if untreated, can lead to joint breakdown. Treatment usually includes drugs, a diet that excludes purine-rich foods, as organ meats, and may include surgery.

graafian follicle /graf′ē-ən/, a baglike structure in the ovary that breaks during ovulation to release an egg. Under the influence of the follicle-triggering hormone one ovarian follicle ripens into a graafian follicle during each menstrual cycle. The cells that form the graafian follicle are arranged in a layer 3 to 4 cells thick around a fluid. Within the follicle the egg triples in size and, when the follicle breaks, is swept into the opening of a fallopian tube. The hollow of the follicle collapses when the egg is released, and the cells enlarge to become the corpus luteum.

graduated bath, a bath in which the temperature of the water is slowly lowered.

GRAE, abbreviation for **generally recognized as effective.**

graft. See **transplant.**

graft-versus-host reaction, a rejection response of certain grafts, especially bone marrow. Rejection signs may include skin lesions with swelling, redness, open sores, scaling, and loss of hair. Such reactions may also affect the joints, the heart, and the blood cells.

grain (gr), the smallest unit of mass in avoirdupois, troy, and apothecaries' weights. It is the same in all and equal to 4.79891 mg. The troy and apothecaries' ounces contain 480 grains; the avoirdupois ounce contains 437.5 grains.

grain itch, a skin condition caused by a mite that lives in grain or straw. The sore is an itchy pimple topped by a tiny blister.

gram (g, gm), a unit of mass in the metric system equal to $\frac{1}{1000}$ of a kilogram, 15.432 grains, and 0.0353 ounce avoirdupois.

gram-molecular weight, the molecule weight of a substance expressed in grams.

Gram's stain, the method of staining microorganisms using a violet stain. It is followed by a counterstain. The retention of either the violet color of the stain (**gram-positive**) or the pink color of the counterstain (**gram-negative**) serves as a means of marking and typing bacteria.

grand mal seizure /gräNmäl′/. See **epilepsy.**

granular /gran′yələr/, **1.** looking or feeling like sand. **2.** appearing under the microscope to have a few or many particles within or on the surface. –**granularity,** *n.*

granulation tissue, soft, pink, fleshy bumps that form during the healing process of some wounds. It consists of many capillaries enclosed by fibrous tissue. Too much growth of granulation tissue results in a lump of flesh (proud flesh) growing above the skin.

granulocyte /gran′yələsīt′/, a white blood cell (leukocyte) containing granule in the cytoplasm. Kinds of granulocytes are **basophil, eosinophil, neutrophil.**

granulocyte transfusion, the use of specially prepared white blood cells to treat an abnormal decrease in granulocytes (neutropenia). The treatment also is used to prevent serious infection in leukemic patients or those receiving cancer chemotherapy. There are the same risks as a blood transfusion.

granulocytopenia /-sī′təpē′nē·ə/. See **neutropenia.**

granulocytosis /-sītō′-/, an abnormal condition of the blood, marked by an increase in the number of granulocytes.

granuloma /gran′yəlō′mə/, a tumor of the pink (granulation) tissue that forms during wound healing. It may result from inflammation, injury, or infection. Granulomas may disappear without treatment, become gangrenous, spread, or remain as a center of infection.

granulomatosis /-mətō′-/, a condition marked by granulomas.

granulosa cell tumor, a fleshy tumor with yellow streaks on an ovary. It may grow to an extremely large size and be linked to the excess production of estrogen. The tumor causes menstrual problems. Also called **folliculoma.**

GRAS, abbreviation for **generally recognized as safe.**

grasp reflex, a reflex brought on by stroking the palm or sole causing the fingers or toes to flex in a grasping motion. The reflex occurs in diseases of brain tissues. In young infants the tonic grasp reflex is normal: When one strokes the infant's palms, the stroking fingers are grasped so firmly that the child can be lifted into the air.

grass-line ligature, a fine cord made of the fibers of a plant. It is used in orthodontics for minor adjustments of the teeth. Its action depends on its ability to shrink when wetted by saliva.

Graves' disease, a disorder of excess thyroid hormone production. It is usually linked to an enlarged thyroid gland and bulging eyes (exophthalmia). Graves' disease, which is more common in women than in men, occurs most often between the ages of 20 and 40 and often follows an infection or physical or emotional stress. Symptoms include nervousness, a small tremor of the hands, weight loss, fatigue, breathlessness, palpitations, heat intolerance, and stomach and intestinal spasms. There may be an enlarged thymus, overgrowth of the lymph nodes, blurred or double vision, and heart and bone disorders. If poorly controlled, infection or stress may cause a life-threatening thyroid storm. Also called **toxic goiter.** See also **goiter.**

gravid, pregnant; carrying fertilized eggs or a fetus.

gravity, the heaviness or weight of an object caused by the universal effect of attraction between any object and any planetary body. The force of the gravity depends on the relative masses of the bodies and on the distance between them.

gray baby syndrome, a condition in premature infants, caused by a reaction to a drug (chloramphenicol). Because the baby's ability to break down and release drugs is not developed, the infant cannot get rid of chloramphenicol. A typical ashen-gray skin color occurs along with bloating of the abdomen, vomiting, difficult breathing, and severe loss of blood circulation.

gray substance, the gray tissue that makes up the core of the spinal cord. It is arranged in two large side-by-side masses linked by a band of fibers. Each portion of the gray substance spreads out, forming the horns of the spinal cord. The horns consist mostly of cell bodies of neurons. The quantity of gray substance varies greatly at different cord levels. In the chest region, the gray substance is small in comparison with surrounding white substance; in the neck and the lower back regions it is larger; and in the tapered end of the cord, its proportion is greatest. Nuclei in the gray matter of the spinal cord function as centers for all spinal reflexes. Also called **gray matter.** See also **spinal cord.**

great auricular nerve, one of the nerves branching from a network of nerves in the neck. One branch spreads to the skin of the face over the parotid gland. The other branch supplies the skin of the mastoid process and the back of the ear.

greater trochanter, a large bulge of the thigh bone (femur), to which are attached various muscles of the thigh.

great saphenous vein, one of the longest veins in the body. It contains 10 to 20 valves along its course through the leg and the thigh before ending in the thigh (femoral) vein.

great vessels, the large arteries and veins going into and coming from the heart. They include the aorta, the pulmonary arteries and veins, and the superior and inferior venae cavae.

greenstick fracture, a break in which the bone is bent but broken only on the outside of the bend. Children are most likely to have greenstick fractures. Keeping the bone rigid is usually effective, and healing is rapid.

grenade-thrower's fracture, a break of the upper arm bone caused by violent muscle shrinking.

Grenz rays, low-energy x-rays used to treat skin conditions. They can not penetrate very far and are usually used by dermatologists.

Grey Turner's sign, bruise of the skin of the side of the back between the ribs and hip bones in a severe disorder of the pancreas.

grid, a device used to absorb radiation scattered during an x-ray examination. A grid absorbs radiation that is not heading along straight lines from the x-ray source to the film.

grief, a pattern of physical and emotional responses to separation or loss. The effects are similar to those of fear, hunger, rage, and pain. The emotions proceed in stages from alarm to disbelief and denial, to anger and guilt, to finding a source of comfort, and, finally, to adjusting to the loss. The way in which a grieving person acts is greatly affected by the culture in which the person has been raised. The group of mind and body symptoms is also called the **grief reaction.** Most serious grief reactions end after four to six weeks, although the period varies and may be much longer, especially in cases of sudden death. **Anticipatory**

grieving is grieving before an actual loss, as contrasted with grief in response to an actual loss. The cause is the knowledge or feeling of the coming loss of an important person in one's life, of one's well-being, or of one's personal possessions.

Grifulvin, a trademark for a drug that fights fungus (griseofulvin).

grinding-in, a corrective grinding of one or more natural or artificial teeth to improve the surfaces.

gripes, severe spasmodic pain in the abdomen caused by an intestinal disorder. Also called **gripping.**

grippe. See **influenza.**

Grisactin, a trademark for an antifungal drug (griseofulvin).

griseofulvin /gris′ē·ōful′vin/, a drug given to treat some infections of the skin, hair, and nails. Patients with liver problems or known allergy to this drug should not take this drug. Side effects include blood disorders, headache, stomach and bowel problems, and rashes.

groin, each of two areas where the abdomen joins the thighs.

Grönblad-Strandberg syndrome /grön′blad-/, an inherited disorder of connective tissue. Symptoms include premature aging and breakdown of the skin, gray or brown streaks on the retina, and blood vessel breakdown with retinal bleeding that causes loss of vision. Heart disease and high blood pressure are common.

groove, a shallow furrow in various structures of the body. For example, grooves along the bones form channels for nerves.

gross, 1. referring to the study of tissue without magnification (macroscopic). 2. large or obese. Compare **microscopic.**

ground, the background of a visual field that can affect the ability of a patient to focus on an object.

ground itch, itching patches, pimples, and blisters of the skin caused by hookworm larvae. It occurs in warm climates. It may be prevented by wearing shoes and by a sanitary disposal of feces. See also **hookworm infection.**

group, a functional division (e.g., air support, salvage, structure protection)

group therapy, the use of psychotherapy in a small group of persons. The group members, usually under the leadership of a psychotherapist, discuss their problems to promote personal growth and change. Group therapy has been found to be very effective in treating addictions. See also **psychotherapy.**

growing fractures, bone break that gradually separates at the edges. The cause often is pressure of soft tissues forcing the edges apart.

G–H

growing pains, **1.** pains that occur in the muscles and joints of children or teenagers. They may result from fatigue, posture problems, and other causes that are not linked to growth. **2.** emotional problems felt during adolescence.

growth, **1.** the normal development of body, organs, and mental powers from infancy to adulthood. In childhood, growth is measured according to age at which physical changes usually appear and at which mental tasks are achieved. Such stages include the prenatal period, infancy, early childhood, middle childhood, and adolescence. There are 2 periods of rapid growth. One is the first 12 months, in which the infant triples in weight and grows up to 50% of the height at birth. The second is in the months around puberty, when the child nears adult height and secondary sexual characteristics emerge. **2.** an increase in the size of an organism or any of its parts.

growth failure, a lack of normal body and mind growth. It may be a result of inherited, diet, disease, mental, or social problems. See also **failure to thrive, maternal deprivation syndrome.**

growth hormone (GH), a substance (hormone) released by the pituitary gland. GH promotes protein building in all cells, increases use of fatty acids for energy, and reduces use of carbohydrate. Growth effects depend on the presence of thyroid hormone, insulin, and carbohydrate. The release of GH, controlled mainly by the central nervous system, occurs in bursts. More than half the total daily amount is released during early sleep. A lack of GH causes dwarfism; an excess results in gigantism or acromegaly. See also **acromegaly, dwarfism, gigantism.**

Grünfelder's reflex /grēn'feldərz/, an automatic curving of the great toe with a fanlike spreading of the other toes. Continued pressure on a membrane behind the ear causes the reflex. It occurs in children who also have middle ear disease.

grunting, abnormal, short loud breaks in breathing out. Grunting is most often heard in a person who has chest pain from pneumonia, fluid in the lungs, or broken ribs.

guaiac test /gwī'ak/, a test using a special solution (guaiac) on feces and urine to detect blood in the intestinal and urinary tracts.

guaifenesin /gwīfen'əsin/, a white-to-slightly-gray powder with a bitter taste and faint odor, widely used in cough medicines. Guaifenesin increases the flow of fluid in the respiratory tract.

guanabenz acetate, a drug given for high blood pressure. Patients allergic to this drug should not take it. It can cause dizziness, sleepiness, and dry mouth.

guanadrel sulfate, a drug given for high blood pressure in patients who have not been helped by a thiazide-type diuretic. Patients who are taking certain other drugs or who

have heart trouble or allergy to this drug should not take it.

guanethidine sulfate, a drug given for mild and severe high blood pressure. Patients who are taking certain other drugs or who have heart trouble or allergy to this drug should not take it. Side effects include low blood pressure, salt and water buildup, slow heart beat, diarrhea, and impotence.

guanine /gwan'ēn/, a basic component of DNA and RNA. It occurs in trace amounts in most cells.

Guérin's fracture /gāraNs'/, a fracture of the upper jaw. Also called **LeFort I fracture.**

Guillain-Barré syndrome /gēyaN'bärā'/, a disorder with inflammation of many nerves. It begins between 1 and 3 weeks after a mild fever linked to a viral infection or with immunization. Pain and weakness affect the arms and legs. Paralysis may develop. The condition may spread and involve the face and chest muscles. There is no treatment other than supportive care.

gum. See **gingiva.**

gumboil, an abscess of the gums and jawbone coming from injury, infection, or tooth decay. The gum is red, swollen, and tender. The abscess may break by itself, or it may require surgery.

gumma. See **granuloma.**

Gunning's splint, a splint used for supporting the jaws in surgery on the jaws.

gunshot fracture, a break caused by a bullet or similar missile.

Gunther's disease /gun'thərz/, an inherited disorder linked to sores brought on by sunlight. See also **porphyria.**

gut, **1.** intestine. **2.** *informal.* stomach and bowels. **3.** thread used in surgery that is made from the intestines of sheep.

Guthrie test, a test for phenylketonuria. A small amount of blood is obtained from an infant and placed with a strain of a bacterium that cannot grow without phenylalanine. The test is positive if the bacteria reproduce. See also **phenylketonuria.**

gutta-percha /gut'ə-pur'chə/, the solid, rubbery sap of various tropical trees. It is used for sealing prepared tooth cavities or to fill a root canal.

gynandrous /gīnan'drəs/, describing a man or a woman who has some of the physical characteristics usually found in the other sex, as a female pseudohermaphrodite. Compare **androgynous.**

gynecologic examination. See **pelvic examination.**

gynecology /gī'nəkol'-, jī'-, jin'-/, a branch of medicine that deals with the health care of women. It is almost always studied and practiced along with obstetrics. See also **interconceptional gynecologic care.**

gynecomastia /gī′nəkōmas′tē·ə/,   an abnormal swelling of one or both breasts in men. The condition is usually temporary and harmless. It may be caused by hormonal imbalance, tumor of the testis or pituitary, drugs containing estrogen or steroids, or failure of the liver to dissolve estrogen in the bloodstream.

Gyne-Lotrimin,   a trademark for a drug that fights fungus (clotrimazole).

gynephobia /gī′nə-/,   a deathly fear of women or an intense dislike of the company of women. It occurs almost only in men.

gyrus /jī′rəs/, *pl.* **gyri** /jī′rī/,   one of the spiral twists of the surface of the brain caused by the folding in of the outer layer.

G–H

H

habit, **1.** a usual way of behaving. **2.** an unwilled pattern of behavior or thought. **3.** the habitual use of drugs or narcotics.

habit training, the process of teaching a child how to adjust to the demands of the outside world by forming certain habits, mainly those related to eating, sleeping, elimination, and dress.

habituation, dependence on a drug, tobacco, or alcohol caused by repeated use, but without the addictive, physiologic need to increase the dose. Compare **addiction.**

habitus /hab′itəs/, a person's looks or physique, as an athletic habitus. See also **somatotype.**

Haemophilus influenzae /hēmof′ələs/, a germ found in the throats of 30% of healthy, normal people. In children and in weak older people harmful inflammation of the throat and lungs may result from infection. It can affect the heart or brain. Secondary infection by *H. influenzae* occurs with the flu and in many other lung diseases. There is an anti-*Haemophilus influenzae* serum available for protection against infection.

hair, a threadlike protein formed in the skin. There are three stages of hair development: **anagen,** the active growing stage; **catagen,** a short pause between the growth and resting phases; and **telogen,** the resting or club stage before shedding. Scalp hair grows at an average rate of 1 mm every 3 days, body and eyebrow hair at a much slower rate. See also **hirsutism, lanugo.**

hairy-cell leukemia, a rare cancer of blood-forming tissues with a gradual onset. It features sudden bruising with severe anemia and a very enlarged spleen. The disease occurs six times more often in men than in women, usually in middle age. Treatment includes removal of the spleen and chemotherapy.

hairy tongue, a dark, colored coating of the tongue that is a harmless and frequent side effect of some antibiotics. The condition improves with no treatment needed. See also **glossitis.**

halcinonide, a drug for use on the skin to reduce inflammation. Viral and fungal diseases of the skin, poor circulation, or known allergies to this drug or to steroid medicines prohibit its use. Side effects include skin rash and illness occurring from too long or excess use.

Halcion, a trademark for a sleeping pill (triazolam).

Haldol, a trademark for a tranquilizer (haloperidol).

Haldrone, a trademark for a hormone that affects blood sugar levels (paramethasone acetate).

half-life (t½), **1.** the time needed for a radioactive substance to lose half of its activity through decay. **2.** the time needed for a drug's level in the bloodstream to go down to one half its beginning level. **3.** the time required for the body to eliminate one half of a dosage of any substance by regular physical processes.

half-sibling, one of two or more children who have at least one parent in common; a half brother or half sister.

halfway house, a special treatment facility, usually for mental patients who no longer need to stay in the hospital but who need some care and time to get used to living on their own.

halitosis /hal′itō′-/, bad breath caused by poor oral hygiene, dental or mouth infections, the eating of certain foods, as garlic or alcohol, use of tobacco, or some diseases, as the odor of acetone in diabetes and ammonia in liver disease.

Hallpike caloric test, a way to check the function of the inner ear in patients with dizzy spells or hearing loss by running cool and warm water or air into the ears. See also **caloric test.**

hallucination, something sensed that is not caused by an outside event. It can occur in any of the senses and is named accordingly: auditory (hearing), gustatory (taste), olfactory (smell), tactile (feeling), or visual hallucination. A **command hallucination** is a psychotic condition in which the patient hears and obeys voices that command him or her to perform certain acts. The hallucinations may cause the patient to behave in dangerous ways. A **hypnagogic hallucination** is one that occurs in the period between wakefulness and sleep. A **lilliputian hallucination** is a false mental image in which things seem smaller than they actually are. **–hallucinate,** *v.*

hallucinogen /həloo′sənəjen′, hal′əsin′əjən/, a substance that excites the brain, causing hallucination, mood change, mistakes in judgments, loss of sense of self, increased pulse, temperature, and blood pressure, and widened pupils. Use of hallucinogens may lead to a habit, as well as possible depression or short-term insanity.

hallucinosis /-ō′sis/, a diseased mental state in which one is aware mainly or only of hallucinations. **Alcoholic hallucinosis** is a mental disorder caused by alcohol. The symptoms are mainly hearing things that are not there, fear, and false feelings of being punished. It is seen with serious alcoholism right after stopping or reducing drinking.

hallux /hal′əks/, *pl.* **halluces** /hal′yəsēz/, the great toe.

hallux rigidus, a painful deformity of the great toe that limits motion at the joint where the toe joins the foot.

hallux valgus, a deformity in which the great toe is bent to the outside toward the other toes; in some cases the great toe rides over or under the other toes.

halo cast, a device used to help keep the neck and head from moving. It involves the trunk, usually with shoulder straps, and a way to fasten pins to a band around the skull. The halo cast is used to help the healing of back injuries and spine dislocations and to keep the back rigid after surgery.

Halog, a trademark for a medicine for use on the skin to reduce inflammation (halcinonide).

halogenated hydrocarbon /haloj′-/, a general anesthetic. Nausea, vomiting, throat spasms and soreness are less severe and frequent when this anesthesia is used. Kinds include enflurane and halothane.

haloperidol /hal′ōper′ədôl/, a tranquilizer used to treat severe mental disorders and to control Gilles de la Tourette's syndrome.

haloprogin, a drug that kills bacteria and fungus, used for infections, as athlete's foot. Known allergy to this drug prevents its use. Side effects include worsening of existing sores, formation of blisters, and itching.

Halotestin, a trademark for a male hormone (fluoxymesterone).

Halotex, a trademark for an antibacterial (haloprogin).

halothane, an anesthetic that is inhaled to bring on and maintain general anesthesia. It is not advised for anesthesia during childbirth unless womb relaxation is needed. Side effects include liver cell death, heart attack, low blood pressure, nausea, and vomiting.

hamate bone /ham′āt/, a bone in the wrist, above the fourth and fifth fingers.

hammertoe, a toe permanently bent at the middle joint, causing a clawlike appearance. It may be present in more than one toe but is most common in the second toe.

hamstring muscle, any one of three muscles at the back of the thigh.

hamstring reflex, a normal deep tendon reflex brought about by tapping one of the hamstring tendons behind the knee. This causes the tendon to contract and the knee to bend. The patient should be lying on his or her back with the knee and hip partly bent and the leg supported by the examiner's hand. See also **deep tendon reflex.**

hamstring tendon, one of the three tendons from the three hamstring muscles in the back of the thigh that connect the hamstring muscles to the knee.

hand, the part of the upper limb below the forearm. It is the most flexible part of the skeleton and has a total of 27 bones.

handblock, a device made of a wood block several inches high with a firm handle that can be gripped by a disabled patient to give a certain amount of body support during activities, as getting into or out of a bed.

hand crew, predetermined individuals who are supervised, organized, and trained principally for clearing brush as a fire suppression measure.

handedness, willed or unwilled preference for use of either the left or right hand. The preference is related to which side of the brain is dominant, with left-handedness occurring when the right side of the brain is dominant and vice versa. Also called **chirality, laterality.**

handicap, referring to an inborn or acquired mental or physical defect that interferes with normal functions of the body or the ability to be self-sufficient. Compare **disability.**

hangman's fracture, a break in the lower neckbones.

hangnail, a piece of partly torn skin of the cuticle or nail fold. Tearing the piece more causes a red, painful, easily infected sore. Early treatment is to trim the hangnail close with nail clippers. For red, sore cases an antibiotic ointment and protective bandage are used.

Hansen's disease. See **leprosy.**

haploid /hap′loid/, having a single set of chromosomes, as in sex cells. Also called **monoploid. See also euploid.** –**haploidy,** *n.*

haptoglobin /hap′təglō′bin/, a blood protein. The amount of haptoglobin is increased in some long-term diseases and disorders with inflammation, and is decreased or absent in some kinds of anemia.

hardening of the arteries, a disease in which arteries thicken and become less elastic (arteriosclerosis).

hard palate, the bony part of the roof of the mouth, behind the soft palate and bounded in front and on the sides by the gums and teeth. Compare **soft palate.**

harelip. See **cleft lip.**

harlequin color, a short-term flushing of the skin on the lower side of the body with paleness of the upward side. Commonly seen in normal infants, it disappears as the child matures.

harlequin fetus, an infant whose skin at birth is completely covered with thick, horny scales that look like armor and are divided by deep red splits. The condition is the most severe form of bony outgrowth of the newborn. The infant is stillborn or dies soon after birth. See also **ichthyosis.**

Harmonyl, a trademark for a high blood pressure medicine (deserpidine).

Harris tube, a tube used to remove pressure from the stomach and intestines. It contains mercury and is passed through the nose and carried through the digestive tract by gravity.

Hartnup disease, an inborn disorder affecting the skin and mental state. Symptoms include dry, scaly skin sores, irritation of tongue and stomach, diarrhea, mental problems, and allergy to the sun. Brief exposure to the sun may cause redness, swelling, and blisters. Treatment focuses on diet.

Haverhill fever. See **ratbite fever.**

haversian system /hāvur′zhən/, a circular section of bone tissue, consisting of plates in the bone around a central canal. **Haversian canal** refers to one of the many tiny lengthwise canals in bone tissue. Each contains blood vessels, connective tissue, nerve fibers, and, sometimes, lymph vessels. The canals are connected to each other and are part of a complex network.

hay fever, *informal.* an acute seasonal allergic irritation of the nose and sinuses caused by tree, grass, or weed pollens. Also called **pollinosis.** See also **allergy, rhinitis.**

hazard, a situation or thing that increases the chance of a loss from some danger that may cause injury or illness. – **hazardous,** *adj.*

hazard analysis, analysis of the hazardous materials present in the community, including their location, quantity, specific history, and risk of release.

hazardous atmosphere, any of the following, which can harm an unprotected fire fighter: heat, flame, smoke, toxic gases, and flashover.

hazardous materials, any substance that jumps out of its container when something goes wrong and hurts or harms the things it touches.

hazardous materials incident, the release, or potential release, of a hazardous material from its container into the environment.

hazardous materials response teams (HMRTs), crews of specially trained and medically evaluated persons responsible for directly managing hazardous materials problems. They may include people from the emergency services, private industry, governmental agencies, or any combination of these. They generally perform more complex and technical functions than the first rescue and EMS companies. Depending on the jurisdiction, HMRTs can function as an advisory group or as actual operations personnel.

hazardous materials specialists, those specially trained and equipped members of the hazardous materials response community who possess both the technical and manipulative skills to function as the hazard sector officer or incident safety officer. These individuals can be considered equivalent to a EMT-P or paramedic. In addition to the functions of the first responder and hazardous materials technician, hazardous materials specialists perform these functions:

1. Identify unknown materials by advanced field screening techniques

2. Perform advanced hazard and risk assessment techniques

3. Demonstrate specialized knowledge of various individual and bulk hazardous materials containers

4. Use all types of chemical and high-temperature personal protective clothing provided by the plant or the community

5. Perform command of all hazard sector and site safety operations as delegated by the incident commander

6. Develop a site safety plan for a hazardous materials incident

hazardous materials technicians, specially trained members of the response community who are responsible for identification, basic hazard and risk assessment, implementation of basic control procedures, use of specialized equipment (including personal protective equipment, and basic decontamination procedures). In addition to the functions of the first responder, hazardous materials technicians perform these functions:

1. Identify unknown materials by simple screening techniques

2. Identify and verify the involved materials

3. Initiate intermediate hazard and risk assessment activities

4. Use nonencapsulating chemical and high-temperature protective clothing as necessary as provided by the plant or community

5. Perform specialized containment and confinement operations on hazardous materials releases (within resource and personal protective equipment capabilities)

6. Implement a site safety plan for an incident

7. Operate field survey instruments as provided by the plant or the community

8. Operate under the requirements of all pertinent local, state, and federal regulations

HCG radioreceptor assay, a urine test to detect pregnancy or missed abortion. The test is negative (within 2 hours) if the patient is not pregnant and positive (within 1 hour) if the patient is pregnant. Also called **pregnancy test.**

headache, a pain in the head from any cause. A **histamine headache** is related to the release of histamine from the body tissues. Symptoms include sudden sharp pain on one side of the head, involving the facial area from the neck to the temple, tearing or watery eyes, and runny nose. Treatment includes the use of antihistamines. A **spinal headache** occurs after spinal anesthesia or a lumbar puncture. It is caused by a loss of spinal fluid, resulting in pressure on the fibers of the spine and skull. A **tension headache** affects the back (occipital) region of the head and neck as the result of overwork or emotional strain. It tenses the body and blocks rest and relaxation. See also **migraine.**

head and neck cancer, any malignant tumor of the upper breathing tract, mouth, throat, facial features, and organs in the neck, appearing as lumps or sores that usually produce early symptoms. Tumors of the mouth, lips, and tongue usually begin as a swelling or nonhealing sore that occur in men over 60 years of age. Long-term alcoholism, heavy use of tobacco, poor oral hygiene, syphilis, and Plummer-Vinson syndrome may help bring on these cancers. Cancers of the nose cause bleeding, blockage in breathing, and facial and dental pain. Upper throat tumors can involve nasal blockage, middle ear problems, and hearing loss. Middle throat tumors cause difficult swallowing and breathing, pain, and lockjaw (trismus). Most lower throat tumors cause hoarseness, difficult swallowing and breathing, cough, and swollen glands. Other cancers can attack the salivary glands, jaw, and ear. Treatment includes surgery, radiation, and chemotherapy. Plastic surgery and artificial parts are often needed to correct deformities and restore functions in patients who have had surgery or radiation on a head or neck tumor. See also specific cancer.

head, eye, ear, nose, and throat (HEENT), a specialty in medicine concerned with the structure, functions, and diseases of the head, eyes, ears, nose, and throat and with the diagnosis and treatment of disorders of those structures.

head injury, any damage to the head resulting from piercing the skull or from the brain knocking too fast against the skull. Blood vessels, nerves, and membranes enclosing the brain are torn; bleeding, pooling of fluid, and blockage of blood flow may result. Infection of the brain's enclosing membranes is a serious result that often follows breaking the bones of the cavities behind the nose. See also **concussion.**

Heaf test. See **tuberculin test.**

healing, the act or process in which the normal, healthy structures and functions are restored to parts of the body that were diseased, damaged, or not functioning.

health, a state of physical, mental, and social well-being and the absence of disease or other disorder. It involves constant change and adaptation to stress. **High-level wellness** is a concept of health that stresses the working together of body, mind, and environment to ensure the highest level of functioning of an individual. See also **homeostasis.**

health assessment, evaluating the health status of a patient by performing a physical examination after obtaining a health history. Various laboratory tests may also be ordered. A major part of care after the health assessment is counseling and education that may explain body functioning and that advises the patient on a healthful way of life.

health behavior, an action taken by a person to maintain, attain, or regain good health and to prevent illness. Health behavior comes from a person's health beliefs. Some common health behaviors are regular exercise, eating a balanced diet, and getting vaccinations on schedule.

health care industry, the many services provided by hospitals and other institutions, nurses, doctors, dentists, government agencies, voluntary agencies, clinics, drug and medical equipment companies, and health insurance companies.

health care system, the complete network of agencies, facilities, and all providers of health care in a certain geographic area. Nurses form the largest number of providers in a health care system.

health certificate, a statement signed by a health care provider that tells the state of health of a person.

health culture, a system that tries to explain and treat sickness and to maintain health. Health cultures are part of the larger culture or tradition of a people. It may be a popular or folk system, or it may be a technical or scientific one.

health education, an educational program directed to the general public that attempts to improve, maintain, and safeguard the health of the community.

health history, (in nursing and medicine) a collection of information obtained from the patient and other sources concerning the patient's physical status and psychologic, social, and sexual functions. The history provides the basis for the diagnosis, treatment, care, and follow-up of the patient. **Complete health history** refers to an account of all of a patient's health patterns. It includes a history of the present illness and of any previous illness. Also listed are social and occupational history, sexual history, and a family health history. The first part of the history, an account obtained during the interview with the patient, describes the **present illness (PI)** as well as any acts or factors that make the symptoms better or worse. The patient is asked what is believed to be the cause of the symptoms and whether or not a similar condition has occurred in the past. The patient's own words often serve as the best description and may be quoted. The second part of the history gives an account of **past health.** This includes past illnesses or inju-

G–H

ries, allergies, operations, vaccinations, stays in the hospital, any pregnancies or mental health history, transfusions, and screening tests. A work history, describing the patient's work and exposure to stress, poisons, radiation, or other work hazards, may be included. The effect of the current illness on the patient's work is also noted. A social history is taken in which the patient's social, cultural, and family settings are outlined, focusing on aspects that might have an effect on the current illness. In some cases a sexual history may be included. Also called **medical history.** See also **occupational history, review of systems, sexual history.**

health maintenance, a program planned to prevent illness, to maintain the best level of function, and to promote health. It is central to health care, especially to nursing care at all levels.

health maintenance, alterations in, a nursing diagnosis that describes the condition in which the patient is unable to identify, manage, or seek help to maintain health. The causes of the problem include the lack of or major changes in communication skills; mental damage or the inability to make careful judgments; damage to or lack of motor skills; lack of money; or the inability to cope. The defining features include a proven lack of knowledge about basic health practices or the inability to take responsibility for meeting those needs, the inability to adapt to changes around one, or a lack of health-seeking behavior.

Health Maintenance Organization (HMO), a type of group health care practice that provides health maintenance and treatment services to members who pay a flat, regular fee that is set without regard to the amount or kind of services received. In addition to diagnostic and treatment services, including hospitalization and surgery, an HMO often offers extra services, as dental, mental, and eye care, and prescription drugs.

health physics, the study of the effects of radiation on the body and the methods for protecting people from the side effects of the radiation. Health physics is concerned with discovering new ways to protect people from these untoward effects. Also called **medical physics.**

health professional, any person who has completed a course of study in a field of health, as a registered nurse, physical therapist, or physician. The person is usually licensed by a government agency or certified by a professional organization.

health provider, any individual who provides health services to health care consumers.

health-related services, services other than medical care, given by a hospital or clinic, that may contribute directly or indirectly to the physical or mental health and well-being of patients. These may include personal or social services.

health resources, all materials, personnel, facilities, funds, and anything else that can be used for providing health care and services.

health risk, a factor that increases one's chances for illness or death. These factors may include social or income levels, certain individual behaviors, family and individual histories, and certain physical changes.

health screening, a program designed to evaluate the health state and potential of an individual. In the process it may be found that a person has a certain disease or condition or is at greater than normal risk of developing it. Health screening may include taking a health history and performing a physical examination, laboratory tests, and x-ray tests. These may be followed by counseling, education, referral, or further testing.

health supervision, health teaching, counseling, or keeping track of the state of the patient's health. This does not include actual physical care. Such supervision occurs in health care agencies, clinics, doctor's offices, or the patient's home.

health systems agency (HSA), an agency established under the terms of the National Health Planning and Resources Development Act of 1974. Health planning agencies are intended to provide health planning and fund raising services in each of several health service areas established by the Act. Health systems agencies are nonprofit and include private organizations, public regional planning bodies, or local government agencies and consumers.

hearing, the special sense that allows sound to be perceived. It is the major function of the ear. Hearing loss can range from mild damage to complete deafness. See also **deafness.**

hearing aid, an electronic device that increases the volume of sound for persons with damaged hearing. The device consists of a microphone, a battery power supply, an amplifier, and a receiver. The receiver is designed, depending on the cause of the hearing loss, to send sound through the outer ear canal or through the skull.

heart, the muscular, cone-shaped organ, about the size of a fist, that pumps blood throughout the body. It beats normally about 70 times per minute by balanced nerve impulses and muscle squeezes. The organ is about 12 cm long, 8 cm wide at its broadest part, and 6 cm thick. The weight of the heart in men averages between 280 and 340 g and in women between 230 and 280 g. The base of the heart is the portion of the heart opposite the tip. The base is tilted to the right side of the body. It forms the upper border of the heart and lies just below the second rib. The layers of the heart, starting from the outside, are the epicardium, the myocardium, and the endocardium. The chambers of the heart include two ventricles with thick muscular walls, making up most of the organ, and two atria with thin muscular walls. An inner wall (septum) separates the ventricles and extends between the atria, dividing the heart into the right and the left sides. The left side of the heart pumps blood with oxygen from the lung veins into the aorta and on to all parts of the body. The right side of the heart pumps blood from which the oxygen has been removed into the lung arteries. Both atria contract almost at the same time, followed quickly by the contraction of the ventricles.

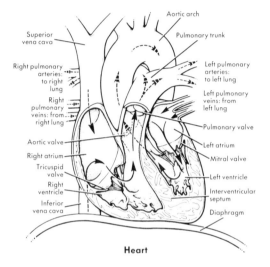

Heart

heart block,   an interference with the normal travel of electric impulses that control activity of the heart muscle. The delay or block can occur in a number of different locations in the heart. **Adams-Stokes syndrome,** a state of sudden fainting, is caused by incomplete heart block. Seizures may also happen. An **atrioventricular (AV) block** occurs at the atrioventricular node, bundle of His, or its branches. An overdose of digitalis, heart disease, or severe heart attack may cause the condition. AV block is a common reason a cardiac pacemaker is inserted. An **intraatrial block** is a delayed or abnormal conduction within an upper heart chamber (atria). An **intraventricular block** occurs in the ventricles. The block can be caused by coronary artery disease, valvular heart disease, ventricular hypertrophy and fibrosis, or other disorders. Outcome depends on the basic heart condition. A kind of intraventricular block is a **bundle branch block.** This is an abnormal conduction of the electric signal through certain fibers in the heart. If many fibers are affected, the heart rate is slowed. For example, a **right bundle branch block** occurs when electric signals that normally travel along fibers on the right side of the heart fail to reach the right lower chamber (ventricle). The cause may be a growth in the right bundle branch of fibers or an enlarged right ventricle of the heart, especially in patients under 40 years of age. In older patients a right bundle branch block is commonly caused by heart blood vessel (coronary artery) disease. Another kind is an **infranodal block,** most often seen in older patients. Symptoms include frequent episodes of fainting and a pulse rate of between 20 and 50 beats per minute. A **sinoatrial (SA) block** is caused by too much stimulation of the vagus nerve, acute infections, and atherosclerosis. SA block may also be a side effect to quinidine or digitalis. A **Mobitz I heart block** may happen after a mild heart attack. Symptoms include weakness, dizziness, and, in some cases, fainting spells. It is usually a temporary condition needing no treatment. **Mobitz II heart block** refers to a loss of conciousness (syncopal attack), occurring without warning when the patient is upright or lying down. It may be temporary or suddenly become a complete block. Treatment for heart block includes drugs and implanting a pacemaker.

heartburn,   a painful burning feeling in the throat (esophagus) just below the breastbone. The condition often comes from stomach contents flowing back (reflux) into the esophagus but may be caused by too much acid in the stomach or peptic ulcer. Antacids relieve the symptoms but do not cure the cause. Also called **pyrosis.** See also **hernia, reflux, ulcer.**

heart disease.   See **congenital heart disease, valvular heart disease.**

heart failure,   a condition in which the heart cannot pump enough blood to meet the needs of body tissues. Extreme exertion may cause heart failure in patients with normal hearts if there is a mismatch between the needs of the body and the volume of blood pumped by the heart. Many patients develop heart failure from more than one cause. Many of the symptoms linked to heart failure are caused by poor function of organs other than the heart, especially the lungs, kidneys, and liver. Heart failure is closely linked to many forms of heart disease and is often diagnosed only after the diagnosis of heart disease. Heart failure in infants and children is usually the result of inherited heart disease. The common causes of heart failure after 40 years of age are hardening of the arteries with clotting of blood inside the heart, high blood pressure, disease of the heart valves, lung disease, and general damage to the heart muscle. Some persons may suffer heart failure caused by a combination of inherited and acquired heart disease. Some causes of heart failure in persons without symptoms are sudden strenuous effort, increased work load, too much salt in the diet, sudden emotional upset, and the giving of excessive volumes of fluids by vein. Most kinds of heart disease first affect the left side of the heart. Heart failures

G-H

are commonly divided into left-sided heart failure and right-sided heart failure. The impairment of one side will eventually affect the other because both sides of the heart are part of a circuit. In failure linked to either side, the pumping action of the heart may be normal, lowered, or raised. **Left-sided heart failure** features reduced ability of the left side of the heart to pump blood to the arteries of the heart. Difficulty in breathing usually occurs with left-sided heart failure. **Right-sided heart failure** is caused by damage of the right side of the heart with clogging and high blood pressure in the veins and small vessels. Swelling of hands and feet occurs with right-sided heart failure. **Atrial failure** refers to the failure of one of the upper heart chambers (atrium) to fill completely with blood. The atria normally provide a pumping function for the heart. In patients with mild heart disease, loss of atrial pumping may not change the amount of blood pumped at rest. However, the amount of blood may decrease during exercise. Heart failure caused by atrial failure may begin with irregular contractions of the upper heart chambers (atrial fibrillation) in patients who have heart disease. **Backward failure** develops when the lower heart chamber (ventricle) cannot empty. Blood backs up in the pulmonary veins and the lungs, causing fluid buildup (pulmonary edema). **Compensated heart failure** refers to a condition in which the body tries to compensate for heart failure. This may include increased nerve stimulation of the heart, increased blood flow to the heart, and enlargement of the heart. **Congestive heart failure (CHF)** refers to circulatory congestion caused by heart disorders. It develops over a length of time and is linked with salt and water balance and kidney function. Sudden CHF may occur after a heart attack. Lung congestion may result. The condition may cause chest pains similar to those of a heart attack. Common symptoms of CHF include difficult breathing, high blood pressure, and swelling of the legs and hands. **Latent heart failure** refers to a heart disease that does not cause problems during rest but produces pain or other symptoms under conditions of increased stress, such as during exercise, fever, and emotional excitement. During stress situations, the heart affected by latent failure is unable to pump enough blood to meet the needs of body tissues and structures. **Left ventricular failure** is a condition in which the left ventricle, the chamber that pumps blood to the body's tissues, fails to contract forcefully enough to maintain a normal output of blood. Fluid accumulates in the lungs because of the weakened blood flow. The heart usually becomes enlarged and develops a sound called a **gallop.** Other signs include breathlessness, pale skin, sweating, and often high blood pressure. The treatment for heart failure commonly involves reducing the workload of the heart, giving certain drugs, as digitalis, to increase heart muscle strength, salt-free diets,

diuretics, and surgery. Many patients with heart failure, especially elderly patients, become constipated and require laxatives, such as mineral oil. The sudden onset of fluid in the lungs (acute pulmonary edema) linked to some cases of heart failure is a life-threatening condition requiring immediate treatment.

heart-lung machine, a machine that takes over the functions of the heart and lungs, especially during heart surgery. The blood is detoured from the veins through an oxygenator, where oxygen is added to the blood, and returned to the arteries.

heart massage, a repeated, rhythmic compression of the heart by outside force. Cardiac massage may be applied directly to the heart during surgery, or through the chest during resuscitation by pressing the chest with force. Cardiac massage is done when the heart stops beating or when an abnormally fast rhythm occurs (ventricular fibrillation). Also called **cardiac massage.** See also **cardiopulmonary resuscitation.**

heart murmur, an abnormal heart sound usually caused when one or more valves fail to function normally. In general, many murmurs heard when the heart contracts are not abnormal. Most murmurs that occur when the heart rests are dangerous. Systolic murmurs are generally less meaningful than diastolic murmurs and are found in many people with no sign of heart disease. Systolic murmurs include ejection murmurs often heard in pregnancy or in patients with anemia, thyroid disease, or heart and lung disease. Pansystolic murmurs are heard in patients with heart valve defects. Also called **cardiac murmur.**

heart rate, the pulse, figured by counting the number of contractions of the heart per unit of time. Tachycardia is a heart rate of more than 100 beats per minute; bradycardia is a heart rate of fewer than 60 beats per minute. See also **pulse.**

heart scan, an image of the heart, obtained after injecting a radioactive material into a vein. It is used for determining the size, shape, and location of the heart, for diagnosing pericarditis, and for viewing the chambers of the heart. See also **cardiography, echocardiogram.**

heart sound, a noise produced within the heart during the heart beat cycle that may reveal abnormal heart structure or function. An example is a low-pitched, extra sound heard with a stethoscope during an **atrial gallop,** an abnormal heart rhythm. It is often heard in heart disease caused by high blood pressure. A **ventricular gallop** is an abnormal heartbeat heard in an older patient with heart disease. The same sound heard in a healthy child or young adult (then called a **physiologic third heart sound**) is not a problem and most often goes away with age. A **click** is an extra heart sound that occurs during heart contraction (systole). An example is an **ejection click.** This may be caused by the sudden swelling of a pulmonary artery, the abrupt widening of the large artery (aorta), or the forceful opening of the aortic valves (cusps).

heart surgery, any surgery involving the heart. It may be done to correct acquired or inherited defects, to replace diseased valves, to open or bypass blocked vessels, or to put an artificial part or a transplant in place. Two major types of heart surgery are done, closed and open. The closed technique is done through a small cut, without using the heart-lung machine. In the open technique the heart chambers are open and fully visible, and blood is detoured around the area by the heart-lung machine. The mortality rate is highest during the first 48 hours after surgery.

heart valve, one of the four structures in the heart that control the flow of blood by opening and closing with each heart beat. The valves permit the flow of blood in only one direction, and any one of the valves may become defective permitting the backflow linked to heart murmurs. The **aortic valve** is between the left lower heart chamber (ventricle) and the aorta. It has three flaps (cusps) that close when the heart beats to prevent blood from flowing back into the heart from the aorta. The **mitral valve,** also called **bicuspid valve,** is between the upper chamber (left atrium) and the lower chamber (left ventricle). It is the only valve with two small cusps. The mitral valve allows blood to flow from the left atrium into the left ventricle. Narrowing of the ventricle forces the blood up against the valve. This closes the two cusps so the flow of blood is moved from the ventricle into the main artery of the body (aorta). The **pulmonary valve** is made up of three cusps that grow from the lining of the pulmonary artery. The cusps close during each heart beat to keep blood from flowing back into the right lower heart chamber (ventricle). The **tricuspid valve** is between the right upper heart chamber (atrium) and the right lower heart chamber (ventricle) of the heart. The tricuspid valve has three cusps. As the right and the left ventricles relax during the relaxation (diastole) phase of the heart beat, the tricuspid valve opens, allowing blood to flow into the ventricle. In the contraction (systole) phase of the heart beat both blood-filled ventricles contract, pumping out their contents, while the tricuspid and mitral valves close to prevent any backflow.

heart cramp, any cramp in the arm, leg, or stomach caused by too little water and salt in the body because of heat exhaustion. It usually occurs after vigorous physical exertion in very hot weather or under other conditions that cause heavy sweating and loss of body fluids and salts.

heat exhaustion, an abnormal condition with weakness, dizziness, nausea, muscle cramps, and fainting. It is caused by low levels of body fluid and salts resulting from exposure to intense heat or the inability to adjust to heat. Body temperature is near normal; blood pressure may drop but usually returns to normal as the person is placed in a lying-down position; the skin is cool, damp, and pale. The person usually recovers with rest and replacement of water and salt. Compare **heatstroke.**

heat rash, tiny blisters and pimples, often red. They are caused by blockage of sweat ducts during periods of heat and high humidity. Tingling and prickling sensations are common. Prevention and treatment include cool, dry temperatures, a good flow of air, and absorbent powders. Also called **miliaria, prickly heat.**

heatstroke, a severe and sometimes fatal condition that results from the failure of the body to regulate its temperature. This is caused by long exposure to the sun or to high temperatures. Lessening or lack of sweating is an early symptom. Body temperature of 105° F or higher, fast pulse rate, hot and dry skin, headache, confusion, blackouts, and convulsions may occur. Treatment includes cooling, resting, and fluid replacement. Also called **heat hyperpyrexia, sunstroke.** Compare **heat exhaustion.**

heaves, *informal.* vomiting and retching.

heavy equipment transport, any ground vehicle capable of transporting a dozer.

heavy metal, a metallic element with a specific gravity five or more times that of water. The heavy metals are antimony, arsenic, bismuth, cadmium, cerium, chromium, cobalt, copper, gallium, gold, iron, lead, manganese, mercury, nickel, platinum, silver, tellurium, thallium, tin, uranium, vanadium, and zinc. Small amounts of many of these elements are common and necessary in the diet. Large amounts of any of them may cause poisoning.

heavy metal poisoning, poisoning caused by the eating, breathing, or absorption of various toxic heavy metals. Kinds of heavy metal poisoning include **antimony poisoning, arsenic poisoning, cadmium poisoning, lead poisoning,** and **mercury poisoning.**

Heberden's node /hē′bərdənz/, an abnormal enlargement of bone or cartilage in a joint of a finger. This most often occurs in wasting diseases of the joints.

Hedulin, a trademark for a blood-thinning drug (phenindione).

heel, the back part of the foot, formed by the largest tarsal bone, the calcaneus.

heel-knee test, a way to check coordination of movements of the legs. In the test the patient, lying face down, is asked to touch the knee of one leg with the heel of the other.

heel-shin test, a way to check coordination of movements of the legs. In the test the patient, lying face down, is asked to pass the heel of one leg slowly down the shin of the other leg from the knee to the ankle.

Hegar's sign, a softening of the uterine cervix early in pregnancy. It is a probable sign of pregnancy.

G–H

height, the measurement of a structure, organ, or other object from bottom to top, when it is placed or viewed in an upright position.

Heimlich maneuver /hīm′lik/, an emergency method for dislodging a piece of food or other object lodged in the windpipe to prevent suffocation. The choking person is grasped from behind by the rescuer, who places a fist, thumb side in, just below the victim's breastbone. The other hand is placed firmly over the fist. The rescuer then pulls the fist firmly and abruptly into the top of the stomach forcing the blockage up the windpipe. If repeated attempts do not free the airway, an emergency cut in the windpipe (tracheotomy) may be necessary. See also **cardiopulmonary resuscitation.**

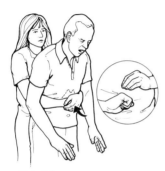

Heimlich maneuver

Heinz bodies /hīns/, oddly shaped bits of altered hemoglobin found in the red blood cells of persons who are allergic to certain chemicals.

helibase, a location within the general incident area for parking, fueling, maintenance, and loading of helicopters.

helibase crew, a crew of three or more individuals who may be assigned to operations or to support helicopter operations.

helicopter tender, a ground service vehicle capable of supplying fuel and support equipment to helicopters.

helispot, a location where a helicopter can take off and land. Some helispots may be used for temporary retardant loading.

helitack, The initial attack phase of fire suppression using helicopters and trained airborne teams to achieve immediate control of wildfires.

helitack foreman, a fire fighter trained in the tactical and logistical use of helicopters for fire suppression.

helitanker, a helicopter equipped with a fixed tank or a suspended bucket-type container that is used for aerial delivery of water or retardants.

helix /hē′liks/, a coiled, spiral-like formation typical of many organic molecules, as deoxyribonucleic acid (DNA).

helminthiasis, a disease caused by invasion of the body by worms (helminths) that may be in the skin, muscles, or intestines. These include flukes, tapeworms, and roundworms. Ascariasis, bilharziasis, filariasis, hookworm, and trichinosis are common forms of the disease.

hemagglutination /hem′əglo͞otinā′shən, hē′mə-/, a clumping together of red blood cells. This is a reaction of the body's defenses and may be caused by antibodies (as **hemagglutinin**), some viruses, and other substances.

hemangioblastoma /hēman′jē·ōblastō′mə/, a brain tumor made up of an excess growth of small blood vessels and vessel-forming cells.

hemangioma /hēman′jē·ō′mə/, a harmless tumor made up of a mass of blood vessels.

hematemesis /hem′ətem′əsis/. See **gastrointestinal bleeding.**

hematocrit /hēmat′əkrit/. See **blood count.**

hematogenous /hem′ətōj′ənəs/, coming from or carried in the blood.

hematology /hem′ətol′-, hē′mə-/, the study of blood and blood-forming tissues. A physician who specializes in the study of blood and its diseases is called a **hematologist.**

hematoma /hem′ətō′mə/, a pooling of blood that escaped from the vessels and became trapped in the tissues of the skin or in an organ. This can result from injury or surgery. First, there is frank bleeding into the space; if the space is limited, pressure slows and eventually stops the flow of blood. The blood clots, forming a mass that can be felt and is often painful. A hematoma may be drained early in the process and bleeding stopped with pressure. If necessary, the bleeding may be stopped by surgically tying off the bleeding vessel. Also called **blood blister.**

hematomyelia /hem′ətōmē′lyə/, the appearance of blood in the fluid of the spinal cord.

hematopoiesis /-pō·ē′sis/, the normal formation and development of blood cells in the bone marrow. In severe anemia and other blood disorders, cells may be produced in organs outside the marrow (extramedullary hematopoiesis).

hematuria /hem′əto͞or′ē·ə/, abnormal presence of blood in the urine. Hematuria can be caused by many kidney diseases and disorders of the genital and urinary systems.

heme /hēm/, the colored, nonprotein part of the hemoglobin molecule in the blood that contains iron. Heme carries oxygen in the red blood cells, releasing it to tissues that give off excess amounts of carbon dioxide (CO_2). See also **hemoglobin.**

hemeralopia /hem′ərəlō′pē·ə/. See **day blindness.**

hemianesthesia /hem'i-/, a loss of feeling on one side of the body.

hemianopia /-anō'pē·ə/, defective vision or blindness in one half of the visual field. **Homonymous hemianopia** is blindness or defective vision in the right or left halves of the visual fields of both eyes. This condition is frequently seen in people who have suffered a stroke.

hemicellulose /-sel'yəlōs/, a type of carbohydrate that makes up most of the stiff portion of the cell walls of plants. It resembles cellulose but is easier to dissolve and to digest. See also **dietary fiber.**

hemicephalia /-səfā'lyə/, a birth defect consisting of the absence of one side of the top layer of the brain. It is caused by the halt of brain growth in the fetus.

hemicrania /-krā'nē·ə/, **1.** a headache, usually migraine, that affects only one side of the head. **2.** a birth defect in which one half of the skull in the fetus is missing.

hemiectromelia /-ek'trəmē'lyə/, a birth defect in which the limbs on one side of the body are not fully formed.

hemignathia /hem'inā'thē·ə/, **1.** a birth defect in which the lower jaw on one side of the face is not fully formed. **2.** a condition of having only one jaw.

hemihyperplasia /-hī'pərplā'zhə/, excessive growth of one half of a specific organ or body part, or of all the organs and parts on one side of the body.

hemihypoplasia /-hī'pōplā'zhə/, partial or incomplete development of one half of a specific organ or body part, or of all the organs and parts on one side of the body.

hemikaryon /-ker'ē·on/, a cell nucleus that contains the halved (haploid) number of chromosomes, or one half of the diploid number, as that of the sex cells.

hemimelia /-mē'lyə/. See **ectromelia.**

hemiparesis /-pərē'-/, muscular weakness of one half of the body.

hemiplegia /-plē'jə/, paralysis of one side of the body. **Cerebral hemiplegia** is caused by a tumor in the brain. **Facial hemiplegia** occurs in the muscles of one side of the face, with the rest of the body not affected. Paralysis of one side of the body in an infant, called **infantile hemiplegia,** may occur at birth from a brain hemorrhage, in the womb from lack of oxygen, or from a fever in infancy. **Spastic hemiplegia** affects one side of the body with increased tendon reflexes and uncontrolled spasms occurring in the affected muscles. Also called **unilateral paralysis.** – **hemiplegic,** *adj.*

hemisphere, **1.** one half of a sphere or globe. **2.** the lateral half of the brain. –**hemispheric, hemispherical,** *adj.*

hemiteras /-ter'əs/, *pl.* **hemiterata,** any patient with a birth defect that is not so severe or disabling as to be called a monstrous (teratic) condition.

hemivertebra, an abnormal birth defect in which a backbone (vertebra) fails to develop completely.

hemochromatosis /hē'məkrō'mətō'-/, a rare disease in which iron deposits build up throughout the body. Enlarged liver, skin discoloration, diabetes mellitus, and heart failure may occur. The disease most often develops in men over 40 years of age and as a result of some anemias requiring multiple blood transfusions.

hemoconcentration, an increase in the number of red blood cells resulting either from a decrease in the liquid content of blood or from increased production of red cells.

hemodialysis /-dī·al'isis/. See **dialysis.**

hemodynamics /-dīnam'-/, the study of factors affecting the force and flow of circulating blood.

Hemofil, a trademark for a human antibleeding medication.

hemoglobin (Hb) /-glō'bin/, a complex protein-iron compound in the blood that carries oxygen to the cells from the lungs and carbon dioxide away from the cells to the lungs. Each red blood cell contains 200 to 300 molecules of hemoglobin. Each molecule of hemoglobin contains several molecules of heme, each of which can carry one molecule of oxygen. **Hemoglobin A (Hb A),** also called adult hemoglobin, is a normal hemoglobin. **Hemoglobin F (Hb F)** is the normal hemoglobin of the fetus, most of which is broken down in the first days after birth and replaced by hemoglobin A. It can carry more oxygen and is present in increased amounts in some diseases, including sickle cell anemia, aplastic anemia, and leukemia. Small amounts are produced throughout life. **Hemoglobin variant** refers to any type of hemoglobin other than hemoglobin A. These variations are determined in the genes and, depending on the kind and extent of change, result in changed physical and chemical function of the red blood cells.

hemoglobin C (Hb C) disease, an inherited blood disorder involving mild but long-term destruction of red blood cells. It is related to the presence of hemoglobin C, an abnormal form of the red-cell-coloring substance.

hemoglobin electrophoresis, a test to identify various abnormal hemoglobins in the blood, including certain inherited disorders, as sickle cell anemia.

hemoglobinopathy /-glō'binop'əthē/, any of a group of inherited disorders known by changes in the structure of the hemoglobin molecule. Kinds of hemoglobinopathies include **hemoglobin C disease** and **sickle cell anemia.** Compare **thalassemia.**

hemoglobin S (Hb S), an abnormal type of hemoglobin that causes sickle cell anemia, a disorder in which the blood cells tend to become sickle-shaped, to move slowly, to clump together, and to break down. See also **sickle cell anemia.**

G–H

hemoglobinuria /-oor'ē·ə/, an abnormal presence in the urine of hemoglobin that is unattached to red blood cells. Hemoglobinuria can result from various diseases of the body's defense system or certain blood disorders. **March hemoglobinuria** occurs after excess physical exercise or prolonged exercise, as marching or long-distance running.

hemolysin /hēmel'isin/, any of the many substances that dissolve red blood cells. Hemolysins are produced by many kinds of bacteria, including some of the staph and strep germs. They are also found in venoms and in some vegetables. Hemolysins appear to aid the bacteria in invading blood cells.

hemolysis /hēmol'isis/, the breakdown of red blood cells and the release of hemoglobin. It occurs normally at the end of the life span of a red cell. However, it may occur under many other circumstances, as when fighting off disease or as a side effect of hemodialysis or artificial heart aids, as pacemakers. Adding too much liquid to the blood by vein can also cause hemolysis. See also **dialysis.** – **hemolytic,** adj.

hemopericardium /-per'ikär'dē·əm/, a buildup of blood within the sac surrounding the heart.

hemoperitoneum /-per'itōnē'əm/, a buildup of blood surrounding the organs in the trunk of the body.

hemophilia /-fil'yə/, a group of hereditary bleeding disorders in which there is a lack of one of the factors needed to clot the blood. The severity of the disorder varies greatly with the extent of the lack. Greater than usual loss of blood during dental work, nosebleeds, blood blisters, and bleeding into the joints are common problems in hemophilia. Severe internal bleeding is less common. **Hemophilia A** is the classic type of hemophilia. **Hemophilia B,** also called **Christmas disease,** is similar to but less severe than hemophilia A. **Hemophilia C,** also called **Rosenthal's syndrome,** is also similar to but less severe than hemophilia A.

hemoptysis /hēmop'tisis/, coughing up of blood from the respiratory tract. Blood-streaked spit often occurs in minor infections of the upper breathing tract or in bronchitis. Heavier bleeding may indicate *Aspergillus* infection, lung abcess, tuberculosis, or cancer. Treatment includes watching the patient for signs of shock, preventing suffocation, and stopping the bleeding. Antibiotics and cough medicines may be given.

hemorrhage /hem'ôrij/, a loss of a large amount of blood in a short period of time, either outside or inside the body. Hemorrhage may be from arteries, veins, or capillaries. A second term often identifies the location. For example, **extradural hemorrhage** refers to bleeding in an area around but outside of the dura mater of the brain or spinal cord. Symptoms are related to shock: rapid pulse, thirst, cold and clammy skin, sighing breaths, dizziness, fainting, paleness, sense of fear, restlessness, and low blood pressure. If bleeding is within a cavity or joint, pain will develop as the cavity is stretched by the rapidly expanding amount of blood. Internal bleeding requires prompt medical attention. The patient is kept warm and quiet. All effort is made to stop a hemorrhage. Pressure is applied directly to a wound or to the proper points. Ice, applied directly to the wound, may slow bleeding by shrinking the blood vessels. Body temperature may be maintained by keeping the person covered and flat. If an arm or leg is wounded, and if the bleeding is severe, a tourniquet may be applied near the wound. A tourniquet is not applied if there is any other way to stop the flow, because the risk is great that the limb will not survive the loss of oxygen caused by blocking the supply of blood. –**hemorrhagic,** adj.

hemorrhagic disease of newborn /hem'ôraj'ik/, a bleeding disorder of newborns that is usually caused by a lack of vitamin K.

hemorrhagic fever, a severe virus infection. The disorder develops rapidly and begins with fever and muscle ache. This is often followed by hemorrhage, blood vessel collapse, shock, and kidney failure. The virus is thought to be carried by mosquitoes, ticks, or mites. Many forms of the disease occur in specific geographic areas. Examples are dengue fever and yellow fever. See specific entry.

hemorrhoid, an enlarged vein in the lower rectum or anus caused by blockage in the veins of the area. Straining to defecate, constipation, and too much sitting may cause hemorrhoids. Pregnancy can help bring on hemorrhoids. Internal hemorrhoids begin above the opening of the anus. If they become large enough to bulge from the anus, they become squeezed and painful.

hemosiderosis /hē'mōsid'ərō'-/, an increased deposit of iron in a variety of tissues, usually without tissue damage. It is often linked to diseases involving long-term, extensive destruction of red blood cells, as thalassemia.

hemostasis /hēmos'təsis, hē'mōstā'sis/, the stopping of bleeding by mechanic or chemical means or by the clotting process of the body. See also **blood clotting.**

hemostatic, having to do with a procedure, device, or substance that stops the flow of blood. Direct pressure, tourniquets, and surgical clamps are mechanic hemostatic measures. Cold packs are hemostatic and include the use of an ice bag on the stomach to halt womb bleeding and washing out the stomach with an iced solution to check stomach bleeding.

hemothorax /-thôr'aks/, a buildup of blood and fluid in the chest cavity, usually because of injury. It may also be caused by small blood vessels that break as a result of inflammation from pneumonia, tuberculosis, or tumors.

Shock from hemorrhage, pain, and breathing failure follows if emergency care is not available.

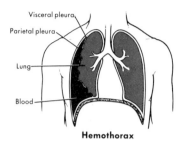

Hemothorax

hemotroph /hē′mətrof/, the food substances that go to the embryo from the mother's bloodstream after the development of the placenta.

Henoch-Schönlein purpura /hen′ok-shān′lĭn/, a short-term allergic disorder of blood vessels, chiefly found in children. Symptoms include bruiselike areas that appear mainly on the lower abdomen, buttocks, and legs, pain in the knees, ankles, or other joints, and bleeding in the stomach and intestines. Blood in the urine is also found. The disease lasts up to 6 weeks and has no long-term effects if kidney involvement is not severe.

heparin /hep′ərin/, a naturally occurring substance that acts in the body to prevent clotting in the veins. It is produced in the connective tissue surrounding capillaries, particularly in the lungs and liver.

heparin sodium, a drug to prevent blood clotting, given for a variety of blood vessel disorders. Known allergy to this drug forbids its use. Side effects include rapid bleeding and disorders involving blood vessel spasms.

hepatic /həpat′ik/, having to do with the liver.

hepatic adenoma, a rapidly growing liver tumor that may become very large and may break, causing deadly internal bleeding. It is sometimes called a ''pill tumor'' because it is often linked to patients who use oral contraceptives.

hepatic coma, a disorder caused by long-term or sudden liver disease. Symptoms include variable consciousness, weakness, slowness, and coma, trembling of the hands, personality change, memory loss, and rapid breathing. Convulsions and death may occur. The disorder occurs because waste that is poisonous to the brain is not removed in the liver before being sent back into the blood flowing to the far ends of the body. Also, substances that the brain requires are not made in the liver and, therefore, are not available to the brain. Treatment in most cases includes cleansing enemas, low-protein diet, and specific treatment for the underlying cause.

hepatic fistula, an abnormal passage from the liver to another organ or body structure.

hepatic node, a lymph gland in one of three groups found in the lower trunk and the pelvic organs supplied by branches of the celiac artery.

hepatitis /hep′ətī′-/, an inflammation of the liver. Symptoms include yellowing of the skin (jaundice), enlarged liver, loss of appetite, stomach discomfort, abnormal liver function, clay-colored stools, and dark urine. The condition may be caused by bacterial or viral infection, worms or other parasites, alcohol, drugs, poison, or transfusion of the wrong type of blood. It may be mild and brief or severe, intense, and life-threatening. The liver usually is able to grow back its tissue, but severe hepatitis may lead to permanent damage. **Anicteric hepatitis** is a mild form of hepatitis in which there is no jaundice. It is mostly seen in infants and young children. Symptoms include loss of appetite, stomach upset, and slight fever. The infection may be mistaken for flu or go unnoticed. **Cholestatic hepatitis** results from infection that causes interruption of the flow of bile in the bile ducts. Symptoms include jaundice and itching. **Viral hepatitis** results from one of the hepatitis viruses, A, B, or non-A, non-B. Symptoms of viral hepatitis include pain over the liver, fever, nausea and vomiting, and diarrhea. The patient should not donate blood. The form caused by the **hepatitis A** virus has a slow onset of symptoms. The virus may be spread by direct contact or through fecal-infected food or water. The infection most often occurs in young adults and is usually followed by complete recovery. The form caused by the **hepatitis B** virus (serum hepatitis) has a rapid onset of symptoms. The virus can be carried in blood products used for transfusion or by the use of unsterile needles and instruments. The infection may be severe and result in prolonged illness, destruction of liver cells, cirrhosis, or death. **Non-A, non-B (NANB) hepatitis** is caused by a virus other than the types that cause hepatitis A or hepatitis B. It is usually milder but is otherwise similar, and treatment is the same as for other forms. More than 90% of the cases of hepatitis in the United States, occurring in patients receiving multiple blood transfusions, is NANB hepatitis. **Recrudescent hepatitis** is a form of viral hepatitis that returns during a time of getting better.

hepatitis B immune globulin (HBIG), a drug to protect one against infection by the hepatitis B virus. Known allergy to the drug or to gamma globulin prohibits its use. Side effects include severe allergic reactions. Pain and swelling at the site of injection also may occur.

hepatization, the changing of lung tissue into a solid mass. In early pneumonia the gathering of red blood cells in the air sacs produce **red hepatization.** In later stages of pneumonia, when white blood cells fill the air sacs, the process becomes **gray hepatization,** or **yellow hepatization** when fat deposits join the process.

hepatocyte /hep'ətōsīt'/, the most basic liver cell that performs all the functions of the liver.

hepatoduodenal ligament /hep'ətōdoo·ədē'nəl, -doo·od'ənəl/, a part of the membrane that lines the abdomen between the liver and the small intestine. A fiberlike capsule between the two layers of the ligament contains the hepatic artery, the common bile duct, the portal vein, lymphatics, and a network of nerves.

hepatojugular reflux /-jug'ələr/, an increase of pressure in the jugular vein when pressure is applied for 30 to 60 seconds over the stomach, suggestive of right-sided heart failure.

hepatolenticular degeneration /-lentik'yələr/. See **Wilson's disease.**

hepatoma /hep'ətō'mə/, a cancer of the liver. Symptoms include pain, low blood pressure, loss of appetite and weight, and fluid buildup in the abdominal cavity. It is most often found together with hepatitis or cirrhosis of the liver. The only useful treatment is to remove the tumor. This is often not possible because the tumors grow rapidly and spread through both lobes of the liver.

hepatomegaly /-meg'əlē/, abnormal enlargement of the liver that is usually a sign of liver disease. It is often found by tapping and feeling the area as part of a physical examination. The liver can easily be felt below the ribs and is tender to the touch. Hepatomegaly may be caused by hepatitis or other infection, alcoholism, obstruction of bile ducts, or cancer.

hepatotoxic /-tok'sik/, destroying liver cells.

hepatotoxicity /-toksis'itē/, the tendency of a substance, usually a drug or alcohol, to have a harmful effect on the liver.

herb bath, a medicinal bath taken in water containing aromatic herbs.

herbicide poisoning, a poisoning caused by eating, breathing, or skin contact with a substance intended for use as a weed killer. Some herbicides can be extremely poisonous, causing burning stomach or throat pain, diarrhea, or other severe symptoms. Many of the commonly used farming weed killers can produce symptoms ranging from skin irritation to low blood pressure, liver and kidney damage, and coma or fits. Death can result from a dose as small as 1 to 10 g. Vomiting or cleansing of the stomach should be induced by eating.

hereditary, having to do with a feature, condition, or disease passed down from parent to offspring; inborn; inherited. Compare **acquired, congenital, familial.**

hereditary disorder. See **inherited disorder.**

hereditary multiple exostoses, a rare disease in which bony outgrowths form on the shafts of the long bones and eventually develop into caps of cartilage covering the ends of the bones. The affected joints lose their ease of move-

ment, and the bones stop growing. The disease begins in childhood and has no cure. Very rarely, the cap of cartilage may become cancerous.

hereditary oral disease, any abnormal, inborn defects of the mouth and its parts, as deformed teeth, tongue, gums, or cleft palate. Many hereditary oral diseases are part of other inherited diseases.

heredity, 1. the process by which particular traits or conditions are passed along from parents to offspring, causing resemblance of individuals related by blood. It involves the division and rejoining of genes during cell division and fertilization. Heredity is affected by events that occur during the development of the embryo. **2.** the total genetic makeup of an individual; the sum of the features inherited from ancestors and the possibilities of passing on these qualities to offspring.

Hering-Breuer reflexes, controlling signals sent by the nerves that maintain the rhythm of breathing and prevent the overfilling of the air sacs in the lungs. These reflexes are well developed at birth. They are brought on by filling up of the airway, increased pressures in the windpipe, or inflation of the lungs. The inflation reflex stops breathing in and stimulates breathing out; the deflation reflex stops breathing out and begins breathing in.

hermaphroditism /hərmaf'rəditizm/, a rare condition in which both male and female sex organs exist in the same person. The condition results from a chromosomal abnormality. Also called **hermaphrodism.** Compare **pseudohermaphroditism.**

hernia, a breakthrough of an organ through a tear in the muscle wall that surrounds it. A hernia may be present at birth, may come from the failure of some structures to close after birth, or may be acquired later in life because of overweight, muscular weakness, surgery, or illness. An **abdominal hernia** is a loop of bowel that bulges through the muscles of the abdomen. This can happen at an old surgical scar. A bulge of part of the stomach through an opening in the diaphragm is a **diaphragmatic hernia.** This occurs most often at the point where the throat passes through the diaphragm. In some cases the intestines may also bulge into the chest. This is one of the most common disorders of the stomach and intestines. It occurs most often in middle-aged and elderly people. A kind of diaphragmatic hernia is **hiatus hernia,** a breakthrough of a portion of the stomach upward through the diaphragm. Symptoms usually include heartburn after meals, when lying down, and on exertion, especially when bending forward. There may be vomiting, difficult swallowing, bloating of the stomach after eating, belching, rumbling in the intestines, rapid breathing, and a dull pain below the breastbone that extends to the shoulder. The continued backup of stomach fluids into the throat may lead to ulcers with bleeding. Treatment includes relieving the discomfort caused by stomach contents backflow. A **femoral hernia** is one in which a loop of intestine moves into the groin. With an **inguinal hernia,** a loop of intestine enters the inguinal canal, sometimes filling, in a male, the entire scrotal sac. An inguinal hernia is usually repaired surgically, to prevent its blocking passage of waste through the bowel. Of all hernias, 75% to 80% are inguinal hernias. An **umbilical hernia** is a soft, skin-covered bulge of intestine through a weakness in the abdominal wall around the belly button (umbilicus). It often closes on its own, but large hernias may need surgery.

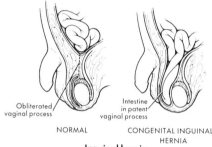

Obliterated vaginal process

Intestine in patent vaginal process

NORMAL   CONGENITAL INGUINAL HERNIA

Inguinal hernia

herniated disk /hur′nē·ā′tid/, a break in the cartilage surrounding a disk in the spine, releasing the substance that cushions the back bones above and below. The central part of each disk between the vertebrae, called the **nucleus pulposus,** is a rubbery substance that loses some ability to recover from strain with age. The nucleus pulposus may be suddenly put under pressure by unusual exercise or by injury, and squeeze out through the cartilage. The resultant pressure on spinal nerve roots may cause considerable pain and damage the nerves. The condition most often occurs in the lower back. Also called **ruptured disk, slipped disk.** See also **cervical disk syndrome.**

herniation, a breakthrough of a body organ or part of an organ through a tear in a membrane, muscle, or other tissue. See also **hernia.**

herniorrhaphy /hur′nē·or′əfē/, the surgical repair of a hernia.

heroin, a morphinelike drug with no currently acceptable medical use in the United States. Heroin is controlled by law in the Comprehensive Drug Abuse Prevention and Control Act of 1970. According to this law, it may not be prescribed to patients but only used for research and teaching use or for chemical analysis by permission from the Drug Enforcement Administration of the Department of Justice. Heroin, like other opium products, can produce relief from pain, slowing of breathing, spasms in the digestive system, and physical dependence. Its major effects are on the brain and spinal cord, the bowel, and the hormone functions and nervous reflexes. Street use of the drug commonly begins with sniffing powdered heroin, which is absorbed through the moist lining of the nose, throat, and breathing tract. Other methods of taking the drug include injecting it under the skin or into a vein. Heroin, which loses much of its pain-killing power when taken by mouth, is more powerful than morphine and acts more rapidly. It is changed into morphine by the body and builds up in the organs, bones, and brain. Repeated use of this drug causes a gradual decrease in the effects felt (tolerance). Physical dependence develops along with tolerance. Withdrawal from heroin after using it even a few times commonly causes severe symptoms. Withdrawal signs usually come shortly before the next planned dose and include anxiety, restlessness, irritability, and craving for another dose. Other withdrawal signs that may appear 8 to 15 hours after the last dose include watery eyes, perspiration, yawning, and restless sleep. On awakening from such sleep, the severely addicted heroin user may experience further withdrawal signs, as vomiting, pain in the bones, diarrhea, convulsions, and heart attack. A variety of liquid substances, as quinine, are used to dissolve street heroin for injection. Impure states of such liquids, together with dirty needles and other unhealthy factors, are responsible for more than half the deaths related to the illegal use of heroin. The most frequent disorders related to injections of impure heroin are tetanus, skin abscesses, infection, and swollen veins. Heroin-connected lung complications include pneumonia, internal bleeding, and tuberculosis. Many nerve disorders may result from the use of street heroin. Women heroin addicts who become pregnant often give birth to premature babies who easily get blood poisoning and may be addicted to heroin at birth. Heroin addicts often return to use of the drug during withdrawal treatment. Withdrawal symptoms, as altered blood pressure and pulse rate, anxiety, and depression, may last for months. Methadone is commonly used as a substitute drug in the treatment of heroin addiction. Many outpatient programs staffed by former opiate users seek to give helpful support for addicts trying to break their drug habits. Some of these programs are Synanon, Daytop Village, and Phoenix House. Research and community-supported mental health projects continue to seek better treatment methods for addicts, many of whom are successfully cured. Denying heroin to addicts in prisons has been much less effective in curing addicts. Most authorities believe that gradual withdrawal under medical care, with counseling, is the most promising approach.

herpangina /hur′panji̇̄′nə/, a viral infection, usually of young children. Symptoms include sore throat, headache, loss of appetite, and pain in the stomach, neck, and arms and legs. Feverish fits and vomiting may occur in infants. Blisters may form in the mouth and throat, which turn into

G–H

shallow sores that heal by themselves. The disease usually runs its course in less than 1 week. Treatment aims to relieve symptoms.

herpes genitalis /hur'pēz/, an infection caused by Type 2 herpes simplex virus (HSV2), usually passed along by sexual contact, that causes painful blisters on the skin and moist lining of the sex organs of males and females. This herpes virus tends to cause repeated attacks. In the male, herpes genitalis infections may resemble penile ulcers. A small group of blisters surrounded by redness of the skin may occur on the tip or foreskin. These turn into surface sores that often heal in 5 to 7 days, although they also may become infected. The sores are painful and often give a burning sensation, urinary problems, fever, illness, and swelling of the lymph nodes in the groin area. The female patient may have similar problems, and members of both sexes may complain of painful sexual intercourse. In the female, herpes genitalis lesions are likely to appear as groups of sores on the surfaces of the cervix, vagina, or perineum. There may be a discharge from the cervix. Vaginal blisters may appear as open sores. Transfer of the virus to the eye results in inflammation of the cornea. Infections that develop in pregnant women may progress to viruses in the blood and a danger of death and illness in the fetus. An attack of herpes within 3 weeks of delivery usually requires that the infant be delivered by cesarean section to avoid dangerous herpesvirus infection of the newborn. Treatment of herpes genitalis sores is with the antibiotic ancyclovir. Untreated, an attack of the disease will generally go away by itself in time. Sores may be cleansed with soap and water, where possible, to prevent secondary infections, and drying medications may be applied to sores that rupture or ooze.

herpes gestationis, a generalized itching or blistering rash appearing in the last 3 to 6 months of pregnancy and disappearing several weeks after delivery. The sores often come back with later pregnancies and are often linked with premature birth and increased fetal death.

herpes simplex, an infection caused by a herpes simplex virus (HSV), which attacks the skin and nervous system and usually produces small, short-lasting, irritating, and sometimes painful fluid-filled blisters on the skin and mucous membranes. HSV1 (oral herpes, herpes labialis) infections tend to occur in the facial area, particularly around the mouth and nose; HSV2 (herpes genitalis) infections are usually limited to the genital area. The first symptoms of a herpes simplex infection usually include burning, tingling, or itching sensations around the edges of the lips or nose within 1 or 2 weeks after contact with an infected person. Several hours later, small red pimples develop in the irritated area, followed by the formation of small fever blisters filled with fluid. Several small blisters may merge to form a larger blister. The blisters generally cause itching, pain, or similar discomfort. Other effects often include a mild fever and enlargement of the lymph nodes in the neck. Within 1 week after the onset of symptoms, thin yellow crusts form on the blisters as healing begins. In skin areas that are moist or protected or in severe cases, healing may be delayed. Once acquired, the virus tends to rest without symptoms in the skin or tissues of the nervous system and may become active from fever, physical or emotional stress, exposure to sunlight, or some foods or drugs. Complications of herpes infections include inflammation of the brain, the cornea of the eye, and gums. In cases involving complications, special treatment may be needed. In uncomplicated cases, the herpes attack usually runs its course in 3 weeks or less. Treatment of herpes simplex is to relieve symptoms. The sores may be washed gently with soap and water to reduce the risk of secondary infection. Applying drying medications to the skin, such as alcohol solutions, although painful, may speed healing.

herpesvirus, any of five related viruses including herpes simplex viruses 1 and 2, varicella-zoster virus, Epstein-Barr virus, and cytomegalovirus.

herpes zoster, a severe infection caused by the varicella-zoster virus (VZV), affecting mainly adults. It causes painful skin blisters that follow the route of nerves infected by the virus. The pain and blisters usually occur on only one side of the body, and any sensory nerve may be affected. The pain, which may be constant or off and on, surface or deep, usually comes before other effects and may mimic other disorders, as appendicitis or pleurisy. Early symptoms may include digestive system disturbances, vague discomfort, fever, and headache. The blisters usually evolve from small red bumps along the path of a nerve, and the skin of the area is overly sensitive. All of the sores may appear within a period of hours or develop gradually over several days. The bumps swell and become thickened with dead cell material. Usually, at the end of the first week, the bumps develop crusts. The symptoms may persist for 2 to 5 weeks. Bed rest is encouraged during the early stages of zoster infection, when fever and other overall effects occur. Preventing direct contact of affected skin areas with irritating fabrics relieves discomfort. Older patients have greatest risk of complications, as exhaustion and jabbing pain (neuralgia) may last for several months after the skin sores have cleared. Other complications include involvement of the ear, eye, face, and soft palate. An attack of herpes zoster does not make one immune to further attacks, but most patients recover without permanent effects except for occasional scarring. Treatment includes calamine lotion or similar medications to relieve itching and aspirin or pain killers for pain symptoms. Cool compresses may be applied to the affected skin areas. Skin medicines that prevent inflammation may be given for severe cases and for elderly patients who may experience jabbing pain along a nerve following a herpes attack. Surgery to remove an affected nerve may be done in cases of severe pain that fail to respond to other treatment. Also called **shingles.** See also **herpes simplex, varicella-zoster virus.**

herpes zoster oticus, a herpes zoster infection causing severe pain in the outer ear structures and pain or paralysis along the facial nerve. Hearing loss and dizziness may also occur. The dizziness is usually short-lived, but the hearing loss and facial paralysis may be permanent. There may be blisters on the ear and in the ear canal. Treatment includes a drug given for dizziness, aspirin for pain, and antiinflammatory medicines for other symptoms.

herpes zoster virus. See **varicella-zoster virus.**

herpetiform /hərpet′ifôrm/, having clusters of blisters; resembling the skin sores of some herpesvirus infections.

Herplex, a trademark for an antiviral drug (idoxuridine).

Hers' disease. See **glycogen storage disease.**

hesperidin /hesper′idin/, a sugar substance occurring in most citrus fruits, especially in the spongy casing of oranges and lemons.

hetastarch, a substance to increase the volume of blood plasma, given to help treat shock and leukophoresis. Severe bleeding, severe heart or kidney problems with excessive or insufficient urination, or known allergy to this drug prohibits its use. Side effects include influenza-like symptoms, muscle pain, fluid retention, and extreme allergic reaction.

heteroallele /het′ərō·əlēl′/, one of a set of genes located at a specific place on similar chromosomes that differs from the other of the pair, resulting in a mutation.

heteroblastic /-blas′-/, developing from different germ layers or kinds of tissue rather than from a single type. Compare **homoblastic.**

heterochromosome, a sex chromosome. See also **heterotypic chromosomes.**

heteroeroticism /-irot′isizm/, sexual feeling or activity directed toward another individual. Also called **alloeroticism.** Compare **autoeroticism.**

heterogamy /het′ərog′əmē/, sexual reproduction in which there is joining of dissimilar sex cells, usually differing in size and structure. The word primarily refers to the reproductive processes of humans and mammals as opposed to certain lower plants and animals.

heterogeneous /het′ərōjē′nē·əs/, **1.** consisting of unlike elements or parts. **2.** not having a uniform quality throughout. Compare **homogeneous.** –**heterogeneity,** *adj.*

heterogenous /het′əroj′ənəs/, derived or developed from another source or from two different sources.

heterologous tumor /het′ərol′əgəs/, a tumor consisting of tissue different from that around it.

heterophil antibody test /het′ərōfil′/, a test for the presence of heterophil antibodies in the blood of patients suspected of having infectious mononucleosis. This antibody eventually appears in the blood of more than 80% of the patients with mononucleosis, hence is a good way to diagnose the disease. See also **Epstein-Barr virus.**

heteroploid /-ploid′/, **1.** an individual, organism, strain, or cell that has fewer or more whole chromosomes in its body cells than is normal for its species. **2.** such an individual, organism, strain, or cell. See also **euploid.**

heterosexual, 1. a person whose sexual desire or preference is for people of the opposite sex. **2.** sexual desire or preference for people of the opposite sex. –**heterosexuality,** *n.*

heterosexual panic, a sudden attack of anxiety resulting in the frantic pursuit of heterosexual activity in response to unconscious or unrecognized homosexual impulses. Compare **homosexual panic.**

heterotopic ossification /-top′ik/, a noncancerous overgrowth of bone, often occurring after a break in the bone, that is sometimes confused with certain bone tumors when seen on x-ray film. Also called **exuberant callus.**

heterotypic chromosomes /-tip′ik/, any unmatched pair of chromosomes, specifically the sex chromosomes.

heterozygous /-zī′gəs/, having two different genes at the same place on matched chromosomes. A person who is heterozygous for a particular trait has inherited a gene for that trait from one parent and the alternative gene from the other parent. For example, a person heterozygous for a disorder caused by a dominant gene, as Huntington's chorea, will show the disease. A person heterozygous for a disorder caused by a recessive gene, as sickle cell anemia, will not show the disease, or will have a milder form of it. The offspring of a heterozygous carrier of a genetic disorder have a 50% chance of inheriting the gene dominant for the trait. Compare **homozygous.**

Hexa-Betalin, a trademark for vitamin B_6 (pyridoxine hydrochloride).

hexachlorophene, a cleanser and antiseptic for external use. It may also be used as an antiseptic scrub and as a disinfectant. Known allergy to this drug prohibits its use. It can be absorbed into the system when used on burns, broken skin, mucous membranes, and infant skin, leading to blood poisoning. The skin should be rinsed thoroughly to prevent absorption of the drug into the bloodstream. Side effects include skin rash and nervous disorders.

G–H

Hexadrol, a trademark for a hormone that affects starch processing in the body (dexamethasone).

hexocyclium methylsulfate, a drug prescribed to help treat ulcers. Narrow-angle glaucoma, asthma, blockage of the genital, urinary, or digestive tract, ulcerative inflammation of the colon, or known allergy to this drug prohibits its use. Side effects include blurred vision, brain and nervous system effects, rapid heart rate, dry mouth, decreased sweating, and allergic reactions.

hiatus /hī·ā′təs/, a usually normal opening in a membrane or other body tissue. –**hiatal,** *adj.*

hiatus hernia. See **hernia.**

hibernoma /hī′bərnō′mə/, a noncancerous tumor, usually on the hips or the back, composed of fat cells that are partly or entirely left over from the fetal stage of growth. Also called **fat cell lipoma.**

hiccup, a sound that is produced by the unintentional squeezing of the diaphragm, followed by rapid closure of the vocal cords. Hiccups have a variety of causes, including indigestion, rapid eating, certain types of surgery, and inflammation of the brain. Most attacks of hiccups do not last longer than a few minutes, but long-lasting or repeated attacks sometimes occur. The condition is most often seen in men. Sedatives are used in extreme cases. Also spelled **hiccough.**

hidrosis /hidrō′-/, sweating. **Anhidrosis** is an abnormal lack of sweating. **Dyshidrosis** is a condition in which abnormal sweating occurs. **Hyperhidrosis** is a state of too much sweating. It is often caused by heat, overactive thyroid, strong emotion, menopause, or infection. Treatment usually includes antiperspirants. It may involve surgery to remove armpit (axillary) sweat glands.

high blood pressure. See **hypertension.**

high-density lipoprotein (HDL). See **lipoprotein.**

high-energy phosphate compound, a chemical compound that fuels muscle contraction, active transport of substances across cell membranes, and the production of many substances in the body.

highest intercostal vein, one of a pair of veins that drain the blood from the upper chest.

high-potassium diet, a diet that contains foods rich in potassium, including all leafy green vegetables, brussels sprouts, citrus fruits, bananas, dates, raisins, beans, meats, and whole grains. It is advised for any condition resulting in the loss of fluid, as acute diarrhea, high blood pressure, and diabetic coma. It is also advised for patients receiving thiazide or corticosteroid therapy.

high-protein diet, a diet that contains large amounts of protein, consisting largely of meats, fish, milk, beans, and nuts. It may be advised in protein loss from any cause, to strengthen a patient before surgery, and in some kidney or liver disorders. It is not advised when added protein could result in harmful levels of urea and other acids in the body.

high-risk infant, any newborn, regardless of birth weight, size, or length of time in the womb, who has a greater than average chance of sickness or death, especially within the first 28 days of life. The cause may be conditions that interfere with the normal birth process or growth and development after birth.

high-vitamin diet, a diet that includes a variety of foods that contain healthful amounts of all of the vitamins necessary for the processes of the body. It is often ordered in combination with other prescribed diets containing larger than usual amounts of protein or calories, especially when treating severe or long-lasting infection, malnutrition, or vitamin deficiency.

hinge axis-orbital plane, a plane that is usually determined by marking three points on the face of the patient. Two of the points, one on each side of the face, are located on the line where the upper and lower jaws are joined. The third point is located on the face at the level of the eye socket just beneath the eye. The hinge axis-orbital plane is used to diagnose and treat misaligned teeth.

hinge joint, a fluid-filled joint in which bone surfaces are closely molded together in a way that permits extensive motion in one plane. The joints of the fingers are hinge joints. Compare **gliding joint, pivot joint.**

hipbone. See **innominate bone.**

hip joint, the ball-and-socket joint of the hip. It consists of the head of the thigh bone (femur) in the cup-shaped hole in the pelvis (acetabulum). These are attached by seven ligaments which permit very extensive movements. Also called **coxal articulation.**

hippocampal commissure /hip′əkam′pəl/, a thin, triangular layer of crosswise fibers that connects the middle edges of the two sides of the hippocampus, a structure in the lower brain.

hippocampal fissure, a division reaching from the lowest point of the corpus callosum to the tip of the temporal lobe of the brain.

hippocampus /-kam′pəs/, *pl.* **hippocampi,** a structure of the brain that functions as an important part of the limbic system. Also called **Ammon's horn.**

Hippocrates /hipok′rətēz/, a Greek physician born about 460 BC on the island of Cos, a center for the worship of Æsculapius. Called the "Father of Medicine," Hippocrates introduced a scientific approach to healing. The **Hippocratic oath** is an oath thought to have come from Hipporates that serves as an ethical guide for the medical profession.

hip replacement, an operation to replace the hip joint with an artificial ball and socket joint. This is done to relieve a constantly painful and stiff hip in serious cases of arthritis, an improperly healed break, or destruction of the joint. Antibiotics are given before the operation, and the patient is taught to walk with crutches. Surgery is done under general anesthesia. After the operation, the patient is placed in traction. The most frequent complications are infection requiring removal of the new joint, or its dislocation. Movement begins gradually, with frequent short walks. Sitting for more than 1 hour is to be avoided, and hip bending beyond 90 degrees may cause dislocation of the new joint. The patient continues an exercise program after release from the hospital to keep the hip moving freely and to strengthen the muscles.

Hiprex, a trademark for a urinary antibacterial (methenamine hippurate).

hirsutism /hur'sootizm/, excessive body hair in a male pattern as a result of heredity, hormonal imbalance, porphyria, or medication. Treatment of the specific cause will usually stop growth of more hair. Excess hair may be removed by electrolysis, chemical removal, shaving, plucking, or rubbing with pumice. Fine facial hair may be most effectively minimized by bleaching.

His-Purkinje system /-pərkin'jē/, a nerve system in the heart tissues that leads from the bundle of His to the Purkinje fibers.

Hispril, a trademark for an antihistamine (diphenylpyraline hydrochloride).

histamine /his'təmin, -mēn/, a compound, found in all cells, produced by the breakdown of histidine. It is released in allergic reactions and causes widening of capillaries, decreased blood pressure, increased release of gastric juice, and tightening of smooth muscles of the bronchi and uterus.

histamine headache. See **headache.**

histidine (His) /his'tidin/, a basic amino acid found in many proteins and the substance from which histamine is produced. It is an essential amino acid in infants.

histiocytic malignant lymphoma /his'tē·ōsī'-/, a tumor on a lymph gland.

histocompatibility antigens, a group of antigens on the surface of many cells. Histocompatibility antigens are the cause of most graft rejections that occur in organ transplants.

histoid neoplasm. See **neoplasm.**

histology /histol'-/, **1.** the science dealing with the microscopic identification of cells and tissue. **2.** the structure of organ tissues, including the makeup of cells and their organization into various body tissues.

histone /his'tōn/, any of a group of proteins, found in the cell nucleus, especially of glandular tissue. They help to regulate gene activity. Histones also interfere with clotting of the blood and have been found in the urine of patients with leukemia and fevers.

histoplasma agglutinin /his'təplaz'mə/, an antibody against fungal lung infections.

histoplasmosis /-plazmō'-/, an infection caused by breathing in spores of the fungus *Histoplasma capsulatum.* It is common in the Mississippi and Ohio valleys. The fungus, spread by airborne spores from soil infected with the droppings of infected birds, acts as a parasite on the cells of the body's defense system.

histotoxin /-tok'sin/, any substance that is poisonous to the body tissues. It is usually produced within the body rather than coming from outside. **–histotoxic,** *adj.*

histrionic personality disorder /his'trē·on'ik/, a disorder having intensely exaggerated behavior, which is typically self-centered and results in severe disturbance in the patient's relationships with others. This can lead to psychosomatic disorders, depression, alcoholism, and drug dependency. Symptoms include emotional excitability, such as irrational angry outbursts or tantrums; abnormal craving for activity and excitement; overreaction to minor events; self-serving threats and gestures; self-centeredness, inconsiderateness; inconsistency; and continuous demand for reassurance because of feelings of helplessness and dependency. A person having this disorder is seen by others as vain, demanding, shallow, self-centered, and self-pampering. The disorder is more common in women than in men and is treated by various psychotherapies. See also **narcissistic personality disorder.**

hives. See **urticaria.**

HMS Liquifilm, a trademark for an eye solution containing an anti-inflammatory hormone (medrysone).

H₂O, symbol for **water.**

Hodgkin's disease /hoj'kinz/, a malignant disorder with painless, steady enlargement of lymph glands, usually first in the neck; enlarged spleen; and the presence of large, unusual white cells (Reed-Sternberg cells). Symptoms include loss of appetite, weight loss, generalized itching, low-grade fever, night sweats, decrease of red blood cells, and increase of white blood cells. The disease affects twice as many males as females, and usually develops between 15 and 35 years of age. Radiation of lymph nodes is the usual treatment for early stages of the disease. Combination chemotherapy is the treatment for advanced disease. In more than one half of the patients treated, the symptoms go away for long periods of time, and 60% to 90% of those with limited spreading of the disease may be cured. Clusters of cases have been reported, but there is no definite evidence of an infectious agent, and the cause of the disease remains a mystery.

G–H

Hoffmann's reflex, an abnormal reflex brought about by sudden, forceful striking of the nail of the index, middle, or ring finger, resulting in bending of the thumb and of the middle and end joints of one of the other fingers. It is a possible sign of motor nerve disease. Also called **Hoffmann's sign.**

holandric inheritance /hōlan'-/. See **inheritance.**

holistic health care, a system of total patient care that considers the physical, emotional, social, economic, and spiritual needs of the patient. It also considers the patient's response to the illness and the impact of the illness on the patient's ability to meet self-care needs. Holistic nursing is the modern nursing practice that expresses this philosophy of care. Also called **comprehensive care.**

holoacardius /hō'lō·əkär'dē·əs/, a separate, grossly defective identical-twin fetus. It is usually composed of a shapeless, nonformed mass in which the heart is absent and the circulation in the womb is provided totally by the heart of the healthy twin through a rerouted blood vessel.

hologynic /-jin'ik/, **1.** designating genes located on attached X chromosomes. **2.** of or pertaining to traits or conditions passed on only from the mother (the maternal line).

holoprosencephaly /-pros'ensef'əlē/, a birth defect caused by the failure of the forebrain to divide into halves during embryonic development. It is known by many midline facial defects, including the development of only one eye in severe cases. It can also be caused by an extra chromosome, being just one of many developmental defects.

Holtzman inkblot technique, a version of the Rorschach test in which many more pictures of inkblots are used, the subject is allowed only one answer to each design, and the scoring is mainly objective rather than subjective.

Homan's sign, pain in the calf that occurs with bending the foot back, indicating blood clots or swollen veins from clots (thrombophlebitis).

homatropine methylbromide, a drug used to prevent blinking and to widen pupils in eye surgery. Narrow-angle glaucoma, asthma, blockage of the genital, urinary, or digestive tract, ulcerative irritation of the colon, or known allergy to this drug prohibits its use. Side effects include blurred vision, central nervous system effects, rapid heart rate, dry mouth, decreased sweating, and allergic reactions.

home care, a health service provided in the patient's home for the purpose of promoting, maintaining, or restoring health or reducing the effects of illness and disability. Service may include medical, dental, or nursing care, speech or physical therapy, the homemaking services of a home health aide, or transportation service. Nursing may be provided by a registered nurse, licensed practical nurse, or a home health aide. Some hospitals have home care

services that include regular visits by a nurse and a physician to patients in their homes.

home health agency, an organization that provides health care in the home. Medicare certification for a home health agency depends on the providing of skilled nursing services and of at least one additional therapeutic service.

homeodynamics /hō'mē·ōdīnam'-/, the process of constantly changing body functions while keeping an overall balance of systems and health.

Homeopathic Pharmacopoeia of the United States /-path'ik/, one of the official drug lists specified in the Federal Food, Drug, and Cosmetic Act. See also **United States Pharmacopoeia.**

homeopathy /hō'mē·op'əthē/, a system of healing based on the theory that "like cures like." The theory was advanced in the late eighteenth century by Dr. Samuel Hahnemann, who believed that a large amount of a particular drug may cause symptoms of a disease and a mild dose may reduce those symptoms; thus, some disease symptoms could be treated by very small doses of medicine. In practice, homeopathists (physicians who practice homeopathy) dilute drugs with milk sugar in ratios of 1 to 10 to achieve the smallest dose of a drug that seems necessary to control the symptoms in a patient. They also prescribe only one medication at a time. Compare **allopathy.** –**homeopathic,** *adj.*

homeostasis /-stā'-/, a relatively constant state within the body, naturally maintained. Various sensing, feedback, and control systems bring about this steady state, especially the reticular formation in the brainstem and the hormone-producing glands. Some of the functions controlled by homeostatic mechanisms are the heart-beat, blood production, blood pressure, body temperature, salt balance, breathing, and glandular secretion. –**homeostatic,** *adj.*

homicide, the death of one human being caused by another human. Homicide is usually intentional and often violent.

homiothermic /hō'mē·ōthur'-/ referring to the ability of warm-blooded animals to keep a relatively stable body temperature regardless of the temperature of the environment. This ability is not fully developed in newborn humans.

homoblastic /hō'mōblas'-/, developing from a single type of tissue. Compare **heteroblastic.**

homogeneous /-jē'nē·əs/, **1.** consisting of similar elements or parts. **2.** having a uniform quality throughout. Compare **heterogeneous.** –**homogeneity,** *adj.*

homogenesis /-jen'əsis/, reproduction by the same process in succeeding generations so that offspring are similar to the parents. Compare **heterogenesis.**

homogenized milk /hōmoj'ənīzd/, pasteurized milk that has been mechanically treated to reduce and spread the fat evenly throughout so that the cream cannot separate and the protein is more digestible.

homogenous /hōmoj′ənəs/, having a likeness in form or structure because of a common ancestral origin. Compare **heterogenous.**

homolateral /-lat′ərəl/, pertaining to the same side of the body.

homolog /hom′əlog/, any organ corresponding in function, origin, and structure to another organ, as the flippers of a seal, corresponding to human hands.

homologous chromosomes /hōmol′əgəs/, any two chromosomes in the doubled set of the body cell that are identical in size, shape, and gene placement. In humans there are 22 pairs of homologous chromosomes and one pair of sex chromosomes, with one member of each pair coming from the mother and the other from the father. Any difference in the size, number, or genetic makeup of the chromosomes leads to defects or disorders from mild to severe in the affected individual.

homologous tumor, a tumor made up of cells resembling those of the tissue in which it is growing.

homoplasty /hō′məplas′tē/, likeness in form or structure because of similar environmental conditions or parallel evolution rather than because of common ancestral origin.

homosexual, **1.** pertaining to, or denoting the same sex. **2.** a person who is sexually attracted to members of the same sex. Compare **heterosexual.** See also **lesbian.**

homosexual panic, a sudden attack of anxiety based on possible unconscious desires and a conscious fear of being homosexual. Compare **heterosexual panic.**

homozygous /-zī′gəs/, having two identical genes at the same place on matched chromosomes. An individual who is homozygous for a particular trait has inherited from each parent one of two identical genes for that trait. A person homozygous for a genetic disease caused by a pair of recessive genes, as sickle cell anemia, shows the disorder, and his or her offspring have a 100% chance of inheriting the gene for the disease. Compare **heterozygous.**

homunculus /hōmung′kyələs/, pl. **homunculi, 1.** a dwarf in which all the body parts are in proportion and in which there is no deformity or abnormality. **2.** (in early theories of development) a minute and complete human being contained in each of the eggs (germ cells) that after fertilization grows from microscopic to normal size; The term was also applied to the human fetus. **3.** (in psychiatry) a little man created by the imagination who possesses magical powers.

hookworm infection, a condition resulting from a spread of hookworms of the genera *Ancylostoma, Necator,* or *Uncinaria* in the small intestine. Infection by *Ancylostoma* is harmful and hard to treat. It is less common than *Necator*

americanus, which is the hookworm most often found in the southern United States. Treatment for hookworm infection is drugs to rid the body of the worms. Blood or iron may be given if the patient is anemic. Infection may be prevented by keeping soil free of fecal matter and by wearing shoes.

hopelessness, a psychologic condition in which one believes that all efforts to change one's life situation will be fruitless.

hordeolum /hôrdē′ələm/. See **sty.**

hormone, a chemical substance produced in one part or organ of the body that starts or runs the activity of an organ or a group of cells in another part of the body. Hormones from the endocrine glands are carried through the bloodstream to the target organ. Release of these hormones is regulated by other hormones, by nerve signals, and by a signal from the target organ indicating a decreased need for the stimulating hormone. This is the basic principle of birth control pills. A steady supply of female hormones in the pills causes a lowered release of the hormones that ordinarily cause the ovary to develop and release the egg, along with the same female hormones (estrogen and progesterone). Other hormones are released by organs for specific reasons, most commonly in the digestive tract.

Horner's syndrome, a nerve condition with narrowed pupils, drooping eyelids, and unusual facial dryness resulting from an injury to the spinal cord, with damage to a neck nerve. When seen in a case of sudden injury, the person is carried flat with as little movement as possible.

horse serum, any vaccine prepared from the blood of a horse, especially tetanus antitoxin. Because many people are allergic to horse serum, a skin test for allergy is usually performed before the vaccine is given. Human tetanus serum is preferred.

horseshoe fistula, an abnormal, semicircular passage in the area around the anus with both openings on the surface of the skin.

hospice /hos′pis/, a system of family-centered care designed to assist the patient with a long-term illness to be comfortable and to maintain a satisfactory life-style through the last phases of dying. Hospice care includes home visits, professional medical help available on call, teaching and emotional support of the family, and physical care of the patient. Some hospice programs provide care in a center, as well as in the home. See also **stages of dying.**

hospitalism, the physical or mental effects of hospitalization or institutionalization on patients, especially infants and children who show this condition through social withdrawal, personality disorders, and stunted growth.

host, 1. an organism that is a victim of parasitic invasion. A **primary** or **definitive host** is one in which the adult parasite lives and reproduces. Humans are definitive hosts for pinworms and tapeworms. A **secondary** or **intermediate host** is one in which the parasite exists in its nonsexual, larval stage. Humans are intermediate hosts for malaria parasites. A **reservoir host** is a primary animal host for organisms that are sometimes parasitic in humans and from which humans may become infected. A **dead-end host** is any animal from which a parasite cannot escape to continue its life cycle. **2.** the recipient of a transplanted organ or tissue. Compare **donor.**

hostility, the tendency of an organism to threaten harm to another or to itself. The hostility may be expressed passively and actively.

hot flash, a short-term feeling of warmth experienced by some women during or after menopause. Hot flashes result from blood flow disturbances caused by hormone changes. The exact cause is not known. Many menopausal women do not experience hot flashes; among those who do, the frequency, length, and strength of flashes vary widely. Though physically harmless, the symptom may be extremely disturbing or, rarely, disabling. Hot flashes may be relieved by the taking of the hormone estrogen in cycles. Also called **hot flush.**

hot line, a means of contacting a trained counselor or specific agency for help with a particular problem, as a rape hot line or a battered-child hot line. The person needing help calls a telephone number and speaks to a counselor who remains nameless and who offers emotional support, advice for action, and referral to other medical, social, or community services. Such services are usually staffed by volunteers who answer phones 24 hours a day, 7 days a week.

hot zone area, area of a hazardous materials incident immediately dangerous to life and health. Requires complete, appropriate protective clothing and equipment. Entry requires approval by the incident commander or a designated sector officer. Complete backup and rescue teams must be in place at the perimeter before operations begin. Only those with a specific job assignment may enter for a limited time.

hourglass uterus, a womb with a segment of circular muscle fibers that contract during labor, causing lack of progress in the birth despite adequate labor contractions. The baby is pushed back in rather than out during contractions.

housemaid's knee. See **bursitis.**

house physician, a physician on call and immediately available in a hospital or other health care facility.

house surgeon, a surgeon on call and immediately available on the premises of a hospital.

housewives' eczema, a common term for skin irritation of the hands caused and worsened by their frequent soaking in water and by the use of soaps and detergents.

Howell-Jolly bodies, round, grainy particles in the red blood cells. They commonly occur in people who have blood diseases, as anemia and leukemia, or no spleen, either from birth or because of surgical removal.

h.s., (in prescriptions) abbreviation for *hora somni,* a Latin phrase meaning bedtime.

Hubbard tank, a large tank in which a patient may be placed to perform underwater exercise. It heats the water and is generally used for exercising the trunk and legs. See also **whirlpool bath.**

Huhn's gland, a gland embedded in tissues on the underneath surface of the tongue.

human bite, a wound caused by the piercing of skin by human teeth. Bacteria are usually present, and serious infection often follows. The area is treated by being thoroughly washed, using an antiseptic, and rinsed well. The wound is examined often and antibiotics given, if necessary.

human chorionic somatomammotropin (HCS), a hormone produced during pregnancy. It regulates carbohydrate and protein processing in the mother to ensure that the fetus receives glucose for energy and protein for growth. HCS may also cause diabetes-like symptoms in the mother.

humanistic existential therapy, a kind of mental therapy that promotes self-awareness and personal growth. It achieves this by stressing current reality and by discovering and changing the patient's usual actions to help make the most of a person's potential. This process may be made easier in a group setting, where problems are revealed through interaction with others. One method is called **client-centered therapy.** In this method the role of the therapist is to listen to the words of the client and then restate them without judging or interpreting them. **Gestalt therapy** is a form that stresses the unity of self awareness, behavior, and experience.

human leukocyte antigen (HLA), a system used to judge the similarity of the tissues of different persons. There are four genetic markers on chromosome 6, with each marker linked to certain diseases or conditions. See also **tissue typing.**

human placental lactogen (HPL), a hormone produced in the placenta that may be lacking in certain abnormalities of pregnancy.

Humatin, a trademark for a drug that fights amebic infections (paromomycin sulfate).

humerus /hyo͞o′mərəs/, *pl.* **humeri,** the largest bone of the upper arm, The lower end has several grooves that connect with the two bones in the lower arm (radius and ulna). Also called **arm bone.** –**humeral,** *adj.*

humidifier lung, a type of allergic lung condition common among workers involved with refrigeration and air conditioning equipment. The cause is a fungus. Symptoms of the short-term form of the disease include chills, cough, fever, difficult breathing, loss of appetite, nausea, and vomiting. The long-term form of the disease is known by fatigue, cough, weight loss, and difficult breathing during exercise. Also called **air conditioner lung.** See also **pneumonitis.**

Humorsol, a trademark for a drug used to treat glaucoma and crossed eyes (demecarium bromide).

Hunter's syndrome. See **mucopolysaccharidosis.**

Huntington's chorea. See **chorea.**

Hurler's syndrome. See **mucopolysaccharidosis.**

Hürthle cell tumor /hur′təl/, a tumor of the thyroid gland composed of large cells (Hürthle cells); it may be harmless (Hürthle cell adenoma) or cancerous (Hürthle cell carcinoma).

Hutchinson's freckle, a tan patch on the skin that grows slowly, becoming mottled, dark, thick, and bumpy. The spot is usually seen on one side of the face of an elderly person. Removal is recommended because it often becomes cancerous. Also called **lentigo maligna.** See also **melanoma.**

hyaline membrane disease /hī′əlīn/. See **respiratory distress syndrome of the newborn.**

hyaloid artery /hī′əloid/, a blood vessel in the embryo that branches to supply the inside of the eye and develops part of the blood supply to the eye lens. The hyaloid artery disappears from the fetus in the ninth month of pregnancy, leaving a leftover, hyaloid canal, which remains in the adult as a narrow passage through the eye.

Hybephen, a trademark for a digestive system drug containing a sedative-hypnotic (phenobarbital).

hybrid /hī′brid/, **1.** an offspring produced from mating plants or animals from different species, varieties, or genotypes. **2.** pertaining to such a plant or animal.

Hycodan, a trademark for a drug used for cough relief.

Hycomine, a trademark for a drug used to treat coughs.

hydantoin /hīdan′tō·in/, any one of a group of medications, similar to the barbiturates, that act to limit epileptic seizures and reduce the spread of the abnormal electric excitation from the point where the seizure starts. The most common hydantoin in current use is phenytoin. See also **phenytoin.**

hydatid /hī′dətid/, a cyst or cystlike structure that usually is filled with fluid.

hydatid cyst, a cyst in the liver that contains larvae of the tapeworm *Echinococcus granulosus,* whose eggs are carried from the intestinal tract to the liver through the blood.

Patients generally lack symptoms, except for a swollen liver and a dull ache over the right upper quarter of the abdomen. A sudden allergic reaction may occur if the cyst ruptures. X-ray tests are used in diagnosis, and because no medical treatment is available, surgical removal of the cyst is required.

hydatid mole. See **molar pregnancy.**

hydatidosis /-ō′sis/, infection with the tapeworm *Echinococcus granulosus*. See also **hydatid cyst.**

Hydeltrasol, a trademark for a drug to treat inflammation (prednisolone sodium phosphate).

Hydeltra TBA, a trademark for a drug to treat inflammation (prednisolone tebutate).

Hydergine, a trademark for a drug used to treat peripheral vein disease.

hydradenitis /hī′dradəni′-/, an infection or inflammation of the sweat glands.

hydralazine, a drug used to treat high blood pressure. Coronary artery disease, rheumatic heart disease, or known allergy to this drug prohibits its use. Side effects include chest pains, rapid or irregular heart beat, loss of appetite, tremors, blood disorders, depression, nausea, and irritation of the nerves.

hydralazine hydrochloride, a drug used to treat high blood pressure. Coronary artery disease, rheumatic heart disease, or known allergy to this drug prohibits its use. Side effects include headache, loss of appetite, rapid heart beat, digestive tract disturbances, and a disorder resembling lupus erythematosus.

hydramnios /hīdram′nē·əs/, an abnormal condition of pregnancy known by an excess of fluid surrounding the fetus. It is linked to maternal disorders, including blood poisoning of pregnancy and diabetes mellitus. Some fetal disorders may interfere with normal exchange of amniotic fluid, resulting in hydramnios. The chances of premature breaking of the water sac, premature labor, and stillbirth are increased. It is diagnosed by feeling, ultrasound, or x-ray examination. Periodic drawing off of fluid may be necessary.

Hydrea, a trademark for an antitumor drug (hydroxyurea).

hydroa /hīdrō′ə/, an unusual blistering skin condition of childhood that comes each summer after exposure to sunlight, sometimes accompanied by itching and thickening of the skin. Hydroa usually disappears soon after puberty. Treatment includes use of sunscreen lotions and the avoidance of exposure to sunlight.

hydrocarbon, any of a group of chemical compounds (organic) that contain hydrogen and carbon only. They are found in living matter, and many are derived from petroleum.

G-H

hydrocele /hī′drəsēl/, a buildup of fluid in any saclike cavity or duct, specifically in the membrane surrounding the testicles or along the spermatic cord. The cause is an inflammation of the sex organs or blackage in the cord. Inborn hydrocele is caused by failure of a canal leading to the scrotum to close completely during prenatal development. In some newborn infants the defect may correct itself. Treatment includes surgery. Drawing off of fluid is only a temporary measure and may cause infection.

hydrocephalus /hī′drōsef′ələs/, a disorder in which an abnormal amount of spinal fluid, usually under high pressure, in the head causes widening of the brain ventricles. The normal flow of cerebrospinal fluid may be prevented by increased release of fluid, blockage in the brain ventricles, or a defect in reabsorption of fluid under the brain lining. These may result from developmental problems, infection, trauma, or brain tumors. The condition may be inborn with rapid onset of symptoms, or it may progress slowly so that neurologic signs do not come until late childhood or even early adulthood. In infants, the head grows at an abnormal rate with bulging softspots and dilated scalp veins. Other signs include irritability, vomiting, leg muscle problems, and failure of normal reflex actions. If the condition progresses, lower brainstem function is disrupted, the skull becomes enormous, and the cortex is destroyed. The infant often does not survive the neonatal period. With a later onset, after the cranial sutures have fused and the skull has formed, symptoms are mainly neurologic and include headache, eye problems, and loss of muscular coordination. In all age groups diagnosis is confirmed by tests, such as spinal fluid examination and a type of x-ray test. Treatment includes surgery to correct the blockage and to shunt the excess fluid away from the head. Parents need to know the signs of shunt malfunction or infection and how to pump the shunt. Outcome depends largely on the cause of the condition. Hydrocephalus is often found with a defect in the spine (myelomeningocele), in which case there is a less favorable outcome.

hydrochloric acid, a compound of hydrogen and chlorine. Hydrochloric acid is secreted in the stomach. It is a main part of gastric juice.

hydrochlorothiazide, a diuretic used to treat hypertension and swelling from fluid buildup. Anuria or allergy to this or similar drugs prevents its use. Side effects include low or high blood sugar, high uric acid, and allergic reactions.

hydrocholeretics /-kō′ləret′-/, drugs that stimulate the making of bile with a low specific gravity, or with a minimal proportion of solid constituents.

Hydrocil, a trademark for a laxative (psyllium hydrophilic muciloid).

hydrocodone bitartrate, a narcotic given to treat cough. Drug dependence or allergy to this drug prevents its use. Side effects include drug dependence and slowing of breathing and circulation.

hydrocortisone /kôr′tisōn/. See **cortisol.**

hydrocortisone valerate, a steroid used on the skin as an antiinflammatory agent. Viral and fungal skin diseases that occur where circulation is slowed or allergy to steroids prevents its use. Side effects include irritation of the skin and various systemic effects that may occur from long or great use.

Hydrocortone, a trademark for a glucocorticoid (hydrocortisone acetate).

Hydro Diuril, a trademark for a diuretic (hydrochlorothiazide).

hydroflumethiazide, a diuretic used to treat hypertension and swelling. Anuria or allergy to this or similar drugs prevents its use. Side effects include blood disorders, low blood pressure, high blood calcium, high blood sugar, high uric acid, and allergic reactions.

hydrogen (H), a gaseous element. It is normally a colorless, odorless, highly inflammable gas. As part of water, hydrogen is crucial in the interaction of acids, bases, and salts in the body and in the fluid balance needed for the body to survive. Hydrogen enables water to dissolve the different substances on which the body depends, as oxygen and food substances.

hydrogen peroxide /pərok′sīd/, an antiinfective used to cleanse open wounds, as a mouthwash, and to aid in removing earwax. Irritations to skin or mucous membranes or allergy to this agent prevent its use. There are no known side effects.

hydromorphone hydrochloride, a narcotic used to treat moderate to severe pain. It is used with caution in many cases, including head injuries, asthma, impaired kidney or liver function, or unstable heart. Allergy to this drug prevents its use. Side effects include drowsiness, dizziness, nausea, constipation, slowed breathing and blood flow, and drug addiction.

hydronephrosis /-nefrō′-/, swelling of parts of the kidney by urine that cannot flow past a blockage in a ureter. The cause may be a tumor, a stone lodged in the ureter, inflammation of the prostate gland, or a urinary tract infection. The person may have pain in the flank. Surgery to remove the blockage may be needed. Prolonged hydronephrosis will result in eventual loss of kidney function.

hydropenia /-pē′nē·ə/, lack of water in the body tissues.

hydrophobia, 1. *nontechnical.* rabies. 2. a morbid, extreme fear of water.

Hydropres, a trademark for a drug containing a diuretic (hydrochlorothiazide) and an antihypertensive (reserpine).

hydrops /hī′drops/, an abnormal amount of clear, watery fluid in a body tissue or cavity, as a joint, a fallopian tube, the middle ear, or the gallbladder. Hydrops in the entire body may occur in infants born with thalassemia or severe Rh sensitization. **Hydrops fetalis** is a massive fluid build-up in the fetus or newborn. Severe anemia occurs. The condition often leads to death, even with immediate exchange transfusions after delivery.

hydroquinone, a bleaching agent. It is given to reduce pigmentation in certain skin conditions in which an excess of melanin causes too much pigment (hyperpigmentation). Sunburn, prickly heat, other skin irritation, or allergy to this drug prevents its use. Side effects include tingling, redness, burning, and severe inflammation of the skin.

hydrosalpinx /-sal′pingks/, an abnormal state of the fallopian tube in which the tube is enlarged and filled with clear fluid. It results from infection that has previously blocked the tube at both ends.

hydrostatic test, a periodic test of breathing-air cylinders to determine whether they can safely contain compressed air.

hydrotherapy, the use of water to treat mental and physical problems. Hydrotherapy may include continuous tub baths, wet sheet packs, or shower sprays.

hydrothorax /-thôr′aks/, a buildup of fluid in the chest cavity, without inflammation.

hydroxyamphetamine hydrobromide, a drug used to dilate the pupil for eye tests and as a diagnostic aid in Horner's syndrome. Narrow-angle glaucoma or allergy to this drug prevents its use. Side effects include high inner eye pressure and light sensitivity.

hydroxyandrosterone /hīdrok′sē·andros′tərōn/, a sex hormone released by the testes and adrenal glands.

hydroxychloroquine sulfate, an antiprotozoal, antirheumatic drug. Allergy to this drug or to other similar drugs prevents its use. It is used with caution in people with alcoholism, blood disease, severe nerve disorder, psoriasis, or porphyria. The drug is not usually recommended in pregnancy. Side effects include eye problems, seizure, and hepatitis. Side effects increase with the dose and length of treatment.

17-hydroxycorticosteroid, any of the hormones, as cortisol, released by adrenal glands, measured in the urine to test adrenal function and diagnose hypoadrenalism or hyperadrenalism.

11-hydroxyetiocholanolone, a sex hormone released by the testes and adrenal glands.

5-hydroxyindoleacetic acid, an acid measured in the blood and urine to diagnose some tumors. It commonly rises above normal levels in whole blood in association with asthma, diarrhea, rapid heart beat, and other symptoms and is elevated in the urine of patients with carcinoid syndrome.

hydroxyprogesterone caproate, a steroid given to treat cancer of the uterus, amenorrhea, and abnormal uterine bleeding caused by hormonal imbalance. Poor liver function, breast cancer, abnormal genital bleeding, blood clotting disorders, or allergy to this drug prevents its use. Side effects include blood clots, stroke, tumors of the eye, loss of appetite, swelling, high blood pressure, jaundice, and depression.

hydroxyproline, an amino acid that is raised in the urine in bone diseases and some genetic disorders, as Marfan's syndrome.

hydroxyurea, A drug used to treat tumors. Bone marrow depression or allergy to this drug prevents its use. It is not to be given to women who are or might become pregnant. Side effects include bone marrow depression, stomach and bowel disturbances, and dermatitis.

hydroxyzine hydrochloride, a minor tranquilizer. It is given to relieve anxiety, nervous tension, hyperkinesis, and motion sickness. Allergy to this drug forbids its use. Side effects include decreased mental alertness.

Hygroton, a trademark for a diuretic (chlorthalidone).

Hylorel, a trademark for a high blood pressure drug (guanadrel sulfate).

hymen /hī′mən/, a fold of mucous membrane, skin, and fibrous tissue at the vagina entrance. It may be absent, small, thin and pliant, or, rarely, tough and dense, completely blocking the entrance. When the hymen is broken, small rounded tabs of membrane remain.

hymenal tag /hī′mənəl/. See **caruncle.**

hymenotomy /-ot′-/, the surgical cutting of the hymen.

hyoscyamine, a drug used to treat hypermotility of the GI and the lower urinary tracts. Narrow-angle glaucoma, asthma, blockage of the urinary or digestive tracts, severe ulcerative colitis, or allergy to this drug prevents its use. Side effects include blurred vision, central nervous system effects, rapid heart rate, dry mouth, decreased sweating, and allergic reactions.

hypalgesia /hī′paljē′sē·ə/, the sense of a painful stimulus to a degree that varies widely from a normal perception of the same stimulus.

Hyperab, a trademark for a passive immunizing agent (rabies immune globulin).

hyperacidity /hī′pərasid′itē/, too much acidity, as in the stomach.

hyperactivity, any abnormally increased activity either of the entire organism or of certain organ, as the heart or thyroid. Compare **hypoactivity.** See also **attention deficit disorder.**

G–H

hyperalimentation /-al'imentā'shən/, overfeeding or the eating of too great an amount of nutrients.

hyperammonemia /-am'ōnē'mē·ə/, too much ammonia in the blood. Ammonia is produced in the intestine and absorbed into the blood, and its poisonous effect is removed (detoxified) in the liver. If there is overproduction of ammonia or a decreased ability to detoxify it, levels in the blood may increase. Untreated, the condition leads to vomiting, coma, and death.

hyperbaric oxygenation /-ber'ik/, giving oxygen at high atmospheric pressure. It is done in special chambers that permit the delivery of pure oxygen at atmospheric pressure that is three times normal. Hyperbaric oxygenation has been used to treat carbon monoxide poisoning, air embolism, smoke inhalation, acute cyanide poisoning, and decompression sickness. It is also used in certain cases of blood loss or anemia.

hyperbilirubinemia /-bil'iroo'binē'mē·ə/, too much of the bile pigment bilirubin in the blood. Symptoms often include yellow skin (jaundice), lack of appetite, and tiredness. The disorder is most often linked to liver disease or blockage of bile. It also occurs when there is too much destruction of red blood cells. Treatment is specific to the underlying condition. When bilirubin levels are high, treatment includes light ray therapy and hydration. **Hyperbilirubinemia of the newborn** is an excess of bilirubin in the blood of the newborn. It is caused by poor liver function. Blood bilirubin levels are up in the normal newborn because infants have a low ability to excrete bilirubin, but above a certain level within the first 24 hours of life it may indicate a serious cause. Severely affected infants also show signs of anemia, which quickly worsen, causing decreased oxygen-carrying capacity that may lead to heart failure and shock. The condition may also harm the nervous system (kernicterus) in severe cases. Aftereffects of kernicterus include mental retardation, cerebral palsy, delayed or abnormal motor development, hearing loss, perceptual problems, and behavioral disorders.

hypercalcemia /-kalsē'mē·ə/, too much calcium in the blood. It most often results from bone loss and release of calcium, as occurs in hyperparathyroidism, spreading bone tumors, Paget's disease, and osteoporosis. Patients with hypercalcemia are confused and have belly pain, muscle pain, and weakness. Extremely high levels of blood calcium may result in shock, kidney failure, and death. Treatment includes diuretics and other drugs.

hypercalciuria /-kal'sēyoōr'ē·ə/, too much calcium in the urine, resulting from conditions such as certain types of arthritis, marked by large amounts of bone loss. Immobilized patients are often hypercalciuric. Some people absorb more calcium than is normal and therefore excrete large amounts into their urine. Concentrated amounts of calcium

in the urinary tract may form kidney stones. Treatment is to correct any underlying disease condition and limit calcium in the diet.

hypercapnia /-kap'nē·ə/, too much carbon dioxide in the blood.

hyperchloremia /-klôrē'mē·ə/, too much chloride in the blood.

hyperchlorhydria /-klôrhid'rē·ə/, too great a release of hydrochloric acid by cells lining the stomach.

hypercholesterolemia /-kōles'tərōle'mē·ə/, too much cholesterol in the blood. High levels of cholesterol and other fats (lipids) may lead to hardening of the arteries. Hypercholesterolemia may be reduced or prevented by avoiding saturated fats, which are found in red meats, eggs, and dairy products.

hyperdynamic syndrome, a cluster of symptoms that signal the onset of shock from germs (septic shock). It often includes a shaking chill, rapid rise in temperature, flushing of the skin, galloping pulse, and alternating rise and fall of the blood pressure. This is a medical emergency that requires expert medical support in a hospital. Emergency measures include keeping the patient warm and elevating the feet to assist blood return. See also **shock.**

hyperemesis gravidarum /-em'əsis/, an abnormal condition of pregnancy marked by long-term vomiting, weight loss, and fluid and electrolyte imbalance. If the condition is severe, brain damage, liver and kidney failure, and death may result. Effective treatment stops vomiting, gives enough fluids and foods, and helps emotions. Fluids, electrolytes, nutrients, and vitamins are given through the veins if the woman is unable to retain fluids by mouth.

hyperemia /-ē'mē·ə/, increased blood in part of the body. It is caused by increased blood flow, as in the inflammatory response, local relaxation of small blood vessels, or blockage of the outflow of blood from an area. Skin in the area usually becomes reddened and warm. –**hyperemic,** *adj.*

hyperextension, (of a joint) a position of maximum extension.

hyperflexia, the forcible overbending of a limb.

hyperfunction, increased function of any organ or system.

hypergenesis /-jen'əsis/, too much growth; overdevelopment. The condition may involve parts of the body or the entire body, as in gigantism. It may even result in the formation of extra parts, as the development of additional fingers or toes. –**hypergenetic,** *adj.*

hyperglycemia /-glīsē'mē·ə/, too much sugar (glucose) in the blood, most often linked to diabetes mellitus. The condition may occur in newborns, after the giving of certain hormones, and with an excess amount of solutions containing glucose given in the vein. Compare **hypoglycemia.**

hyperhidrosis /-hīdrō'-/.   See **hidrosis.**

hyperimmune,   having an unusual abundance of antibodies, producing a greater than normal immunity.

hyperinsulinism /-in'sŏŏlinizm/,   too much insulin in the body, as may occur when a greater than required dose is given.

hyperkalemia /-kəlē'mē·ə/,   too much potassium in the blood. This condition often occurs in kidney failure. Symptoms include nausea, diarrhea, muscle weakness, and heart irregularlies. Treatment includes the intravenous giving of sodium bicarbonate, calcium salts, and dextrose. Hemodialysis is used if these measures fail.

hyperkeratosis /-ker'ətō'-/,   formation of skin overgrowth. See also **callus, corn.**

hyperlipidemia /-lip'ide'mē·ə/,   an excess of fats or fat-like substances (lipids) in the blood.

hyperlipoproteinemia /-lip'ōprō'tēnē'mē·ə/,   any of a group of disorders that feature too much of certain protein-bound fats lipids and other fatty substances in the blood. Type I hyperlipoproteinemia. See also **lipoprotein.**

hypermagnesemia /-mag'nēsē'mē·ə/,   too much magnesium in the blood. This occurs in kidney failure and in use of a large quantity of drugs containing magnesium, as antacids. Irregular heart beat and depression of deep tendon reflexes and breathing result. Treatment often includes intravenous fluids, a diuretic, and hemodialysis.

hypermetria /-mē'trē·ə/,   an abnormal condition of lessened power to control the range of muscular action, causing movements that overreach the intended goal of the affected person. Compare **hypometria.**

hypermorph /hī'pərmôrf/,   **1.** a person whose arms and legs are too long in relation to the trunk. **2.** (in genetics) a mutant gene that shows increased activity in the expression of a trait.

hypernatremia /-natrē'mē·ə/,   too much sodium in the blood, caused by an excess loss of water and electrolytes resulting from diarrhea, excessive sweating, or too little water intake. When water loss is caused by poor kidney function, urine is profuse and dilute. If water loss is not through the kidneys, as in diarrhea and excess sweating, the urine is scanty and highly concentrated. People with hypernatremia may become mentally confused, have seizures, and lapse into coma. Treatment includes restoring fluid and electrolyte balance by mouth or by slow injections into the veins. See also **diabetes insipidus.**

hyperopia /-ō'pē·ə/.   See **farsightedness.**

hyperosmia /-oz'mē·ə/,   an abnormally high sensitivity to odors. Compare **anosmia.**

hyperparathyroidism /-per'əthī'roidizm/,   overactivity of one or more of the four parathyroid glands. Too much parathyroid hormone (PTH) is made. Calcium is drawn from the bones, and much of it is then absorbed by the kidneys, stomach, and intestines. Disorders occur in most systems of the body. Kidney failure, peptic ulcers, bone fractures, and weak muscles may develop. Other symptoms may include belly pain, nausea, loss of appetite, abnormal behavior, and coma. Treatment includes surgery to remove a tumor if that is the cause, or removal of part of the glands, and limiting intake of calcium. During treatment, the amounts of calcium, phosphorus, potassium, and magnesium in the blood are regularly measured. Fluid may be given through the veins to dilute the calcium buildup. Mild exercise is painful but promotes healing of bones.

hyperphenylalaninemia /-fen'ilal'əninē'mē·ə/,   an abnormally high amount of the amino acid, phenylalanine, in the blood. This may result from one of several defects in the process of breaking down phenylalanine. See also **phenylketonuria.**

hyperphoria /-fôr'ē·ə/,   the tendency of an eye to deviate upward.

hyperpigmentation /-pig'məntā'shən/,   unusual darkening of the skin. Causes include heredity, drugs, exposure to the sun, and too little adrenaline. Compare **hypopigmentation.**

hyperplasia /-plā'zhə/,   an increase in the number of cells of a body part. Compare **hypertrophy.**

hyperploidy /-ploi'dē/,   any increase in chromosome number that involves individual chromosomes rather than entire sets, resulting in more than the normal number characteristic of the species, as in Down's syndrome. The unbalanced sets of chromosomes are referred to as hyperdiploid, hypertriploid, hypertetraploid, and so on, depending on the number of multiples of the basic number of chromosomes they contain. Compare **hypoploidy.** See also **euploid.**

hyperpnea /-pnē'ə/.   See **respiratory rate.**

hyperprolactinemia /-prōlak'tinē'mē·ə/,   too much of the hormone prolactin in the blood. The condition is caused by a hypothalamic-pituitary problem. In women it is usually linked to breast problems; in men it may be a factor in decreased sexual interest and impotence. It may be a result of endocrine side effects related to certain tranquilizers.

hyperpyrexia /-pīrek'sē·ə/,   an extremely high temperature sometimes occurring in serious infectious diseases, especially in young children. Malignant hyperpyrexia, marked by a rapid rise in temperature, rapid heart beat, rapid breathing, sweating, rigidity, and blotchy blue skin (cyanosis) occasionally occurs in patients under general anesthesia. A high temperature may be reduced by sponging the body with tepid water and alcohol, by giving a tepid tub bath, or by giving aspirin or acetaminophen. See also **fever.**

hyperreflexia /-riflek'sē·ə/,   a neurologic condition marked by increased reflex reactions.

G–H

hypersensitivity, an abnormal condition marked by an overreaction to a particular stimulus. See also **allergy.** – **hypersensitive,** *adj.*

hypersensitvity pneumonitis, lung inflammation caused by exposure to a foreign substance (allergen). The allergen may be from a fungus, bird droppings, animal fur, or wood dust. It may also result from a side effect of a drug. Symptoms include fever, difficulty in breathing, fatigue, muscle aches, and fluid in the lungs. The symptoms usually develop 4 to 6 hours after exposure.

hypersensitivity reaction, an excessive response of the immune system to a sensitizing antigen. The antigenic stimulant is an allergen. Several factors fix the strength of an allergic response: the responsiveness of the host to the allergen, the amount of allergen, the kind of allergen, its way into the body, the timing of the exposures, and the site of the allergen-immune mediator reaction.

hypersomnia /-som′nē·ə/, **1.** very deep or long sleep, usually caused by mental rather than physical factors and with confusion on waking. **2.** great drowsiness.

hypersplenism /-splē′nizm/, a disorder consisting of a large spleen and a lack of one or more types of blood cells. Causes include tumors, anemia, malaria, tuberculosis, and various connective tissue and inflammatory diseases. Symptoms include stomach pain on the left side and a feeling of fullness after very little food, because the large spleen is pressing on the stomach. Treatment of the cause may cure the disorder. The spleen is removed (splenectomy) only in certain cases. See also **splenectomy.**

Hyperstat, a trademark for a drug that dilates vessels.

hypertelorism /-tel′ərizm/, a developmental defect marked by an abnormally wide space between two organs or parts. For example, **ocular hypertelorism** is a birth defect marked by a very wide bridge of the nose and more distance between the eyes. The condition is often linked to other head and face problems and some mental retardation. Compare **hypotelorism.**

hypertension, a common disorder, often without symptoms, marked by high blood pressure persistently exceeding 140/90. **Essential hypertension,** also called **primary hypertension,** the most frequent kind, has no one known cause, but its risk is increased by overweight, a high sodium level in the blood, a high cholesterol level, and a family history of high blood pressure. **Secondary hypertension** is linked to diseases of the kidneys, lungs, glands, and vessels. For example, **pulmonary hypertension** is a condition of abnormally high pressure within the arteries and veins of the lungs. **Renal hypertension** results from kidney disease, as kidney cancer and kidney stones. Excess use of painkillers and some drug side effects may also result in renal hypertension. Other known causes of hyper-

tension include adrenal problems, overactive thyroid gland, and certain pregnancies. Hypertension is more common in men than in women and is twice as great in blacks as in whites. Persons with mild or moderate hypertension may have no symptoms or may experience headaches, especially on rising, ringing in the ears, lightheadedness, and easy tiredness. With sustained hypertension artery walls become thickened and resistant to blood flow, and, as a result, the blood supply to the heart may be reduced causing angina or heart attack. High blood pressure is often accompanied by anxiety attacks, rapid or irregular heart beat, profuse sweating, pale skin, nausea, and, in some cases, fluid in the lungs. **Malignant hypertension** is the most life-threatening form of high blood pressure. It features very high blood pressure (a diastolic pressure higher than 120) that may damage the tissues of small vessels, the brain, the eyes (retinas), the heart, and the kidneys. Symptoms include severe headaches, blurred vision, and confusion. It may result in heart attack or stroke. A variety of factors, as stress, a family history of the disease, being overweight, tobacco, birth control pills, high intake of table salt (sodium chloride), inactive life-style, and aging may cause it. Many drugs are used to treat hypertension. Persons with high blood pressure are advised to follow a low-sodium, low-saturated fat diet, to reduce calories to control obesity, to exercise, to avoid stress, and to take adequate rest. See also **blood pressure.**

hypertensive crisis, a sudden severe increase in blood pressure to a level exceeding 200/120, occurring most often in untreated hypertension and in patients who have stopped taking prescribed antihypertensive medication.

hypertensive encephalopathy, a set of symptoms, including headache, convulsions, and coma, linked with a type of kidney disease (glomerulonephritis).

hyperthermia /-thur′mē·ə/, a much higher than normal body temperature. It may be produced by the patient's physician as treatment or accidently as a byproduct of treatment, or may occur from other causes. **Habitual hyperthermia** is a condition of unknown cause that occurs in young females, in which body temperatures of 99° to 100.5° F occur off and on for years. Fatigue, sadness, vague aches and pains, loss of sleep, bowel problems, and headaches also occur. No organic cause can be found; the diagnosis is usually made only after a long period of observing the patient. **Introperative hyperthermia** is heat delivered to internal sites that have been exposed by surgery. After heating the patient is "closed." **Malignant hyperthermia** is an inherited disorder that features an often fatal high body temperature, with rigid muscles occurring in affected patients exposed to certain anesthetic drugs. Patients who have malignant hyperthermia are informed of their condition and told that many of their close relatives are likely to have the same chance of getting the disorder.

hyperthyroidism /-thī'roidizm/, a disorder with too much activity of the thyroid gland. The gland is usually swollen, releasing greater than normal amounts of thyroid hormones, which speeds up the body processes. Symptoms include nervousness, bulging of the eyeballs, tremor, constant hunger, weight loss, fatigue, heat intolerance, rapid and irregular heart beat, and diarrhea. Antithyroid drugs are usually given. Surgical removal of the gland is sometimes necessary. Untreated hyperthyroidism may lead to death because of heart failure.

hypertrophic catarrh /-trof'ik/, a chronic condition marked by inflammation and discharge from a mucous membrane, with thickening of the mucous and submucous tissue.

hypertrophy /hīpur'trəfē/, an increase in the size of an organ caused by an increase in the size of the cells rather than the number of cells. Compare **atrophy**. **–hypertrophic,** *adj.*

Hypertussis, a trademark for an immunizing agent (pertussis immune globulin).

hyperventilation, a breathing rate that is greater than needed for the exchange of oxygen and carbon dioxide. Symptoms include chest pain, dizziness, faintness, and numbness of the fingers and toes. Causes of hyperventilation include asthma, exercise, fever, hyperthyroidism, infections, head injuries, some hormones and drugs, and mental factors, as anxiety or pain. **Central neurogenic hyperventilation (CNHV)** is a pattern of rapid and regular breathing at a rate of about 25 per minute. This occurs in patients who are in coma. Increasing regularity, rather than rate, shows a greater depth of coma. Compare **hypoventilation**. See also **respiratory center.**

hypervitaminosis, an abnormal condition resulting from intake of dangerous amounts of one or more vitamins, especially over a long period of time. Serious effects may result from overdoses of vitamins A, D, E, or K, but rarely with the water-soluble B and C vitamins. Compare **avitaminosis**. See also specific vitamins.

hypervolemia /-vōlē'mē·ə/, an increase in the amount of fluid outside the cells, particularly in the volume of circulating blood.

hypesthesia /hī'pesthē'zhə/, abnormally low level of feeling in response to stimulation of the sensory nerves. Touch, pain, heat, and cold are poorly perceived.

hyphema /hīfē'mə/, a bleeding into the front chamber of the eye, usually caused by a blow to the eye. Bed rest is required. The patient should be treated by an ophthalmologist who can decide the need for removing the blood, and the need for medication. Glaucoma may result from recurrent bleeding.

hypnagogue /hip'nəgog/, an agent or substance that tends to induce sleep or the feeling of dreamy sleepiness, as occurs before falling asleep. See also **hypnotics**. **–hypnagogic,** *adj.*

hypnosis, a passive, trancelike state that resembles normal sleep during which perception and memory are changed, resulting in increased responsiveness to suggestion. The condition is usually caused by the monotonous repetition of words and gestures while the person is completely relaxed. Hypnosis is used in some forms of psychotherapy and psychoanalysis, in behavior-changing programs, or in medicine to reduce pain and aid relaxation.

hypnotics, a class of drugs often used as sedatives.

hypnotism, the study or practice of producing hypnosis. One who practices hypnotism is a **hypnotist.**

hypoacidity /hī'pō·asid'itē/, a lack of acid.

hypoactivity, any abnormally low activity of the body or its organs, as lowered heart output, thyroid gland activity, or intestinal activity.

hypoadrenalism /-adrē'nəlizm/. See **Addison's disease.**

hypocalcemia /-kalsē'mē·ə/, too little calcium in the blood. Severe hypocalcemia features irregular heart beat, muscle spasms, and burning or prickling feelings of the hands, feet, lips, and tongue. Causes include hypoparathyroidism, too little vitamin D consumption, kidney failure, severe inflammation of the pancreas, or too little magnesium and protein in the blood. The underlying disorder is diagnosed and treated, and calcium is given by mouth or through the veins. Hypocalcemia is also seen in immature newborn babies, in infants born of mothers with diabetes, or in normal babies delivered by normal mothers after a long or hard labor and delivery. It is marked by vomiting, twitching of arms and legs, poor muscle tone, high-pitched crying, and difficulty in breathing. See also **tetany**. **–hypocalcemic,** *adj.*

hypochlorhydria /-klôrhid'rē·ə/, too low a level of hydrochloric acid in the stomach.

hypochondria /-kon'drē·ə/, a condition with extreme anxiety, depression, and the belief that certain real or imagined physical symptoms are signs of a serious illness or disease despite medical evidence that this is not the case. The cause is some unsolved mental problem and may involve a specific organ, as the heart, lungs, or eyes, or several body systems at various times or at the same time. In severe cases, the distorted body-mind relationship is so strong that actual symptoms and disease may develop. Treatment may consist of psychotherapy to uncover the underlying emotional conflict.

hypochromic /-krō'mik/, having less than normal color, usually describing a red blood cell and characterizing anemias linked to decreased making of hemoglobin. See also **anemia.**

G–H

hypodermic needle /-dur′mik/, a short, thin, hollow needle that attaches to a syringe for injecting a drug under the skin or into vessels or for withdrawing a fluid, as blood, for examination.

hypodermoclysis /-dərmok′lisis/, the injection of a solution beneath the skin to supply a continuous and large amount of fluid, nutrients and other important substances. It replaces the loss or too little intake of water and salt during illness or surgery or after shock or excessive bleeding and is done only when the patient is unable to take fluids through the veins, mouth, or rectum. The process takes a long time.

hypofibrinogenemia /-fī′brōjənē′mē·ə/, too little fibrinogen, a blood clotting factor, in the blood. The condition may occur as a side effect of early detachment of the placenta in pregnancy.

hypogammaglobulinemia /-gam′əglob′yəlinē′mē·ə/, a less than normal amount of gamma globulin in the blood, usually the result of increased protein breakdown or the loss of protein through urination. The condition is associated with a decreased resistance to infection.

hypogenitalism /-jen′ətəlizm/, a condition of retarded sexual development caused by a defect in male or female hormone production in the testicles or ovaries.

hypoglossal nerve /-glos′əl/, either of a pair of nerves in the head needed for swallowing and for moving the tongue.

hypoglycemia /-glīsē′mē·ə/, a less than normal amount of sugar in the blood, usually caused by being given too much insulin, excessive release of insulin by the pancreas, or low food intake. Symptoms include weakness, headache, hunger, problems with vision, loss of muscle coordination, anxiety, personality changes, and, if untreated, delirium, coma, and death. Treatment includes giving sugar in orange juice by mouth if the person is conscious or through the veins if the person is unconscious.

hypoglycemic agent, any of a large group of quite different drugs, including insulin, prescribed to decrease the amount of sugar in the blood.

hypoglycemic shock treatment. See **insulin shock treatment.**

hypokalemia /-kəlē′mē·ə/, a condition in which too little potassium is found in the blood. There is an abnormal ECG, weakness, and non-rigid paralysis. Causes include starvation, treatment of diabetes or adrenal tumor, or taking diuretics. Mild hypokalemia may go away when the underlying condition is corrected. Severe hypokalemia may be treated by giving potassium chloride and by a diet high in potassium. Compare **hyperkalemia.** See also **electrolyte balance.**

hypolipoproteinemia /-lip′ōprō′tēnē′mē·ə/, a group of defects in fatty protein (lipoprotein) that result in varying signs. Primary, or hereditary, hypolipoproteinemia factors include abnormal depositing of fats in the body, especially in the kidneys and liver. There is also abnormal transport of certain fats (triglycerides) in the blood, low levels of high-density lipoproteins, and high levels of low-density lipoproteins. Effects in the eye, intestines, and nerves may also be present. The condition may also accompany anemia or malnutrition.

hypomagnesemia /-mag′nēsē′mē·ə/, abnormally low magnesium in the blood. Symptoms include nausea, vomiting, muscle weakness, tremors, and muscle spasms. A mild case usually results from too little absorption of magnesium in the kidney or intestine, although it is also seen after long term feeding by injection and during nursing. A more severe form is linked with intestinal problems, protein malnutrition, and parathyroid disease. Magnesium salts to correct the condition may be given orally or through the veins.

hypomania, a mentally unhealthy state of optimism, excitability, a marked hyperactivity and talkativeness, heightened sexual interest, quick anger and irritability, and a decreased need for sleep.

hypometria /-mē′trē·ə/, an abnormal state with an inability to control the range of muscular action, resulting in movements that fall short of the intended goals of the affected person. Compare **hypermetria.**

hypomorph /hī′pōmôrf/, **1.** a person whose legs are too short in relation to the trunk and whose sitting height is too great a fraction of standing height. **2.** (in genetics) a mutant gene that has a reduced effect on the expression of a trait but at a level too low to result in abnormal development. Also called **leaky gene.**

hyponatremia /-natrē′mē·ə/, less than the normal amount of sodium in the blood, caused by too little excretion of water or by too much water in the bloodstream. In a severe case, the person may develop water intoxication leading to muscle spasms, convulsions, and coma. Treatment includes injecting a balanced solution into the veins.

hypoparathyroidism /-per′əthī′roidism/, a condition of lowered parathyroid function, which can be caused by a problem in the gland itself or by raised blood calcium levels.

hypophosphatasia /-fos′fətā′zhə/, inherited absence of an enzyme essential to the build-up of calcium in bone tissue (alkaline phosphatase). Affected newborns vomit, grow slowly, and often die in infancy. Children who survive have many skeletal deformities. There is no known treatment.

hypophysectomy /hīpof′əsek′-/, surgical removal of the pituitary gland. It may be done to slow the growth and spread of cancer of the breast, ovary, or prostate gland, to halt the breakdown of the retina in diabetes, or to remove a pituitary tumor. The gland is removed only if other treatment, as x-ray therapy, radioactive implants, or freezing fails to destroy all pituitary tissue.   **–hypophysectomize,** *v.*

hypopigmentation /-pig'məntā'shən/, unusual lack of skin color, seen, e.g., in albinos. Compare **hyperpigmentation.**

hypopituitarism /-pityoo'itərizm/, an abnormal condition caused by weak activity of the pituitary gland. There are large deposits of fat and adolescent characteristics.

hypoplasia /-plā'zhə/, incomplete or underdeveloped organ or tissue, usually the result of a decrease in the number of cells. See also **cartilage-hair hypoplasia.**

hypoploidy /-ploi'dē/, any decrease in chromosome number that involves individual chromosomes rather than entire sets, resulting in fewer than the normal number characteristic of the species, as in Turner's syndrome. The unbalanced sets of chromosomes are referred to as hypodiploid, hypotriploid, hypotetraploid, and so on, depending on the number of multiples of the basic number of chromosomes they contain. Compare **hyperploidy.** See also **euploid.**

hypopnea /-pnē'ə/.   See **respiratory rate.**

hypoproteinemia /-prō'tēnē'mē-ə/, a disorder with a decrease in the amount of protein in the blood to an abnormally low level. Symptoms include swelling of the tissues, nausea, vomiting, diarrhea, and abdominal pain. It may be caused by too little protein in the diet, by certain intestinal diseases, or by kidney failure.

hypoprothrombinemia /-prōthrom'binē'mē-ə/, an abnormal reduction in the amount of prothrombin (factor II) in the blood. There is poor clot formation, longer bleeding time, or uncontrolled bleeding. The condition is usually the result of inadequate making of prothrombin in the liver from a low vitamin K level caused by severe liver disease or by anticoagulant therapy with a drug (dicumarol). See also **blood clotting.**

hypoptyalism /hī'pōtī'əlizm/, a condition with a decrease in the amount of saliva released by the salivary glands.

hypopyon /hīpō'pē·on/, a gathering of pus in the front chamber of an eye, appearing as a gray fluid between the cornea and the iris. It may occur as a side effect of conjunctivitis, herpetic keratitis, or corneal ulcer.

hyposalivation /-sal'ivā'shən/, a low rate of saliva flow that may be linked with excess loss of body fluids, radiation therapy of the salivary gland regions, anxiety, the use of drugs, as atropine and antihistamines, vitamin deficiency, saliva gland infections, or various disorders.

hypospadias /-spā'dē·as/, an inherited defect in which the urinary opening is on the underside of the penis. Incontinence does not occur. An operation is done if needed. A corresponding defect in women is rare but recognized by the location of the urinary opening in the vagina. Compare **epispadias.**

hypotelorism /-tel'ərizm/, a condition with an abnormally decreased distance between two organs or parts. For example, **ocular hypotelorism** is a birth defect with a narrowing of the bridge of the nose and an abnormally small distance between the eyes. It results in a form of cross eye (convergent strabismus). The condition is often linked to badly formed parts of the head and face, and some slow mental growth (mental retardation).

hypotension,   an abnormal condition in which the blood pressure is too low for normal functioning. **Deliberate hypotension** refers to a process in which a drug is given to reduce blood pressure briefly during surgery. This reduces bleeding, making vessels and tissues more visible to the surgeon. **Orthostatic hypotension,** or postural hypotension, occurs when a patient stands after sitting or lying down. The falling blood pressure may cause the patient to faint. **Supine hypotension** occurs when a pregnant woman is lying on her back. It is caused by lessened vein flow that results from pressure of the heavy womb and fetus on the vena cava.

hypothalamus /-thal'əməs/, a portion of the brain, forming the floor and part of the side wall of the third ventricle. It activates, controls, and integrates part of the nervous system, the endocrine processes, and many bodily functions, as temperature, sleep, and appetite.   **–hypothalamic,** *adj.*

hypothermia /-thur'mē-ə/, **1.** a dangerous condition in which the temperature of the body is below 95° F (35° C). The cause is usually long exposure to cold. Breathing is shallow and slow, and the heart rate is faint and slow. The person is very pale and may appear to be dead. People who are very old or very young, people who have heart or circulation problems, and people who are hungry, tired, or under the influence of alcohol are most likely to get hypothermia. Treatment includes slowly warming the person. Hospitalization is necessary. **2.** purposely lowering body temperature with cooling mattresses or ice to prepare for surgery.

hypothermia therapy,   lowering a patient's body temperature to counteract long-term high fever caused by certain diseases, or, less often, as an aid to anesthesia in heart or brain surgery. Hypothermia may be produced by placing crushed ice around the patient, or by placing the body in ice water. Most commonly it is done by applying cooling blankets or vinyl pads containing coils through which cold water and alcohol are pumped. At the end of treatment, the cooling blanket is replaced by regular blankets, and the patient usually warms at his or her own rate.

hypothyroidism /-thī'roidism/, a condition of decreased thyroid gland activity. It is sometimes caused by surgical

G–H

removal of all or part of the gland. An overdose of anti-thyroid medicine, release of thyroid-stimulating hormone by the pituitary gland, or atrophy of the thyroid gland itself can also be responsible. Weight gain, sluggishness, dryness of the skin, constipation, arthritis, and slowing of the processes of the body may occur. Untreated, hypothyroidism leads to coma and death. Treatment includes the deficient hormone.

hypoventilation, an abnormal condition of the lungs. Symptoms include turning blue, clubbing of the fingers, increase in red cell mass in the blood, and increased carbon dioxide pressure in the arteries. Lowered breathing rate also results when the amount of air that enters the lungs and takes part in gas exchanges is not enough for body needs. The cause may be uneven distribution of air breathed in (as in bronchitis), obesity, disease of the bones, nerves, or muscles affecting the chest, less response of the breathing center to carbon dioxide, and reduced functional lung tissue, as in emphysema. Treatment includes weight reduction for obesity, artificial respiration, and surgically opening the windpipe (trachea). Compare **hyperventilation.**

hypovolemia /-vōlē′mē·ə/, an abnormally low circulating blood volume.

hypovolemic shock. See **shock.**

hypoxemia /hī′poksē′mē·ə/, an abnormal lack of oxygen in the blood in the arteries. Symptoms of acute hypoxemia include turning blue, stupor, coma, increased blood pressure, too rapid heart beat, and an increase in heart output that later falls, resulting in low blood pressure and irregular heart beat or heart stoppage. Chronic hypoxemia stimulates red blood cell making by the bone marrow, leading to an excess of red cells. Oxygen therapy treats decreased oxygen pressure in the blood or too little oxygen intake. Hypoxemia resulting from shunting of blood from the right side of the heart to the left side of the heart without exchange of gases in the lungs is treated with bronchial hygiene and breathing therapy.

hypoxia /hīpok′sē·ə/, too little oxygen in the cells. Symptoms include turning blue, too fast a heart rate, high blood pressure, contractions of blood vessels, dizziness, and mental confusion. Mild hypoxia increases heart and breathing rates. Severe hypoxia leads to irregular breathing, failure to breathe, and heart failure. Increased sensitivity to the effect of certain drugs that reduce breathing is common in chronic hypoxia, resulting in severe depression or failure of breathing when relatively small doses are taken. The tissues most sensitive to hypoxia are the brain, heart, vessels of the lungs, and liver. Treatment includes heart and lung stimulant drugs, oxygen therapy, mechanic ventilation, and frequent analysis of blood gases. Compare **hypoxemia.** See also **anoxia.**

hypsibrachycephaly /hip′sibrak′ēsef′əlē/, having a skull that is high with a broad forehead. See also **brachycephaly, oxycephaly.**

hysterectomy /-ek′-/, removal of the uterus by surgery, done to remove tumors of the uterus or to treat chronic pelvic inflammation, uterine bleeding, and cancer of the uterus. Types of hysterectomy include **total hysterectomy,** in which the uterus and cervix are removed, and **radical hysterectomy,** in which ovaries, fallopian tubes, and lymph glands are removed with the uterus and cervix. Menstruation ceases after either type is performed. In an **abdominal hysterectomy,** the uterus is removed through the abdomen. A kind of hysterectomy is a **cesarean hysterectomy** in which the uterus is removed at the time of cesarean section. It is done most often for complications of cesarean section, usually severe bleeding. Less often it treats a disease, as a cancer. It is rarely done for sterilization because the danger of bleeding is greater when both operations are done together. **Colpohysterectomy** refers to removal of the uterus (hysterectomy) by way of the vagina. A **panhysterectomy** is the removal of the uterus and cervix. Treatment after a hysterectomy includes prevention of circulation problems because inflammation of the blood vessels of the pelvis and upper thigh is a frequent complication. Low back pain or scanty urine may indicate a blocked ureter.

hysteria, a state of tension or excitement in a person or group, marked by unmanageable fear and short-term loss of control over the emotions.

hysteric neurosis, an emotional disorder (neurosis) in which extreme excitability and anxiety caused by a conflict are changed into physical symptoms having no organic basis or into states of changed consciousness or identity. For example, **hysteric fever** is an abnormal rise in body temperature without general symptoms, often seen in hysteric neurosis. Kinds include **conversion disorder** and **dissociative disorder.**

hysterosalpingogram /his′tərōsalping′gōgram′/, an x-ray film of the uterus and the fallopian tubes to see the cavity of the uterus and the passageway of the tubes. The x-ray record is made after injecting a dye in the uterine cavity. A blockage of a structure is shown on the film because the dye cannot pass to the farther structures. A group of these films (serial hysterosalpingograms) are used in the diagnosis of the cause of infertility.

hysterosalpingo-oophorectomy /-salping′gō-ō′əfôrek′-/, surgery to remove one or both ovaries and fallopian tubes along with the uterus. It is done to treat cancer of the reproductive tract and chronic endometriosis. To avoid the severe symptoms of sudden menopause, a portion of one ovary is left, unless there is cancer. If both ovaries are removed and there is no cancer, estrogen replacement therapy is often begun right away. Inflammation of the blood vessels of the pelvis or thigh is a frequent complication. Elastic stockings or bandages are used on the legs to prevent this. The patient is instructed to avoid sharply flexing the thighs or knees. Low back pain or scanty urine may indicate a blocked ureter. Compare **hysterectomy.**

hysteroscopy /his′təros′kəpē/,   direct visual inspection of the cervical canal and uterine cavity with an instrument (hysteroscope) passed through the vagina and into the uterus. It is done to examine the lining of the uterus (endometrium), to secure a sample for biopsy, to remove an intrauterine device, or to remove cervical polyps. The surrounding tissues are examined. The procedure is not done in cases of pregnancy, acute pelvic inflammation, chronic upper genital tract infection, recent uterine perforation, and known or suspected cervical cancer.

hysterotomy /-ot′-/,   surgical cutting of the uterus, done as an abortion method in a pregnancy beyond the first three months (trimester). The lower part of the uterus is cut, and the products of conception are withdrawn. Later care includes close observation for too much vaginal bleeding.

Hytakerol,   a trademark for a calcium regulator (dihydrotachysterol).

Hytone,   a trademark for a steroid (hydrocortisone), used in a topical ointment for the relief of inflammation of the skin.

G–H

I

iatrogenic /ī′atrōjen′ik, yat′-/, caused by treatment or diagnostic procedures. An iatrogenic disorder is a condition caused by medical personnel or procedures or through exposure to the environment of a health care facility.

ibuprofen, a nonsteroidal antiinflammatory agent prescribed in the treatment of rheumatoid and osteoarthritis conditions. Kidney, stomach, or intestinal disorders, or known allergy to this or similar drugs or to aspirin prohibits its use. Side effects include stomach trouble, gastric or duodenal ulceration, dizziness, skin rash, and ringing in the ear. Ibuprofen may interact with other drugs.

ichthammol, a local antiinfective to treat some skin diseases.

ichthyosis /ik′thē·ō′-/, any of several inherited skin conditions in which the skin is dry and cracked, like fish scales. It usually appears at or shortly after birth and may be part of several rare disorders. Also called **fish skin disease, xeroderma.**

ictal, referring to a sudden, sharp onset, as convulsions of an epileptic seizure.

icterus index /ik′tərəs/, a liver function test. When liver disease is present, the index usually has a high value; with various anemias, low values are found.

ICU, abbreviation for **intensive care unit.**

id, (in psychoanalysis) the part of the psyche working in the unconscious that is the source of instinctive energy and has strong tendencies to self-preservation.

ID number, the four-digit identification number assigned to a hazardous material by the Department of Transportation: may include the prefix UN (United Nations) or NA (North American).

idea, thought, concept, intention, or impression that is in the mind as a result of awareness or understanding. An example is an **autochthonous idea** that begins in the unconscious and arises in the mind, independent of any conscious train of thought. A returning, irrational thought that persists in the mind is called a **compulsive idea.** It often results in a compelling need to do some improper act. A **fixed idea** is a continuous, single-minded thought or one that controls mental activity and continues despite evidence or logical proof that it is false. An **idea of influence** is an obsessive delusion, often seen in paranoid disorders, that external forces or persons are controlling one's thoughts, actions, and feelings. An **idea of persecution,** seen often in paranoid disorders, is a belief that one is threatened, discriminated against, or mistreated by others or by outside forces. An **idea of reference** is an obsessive delusion that the statements or actions of others refer to oneself, usually viewed as negative.

ideational apraxia. See **apraxia.**

identical twins. See **twin.**

identification, an unconscious defense mechanism by which a person patterns his or her personality on that of another person, assuming the person's nature and actions. The process is a normal function of personality growth and learning. It adds to the gaining of interests and ideals. **Competitive identification** is done in order to outdo the other person. **Positive identification** is a patterning of one's personality on that of another for whom one has much respect.

identity crisis, a time of being confused about one's sense of self and role in society, occurring most often in the change from one stage of life to the next. During adolescence, the person may be confused about personal worth, abilities, values, goals, choice of career, and place in the world. The erosion of family life, mobility of the population, and changes in the relation between the sexes all cause a higher rate of identity crises. Although confusion regarding one's identity is usually considered an adolescent problem, it also is common among old people who lose their status in the community and their place as head of a family.

ideophobia /ī′dē·ō-/, an anxiety disorder marked by the irrational fear or distrust of ideas or reason. See also **phobia.**

idiopathic disease /id′ē·ōpath′ik/, a disease that develops without an apparent or known cause although it may have a recognizable pattern of signs and symptoms and may be curable.

idiopathic scoliosis. See **spinal curvature.**

idiopathy /id′ē·op′əthē/, any primary disease with no apparent cause. –**idiopathic,** *adj.*

idiosyncrasy /id′ē·ōsin′krəsē/, **1.** a physical or behavioral feature unique to a person or group. **2.** an person's unique allergy to a drug, food, or other factor. See also **allergy.** –**idiosyncratic,** *adj.*

idiot, an out of date term for a very retarded person with an IQ below 20, unable to develop past the mental age of 3 or 4 years. See also **mental retardation.**

idiot savant /ēdē·ō′sävän′, savant′/, a person with severe mental retardation who is able to perform some unusual mental feats, mainly those involving music, puzzle-solving, or the use of numbers.

idoxuridine, an eye drug given for herpes simplex keratitis. Deep ulcers in the cornea or known allergy to this drug forbids its use. Side effects include visual problems and eye discomfort.

id reaction, an allergy caused by a fungal infection. There are very itchy skin and blisters that are usually distant from the primary fungus infection.

Ig, abbreviation for **immunoglobulin.**

ignition (auto ignition) temperature, the minimum temperature required to ignite gas or vapor without the presence of a spark or flame.

ileal conduit /il′ē·əl/, a way to route urine through intestinal tissue. Tubes are put in a piece of detached intestine, which is then sewed to a hole in the abdominal wall where a collecting device is fixed.

ileitis /il′ē·ī′-/, inflammation of the lowest part of the small intestine. See also **Crohn's disease.**

ileocecal valve /il′ē·ōsē′kəl/, the valve between the lowest part of the small intestine and the start of the large intestine. The valve has two flaps that project into the large intestine, allowing the contents of the intestine to pass only in a forward direction.

ileocystoplasty /-sis′təplas′tē/, surgery in which the bladder is rebuilt with a piece of intestine.

ileostomy /il′ē·os′-/, surgery to form an opening of the ileum onto the surface of the abdomen, through which fecal matter is emptied. The operation is used for ulcerative colitis, Crohn's disease, or cancer of the large bowel. The diseased portion of the large bowel is removed in a permanent ileostomy; sometimes segments of bowel may be reconnected after healing. After surgery, the patient wears a temporary disposable bag. A pouch may be made with part of the intestine, called a **continent ileostomy.** Body waste gathers in this pouch and is then drained from the body when it is full. The patient is able to do this without help. A continent ileostomy has several advantages. These include the lack of unpleasant odors and the convenience of not having a drainage bag outside the body. See also **colostomy, enterostomy, ostomy.**

ileum /il′ē·əm/, *pl.* **ilea,** a portion of the small intestine. It opens into the large intestine. –**ileac, ileal,** *adj.*

ileus /il′ē·əs/, a blockage of the intestines. It may occur when the bowels don't move, or with something in the way.

illness, an abnormal state in which the social, physical, emotional, or mental function of a person is reduced, compared with that person's previous state.

illness experience, the process of being ill, in five stages: phase I, noticing a symptom; phase II, taking on a sick role; phase III, making contact for health care; phase IV, being dependent (a patient); and phase V, getting well or being rehabilitated. Each stage is marked by certain decisions, behaviors, and end points. During phase I, the person decides something is wrong and tries to improve it. Phase I ends with the person accepting the reality of the symptom, no longer delaying any act to find help or denying the symptom. During phase II the person decides that the illness is real and that care is needed. The outcome of this phase is acceptance of the role — or denial of its necessity. In phase III professional advice is sought. The person usually asks for help and treatment. Denial may still occur, and the patient may ''shop'' more for medical care or may accept the illness, the medical authority, and the plan for treatment. In phase IV professional treatment is accepted by the person, who is now seen as a patient. At any time during this phase the dependent patient may develop mixed feelings and decide to reject treatment. More often, care is accepted with mixed feelings. The patient needs to be informed and given emotional support during this phase. During phase V, the patient resumes the usual tasks and roles as much as possible. Some people do not willingly give up the sick role. Most people accept the recovery and work toward rehabilitation.

illusion, a false understanding of an external sensory stimulus, usually visual or auditory, as a mirage in the desert or voices on the wind. Compare **delusion, hallucination.**

Ilopan, a trademark for a precursor of coenzyme A (dexpanthenol).

Ilosone, a trademark for an antibacterial (erythromycin estolate).

Ilozyme, a trademark for a digestant (pancrelipase).

image, 1. a visual reproduction of the likeness of someone or something, as a photograph. 2. a representation of an object, as that made by a reflection. 3. a person or thing that looks like another. 4. a mental picture, idea, or concept of an objective reality. 5. (in psychology) a mental representation of something seen before and later changed by other events. See also **body image, eidetic image, tactile image.**

imagery /im′ijrē′/, (in psychiatry) the forming of mental concepts, figures, ideas; any product of the imagination. In mentally ill persons these images are often bizarre and delusional.

I–J

imagination, **1.** the ability to form or the act or process of forming mental images or concepts of things that are not directly available to the senses. **2.** (in psychology) the ability to reproduce images or ideas in the memory to form new images and ideas concerned with a goal or problem.

imago /imā′gō/, (in analytic psychology) an unconscious, usually idealized mental image of an important person, for example, one's mother, in a person's youth.

imbalance, lack of balance, such as between opposing muscle groups, or fluid and electrolytes in the body tissues, or subjects in a population group, as an only girl in a large family of boys.

imbecile, an out-of-date term for a moderately retarded person having an I.Q. of 20 to 49, unable to develop past a mental age of 7 or 8 years. See also **mental retardation.**

imbricate /im′brikāt/, to build a surface with overlapping layers of material. Surgeons may imbricate with layers of tissue when closing a wound or other opening in a body part.

Imferon, a trademark for an injectable red blood builder (iron dextran).

imipramine hydrochloride, an antidepressant that is slow to start acting. It is given to treat mental depression. This should not be used by patients who are also taking monoamine oxidase inhibitors, have had recent heart trouble or seizures, or known allergy to this drug. Side effects include sedation, stomach or intestinal troubles, and heart and neurologic reactions. It should not be stopped quickly. This drug interacts with many other drugs.

immature baby, a term sometimes used for an infant weighing less than 1134 g (2.5 lb) and quite underdeveloped at birth.

immediately dangerous to life and health (IDLH), any atmosphere that poses an immediate hazard to life or produces immediate, irreversible, debilitating effects on health. IDLH concentrations represent concentrations at which respiratory protection is required. IDLHs are expressed in parts per million or milligrams per cubic meter.

immersion, the placing of a body or an object into water or other liquid so that it is completely covered by the liquid. –**immerse,** *v.*

immersion foot, an abnormal state of the feet with damage to the muscles, nerves, skin, and blood vessels. It is caused by long exposure to dampness or by long immersion in cold water.

immiscible /imis′ibəl/, not being able to be mixed, as oil and water.

immune complex hypersensitivity, a sudden allergy (IgG or IgM dependent) to certain substances. A skin test results in redness and swelling in 3 to 8 hours. It is seen in serum sickness, Arthus reaction, and glomerulonephritis. See also **immunoglobulin.**

immune gamma globulin, passive immunizing agents obtained from pooled human plasma. It is given for immunization against measles, poliomyelitis, chickenpox, serum hepatitis after transfusion, hepatitis A, and other disorders. Known allergy to gamma globulins prevents its use. Side effects include pain and inflammation at the site of injection and allergic reactions.

immune human globulin, a sterile solution of globulins from adult human blood used to immunize.

immune system, a related group of responses of various body organs that protects the body from disease organisms, other foreign bodies, and cancers. The main organs of the immune response system are the bone marrow, the thymus, and the lymphoid tissues. The system uses other organs too, as the lymph nodes, the spleen, and the lymphatic vessels. The system includes the humoral immune response and the cell-mediated response. **Humoral response** refers to a broad category of allergic reactions. It is especially effective against bacterial and viral invasions. **Cell-mediated immune response** is the response of special white blood cells rather than by antibodies. It causes an allergy that does not show up right away. A common type of this response is skin rash from poison ivy. It is also the main reaction that works to reject organ transplants. When this occurs, certain methods, such as drugs and radiation, must be used to stop rejection of transplants. One protein of the immune response is interferon. It is made by body cells after a virus invades. It fights and may slow the growth of cancer cells. The immune system also protects the body from invasion by making local barriers and inflammation. The humoral response and the cell-mediated response develop if these first defenses fail to protect the body.

immunity, the quality of being unaffected by a certain disease or condition. **Natural immunity** is a usually inborn and permanent form of immunity to a specific disease. Kinds of natural immunity include individual, racial, and species immunity. **Individual immunity** is rare and not shared by other members of the race and species. It may occur because the person has an infection that goes unnoticed. **Racial immunity** is a form shared by most members of a genetically related group. **Species immunity** is shared by all members of a species. **Acquired immunity** is any form of protection that is gotten after birth. It may be natural or not. With **naturally acquired immunity** the body is able to fight off infections successfully after having the disease. Immunity can come from the mother during pregnancy. The mother can also pass this immunity to a baby through her milk. **Artificially acquired immunity** is gotten by vaccination. **Active immunity** is a form of long-term, gained immunity. It protects the body from new infection. **Passive immunity** is not permanent and does not last as long as active immunity. It results from antibodies that are carried through the placenta to a fetus or through a breast substance (colostrum) from a mother to an infant. Passive immunity is also caused by injecting a drug (antiserum) for treatment or prevention. **Autoimmunity** is an abnormal condition in which the body reacts against its own tissues. Autoimmunity may result in allergy and autoimmune disease. **Cellular immunity** refers to the growth of special white blood cells (T lymphocytes) after exposure to a foreign substance (antigen). These T cells go to work each time they meet the same substance. Cellular immunity helps the body to resist infection caused by viruses and some bacteria. For example, a person who has had chickenpox will not get the disease a second time. Cellular immunity also plays a role in delayed allergic responses. It is involved in resistance to cancer, some diseases of the immune system, graft rejection, and some allergies. **Humoral immunity** results from the development and the continuing presence of circulating antibodies which are produced by the body's defense system.

immunization,   a process by which resistance to an infectious disease is caused or increased.

immunodeficient,   an abnormal state of the immune system in which immunity is too low and resistance to infection is decreased.

immunogen /imyoo′nəjən/,   any agent or substance able to provoke an immune response or cause immunity.

immunoglobulin /im′yoōnōglob′yəlin/,   any of five distinct antibodies in the serum and external secretions of the body. In response to certain antigens, immunoglobulins are formed in the bone marrow, spleen, and all lymphoid tissue of the body except the thymus. **Immunoglobulin A (IgA)** is one of the five classes of antibodies made by the body and one of the most common. It is found in all secretions of the body and is the major antibody in the mucous membrane of the intestines, bronchi, saliva, and tears. IgA combines with protein in the mucosa and defends body surfaces against invading microorganisms. It protects body tissues by seeking out foreign microororganisms and starting an antigen-antibody reaction. **IgA deficiency** is the most common type of immunoglobulin deficiency, appearing in about 1 in 400 persons. The age of onset varies. The IgA deficiency is common in patients with rheumatoid arthritis. Symptoms include allergies linked to chronic lung infection, stomach and intestinal diseases, autoimmune diseases, as rheumatoid arthritis, systemic lupus erythematosus, and chronic hepatitis, and malignant tumors. Symptoms of IgA deficiency are often lacking in patients whose immune systems may be making up for low IgA

with extra amounts of IgM to assure adequate defenses. Diagnoses of IgA-deficient patients depend on the results of tests that commonly show normal IgE and IgM levels while IgA levels are low. The IgA deficiency is lifelong, and patients need to watch for symptoms and to seek treatment promptly. There is no known cure; treatment usually involves the effort to control associated diseases. **Immunoglobulin D (IgD)** is a specialized protein found in small amounts in serum tissue. The precise function of IgD is not known, but it increases in quantity during allergic reactions to milk, insulin, penicillin, and various toxins. **Immunoglobulin E (IgE)** is concentrated in the lung, the skin, and the cells of mucous membranes. It provides the main defense against antigens from the environment and is believed to be stimulated by immunoglobulin A. IgE reacts with certain antigens to release certain chemicals that cause reactions such as reddening of the skin. **Immunoglobulin G (IgG)** is a specialized protein produced by the body in response to invasions by bacteria, fungi, and viruses. In pregnancy, IgG crosses the placenta to the fetus and protects against red cell and white cell antigens. **Immunoglobulin M (IgM)** is the largest in structure. It is the first immunoglobulin the body makes when challenged by antigens and is found in circulating fluids. IgM triggers the increased production of immunoglobulin G and the important acitivities needed for effective antibody response.

immunologic tests,   tests based on the principles of antigen-antibody reactions.

immunology /-ol′-/,   the study of the reaction of tissues of the immune system of the body to stimulation by antigens. A specialist in immunology is called an **immunologist.**

immunomodulator /-mod′yəlā′tər/,   a substance that acts to change the body's immune response by increasing or decreasing the ability of the immune system to produce modified blood antibodies or cells that recognize and react with the antigen that caused their production. Some immunomodulating substances are naturally present in the body. Some of these are available in various prescription drugs. **–immunomodulation,** *n.*

immunosuppression,   **1.** the giving of agents that reduce the ability of the immune system to respond to stimulation by antigens. Immunosuppression may be deliberate, as when preparing for bone marrow or other transplants to prevent rejection of the donor tissue, or an accidental byproduct, as often results from chemotherapy for the treatment of cancer. **2.** an abnormal condition of the immune system that features a markedly lowered ability to respond to stimulation by antigens.

immunosuppressive,   pertaining to a substance or procedure that lessens or prevents an immune response.

immunotherapy,   a treatment for allergies. Increasingly large doses of the offending allergens are given to gradu-

I–J

ally develop immunity. The more exposed the person is to the offending allergen, the more blocking antibody is developed. Low doses of the offending allergen are gradually increased throughout the year or during a 3- to 6-month period before the allergy season starts; it usually continues until the patient shows no allergic response for 2 to 5 years. Also called **hyposensitization.**

Imodium, a trademark for a drug (loperamide hydrochloride) used as an antidiarrheal agent.

Imovax, a trademark for a rabies virus vaccine (rabies human diploid cell vaccine).

impacted, tightly or firmly wedged in too limited a space.

impacted fracture, a bone break in which the adjacent ends of the fractured bone are wedged together.

impacted tooth, a tooth so positioned against another tooth, bone, or soft tissue that its full emergence is impossible or unlikely.

impaired glucose tolerance (IGT), a condition in which blood glucose levels after fasting are higher than normal but lower than those for diabetes. In some patients this represents a stage in the natural history of diabetes, but in many persons IGT either does not progress or goes back to normal. See also **diabetes.**

impairment, any disorder in structure or function resulting from abnormalities that interfere with normal activities.

imperforate /impur'fərit/, lacking a normal opening in a body organ or passageway. An infant may be born with an imperforate anus.

imperforate anus, any of several inborn defects of the anus. The common form is a condition in which the rectal pouch ends before reaching the surface (anal agenesis). An abnormal canal to the surface is present in 80% to 90% of cases. Other forms include a defect in which the anal opening is small (anal stenosis) and one in which the anal membrane covers the opening creating an obstruction (anal membrane atresia). The defect is often found at birth.

impermeable, (of a tissue, membrane, or film) preventing the passage of a substance through it.

impetigo /im'pəti'gō/, an infection of the skin beginning as a redness and progressing to itching blisters, breakdown of the skin, and honey-colored crusts. Lesions usually form on the face and spread locally. The disorder is highly contagious by contact with the discharge from the lesions. Acute kidney trouble is an occasional complication.

implant, 1. a radioactive substance placed in tissue for therapy. Seeds containing iodine 125 may be implanted permanently in prostate and chest tumors. Seeds of iridium 192 in ribbons or wire may be placed temporarily in head and neck cancers. Sealed sources of cesium 137 or radium 226 may be implanted in the body cavity temporarily in the treatment of cancers of the female organs. Strontium 90 in sealed sources may be placed for a brief period (usually less than 2 minutes) in treating eye tumors. Needles containing radium 226 may be used as temporary implants. Patients with radioactive implants are usually isolated from other patients. 2. (in surgery) material inserted or grafted into an organ or structure of the body. The implant may be of tissue, as in a blood vessel graft, or of an artificial substance, as an artificial hip, a pacemaker, or a container of radioactive material.

implantation dermoid cyst, a tumor derived from embryo tissues, caused by an injury that forces part of the outer germ layer of the embryo into the embryo's body.

implosive therapy. See **flooding.**

impotence, 1. weakness. 2. inability of the adult male to achieve erection or, less commonly, to ejaculate having achieved an erection. Several forms are recognized. **Functional impotence** has a psychologic basis. **Anatomic impotence** results from faulty genitals. **Atonic impotence** involves disturbed neuromuscular function. Poor health, age, drugs, and fatigue can inhibit normal sexual function. Also called **impotency.** –**impotent,** adj.

impregnate, 1. to make pregnant; to fertilize. 2. to saturate or mix with another substance. –**impregnable,** adj., **impregnation,** n.

impression, 1. (in dentistry and prosthetic medicine) a mold of a part of the mouth or other part of the body from which a replacement part may be formed. 2. (in the medical record) the examiner's diagnosis or assessment of a problem, disease, or condition. 3. a strong sensation or effect on the mind or feelings.

impulse, a sudden, strong, often irrational drive, urge, desire, or action resulting from a particular feeling or mental state. See also **nerve impulse.** –**impulsive,** adj.

Imuran, a trademark for an immunosuppressive (azathioprine).

inactive colon, decreased tone of the bowel resulting in fewer contractions and propelling movements. It causes delay in the normal 12-hour time it takes the contents to pass through the intestine and colon. Colon inactivity may result from an oversized colon, aging, depression, faulty bowel habits, not enough fluid intake, lack of exercise, a low-residue or starvation diet, prolonged bed rest, or a nerve disease. Normal function of the colon is often reduced by the continued use of laxatives. A too large, inactive colon with chronic constipation may be inborn or acquired. Treatment of inactive colon includes a training program to establish regular bowel habits, the use of stool softeners, and a diet with adequate roughage.

inadequate personality, a personality that features a lack of physical stamina, immature emotions, social instability, poor judgment, reduced drive, and an inability to adapt or react well to new or stressful situations.

inanition /in'ənish'ən/, **1.** an exhausted condition from lack of food and water or a defect in digestion; starvation. **2.** a slow-moving state from a loss of vitality or vigor.

inanition fever, a temporary, mild fever in the newborn in the first few days after birth, usually caused by water loss.

inborn, acquired or occurring during life in the uterus; innate. See also **congenital, hereditary.**

inborn error of metabolism, one of many abnormal conditions caused by an inherited defect of an enzyme or other protein. People with such diseases are each defective in only protein, but generally have a large number of physical signs showing the genetic trait. The diseases are rare. Kinds of inborn errors of metabolism include **phenylketonuria, Tay-Sachs disease, galactosemia.**

inbreeding, the production of offspring by the mating of closely related persons, organisms, or plants. Self-fertilization is the most extreme form. It normally occurs in certain plants and lower animals. The practice provides a greater chance for both desirable and undesirable recessive traits to show up in the offspring. In humans, the amount of inbreeding in a specific population is largely controlled by tradition and cultural practices.

incarcerate /inkär'sərāt/, to trap, imprison, or confine, as a loop of intestine in a hernia. See also **hernia.**

incest, sexual intercourse between members of the same family. Intercourse with distant relatives does not count. Intercourse is incest only when those participating could not legally marry. −**incestuous,** adj.

incidence, **1.** the number of times an event occurs. **2.** (in epidemiology) the number of new cases in a particular period of time.

incident, an occurrence or event, caused either by humans or natural phenomena, that requires action by emergency service personnel to prevent or minimize loss of life or damage to property and/or natural resources.

incident action plan, the incident action plan, which is initially prepared at the first meeting, contains general control objectives reflecting the overall incident strategy and specific action plans for the next operational period. When complete, the incident action plans will have a number of attachments.

incident base, that location at which the primary logistics functions are coordinated and administered. (Incident name or other designator will be added to the term ''base.'') The incident command post may be colocated with the base. There is only one base per incident.

incident commander (IC), the individual responsible for establishing and managing the overall operational plan at a fire rescue or hazardous materials incident. This process includes developing an effective organizational structure, allocating resources, making appropriate assignments, managing information, and continually attempting to achieve the basic command objectives. The individual responsible for the management of all incident operations.

incident command post (ICP), that location at which the primary command functions are executed and usually colocated with the incident base.

incident command system (ICS), the combination of facilities, equipment, personnel, procedures, and communications operating within a common organizational structure with responsibility for the management of assigned resources to effectively accomplish stated objectives pertaining to an incident.

incidental additives, food additives caused by pesticides, herbicides, or chemicals used in food processing.

incipient, beginning to appear, as a symptom or disease; coming into existence.

incision, a cut made surgically by a sharp instrument creating an opening into an organ or space in the body.

incisor, one of the eight front teeth, four in each dental arch. They first appear as milk teeth during infancy. They are replaced by permanent incisors during childhood. They last until old age. The crown of the incisor is chisel shaped and has a sharp cutting edge. The upper incisors are larger and stronger than the lower and are directed at a slant downward and forward.

inclusion, **1.** the act of enclosing or the state of being enclosed. **2.** a structure within another, as inclusions inside of the cells.

inclusion bodies, microscopic objects of various shapes and sizes observed in the blood cells or other tissue cells, depending on the type of disease.

inclusion dermoid cyst, a tumor derived from embryo tissues, caused by a foreign tissue being enclosed when a developmental cleft closes.

incoherent, **1.** disordered; without logical connection. **2.** unable to express one's ideas in an orderly, clear way, usually as a result of emotional stress.

incompatible, unable to coexist. A tissue transplant may be rejected because recipient and donor antibody factors are incompatible.

incompetence, lack of ability. Body organs that do not function adequately may be described as incompetent. −**incompetent,** adj.

incompetent cervix, (in obstetrics) a condition in which the uterus opens at the cervix before term without labor or contractions of the uterus. Miscarriage or premature delivery may result. Treatment includes holding the uterus closed with a suture.

I−J

incomplete fracture, a bone break in which the crack in the bone tissue does not completely go across the width of the affected bone.

incontinence, the inability to control urination or defecation, common in the aged. Treatment includes bladder retraining, implanting of an artificial sphincter, and the use of internal or external drainage devices. Stress incontinence is caused by coughing, straining, or heavy lifting. It occurs more often in women than in men. Mild cases may be treated by exercises or they may respond to drug therapy. Severe cases may require surgery to correct the defect. Bowel incontinence may result from relaxation of the anal sphincter or by central nervous system or spinal cord disorders and may be treated by a program of bowel training. See also **bowel training, Kegel exercises. –incontinent,** *adj.*

increment, an increase or gain, such as the amount of an increase or gain in pressure in the uterus as contractions begin in labor. **–incremental,** *adj.*

incrustation, hardened fluid discharge, scale, or scab.

incubation period, 1. the time between exposure to a disease-causing organism and the onset of symptoms of a disease. **2.** the time required for the growth of an embryo in an egg or for the growth and reproduction of tissue cells or microorganisms being grown in a special laboratory environment.

incubator, an apparatus used to provide a controlled environment, especially a certain temperature. Other conditions, such as darkness, light, oxygen, moisture, or dryness, may also be provided. An example is an **isolation incubator,** an inclosed bed kept for premature or other infants who require special treatment.

incudectomy /in′kyo͞odek′-/, surgical removal of the "anvil" (incus) of the ear. This is done to treat deafness resulting from decay of the tip of the anvil. The defective anvil is removed and replaced with a bone chip graft so that sound vibrations are again transmitted.

incus /ing′kəs/, *pl.* **incudes** /ing-ko͞o′dēz/, one of the three small bones in the middle ear. It communicates sound vibrations. See also **ear.**

indandione derivative, an oral anticoagulant designed for long-term use in patients who cannot tolerate most oral anticoagulants. The indandiones are difficult to control and may cause grave side effects, including severe kidney and liver problems. For this reason coumarin derivatives are preferred. Extreme fatigue, sore throat, chills, and fever are signs of impending toxicity and require stopping the drug. Compare **coumarin.**

indentation, a notch, pit, or depression in the surface of an object, as toothmarks on the tongue or skin. **–indent,** *v.*

Inderal, a trademark for a beta-adrenergic blocking agent (propranolol).

indican, a substance produced in the intestine by the breakdown of the amino acid tryptophan, absorbed by the intestinal wall, and passed in the urine. It may be high in the urine of persons on high-protein diets.

indication, a reason to prescribe a medication or perform a treatment. For example, a bacterial infection may be an indication for prescribing a specific antibiotic. **–indicate,** *v.*

indigenous /indij′ənəs/, native to or found naturally in a specified area or environment, as certain species of bacteria in the human digestive tract.

indigestion. See **dyspepsia.**

Indocin, a trademark for an agent (indomethacin) that reduces inflammation.

Indoklon, a trademark for an inhaled anesthetic (flurothyl).

indomethacin, a nonsteroid agent for reducing inlammation. It is prescribed in the treatment of arthritis and other conditions with pain, redness, or swelling.

induce, to cause or stimulate the start of an activity, as an enzyme induces a metabolic activity. **–inducer, induction,** *n.*

induction of labor, an obstetric procedure in which labor is begun artificially by rupturing the fetal membranes or giving a drug. It is done because the condition of the fetus or mother requires it or for the convenience of the mother or the obstetrician.

induration, hardening of a tissue, particularly the skin, because of excess fluid retention, inflammation, or growth of a tumor. **–indurated,** *adj.*

inert /inurt′/, **1.** not moving or acting, as inert matter. **2.** (of a medical ingredient) not medically active; serving only as a bulking, binding, or sweetening agent or other nonmedical use in a drug. **3.** (of a chemical substance) not taking part in a chemical reaction or acting as a catalyst, as an inert gas.

inertia /inur′shə/, **1.** the tendency of a body at rest or in motion to remain at rest or in motion in the same direction unless acted on by an outside force. **2.** an abnormal state of general inactivity or sluggishness in an organ or body part.

infant, a child who is in the earliest stage of life outside the womb. Infancy covers the time extending from birth to about 12 months of age, when the baby is able to assume an erect posture. Some extend the period to 24 months of age.

infant death, the death of a live-born infant before 1 year of age.

infant feeder, a device for feeding small or weak infants who cannot suck hard enough to nurse from the breast or to get milk from a bottle. The feeder looks like a bulb syringe with a long soft nipple on the end. It permits the baby to suck and swallow without great effort and prevents the escape of fluid into the infant's windpipe.

infanticide /infan'tisīd/, the killing of an infant or young child. The act is often a psychotic reaction linked with severe depression. Infanticide may become a neurotic obsession in mothers who do not want the baby or who do not feel physically, mentally, or emotionally capable of caring for or coping with it.

infantile, 1. relating to or typical of infants or infancy. 2. lacking maturity, or reasonableness. 3. being in a very early stage of development.

infantile paralysis. See **poliomyelitis.**

infantilism /in'fantəlizm, infant'-/, 1. a condition in which various body and mental traits of childhood persist in the adult. It features mental retardation, underdeveloped sex organs, and, usually, small stature. 2. a condition, usually of psychologic rather than organic origin, with speech and voice patterns in an older child or adult that are typical of very young children.

infant mortality, the statistic rate of infant death during the first year after live birth. It is expressed as the number of such births per 1000 live births in a given geographic area in a given period of time. Neonatal mortality accounts for 70% of infant mortality.

infant of addicted mother. See **drug addiction.**

infant psychiatry, the branch of psychiatry that specializes in the diagnosis and treatment of the psychological disorders and symptoms of infants, such as poor infant-parent attachment, and disturbances in sleeping, eating, and elimination.

infarct /infärkt'/, an area of decay in a tissue, vessel, organ, or part resulting from an interruption in the blood supply to the area, or, less often, by the blockage of a vein that carries blood away from the area. An infarct may resemble a red swollen bruise, because of bleeding and a buildup of blood in the area. Some infarcts are pale and white, caused by a lack of blood to the area. –**infarcted,** *adj.*

infarct extension, a decay in heart tissue that has spread beyond the original area, usually as a result of the death of neighboring cells.

infarction /infärk'shən/, the development and formation of an infarct. See also **myocardial infarction.**

infect, to transmit a germ that may cause an infectious disease in another person.

infection, 1. the invasion of the body by germs that reproduce and multiply, causing disease by local cell injury, release of poisons, or germ-antibody reaction in the cells. **Endogenous infection** is caused by an organism that has remained in the body from a previous illness. After a time of being dormant, it has become active again. An example is tuberculosis, which often occurs again. **Mixed infection** is caused by several different microorganisms, as in some open sores, pneumonia, and infections of wounds. Many combinations of bacteria, viruses, and fungi may be involved. **Retrograde infection** spreads along a tube or duct against the flow of fluids or wastes, as in the urinary and lymph systems. **Secondary infection** is caused by a microorganism that comes after another kind of organism. 2. a disease caused by the invasion of the body by germs. Compare **infestation.**

infectious, 1. capable of causing an infection. 2. caused by an infection.

infectious mononucleosis, an acute herpesvirus infection caused by the Epstein-Barr virus (EBV). Symptoms include fever, sore throat, swollen lymph glands, abnormal liver function, and bruising. The disease is usually transmitted by droplet infection. Young people are most often affected. In childhood, the disease is mild and usually unnoticed. The older the person, the more severe the symptoms are likely to be. Infection gives permanent immunity. Treatment include bed rest to prevent serious complications of the liver or spleen, analgesics to control pain, and salt gargles for throat discomfort. Rupture of the spleen may occur, requiring immediate surgery and blood transfusion.

inferior, 1. below or lower than a given point of reference, as the feet are inferior to the legs. 2. of poorer quality or value. Compare **superior.**

inferior aperture of minor pelvis, an irregular opening in the bone structure at the rear of the pelvis.

inferior aperture of thorax, an irregular opening in the bone structure at the center of the front of the chest.

inferiority complex, 1. a feeling of fear and resentment resulting from a sense of being inadequate. It features a variety of abnormal behaviors. 2. (in psychoanalysis) a striving for unrealistic goals because of an unresolved Oedipus complex.

inferior mesenteric vein, the vein in the lower body that returns the blood from the rectum and the colon. Compare **superior mesenteric vein.**

inferior phrenic artery, a small branch of the abdominal aorta, arising from the aorta itself, the renal artery, or the main abdominal artery. It supplies the diaphragm with blood.

inferior radioulnar joint, the pivotlike joint connecting the two bones of the lower arm (ulna and radius) at the wrist. The joint allows the wrist to rotate the lower arm.

inferior sagittal sinus, a vein path that drains blood from the brain into the internal jugular vein.

inferior thyroid vein, a vein that drains blood from a network of veins (plexus) on the thyroid gland.

I–J

inferior ulnar collateral artery, one of a number of branches of the deep brachial arteries in the arm, arising near the elbow and carrying blood to the muscles of the forearm.

infertile /infur′təl/, not being able to produce offspring. This condition may be present in one or both sex partners. It may be temporary and reversible. The cause may be physical, including immature sex organs, abnormalities of the reproductive system, hormone imbalance, and trouble in other organ systems. It may result from psychologic or emotional problems. The condition is classified as primary, if pregnancy has never occurred, and secondary, when there have been one or more pregnancies. Compare **sterile.** –**infertility,** n.

infest, to attack, invade, and live on the skin or in the organs of a body. Compare **infect.**

infestation, the presence of animal parasites in the environment, on the skin, or in the hair.

infiltration, the process whereby a fluid passes into the tissues, as when an intravenous fluid catheter comes out of the vein.

inflammation, the response of the tissues of the body to irritation or injury. Inflammation may be acute or chronic. Its chief signs are redness, heat, swelling, and pain, accompanied by loss of function. The severity of any inflammation depends on the cause, the area affected, and the condition of the person.

inflammatory fracture, a fracture of bone tissue weakened by inflammation.

influenza, a highly contagious infection usually of the lungs caused by a virus and transmitted by airborne particles. Symptoms include sore throat, cough, chills, fever, muscular pains, and weakness. The incubation period is brief (from 1 to 3 days), and the onset is usually sudden. Three main strains of influenza virus have been recognized: type A, type B, and type C. New strains of the virus emerge at regular intervals and are named according to their geographic origin. For example, Asian flu is a type A influenza. Treatment includes bed rest, aspirin, and drinking of fluids. Complete recovery in from 3 to 10 days is the rule. However, complications such as bacterial pneumonia may occur among high-risk patients, as the elderly, the very young, and people who have chronic diseases of the lungs. Yearly vaccination with the currently prevalent strain of influenza virus is recommended for elderly or weak persons. Also called **grippe,** (informal) **flu.**

influenza-virus vaccine, an active immunizing agent, prescribed for immunization against influenza. Acute infection or allergy to eggs prohibits its use.

informed consent, permission obtained from a patient to perform a specific test or procedure, i.e., actual consent given after the patient is made aware of your level of training and what you are planning to do. Informed consent is required before surgery. The document used must be written in a language understood by the patient. It must be dated and signed by the patient and at least one witness. Included in the document are clear statements that describe the procedure or test. They must also clarify the expected benefits and the risk to the patient, the expected consequences of not allowing the test or procedure, and the other procedures or diagnostic aids that are available. Also required is a statement that care will not be withheld if the patient does not consent. Informed consent is voluntary. By law, informed consent must be obtained more than some specified number of days or hours before certain procedures, including therapeutic abortion and sterilization. It must always be obtained when the patient is fully competent.

infraction fracture, a bone fracture with a small line that shows up in x-ray examination. It is most commonly associated with a disorder of metabolism.

infranodal block /in′frənō′dəl/. See **heart block.**

infraradian rhythm /-rā′dē·ən/, a rhythm in the body that repeats in patterns greater than 24-hour periods.

infrared (IR), a heat detection system used for fire detection, mapping, and hot spot identification.

infrared groundlink, a capability through the use of a special mobile ground station to receive air to ground infrared imagery for interpretation.

infrared therapy, treatment by exposure to various wavelengths of infrared radiation (radiant heat).

infusion, 1. the introduction of a substance, as a fluid, nutrient, or drug, directly into a vein by means of gravity flow. Compare **injection, instillation, insufflation. 2.** the substance introduced into the body by infusion. **3.** the steeping of a substance, as an herb, in order to extract its medicinal properties. **4.** the extract obtained by the steeping process. –**infuse,** v.

infusion pump, an apparatus that delivers measured amounts of a drug through injection over a period of time. Some kinds of infusion pumps can be implanted surgically.

ingestion, the introduction of a chemical into the body through the mouth. Inhaled chemicals may be trapped in saliva and swallowed. Exposed personnel should be prohibited from smoking, eating, or drinking except in designated rest areas after being decontaminated.

ingredient statement, all pesticide labels must have statements that break down the chemical ingredients by their relative percentages or as pounds per gallon of concentrate. ''Active'' ingredients are the active chemicals within the mixture. They must be listed by chemical name, and their common name may also be shown. ''Inert'' ingredients have no pesticide activity and are usually not broken into specific components, only total percentage. A number of pesticide products, particularly those used in the home, use flammable products only as the inert ingredients, which may not be easy to identify.

ingrown hair, a hair that fails to follow the normal channel to the surface. The free end becomes embedded in the skin. Inflammation and pus formation follow.

ingrown toenail, a toenail with a top edge that grows or is pressed into the skin of the toe, causing an inflammation. Infection is common. Treatment includes wider shoes, proper trimming of the nail, and surgery to narrow the nail.

inguinal /ing′gwinəl/, pertaining to the groin.

inguinal canal, the tubular passage through the lower layers of the belly wall. It is a common site for hernias. **Inguinal ring** refers to either of the two openings of the inguinal canal.

inguinal falx, a tendon that helps to strengthen the front wall of the groin. The width and the strength of the inguinal falx vary. Also called **conjoined tendon.**

inguinal hernia. See **hernia.**

inguinal node, a lymph node in the upper thigh.

inhalation, the introducton of chemical vapors or toxic products of combustion into the body by way of the respiratory system. Toxins may be absorbed into the bloodstream and carried to other internal organs, or they may affect the upper and/or lower respiratory tract. Resulting respiratory injuries include pulmonary edema and respiratory congestion. Inhalation is the most common exposure route and often the most damaging.

inhalation administration of medication, giving a drug by inhalation of the vapor released from a small, fragile glass container packed in a fine mesh that is crushed for immediate use. Amyl nitrate and ammonia act quickly and are often used in this way. The drug is absorbed into the blood through the mucous membrane of the nasal passages. Vaporized drugs are also given by inhalation. See also **inhalation therapy.**

inhalation analgesia, giving anesthetic gas during the second stage of labor to reduce pain. Consciousness is retained to allow the woman to follow instructions and to avoid the unwelcome effects of general anesthesia.

inhalation therapy, a treatment in which a substance is introduced into the lungs by breathing. Oxygen, water, and various drugs may be given using methods of inhalation therapy. Treatment goals include improving strength of breathing in a bedridden patient, opening air passages in an asthmatic, or loosening mucus in a person with chronic lung disease.

inhale, to breathe in or to draw in with the breath. – **inhalation,** *n.*

inherent, inborn, innate; natural to an environment.

inheritance, the acquiring by an offspring of genetic material from its parents; the total genetic makeup of the fertilized ovum. Traits or conditions are transmitted in this way from one generation to the next. See also **autosomal dominant inheritance, autosomal recessive inheritance, X-linked dominant inheritance, X-linked recessive inheritance.**

inherited disorder, any disease or condition that is genetically determined. Also called **genetic disorder, hereditary disorder.**

inhibition, 1. the act or state of inhibiting or of being inhibited, restrained, prevented, or held back. 2. (in psychology) the unconscious restraint of a certain behavior, usually resulting from the social or cultural forces; the condition causing this restraint. 3. (in psychoanalysis) the process in which the superego prevents the conscious expression of an unconscious instinctual drive, thought, or urge. 4. (in physiology) restraining, checking, or arresting the action of an organ or cell. 5. (in chemistry) the stopping or slowing down of the rate of a chemical reaction.

inhibitory, tending to stop or slow a process, as a neuron that lowers the intensity of a nerve impulse. Compare **induce.**

inion /in′ē·on/, the most prominent point of the back of the head, where the occipital bone bulges the farthest.

initial attack, resources initially committed to an incident.

injection, 1. the act of forcing a liquid into the body with a syringe. Injections are named according to where they are given. See also **injection technique. 2.** the substance injected. **3.** redness and swelling observed in the physical examination of a part of the body, caused by enlargement of the blood vessels from inflammation or infection. – **inject,** *v.*

injection technique, the various ways that a hypodermic needle is inserted to leave a substance, as a serum or vaccine. The site is first cleaned with alcohol or acetone. The needle is put in with a quick thrust. The solution is slowly introduced by pushing the plunger of the syringe, the needle is withdrawn quickly, and the site is massaged. When put into the skin, it is an **intradermal injection.** An **intramuscular injection** is put into a muscle. An **intrathecal injection** is put in a narrow space between membranes of the brain and spine (subarachnoid space) to spread a substance through the spinal fluid. An **intravenous injection** is put into a vein. A **subcutaneous injection** is put into the tissue beneath the skin, usually on the upper arm, thigh, or abdomen.

inlay splint, a casting for fixing or supporting one or more adjacent teeth. It is composed of two or more inlays soldered together or a single casting.

I–J

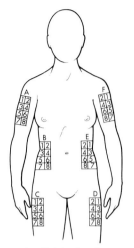

Insulin injection sites

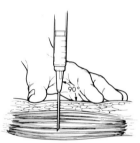

Intramuscular injection

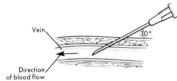

Intravenous injection (note bevel direction of needle)

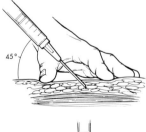

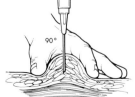

Subcutaneous injection

inlet, a passage leading into a cavity, as the pelvic inlet that marks the brim of the pelvic cavity.

in loco parentis /in lō′kō pəren′tis/, a Latin phrase meaning ''in the place of the parent'': the taking on by a person or institution of the parental obligations of caring for a child without adoption.

innate, 1. existing in or belonging to a person from birth; inborn; hereditary; congenital. **2.** referring to a natural and essential trait of something or someone. **3.** originating in or produced by the mind.

inner cell mass, a cluster of cells around a central part of a fertilized ovum. The embryo develops from it. See also **trophoblast.**

innervation, the distribution or supply of nerve fibers or nerve impulses to a part of the body.

innocent, benign, or healthy; not malignant, as an innocent heart murmur.

innominate artery /inom′ināt/, one of the three arteries that branch from the arch of the aorta. It divides into the right common carotid and the right subclavian arteries.

innominate bone, the hipbone. It consists of the ilium, ischium, and pubis. It joins with the sacrum and coccyx to form the pelvis.

innominate vein, a large vein on either side of the neck. It is formed by the union of the internal jugular and subclavian veins. The two veins drain blood from the head and neck.

inoculate /inok′yəlāt/, to introduce a substance into the body to cause or to increase immunity to a disease or condition. It is introduced by making multiple scratches in the skin after placing a drop of the substance on the skin, by puncture of the skin with an implement bearing multiple short tines, or by injection.

inoculum /inok′yələm/, *pl.* **inocula,** a substance introduced into the body to cause or to increase immunity to a given disease or condition. Also called **inoculant.** See also **immunity.**

inosine /in′əsēn/, a substance, derived from animal tissue, especially intestines, originally used in food processing and flavoring. It has also been used in the treatment of heart disorders. **Inosiplex** is a form of inosine that acts as a stimulator of the immune system. They are now under investigation for use in cancer therapy and in the treatment of virus infections.

inositol, a form of sugar (glucose) that occurs widely in plant and animal tissues.

inotropic /in′ōtrop′ik/, pertaining to the force of muscle contractions, particularly contractions of the heart muscle. An inotropic agent increases the ability of the heart tissue to contract easily.

inpatient, a patient who has been admitted to a hospital or other health care facility for at least an overnight stay. It also refers to the treatment or care of such a patient.

insanity, *informal.* a severe mental disorder or defect. It is more a legal term than a medical one. It refers to those mental illnesses that are so serious as to interfere with one's ability to function within the legal limits of society and to look after one's personal affairs. When a person is classified as insane, various legal actions can take place, as commitment to an institution. See also **psychosis.**

insect bite, the bite of any arthropod, such as a louse, flea, mite, tick, and spider. Many arthropods inject venom that produces poisoning or severe local reaction. Others inject saliva that may contain viruses, or substances that produce mild irritation. The degree of irritation of an insect's bite is affected by the shape of its mouth parts. A horsefly, for example, makes a short lateral and coarse wound, while a tick takes hold with its backward curved teeth, making its removal difficult. Spiders inflict a sharp pinprick bite that may remain unnoticed until the injected venom has begun to produce a painful reaction. Treatment of a bite depends on the species of insect, the reaction to the bite, and the risk of further trouble developing from it. First aid treatment generally includes ice or cold packs, careful cleaning of the wound, and antihistamines or specific antivenin as necessary.

insecticide poisoning, poisoning resulting from inhaling, swallowing, or absorbing through the skin insecticides with chlorophenothane, as DDT, heptachlor, dieldrin, and chlordane. Symptoms include vomiting, weakness, convulsions, tremors, rapid heart beats, breathing failure, and fluid in the lungs.

insertion, (in anatomy) the place of attachment, as of a muscle to the bone it moves.

insidious /insid′ē·əs/, describing a change that is gradual, subtle, or not noticed. Certain chronic diseases, as glaucoma, can develop insidiously. Their symptoms are not detected by the patient until the disorder is established. Compare **acute.**

insight, **1.** the capacity of grasping the true nature of a situation or a deep truth. **2.** an instance of penetrating or comprehending a deep truth, primarily through intuitive understanding. **3.** (in psychology) a type of self-understanding. Insight is one of the most important goals of psychotherapy. Along with integration, it leads to change in faulty behavior. See also **integration.**

in situ /in sī′tōō, sit′ōō/, **1.** in the natural or usual place. **2.** describing a cancer that has not spread or invaded neighboring tissues, as carcinoma in situ.

insomnia, chronic inability to sleep or to remain asleep through the night. The condition is caused by a variety of physical and psychologic factors. These include emotional stress, physical pain and discomfort, disorders in brain function, drug abuse and drug dependence, and other problems that produce anxiety and tensions. Treatment may include sedatives, tranquilizers, psychotherapy, and exercise.

inspiration, the act of drawing air into the lungs in order to exchange oxygen for carbon dioxide; breathing in. The major muscle of inspiration is the diaphragm, the contraction of which creates a low pressure in the chest, causing the lungs to expand and air to flow inward. Since expiration is usually a passive process, the muscles of inspiration alone perform normal breathing. Compare **expiration.**

inspiratory capacity (IC) /inspī′rətôr′e/, the maximum volume of air that can be inhaled into the lungs from the normal resting position after exhaling. It is measured with a device called a spirometer.

inspiratory reserve volume, the maximum volume of air that can be further inspired from the normal resting position after inhaling.

instillation, a way in which a fluid is slowly put into a cavity of the body and allowed to remain for a specific length of time before being withdrawn. It is done to expose the tissues of the area to the solution, to warmth or cold, or to a drug or substance in the solution. Compare **infusion, injection, insufflate.** −**instill,** *v.*

instrument, a surgical tool or device designed to perform a specific function, as cutting, grasping, or suturing. Surgical instruments are usually made of steel. Proper care of surgical instruments includes correct use, careful handling, inspection for defects, adequate and appropriate sterilization, and proper storage.

instrumentation, the use of instruments for treatment and diagnosis.

insufficiency, inability of an organ or other body part to perform a necessary function adequately. A kind of insufficiency is **vascular insufficiency.**

insufflate /insuf′lāt/, to blow a gas or powder into a tube, cavity, or organ. It is done to allow visual examination, to remove an obstruction, or to apply medication. −**insufflation,** *n.*

insulin /in′soolin, in′syəlin/, **1.** a naturally occurring hormone released by the pancreas in response to increased levels of sugar in the blood. The hormone acts to regulate the body's use of sugar and some of the processes involved with fats, carbohydrates, and proteins. Insulin lowers blood sugar levels and promotes transport and entry of sugar into the muscle cells and other tissues. Inadequate secretion of insulin results in too much blood sugar (hyperglycemia) and in the signs of diabetes mellitus. Uncorrected severe deficiency of insulin causes death. **2.** a preparation of the hormone given in treating diabetes mellitus. The preparations of insulin available for prescription vary in promptness, intensity, and duration of action. They are termed rapid-acting, intermediate-acting and long-acting. **Rapid-acting insulin,** also called short-acting insulin, is one of a group of insulin drugs in which the start of action is fast, about 1 hour, and lasts about 6 to 14 hours. **Prompt insulin-zinc suspension** is a rapid-acting insulin used to treat diabetes mellitus when a quick response is needed. Its action is only slightly slower than a shot of insulin. **Long-acting insulin** takes effect within 8 hours, reaches a peak of action in 16 to 24 hours, and lasts more than 36 hours. **Extended insulin-zinc suspension** and **protamine zinc insulin suspension** are both long-acting insulin and are absorbed slowly at a steady rate. **Isophane insulin suspension** is a modified form of protamine zinc insulin suspension. **Human insulin** is made from bacteria found naturally in the human digestive tract. Human insulin does not cause the allergic reactions that animal insulins do, especially in patients who only require insulin on a short-term basis. **Intermediate-acting insulin** has a range of action between the rapid-acting and long-acting forms. Most forms of insulin drugs are given by subcutaneous injection. Many drugs interact with insulin. Fever, stress, infection, pregnancy, surgery, and hyperthyroidism may increase insulin requirements. Liver or kidney disease, hypothyroidism, and vomiting may decrease them.

insulin-dependent diabetes mellitus (IDDM). See **diabetes mellitus.**

insulin injection, the use of a hypodermic needle to give insulin, either under the skin (subcutaneous) or into a vein (intravenous).

insulin kinase, an enzyme, assumed to be present in the liver, that activates insulin.

insulinoma /-ō′mə/, a benign tumor of the insulin-secreting cells of the pancreas. Treatment may include surgical removal of the tumor.

insulin reaction, the ill effects caused by too high levels of circulating insulin.

insulin shock, a form of shock caused by an overdose of insulin, a decreased intake of food, or too much exercise. There is a serious lack of sugar (glucose) in the blood. Symptoms include sweating, trembling, chilliness, nervousness, irritability, hunger, hallucination, numbness, and pale skin. Uncorrected, it will progress to convulsions, coma, and death. Treatment requires an immediate dose of glucose (sugar). Compare **ketoacidosis.**

insulin shock treatment, the injection of large, convulsion-producing doses of insulin. It is given as a treatment in psychoses, especially schizophrenia. Electric shock therapy is currently given more commonly than insulin shock. Also called **hypoglycemic shock treatment.**

insulin tolerance test, a test of the body's ability to use insulin. Insulin is given, and blood glucose is measured at regular intervals. Thirty minutes after the insulin is given, blood glucose is usually lower but not less than half of the fasting glucose level. Glucose levels usually return to normal after about 90 minutes. In people with hypoglycemia, the glucose levels may drop lower and be slower to return to normal.

Intal, a trademark for an antiasthmatic (cromolyn sodium).

integral dose, (in radiotherapy) the total amount of energy absorbed by a patient or object during exposure to radiation. Also called **volume dose.**

integrating dose meter, (in radiotherapy) a meter, usually designed to be placed on the patient's skin, with a system for determining the total radiation given during an exposure.

integration, 1. the act or process of unifying or bringing together. 2. (in psychology) the organization of all elements of the personality into a functional whole, one of the primary goals in psychotherapy. See also **insight.** –**integrate,** v.

integration of self, one of the factors in high-level health. It is necessary for maturity and is marked by the integration of mind, body, and spirit into one smoothly working unit.

integument /integ′yəmənt/, a covering or skin. –**integumentary,** adj.

integumentary system, the skin and its extensions, hair, nails, and sweat and sebaceous glands.

integumentary system assessment, an evaluation of the general condition of a patient's skin and of factors that may contribute to the presence of a skin disorder.

intellect, 1. the power and ability of the mind to know and understand. Intellect is contrasted with feeling or with willing. 2. a person having a great capacity for thought and knowledge. –**intellectual,** adj., n.

intellectualization, (in psychiatry) a defense mechanism in which reasoning is used to block an unconscious conflict and the emotional stress linked to it.

intelligence, the ability to acquire, retain, and apply experience, understanding, knowledge, reasoning, and judgment in coping with new experiences.

intelligence quotient (IQ), a numeric expression of one's intellectual level as measured against the average of one's own group. On several scales it is found by dividing mental age, derived through psychologic testing, by the chronologic age and multiplying the result by 100. Average IQ is considered to be 100.

intelligence test, any test standarized to determine a person's mental age by measuring capacity to absorb information and to solve problems. These tests are used by the medical profession to diagnose mental retardation and to aid in the planning of treatment programs.

intensive care, health care given for various acute life-threatening conditions, as multiple injury, severe burns, or heart attack. It is also given after some kinds of surgery. Such care is most often given in an intensive care unit. Also called **critical care.**

intensive care unit (ICU), a hospital unit in which patients needing close monitoring and intensive care are housed for as long as needed. An ICU contains highly technical monitoring devices and equipment. The staff in the unit is trained to give critical care as needed by the patients. A **neonatal intensive care unit (NICU)** is a hospital unit with special equipment for the care of premature and seriously ill newborn infants. See also **coronary care unit.**

intention, a kind of healing process. Healing by **first intention** is the union of the edges of a wound to complete healing without scar formation or a kind of fibrous tissue (granulation). Healing by **second intention** is wound closure in which the edges are separated, granulation develops to fill the gap, and, finally, tissue quickly grows in over the granulations, producing a thin scar. Healing by **third intention** is wound closure in which granulation fills the gap with tissue growing over the granulation at a slower rate and producing a larger scar.

intercapillary glomerulosclerosis /in′tərkap′iler′ē/, a disorder in which certain parts of the kidney (the renal glomeruli) break down. It is linked with diabetes. It often produces high blood pressure.

intercellular /-sel′yələr/, between or among cells.

interconceptional gynecologic care, health care of a woman during her reproductive years, except during pregnancies, and within 6 weeks after delivery. Testing for cervical cancer, breast and pelvic examinations, and evaluation of general health are routine. Testing and treatment for pelvic, vaginal, or genital infections may be required. A contraceptive method may also be provided. The basic examination is usually done annually. Infections or other complaints are diagnosed and treated as symptoms appear.

intercondylar fracture /-kon′dilər/, a fracture of the tissue between the round lumps at the end of a bone (condyles).

intercostal /-kos′təl/, pertaining to the space between two ribs.

intercostal bulging, the visible bulging of the soft tissues of the intercostal spaces that occurs when it is harder to exhale, as in asthma, cystic fibrosis, or blocking of a breath passage by a foreign body.

intercostal node, a lymph node in one of three groups near the back parts of the intercostal spaces. Such nodes are associated with lymphatic vessels that drain the rear sides of the chest. See also **lymph node.**

intercourse, *informal.* sexual intercourse. See **coitus.**

interior mesenteric artery /mes′enter′ik/, a branch of the abdominal aorta. It arises just above the division into the common iliacs and supplies much of the colon and rectum.

interlobular duct /-lob′yələr/, any duct connecting or draining the small lobes of a gland.

intermediate care facility, a health facility that provides intermediate care, a level of medical care for certain chronically ill or disabled individuals. Medical-related services are offered to persons with a variety of conditions requiring institutional facilities. The degree of care is less than what is provided by a hospital or skilled nursing facility. An example is a health care facility for mentally retarded persons.

intermediate cuneiform bone, the smallest of the three wedge-shaped (cuneiform) bones of the foot.

intermediate host. See **host.**

intermenstrual, pertaining to the time between menstrual periods.

intermenstrual fever, the normal, slight rise in temperature that marks ovulation. It usually occurs about 14 days before the onset of menstruation.

intermittent, alternating between periods of activity and inactivity, as rheumatoid arthritis, which is marked by periods of symptoms and periods of remission.

intermittent mandatory ventilation (IMV), a method of breathing therapy in which the patient is allowed to breathe independently and then, at certain intervals, a ventilation machine forces him to take a breath under pressure. See also **respiratory therapy.**

intern, a doctor in the first postgraduate year, learning medical practice under supervision before starting a residency.

internal, within or inside. **–internally,** *adv.*

internal ear. See **ear.**

internal exposure or **hazard,** exposure to radiation from radioactive materials that have entered the body.

internal fixation, any method of holding together pieces of fractured bone without using appliances outside the skin. Various devices, such as smooth or threaded pins, wires, screws, or plates, may be used to stabilize the fragments. Sometimes the device is removed at a later operation, or it may just remain. Compare **external pin fixation.**

internalization, the process of adopting, either unconsciously or consciously, the attitudes, beliefs, values, and standards of someone else or, more generally, of the society or group to which one belongs.

internal jugular vein, one of a pair of veins in the neck. Each vein collects blood from one side of the brain, the face, and the neck. At the base of the skull, in some peo-

I–J

ple, the vein forms a jugular bulb. Compare **external jugular vein.**

internal medicine, the branch of medicine concerned with study of the physiology and pathology of internal organs and with medical diagnosis and treatment of disorders of organs.

International Red Cross Society, an international charity organization, based in Geneva, Switzerland. It provides humane treatment to victims of war and disaster. It assures neutral hospitals and medical personnel during war. See also **American Red Cross.**

International System of Units, the standardization of measurement of substances, including some antibiotics, vitamins, enzymes, and hormones. An **International Unit (IU)** of substance is the amount that produces a specific biologic result. Each IU of a substance has the same strength and action as another unit of the same substance. See also **centimeter-gram-second system, SI units.**

internist, a doctor specializing in internal medicine.

interoceptor /in′tərōsep′tər/, any sensory nerve ending in cells in the internal organs that responds to stimuli from within the body regarding their function, such as digestion, excretion, and blood pressure.

interperiosteal fracture /-per′ē·os′tēəl/, a fracture in which the bone covering (periosteum) is not disrupted.

interpersonal therapy, psychotherapy that views faulty communications, actions, and relationships between people as basic factors in behavior problems.

interphase, the stage in the cell cycle when the cell is not dividing.

intersexuality, the state in which a person has male and female body features to varying degrees or in which the appearance of the external genitals is unclear or differs from the gonadal or genetic sex. Some conditions are seen at birth, but others may not be seen until later as resulting from delayed development or infertility.

interstitial /-stish′əl/, referring to the space between tissues.

intertrigo /-trī′gō/, an irritation of opposing skin surfaces caused by friction. Common sites are the armpits, the folds beneath large breasts, and the inner thighs. Infection may occur if the area is also warm and moist. Prevention is by weight reduction, powdering, cleansing, and antifungal medication when necessary.

intertrochanteric fracture /-trō′kənter′ik/, a fracture marked by a crack in the tissue below the neck of the thigh bone (femur).

intervention, any act to prevent harm to a patient or to improve the mental, emotional, or physical function of a patient.

intervertebral /-vur′təbrəl/, of the space between any two vertebrae, such as the disks.

intervertebral disk, one of the fibrous disks found between spinal vertebrae. The disks vary in size, shape, thickness, and number depending on location in the back and on which vertebrae they separate.

intestinal apoplexy /intes′tinəl/, the sudden blockage of one of the three main arteries to the intestine by an embolism or a thrombus. This state leads rapidly to death of intestinal tissue and is often fatal. Treatment is often surgery. The blockage is removed, and often the affected portion of the bowel is corrected.

intestinal fistula, an abnormal passage from the intestine to an outside abdominal opening. It may also refer to one created surgically for the exit of feces after removal of a malignant or severely ulcerated segment of the bowel. See also **colostomy.**

intestinal flu, a disorder (gastroenteritis) often caused by a virus. Symptoms include cramps, diarrhea, nausea, and vomiting. The disease usually is mild. Treatment includes control of diarrhea with medicine and a diet of clear fluids. See also **gastroenteritis.**

intestinal juices, the secretions of glands lining the intestine.

intestinal obstruction, any blockage that causes failure of the intestinal contents to pass through the bowel. Common causes include scar tissue (adhesions), impacted feces, tumor of the bowel, hernia, and bowel disease with inflammation. Small bowel blockage may cause severe pain, vomiting of fecal matter, dehydration, and a drop in blood pressure. Colon blockage causes less severe pain, marked stomach swelling, and constipation. X-ray tests show the level of obstruction and its cause. Treatment includes the emptying of intestinal contents by an intestinal tube. Surgery is sometimes needed. Fluid and electrolyte balance are restored by intravenous infusion. Nonnarcotic analgesics are often given. Also called *(informal)* **ileus.** See also **hernia, intussusception, volvulus.**

intestinal strangulation, stopping of blood flow to the bowel, causing swelling, cyanosis, and gangrene of the affected loop of bowel. This state is often caused by a hernia, intussusception, or volvulus. Early signs of intestinal strangulation are like those of intestinal obstruction, but peritonitis, shock, and the presence of a tender mass in the abdomen are important in making a correct diagnosis. Treatment includes the immediate correction of fluid and electrolyte imbalance, and surgery. Also called **intestinal infarction.**

intestine, the portion of the food canal from the stomach to the anus. The **large intestine** is the portion of the digestive tract made up of the cecum, the appendix, the ascending, transverse, and descending colons, and the rectum. The ileocecal valve separates the cecum from the ileum, preventing a reverse flow into the small intestine. The

small intestine is the longest part of the digestive tract, extending for about 7 m (23 feet) from the top opening of the stomach to the anus. It is divided into the duodenum, jejunum, and ileum. Decreasing in width from beginning to end, it is found in the middle and back part of the lower body, surrounded by large intestine. **–intestinal,** *adj.*

intolerance, a state marked by an inability to absorb or make use of a nutrient or medicine. Exposure to the substance may cause an adverse reaction, as in lactose intolerance. Compare **allergy.**

intoxication, **1.** the state of being poisoned by a drug or other substance. **2.** the state of being drunk because of drinking too much alcohol. **3.** a state of high mental or emotional excitement, usually happiness.

intraaortic balloon pump /in′trə-ā-ôr′-/, a device that assists in the management of heart failure (left ventricular). The balloon is attached to a catheter inserted in the aorta and is automatically inflated and deflated to aid in pumping blood.

intraarticular /-ärtik′yələr/, in a joint.

intraarticular fracture, a fracture within the joint surfaces of a bone.

intraarticular injection, the injection of medicine into a joint space, usually to reduce inflammation, as in bursitis. With the same method, fluid may be drawn from the joint space in a buildup of fluid in a joint, caused by injury or inflammation.

intraatrial /-ā′trē-əl/, in an atrium in the heart.

intraatrial block. See **heart block.**

intracapsular fracture /-kap′sōōlər/, a fracture in the capsule of a joint.

intracellular fluid /-ser′yələr/, a fluid in cell membranes in most tissues, with dissolved substances essential to healthy functioning of the body.

intracerebral /-ser′əbrəl/, in the brain tissue, inside the bony skull.

intracranial pressure /-krā′nē-əl/, pressure in the skull (cranium).

intractable, having no relief, as a symptom or disease that is not helped by treatment.

intracutaneous /-kōōtā′nē-əs/, in the layers of the skin.

intradermal test /-dur′məl/. See **allergy testing.**

intraductal carcinoma /-duk′təl/, a tumor, usually large and occuring most often in the breast ducts.

intradural lipoma /-dōōr′əl/, a fatty tumor of the spine, causing pain and poor function.

intraepidermal carcinoma /-ep′idur′məl/, a tumor of skin cells that often occurs at many sites at the same time. The lesions grow slowly without healing at the center. They resist chemotherapy and radiation.

intraocular /-ok′yələr/, referring to the eyeball.

intraocular pressure, the internal pressure of the eye, regulated via a fine sieve (the trabecular meshwork). In older persons, the meshwork may be blocked, causing higher intraocular pressure. See also **glaucoma.**

intrapartal care, care of a pregnant woman from the start of labor to the end of the third stage of labor with the release of the placenta.

intraperiosteal fracture /-per′ē-os′tē-əl/, a fracture that does not rupture the bone cover.

intrathecal /-thē′kəl/, referring to a structure, process, or substance in a sheath, as the spinal fluid in the theca of the spinal canal.

intrauterine device (IUD) /-yōō′tərin/, a birth control device consisting of a bent strip of plastic or other material that is put in the uterus to prevent pregnancy. It is put in during or just after menstruation, which assures that a pregnancy does not exist, and when the cervix is slightly open. The tail string of the IUD hangs from the cervix, by which the wearer can be sure the device is in place. The string also gives a way to remove the IUD. IUDs can cause problems. Infection is the most serious. Such infections in pregnancy may be lethal; so the IUD is removed if pregnancy is suspected. Other complications include perforation of the uterus, an infection (salpingitis) causing sterility, embedding of the device in the wall of the uterus, bleeding, pain, cramping, undetected expulsion, and irritation of the penis. Women without problems using an IUD are commonly able to retain the device safely for several years, or indefinitely. Also called **intrauterine contraceptive device (IUCD),** *(informal)* **coil, loop.**

intrauterine fracture, a fracture during fetal life.

intrauterine growth retardation, an abnormal process in which the development of the fetus is delayed by genetic factors, maternal disease, or fetal malnutrition. See also **birth weight.**

intravascular coagulation test /-vas′kyələr/, a test for finding internal blood clotting.

intravenous (IV) /-vē′nəs/, referring to the inside of a vein, as of a blood clot, an injection, or a catheter.

intravenous bolus, a large dose of medication given in the vein. The IV bolus is often used when medicine is needed quickly, as in an emergency, when drugs are given that cannot be diluted, such as many cancer drugs, and when a peak drug level is needed in the bloodstream of the patient. The IV bolus is not used when the medicine must be diluted or when the rapid giving of the medicine, as potassium chloride, could cause death. The IV bolus site is prepared with an antiseptic. If a primary IV line is already in, the IV bolus is given by mixing the prescribed drug with the right amount of IV solution. Also called **intravenous push.**

I–J

intravenous controller, any device that automatically delivers IV fluid at selectable flow rates, usually between one and 69 drops per minute.

intravenous DSA (IV-DSA), a form of angiography in which dye is in a vein rather than an artery.

intravenous fat emulsion, a preparation of 10% fat given by vein to keep up the weight or growth of patients. Such fat emulsions are made from soybean oil and egg-yolk. Immediate side effects or those soon after the onset of the infusion may include temperature rise, flushing, sweating, pressure sensations over the eyes, nausea, vomiting, headache, chest and back pains, dyspnea, and cyanosis. Delayed side effects may also occur.

intravenous feeding, the giving of nutrients through a vein.

intravenous infusion, a solution given in a vein or the process of giving a solution in a vein. This is done to maintain the right amount of fluids in the body, increase the amount of blood, replace lost substances (electrolytes) such as potassium or sodium, or provide some nutrition. A needle is put into a vein, usually in the patient's arm or leg. A tube connects the needle to a bottle of germ-free solution. The fluid is made to run into the vein slowly. While the fluid is given, the entire IV system is kept closed so that it stays sterile. The flow rate and amount of solution is watched closely, and the area where the needle is put in is checked often. Infants, aged patients with blood flow problems or kidney disease, and burn patients need special attention.

intravenous peristaltic pump, any of several devices for giving IV fluids by pressure on the IV tubing rather than on the fluid itself. An alarm sounds when the infusion does not flow at the right rate.

intravenous piston pump, any of several devices that control the infusion of IV fluids by piston action. The pump stops the IV fluid if the IV line is clogged or if fluid leaking into tissues is detected. Compare **intravenous controller, intravenous peristaltic pump, intravenous syringe pump.**

intravenous syringe pump, any of several devices that automatically compress a syringe plunger at a certain rate. Such devices are used with disposable syringes that can deliver blood, medications, or nutrients by IV, arterial, or subcutaneous routes. IV syringe pumps are often used to treat infants and ambulatory patients.

intravenous therapy, the giving of fluids or drugs in the general circulation through a vein punctured by a sharp instrument attached to a syringe or catheter.

intraventricular /-ventrik′yələr/, referring to the space in a ventricle.

intraventricular block. See **heart block.**

intrinsic, 1. natural or inherent. **2.** coming from or in an organ or tissue.

intrinsic factor, a substance released by the stomach lining (gastric mucosa). It is needed for the absorption of vitamin B_{12} and the normal growth of red blood cells. Pernicious anemia is caused by the absence of intrinsic factor. The lack may result from gastrectomy, a severe thyroid problem, or atrophy of the gastric mucosa. See also **nutritional anemia.**

introjection, an unconscious mechanism in which someone builds into his own ego structure the qualities of someone else.

Intropin, a trademark for an adrenergic (dopamine hydrochloride).

introspection, 1. the act of examining one's own thoughts and emotions by focusing on the inner self. **2.** a tendency to look inward at the inner self. –**introspective,** *adj.*

introversion, the tendency to direct one's interests, thoughts, and energies inward or to things concerned only with the self. Compare **extroversion.**

introvert, a person whose interests are directed inward and who is shy, withdrawn, emotionally reserved, and self-absorbed. Compare **extrovert.**

intubation /in′tyoobā′shən/, passing a tube into a body aperture, as putting a breathing tube through the mouth or nose or into the throat to provide an airway for anesthetic gas or oxygen. **Blind intubation** is putting a breathing tube in without using a laryngoscope. Kinds of intubation are **endotracheal intubation** and **nasogastric intubation.**

intussusception /in′təsusep′shən/, the sinking of one part of the bowel into the next, like a telescope effect. Such intestinal blockage may involve the small intestine, colon, or ileum. Intussusception occurs most often in infants and small children. It features intestinal pain, vomiting, and bloody mucus in the stool. Surgery is often needed to clear the blockage. See also **intestinal obstruction.**

inulin clearance /in′yəlin/, a kidney function test of the rate a starch, inulin, filters through the kidney. Inulin is given by mouth.

inunction /inungk′shən/, **1.** the rubbing of a drug mixed with oil or fat into the skin, with absorption of the active agent. **2.** any compound so applied.

invagination /invaj′inā′shən/, **1.** a state in which one part of a structure telescopes into another, as the intestine during peristalsis. If the invagination is extensive or involves a tumor or polyps, it may cause intestinal blockage. Then surgery is needed. **2.** surgery to fix a hernia by replacing the contents of the hernial sac in the abdominal cavity. See also **hernia, intestinal obstruction, peristalsis.** –**invaginate,** *v.*

invasion, the process by which cancer cells move into deeper tissue and into blood vessels and lymph channels.

invasive, marked by a tendency to spread. An example is **invasive carcinoma,** a cancerous growth with cells that destroy surrounding tissues.

Inversine, a trademark for a nerve blocking drug (mecamylamine hydrochloride).

inverse square law, the relationship that the radiation intensity is inversely proportional to the square of the distance from the source.

inversion, 1. an abnormal state in which an organ is turned inside out, as a uterine inversion. 2. a chromosomal defect in which two or more parts of a chromosome break off and separate. They rejoin the chromosome in the wrong order.

invert, 1. a homosexual. 2. to turn something upside down or inside out.

investigational new drug (IND), a drug not yet approved by the Food and Drug Administration, only for use in experiments to see its safety and effectiveness.

in vitro /in vē′trō/, (of a biologic reaction) occurring in laboratory apparatus.

in vivo /in vē′vō/, (of a biologic reaction) occurring in a living organism.

in vivo tracer study, (in nuclear medicine) a diagnostic procedure in which a series of radiograms of a given radioactive tracer show structures or processes.

involuntary, without conscious control or direction.

involution, a normal process marked by decreasing size of an organ, as involution of the uterus after birth.

involutional melancholia, a state of depression during menopause. The problem starts slowly and is marked by pessimism, irritability, insomnia, loss of appetite, feelings of anxiety, and an increase in motor activity, ranging from mere restlessness to extreme agitation. Treatment may include antidepressant drugs. Also called **climacteric melancholia.** See also **depression.**

iodine (I) /ī′ōdīn/, an essential trace element. Almost 80% of the iodine present in the body is in the thyroid gland. A lack of iodine can result in goiter or cretinism. Iodine is found in seafoods, iodized salt, and some dairy products. Radioisotopes of iodine are used to treat thyroid cancer.

iodism /ī′ōdizm/, a state caused by too much iodine. It features increased saliva, runny nose (rhinitis), weakness, and skin eruption.

iodize /ī′ōdīz/, to treat or saturate with iodine. Table salt is iodized to prevent goiter in areas with too little iodine in the drinking water or food.

iodochlorhydroxyquin, a drug given to treat eczema, athlete's foot, and other fungal infections. Tuberculosis or viral skin conditions or allergy to this drug or to iodine prohibits its use. Side effects include irritation to sensitive skin.

iododerma /ī′ōdōdur′mə/, a skin rash caused by an allergy to iodides in the diet.

iodoform /ī·ō′dōfôrm/, a surface antiinfective used as an antiseptic.

iodophor /ī·ō′dōfôr/, an antiseptic or disinfectant that combines iodine with something else, as a detergent.

iodoquinol, drug to treat intestinal amebas. Liver disease and allergy to iodine or 8-hydroxyquinolines prevents use. Side effects include dizziness, swollen thyroid gland, and eye problems.

ion /ī′on, ī′ən/, an atom or group of atoms with an electric charge.

Ionamin, a trademark for an anoretic (phentermine).

ionization /ī′ōnīzā′shən/, the process in which a neutral atom or molecule gains or loses electrons. Ionization can cause cell death or change.

ionization chamber, a device that consists of two oppositely charged electrodes and that is used to measure radioactivity.

ionizing radiation, electromagnetic radiation (x-ray and gamma ray photons) or particulate radiation (alpha particles, beta particles, electrons, positrons, protons, neutrons, and heavy particles) capable of producing ions by direct or secondary processes.

iontophoretic pilocarpine test /ī·on′tōfôret′ik/, a sweat test for cystic fibrosis. Sweat is caused with a drug (pilocarpine) and is absorbed from the forearm in a weighed gauze pad. The sweat sample is then analyzed for sodium and chloride electrolytes.

ipecac /ip′əkak/, a drug to cause vomiting in some poisonings and drug overdoses. Allergy to this drug prevents its use. It is not for unconscious patients or for poisoning by petroleum distillates, strong alkalis, acids, or strychnine. Side effects include heart poisoning if vomiting does not occur and the drug is retained. If vomiting does not occur, the ipecac is removed by washing out the stomach.

IPPB (intermittent positive pressure breathing), a form of assisted breathing with a device (ventilator) in which compressed gas is delivered to the person's airways until a preset pressure is reached. The patient closes the lips on the mouthpiece and does not allow air to escape from the nose or mouth during inspiration. The patient lets the lungs be filled by the machine. Passive exhalation is allowed through a valve, and the cycle starts again. Ventilation may be improved by the use of the device. Secretions may be thinned and cleared, and the passages may be humidified. Also called **(IPPV) intermittent positive pressure ventilation.**

IQ, abbreviation for **intelligence quotient.**

I–J

iridectomy /i′ridek′-/, surgery to remove part of the iris of the eye, often to restore drainage of the fluid to treat glaucoma or to remove a foreign body or tumor. After surgery the patient is watched for hemorrhage or excessive pain.

iridotomy /i′ridot′-/, a cut in the iris of the eye, to relieve blockage of the pupil, to enlarge the pupil in cataract extraction, or to treat glaucoma. Atropine and an antibiotic are given. A dressing and shield are applied. Great pain is abnormal.

iris /ī′ris/, a circular, contracting disc suspended between the cornea and the crystalline lens of the eye. Dark pigment cells under the clear tissue of the iris produce different colored irises. Albinos have no pigment. In blue eyes the pigment cells are only on the back surface of the iris, but in gray eyes, brown eyes, and black eyes the pigment cells appear in the front layer.

iritis /īrī′-/, an inflammatory condition of the iris of the eye. Symptoms include pain, tearing, sensitivity to light, and, if severe, lessened visual sharpness. On examination the eye looks cloudy, the iris bulges, and the pupil is contracted. A steroid may be given to reduce inflammation.

iron (Fe), a common metallic element needed to make hemoglobin. **Total iron** refers to the total iron concentration in the blood.

iron deficiency anemia. See **nutritional anemia.**

iron dextran, a drug to treat iron deficiency anemia not helped by oral iron therapy. Early pregnancy, anemias other than iron deficiency anemia, or allergy to this drug prevents its use. Side effects include severe allergic reactions, inflammation or phlebitis at the site of injection, headache, bowel distress, and fever.

iron metabolism, processes involved in the entry of iron in the body through its absorption, its transport and storage, its formation of hemoglobin, and its eventual excretion.

iron-rich food, any nutrient with a lot of iron. The best source of dietary iron is liver, with oysters, clams, heart, kidney, lean meat, and tongue as second choices. Leafy green vegetables are the best plant sources.

iron salts poisoning, poisoning caused by overdose of ferric or ferrous salts, marked by vomiting, bloody diarrhea, blue skin, and stomach pain. Therapy includes washing out the stomach, emetics, deferoxamine, and supportive therapy.

iron saturation, the capacity of iron to saturate transferrin, measured in the blood to detect iron excess or deficiency.

irradiation, exposure to radiant energy, such as heat, light, or x-ray. Radioactive sources of radiant energy, such as isotopes of iodine or cobalt, are used to examine internal body structures. Radioactivity destroys microorganisms or cells that are cancerous. Infrared or ultraviolet light produce heat in tissues to relieve pain and soreness or to treat acne, psoriasis, or other skin ailments. Ultraviolet light is also used to identify some bacteria and toxic molds. –**irradiate,** *v.*

irreducible, unable to be returned to the normal position or state, as an irreducible hernia. See also **incarcerate.**

irrigation, the process of washing out a body cavity or wounded area with a stream of water or other fluid. It is also used to cleanse a tube or drain in the body, as an indwelling catheter. The process is often done on the eye, ear, throat, vagina, and urinary tract. Gentle pressure is used in starting the fluid, except in the cleaning of wounds. The solution is removed from internal cavities through suction or by drainage. See also **lavage.** –**irrigate,** *v.*

irrigator, an apparatus with a flexible tube for flushing or washing out a body cavity.

irritable bowel syndrome, abnormally increased movement of the small and large intestines, often found with emotional stress. Young adults are often affected. Symptoms include diarrhea and, sometimes, pain in the lower abdomen. The pain is often stopped by moving the bowels. Also called **mucous colitis, spastic colon.**

ischemia /iskē′mē·ə/, poor blood supply to an organ or part, often marked by pain and organ disorder, as in ischemic heart disease. Some causes of ischemia are blood clots in arteries, atherosclerosis, and narrowing of veins. Poor blood flow may also be caused by tight orthopedic casts or injury. **Ischemic pain** refers to the unpleasant, often very painful feeling associated with ischemia. Ischemic pain caused by blocked arteries is often severe and may not be relieved, even with narcotics. The ischemic pain of partial vessel blockage is not as severe as the abrupt pain of a completely blocked artery, as by an embolism. The person with vessel disease may have ischemic pain only while exercising because the demands for oxygen cannot be met by the low blood flow. The ischemic pain caused by the pressure of a cast is difficult to distinguish from the sharp pain caused by surgery, because both types of pain may be local rather than spread out, as is the pain caused by injury.

Ishihara color test /ish′ēhä′rä/, a test of color vision using a series of plates on which are printed round dots in many colors and patterns. People with normal color vision can discern specific numbers or patterns on the plates; the inability to pick out a given number or shape means a specific lack in color perception.

islands of Langerhans, pancreas cells that make insulin, glucagon, and pancreatic polypeptide. Their secretions are important regulators of sugar metabolism. Also called **islets of Langerhans.**

islet cell tumor, any tumor of the islands of Langerhans.

Ismelin, a trademark for high blood pressure drug (guanethidine sulfate).

isocarboxazid, a drug to treat mental depression. Liver or kidney dysfunction, congestive heart failure, an adrenal gland tumor (pheochromocytoma), use of a nervous system drug or foods high in tryptophan or tyramine, or allergy to this drug prevents its use. Side effects include hyperactivity, irregular heart beat, low blood pressure, vertigo, and blurred vision. Monoamine oxidase inhibitors cause many bad drug interactions.

isoetharine mesylate, a drug for bronchial asthma, bronchitis, and emphysema. A history of irregular heart beat or allergy to this drug or to sympathomimetic drugs prevents its use. Side effects include irregular or rapid heart rate, dizziness, nervousness, and headache.

isoimmunization /ĩsō-/, the development of antibodies in a species with antigens from the same species, such as the development of anti-Rh antibodies in an Rh-negative person.

isoflurophate, a drug for open-angle glaucoma and esotropia. Eye inflammation or allergy to this drug or to other like drugs prohibits its use. Side effects include nervous system effects, sight problems, a rise in inner eye pressure, and, with long-term use, growth of cataracts.

isogenesis /-jen′əsis/, development from a common origin and according to similar processes.

isolation, the separation of a seriously ill patient from others to stop the spread of infection or protect the patient from irritating factors. A patient given radiation implant therapy may be isolated to reduce exposing others to radioactivity.

Isolette, a trademark for a self-contained incubator that has a controlled heat, humidity, and oxygen area for the isolation and care of premature and low-weight newborns. See also **incubator.**

isoleucine (Ile) /-loo′sēn/, an amino acid in most dietary proteins. It is needed for proper growth in infants and nitrogen balance in adults. See also **amino acid.**

isometheptene hydrochloride, a drug in some fixed-combination drugs for migraine.

isometric exercise, a form of exercise that raises muscle tension by putting pressure against stable resistance. This may be done by opposing different muscles in the same person, as by pressing the hands together or by making a limb push or pull against an immovable object. Compare **isotonic exercise.** See also **exercise.**

isoniazid, a drug used to treat tuberculosis. Liver disease, a previous negative reaction to isoniazid, or allergy to this drug prevents its use. Side effects include liver disease, nervous system disorders, rashes, fever, and central nervous system effects. Also called **INH (isonicotinic acid hydrazide).**

isopropamide iodide, a drug used to treat ulcers. Glaucoma, asthma, obstruction of the genitourinary or intestinal tract, ulcerative colitis, or allergy to this drug prevents its use. Side effects include blurred vision, central nervous system effects, rapid heart rate, dry mouth, less sweat, and allergic reactions.

isopropyl alcohol /-prō′pil/, a clear, colorless, bitter aromatic liquid that can be mixed with water, ether, chloroform, and ethyl alcohol. A solution of 70% isopropyl alcohol in water is used as a rubbing compound. See also **alcohol.**

isoproterenol hydrochloride, a bronchodilator and a cardiac stimulant. Irregular heart beat or allergy to this drug prevents its use. Side effects include heart problems and low blood pressure.

Isoptin, a trademark for a slow channel blocker or calcium ion antagonist (verapamil).

Isopto Atropine, a trademark for a nervous system drug (atropine sulfate).

Isopto Carbachol, a trademark for a nervous system drug (carbachol).

Isopto Carpine, a trademark for a nervous system drug (pilocarpine hydrochloride).

Isopto Cetamide, a trademark for an antibacterial (sulfacetamide sodium).

Isopto Homatropine, a trademark for a nervous system drug (homatropine hydrobromide).

Isopto Hyoscine, a trademark for a nervous system drug (scopolamine hydrobromide).

Isordil, a trademark for a drug used to stop chest pain (isosorbide dinitrate).

isosorbide dinitrate, a drug used to stop chest pain. It is used as a coronary vasodilator in the treatment of some heart problems. Known allergy to this drug prohibits its use. Side effects include occasional low blood pressure, flushing, headache, and dizziness.

isotonic exercise, a form of exercise in which the muscle contracts and causes movement. There is little change in the resistance so the force of the contraction remains constant. Compare **isometric exercise.** See also **exercise.**

isotope /ī′sətōp/, any of different forms of a chemical element having almost the same properties. Radioactive isotopes are used in many diagnostic and therapeutic procedures.

isotopic tracer /-top′ik/, an isotope of an element put into a sample to permit observation of the course of the element through a chemical, physical, or biologic process.

isotretinoin, an antiacne drug given for cystic acne.

isoxsuprine hydrochloride, a drug to improve blood flow in the brain and in hardening of the arteries, Raynaud's disease, and Buerger's disease. Allergy to this drug prohibits its use. Side effects include rapid heart rate, low

I–J

blood pressure, and skin problems. See also **Buerger's disease, Raynand's phenomenon.**

Isuprel, a trademark for a beta-adrenergic stimulant (isoproterenol).

itch, a tingling, annoying feeling on the skin that makes one want to scratch it, such as may be caused by a mosquito bite, or an allergic reaction.

IU, I.U., abbreviation for **International Unit.**

IUD, abbreviation for **intrauterine device.**

IV, abbreviation for **intravenous,** referring to the giving of fluids or drugs by injection in a vein.

IV push, a method in which a large amount of drug or IV fluid is given rapidly via IV injection or infusion. See also **injection.**

Ixodes /iksō′dēz/, parasitic hard-shelled ticks that carry infections, as Rocky Mountain spotted fever.

J

jackknife position, position in which the patient is placed on the back in a semisitting position, with the shoulders elevated and the thighs flexed at right angles to the abdomen. Examination of the male urethra is aided by this position.

Jacquemier's sign /zhäkmē·āz′/, a deepening of the color of the mucous membrane of the vagina just below the outlet of the urethra. It may be noted after the fourth week of pregnancy, but it is not a reliable sign of pregnancy.

jamais vu /zhämävY′, -vē′, -vōō′/, the feeling of being a stranger when with a person one knows or when in a familiar place. It occurs sometimes in normal people but more often in people who have epilepsy (temporal lobe). The French phrase means "never seen." Compare **déjà vu.**

Janeway lesion, a small red blemish on the palms or soles. It is sometimes a sign of an infection of the heart (subacute bacterial endocarditis).

Jarisch-Herxheimer reaction, a sudden passing fever and worsening of skin lesions seen a few hours after the giving of penicillin or other antibiotics to treat spirosis, or relapsing fever. It lasts less than 24 hours and needs no treatment.

Jarvik-7. See **artificial heart.**

Jarotzky's treatment, the use of a bland diet of egg whites, fresh butter, bread, milk, and noodles to treat gastric ulcer.

jaundice, a yellow discoloring of the skin, mucous membranes, and eyes, caused by too much bile pigment (bilirubin) in the blood. Persons with jaundice may also have nausea, vomiting, and stomach pain and may pass dark urine. Jaundice is a symptom of many disorders, including liver diseases, biliary obstruction, and some anemias. See also **hepatitis.**

jaw, a common term used to describe the large bones (maxillae and mandible) forming the mouth and the soft tissue that covers these structures. The **jaw relation** is any fitting together of the lower (mandible) to the upper (maxillae) jaw.

jaw reflex, an abnormal reflex elicited by tapping the chin with a rubber hammer while the mouth is half open and the jaw muscles are relaxed. A quick snapping shut of the jaw implies damage to part of the cerebral cortex.

Jefferson fracture, a fracture marked by bursting of the atlas ring of the spine.

jejunum /jəjōō′nəm/, one of the three portions of the small intestine, connecting with the duodenum and the ileum. The jejunum has a slightly larger diameter, a deeper color, and a thicker wall than the ileum. Compare **ileum.** –**jejunal,** adj.

jellyfish sting, a wound caused by skin contact with a jellyfish, a sea animal with a bell-shaped jellylike body and many long tentacles with stingers. In most cases a tender, red welt forms on the affected skin. Treatment involves carefully removing tentacles and applying a compress of alcohol and aromatic spirits of ammonia.

Jendrassik's maneuver /yendrä′shiks/, a method used in testing reflexes of the arms and hands. The patient hooks the flexed fingers of the two hands together and tries to pull them apart.

jet lag, a condition marked by fatigue, sleeplessness, and sluggish body functions caused by disruption of the normal biologic clock (circadian rhythm) because of air travel across several time zones.

jock itch, a fungal infection of the groin. It is most common in the tropics and among males. Topical antifungals, as miconazole and clotrimazole, are often given. The antibiotic griseofulvin is used only for severe, resistant cases. Also called **tinea cruris.**

Jod-Basedow phenomenon, excess thyroid hormone production when dietary iodine is given to a patient with endemic goiter in an area of environmental iodine deficiency. It is presumed that iodine deficiency protects some patients with endemic goiter from this condition. The disorder may also occur when large doses of iodine are given to patients with nontoxic goiter in areas with enough environmental iodine.

jogger's heel, a painful problem common among joggers and distance runners. Symptoms include bruising, bursitis, or bony spurs, caused by repetitive and forceful strikes of the heel on the ground. Rest, heat, or corticosteroid medication or aspirin may be used.

joint, any of the connections between bones. Each is classified according to structure and movability as fibrous, cartilaginous, or synovial. A **cartilaginous joint** is one that can move slightly. In it, the cartilage joins the bone. Typical slightly movable joints connect the vertebrae and the pubic bones. A **fibrous joint** is an immovable joint, as those of the skull segments, in which a fiberlike tissue may connect the bones. A **synovial joint** is a freely movable joint in which touching bony surfaces are covered by cartilage and connected by ligaments lined with synovial membrane. Kinds of synovial joints are **ball and socket joint, condyloid joint, gliding joint, hinge joint, pivot joint, saddle joint, uniaxial joint.** Most of the joints in the body are freely movable. Also called **articulation.**

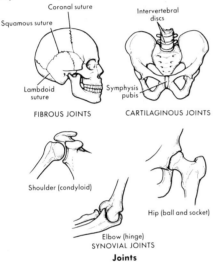

Joints

joint capsule. See **capsule.**

joint chondroma, a mass of cartilage that develops in the synovial membrane of a joint.

joint fracture, a break in the articular surfaces of the bony structures of a joint.

judgment, (in psychiatry) seeing the relation of ideas and forming right conclusions from them and experience.

juice, any fluid secreted by the tissues of animals or plants. In humans, it often refers to those released by the digestive glands. Kinds of juices include **gastric juice, intestinal juice, pancreatic juice.**

junction nevus, a hairless, flat or slightly raised, brown skin blemish. A junction nevus may be found anywhere on the body. Cancerous change may be signaled by increase in size, hardness or darkening, bleeding, or the appearance of darkening around the nevus. Junction nevi with these changes should be removed.

jurisdictional agency, the agency having jurisdiction and responsibility for a specific geographical area.

juvenile, **1.** a young person; child. **2.** referring to or suitable for a young person; youthful. **3.** physiologically immature.

juvenile alveolar rhabdomyosarcoma, a quickly growing muscle tumor in children and adolescents.

juvenile delinquency, antisocial or illegal acts by children or adolescents that cannot be controlled by parents, endanger others, and concern law enforcement agencies. Such behavior is marked by aggression, destruction, hostility, and cruelty. It occurs more often in boys than girls. **Juvenile delinquent** refers to a person who acts illegally and who is not old enough to be treated as an adult under the laws of the community.

juvenile rheumatoid arthritis. See **rheumatoid arthritis.**

K

Kahn test, **1.** a blood test for syphilis. **2.** a test for the presence of cancer by measuring the amount of a protein in a blood sample.

Kallmann's syndrome, a condition with the absence of the sense of smell and poorly developed reproductive glands.

kanamycin sulfate, an antibiotic for some severe infections and those resistant to other antibiotics. Known allergy to this drug or related antibiotics prohibits its use. Drugs that can cause damage to the ears may interact. It is used with caution in patients with impaired kidney function and in the elderly. Side effects include kidney disorders, loss of hearing and sense of balance, paralysis, and allergic reactions.

Kantrex, a trademark for an antibiotic (kanamycin sulfate).

Kanulase, a trademark for a drug that reduces intestinal gas.

Kaochlor, a trademark for a mineral replacement remedy (potassium chloride).

kaolin /kā′əlin/, a fine white clay taken orally to treat diarrhea, often with a softening agent, pectin. Kaolin in an ointment base is also used on the skin as a protective cream.

Kaon, a trademark for a mineral replacement remedy (potassium chloride).

Kaopectate, a trademark for a drug to treat diarrhea containing an adsorbent (kaolin) and a softening agent (pectin).

Kaposi's sarcoma /kap′əsēz/, a cancer that begins as soft, brownish or purple pimples on the feet and slowly spreads through the skin to the lymph nodes and abdominal organs. It occurs most often in men and is occasionally associated with AIDS (aquired immune deficiency syndrome), diabetes, lymph cancer, or other disorders. Radiation therapy and drugs are used to treat the cancer.

karaya powder /kär′äyä/, a dried form of a gummy plant secretion used as a bulk laxative. Because of its ability to absorb water, karaya powder may also be used in treating acute diarrhea, or as a drying agent in preparing the skin for dressings around bedsores.

karyon /ker′ē·on/, the nucleus of a cell.

karyosome /ker′ē·əsōm′/, a dense, irregular mass of genetic material in the cell nucleus that may be confused with the nucleolus.

karyotype /-tīp′/, **1.** the total portrait of the chromosomes in a body cell of an individual or species, as photographed through a microscope lens. It shows the number, form, size, and arrangement of chromosomes within the nucleus. **2.** a diagram of the chromosomes in a body cell of an individual or species, arranged in pairs in descending order of size. See also **chromosome.**

KayCiel, a trademark for a mineral replacement drug (potassium chloride).

Keflex, a trademark for an antibiotic (cephalexin).

Keflin, a trademark for an antibiotic (cephalothin).

Kegel exercises, a system of exercises in which a woman strengthens the muscles of her pelvic diaphragm and pubic area, particularly after childbirth.

keloid /kē′loid/, overgrowth of scar tissue at the site of a wound of the skin. The new tissue is elevated, rounded, and firm, with irregular, clawlike margins. Young women and blacks are most likely to develop keloids. **Keloidosis** is a condition of habitual or multiple formation of keloids.

Kemadrin, a trademark for a skeletal muscle relaxant (procyclidine hydrochloride).

Kenacort Diacetate, a trademark for an adrenal hormone (triamcinolone diacetate).

Kenalog, a trademark for an adrenal hormone (triamcinolone acetonide).

Kennedy classification, a method of classifying conditions of missing teeth and partial dentures, based on the position of the spaces between the remaining teeth.

keratectomy /ker′ətek′-/ surgical removal of a portion of the cornea of the eye. The tissue is cut out using local anesthesia. An antibiotic and a light dressing are then applied. New corneal tissue grows rapidly, filling a small cut area in about 60 hours.

keratin /ker′ətin/, a fibrous, sulfur-containing protein found in human skin, hair, nails, and tooth enamel. Gastric juice of the stomach does not dissolve the protein. For this reason it is often used as a coating for pills that must pass through the stomach unchanged to be dissolved in the intestines.

keratinization, a process by which skin cells exposed to the environment lose their moisture and are replaced by horny tissue.

keratinocyte /ker′ətinōsīt′/, a cell of the outer layer of the skin (epidermis) that produces keratin and other proteins.

keratitis /ker′ətī′-/, any inflammation of the cornea of the eye.

keratoacanthoma /ker′ətō·ak′anthō′mə/, a fast-growing, benign, ''flesh''-colored pimple with a central plug of keratin. The lesion usually occurs on the face or the back of hands and arms. It disappears spontaneously.

keratoconjunctivitis /-konjungk′tivi′-/, inflammation of the cornea and the mucous membrane lining the eyelid (conjunctiva). One form of the disorder (**phlyctenular keratoconjunctivitis**) causes tiny bumpy sores on the surface of the cornea from allergic material in germs or parasites. Children get it most often. A lack of vitamins may be a factor. Treatment is with hormone drugs, but scars may remain on the eye.

keratoconjunctivitis sicca, dryness of the cornea because of a lack of tear secretions. The eye feels gritty and irritated.

keratoconus /-kō′nəs/, a conelike bulge on the cornea of the eye. It may result in severe astigmatism.

keratolysis /ker′ətol′isis/, an abnormal loosening and shedding of the outer layer of the skin, which usually involves the palms of the hands or soles of the feet.

keratomalacia /-məlā′shə/, an eye condition with dryness and ulceration of the cornea, resulting from severe vitamin A deficiency. Diseases such as ulcerative colitis or cystic fibrosis may cause the deficiency. Symptoms include night blindness, sensitivity to light, and swelling and redness of the eyelids. Without adequate treatment, the cornea eventually softens and develops holes, resulting in blindness. See also **vitamin A.**

keratopathy /ker′ətop′əthē/, any disease of the cornea without inflammation. Compare **keratitis.**

keratosis /ker′ətō′-/, any skin condition in which there is overgrowth and thickening of the outer skin layers.

kerion /kir′ē·on/, an inflamed, boggy tumor that develops as a reaction to a fungus infection of the skin. It may accompany ringworm of the scalp. The lesion heals within a short time without treatment.

kernicterus /kernik′tərəs/, an abnormal buildup in central nervous system tissues of bilirubin, a yellowish pigment normally present in bile. An excessive amount of the pigment circulating in blood causes it.

kerosene poisoning. See **petroleum distillate poisoning.**

ketoacidosis /kē′tō·as′idō′-/, acidosis, an excessive level of acid in the blood, accompanied by ketosis, an increase of ketones in blood. Ketones are substances normally processed by the liver from fats. The condition may occur as a complication of diabetes mellitus. Symptoms are a fruity odor of the breath, mental confusion, breathing distress, nausea, vomiting, dehydration, weight loss, and, if untreated, coma. Emergency treatment includes administrating insulin, intravenous fluids, and correcting the body's acid-base balance. **Alcoholic ketoacidosis** refers to the condition as seen in alcoholics.

ketoaciduria /-as′idoor′ē·ə/, presence in the urine of excessive amounts of ketones, substances processed by the liver from fats. It results from uncontrolled diabetes mellitus, starvation, or any other condition in which fats are consumed as body fuel instead of carbohydrates. Also called **ketonuria.** See also **ketosis.**

ketoconazole, an antifungal agent prescribed for the treatment of candidiasis, histoplasmosis, and other fungal diseases. Known allergy to this drug prohibits its use. Side effects include liver disorders.

ketone bodies /kē′ton/, a group name for ketones, substances produced in the body through a normal change fats undergo in the liver. Also called **acetone bodies.**

ketosis /kētō′-/, an abnormal buildup of ketones in body tissues and fluid. This state occurs in starvation, sometimes in pregnancy, and, most often, in diabetes mellitus. Symptoms are ketones in urine, loss of potassium in urine, and a fruity odor on the breath. Untreated, ketosis may progress to ketoacidosis, coma, and death.

kg, abbreviation for **kilogram.**

kidney, one of a pair of bean-shaped urinary organs in the back of the abdomen on each side of the spine. The tops of the kidneys are on a level with the border of the lowest ribs. Each kidney is about 11 cm long, 6 cm wide, and 2.5 cm thick. Each kidney weighs from 115 to 170 g. The kidneys produce and eliminate urine through a complex system with more than 2 million tiny filters (nephrons). The nephrons filter blood under high pressure, removing urea, salts, and other soluble wastes. These wastes are then sent from the body as urine. Collecting tubules take urine into the renal pelvis, which is at the center of the kidney. The collecting tubules are important in keeping the fluid balance of the body by letting water seep through their membranes. The kidneys return the purified fluid to the blood. All of the blood in the body passes through the kidneys about 20 times every hour but only about one fifth is filtered by the nephrons during that period. Hormones control the function of the kidneys in regulating the water content of the body. The pituitary gland produces the most important, the antidiuretic hormone (ADH). ADH stimulates the reabsorption of water into the blood. If this hormone is not present in the blood, the kidney membranes do not allow the water to pass.

kidney cancer, a malignant tumor of the kidney's filtration tissue or of the renal pelvis, the urine-collecting system attached to the kidney. Cancer of the filtration tissue accounts for 80% of kidney tumors. Causes identified with the disease are exposure to chemicals such as benzene, tobacco smoke, and the use of drugs containing phenacetin. Symptoms include bloody urine, back pain, and fever. Surgery to remove the cancerous kidney is the usual treatment. The remaining kidney, if healthy, can generally make up for the loss.

kidney dialysis. See **hemodialysis.**

kidney disease, any of a large group of conditions including infectious, inflammatory, obstructive, circulatory, and cancerous disorders of the kidney. Signs and symptoms of kidney disease include bloody urine, persistent protein in urine, pus in urine, edema, difficult urination, and pain in the back. Specific symptoms vary with the type of disorder. For example, bloody urine with severe, colicky pain suggests obstruction by a kidney stone. Bloody urine without pain may indicate kidney cancer. Protein in urine is generally a sign of disease in the filtration units of the kidney. Pus in urine indicates infectious disease. Treatment depends on the type of kidney disease diagnosed. Some forms may lead to kidney failure, coma, and death unless hemodialysis is started.

kidney failure, the inability of the kidneys to work. The condition may be short-term (acute) or long-term (chronic). **Acute kidney failure** features very low amounts of urine and a rapid buildup of nitrogen wastes in the blood. It is caused by bleeding, injury, burns, poisoning, acute infection, or a blocked urinary tract. Many forms of acute renal failure are cured after the cause has been found. **Chronic kidney failure** may result from many diseases. The early signs are fatigue and mental dullness. Later, a lack of urine, seizures, bleeding in the digestive tract, poor diet, and many nerve disorders may occur. The skin may turn yellow-brown and become covered with a crystal-like substance (uremic frost). Congestive heart failure and high blood pressure are problems that may occur. There is a constant amount of urine no matter how much water the patient drinks. Anemia often occurs. Treatment for either form of kidney failure may include the use of antibiotics and fluid-releasing drugs (diuretics) and restricting the amount of water and protein taken in. When medical measures no longer work, long-term kidney filtering (dialysis) is often begun, and a kidney transplant is considered. Also called **renal failure.**

kidney stone, a mineral buildup (stone) in the kidney. If the stone is large enough to block the tube (ureter) and stop the flow of urine from the kidney, it must be removed by surgery or other methods. Also called **renal calculus.**

kilogram (kg) /kil′əgram/, a unit for the measurement of mass in the metric system. One kilogram is equal to 1000 grams or to 2.2046 pounds avoirdupois.

kilogram calorie. See **calorie.**

kinematics /kin′əmat′-, kī′nə-/, the study of the motion of the body without regard to the forces acting to produce the motion. Kinematics considers the motions of all body parts relative to the part involved in the motion. Kinematics is especially important in the diagnosis and treatment of joint disorders. Compare **kinetics.**

kinesics /kinē′siks/, the study of body position and movement in communication between people. It is used especially in mental health examinations.

kinesiology /kinē′sē·ol′-/, the scientific study of muscular activity and of the anatomy, physiology, and mechanics of body movement.

kinetics /kinet′-/, the study of the forces that produce, stop, or modify motions of the body. Compare **kinematics.**

kinetotherapeutic bath /kinet′ō-/, a bath in which underwater exercises are performed to strengthen weak or partially paralyzed muscles.

kiting, *informal.* illegal altering of a drug prescription to indicate that more of a drug was prescribed than actually ordered by a physician. Kiting may be done by a patient seeking greater quantities of drugs, especially narcotics, or may be done by a pharmacist to increase reimbursement from a third party, such as an involved insurance company.

Klebsiella /kleb′zē·el′ə/, a kind of bacteria that causes several respiratory diseases.

Kleine-Levin syndrome /klīn′-/, a disorder often associated with psychotic conditions, with symptoms of abnormal drowsiness, hunger, and excessive activity. There is no specific treatment. Compare **narcolepsy.**

kleptolagnia /klep′tālag′nē·ə/, sexual excitement or satisfaction produced by stealing.

kleptomania /klep′tə-/, a neurosis with an abnormal, uncontrollable, and repeated urge to steal. Objects are not taken for their monetary value, immediate need, or use but for their symbolic meaning, which may be associated with an emotional conflict. **–kleptomaniac,** *n.*

Klinefelter's syndrome /klīn′feltərz/, an abnormal condition of male sexual characteristics in which the body cells contain one or more extra X chromosomes (female sex chromosomes). Characteristics include small, firm testicles; long legs; femalelike breasts, and varicose veins. The severity of the abnormalities increases with greater numbers of X chromosomes. The most common abnormality is a 47,XXY karyotype. The man may appear generally normal, although he is infertile. See also **karyotype.**

K–L

Klor, a trademark for a mineral replacement drug (potassium chloride).

Klorvess, a trademark for a mineral supplement (potassium chloride).

knee, a joint with a group of parts that connects the thigh with the lower leg. It consists of three rounded bone surfaces (condyloid joints), 12 bands of fibrous tissue (ligaments), 13 fluid-filled sacs (bursae), and the kneecap (patella). The largest bursa is the prepatellar (kneecap) bursa between the patellar ligament and the skin.

knee-ankle interaction, one of the major factors that control leg motion in walking. It helps to minimize the change in the body's center of gravity during walking. The diagnosis and treatment of various bone and joint diseases often includes observing knee-ankle interaction.

kneecap, a flat, triangle-shaped bone at the front of the knee joint. Also called **patella.**

knee-chest position. See **body position.**

knee-hip flexion, a body movement that allows the passage of body weight over the supporting leg during walking. Knee-hip flexion may be used in the diagnosis and treatment of various bone and joint diseases.

knee-jerk reflex. See **deep tendon reflex.**

knee joint, the complex, hinged joint at the knee that, with its ligaments, permits movements, such as flexion, extension, and, in certain positions, rotation of the leg. It is a common site for sprains and dislocations.

knee replacement, the surgical insertion of a hinged artificial joint. It relieves pain and restores motion to a knee affected by arthritis or injury. The diseased bone surfaces are removed and a two-piece metallic hinge is cemented into the cavities of the upper and lower leg bones (femur and tibia).

knife needle, a surgical knife with a needle point, used to remove a cataract and in other eye operations, such as glaucoma surgery.

knock-knee, a deformity in which the legs are curved in so that the knees are close together, knocking as the person walks. Also called **genu valgum.**

Knoop hardness test, a method of measuring tooth surface hardness by resistance of the tooth to a tool made of diamond.

knot, lacing together the surgical ligature or suture ends so that the material used, such as silk or wire, remains in place.

Koebner phenomenon /kōb′nər/, skin lesions that develop at the site of an injury resulting in psoriasis, or a similar kind of skin disease. See also **psoriasis.**

koilonychia /koi′lōnik′ē·ə/, spoon nails; a condition in which fingernails are thin and curved inwardly from side to side. Usually inherited, it may also occur with iron deficiency anemia and Raynaud's phenomenon.

Konȳne, a trademark for a blood coagulating drug (factor IX complex).

Koplik's spots, small red spots with bluish-white centers found on the inside of the mouth of persons with measles. The rash of measles usually erupts 1 or 2 days after the appearance of Koplik's spots.

Korotkoff sounds /kôrot′kôf/, sounds of blood flow heard during a blood pressure reading with a sphygmomanometer (blood pressure gauge) and stethoscope. See also **blood pressure, diastole, sphygmomanometer, systole.**

Korsakoff's psychosis /kôr′səkôfs/, a form of memory loss often seen in chronic alcoholics. The person is usually disoriented and gives false information to conceal the condition.

kosher /kō′shər/, conforming to or prepared in accordance with the dietary or ceremonial laws of Judaism.

Krabbe's disease, an inherited disease of the body's use of fats (lipids), present at birth. Infants become paralyzed, blind, deaf, and increasingly retarded, and eventually die of paralysis. There is no known treatment for the disease, but it can be detected by a prenatal test (amniocentesis). See also **lipidosis.**

kraurosis /krôrō′-/, a thickening and shriveling of the skin. **Kraurosis vulvae** refers to a condition of dryness, itching, and atrophy of the vulva. It occurs in aged women and often leads to cancer.

Krause's corpuscles, nerve endings that are sensitive to temperature.

Krebs' citric acid cycle /krebz/, a series of enzyme reactions in which the body uses carbohydrates, proteins, and fats to yield carbon dioxide, water, and energy.

Krukenberg's tumor, a tumor of the ovary that has spread from cancer cells of the stomach or intestines.

Küntscher nail /kōōn′chər/, a stainless steel nail used in bone surgery to repair fractures of the long bones, especially the femur, the long bone of the thigh.

Kupffer's cells /kōōp′fərz/, liver cells that filter bacteria and other small, foreign proteins out of the blood.

Kussmaul breathing /kōōs′moul/, abnormally deep, very rapid breathing with sighing. It occurs in diabetic acidosis, a condition of too much acid in the blood.

Kussmaul's sign, **1.** a pulse that rises in rate when exhaling and falls when inhaling. It occurs in certain heart and chest disorders. **2.** convulsions and coma associated with a disorder of the stomach and intestines caused by swallowing a poison.

Kwell, a trademark for a drug that destroys lice and mites (gamma benzene hexachloride).

kymography /kīmog′rəfē, kē-/, a method for recording motion pictures of body organs.

kyphoscoliosis /kī′fōskō′lē·ō′-/. See **spinal curvature.**

kyphosis /kīfō′-/. See **spinal curvature.**

L

L, symbol for **liter.**

label, a substance, usually radioactive, with a special attraction for a specific organ, tissue, or cell, in which it may become deposited. The radioactivity gives a signal that can be followed through various body processes, making it useful in diagnosis, such as in locating a tumor.

label, see **shipping package label warning.**

labeling, providing information on a drug, food, device, or cosmetic to the purchaser or user. The information may be given as printing on a carton, adhesive label, or package insert. Regulations for labeling are decided by the Food and Drug Administration. The label must contain directions for use, unless such directions are exempted by regulation, as well as warnings. It may not contain false or misleading information.

labia /lā′bē·ə/, *sing.* **labium,** the fleshy, liplike edges of an organ or tissue, such as the folds of skin at the opening of the vagina.

labia majora /majôr′ə/, *sing.* **labium majus,** two long lips of skin, one on each side of the vaginal opening, that form the border of the vulva. Each labium contains connective tissue, fat, and a thin layer of muscle. In some women the outer surface of each lip may be covered with coarse pubic hair. The labia majora and the pouch of skin (scrotum) containing the male testes are derived from the same tissues of the embryo.

labia minora /minôr′ə/, *sing.* **labium minus,** two folds of skin between the labia majora, extending from the clitoris backward on both sides of the vaginal opening. Each labium divides into an upper and a lower division.

labile /lā′bil/, **1.** unstable; having a tendency to change or to be easily altered. **2.** describing a personality with rapidly shifting or changing emotions.

labor, the time and processes that occur during childbirth from the beginning of cervical dilatation to the delivery of the placenta, or afterbirth. In the early stage of childbirth, called the **latent phase** or **prodromal labor,** there are irregular, few, and mild contractions of the uterus. Little or no dilation of the cervix or descent of the fetus occurs. During the **active phase** of labor, the cervix widens from about 5 cm to 10 cm (2 to 4 inches). The **acceleration phase** is the first part of active labor. The cervix opens more quickly during this time. Called **transition,** the last phase of the first stage of labor is sometimes shown by the cervix dilating 8 to 10 cm. When the cervix is fully widened, the contractions occur every 1½ to 3 minutes and last from 40 to 90 seconds, the time between contractions tends to lessen, and the length and intensity of the contractions tend to increase. **Engagement** refers to the point in childbirth when the part of the fetus descending first comes down into the mother's pelvis. This occurs roughly halfway through labor. The **expulsive stage of labor** is the second stage, during which contractions or the uterus are accompanied by an urge to bear down. It begins after the cervix is completely widened. This stage ends with the complete delivery of the infant. **Premature labor** refers to labor that occurs earlier in pregnancy than normal, either before the fetus has reached a weight of 2000 to 2500 grams (5 to 5.5 pounds) or before the thirty-seventh week of pregnancy. If premature labor itself threatens the fetus, the outcome of pregnancy may be helped if labor can be put off. Misdiagnosis of the age of the fetus may lead to inducing labor that is premature. **Cardinal movements of labor** refers to the sequence of movements by the infant as it comes down through the pelvis during labor and birth. **Dry labor** refers to labor in which the water (amniotic fluid) has already escaped. See also **birth.**

laboratory, a facility, room, or building in which scientific research, experiments, or tests are carried out.

laboratory medicine, the branch of medicine in which specimens of tissue, fluid, or other body substance are examined in the laboratory.

laboratory test, a procedure, usually conducted in a laboratory, that is intended to detect, identify, or measure one or more important substances, evaluate organ functions, or establish the nature of a disease. Laboratory tests range from quite simple to extremely complex. They are commonly used to help establish or confirm a diagnosis and often aid in managing a disease.

labor coach, a person who assists a woman in labor and delivery. The coach, often the father of the baby, encourages the woman to use ways that were taught in a program of preparation for childbirth. The goal is to minimize the need for drugs for relieving pain.

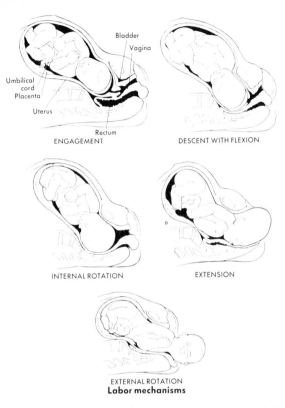

ENGAGEMENT   DESCENT WITH FLEXION

INTERNAL ROTATION   EXTENSION

EXTERNAL ROTATION
Labor mechanisms

labored breathing, increased effort in breathing, including use of the muscles of the chest wall, noisy breathing, grunting, or flaring of the nostrils.

labyrinth. See **ear.**

labyrinthitis /lab′ərinthī′-/, inflammation of the fluid-filled canals of the inner ear, resulting in dizziness.

laceration /las′ərā′shən/, a torn, jagged wound. **–lacerate,** *v.,* **lacerated,** *adj.*

lacrimal /lak′riməl/, pertaining to tears.

lacrimal bone, one of the smallest bones of the face, located at the front of the inner wall of the eye socket.

lacrimal duct, one of two channels through which tears pass from the inner corner of the eye to the lacrimal sac. See also **lacrimal sac.**

lacrimal fistula, an abnormal channel from a tear duct to the surface of the eye or eyelid.

lacrimal gland, one of a pair of oval-shaped glands about the size of an almond situated above the eye. The watery secretion from the gland consists of the tears, slightly alkaline and salty, that moisten the eye. The **lacrimal papilla** is the small elevation on the margin of each eyelid, through which tears emerge from the lacrimal gland.

lacrimal sac, one of two sacs lodged in a deep groove formed by the face bones between the inner corners of the eyes and the nose. Tears from the eyes fill the sacs, and

drain down small tubes (nasolacrimal ducts) into the cavity of the nose.

lacrimation /lak′rimā′shən/, **1.** the normal continuous secretion of tears by the lacrimal glands above the eyes. **2.** an excessive amount of tear production, as in crying or weeping.

lactalbumin /lak′talbyoo′min/, a highly nutritious protein found in milk. It is similar to serum albumin. See also **serum albumin.**

lactase /lak′tās/, an enzyme that increases the rate of the change of milk sugar (lactose) to glucose and galactose, carbohydrates needed by the body for energy. Lactase is concentrated in the kidney, liver, and intestinal lining.

lactase deficiency, an abnormal lack in the amount of the enzyme lactase in the body. This results in the inability to digest milk sugar (lactose). See also **lactose intolerance.**

lactation, the process of the making and release of milk from the breasts for the feeding of an infant. See also **breast feeding.**

lacteal /lak′tē·əl/, pertaining to milk.

lacteal fistula, an abnormal passage opening into a milk duct in the breast.

lacteal gland, one of the many lymph capillaries in the fingerlike bumps (villi) of the small intestine wall. The capillary is filled with a fluid (chyle) that turns milky white during the absorption of fat.

lactic, referring to milk and milk products.

lactic acid, an organic acid normally present in tissue. One form of lactic acid in muscle and blood is a product of the change of the carbohydrates, glucose and glycogen, to energy during physical exercise. Lactic acid is also found in the stomach, in sour milk, and in some foods, such as sauerkraut.

Lactinex, a trademark for a drug containing bacteria *(Lactobacillus)* used for gastrointestinal disorders.

Lactobacillus, any of a group of rod-shaped bacteria that produce lactic acid from carbohydrates. Some species are normally found in the human intestinal tract and vagina.

lactogen /lak′təjən/, a drug or other agent that stimulates the making and release of milk. **–lactogenic,** *adj.*

lacto-ovovegetarian /-ō′vōvej′-/, one whose diet consists mainly of vegetables and also includes eggs *(ovo),* milk, and cheese *(lacto),* but no meat, fish, or poultry. Also called **ovo-lactovegetarian.**

lactose /lak′tōs/, a sugar found in the milk of all mammals. Lactose is used as a laxative or a diuretic, and in some formulas for infant feeding. Also called **milk sugar.**

lactose intolerance, a disorder resulting in the inability to digest milk sugar (lactose) because of an enzyme, lactase, deficiency. Symptoms include bloating, intestinal gas, nausea, diarrhea, and cramps. The diet restricts such foods as milk, cheese, butter, margarine, and any other products containing milk. See also **lactase deficiency.**

lactosuria /-ōōr′ē∙ə/, the presence of milk sugar (lactose) in the urine. This may occur in late pregnancy or during breast milk production (lactation).

lactovegetarian, one whose diet consists of milk and milk products (*lacto*) in addition to foods of vegetable origin but does not include eggs, meat, fish, or poultry.

lactulose /lak′tyəlōs/, a synthetic sugar not absorbed by the body and used as a laxative in chronic constipation. Its ability to increase fecal water content, however, may also cause diarrhea.

Laetrile /lā′ətril/, a substance composed mainly of amygdalin, a cyanide-producing chemical derived from apricot pits. Laetrile has been offered as a cancer drug despite studies by the National Cancer Institute that failed to show benefits from its use. It is claimed that amygdalin is changed by enzymes in cancer cells to substances that kill the cancer cells. See also **amygdalin.**

lagophthalmos /lag′ofthal′məs/, an abnormal condition in which an eye cannot be fully closed because of a nervous system or muscle disorder. Also called **hare's eye.**

laked blood /lākt/, blood in which breakdown of the red blood cells has occurred, as may happen in poisoning or severe burns.

lallation /lalā′shən/, **1.** babbling, repetitive, unintelligible speech, like that of an infant. **2.** a speech disorder with a defective pronunciation of words containing the sound /l/ or the use of the sound /l/ in place of the sound /r/.

Lamaze method /ləmäz′/, a system of preparation for childbirth developed in the 1950s by a French obstetrician, Fernand Lamaze. The Lamaze method has become the most often used means of teaching natural childbirth, without the use of drugs. It requires classes, practice at home, and coaching during labor and delivery, often by a trained coach called a ''monitrice.'' The classes, given during pregnancy, teach exercises to develop strength and control in the abdominal muscles and those of the vaginal area, and methods of breathing and relaxation. Compare **Bradley method, Read method.** See also **natural childbirth.**

lamella /ləmel′ə/, *pl.* **lamellae, 1.** a thin leaf or plate, as of bone. **2.** a medicated disk, prepared from glycerin to place under the eyelid, where it dissolves and is absorbed.

lamina /lam′inə/, *pl.* **laminae,** a thin, flat plate or layer, such as the lamina of the thyroid cartilage that overlays the structure on each side.

laminaria tent /lam′iner′ē∙ə/, a cone of dried seaweed that swells as it absorbs water and is sometimes used to

dilate the cervix in preparation for induced abortion or labor.

laminectomy /lam′inek′-/, the surgical chipping away of the thin bony arches (laminae) of one or more vertebrae, done to relieve compression of the spinal cord. The cause may be a bone displaced in an injury or the breakdown of a cartilage disk. Fusion of some vertebrae may be necessary for stability of the spine if several laminae are removed. –**laminectomize,** *v.*

lanatoside C /lanat′əsīd/, a heart tonic used for congestive heart failure and heart beat abnormalities. Rapid heart beat or known allergy to this drug prohibits its use. Side effects include irregular or slow pulse, nausea, tiredness, and loss of appetite.

lance, to puncture a pus-forming lesion to release accumulated matter. A deep infection may need a drainage tube. If a boil is on the face, an antibiotic is given to prevent infection from spreading into the brain. Infected matter from the lesion must be kept off surrounding skin to prevent a recurrence.

lancet, a short, pointed blade used to obtain a drop of blood for a blood sample.

lancinating, pertaining to a sensation that is sharply piercing or tearing, as a pain may be.

Landau reflex /lan′dou/, a normal response of infants when lying on the back to maintain an arc with the head raised and the legs slightly flexed. The reflex is poor in those with floppy infant syndrome and exaggerated in certain other disorders.

lanolin /lan′ōlin/, a fatlike substance from the wool of sheep. It contains about 25% water as a water-in-oil emulsion and is used as an ointment base and a softening agent for the skin.

Lanoxin, a trademark for a heart tonic (digoxin).

lanugo /lanōō′gō, lanyōō′gō/, **1.** the soft, downy hair covering a normal fetus, beginning with the fifth month of life in the uterus and almost entirely shed by the ninth month. **2.** the fine, soft hair covering all parts of the body except palms, soles, and areas where other types of hair are normally found. Also called **vellus hair.**

laparoscopy /lap′əros′kəpē/, the examination of the abdominal cavity. An instrument consisting of a lighted tube with magnifying lenses (laparoscope) is inserted through a small cut in the abdominal wall. The method is also used for examining the ovaries and fallopian tubes. Also called **abdominoscopy.**

laparotomy /-ot′-/, a surgical cut into a cavity of the abdomen. Some kinds of laparotomy are **appendectomy, cholecystectomy, colostomy.**

large intestine. See **intestine.**

large quantity, an amount of radioactive material that exceeds the type B quantity limitations.

K–L

Largon, a trademark for a sedative (propiomazine hydrochloride).

Larodopa, a trademark for an antiparkinsonian drug (levodopa).

laryngeal cancer /lerin′jē·əl/, a malignant tumor arising from the lining of the voicebox (larynx). Persistent hoarseness is usually the first sign. Advanced lesions may cause a sore throat, breathing and swallowing difficulties, and swelling of the lymph glands in the neck. Laryngeal tumors are more common in men than in women and occur most frequently between 50 and 70 years of age. Chronic alcoholism and heavy use of tobacco increase the risk of developing the cancer. Treatment for small lesions is usually radiation. Surgical removal (laryngectomy), often combined with radiation, is indicated for extensive lesions.

laryngeal prominence. See **Adam's apple.**

laryngectomy /ler′injek′-/, surgical removal of the voicebox (larynx) to treat cancer. An opening called a tracheostomy is made from the outside of the throat to the windpipe (trachea) to ensure an adequate airway for breathing. In a partial laryngectomy only the vocal cords are removed, and the tracheostomy is closed within several days. If the cancer is extensive, the entire larynx, the Adam's apple, and a tissue flap (epiglottis) that closes the windpipe when a person swallows are all removed. The tracheostomy becomes permanent after surgery. A laryngectomy tube, which remains in the throat for about 1 month, is inserted. Following the operation, many persons with laryngectomies learn esophageal speech, some use an electric voicebox, and a few undergo surgical reconstruction. –**laryngectomize,** v.

laryngismus /-jiz′məs/, a condition of uncontrolled spasms of the voicebox (larynx). A crowing sound is made on taking a breath. The skin may become bluish from a lack of oxygen. The condition occurs in inflammation of the larynx and with rickets. The larynx of the infant and young child is particularly affected by spasms when infected or irritated and may become obstructed.

laryngitis /-jī′-/, inflammation of the mucous membrane lining the voicebox (larynx), accompanied by swelling of the vocal cords with hoarseness or loss of voice. It may be caused by a cold, irritating fumes or sudden temperature changes. Chronic laryngitis may result from excessive use of the voice or heavy smoking. In acute laryngitis, there may be a cough, and the throat usually feels scratchy and painful. Acute laryngitis may cause serious breathing problems in children under 5 years of age. The child may develop a hoarse, barking cough and noisy breathing, become restless, and gasp for air. Treatment includes providing large amounts of vaporized cool mist. Chronic laryngitis may be treated by removing irritants, avoiding smoking, voice rest, correcting faulty voice habits, cough medica-

tion, steam inhalations, and spraying the throat with medications recommended by the physician.

laryngopharyngitis /lering′gōfer′injī′-/, inflammation of both the voicebox (larynx) and throat (pharynx). See also **laryngitis, pharyngitis.**

laryngopharyngography /-fer′ingog′rəfē/, the x-ray examination of the voicebox (larynx) and the throat (pharynx). Also called **laryngography.**

laryngoscope /lering′goskōp/, an instrument with a light and magnifying lenses for examining the larynx.

laryngospasm /-spazm/, a sudden, temporary closure of the larynx. See also **laryngismus.**

laryngotracheobronchitis (LTB) /-trā′kē·ōbrongkī′-/, an inflammation of the throat and bronchial tubes leading to the lungs. Symptoms are hoarseness, a dry cough, and breathing difficulty. Among the causes are infection by certain viruses, and the bacteria associated with bronchitis, influenza, and diptheria. Treatment includes steam inhalations, cough suppressants, and sometimes antibiotics. See also **croup.**

larynx /ler′ingks/, the voicebox that is part of the air passage connecting the throat with the windpipe (trachea) leading toward the lungs. It produces a large bump in the neck called the Adam's apple, which becomes larger in men than in women. The larynx, lined with mucous membrane, forms the bottom portion of the front wall of the throat. It is composed of rings of cartilages, all connected together by ligaments and moved by various muscles. – **laryngeal,** adj.

Lasan, a trademark for an ointment (anthralin) to treat a skin disease, psoriasis.

laser, acronym for light amplification by stimulated emission of radiation, a source of intense radiation of the visible, ultraviolet, or infrared portions of the light spectrum. Lasers are used in surgery to divide or weld tissues or to destroy tissue cells.

Lasix, a trademark for a water pill or diuretic (furosemide).

latency stage /lā′tənsē/, a period in psychosexual development occurring between early childhood and puberty.

latent, pertaining to a condition that is inactive or existing as a potential problem, as tuberculosis may be latent for a long period of time and then become active under certain conditions.

latent period, an interval between the time of exposure to an injurious dose of radiation and the response of the body tissues to the radiation.

lateral, 1. on the side. 2. away from the middle of the body or body part or organ.

lateral pelvic displacement, one of the major leg muscle actions produced by the horizontal shift of the pelvis. It helps to synchronize the movements of walking. It is often used in the diagnosis and treatment of various bone or joint diseases and deformities.

lateral rocking,   a sideways rocking of the body used to move the body forward or backward when normal muscle action is not possible. The method is used by some disabled persons to move to or from the edge of a chair or to another sitting position on a bed. The rocking is done while leaning the trunk forward with the arms in front.

latex fixation test,   a blood test used in the diagnosis of rheumatoid arthritis.

latissimus dorsi,   one of a pair of large triangular muscles of the back. The base of the triangle is at the level of the lower four ribs. The latissimus dorsi moves the arm, draws the shoulder back and down, and helps draw the body up when climbing.

laughing gas,   *informal.* nitrous oxide, a side effect of which is laughter or giggling when given in less than anesthetizing amounts.

lavage /ləväzh′/,   the process of washing out an organ, usually the bladder, bowel, sinuses, or stomach, for treatment, as when a poison has been swallowed. **Blood lavage** removes poisons from the blood by injecting blood into the veins. **Gastric lavage** is the washing out of the stomach with sterile water or a salt fluid. This is done before and after surgery to remove irritants and swallowed poisons or to prepare the stomach to have instruments placed in it. See also **dialysis, irrigation.**

law enforcement,   those individuals who are legally empowered to manage the location and activities of the general public. Generally they will be police officers, but this category may also include the private security guards found at many fixed facilities.

laxative,   1. pertaining to a substance that causes evacuation of the bowel by a mild action. **2.** a laxative agent that promotes bowel evacuation by increasing the bulk of the feces, by softening the stool, or by lubricating the intestinal wall. Compare **cathartic.**

LD-50 or **LD₅₀ dose,**   the dose of radiation needed to kill, within a specified time period, 50% of the individuals in a large group of animals or organisms. This is about 300 to 500 rad for humans.

lead /lēd/,   an electric connection attached to the body to record electric activity, especially of the heart or brain. An example is an **esophageal lead,** which is placed within the esophagus. This helps to identify heart irregularities. An **intracardiac lead** is one in which the exploring electrode is placed in a heart chamber. See also **electrocardiograph, electroencephalograph.**

lead pipe fracture /lĕd/,   a fracture that compresses the bony tissue at the point of impact and creates a straight-line (linear) fracture on the opposite side of the same bone.

lead poisoning /lĕd/,   an abnormal condition caused by swallowing or breathing substances containing lead. Many children have developed the condition as a result of eating flakes of lead paint peeling from walls or furniture. Poisoning also occurs from drinking water carried in lead pipes, lead salts in some foods and wines, the use of pewter or earthenware dishes covered with lead glaze, and the use of leaded gasoline. Breathing of lead fumes is common in industry. Symptoms of chronic lead poisoning are extreme irritability, loss of appetite, and anemia. Symptoms of the acute form of lead poisoning are a burning sensation in the mouth and esophagus, colic, constipation or diarrhea, mental disturbances, and paralysis of the arms and legs, followed in severe cases by convulsions and muscular collapse. If lead is swallowed, treatment includes washing out the stomach with magnesium or sodium sulfate. Brain disease must be anticipated in children with lead poisoning.

learning disability,   an abnormal condition often affecting children of normal or above-average intelligence. There is difficulty in learning such fundamental procedures as reading, writing, and arithmetic. The condition may result from medical and psychologic causes.

leather bottle stomach,   a thickening of the wall of the stomach, resulting in a rigid, shrunken organ. Causes include cancer, syphilis, and Crohn's disease involving the stomach.

Leboyer method of delivery /leboiyā′/,   a method of childbirth developed by the French obstetrician Charles Leboyer. It has four basic features, including: (1) a gentle, controlled delivery in a quiet, dimly lit room; (2) avoiding pulling on the infant's head; (3) avoiding overstimulating the infant's nervous system; and (4) encouraging maternal-infant bonding. The goal is to minimize the shock of birth by gently introducing the newborn to life outside of the womb. Following delivery, the baby is laid on the mother's abdomen. The infant's back is massaged as the umbilical cord stops pulsating, and, when regular breathing is established, the baby is gently supported in a warm tub of water. Some studies have claimed superior psychologic, social, and intellectual development in children delivered by this method. Compare **Bradley method, Lamaze method, Read method.**

lecithin /les′ithin/,   any of a group of phosphorus-rich fats common in plants and animals. Lecithins are found in the liver, nerve tissue, semen, bile, and blood. They are essential for transforming fats in the body. Rich dietary sources are soybeans, egg yolk, and corn. Deficiency leads to liver and kidney disorders, high serum cholesterol levels, atherosclerosis, and arteriosclerosis.

Ledercillin VK,   a trademark for an antibiotic (penicillin V potassium).

left-handedness.   See **handedness.**

K–L

left-heart failure. See **heart failure.**

left pulmonary artery, the shorter and smaller of two arteries conveying blood from the heart to the lungs.

left ventricular assist device (LVAD), a mechanical pump that is used to aid the natural pumping action of the left ventricle of the heart.

left ventricular failure. See **heart failure.**

leg cylinder cast, a device of plaster of paris or fiberglass to hold the leg in treating fractures in the legs from the ankle to the upper thigh. The foot is not encased. It is also used for knee disorders, soft tissue injury, and correcting deformities.

Legionnaires' disease, an acute pneumonia caused by infection with a germ (*Legionella pneumophilia*). There is an influenza-like illness followed shortly by inflammation of the membrane covering the lungs (pleurisy). Symptoms include high fever, chills, muscle aches, headache, dry cough, and diarrhea. Usually the disease is self-limited, but the death rate has been 15% to 20% in a few localized epidemics. Contaminated air conditioning cooling towers and moist soil may be a source of organisms. Person-to-person spread has not occurred. The risk of infection increases with the presence of other conditions, as heart and lung diseases. Treatment includes supportive care of symptoms and antibiotics.

leiomyofibroma /lī′omī′ōfībrō′mə/, a tumor of smooth muscle cells and fibrous connective tissue.

leiomyoma /-mī·ō′mə/, a noncancerous smooth muscle tumor most commonly occurring in the stomach, esophagus, or small intestine. Surgery is necessary if the tumor causes sudden and possibly severe bleeding.

leiomyoma cutis, a tumor of the smooth muscles that raise the hair. The lesion features many small, tender, red masses of tissue.

leiomyoma uteri. See **fibroids.**

leishmaniasis /lēsh′mənī′əsis/, infection with a protozoan parasite of the *Leishmania* group that is transmitted to humans by sand flies. The diseases caused by these microorganisms may involve the skin or abdominal organs, causing ulcers or a skin disorder that resembles leprosy.

length of stay (LOS), the period of time a patient remains in a hospital or other health care facility as an inpatient.

lens of the eye. See **crystalline lens.**

lens implant, an artifical eye lens of clear plastic that is usually put in an eye at the time a clouded or opaque lens (cataract) is removed. It may also be used for patients with extreme nearsightedness or other visual problems. The operation may be performed with a local anesthetic, but general anesthesia is used more often. The plastic lens is inserted through a cut in the cornea.

Lente Insulin, a trademark for an antidiabetic agent (insulin zinc suspension).

lentigo /lentī′gō/, *pl.* **lentigines** /lentij′ənēz/, a tan or brown spot on the skin brought on by sun exposure, usually in a middle-aged or older person. Another variety, called **juvenile lentigo** and unrelated to sunlight, appears in children 2 to 5 years of age. The colored material in a lentigo is at a deeper level of the skin than in a freckle. Both types are noncancerous, and no treatment is necessary. Compare **freckle.**

lepromin test /leprō′min/, a skin sensitivity test used to distinguish between two forms of leprosy.

leprosy /lep′rəsē/, a chronic disease, caused by *Mycobacterium leprae,* that may take either of two forms. **Tuberculoid leprosy,** seen in those with high resistance to the disease-causing bacteria, appears as a thickening of nerves of the skin with saucer-shaped skin lesions. **Lepromatous leprosy,** seen in those with little resistance, involves many systems of the body, with widespread skin lesions, eye inflammation, destruction of nose cartilage and bone, and atrophy of the testicles. Blindness may result. Death from leprosy is rare unless tuberculosis or another disease occurs at the same time. Contrary to common belief, leprosy is not very contagious. Prolonged, intimate contact is required for it to be spread between persons. Children are more susceptible than adults. Treatment with sulfa drugs usually results in improvement of skin lesions, but recovery from nerve impairment is limited. Plastic surgery and physical therapy are often necessary. The disease occurs mostly in undeveloped tropical and subtropical countries. In the United States, patients may be sent to the U.S. Public Health Service leprosarium in Carville, Louisiana. Also called **Hansen's disease.**

leptocytosis /lep′tōsītō′-/, a condition in which abnormal red blood cells that resemble ''bull's-eye'' targets are present in the blood. A form of anemia (thalassemia), some kinds of liver disease, and absence of the spleen are linked with leptocytosis.

leptospirosis /-spīrō′-/, an acute infectious disease caused by a microorganism, *Leptospira interrogans,* transmitted through infected animals, especially rodents or dogs. Human infections come from direct contact with the urine or tissues of the infected animal or indirectly from contact with contaminated water or soil. Symptoms include jaundice, bleeding into the skin, fever, chills, and muscular pain. Antibiotics are used in treatment. Severe infections can damage the kidneys and the liver. The most serious form is called **Weil's disease.**

Leriche's syndrome /ləreshs′/, a disorder with gradual blockage of the abdominal aorta, the artery that supplies blood to the stomach, liver, and spleen. Symptoms include pain in buttocks, thighs, or calves, absence of pulsation in leg arteries, pale, cold legs, gangrene of the toes, and impotence in men. Treatment may include removal of the blockage or surgery to install a synthetic bypass graft.

lesbian, 1. a female homosexual. **2.** referring to the sexual preference or desire of one woman for another. – **lesbianism,** *n.*

Lesch-Nyhan syndrome /lesh'-nī'han/, a hereditary disorder affecting males, in which there is an excess production of uric acid, normally present in blood and urine. Symptoms include mental retardation, self-mutilation of the fingers and lips by biting, impaired kidney function, and abnormal physical development.

lesion, 1. a wound, injury, or other damage in body tissue. **2.** any visible, local abnormal area of skin, as a wound, sore, rash, or boil. A lesion may be described as benign (noncancerous), malignant (cancerous), gross (visible), occult (of unknown cause), or primary (first).

lesser occipital nerve, one of a pair of nerves that runs along the side of the head behind the ear.

let-down, a sensation in the breasts of women who are breast feeding an infant that often occurs as the milk flows into the ducts.

lethal /lē'thəl/, capable of causing death.

lethal concentrations, 50% kill (LC-50), the concentration of an inhaled substance that results in the death of 50% of the test population. LC-50 is an inhalation exposure expressed in parts per million (ppm), milligrams per liter, or milligrams per cubic meter. (The lower the value, the more toxic the substance.)

lethal dose, 50% kill (LD-50), the concentration of an ingested or infected substance that results in the death of 50% of the test populations. LD-50 is an oral or dermal exposure expressed in milligrams per kilogram. (The lower the dose, the more toxic the substance.)

lethal gene. See **gene.**

lethargy /leth'ərjē/, **1.** the state or quality of being indifferent or sluggish. An example is **lucid lethargy,** a state in which there is a loss of will and an inability to act, even though the patient is conscious and has normal thinking function. **2.** stupor or coma resulting from disease or hypnosis. A trancelike state produced during hypnosis is called **induced lethargy.**

leucine (Leu) /lōo'sin/, an amino acid essential for best growth in infants and nitrogen balance in adults. It cannot be synthesized by the body and is obtained by the conversion of protein during digestion. An inherited inability of the body to use leucine properly is called maple syrup urine disease. See also **amino acid.**

leucovorin calcium, an antianemic drug given to treat an overdose of a folic acid antagonist, as methotrexate drugs, and certain other types of anemia. Anemia caused by vitamin B_{12} or known allergy to this drug prohibits its use. Allergic reactions may occur.

leukapheresis /lōo'kəfərē'-/, a process by which blood is withdrawn from a vein, white blood cells are selectively removed, and the remaining blood is recycled back into the donor. The white cells may be used for treating patients with blood deficiencies.

leukemia, a cancer of blood-forming tissues. Replacement of bone marrow with immature white blood cells (leukocytes) occurs, and abnormal numbers and forms of immature white cells appear in circulation. Acute leukemia usually begins suddenly. It rapidly progresses from early symptoms, such as fatigue, pale skin, weight loss, and easy bruising, to fever, bleeding, extreme weakness, bone or joint pain, and repeated infections. Chronic leukemia develops slowly. Signs similar to those of the acute form of the disease may not appear for years. Leukemia is the most common cancer in children, particularly those between 2 and 5 years of age. The disease causes about 15,900 deaths a year. Males are affected twice as frequently as females. The cause of leukemia is not clear, but it may result from exposure to radiation or chemicals that are toxic to bone marrow. The risk of the disease is increased in persons with other diseases, as Down's syndrome. The risk is also higher in an identical twin of a leukemia patient. Leukemia is classified according to the kinds of abnormal cells, the course of the disease, and the duration of the disease. The two major types of leukemia are **acute lymphocytic leukemia (ALL)** and **acute myelocytic leukemia (AML).** ALL is usually a disease of children, whereas AML occurs in all age groups. ALL features many not fully-formed white blood cells that collect in the bone marrow, blood, lymph nodes, spleen, liver, and other organs. The number of normal blood cells is reduced. With AML, there occurs rapid growth of not fully-formed granular leukocytes, a type of white blood cell. The symptoms may begin quickly or not. Typical symptoms include spongy bleeding gums, iron-poor blood, fatigue, fever, shortness of breath, large spleen, joint and bone pains, and many infections. Greenish tumors (chloromas) may develop in bone or soft tissue. AML may occur at any age, but it usually affects young adults. **Acute promyelocytic leukemia** is a form of this kind of cancer. **Chronic lymphocytic leukemia (CLL)** is rare under the age of 35 and is more common in men than in women. Symptoms begin slowly with fatigue, loss of appetite, weight loss, night sweating, and enlarged spleen. Most patients can continue normal activities for years. **Chronic myelocytic leukemia (CML)** occurs most often in mature adults and begins slowly. Symptoms include fatigue, heat intolerance, bleeding gums, skin sores, weight loss, and upset stomach. **Mixed leukemia** features an excess of many different kinds of white blood cells, in contrast to a single type of white cell, as in lymphocytic or myelocytic leukemia. Diagnoses of acute and chronic

K–L

forms of leukemia are made by blood tests and bone marrow studies. The most effective treatment includes intensive chemotheraphy, using antibiotics to prevent infections, and blood transfusions. Other treatments for prolonging remission include BCG vaccine or bone marrow transplant. A child is usually put in the hospital because of the side effects of the drugs and the high risk of problems. In small children radiation is limited to the skull to prevent stunted growth, but older children may have radiation to the skull and spine.

leukemia cutis, a condition, usually affecting the skin of the face, in which yellowish, red, or purple lesions and large accumulations of white (leukemic) blood cells develop.

leukemoid reaction, an abnormal condition resembling leukemia in which the white blood cell count rises in response to an allergy, inflammatory disease, infection, poison, hemorrhage, burn, or other causes of severe physical stress.

Leukeran, a trademark for an anticancer drug (chlorambucil).

leukocyte /loo′kəsīt/, a white blood cell. There are five types of leukocytes, classified by the presence or absence of small particles (granules) in the cytoplasm, the main substance of the cell. The agranulocytes, or those without granules, are lymphocytes and monocytes. The granulocytes, white cells with granules, are called neutrophils, basophils, and eosinophils. Leukocytes are larger than red blood cells (erythrocytes). A cubic millimeter of normal blood usually contains 5000 to 10,000 leukocytes. Among the most important functions of the leukocytes are the destruction of bacteria, fungi, and viruses, and rendering harmless poisonous substances that may result from allergic reactions and cell injury.

leukocytosis /-sītō′-/, an abnormal increase in the number of circulating white blood cells. This often accompanies bacterial, but not usually viral, infections. Leukemia may be associated with a white blood cell count as high as 500,000 to 1 million per cubic millimeter of blood.

leukoderma /-dur′mə/, loss of skin pigment, especially in patches, caused by a number of disorders. Compare **vitiligo.**

leukonychia /-nik′ē·ə/, a harmless condition in which white patches appear under the nails. Injury or infection can cause white spots or streaks on nails. A common cause is the presence of air bubbles under the nails.

leukopenia /-pē′nē·ə/, an abnormal decrease in the number of white blood cells to fewer than 5000 cells per cubic millimeter. It may be caused by an adverse drug reaction, radiation poisoning, or another abnormal condition and may affect one or all kinds of white blood cells.

leukoplakia /-plā′kē·ə/, a precancerous, slowly developing change in the normal tissue of a mucous membrane. Thickened, white patches that are slightly raised appear. They may occur on the penis or vulva. Those on the lips and inside surface of the cheeks are linked with pipe smoking.

leukorrhea /-rē′ə/. See **vaginal discharge.**

leukotoxin /-tok′sin/, a substance that can inactivate or destroy white blood cells. **–leukotoxic,** adj.

leukotrienes, a group of chemical compounds that occur naturally in white blood cells (leukocytes). They are able to produce allergic and inflammatory reactions, and may take part in the development of asthma and rheumatoid arthritis.

levator /ləvā′tər/, pl. **levatores** /lev′ətôr′ēz/, a muscle that raises a structure of the body. The **levator ani** is one of a pair of muscles of the pelvis that stretches across the bottom of the pelvic cavity like a hammock, supporting the pelvic organs. The **levator palpebrae superioris** is a muscle of the upper eyelid that raises the eyelid. The **levator scapulae** is a muscle of the back and sides of the neck that raises the scapula of the shoulder.

LeVeen shunt, a tube (shunt) that is surgically implanted to drain a fluid buildup in the abdominal cavity caused by cirrhosis of the liver, right-sided heart failure, or cancer of the abdomen.

lever, any bone and associated joint of the body that act together so that force applied to one end of the bone will lift a weight at another point. An example is the action of muscles that move the forearm at the elbow joint.

Levin tube, a plastic catheter that is inserted through the nose and throat and into the stomach. See also **nasogastric intubation.**

levitation, a hallucination that one is floating or rising in the air. The sensation may also occur in dreams. **–levitate,** v.

levodopa, a drug prescribed in the treatment of Parkinson's disease, juvenile forms of Huntington's disease, and chronic manganese poisoning.

Levo-Dromoran, a trademark for a narcotic painkiller (levorphanol tartrate).

Levophed Bitartrate, a trademark for a drug used to raise blood pressure (norepinephrine bitartrate).

Levoprome, a trademark for an analgesic drug (methotrimeprazine).

levorphanol tartrate, a narcotic analgesic drug prescribed for pain relief, particularly before an operation. Alcoholism, asthma, depressed breathing, oxygen lack, or known allergy to this drug prohibits its use. Side effects include drug dependence, falling blood pressure, irregular heart beat, and retention of urine.

Levsinex, a trademark for a peptic ulcer drug (hyoscyamine sulfate).

levulose /lev'yəlōs/. See **fructose.**

Leydig cells /lī'dig/, cells of the testes that secrete testosterone, a male sex hormone.

Leydig cell tumor, a generally noncancerous tumor of a testis. It may cause breast development in men and premature sexual development if the tumor occurs before puberty.

Lhermitte's sign /ler'mits/, sudden, temporary, electric-like shocks spreading down the body when the head is flexed forward. It occurs chiefly in multiple sclerosis but also in compression disorders of the spinal cord in the neck.

liberation, 1. the process of drug release into a body organ or system from the dosage given. 2. the activation of an enzyme or chemical reaction.

libido /libē'dō, libī'dō/, the psychic energy or instinctual drive associated with sexual desire, pleasure, or creativity.

Librax, a trademark for a gastrointestinal drug containing a sedative (chlordiazepoxide hydrochloride).

Libritabs, a trademark for an antianxiety agent (chlordiazepoxide hydrochloride).

Librium, a trademark for an antianxiety agent (chlordiazepoxide hydrochloride).

licensed practical nurse (LPN), a person trained in basic nursing techniques and direct patient care who practices under the supervision of a registered nurse.

lichenification /līken'ifikā'-/, a thickening and hardening of the skin, often resulting from irritation caused by repeated scratching of an itching lesion. –**lichenified,** *adj.*

lichen nitidus /lī'kən/, a skin disorder in which numerous small, flat, pale, glistening pimples form. Also called **Pinkus' disease.**

lichen planus, an itching skin disease of unknown cause. There are small, flat, purplish pimples or patches with fine, gray lines on the surface. Common sites are wrists, forearms, ankles, abdomen, and lower back. On mucous membranes the lesions appear gray and lacy. Nails may have ridges running lengthwise.

lichen sclerosis et atrophicus, a chronic skin disease. White, flat pimples with a red outer ring and black, hard plugs occur on the trunk and lower part of the body. In advanced cases, the pimples tend to merge into large, white patches of thin, itching skin.

lichen simplex chronicus, a skin disease in which a patch of itching pimples forms. Emotional factors and injury, such as scratching of lesions, prolong the symptoms.

Lidaform-HC, a trademark for a skin disease drug containing an adrenal gland hormone (hydrocortisone acetate),
an infection preventive (iodochlorhydroxyquin), and a local anesthetic (lidocaine).

Lidex, a trademark for an adrenal gland hormone (fluocinonide).

lidocaine hydrochloride, a local anesthetic agent prescribed for skin or mucous membranes, and also used internally as an antiarrhythmic agent.

lie detector, an electronic instrument used to detect suspected lying or anxiety in regard to specific questions. A commonly used lie detector is the polygraph recorder that records pulse, breathing rate, blood pressure, and perspiration.

lienal vein /lē·ē'nəl/, a large vein of the lower body that is important in circulating blood from the spleen.

life island, a plastic bubble enclosing a bed, used to provide a germ-free environment for a patient.

life space, a term used by American psychologists to describe all of the influences existing at the same time that may affect individual behavior. The total of the influences make up the life space.

life-style-induced health problems, diseases with histories that include known exposure to certain health-threatening or risk factors. An example is heart disease associated with cigarette smoking, poor eating habits, lack of exercise, and psychologic stress.

ligament /lig'əmənt/, 1. a white, shiny, flexible band of fibrous tissue binding joints together and connecting various bones and cartilages. When part of a joint membrane, they are covered with fibrous tissue that blends with surrounding connective tissue. Yellow elastic ligaments connect certain parts of adjoining vertebrae. They help to hold the body erect. Compare **tendon.** 2. a layer of membrane with little or no stretching ability, extending from one abdominal organ to another. See also **broad ligament.**

ligamental tear, a tear of the fibers of a ligament connecting and surrounding the bones of a joint. An injury to the joint, such as from a sudden twisting motion, causes torn ligaments. This may occur at any joint but is most common in the knees, and is often linked with sports injuries.

ligation /līgā'shən/, tying off a blood vessel or duct with a suture or wire to stop or prevent bleeding during surgery, to stop bleeding from an injury, or to prevent passage of material through a duct, as in ligation of the fallopian tubes to sterilize a woman. See also **vein ligation and stripping.**

ligature /lig'əchər/, 1. a suture. 2. a wire, such as used in orthodontia to straighten teeth.

light, radiant energy of the wavelength and frequency that stimulate visual receptor cells in the retina of the eye to produce nerve impulses that are perceived in the brain as vision.

K–L

light bath, the exposure of uncovered skin to the sun or to ultraviolet light rays from an artificial source for healing purposes.

light diet, a diet for convalescent or bedridden patients taking little or no exercise. It consists of simple, moderate amounts of soft-cooked and easily digested foods, including meats, potatoes, rice, eggs, pasta, some fruits, refined cereals, and breads. It avoids all highly seasoned and fried foods.

lightening, a sensation felt by many women late in pregnancy as the fetus settles lower in the pelvis, leaving more space in the upper abdomen. The diaphragm, no longer restricted by pressure of the uterus beneath it, can move down more fully, allowing deeper breaths to be taken. The stomach, also less compressed, can hold more food at each meal. The profile of the abdomen changes, because the round, full uterus is visibly lower. The fetus is then said to have ''dropped.''

light reflex, the mechanism by which the pupil of the eye reacts to changes in light and darkness. The **consensual reaction to light** is the narrowing of the pupil of one eye when the other eye is exposed to light.

lignin /lig′nin/, a type of cellulose that forms the cell walls of plants. It provides bulk in the diet necessary for proper functioning of the stomach and intestines. See also **dietary fiber.**

limb, a body part, such as an arm or leg, or a branch of an internal organ.

limbic system, a group of related nervous system structures within the midbrain that are linked with various emotions and feelings, as anger, fear, sexual arousal, pleasure, and sadness. The function of the system is poorly understood.

limited quantity, an amount of radioactive material that is exempted from specification packaging, marking, and labeling because of low radiological hazard. Includes small quantities and certain manufactured articles.

limp, an abnormal pattern of walking, often favoring one leg.

Lincocin, a trademark for an antibiotic drug (lincomycin).

lincomycin hydrochloride, an antibiotic drug prescribed in the treatment of certain infections. Known allergy to this drug or to similar drugs prohibits its use. Side effects include blood disorders, diarrhea, and digestive tract infections.

lindane, a drug prescribed in the treatment of pediculosis and scabies, skin diseases caused by lice and mites. It is not usually given to infants or pregnant women and is not applied to the face. Known allergy to this drug prohibits its use. Side effects include nerve damage, anemia, and irritation of eyes, skin, and mucous tissues.

line, a stripe, streak, or narrow ridge, often imaginary, that connects areas of the body or that separates various parts of the body, as the hair line or nipple line. Also called **linea.**

linea alba /lin′ē·ə/, a seam that runs along the middle line of the abdomen beneath the skin, formed by a tendon extending from the breastbone to the pubic area. It contains the navel.

linea nigra, a dark line appearing on the abdomen of a pregnant woman during the latter part of the pregnancy. It usually extends from the pubic area to the navel.

linear fracture, a fracture that runs along the length of a bone.

lingual artery /ling′gwal/, one of a pair of arteries that branch along the sides of the neck and head to supply the tongue and surrounding muscles.

lingual crib, an orthodontic device consisting of a wire frame suspended on the inner surface of the upper front teeth. It discourages undesirable thumb and tongue habits that can produce malocclusions in children.

lingual frenum, a band of tissue that extends from the floor of the mouth to the underside of the tongue and causes tongue-tie, a speech impediment.

liniment /lin′imənt/, a remedy, usually containing an alcoholic, oily, or soapy substance, that is rubbed on the skin, producing an inflammatory reaction to reduce one elsewhere.

linoleic acid /lin′ōlē′ik/. See **fatty acid.**

linolenic acid /-len′ik/. See **fatty acid.**

Lioresal, a trademark for an antispastic and muscle-relaxant agent (baclofen).

liothyronine sodium, a synthetic thyroid hormone prescribed in the treatment of thyroid deficiency, simple goiter, or cretinism. Excessive thyroid hormone, heart disorders, or known allergy to this drug prohibits its use. It is used with caution in patients with diabetes mellitus. Side effects, usually caused by overdosage, include thyroid toxicity, nausea, high blood pressure, nervousness, and loss of weight.

liotrix, a mixture of the thyroid hormones T_3 and T_4 used to treat hypothyroid conditions. Abnormal conditions of the heart or known allergy to this drug prohibits its use. Side effects include rapid heart beat, nervousness, insomnia, and fever.

lip, any rimlike structure bordering a cavity or groove, such as that surrounding the opening of the mouth.

lipase /lī′pās/, any of several digestive system enzymes that increase the breakdown of fats (lipids).

lipectomy /lipek′-/, surgical removal of fat beneath the skin, as from the abdominal wall.

lipid, any of the various fats or fatlike substances in plant or animal tissues. Lipids are insoluble in water but soluble in alcohol and other organic solvents. They are stored in the body and serve as an energy reserve, but may be elevated in certain diseases, such as atherosclerosis. A **derived lipid** comes from the breakdown of other fats, including fatty acids. Kinds of lipids include **cholesterol, fatty acids, phospholipids, triglycerides.**

lipidosis /lip′idō′-/, any disorder that involves the buildup of abnormal levels of certain fats (lipids) in the body. Kinds of lipidoses are **Gaucher's disease, Krabbe's disease, Niemann-Pick disease, Tay-Sachs disease.**

lipodystrophy /lip′ōdis′trəfē/, any abnormality in the use of fats in the body, particularly one in which the fat deposits under the skin are affected.

lip of hip fracture, a fracture of the lip of the hip socket, often associated with hip displacement.

lipoid /lip′oid/, any substance that resembles a fat.

lipoma /lipō′mə/, a tumor consisting of fat cells. A **lipoma arborescens** is a fatty tumor of a joint, with a treelike distribution of fat cells. A **lipoma capsulare** is in the capsule of an organ, such as the capsule or sheath covering the kidney. A **lipoma fibrosum** contains masses of fibrous tissue.

lipomatosis /-mətō′-/, abnormal tumorlike accumulations of fat in body tissues. **Multiple lipomatosis** is an inherited disorder. The deposits of fat are not available for use by the body, even in starvation. With **lipomatosis dolorosa,** there are painful or tender fat deposits.

lipomatous myxoma /lipō′mətəs/, a tumor containing fatty tissue that begins in connective tissue.

lipoprotein /lip′ōprō′tēn/, a protein in which fats (lipids) form a part of the molecule. Practically all of the lipids in human blood are present as lipoproteins. Lipoproteins are classified by their size or density. See also **cholesterol, triglyceride.**

liposarcoma /-särkō′mə/, a cancerous growth of fat cells.

Liquaemin Sodium, a trademark for a blood anticoagulant (heparin sodium).

liquid, a state of matter between solid and gas, in which the substance flows freely and assumes the shape of the vessel in which it is contained.

liquid diet, a diet consisting of foods that can be served in liquid or strained form plus custard, ice cream, pudding, tapioca, and soft-cooked eggs. It is prescribed in acute infections, in acute inflammatory conditions of the gastrointestinal tract, and for patients unable to consume soft or semifluid foods, usually following surgery. A **full-liquid diet** is made up only of liquids and foods that turn to liquid at body temperature. It includes milk, milk drinks, carbonated beverages, coffee, tea, strained fruit juices, broth, strained cream soup, raw eggs, cream, infant cereals in milk, thin custards, gelatin desserts, and ice cream. The diet is given following surgery, in some infections, in some stomach disorders, and for patients too ill to chew.

Lisfranc's fracture /lisfrangks′/, a fracture dislocation of the foot in which one or all of the toe bones are displaced.

listeriosis, a disease caused by a germ that infects shellfish, birds, spiders, and mammals in all areas of the world. It is transmitted to humans by direct contact with infected animals, by breathing of dust, or by contact with contaminated sewage or soil. All secretions from an infected person may contain the organism. The signs of infection are circulatory collapse, shock, heart inflammation, enlarged liver and spleen, and a dark, red rash over the trunk and the legs.

Lithane, a trademark for an antimanic drug (lithium carbonate) for use in manic-depressive psychosis.

lithiasis /lithī′əsis/, the formation of stones (calculi) from mineral salts in the hollow organs or ducts of the body. This occurs most commonly in the gallbladder, kidney, and lower urinary tract. The condition can irritate or obstruct the organ, and is extremely painful. Surgery may be necessary if the stones cannot be excreted. Lower urinary tract stones often can be dissolved.

lithium carbonate, an antimanic agent prescribed in the treatment of manic episodes of manic-depressive disorder. It is used with caution in the presence of kidney or heart disease and is not recommended for children under 12 years of age. Known allergy to this drug prohibits its use. Side effects include kidney damage, excessive thirst and urination, and impairment of mental and physical abilities. Retention of sodium and fluid in the body tissues may occur.

Lithonate, a trademark for an antimanic agent (lithium carbonate) used in manic-depressive psychosis.

lithotomy /lithot′-/, the surgical removal of a stone (calculus), especially one from the urinary tract.

lithotomy position. See **body position.**

live birth, the birth of an infant that exhibits any sign of life, such as breathing, heart beat, umbilical cord pulsation, or movement of voluntary muscles. Length of pregnancy of the mother is not considered. A live birth is not always one in which the infant is capable of continuing life (viable).

livedo /livē′dō/, a blue or reddish blotching of the skin. It worsens in cold weather and probably is caused by a spasm of small arteries (arterioles).

liver, the largest gland of the body and one of its most complex organs. Located in the upper right portion of the abdominal cavity, the liver attaches to the diaphragm by two ligaments. It is completely covered by a membrane

K–L

(peritoneum) except where it attaches to a ligament. The liver is divided into four lobes, with the right lobe much larger than the others. The hepatic artery conveys oxygenated blood from the heart to the liver. The hepatic portal vein conveys nutrient-filled blood from the stomach and the intestines. At any given moment the liver holds about 1 pint of blood or about 13% of the total blood supply of the body. Dark reddish-brown in color, it has a soft, solid consistency shaped like an irregular hemisphere. Some of its major functions are producing bile by liver cells; processing glucose, proteins, vitamins, fats, and most of the other compounds used by the body; producing hemoglobin for vital use of its iron content in red blood cells; and converting poisonous ammonia to urea. It also renders harmless numerous substances, such as alcohol, nicotine, and other poisons, as well as various harmful substances produced by the intestine. Bile from the liver is stored in the gallbladder and in blood vessels. See also **gallbladder.**

liver biopsy, a method in which a special needle is introduced into the liver using local anesthesia to obtain a sample for laboratory examination.

liver cancer, a malignant tumor of the liver. It occurs most often by the spread of cells from another cancer in the body. Symptoms include abdominal bloating, loss of appetite, weakness, a dull upper abdominal pain, fluid buildup, mild jaundice, and a tender enlarged liver. Primary liver cancer (one that originates in the liver) is relatively uncommon in the United States. Primary tumors occur more often in men than in women, develop most often in the sixth decade of life, and are linked with cirrhosis of the liver in 70% of the cases. Other risk factors include an excess of iron in the liver, infection from the fluke parasite, exposure to chemicals such as vinyl chloride or arsenic, and nutritional deficiencies. Although alcoholism may be a factor, nonalcoholic cirrhosis is a greater risk than alcoholic cirrhosis. Aflatoxins, cancer-causing substances produced by fungus in moldy grain and peanuts, appear to be linked to high rates of liver cancer in tropical areas. Primary liver cancers migrate to lymph nodes, the lungs, brain, and other sites. Treatment includes surgical removal of a liver lobe and anticancer drugs. Because the liver is able to regenerate itself, 80% of it may be removed.

liver disease, any of a group of liver disorders. The most important diseases in this group are cirrhosis, bile problems (cholestasis), and hepatitis. Characteristics of liver disease are jaundice, loss of appetite, enlarged liver, fluid buildup, and impaired consciousness. See also **cholestasis, cirrhosis, hepatitis.**

liver function test, a test used to evaluate various functions of the liver, such as metabolism, storage, filtration, and excretion.

liver scan, a method of making an image of the liver by injecting into a vein a radioactive compound that is taken up in the cells of the liver. The radiation emitted by the compound is recorded by a radiation detector and can be photographed with a special camera or filmed with x-rays. Liver scans can locate abscesses or tumors.

liver spot, *nontechnical.* a brown or black slightly raised lesion seen on older persons.

living-in unit, a room provided in some hospitals for mothers who want to assume immediate care of their newborn infants under the supervision of nursing personnel.

living will, a written agreement between a patient and physician to withhold heroic measures if the patient's condition is found to be terminal.

lizard bite, a bite of the large Gila monster of Arizona, New Mexico, and Utah, and the beaded lizard of Mexico. They are the only lizards known to be venomous. The symptoms of their bites and the recommended treatment are similar to those of the bites from moderately poisonous snakes.

lobar pneumonia. See **pneumonia.**

lobe, a partly detached portion of any organ, outlined by clefts, furrows, or connective tissue, as the lobes of the brain, liver, and lungs. –**lobar, lobular,** *adj.*

lobectomy /lōbek'-/, chest surgery in which a lobe of a lung is removed. A lobectomy may be done to remove a cancer and to treat uncontrolled inflammation, an injury with severe bleeding, or tuberculosis. Before surgery, any respiratory infection is cleared and smoking is forbidden. The chest cavity is entered through a long back-to-front cut to remove the diseased lobe. The remaining lung tissue overexpands to fill the new space.

lobotomy /lōbot'-/, brain surgery in which nerve fibers in the frontal lobe of the brain are cut. Severe, difficult-to-treat depression and pain are among the reasons for the operation. It is rarely done now because it has many unpredictable and undesirable effects, including loss of bladder and bowel control, personality change, and socially unacceptable behavior.

lobular carcinoma /lob'yələr/, a tumor that often forms a widely spread mass and accounts for a small number of breast tumors.

local, **1.** pertaining to a small, defined area of the body. **2.** pertaining to a treatment or drug applied locally to a small area, as a local anesthetic.

local anesthesia, the direct giving of a local anesthetic agent to cause the loss of feeling in a small area of the body. Brief surgical or dental procedures are the most common reasons for using local anesthesia. The anesthetic may be applied to the surface of the skin or membrane or injected through or under the skin. Drawbacks to use include allergic reactions to some anesthetics and occasional difficulty in deadening the local nerves. The advantage is that a conscious patient can cooperate and does not require breathing support. To avoid general anesthesia, some major surgical procedures are occasionally performed using local anesthesia. **Caudal anesthesia** uses a local drug to numb the senses in the lower part of the spinal canal. It is used during labor and childbirth, and for surgery on the rectum, genitals, or urinary tract. **Saddle block anesthesia** is a form that affects the parts of the body that would touch a saddle if the patient were riding a horse. Saddle block anesthesia is common in some places for anesthesia during childbirth. Compare **general anesthesia, regional anesthesia, topical anesthesia.**

local anesthetic, a substance used to reduce or eliminate nerve sensation, specifically pain, in a limited area of the body. Local anesthetics act by blocking transmission of nerve impulses. More than 100 drugs are available for local anesthesia. Any substance potent enough to induce local anesthesia can also cause adverse side effects, ranging from easily reversible skin disorders to fatal sensitivity reactions or both lung and heart arrest.

lochia /lō′kē·ə/, the discharge that flows from the vagina following childbirth. During the first few days, the lochia is red and consists of blood, discarded cells from the uterus and placental tissue, and fetal body matter, such as hair or fat from the skin covering. After the third day, the amount of blood lessens, the lochia becomes darker and thinner, and then watery. During the second week, white blood cells and bacteria appear in large numbers along with fatty material, causing the lochia to appear yellow. The flow of lochia stops at about 6 weeks.

locking point, a point on the body at which light pressure can be applied to help a weak or debilitated person maintain a certain posture or position. A basic locking point is the body's center of gravity, at the level of the sacral vertebra in the lower back area, where mild pressure can assist a person in standing or walking erect.

lockjaw. See **tetanus.**

locus, a specific place or position, as the locus of a particular gene on a chromosome, or the locus of infection, a site in the body where an infection originates.

Lodrane, a trademark for a smooth muscle relaxant (theophylline).

Loestrin, a trademark for an oral contraceptive containing an estrogen (ethinyl estradiol) and a progestin (norethindrone acetate).

Lofenalac, a trademark for a commercial milk-substitute formula that is low in an amino acid (phenylalamine) and used for infants with phenylketonuria. It is made from a milk protein (casein) and supplemented with an amino acid (tyrosine) and fortified with added fat, carbohydrate, minerals, and vitamins to balance the formula. See also **phenylketonuria.**

log-roll, a way to turn a bedridden person from one side to the other or completely over without flexing the spinal column. The arms of the patient are folded across the chest, and the legs are extended. A draw sheet under the person is used to make it easier.

loin, a part of the body on each side of the spinal column between the lowest ribs and the hip bones.

Lomotil, a trademark for an antidiarrheal drug.

lomustine, an anticancer agent prescribed in the treatment of a variety of malignant tumor diseases. Known allergy to this drug prohibits its use. Side effects include bone marrow disorders, nausea, and vomiting.

Lonalac, a trademark for a low sodium, nutritional supplement.

long-acting drug, a remedy with a prolonged effect. It may result from the slow release of the drug or depend on a gradual absorption of small amounts of the drug over an extended period of time.

long-acting thyroid stimulator (LATS), a natural substance, probably an antibody, that causes prolonged stimulation of the thyroid gland. Rapid growth of the gland and excess activity of thyroid function results in hyperthyroidism. It is found in the blood of 50% of patients affected with Graves' disease.

longitudinal, referring to a measurement in the direction of the long axis of an organ, object, or body, such as an imaginary line from head to toe.

long-term care, the provision of medical care services on a repeated or continuing basis to persons with chronic physical or mental disorders. The care may be given in various settings.

long tract signs, signs of nervous system disorders, such as repeated involuntary muscle contractions or loss of bladder control. They usually indicate a lesion in the middle or upper part of the spinal cord or in the brain, disrupting nerve impulses normally transmitted over long nerve tracts.

Loniten, a trademark for a high blood pressure drug (minoxidil).

loop. See **intrauterine device.**

loop colostomy. See **colostomy.**

loosening, a psychologic disturbance in which the association of ideas become vague and unfocused. The condition is frequently a symptom of schizophrenia.

Lo/Ovral, a trademark for an oral contraceptive containing an estrogen (ethinyl estradiol) and a progestin (norgestrel).

loperamide hydrochloride, a drug prescribed in the treatment of diarrhea. Known allergy to this drug prohibits its use. It is not given to patients in whom constipation must be avoided. Side effects include abdominal pain, constipation, nausea, and vomiting.

Lopid, a trademark for a fat-metabolism-regulating agent (gemfibrozil).

Lopressor, a trademark for a drug used to treat high blood pressure (metoprolol tartrate).

Loprox, a trademark for a drug used to treat fungus infections (ciclopirox olamine).

lordosis. See **spinal curvature.**

Lorelco, a trademark for a cholesterol-reducing drug (probucol).

lotion, a liquid preparation applied to protect the skin or to treat a skin disorder.

Lotrimin, a trademark for a drug used to treat fungus infections (clotrimazole).

Lotusate, a trademark for a barbiturate sedative (talbutal).

Lou Gehrig's disease. See **amyotrophic lateral sclerosis.**

Louis-Bar syndrome. See **ataxia-telangiectasia.**

loupe /lo͞op/, a magnifying lens mounted in a frame worn on the head by an examining physician, and used to examine the eyes.

louse bite, a tiny puncture wound produced by a louse, a small, wingless insect. Diseases such as typhus and relapsing fever may be transmitted by lice. Head and body lice are common parasites and often found among school children. The bite may cause intense itching, resulting in infection from scratching. Bathing, applying an approved insecticide, and cleaning clothes and bed linens are recommended ways to treat and prevent the spread of lice.

low back pain, pain at the base of the spine that may be caused by a muscle sprain or strain, arthritis, a tumor, or a ruptured cartilage disk between vertebrae. Other causes are poor posture, obesity, enlarged prostate gland, sagging abdominal muscles, sitting for prolonged periods of time, or excessive physical effort involving the back muscles. The pain may be accompanied by muscle weakness or spasms. It may radiate down the back of one or both legs, as in sciatica. It may be started or increased by coughing, sneezing, rising from a seated position, lifting, stretching, bending, or turning. To guard against the pain, the patient may decrease the range of motion of the spine. The low back pain patient should sleep on a firm mattress with the knees flexed and supported. Painkillers, muscle relaxants, and tranquilizers may help, as may applying dry or moist heat. A corset or back brace may be required.

low birth weight (LBW) infant, an infant whose weight at birth is less than 2500 grams (5.5 pounds). These babies are at risk for developing oxygen starvation during labor, low blood sugar after birth, and growth retardation in childhood, especially if the low birth weight is the result of a prolonged deficiency before birth, maternal malnutrition, or the mother's drug or alcohol addiction. Many low birth weight infants have no problems and develop normally.

low calcium diet, a diet that restricts the use of calcium and eliminates most of the dairy foods, all breads made with milk, fresh or dry, and deep-green leafy vegetables. It is prescribed for patients who form kidney stones. Meats, including beef, lamb, pork, veal, and poultry, fish, vegetables, legumes, and fruits are recommended.

low caloric diet, a diet that limits the intake of calories, usually to cause a reduction in body weight. Such diets may be designated as 800 calorie, 1000 calorie, or other specific numbers of calories. Exchange lists may be used to allow patients to select foods they like from groups of foods that are sources of carbohydrates, proteins, and fats.

low cholesterol diet, a diet that restricts foods containing animal fats, such as egg yolk, cream, butter, milk, muscle and organ meats, and shellfish and recommends poultry, fish, vegetables, fruits, cottage cheese, and fats from plant sources (polyunsaturated). The diet is for patients with high serum cholesterol levels, heart disorders, obesity, and excessive blood fats. Also called **low saturated fat diet.**

low-density lipoprotein (LDL). See **lipoprotein.**

low fat diet, a diet with limited amounts of fat and consisting chiefly of easily digestible foods with a high carbohydrate content. Included are all vegetables, lean meats, fish, fowl, pasta, cereals, and whole wheat or enriched bread. Egg yolk and fatty meats are restricted. The diet may be recommended for gallbladder disease and malabsorption disorders.

low fat milk, milk containing 1% to 2% fat, intermediate in fat content between whole and skimmed milk.

Lown-Ganong-Levine syndrome (LGL) /lōn'-genôN'-ləvēn'/, a disorder of the muscle contraction signal of the heart (atrioventricular conduction system). Treatment includes drugs and a pacemaker. See also **heart block.**

low-residue diet, a diet that leaves a minimal residue of feces in the bowels after digestion and absorption. It consists of tender meats, poultry, fish, eggs, white bread, pasta, simple desserts, clear soups, tea, and coffee. Omitted are highly seasoned or fried foods, all fruits and fruit juices, raw vegetables, whole grain cereals and bread, nuts, jams, and, usually, milk. The diet is prescribed in cases of pouchlike formations in the intestinal wall (diverticulosis) and inflammation of the pouches (diverticulitis) and before and after bowel surgery. Because it is lacking in calcium, iron, and vitamins, the diet should be used only for a limited period of time.

low salt diet. See **low sodium diet.**

low saturated fat diet. See **low cholesterol diet.**

low sodium diet, a diet that restricts the use of table salt (sodium chloride) and other compounds or food additives containing sodium, as baking powder, monosodium glutamate, and sodium sulfate. It is prescribed for high blood pressure, for fluid buildup in tissues (edema), especially when linked with heart, kidney, or liver disease, and during treatment with steroid hormones. The degree of restriction depends on the severity of the condition. Included in the diet are eggs, skimmed milk, beef, poultry, lamb, pork, veal, fish, potatoes, green beans, broccoli, asparagus, peas, salad ingredients, and fresh fruits. Foods avoided include all salty fish and meats, cheese, salted butter or margarine, any breads or cereals made with salt, beets, carrots, celery, sauerkraut, spinach, and most canned or frozen foods — unless prepared without sodium. Also to be avoided are many drugs, as laxatives and alkalizers, that contain sodium, and drinking water from a source using a water softener that adds sodium to replace calcium in the water. Also called **low salt diet, salt-free diet, sodium-restricted diet.**

low-specific activity (LSA) material, material containing uniformly distributed radioactive material in low concentrations. This type of material does not constitute a radiological safety hazard.

loxapine, a tranquilizer used to treat a severe mental disorder (schizophrenia). Parkinson's disease, taking sedatives or tranquilizers at the same time, liver or kidney disorders, low blood pressure, or known allergy to this drug forbids its use. Side effects include low blood pressure, liver problems, and a variety of nervous system and allergic reactions.

Loxitane, a trademark for a tranquilizer (loxapine succinate).

lozenge /loz′ənj/. See **troche.**

lucid /lōō′sid/, clear, rational, and able to be understood. A **lucid interval** refers to a period of relative mental clarity between periods of irrationality, especially in organic brain disorders, as delirium or dementia.

Ludiomil, a trademark for an antidepressant drug (maprotiline hydrochloride).

Ludwig's angina /lōōd′viks/, an acute streptococcal infection of the floor of the mouth and parts of the neck. It causes the tongue to become swollen, thereby blocking the airway to the lungs. It is treated with penicillin.

Lufyllin, a trademark for a smooth muscle relaxant (dyphylline).

lumbago /lumbā′gō/, pain in the lower back (lumbar region) caused by muscle strain, rheumatoid arthritis, osteoarthritis, or a ruptured spinal disk. **Ischemic lumbago** features pain in the lower back and buttocks, caused by poor blood circulation to the area.

lumbar /lum′bär/, pertaining to the part of the body between the chest and the pelvis, particularly the lower back area.

lumbar nerves, the five pairs of spinal nerves in the lumbar region. The **lumbar plexus** is a network of nerves formed by divisions of the lumbar nerves. It is located on the inside of the back abdominal wall.

lumbar puncture (LP), putting a hollow needle into the lumbar portion of the spine. Lumbar puncture is often done to get samples of fluid for diagnostic purposes, and also done for treatment reasons. Fluid is drawn from a space outside the spinal cord, between the third and fourth lumbar vertebrae. Diagnostic purposes include obtaining cerebrospinal fluid for laboratory analysis; evaluating the canal for the presence of a tumor; and injecting a dye for x-rays of the nervous system structures, as the spinal canal and brain. Treatment reasons for lumbar puncture include removing blood or pus from the canal space; injecting drugs; withdrawing cerebrospinal fluid to reduce pressure in the skull; and spinal anesthesia. Lumbar puncture is not done if a brain tumor is suspected, or if there are signs of infection at the site of puncture. Infection, leakage of cerebrospinal fluid, headache, nausea, vomiting, or urination difficulty occur in approximately 25% of patients.

lumbar subarachnoid peritoneostomy, an operation to drain cerebrospinal fluid (CSF) in hydrocephalus, usually in the newborn. It may be done when a temporary shunt is needed. See also **hydrocephalus.**

lumbar subarachnoid ureterostomy, an operation to drain excess cerebrospinal fluid (CSF) though the ureter to the bladder in hydrocephalus, usually in the newborn. See also **hydrocephalus.**

lumbar veins, four pairs of veins that collect blood by dorsal tributaries from the loins and by abdominal tributaries from the walls of the abdomen.

lumbar vertebra. See **vertebra.**

lumbosacral plexus /lum′bōsā′krəl/, a network of lumbar, sacral, and coccygeal nerves that supply the legs and pelvic area.

lumen /lōō′mən/, a cavity or the channel within any organ or structure of the body.

Luminal, a trademark for an anticonvulsant and sedative-hypnotic drug (phenobarbital).

lumpectomy /lumpek′-/, surgical removal of a breast tumor without removing large amounts of surrounding tissue or adjacent lymph nodes. See also **breast cancer, mastectomy.**

lunate bone /lōō′nāt/, one of the bones of the wrist.

lung, one of a pair of light, spongy organs in the chest. The lungs provide the mechanisms for inhaling air from which oxygen is extracted and for exhaling carbon dioxide, a waste product of the body. The pulmonary arteries bring

K–L

blood to the lungs where the oxygen is replaced. The bronchial arteries supply blood to nourish the lung tissues. Most of this blood returns to the heart through the pulmonary veins. The surfaces of the lungs cradle the heart. The peak of the lung extends into the root of the neck above the first rib. The base rests on the surface of the diaphragm, and moves with the diaphragm, down during inhaling and up during exhaling. The lungs are composed of lobes that are smooth and shiny on their surface. The right lung contains three lobes; the left lung, two lobes. Each lung is covered with a thin, moist (pleural) membrane. An inner fibrous layer contains secondary small lobes (lobules) divided into primary lobules, each of which consists of blood vessels, lymph vessels, nerves, and a duct (alveolar) connecting with air spaces. The color of the lungs at birth is pinkish-white, and darkens in later life from carbon granules that are inhaled from the atmosphere.

lung cancer, a malignant disorder that develops most often in scarred or diseased lungs, and is usually far advanced when detected. Symptoms include persistent cough, breathing difficulty, pus or blood-streaked sputum, chest pain, and repeated attacks of bronchitis or pneumonia. The cause is linked to cigarette smoking in 75% of cases. Other causes are exposure to asbestos, arsenic, coal products, radiation, iron oxide, petroleum, and various other chemicals. Lung cancers spread widely to other organs. Oat-cell carcinomas, which resemble tiny oat seeds, usually invade bone marrow. Large-cell lung cancers spread to lymph nodes in the chest and the gastrointestinal system. Surgery is the most effective treatment, but only one half of the cases can be treated by surgery by the time the disease is detected. Surgery is not done if cancer cells are found in nearby lymph nodes. Radiation is used to treat cancers untreatable by surgery. Chemotherapy is especially prescribed for oat-cell carcinoma.

lung scan, an x-ray examination of a lung and its function.

lunula /loon′yələ/, *pl.* **lunulae,** the crescent-shaped pale area at the base of a fingernail or toenail.

lupus erythematosus /loo′pəs er′ithē′mətō′səs/, a long-term inflammatory disorder that occurs in two forms. The cause is uncertain.

lupus erythematosus preparation (LE prep), a laboratory test for lupus erythematosus in which white blood cells are mixed with a specimen of the patient's blood serum. Large granules appear within the white cells if the patient has lupus erythematosus.

lupus vulgaris, a form of skin tuberculosis in which areas of the skin become ulcerated and heal slowly, leaving deeply scarred tissue. The disease is not related to lupus erythematosus.

Luride, a trademark for a chemical (sodium fluoride) that reduces tooth decay and cavities.

luteal /loo′tē·əl/, pertaining to the corpus luteum of the female ovary or its functions or effects.

luteinizing hormone (LH) /loo′tē·ini′zing/, a hormone produced by the pituitary gland. In men, it stimulates the secretion of the male sex hormone (testosterone) by the testes. Testosterone, together with follicle stimulating hormone (FSH), stimulates the testes to produce sperm. In females, luteinizing hormone, working together with FSH, stimulates the tiny cavities (follicles) containing ova, or egg cells, in the ovary to secrete estrogen, the female sex hormone.

lying-in, **1.** designating the time before, during, and after childbirth. **2.** designating a hospital that provides care for women in childbirth.

Lyme arthritis, an acute inflammatory disease, involving one or more joints, believed to be transmitted by a tick-borne disease organism. The condition was first found in Lyme, Connecticut, but has also been reported in other parts of the United States. Symptoms include chills, fever, headache, discomfort, a skin eruption, and inflammation with swelling of joints. Knees, other large joints, and jaw (temperomandibular) joints are most commonly involved.

lymph, a thin, clear, slightly yellow fluid originating in many organs and tissues of the body. It circulates through the lymphatic vessels and is filtered by the lymph nodes. Its composition varies depending on the organ or tissue it is in, but generally contains about 95% water, a few red blood cells, and variable numbers of white blood cells. It is similar to blood plasma except for a lower amount of protein material. See also **chyle.**

lymphadenitis /limfad′əni′-/, an inflammatory condition of the lymph nodes, usually the result of circulating cancer cells, a bacterial infection, or other inflammatory condition. The nodes may be swollen, hard, smooth or irregular, or red, and may feel hot. The location of the affected node is usually related to the site or origin of disease.

lymphangiography /limfan′je·og′rəfē/, the x-ray examination of lymph glands and lymphatic vessels after an injection of a dye. Also called **lymphography.**

lymphangioma /-je·ō′mə/, a yellowish-tan tumor on the skin, composed of a mass of dilated lymph vessels. It is often removed by surgery or a form of surgery using an electric current (electrocoagulation) for cosmetic reasons.

lymphangitis /lim′fanji′-/, an inflammation of one or more lymphatic vessels, often resulting from an acute streptococcal infection caused by an insect or animal bite in an arm or leg. Fine red streaks may extend from the infected area to the armpit or groin. Other signs are fever, chills, headache, and muscle ache. The infection may spread to the bloodstream. Antibiotics and hot soaks are usually prescribed as treatment.

lymphatic /limfat′ik/,   pertaining to the lymphatic system of the body.

lymphatic system,   a vast, complex network of capillaries, thin vessels, valves, ducts, nodes, and organs. It helps to protect and maintain the fluid environment of the body by producing, filtering, and conveying lymph and by producing various blood cells. The lymphatic network transports fats, proteins, and other substances to the blood system. It also restores 60% of the fluid that leaks out of cells into spaces between cells. Small valves help to control the flow of lymph and prevent blood from flowing into the lymphatic vessels. Usually, two valves of equal size are found opposite each other. Most are found near the lymph nodes and there are more in the neck and arms than in the legs. The lymph collected throughout the body drains into the blood through two ducts situated in the neck. Various body movements combine to squeeze the lymph through the lymphatic system. The thoracic duct on the left side of the neck is the major vessel of the lymphatic system and conveys lymph from the whole body, except for the upper right side, which is served by the right lymphatic duct. Lymphatic vessels resemble veins but have more valves, thinner walls, and contain lymph nodes. The lymphatic capillaries, which are the beginning of the system, form a continuous network over the entire body, except for the cornea of the eye. The system also includes specialized lymphatic organs, such as the tonsils, thymus, and spleen. The lymphatics of the intestine contain a special milky substance called chyle. See also **chyle, lymph, lymph node, spleen, thymus.**

lymphedema /lim′fədē′mə/,   a disorder in which lymph accumulates in soft tissue with swelling caused by inflammation, obstruction, or removal of lymph vessels. Congenital lymphedema (Milroy's disease) is a hereditary disorder with blockage of the lymph vessels. Lymphedema praecox occurs in adolescence, chiefly in women, and causes swelling of the lower limbs. Secondary lymphedema may follow surgical removal of lymph channels with the breast in mastectomy. Tumors or worm parasites may block lymph drainage. Lymphedema of the lower limbs begins with mild swelling of the foot and gradually extends to the entire leg. Long standing, pregnancy, obesity, warm weather, and the menstrual period aggravate the condition. Lymph drainage from the leg can be improved by sleeping with the foot of the bed slightly elevated, elastic stockings, and moderate, regular exercise. Light massage in the direction of the lymph flow and diuretics may be prescribed. Surgery may also be done.

lymph node,   one of many small oval structures that filter the lymph, fight infection, and in which there are formed white blood cells and blood plasma cells. Lymph nodes are of different sizes, some as small as pinheads, others as large as beans. Each node is enclosed in a fibrous capsule, and consists of closely packed white cells (lymphocytes), connective tissue, and lymph pathways. Most lymph nodes are clustered in specific areas, as the mouth, neck, lower arm, armpit, and groin. For example, a **visceral lymph node** filters lymph circulating in the lymphatic vessels of the viscera of the chest, lower body, and the pelvis. The lymphatic network and nodes of the breast are especially crucial in the diagnosis and treatment of breast cancer in women. Also called **lymph gland.**

lymphocyte /lim′fəsīt/,   one of two kinds of small white blood cells (leukocytes). Lymphocytes normally include 25% of the total white blood cell count but increase in number in response to infection. They occur in two forms: **B cells** and **T cells.** Each has its own function. The function of the B cell is to search out, identify, and bind with specific intruders (allergens or antigens). B cells create antibodies for insertion into their own cell membranes. When exposed to a specific allergen or antigen, the B cell is activated. It travels to the spleen or to the lymph nodes, and rapidly produces special cells that create and secrete large amounts of antibody. T cells are lymphocytes that have circulated through the thymus gland and have become thymocytes. When exposed to an antigen, they divide rapidly and produce large numbers of new T cells sensitized to that antigen. T cells are often called ''killer cells'' because they secrete special chemical compounds and assist B cells in destroying foreign protein. T cells also appear to play a significant role in the body's resistance to the growth and spread of cancer cells.

lymphocytic choriomeningitis /-sit′ik/,   a virus infection of the brain and spinal cord membranes and fluid. Symptoms include fever, headache, and stiff neck. The infection occurs mainly in young adults, most often in the fall and winter months. Recovery usually takes place within 2 weeks.

lymphocytopenia /-sī′təpē′nē·ə/,   a smaller than normal number of white cells (lymphocytes) in the blood. This may occur as a blood disorder or with nutritional deficiency, cancer, or infectious mononucleosis.

lymphogranuloma venereum (LGV) /-gran′yəlō′mə/,   a sexually transmitted disease caused by a strain of the germ *Chlamydia trachomatis.* Signs are genital lesions, swelling of the lymph nodes in the groin, headache, and fever. Ulcers of the rectum occur less commonly. Antibiotics are usually prescribed for the patient and for any person with whom there has been sexual contact. See also Chlamydia.

lymphoma /limfō′mə/,   a tumor of lymphoid tissue that is usually cancerous. Lymphoid tissue is netlike and holds lymphocytes, a type of white blood cell, in its spaces. The various lymphomas differ in degree of structure and content, but their effects are similar. The appearance of one or more painless, enlarged lymph nodes in the neck is followed by weakness, fever, weight loss, and anemia. The greater the amount of involved lymph tissue, the more effects will occur. The spleen and liver may enlarge. Gastrointestinal problems and bone lesions often develop. Men are more likely than women to develop lymphoid tumors. **Non-Hodgkin's lymphoma** refers to any kind of cancer of the lymph tissues other than Hodgkin's disease. **Undifferentiated malignant lymphoma** describes one having many large cells with large nuclei, small amounts of pale cytoplasm, and poorly defined borders. Treatment for lymphoma includes radiation and drugs. **Lymphoma staging** is a system for classifying lymphomas according to the stage of the disease for the purpose of appropriate treatment. Stage I involves a single lymph node region. Stage II includes two or more lymph node regions on the same side of the diaphragm. In Stage III, lymph nodes on both sides of the diaphragm are affected. There may be involvement of the spleen or of another organ or site. Stage IV is typified by widespread involvement of one or more body organs or sites with or without lymph node involvement.

lymphosarcoma cell leukemia /-särkō'mə/, a cancer of blood-forming tissues. Many lymphoma cancer cells in the blood infiltrate surrounding tissues. The disease may occur with lymphoma or exist separately with more bone marrow involvement than is found in lymphoma. See also **leukemia.**

lypressin, an antidiuretic nasal spray prescribed in diabetes insipidus to decrease urine loss. Blood vessel disease or known allergy to this drug prohibits its use. Side effects include chest pains in patients with heart disease, nausea, and cramping.

lysergide /līsur'jīd/, a drug derived from ergot, a fungus of cereal grains, that causes hallucinations. The potent drug can cause eye pupil dilation, increased blood pressure, tremors, muscle weakness, increased body temperature, and hallucinations. Depending on dose size, there may also be dizziness, drowsiness, numbness, tingling sensations, and euphoria or discomfort. Also called **LSD, lysergic acid diethylamide,** (slang) **acid.** See also **hallucinogen.**

lysine (Lys) /lī'sin/, an essential amino acid needed for proper growth in infants and for maintenance of nitrogen balance in adults. See also **amino acid, protein.**

lysinemia /-ē'mē·ə/, an inborn disorder that causes the inability of the body to use the essential amino acid lysine. This results in muscle weakness and mental retardation. Treatment consists of a diet that controls the intake of lysine by reducing proteins, such as milk and meats, and includes more fruits, vegetables, and rice.

lysis /lī'sis/, destruction, as of a cell through the action of an enzyme or antibody.

Lysodren, a trademark for an anticancer drug (mitotane).

lysosome /lī'səsōm/, a particle in a cell that contains enzymes capable of destroying the cell. It is believed that lysosomes may play an important role in certain self-destructive diseases in which the wasting of tissue occurs, such as muscular dystrophy.

lysozyme /-zīm/, an enzyme with antiseptic actions that destroys some foreign organisms. It is found in white blood cells and is normally present in saliva, sweat, breast milk, and tears.

lytic cocktail /lit'ik/, informal. an anesthetic compound of chlorpromazine, meperidine, and promethazine that blocks the autonomic nervous system, depresses the circulatory system, and induces paralysis of nerve activity. See also **analgesic cocktail.**

Lytren, a trademark for a nutritional supplement containing various electrolytes.

M

m, abbreviation for **meter.**

macerate /mas′ərāt/, to soften something solid by soaking. **–maceration,** *n.*

macrocephaly /mak′rōsef′əlē/, a birth defect marked by a head and brain that are too large in relation to the body. It is linked to some degree of mental defect and slowed growth. The face is usually normal. Macrocephaly is different from hydrocephalus, in which the growth of the head is caused by too much fluid of the brain and spine, usually under increased pressure. Tests may be needed to tell the two conditions apart.

macrocyte /mak′rəsīt/, an unusually large, mature red blood cell.

Macrodantin, a trademark for an antibiotic (nitrofurantoin).

Macrodex, a trademark for a blood plasma expander (dextran).

macrogenitosomia /mak′rōjen′itōsō′mē·ə/, a condition in which the sex organs of males are prematurely large. It results from an excess of a male sex hormone (androgen) during fetal growth. In females, there is some outer male genital appearance (pseudohermaphroditism).

macroglossia /-glos′ē·ə/, a birth defect with a large size of the tongue, as seen in Down's syndrome.

macrognathia /-nā′thē·ə/, an abnormally large growth of the jaw.

macronutrient /-noo′trē·ənt/, a chemical element needed in large amounts for the body. Macronutrients include carbon, hydrogen, oxygen, nitrogen, potassium, sodium, calcium, chloride, magnesium, phosphorus, and sulfur. Also called **major element.** Compare **micronutrient.**

macrophage /mak′rəfāj/, any large cell that can surround and digest foreign substances in the body, as protozoa or bacteria. They are found in the liver, spleen, and in the loose connective tissue.

macula /mak′yələ/, *pl.* **maculae,** a small colored area or a spot. It may be permanent. For example, the **macula lutea** is a small, oval, yellow area of the retina of the eye. Near the optic nerve, it has special cones at its center. Accurate sight occurs when an image is focused on this special part of the macula lutea.

Madelung's neck, an accumulation of fat around the neck that is not a true fat tumor. Also called **lipoma annulare colli.**

mafenide acetate, a drug given to treat burns. It prevents infections. Allergy to this drug or to sulfonamide prohibits its use. Side effects include allergic reactions and new infections, particularly by *Candida albicans.* See also **sulfonamide.**

magaldrate, an antacid given for stomach upset linked to heartburn, sour stomach, or acid indigestion. It may change absorption of other drugs, as tetracyclines. There may be a change in bowel function.

magnesium (Mg), a silver-white mineral. Magnesium is needed for many chemical activities of the body and is important for nerves and muscles. About 50% of the body's magnesium is in the bones.

magnesium sulfate, a salt of magnesium given by injection to prevent seizures, especially in preeclampsia of pregnancy. It is also given by mouth to treat constipation and heartburn and to correct a lack of magnesium in the body. It is used with care in kidney disease or if the patient is allergic to the drug. Difficulty in breathing, severe heart problems, or symptoms of appendicitis or constipation prohibits its use. Side effects include a shutdown of the blood flow from too much magnesium in the blood, difficulty in breathing, confusion, and muscle weakness. Also called **Epson salts.**

Majocchi's granuloma /məjok′ēz/, a ringworm that affects mainly the lower legs. A fungus (*Trichophyton*) infects the hairs of the affected site and raises spongy tumors. The tumors last for 3 to 4 months and are slowly absorbed. They may also decay, often leaving deep scars. Also called **trichophytic granuloma.**

major medical insurance, insurance coverage developed to offset the costs of lengthy or major illness and injury. Most major medical insurance policies are written to pay a certain amount of costs up to a certain figure, beyond which payment is made in full up to a maximum amount. After the maximum amount, payment stops. Many policies require the insured to pay a deductible.

major surgery, any surgery that needs general anesthesia or help in breathing or both.

mal /mal, mäl/, an illness or disease, as grand mal or petit mal.

malabsorption, a failure of the intestines to absorb nutrients. It may result from a birth defect involving the digestion, malnutrition, or any abnormal condition of the digestive system that prevents needed food elements from being absorbed.

malabsorption syndrome, a group of symptoms resulting from disorders in the intestines' ability to absorb nutrients from foods eaten. It may lead to loss of appetite, weight loss, swollen abdomen, muscle cramps, bone pain, and fat in the feces. Anemia, weakness, and tiredness can occur because iron, folic acid, and vitamin B_{12} are not absorbed in right amounts. Among the many conditions causing this syndrome are stomach or small bowel surgery, celiac disease, tropical sprue, cystic fibrosis, Whipple's disease, and intestinal lymphangiectasia, a disease involving the grouping of the lymph ducts in the intestines. Treatment and its result depend on the specific condition.

malacia /məlā′shə/, an abnormal softening or a sponginess in any part or any tissue of the body.

malaise /malāz′/, a vague feeling of body weakness or discomfort, often indicating the beginning of disease.

malalignment /mal′əlīn′mənt/, a failure of parts of the body to line up normally, as teeth that do not conform to the dental arch.

malaria /məler′ē·ə/, an infection caused by one or more of at least four different species of the protozoan organism *Plasmodium,* carried by a mosquito bite. Malaria can also be spread by blood transfusion or by the use of an infected needle. Symptoms include chills, fever, anemia, and a large spleen. Malaria tends to become a lifelong disease. Because the life cycle of the infecting parasite changes with the species, the patterns of chills and fever differ, as do the length and seriousness of the disease. The disease is mostly found in tropical areas. However, a number of new cases are brought to North America by refugees, military personnel, and travelers. *Plasmodium* parasites enter the red blood cells of the infected human, where they mature and reproduce. Malaria attacks (paroxysms) occur at regular intervals. Prevention with antimalarial drugs is important for those visiting areas where infection is possible. **−malarial,** *adj.*

malathion poisoning /mal′əthī′on/, məlā′thē·ən/, a toxic condition caused by swallowing malathion or by absorbing it through the skin. Malathion is an organophosphorus insecticide. It is a chemical cousin of military nerve gas. Symptoms of poisoning include vomiting, nausea, stomach cramps, headache, dizziness, weakness, confusion, convulsions, and breathing problems. Treatment includes immediately giving atropine by injection, an insecticide antidote, flushing the stomach with water, giving a salt water enema, help in breathing, and oxygen. Malathion is much less toxic than parathion, an agricultural insecticide. It is the only organophosphorus insecticide approved for household use.

male, 1. referring to the sex that produces sperm cells and fertilizes the female to have offspring; masculine. **2.** a male person.

male reproductive system assessment, an evaluation of the condition of the patient's sex organs, past and present genital or urinary infections and disorders, and reproductive history. Questions concern the frequency or difficulty in urinating, discharge from the penis, hernia, genital sores, discomfort or pain in the groin, lower back, or legs, and past treatment for an inflammation (epididymitis), gonorrhea, genital herpes, swollen scrotum (hydrocele), nonspecific disease of the urethra (urethritis), undescended testicle (orchitis), disease of the prostate (prostatitis), syphilis, and varicose testicular veins (varicocele).

malformation, an abnormal structure in the body. See also **birth defect.**

malignant /məlig′nənt/, **1.** tending to become worse and possibly cause death. **2.** describing a tumor that is cancerous, involving many organs, and spreading. **−malignancy,** *n.*

malignant neoplasm. See **neoplasm.**

malingering, a conscious faking of the symptoms of a disease or injury to gain some desired end.

malleolus /məlē′ələs/, *pl.* **malleoli,** a rounded bony structure, as the bump on each side of the ankle.

malleus /mal′ē·əs/, one of the three tiny bones (ossicles) in the middle ear, resembling a hammer or mallet. It is connected to the eardrum and carries sound vibrations to the anvil (incus). See also **ear.**

Mallory-Weiss syndrome, a condition in which heavy bleeding follows a break in the mucous membrane of the esophagus at its connection with the stomach. The break is usually caused by repeated vomiting. Surgery is usually needed to stop the bleeding. After repair, the chance for recovery is excellent.

malnutrition, any disorder concerning nutrition. It may result from an unbalanced diet or from eating too little or too much food. It may also result from improper body use of foods. Compare **deficiency disease.**

malocclusion /mal′əkloo′zhən/, abnormal contact of the teeth of the upper jaw with the teeth of the lower jaw. See also **occlusion.**

malpractice, a professional mistake that is a direct cause of injury or harm to a patient. It may result from a lack of knowledge, experience, or skill that can be expected in others in the profession. It may also result from a failure to use reasonable care or judgment.

mammary gland, one of two half-sphere-shaped glands on the chest of mature females. It is also seen in simple form in children and in males. Gland tissue forms a ring of lobes with small sacs (alveoli). Each lobe has a system of ducts for the passage of milk from the alveoli to the nipple. The inner portion of the breast is filled with gland tissue. The outer portion is made up mostly of fatty tissue. The left breast is usually larger than the right. Also called **breast.**

mammogram, an x-ray film of the soft tissues of the breast made to identify various lumps (cysts or tumors).

mammoplasty, surgical reshaping of the breasts. It is done to reduce or lift large or sagging breasts, to enlarge small breasts, or to reconstruct a breast after removal of a tumor. To reduce the size of the breasts and raise them, excess tissue is removed from the bottom of the breasts. To enlarge a breast, a thin plastic sac of silicone fluid may be inserted in a pouch formed beneath the breast on the chest wall. The complications after surgery are infection and, with the use of implants, rejection by tissues of the foreign body.

mammothermography /mam′ōthər mog′rə fē/, a way in which a special test (infrared thermography) is used for examining the breast to detect abnormal growths. It is done by outlining hot and cold tissue areas. Compare **mammography.** See also **thermography.**

management by objective (MBO), top down management so that all involved know and understand the objectives of the operation.

Mandelamine, a trademark for an antibiotic (methenamine mandelate).

mandible /man′dibəl/, a large bone forming the lower jaw. It consists of a horizontal part that has the lower teeth and two vertical parts that form a joint with the upper jaw (maxilla).

mandibular sling /mandib′yələr/, the connection between the lower jaw (mandible) and the upper jaw (maxilla), formed by the two face muscles. The mouth is opened and closed as the mandible moves with the help of the mandibular sling.

Mandol, a trademark for an antibiotic (cefamandole nafate).

maneuver, in obstetrics, moving the fetus to aid in childbirth.

mania, a mood disorder with too much excitement, excess elation, overactivity, nervousness, talking too much, flight of ideas, and not paying attention. Violent, destructive, or self-destructive behavior occurs at times. It is seen in the major mental disorders, as the manic phase of bipolar disorder, and in certain organic brain diseases, as dementia. **Transitory mania** features a sudden onset of excessive reactions that only last a short time, usually from 1 hour to a few days. **Hysteric mania** has combined symptoms of hysteria and mania. **Puerperal mania** is a severe mental disorder that sometimes occurs in women after childbirth. It is a severe reaction of depression and then excitement. −**maniac,** *n., adj.,* **maniacal,** *adj.*

manic depressive, a patient with or showing the symptoms of bipolar disorder.

manipulation, the skillful use of the hands in therapy or diagnosis, as feeling with the hands, resetting a dislocation, turning the unborn, or some treatments in physical therapy and bone therapy (osteopathy). See also **massage.**

Mantadil, a trademark for a skin cream with an adrenal hormone (hydrocortisone acetate) and an antihistamine (chlorcyclizine hydrochloride).

Mantoux test. See **tuberculin test.**

manual rotation, a maneuver in which a baby's head is turned by the hand of a physician in the birth canal to make childbirth easier. Compare **forceps rotation.**

MAO inhibitor. See **monoamine oxidase inhibitor.**

Maolate, a trademark for a skeletal muscle relaxant (chlorphenesin carbamate).

maple bark disease, a type of lung disease (pneumonitis) caused by a mold *Cryptostroma corticale,* found in the bark of maple trees. In a sensitive patient the condition may be sudden, with fever, cough, and vomiting. It also may be long term, with weakness, weight loss, uncomfortable breathing when exercising, and coughing up sputum.

maple syrup urine disease, an inherited disorder in which an enzyme needed for the breakdown of three amino acids (valine, leucine, and isoleucine) is lacking. The disease is usually discovered in infancy. It is recognized by the typical maple syrup odor of the urine and by unnatural reflexes. Stress, fever, infection, and taking in lysine, leucine, or isoleucine make the condition worse. Treatment includes a diet avoiding these amino acids. Kidney dialysis or blood transfusion are seldom given. Also called **branched chain ketoaciduria.**

maprotiline hydrochloride, an antidepressant similar to the tricyclics. It is given for the treatment of depression. See also **tricyclic compound.**

marasmus /məraz′məs/, a condition of excess malnutrition and wasting, mostly in young children. It results from a lack of enough calories and proteins. Marasmus is seen in failure to thrive children and in starvation. Less commonly, it occurs as a result of an inability to absorb or use protein. See also **failure to thrive, kwashiorkor.**

Marax, a trademark for a respiratory drug containing a smooth muscle relaxant (theophylline), a stimulant (ephedrine sulfate), and a tranquilizer (hydroxyzine hydrochloride).

M−N

Marcaine Hydrochloride,   a trademark for a local anesthetic (bupivacaine hydrochloride).

march foot,   an abnormal condition of the foot. It is caused by excess use, as in a long march. The forefoot is swollen and painful. One or more of the foot bones may be broken. See also **stress fracture.**

Marcus Gunn pupil sign,   a test for disease of the optic nerve or retina of the eye. In a dark room a beam of light is moved from one eye to the other. Normal narrowing of the pupil of an affected eye occurs when the beam is directed at the opposite eye. As the light is moved to the abnormal eye, the direct reaction to light is weaker and both pupils appear to widen. It indicates poor conduction by the optic nerve fibers. Also called **swinging light test.**

Marezine Hydrochloride,   a trademark for a motion sickness drug (cyclizine hydrochloride) that can be injected.

Marfan's syndrome,   an inherited condition with excess length of the bones, often linked with problems of the eyes, heart, and circulation. The disease causes major muscle and bone disorders, as underdeveloped muscles, weak ligaments, excess joint movements, and long bones. Changes of the heart and the circulation include breaking of the fibers in the walls of the major heart artery (aorta). Visual changes include many disorders, as dislocation of the lens of the eye. The disease affects men and women equally. It lengthens the legs so that most adult patients with the disease are over 6 feet tall. The skulls are usually uneven in shape or size. A curved spine may develop and increase during adolescence. No specific treatment is known. Many of the problems may be treated with surgery.

marijuana.   See **cannabis.**

Marplan,   a trademark for an antidepressant (isocarboxazid).

Marshall-Marchetti operation,   surgery done to correct the inability to urinate. The surgery puts the urethra and bladder into their normal position.

masculine,   having the physical characteristics of a male. –**masculinize,** v.

masculinization,   the normal development of male sex properties. See also **virilism.**

mask,   a cover worn over the nose and mouth to prevent breathing in toxic or irritating materials, to control delivery of oxygen or anesthetic gas, or to protect a patient from germs exhaled by medical personnel.

masking,   1. concealing a disorder by a second condition, as when a person begins a weight-loss diet while an undiagnosed wasting disease, as cancer, has developed. The loss of body weight is considered to be the result of the diet. This delays diagnosis and treatment. 2. the unconscious display of a personality trait that hides a behavior disorder.

masking agent,   a cosmetic preparation for covering moles, surgical scars, and other marks. Masking agents are generally made up of a ''flesh''-colored dye in a lotion or cream base.

masochism /mas'əkizm/,   pleasure gotten from receiving physical, mental, or emotional abuse. The abuse may be given by another person or by oneself. Compare **sadism.**

mass,   1. a group of cells clumped together as a tumor. 2. the physical condition of matter that gives it weight and inertia.

massage,   the manipulation of the soft tissue of the body. The purpose is to increase circulation, to improve muscle tone, and to relax the patient. It is done either with bare hands or through mechanical means, as a vibrator. The most common sites for massage are the back, knees, elbows, and heels. Care is taken not to massage inflamed areas (particularly of the legs, because of the danger of loosening blood clots), open wounds and areas of rash, or tumors. Massage is done with the patient lying face down or on the side, in a comfortable position. Lotion or cream is put on the area to be massaged. **Clapping** is a form alternating the cupped palms in a series of rapid, sharp blows. Strong circular movements of the hand in which deeper tissues are stroked or rubbed is called **friction. Effleurage** uses long, light, or firm strokes, usually over the spine and back. **Fingertip effleurage** is done with the tips of the fingers in a circle pattern over one part of the body or in long strokes over the back or an arm, leg, hand or foot. **Rolling effleurage** is a circular rubbing stroke done with the hand flat, the palm and fingers acting as a unit. **Frôlement** uses a light brushing stroke with the hand. **Kneading** is a grasping, rolling, and pressing movement used in massaging the muscles. **Pétrissage** is a type of massage in which the skin is gently lifted and squeezed. With **tapotement,** the body is tapped in a rhythmic manner with the tips of the fingers or the sides of the hands. It is often used on the chest wall of patients with inflammation of the bronchi (bronchitis) to help loosen the mucus in the air passages. **Vibration** is done by quick tapping with the fingertips, alternating the fingers in a rhythmic way, or by a mechanic device.

masseter /masē'tər/,   the thick, rectangular muscle in the cheek that closes the jaw. It is one of four muscles used in chewing.

mass reflex,   a disorder seen in patients with a cut spinal cord caused by a widespread nerve discharge. This results in muscle spasms, involuntary urination and defecation, high blood pressure, and heavy sweating. A mass reflex may occur from scratching or other painful stimulation of the skin, a bloated bladder or intestines, cold weather, sitting for too long, or emotional stress. Muscle spasms may be so violent as to throw the patient off a bed. Drugs to reduce mass reflexes and exercises in warm water help. Surgery on the brain and nerves may be necessary.

MAST, medical anti-shock trousers (garment).

mastalgia /mastal′jə/, pain in the breast caused by clogging or ''caking'' during milk release, an infection, a breast disease including cysts, menstruation, or advanced cancer. –**mastalgic,** *adj.*

mastectomy /mastek′-/, removing through surgery one or both breasts to treat a cancer. In a **simple mastectomy,** only breast tissue is removed. The underlying muscles and nearby lymph nodes are left intact. In a **modified radical mastectomy,** the large muscles of the chest that move the arm are saved and some of the nearby lymph nodes. The operation treats early and easily spotted cancers of the breast. It is reported to be as successful as the more complicated radical mastectomy. **Radical mastectomy** is removal of an entire breast, with the chest (pectoral) muscles, armpit (axillary) lymph nodes, all fat, and other nearby tissues. Swelling of the arm on the affected side occurs because the armpit structures that drain the lymph from the arm are removed during surgery. Lung collapse may develop if deep breathing and coughing are not regularly done. A pressure dressing is most often applied to the cut and left in place until bleeding and draining have stopped. A drain is often left in the wound for many days. Health care includes arm and shoulder exercises that get more complex over time. A volunteer service, Reach to Recovery, may help to counsel and support the woman before and after surgery. Chemical and radiation treatments may continue after surgery. The woman is told never to allow blood to be drawn from the affected arm. The use of injecting fluids or foods into the veins is also to be avoided in that arm, which will lack lymph nodes. Blood pressure measurement, vaccination, and other injections should be done on the other arm. In a **subcutaneous mastectomy,** all the breast tissue of one or both breasts is removed leaving the skin, areola, and nipple intact. The nearby lymph nodes and the underlying muscles are not removed. It may be done on women who are at great risk of getting breast cancer. Reconstruction of the breasts is done by a plastic surgeon, through inserting prostheses to return the normal shape to the breasts. See also **breast cancer, lumpectomy, postmastectomy exercises.**

mastication, chewing, tearing, or grinding food with the teeth while it becomes mixed with saliva. See also **bolus, digestion, ptyalin.**

masticatory system /mas′tikətôr′ē/, the group of organs, structures, and nerves used in chewing. It includes the jaws, the teeth and their supporting structures, the hinge (temporomandibular) joints, the tongue, lips, and cheeks. Also called **masticatory apparatus.**

mastitis /mastī′-/, an inflamed breast. It is usually caused by bacterial infection. **Acute mastitis** is most common in the first 2 months of breast feeding. There is pain, swelling, redness, lymph gland disorders, and fever. If not properly treated, sores may form. Antibiotics, rest, painkillers, and warm soaks are usually prescribed. Usually breast feeding may continue. **Chronic tuberculous mastitis** is a rare spread of tuberculosis from the lungs and ribs beneath the breast.

mastoidectomy /mas′toidek′-/, removing with surgery a portion of the mastoid bone at the side of the skull. It may be done to treat long-term pus-forming, middle ear infection (otitis media) or mastoid bone inflammation (mastoiditis) when antibiotics are not useful. Entry is made through the ear canal or from behind the ear. In a simple mastoidectomy, infected bone cells are removed. The eardrum is cut to drain the middle ear. Antibiotics are then put in the ear. In a radical operation, the eardrum and most middle ear structures are removed. After surgery a hearing aid may be used.

mastoiditis /-dī′-/, an infection of one of the mastoid bones, usually an extension of a middle ear infection. It features earache, fever, headache, and discomfort. Children are most often affected. Treatment includes antibiotics, often given by injection for several days. Some hearing loss may follow the infection.

mastoid process, a bulge of a portion of the temporal bone at the side of the skull where various muscles attach. A hollow section of the mastoid process has air cells. They are the site of infections that spread from the ear. See also **temporal bone.**

masturbation, sexual activity in which the penis or clitoris is stimulated by means other than sexual intercourse. It leads usually to an orgasm. It is done, at least once in a while, by most people. It is considered to be normal and harmless. Also called, in men, **onanism.**

materia medica, 1. the study of drugs and other substances used in medicine, their origins, preparation, uses, and effects. **2.** a substance or a drug used in medicine.

Materna 1.60, a trademark for a multivitamin supplement with calcium and iron for pregnant women.

maternal and child health (MCH) services, various services and programs organized for the purpose of giving medical and social services for mothers and children. Medical services include care before and after birth, family planning care, and child care in infancy.

maternal deprivation syndrome, a condition in which slowed growth occurs as a result of a lack of physical or emotional stimulation. It is seen most often in infants. Symptoms include a lack of physical growth, with weight abnormally low for age and size, malnutrition, withdrawal, silence, and irritability. The child also has an unnatural

M–N

stiffness. Causes include factors such as parents not caring, insecurity of the mother, or lack of mother-child bonding. Other factors are unreal expectations and disappointment about the sex or appearance of the child, and unfavorable conditions within the family. Treatment may require hospitalization, especially in cases of severe malnutrition. Emotionally deprived children often are slow in intellectual development, fail to learn normal social behavior, and are unable to form trusting, meaningful relationships with others. See also **failure to thrive.**

maternal-infant bonding. See **bonding.**

maternity cycle, the prebirth (antepartal), birth (intrapartal), and postbirth (postpartal) periods of pregnancy and the return of reproductive organs to normal (puerperium). The cycle lasts from conception to 6 weeks after birth.

matrifocal family /mat'rifō'kəl/, a family unit made up of a mother and her children. Biologic fathers have a temporary place in the family during the first years of the children's lives. They have a more permanent position in their own original families.

matrix, 1. a substance found between tissue cells. **2.** also called **ground substance.** a basic substance from which a specific organ or kind of tissue develops.

matter, 1. anything that has mass and occupies space. **2.** any substance not otherwise identified as to its parts, as gray matter, pus, or blood serum oozing from a wound.

Matulane, a trademark for an anticancer drug (procarbazine hydrochloride).

maturation, 1. the process or condition of coming to complete development. **2.** the final stages in the formation of germ cells (ova or spermatazoa) in which the number of chromosomes in each cell is reduced to the number needed for reproduction.

mature, to become fully developed; to ripen.

maturity, 1. a state of complete growth or development, usually the period of life between adolescence and old age. **2.** the stage at which an organism can reproduce.

Maxibolin, a trademark for a body-building hormone (ethylestrenol).

Maxidex, a trademark for an adrenal hormone drug (dexamethasone).

maxilla /maksil'ə/, pl. **maxillae,** one of a pair of large bones that form the upper jaw.

maxillary sinus /mak'siler'ē/. See **nasal sinus.**

maximal breathing capacity (MBC), the amount of oxygen and carbon dioxide that can be exchanged per minute at the greatest rate and depth of breathing by a person.

maximal expiratory flow rate (MEFR), the rate of the most rapid flow of carbon dioxide from the lungs possible when a person exhales or breathes out.

maximum oxygen uptake, the greatest amount of oxygen that can be moved by the bloodstream from the lungs to the working muscle tissue.

Maxitrol, a trademark for an eye medication. It contains an adrenal hormone (dexamethasone) and antibiotics (neomycin sulfate and polymyxin B sulfate).

mazindol, a drug used to decrease the appetite. It is given to reduce food intake in the case of overweight caused by overeating. Glaucoma, history of drug abuse, use of a monoamine oxidase inhibitor at the same time, or known allergy to this drug prohibits its use. Side effects include inability to sleep, irregular heart beats, dizziness, dry mouth, rapid heart beat, and allergic reactions.

McArdle's disease. See **glycogen storage disease.**

McBurney's point, a place on the stomach that is very sensitive in acute appendicitis, about 2 inches from the edge of the right hipbone on a line between that bone and the navel. See also **appendicitis.**

mcg, abbreviation for **microgram.**

McMurray's sign, a click heard when moving the lower leg bone (tibia) on the upper leg bone (femur), showing injury to cartilage in the kneecap.

M.D., abbreviation for *Doctor of Medicine.* See **physician.**

Meals on Wheels, a program that takes hot meals to elderly, physically disabled, or other persons who cannot give themselves nutritionally adequate warm meals daily.

measles, an acute, highly contagious, viral disease that occurs foremost in young children who have not been vaccinated. Measles is carried by direct contact with droplets spread from the nose, throat, and mouth of infected patients, usually in the early stage of the disease. An inactive period of 7 to 14 days is followed by the beginning stage of the disease. Symptoms include fever, discomfort, runny nose, cough, eye irritation, sensitivity to light, and loss of appetite. Diagnosis is based on laboratory tests or on identifying small red spots (Koplik spots) inside of the cheeks, which appear 1 to 2 days before the appearance of the rash. Throat inflammation develops. The temperature may rise to 103° or 104° F. The rash first appears as irregular brownish-pink spots around the hairline, the ears, and the neck. It spreads rapidly to the body, arms, and legs. The red and dense patches give the skin a blotchy appearance. Within 3 to 5 days, the fever decreases, the spots flatten, turn a brownish color, and begin to fade. Treatment includes bed rest, antifever drugs, and antibiotics to control bacterial infection. Calamine lotion or corn starch solution are used to relieve itching. Preventive measures include vaccinating with measles virus vaccine after the child is 1 year of age. Passive immunization with immune serum globulin is advised for unvaccinated individuals exposed to the disease. Complications sometimes occur, such as middle ear infection (otitis media) and pneumonia. Also called **rubeola.**

measles and rubella virus vaccine live, an active immunizing agent. It is given to prevent measles and rubella. Suppressed natural resistance, use of costeroid drugs at the same time, tuberculosis, known or suspected pregnancy, and allergy to neomycin prohibit its use. Tumors of the lymphatic system or bone marrow, or active disease infection also prohibits its use. It should not be given for 3 months after use of whole blood, plasma, or immune serum globulin. It also should not be given for 1 month before or after vaccination with other live virus vaccines, except mumps vaccine. Side effects include a strong allergic reaction.

measles, mumps, and rubella virus vaccine live (MMR), an active immunizing agent. It is given for simultaneous vaccination against measles, mumps, and rubella. Suppressed natural resistance, simultaneous use of steroid drugs, tuberculosis, and allergy to neomycin prohibits its use. Tumors of the lymph system or bone marrow, known or suspected pregnancy, or severe infection also prohibits its use. It is not given for 3 months after use of whole blood, plasma, or immune serum globulin. It is also not given for 1 month before or after vaccination with other live virus vaccines. Side effects include a strong allergic reaction.

meatus /mē·ā′təs/, an opening or tunnel through any part of the body, as the external acoustic meatus that leads from the outer ear to the eardrum (tympanic membrane).

Mebaral, a trademark for an anticonvulsant and sedative drug (mephobarbital).

mebendazole, an antiworm (anthelmintic) drug given to treat pinworm, whipworm, roundworm, and hookworm infestations. Pregnancy or known allergy to this drug prohibits its use. Side effects include intestinal pain and diarrhea.

mechanical stress, the result of a transfer of energy when one subject physically contacts or collides with another. Indications are punctures, gouges, breaks, or tears in the container. A container may also be weakened but have no visible signs of potential release.

mechlorethamine hydrochloride, an anticancer drug given to treat a variety of tumors. Bone marrow disorders, pregnancy, infection, or known allergy to this drug prohibits its use. Side effects include bone marrow problems, inflammation at the injection site, nausea, vomiting, and hair loss. Also called **nitrogen mustard.**

Meclan, a trademark for an antibiotic (meclocycline sulfosalicylate).

meclizine hydrochloride, an antihistamine given to prevent and treat motion sickness. Newborn infants and nursing mothers are not given this drug. Asthma or known

allergy to this drug prohibits its use. Side effects include drowsiness, skin rash, allergic reactions, dry mouth, rapid heart beat, and nervousness.

meclofenamate sodium, an antiinflammatory drug given in the treatment of rheumatoid arthritis and osteoarthritis.

Meclomen, a trademark for an antiinflammatory drug (meclofenamate sodium).

meconium /məkō′nē·əm/, a material that collects in the intestines of a fetus. It forms the first stool of a newborn. Thick and sticky, it is usually greenish to black in color. Meconium is composed of secretions of the intestinal glands, some amniotic fluid, and debris, as bile dyes, fatty acids, skin cells, mucus, fine hair, and blood. Meconium in the amniotic fluid during labor may mean the baby is in distress. The breathing in of meconium by the baby from the amniotic fluid can block the air passages and result in failure of the lungs to expand or cause other breathing problems, as pneumonia.

meconium ileus, blockage of the small intestine in the newborn with thick, dry meconium. Symptoms include a swollen abdomen, vomiting, failure to pass meconium within the first 24 to 48 hours after birth, and rapid loss of fluids. It is caused by lack of pancreatic enzymes and is the earliest sign of cystic fibrosis. In simple cases, the blockage may be dislodged by giving enemas. If enemas do not dislodge the blockage, surgery is necessary. See also **cystic fibrosis.**

meconium plug syndrome, blockage of the large intestine in the newborn. It is caused by thick, rubbery meconium that may fill the whole colon and part of the small intestine. Symptoms include failure to pass meconium within the first 24 to 48 hours following birth, a swollen abdomen, and vomiting if complete intestinal blockage occurs. A barium enema will reveal the plug and in most cases will dislodge it from the bowel wall. Additional gentle saltwater (saline) enemas may be needed to expel the plug. The condition may be a sign of Hirschsprung's disease or cystic fibrosis.

medial /mē′dē·əl/, placed near the middle of the body.

medial cuneiform bone, the largest of the wedge-shaped (cuneiform) bones of the foot. It links the toes to the ankle bones.

median effective dose (ED$_{50}$), the dose of a drug that causes a specific effect in one half of the patients to whom it is given.

median nerve, a nerve that extends along the forearm and the hand and supplies various muscles and the skin of these parts.

mediastinum /mē′dē·əstī′nəm/, a part of the space in the middle of the chest, between the sacs containing the two lungs. It extends from the breastbone (sternum) to the

M–N

spine. It contains all of the chest organs, except the lungs.

Mediatric, a trademark for a food supplement with multivitamins, minerals, hormones, and a central nervous system stimulant (methamphetamine hydrochloride).

Medicaid, a federally paid, state operated program of medical assistance to patients with low incomes. It is authorized by Title XIX of the Social Security Act. Under broad federal guidelines, the individual states determine benefits, eligibility, rates of payment, and methods of distribution. The **Early and Periodic Screening Diagnosis and Treatment (EPSDT)** is a section of the Medicaid program that requires all states to run a program to determine the physical and mental defects of persons under 21 who are covered by the program and to provide short- and long-range treatment.

medical center, 1. a health care facility. 2. a hospital, especially one staffed and set up to care for many patients and for a large number of diseases and disorders, using modern technology.

medical consultation, a procedure whereby, on request by one physician, another physician reviews a patient's medical history, examines the patient, and makes suggestions about care and treatment. The medical consultant often is a specialist with experience in a specific field of medicine.

medical history. See **health history.**

Medical Practices Act, laws requiring an individual to be licensed or certified to practice medicine or to provide certain levels of care.

Medicare, federally paid national health insurance. It is for certain persons over 65 years of age. The program is divided into two parts. Part A protects against costs of medical, surgical, and mental hospital care. Part B is a voluntary medical insurance program paid in part from federal funds and in part from premiums paid by persons enrolled in the program. Medicare enrollment is offered to persons 65 years of age or older who can receive Social Security or railroad retirement benefits. Other persons over 65 years of age, as federal employees and aliens, may not be permitted to join. Medicare was set up by Title XVIII of the Social Security Act of 1965.

medicated tub bath, a bath in which a drug is put in water, usually to treat skin disorders, as psoriasis. The water temperature is usually between 96° F (35.6° C) and 100° F (37.8° C). The temperature may be as high as 103° F (39. Most medicated baths are half-hour treatments. A folded towel or waterproof pillow is placed behind the head. A towel is draped over the shoulders for comfort. In certain conditions, the patient may scrub the affected skin areas with a brush and washcloth. In others, the physician may advise that the skin should not be scrubbed at all.

After the bath the skin is patted dry. Ointment, cream, or other skin medication is applied.

medication, a drug or other substance that is used as a drug or remedy for illness.

medicine, 1. a drug or a remedy for illness. 2. the art and science of the diagnosis, treatment, and prevention of disease and keeping good health. 3. the art of treating disease without surgery.

Medihaler-Epi, a trademark for a stimulant (epinephrine bitartrate).

Medihaler-Ergotamine Aerosol, a trademark for a painkiller (ergotamine tartrate).

meditation, a state of consciousness in which the individual tries to stop awareness of the surroundings so the mind can focus on a single thing, as a sound, key word, or image. It leads to a state of rest and relief from stress. A wide variety of meditation therapies are used to clear the mind of stressful outside disturbances.

medium, *pl.* **media,** a substance through which something moves or through which it acts. For example, a **contrast medium** is a substance, as a dye, that has a different quality than body tissues. It causes contrasts of body structures when used with x-ray films.

Medrol, a trademark for an adrenal hormone drug (methylprednisolone disodium phosphate).

Medrol Acetate, a trademark for an adrenal hormone drug (methylprednisolone acetate).

medroxyprogesterone acetate, a female sex hormone, progestin. It is given to treat menstrual disorders caused by unbalanced hormones. Known or suspected pregnancy, blood clots, stroke, liver problems, cancer of the breast or genitals, abnormal vaginal bleeding, missed abortion, or known allergy to this drug prohibits its use. Side effects include blood clots, stroke, and liver disease (hepatitis).

medulla /mədul′ə/, the most inner part of a structure or organ, as the adrenal medulla, or inner part of the adrenal gland.

medulla oblongata. See **brain.**

medullary carcinoma /med′yəler′ē/, soft cancer of a thin layer of cells covering various body parts (epithelium) containing little or no fiberlike tissue. A small percentage of breast and thyroid tumors are medullary carcinomas.

medullary cystic disease, a lifelong disease of the kidney. It is marked by the slow beginning of excess urea in the body (uremia). The disease appears in young children or adolescents, who pass large volumes of watered-down urine with greater than normal amounts of salt (sodium). Kidney dialysis is the usual treatment for the disease as the uremia continues and becomes worse. See also **uremia.**

medullary sponge kidney, a birth defect of the kidney. It leads to widening of the tubes that collect urine in the kidney. Patients with this defect often develop a kidney stone or an infection of the kidney because the urine flow is reduced or stopped. Treatment includes drugs to increase the acid in the urine. A diet low in calcium and high in fluids must be followed to reduce the danger of forming stones.

medulloblastoma /med′yəlōblastō′mə/, a brain cancer that develops from leftover embryonic nerve cells. It occurs most often between 5 and 9 years of age and affects more boys than girls. Although medulloblastomas can be treated with radiation, they grow rapidly, and radiotherapy usually allows one to live for only 1 or 2 years longer.

mefenamic acid /mef′ənam′ik/, a drug given to treat mild to moderate pain. Stomach and intestinal ulcers or inflammation, kidney problems, or known allergy to this drug prohibits its use. It is used carefully in patients with asthma. Side effects include blood disorders, stomach upset, diarrhea, dizziness, drowsiness, or skin rash.

Mefoxin, a trademark for an antibiotic (cefoxitin sodium).

megacaryocyte /me′gəker′ē·əsīt′/, a very large bone marrow cell. Megacaryocytes are needed to make platelets in the marrow. They are normally not in the blood circulation. See also **platelet.** –**megacaryocytic,** *adj.*

megacaryocytic leukemia /-sit′ik/, a cancerous disease of blood-forming tissue in which megacaryocytes increase abnormally in the bone marrow and move in the blood in large numbers.

Megace, a trademark for a female sex hormone used as an anticancer drug (megestrol acetate).

megacolon /-kō′lən/, massive, abnormal widening of the large intestine (colon) that may be inborn or may develop later in life. **Congenital megacolon** (Hirschsprung's disease) is caused by the lack of autonomic nerve centers in the smooth muscle wall of the colon. **Toxic megacolon** is a serious result of ulcerative colitis and may lead to a tear in the colon, blood poisoning, and death. Surgery is the usual treatment for toxic and inborn megacolon. **Acquired megacolon** is the result of a long-term inability to defecate. It usually occurs in children who are psychotic or mentally retarded. The colon is widened by being overfilled with feces. Laxatives, enemas, and psychiatric treatment are often necessary. See also **Hirschsprung's disease.**

megaesophagus /-ēsof′əgəs/, abnormal widening of the lower parts of the esophagus. It results from the failure of the muscle at the opening to the stomach to relax and allow food to pass from the esophagus into the stomach.

megalencephaly /meg′əlensef′əlē/, a condition with an abnormal overgrowth of brain tissue. In some cases brain tissue overgrowth is linked to mental retardation or a central nervous system disorder, as epilepsy.

megaloblastic anemia /meg′əlōblas′-/. See **nutritional anemia.**

megalocystis /-sis′-/, an abnormal condition of a large and thin-walled bladder occurring mostly in girls. Surgery may be done to reduce the size of the bladder or change the flow of urine through the small intestine.

megalomania, an abnormal mental state with delusions of grandeur in which one believes oneself to be a person of great power, fame, or wealth. See also **mania.**

megaloureter /-yŏŏr′ətər/, an abnormal condition with great widening of one or both ureters leading from the kidney to the bladder. It results from failure of the smooth muscle in the ureters. Treatment includes surgery.

megestrol acetate /məjes′trōl/, a hormone anticancer drug given to treat cancer of the uterus and to relieve symptoms of the late stages of uterine and breast cancer. Known allergy to the drug or pregnancy prohibits its use. Side effects include hair loss and blood clots.

meibomian gland /mībō′mē·ən/, one of several oil glands that release a fatty material (sebum) from their ducts on the outer side of each eyelid. The glands are in the supporting tissues of each eyelid.

Meigs' syndrome /megz/, a pooling of fluid in the chest linked to a tumor of the ovaries or other pelvic tumor.

meiosis /mī·ō′-/, dividing a sex cell, as it matures, into two, then four ova or spermatozoa (gametes). The nucleus of each gamete receives one half of the number of chromosomes in the body cells of the species. In humans, meiosis results in gametes each containing 23 chromosomes, including one sex chromosome. Compare **mitosis.**

melancholia /mel′angkō′lē·ə/, excess sadness; melancholy.

melanin /mel′ənin/, a black or dark brown color that occurs naturally in the hair, skin, and in the iris and choroid membrane of the eye. See also **melanocyte.**

melanocyte /mel′ənōsīt′/, a body cell able to make the color of skin, hair, and eyes (melanin). Such cells are found throughout the bottom (basal) cell layer of the skin. They form melanin color from an amino acid (tyrosine). A hormone (**melanocyte stimulating hormone**), released by the pituitary gland, controls the amount and appearance of melanin color in skin cells.

melanoderma /-dur′mə/, any abnormal darkening of the skin caused by large amounts of melanin or by chemical compounds of iron or silver.

melanoma /mel′ənō′mə/, any of a group of skin tumors (benign or malignant) that are made up of melanocytes. Most melanomas form flat dark skin patches over several months or years. They occur most often in fair-skinned people having light-colored eyes. Any black or brown spot having an irregular border, and color appearing to move beyond that border may mean a melanoma. Compare **blue nevus.** See also **choroidal malignant melanoma, Hutchinson's freckle.**

M–N

melatonin /-tō′nin/, a hormone released into the blood by the pineal gland in the brain. It follows a 24-hour rhythm with blood levels up to ten times greater at night than during the day. The hormone seems to stop a number of endocrine gland functions, including the gonadotropic hormones. Decreases in melatonin can result in too early puberty or in sex gland problems.

melena /məlē′nə/. See **gastrointestinal bleeding.**

Mellaril, a trademark for a tranquilizer (thioridazine).

melphalan, an anticancer drug. It is given to treat cancer tumors, including multiple myeloma. Pregnancy, recent use of anticancer drugs or having radiation treatment, or known allergy to this drug prohibits its use. Side effects include bone marrow disorders, nausea, and vomiting.

melting point, the temperature at which a solid changes to a liquid. This temperature is also the freezing point, depending on the direction of the change. For mixtures, a melting point range may be given.

membrana tectoria, the broad, strong ligament helping to connect the spinal column to the skull.

membrane, a thin layer of tissue that covers a surface, lines a space, or divides a space, as the stomach membrane that lines the stomach wall. See also **mucous membrane, serous membrane, skin, synovial membrane.**

membranous labyrinth /mem′brənəs/, a network of three fluid-filled, membrane-lined ducts hanging in the bony half-circle canals of the inner ear. They are linked to the sense of balance. The ducts contain a fluid called endolymph.

memory, the ability or power that enables one to remember and to recall, through unconscious means of association, previous sensations, ideas, or information that has been consciously learned. **Anterograde memory** is the memory of events of long ago but not of those that happen recently. **Long-term memory** is the ability to recall sensations, events, ideas, and other information for long periods of time without apparent effort. **Short-term memory** is memory of recent events.

menarche /menär′kē/, the first menstruation and the beginning of the menstrual cycle in females. It usually occurs between 9 and 17 years of age. See also **pubarche.**

Mendel's laws, basic laws of inheritance of physical traits. They are based on the breeding experiments of garden peas by the nineteenth-century Austrian monk Gregor Mendel.

Mendelson's syndrome, a kind of chemical pneumonia resulting from breathing stomach acid into the lungs. It usually occurs when a person vomits while drunk, is drowsy from anesthesia, or is unconscious.

Menest, a trademark for a form of estrogen.

Meniere's disease /mānē·erz′/, a disease of the inner ear with periods of dizziness (vertigo), nerve deafness, and buzzing or ringing in the ear (tinnitus). The cause is not known. Occasionally the condition shows up after middle ear infection or a head injury. There also may be nausea, vomiting, and heavy sweating. Sudden movements often worsen the dizziness. The patient should have help while walking. Attacks last from a few minutes to several hours. Treatment includes a low-salt diet and antihistamines or other drugs. In very bad cases, surgery on the labyrinth or vestibular nerve linked to the sense of balance may be required.

meninges /minin′jēz/, *sing.* **meninx** /mē′ningks, men′-/, any one of the three membranes that cover the brain and the spinal cord. They are the tough outer layer (dura mater), a thin inner layer (pia mater), and a spiderweb-like middle layer (arachnoid). The pia mater and the arachnoid can become inflamed by a bacterial infection. This may cause life-threatening problems. –**meningeal,** *adj.*

meningioma /minin′jē·ō′mə/, a tumor of the meningeal membranes covering the brain and spinal cord. Meningiomas often grow slowly. They usually contain blood vessels. The tumors may vary in shape and structure. They may invade the skull, causing weakening of the bones and pressure on the brain tissue. A meningioma usually occurs in adults. It follows in some cases after a head injury.

meningitis /men′injī′-/, any infection or inflammation of the membranes covering the brain and spinal cord. Usually pus-forming, it involves the fluid of the brain and spine in the space between the membranes that cover the brain. Symptoms vary depending on the cause. They may include fever, headache, stiff neck and back, nausea, and skin rash. The most common causes are bacterial infection with *Streptococcus pneumoniae, Neisseria meningitidis,* or *Haemophilus influenzae.* **Aseptic meningitis** may be caused by other kinds of bacteria, chemical irritation, tumor, or viruses including coxsackieviruses, nonparalytic polio viruses, echoviruses, and mumps. Yeasts as *Candida* and fungi as *Cryptococcus* may cause a harsh, often fatal, meningitis. Tuberculous meningitis, almost always fatal if untreated, may result in many nervous system problems. Meningitis is especially common in children during the late summer and early fall. In about one third of the children, no organism can be found. The fluid of the brain and spinal cord shows white blood cells but no bacteria. Complete recovery, without complication or lasting problems, is usual. Except for adenine arabinoside, advised for herpes simplex meningitis, there is no specific treatment for viral infections of the meninges. Antifungus drugs given for several weeks may prevent death from fungal meningitis. Bacterial meningitis is treated with antibiotics.

meningocele /mining'gōsēl'/, a saclike bulge of either the brain or spinal membranes (meninges) through a defect in the skull or the spinal column. It forms a lump (hernial cyst) that is filled with fluid from the brain and the spine. It does not contain nerve tissue. Treatment includes surgery. See also **neural tube defect.**

meningococcal polysaccharide vaccine /-kok'əl/, either of two active drugs used to fight meningococcal disease bacteria. It is used for vaccination against meningococcal meningitis. Reduction of the natural resistance to disease or sudden infection prohibits its use. Side effects include a severe allergic reaction.

meningococcemia /-koksē'mē·ə/, a disease caused by bacteria (*Neisseria meningitidis*) in the blood. Symptoms include chills, pain in the muscles and joints, headache, pinhead-sized spots of bleeding under the skin, sore throat, and collapse. Other symptoms are rapid heart beat with fast breathing and pulse rate. Body temperature may rise and fall. Treatment includes antibiotics.

meningococcus /-kok'əs/, a germ (bacterium) often found in the nose and throat of persons who are carriers, but not ill themselves. The organism may cause blood poisoning or spinal meningitis. Crowded conditions, as may be found in army camps, group the number of carriers together and reduce some people's ability to resist the disease. Bleeding beneath the skin is a major clue to the diagnosis. Treatment includes antibiotics. Several meningococcal vaccines are available. See also **meningitis.** –**meningococcal,** *adj.*

meningoencephalocele /-ensef'əlōsēl'/, a saclike lump (cyst) that contains brain tissue, cerebrospinal fluid, and the brain's covering (meninges). It pushes through a defect in the skull. The condition is often linked to other defects in the brain. See also **neural tube defect.**

meniscectomy /men'isek'-/, an operation to remove the crescent-shaped cartilage of the knee joint. Long-term pain from a torn cartilage and unstable or locking of the joint are the usual reasons for surgery.

meniscus /minis'kəs/, a curved part of cartilage in the knees and other joints. A **discoid meniscus** is an abnormal condition in which the meniscus of the knee is shaped like a disk rather than the normal half-moon. The outside of the cartilage is most often affected, although the inner part may also be involved. The condition occurs more often in children between 6 and 8 years of age. Common complaints are that a ''clicking'' occurs in the knee joint or that the knee joint gives way.

Menke's kinky hair syndrome /men'kēz/, a disorder affecting the normal absorption of copper from the intestine. It features the growth of sparse, kinky hair. Infants with the disorder have brain problems, slowed growth, and early death. Early diagnosis and injections of copper may stop brain damage.

menometrorrhagia /men'ōmet'rôrā'jə/, excess menstrual and uterine bleeding that is not caused by menstruation. It may be a sign of cancer, especially cancer of the cervix.

menopause /men'əpôz/, the end of menstruation, generally meaning the period ending the female reproductive phase of life (climacteric). Menses stop naturally with the decline of monthly hormonal cylces between 45 and 60 years of age. It may stop earlier in life as a result of illness or the surgical removal of the uterus or both ovaries. As the production of estrogen by the ovaries and pituitary gonad stimulating hormones decreases, ovulation and menstruation happen less often and eventually stop. Variations in the circulating levels of the hormones occur as the levels decline. Hot flushes are the only general symptom of menopause that nearly every woman has. They can often be controlled with estrogen but will stop in time without hormonal treatment. Occasionally, heavy irregular bleeding occurs at this time, usually linked to fiberlike tumors or other uterine disorders. Estrogens may be effective.

menorrhagia /men'ôrā'jə/, abnormally heavy or long menstrual periods. Menorrhagia occurs sometimes during the reproductive years of most women's lives. If the condition becomes long-term, anemia may result. Abnormal bleeding after menopause always needs to be checked to rule out cancer. Menorrhagia often results from fiberlike tumors of the uterus.

menostasis /mənos'təsis/, an abnormal condition in which the products of menstruation cannot leave the uterus or vagina because of a blockage of the cervix or the opening of the vagina.

menotropins /men'ətrop'ins/, a preparation of gonad-stimulating hormones from the urine of women who have gone through menopause. They are given with chorionic gonadotropin to cause ovulation in women and to make sperm (spermatogenesis) in men. High gonad-stimulating hormone levels in the urine, thyroid or adrenal gland problems, pituitary gland tumor, abnormal bleeding, ovarian lumps (cysts), pregnancy, or known allergy to this drug prohibits its use. Side effects include too much stimulation of the ovaries, blood clots, multiple pregnancies, and possible birth defects.

Menrium, a trademark for a drug for menopause symptoms. It contains estrogens and a sedative (chlordiazepoxide).

menses /men'sēz/, the normal flow of blood and cast-off uterine cells that occurs during menstruation. The first day of the flow of the menses is the first day of the menstrual cycle.

menstrual age, the age of an embryo or fetus as counted from the first day of the last menstrual period.

M–N

menstrual cycle, the repeating cycle of change in the membrane lining (endometrium) of the uterus. The temporary layer of the endometrium sheds during menstruation. It then regrows, thickens, is kept for several days through ovulation, and sheds again at the next menstruation. The average length of the cycle, from the first day of bleeding of one cycle to the first of another, is 28 days. However, the length and character vary greatly among individual women. Menstrual cycles begin at puberty. They end with the menopause. There are three phases of the cycle. The **proliferative phase** is the one following menstruation when the lining of the uterus becomes thick and rich in blood supply. The phase ends with releasing of the egg (ovulation). The **secretory phase** follows the release of the egg (ovum) from the ovaries. The **menstrual phase,** the last of the three phases, is the one in which menstruation occurs. The cast off lining of the endometrium is shed and bleeding occurs, leaving the permanent layer (stratum basale). The days of the menstrual cycle are counted from the first day of the menstrual phase.

menstruation, the periodic discharge through the vagina from the nonpregnant uterus. It is made up of a bloody mass containing cast-off tissue from the shedding of the membrane lining (endometrium). The average length of menstruation is 4 to 5 days. **Anovular menstruation** is menstrual bleeding that occurs even though an egg has not been released from the ovary (ovulation). The egg (ovum) either stays in the follicle and breaks down or in rare cases is fertilized. This causes an ovarian pregnancy. **Retrograde menstruation** is a backflow of menstrual fluids through the uterine space and the fallopian tubes into the abdomen space. Pieces of matter from the uterus may become joined to the ovaries or other organs, causing endometriosis. **Vicarious menstruation** refers to bleeding from a site other than the uterus at the time when menstruation is normally expected. Such bleeding is caused by the small blood vessels releasing more blood during menstruation. See also **menstrual cycle.** –**menstruate,** v.

mental, relating to, or characteristic of, the mind (psyche).

mental handicap, any mental defect resulting from a birth defect, serious injury, or disease that causes thinking problems and prevents a person from taking part in activities normal for a particular age group. See also **mental retardation.**

mental health, a state of mind in which a person who is healthy is able to cope with and adjust to the stresses of everyday living.

mental illness, any disorder of emotional balance, as shown in abnormal behavior or mental problems. It is caused by genetic, physical, chemical, biologic, mental, or social and cultural factors.

mental retardation, a disorder marked by less than average general intellectual function with problems in the ability to learn and to act socially. The disorder is twice as common among males as among females. It may be named according to the intelligence quotient as: borderline, IQ 71 to 84; mild, IQ 50 to 70; moderate, IQ 35 to 49; severe, IQ 20 to 34; and profound, IQ below 20. Treatment is made up of educational programs and training according to the level of retardation. Emphasis is placed on prevention, as genetic counseling, and checking the amniotic fluid for defects (amniocentesis).

menthol, a drug with a cooling effect that relieves discomfort and itching. It is part of many skin creams and ointments.

mentholated camphor, a mixture of equal parts of camphor and menthol used in drugs. It causes a surface inflammation so as to relieve one on a deeper level (counterirritant).

mepenzolate bromide, a drug used to treat stomach and intestine problems, and peptic ulcer. Narrow-angle glaucoma, asthma, blockage of the urinary or stomach and intestinal tracts, severe ulcerative colitis, or known allergy to this drug prohibits its use. Side effects include blurred vision, rapid heart beat, dry mouth, and allergic reactions.

Mepergan, a trademark for a central nervous system drug. It contains a narcotic (meperidine hydrochloride) and an antihistamine (promethazine hydrochloride).

meperidine hydrochloride, a narcotic painkiller used to treat moderate to severe pain. It is also used before surgery to relieve pain and anxiety. Head injuries, asthma, kidney or liver problems, unstable heart condition, simultaneous use of a monoamine oxidase inhibitor, or known allergy to this drug prohibits its use. Side effects include drowsiness, dizziness, nausea, constipation, sweating, difficulty in breathing, slowed blood circulation, and drug addiction.

mephenytoin, a drug used to control seizures in epilepsy when less dangerous drugs have not been effective. It is seldom used during pregnancy. Known allergy to this drug or to any hydantoin prohibits its use. Side effects include rash, fever, liver disorders, and various blood problems. The frequency of side effects limits the use of this drug.

mephobarbital, a sedative drug used to fight convulsions. It is given to treat anxiety, nervous tension, inability to sleep, and epilepsy. An inherited disorder (porphyria) or known allergy to this drug or to barbiturates prohibits its use. Side effects include drug addiction, lack of vitamin D, excitement, skin rash, and stomach upset.

Mephyton, a trademark for a vitamin K product (phytonadione).

meprobamate, a sedative used to treat anxiety and tension and as a muscle relaxer.

meralgia paresthetica /meral'jə per'əsthet'ikə/, a condition with pain, tingling, and numbness on the surface of the thigh. The cause is that a nerve is trapped in the inguinal ligament, which extends from the hipbone to the pubic bone.

mercaptopurine, an anticancer and immune-suppressing drug used to treat many cancers, including acute lymphocytic leukemia.

mercurial diuretic, any one of several drugs that have mercury. Mercurial diuretics prevent sodium and chloride from being reabsorbed and potassium from being released through the kidney. The main use for the drugs is to treat fluid pooling from heart disease, cirrhosis of the liver, or lack of urine in kidney disease. Side effects include blood disorders, mercury poisoning, harsh allergic reactions, flushing, hives, fever, nausea, and vomiting.

mercury (Hg), a metal element used in dental devices, thermometers, and blood pressure measuring instruments. It forms many poisonous compounds.

mercury poisoning, a serious condition caused by swallowing or breathing mercury or a mercury compound. A long-term form results from breathing the vapors or dust of mercury compounds or from repeated swallowing of very small amounts. It leads to irritability, excess saliva, loosened teeth, gum disorders, slurred speech, trembling, and staggering. Symptoms of sudden mercury poisoning include a metal taste in the mouth, thirst, nausea, vomiting, severe stomach pain, bloody diarrhea, and kidney failure that may result in death. Treatment includes flushing the stomach with milk and egg white or baking soda (sodium bicarbonate), and drugs that help release the poison from the body. Free mercury, as in thermometers, is not absorbed by the stomach or intestines. Mercury compounds are found in farming chemicals and in certain antiseptics and dyes. They are used heavily in industry. Industrial wastes containing mercury have been located in some areas. Seafood from contaminated waters has caused serious public health problems.

mercy killing. See **euthanasia.**

Merthiolate, a trademark for a drug for skin infections (thimerosal).

Meruvax, a trademark for an active vaccinating drug (live rubella virus vaccine).

Mesantoin, a trademark for a drug to control convulsions (mephenytoin).

mescaline /mes'kəlēn/, a mind-altering, poisonous alkaline drug. It comes from the flowering heads of a cactus. Closely related chemically to epinephrine, mescaline causes an irregular heart rate, sweating, widened eye pupils, anxiety, and hallucinations of sight. Also called **peyote.**

mesencephalon /mes'ensef'əlon/. See **brain.**

mesenteric node /mes'enter'ik/, a lymph gland in in one of three groups serving parts of the intestine. The mesenteric nodes receive lymph from the small and large intestine and the appendix.

mesentery proper /mes'enter'ē/, a broad, fan-shaped fold of stomach wall membrane (peritoneum). It connects the membranes of the small intestine (jejunum and ileum) with the back wall of the abdomen. It holds the small intestine and various nerves and arteries of the abdomen.

mesioversion /mē'zē·ō·vur'zhən/, **1.** a condition in which one or more teeth are closer than normal to the middle. **2.** a condition in which the upper or lower jaw is farther forward than normal.

mesoderm /mes'ōdrum/. See **embryonic layer.**

mesomorph /-môrf/. See **somatotype.**

mesonephric duct /-nef'rik/, a duct of the human embryo. It creates in the male the passageways of the reproductive system. In the female, it becomes part of the ligament of the ovaries.

mesoridazine besylate, a tranquilizer used to treat psychotic disorders, behavior problems in mental diseases, and alcoholism. Parkinson's disease, use at the same time of central nervous system depressant drugs, liver or kidney problems, falling blood pressure, or known allergy to this drug or similar drugs prohibits its use. Side effects include low blood pressure, liver problems, many nerve and brain reactions, blood disorders, and allergic reactions.

mesothelioma /-thē'lē·ō'mə/, a cancer of the membranes of the lungs, heart, or stomach. It is linked to earlier contact with asbestos. The tumor may form thick sheets covering the internal organs. The outlook for recovery is poor.

mesothelium /-thē'lē·əm/, a layer of cells that lines the body cavities of the embryo. It continues after birth as a covering on membranes, as the pleura of the chest and pericardium of the heart.

message center, part of the communications center and collocated or placed adjacent to it. It receives, records, and routes information about resources reporting to the incident, resource status, and administration and tactical traffic.

messenger RNA. See **ribonucleic acid.**

Mestinon, a trademark for a nerve and muscle blocking drug (pyridostigmine). It is used as an aid to anesthesia and to treat myasthenia gravis.

mestranol /mes'trənōl/, an estrogen combined in some drugs with a progestin as a birth control pill.

metabolic /met'əbol'ik/, referring to **metabolism.**

metabolic acidosis. See **acidosis.**

metabolic alkalosis. See **alkalosis.**

metabolic disorder, any disorder that interferes with normal digestion and use of food in the body.

M–

metabolic equivalent (MET), the amount of oxygen taken in per kilogram of body weight per minute when a person is at rest.

metabolic rate, the amount of energy released or used in a given unit of time. The metabolic rate is listed in calories as the amount of heat released during metabolism at the cell level.

metabolism /mətab′əlizm/, the sum of all chemical processes that take place in the body as they relate to the movement of nutrients in the blood after digestion, resulting in growth, energy, release of wastes, and other body functions. Metabolism takes place in two steps. The first step is the constructive phase (anabolism). Smaller molecules (amino acids) are converted to larger molecules (proteins). The second step is the destructive phase (catabolism). Larger molecules (as glycogen) are converted to smaller molecules (as glucose). Exercise, body temperature, hormone activity, and digestion can increase the rate of metabolism. **Carbohydrate metabolism** refers to the sum of the building up and breaking down of carbohydrates in the body. This mainly involves galactose, fructose, and glucose. **Cholesterol metabolism** refers to the chemical processes involving cholesterol in the body. Cholesterol is quickly absorbed from foods. It is also made in the liver and most other tissues in the body. As more cholesterol is eaten, less is produced. See also **acid-base metabolism, anabolism, basal metabolism, catabolism.** –**metabolic,** *adj.*

metabolite /-līt/, a substance made by metabolic action or one necessary for a metabolic process. An essential metabolite is one needed for an important metabolic process. For example, urea and ammonia are metabolites of proteins.

metacarpus /me′təkär′pəs/, the middle portion of the hand. It consists of five slender bones numbered from the thumb side, metacarpals I through V. –**metacarpal,** *adj., n.*

Metahydrin, a trademark for a diuretic used in the treatment of high blood pressure (trichlormethiazide).

metal fume fever, a job-related disorder caused by breathing fumes of metal compounds. Symptoms are similar to those of influenza. Treatment of the symptoms usually relieve the condition.

metamorphopsia /-môrfop′sē·ə/, a defect in seeing. Objects are seen as distorted in shape, resulting from a disease of the retina, as a fluid leak at the back of the eye.

Metandren, a trademark for an androgen (methyltestosterone).

metaphyseal dysplasia /-fiz′ē·əl/, an abnormal condition of defective growth of the long bones. The ends of the affected bone (most often the femur or the tibia of the legs) become large and the middle becomes smaller.

metaproterenol sulfate, a bronchial tube widening drug. It is given in the treatment of bronchial asthma. Irregular heart rhythms linked to rapid heart beat or known allergy to this drug prohibits its use. Side effects include rapid heart beat, high blood pressure, and heart attack.

metaraminol bitartrate, a drug used to restore blood pressure. It is given to treat very low blood pressure and shock that may occur after surgery. Known allergy to this drug prohibits its use. Side effects include irregular heart rhythms, tissue damage at the injection site, high blood pressure, tremors, and nausea.

metastasis /mətas′təsis/, *pl.* **metastases,** the tumor or the process by which tumor cells are spread to distant parts of the body. Because cancers have no enclosing capsule, their cells may escape and be transported by the lymph circulation or the bloodstream to hook onto lymph nodes and other organs far from the original tumor. –**metastatic,** *adj.,* **metastasize,** *v.*

metatarsalgia /-tärsal′jə/, a painful condition around the foot bones. It is caused by new calcium formations or another abnormality of the foot.

metatarsus /-tär′səs/, a part of the foot, made up of five bones numbered I to V, from the large toe. Each bone has a long, slender body, and connects with the first row of toe bones (phalanges) at the outer end. –**metatarsal,** *adj.*

Metatensin, a trademark for a heart drug. It contains a diuretic (trichlormethiazide) and a high blood pressure drug (reserpine).

meteorism, gathering of gas in the stomach or the intestine, usually with a bloated abdomen.

meteorotropism /mē′tē·ərətrō′pizm/, a body reaction to influences of climate shown by biologic occurrences, as sudden death, attacks of arthritis, and chest pain (angina) during weather changes. –**meteorotropic,** *adj.*

meter (m), a metric unit of length equal to 39.37 inches.

methacycline hydrochloride, an antibiotic given to treat many infections. Kidney or liver disease, pregnancy, early childhood, or known allergy to this drug or similar drugs prohibits its use. Side effects include stomach and intestinal problems, sensitivity to light, additional infections, and allergic reactions. Discoloration of teeth may occur in children exposed to the drug before 8 years of age.

methadone hydrochloride, a narcotic drug used for anesthesia or as a substitute for heroin. It allows withdrawal without severe reactions. It is not given to pregnant women or to patients with liver disease.

methanol, a clear, colorless, toxic, liquid distilled from wood. Drinking methanol paralyzes the eye nerve. It may cause death. Also called **wood alcohol.**

metharbital, drug used to treat epilepsy. Known allergy to barbiturates prohibits its use. It is used with care in pregnancy or liver disease. Side effects include loss of voluntary muscle control, irritability in children, confusion in elderly patients, rashes, and other allergic reactions.

methazolamide, a diuretic drug given to treat glaucoma.

methdilazine, an antihistamine. It is given to relieve itching. Asthma, glaucoma, or known allergy to this drug or similar drugs prohibits its use. It is not given to newborn infants or nursing mothers. Side effects include bone marrow disorders, involuntary muscle movements, dry mouth, and drowsiness.

methemoglobin /met·hē′məglō′bin/, a form of hemoglobin in which the iron is changed so it cannot carry oxygen and thus does not help the normal breathing of body tissues. See also **hemoglobin.**

methenamine, an antibiotic given to treat urinary tract infections. Liver or kidney disease or known allergy to this drug or to similar drugs prohibits its use. Side effects include severe stomach and intestinal disturbances and rashes.

Methergine, a trademark for a drug that causes the uterus to contract, to control bleeding after childbirth (methylergonovine maleate).

methicillin sodium, an antibiotic given mostly in the treatment of severe penicillin-immune staphylococcal infections. Known allergy to this drug or to any penicillin prohibits its use. Side effects include vein inflammation at the injection site, kidney problems, and allergic reactions.

methionine (Met), amino acid needed for proper growth in infants and for nitrogen balance in adults. It is also given in the treatment of liver diseases.

methocarbamol, a drug used to treat skeletal muscle spasms. Kidney disease, central nervous system defects, or known allergy to this drug prohibits its use. Side effects include low blood pressure, rapid heart beat, drowsiness, dizziness, and nausea.

method, a technique or procedure for creating a desired effect, as a surgical procedure, a laboratory test, or a diagnostic technique.

methotrexate, an anticancer drug used to treat severe skin inflammation (psoriasis) and many cancers.

methoxsalen, a drug applied to the skin to increase skin darkening (pigmentation). It is also given for repigmentation in loss of skin color (vitiligo). Liver disease, use at the same time of any drug that may cause light sensitivity reactions, or known allergy to this drug prohibits its use. Side effects include central nervous system effects, skin burns, stomach and intestinal discomfort, and allergic reactions.

methscopolamine bromide, a drug used to treat overactivity of the stomach and intestines and to treat peptic ulcer. Glaucoma, asthma, blockage of the tract or of the stomach or intestines, severe ulcerative colitis, or known allergy to this drug prohibits its use. Side effects include blurred vision, central nervous system effects, rapid heart beat, dry mouth, little sweating, or allergic reactions.

methsuximide, a drug used to treat convulsions in petit mal epilepsy. Known allergy to this drug or to any similar drug prohibits its use. Side effects include blood disorders, liver and kidney damage, and a nervous system disease (systemic lupus erythematosus).

methyclothiazide, a diuretic and high blood pressure drug. It is given to treat high blood pressure and pooling of fluid (edema).

methylbenzethonium chloride, an antiinfective skin medication. It is given for the prevention and treatment of diaper rash and other skin disorders. Known allergy to this drug prohibits its use. Local skin irritation may occur.

methylcellulose, a bulk-forming laxative given to treat constipation. Appendicitis, serious disease of the stomach, intestine problems, intestine blockage or stomach ulcer, or known allergy to this drug prohibits its use. Side effects include blockage of the intestines and more constipation if not enough fluids are drunk.

methyldopa, a drug given to reduce high blood pressure.

methylergonovine maleate, an drug given to prevent or to treat failure of the uterus to return to normal size, bleeding, or other problems after childbirth. It is not given during pregnancy or given by injection into a vein, except in life-threatening situations. High blood pressure, general body poisoning, or known allergy to ergot alkaloid drugs prohibits its use. Side effects include high blood pressure, nausea, blurred sight, headaches, convulsions, and death. Side effects are more common after giving the drug by intravenous (IV) injection.

methylphenidate hydrochloride, a central nervous system stimulating drug. It is given to treat overactivity in children and to treat a sleep disorder (narcolepsy) in adults. Glaucoma, severe anxiety, tension, mental depression, or known allergy to this drug prohibits its use. It is not given to children under 6 years of age. Side effects include nervousness, inability to sleep, loss of appetite, allergic reactions, and rapid heart beat.

methylprednisolone, an adrenal hormone given to treat inflammatory conditions, including rheumatic fever and rheumatoid arthritis.

methyltestosterone, a male sex hormone given to treat a lack of testosterone, bone weakening (osteoporosis), and female breast cancer. It is also given to stimulate growth, weight gain, and the making of red blood cells. Cancer of the male breast or prostate, heart, kidney, or liver disease, excess blood calcium, known or suspected pregnancy, breast feeding, or known allergy to this drug prohibits its

M–N

use. Side effects include excess blood calcium, the pooling of fluids, male features in female patients, and liver disease (jaundice).

methyprylon, a sedative and hypnotic drug used to treat an inability to sleep (insomnia). Known allergy to this drug prohibits its use. Side effects include dizziness, excitability, headache, rash, and stomach upset.

methysergide maleate, a blood vessel relaxing drug used to relieve migraine headache. Pregnancy, severe infection, liver or kidney disorders, heart, lung, or circulation system disease, or known allergy to this drug prohibits its use. It is not to be given to children. Side effects includee mild upset stomach and heartburn.

Meticorten, a trademark for an adrenal hormone (prednisone).

metoclopramide hydrochloride, a stomach and intestinal stimulating drug. It is given to stimulate stomach activity, to increase the strength of stomach contractions and to stop vomiting. Epilepsy, use at the same time of drugs that cause nervous system reactions, adrenal gland disorders, stomach bleeding, blockage, or ulcer, or known allergy to this drug prohibits its use. Side effects include central nervous system reactions, usually in children, stomach and intestinal disturbances, drowsiness, and allergic reactions.

metolazone, a drug used to treat fluid pooling (edema) and high blood pressure.

metoprolol tartrate, a nerve signal blocker drug. It is given to treat high blood pressure. Slow heart rate, heart diseases, breathing disorders, or known allergy to this drug prohibits its use. Side effects include fatigue, abnormally slow heart rate, lung spasms, and stomach upset.

metralgia /mətral′jə/, tenderness or pain in the uterus.

Metreton, a trademark for an adrenal hormone (prednisolone sodium phosphate).

metric equivalent, any value in metric units of measurement that equals the same value in English units, as 2.54 centimeters equal 1 inch or 1 liter equals 1.0567 quarts.

metric system, a decimal system of measurement based on the meter (39.37 inches) as the unit of length. The gram (15.432 grains) is the unit of weight or mass. The liter (0.908 US dry quart or 1.0567 US liquid quart) is the unit of volume.

metritis /mətrī′-/, inflammation of the walls of the uterus. Kinds of metritis are **endometritis** and **parametritis.**

metronidazole, an drug given to treat infections from amebas, certain bacteria, and *Trichomonas.* First three months of pregnancy, blood disorders, central nervous system disorders, or known allergy to this drug prohibits its

use. Side effects include severe stomach and intestinal distress, dizziness, blood disorders, nervous system problems, and a metal taste in the mouth.

metrorrhagia /met′rôrā′jə/, uterine bleeding other than that caused by menstruation. It may be caused by tumors in the uterus or may be a sign of a cancer of the urinary and genital glands, especially cervical cancer.

Metubine, a trademark for a neuromuscular blocking drug (metocurine iodide). It is used to assist in anesthesia.

metyrapone, a diagnostic test drug. It is used to test hypothalamus and pituitary gland functions.

metyrosine, a high blood pressure drug. It is given to treat an adrenal gland disorder. Known allergy to this drug prohibits its use. Side effects include central nervous system reactions, drowsiness, diarrhea, and anxiety.

Meynet's node /mānāz′/, any of the many small bumps that may develop in the capsules surrounding joints and in tendons affected by rheumatic diseases, especially in children.

Mezlin, a trademark for a partly artificial penicillin antibiotic (mezlocillin sodium).

mezlocillin sodium, an antibiotic given for respiratory, abdominal, urinary tract, gynecologic, and skin infections. It is also given for bacterial blood poisoning. Allergy to any of the penicillins prohibits its use. Side effects include excess sensitivity, convulsions, abdominal pain, blood disorders, and changes in liver and kidney functions.

mg, abbreviation for **milligram.**

miconazole nitrate, an antifungus drug used to treat certain fungus infections of the skin and vagina. It is also injected to treat systemic fungus infections. Known allergy to this drug prohibits its use. Side effects of skin or vaginal use are irritation and burning. When used by injection, nausea, itching, vein inflammation, and anemia may occur.

microangiopathy /mī′krō·an′jē·op′əthē/, a disease of the small blood vessels in which a membrane of capillaries thickens (diabetic microangiopathy) or in which clots form in the arterioles and the capillaries (thrombotic microangiopathy).

microbe /mī′krōb/, a microorganism. –**microbial,** *adj.*

microcephaly /-sef′əlē/, a birth defect with an abnormally small head in relation to the rest of the body. It leads to slowed growth of the brain with some degree of mental retardation. The face is generally normal. The cause may be heredity, an accident while an embryo or fetus, as exposure to irradiation, chemical agents, or mother's infection, or an injury, especially during the last 3 months of pregnancy.

microcheiria /-kī′rē·ə/, a birth defect with abnormally small hands. The condition is often linked to bone and muscle disorders.

microcurie, a one-millionth part of a curie (see **curie**) or 37,000 disintegrations per second. Abbreviation: μCi.

microcyte /mī′krəsīt/, an abnormally small red blood cell. It often occurs in iron deficiency and other anemias.

microdactyly /-dak′tilē/, a birth defect with abnormally small fingers and toes. The condition is usually linked to bone and muscle disorders.

micrognathia /-nā′thē·ə/, slowed growth of the jaw, especially the lower jaw.

micromelic dwarf /-mel′ik/, a dwarf whose arms and legs are abnormally short.

Micronor, a trademark for a birth control pill. It contains a progestin (norethindrone).

micronutrient /-noo′trē·ənt/, an organic compound, as a vitamin, or a chemical element, as zinc or iodine. Micronutrients are needed only in small amounts for the normal processes of the body. Also called **trace element.**

microorganism, a tiny animal or plant able to carry on living processes. It may or may not be a cause of disease. Kinds of microorganisms include **bacteria, fungi, protozoa, viruses.**

microphage /mī′krəfāj/, a white blood cell able to take in and digest small things, as bacteria.

microphthalmos /mī′krofthal′məs/, a birth defect with abnormal smallness of one or both eyes.

micropodia /-pō′dē·ə/, a birth defect with abnormal smallness of the feet. The condition is often linked to other defects or to bone disorders.

micropsia /mīkrop′sē·ə/, an abnormal condition of seeing, in which objects are seen as smaller than they really are. It often occurs during hallucinations. –**microptic,** *adj.*

microscopic, referring to very small objects, visible only when seen with a microscope.

microsomia /-sō′mē·ə/, a condition of an abnormally small and underdeveloped, yet otherwise perfectly formed body with normal relationships of the various parts.

microthermy /-thur′mē/, a treatment in which heat is given off by radio waves. It is used in physical therapy.

micturition reflex /mik′tərish′ən/, a normal reaction to a rise in fluid pressure within the urinary bladder. It causes the bladder wall to contract and a circular band of muscle (sphincter) to relax and open the urethra. This results in a flow of urine. Voluntary control of this reflex normally prevents undesired urination, as occurs in infancy.

Midamor, a trademark for a diuretic (amiloride hydrochloride).

middle cardiac vein, one of five blood veins of the heart muscle.

middle ear. See **ear.**

middle lobe syndrome, a local collapse of the middle lobe of the right lung. It is linked to a long-term infection, cough, wheezing, and inflammation of the lung. Blockage of the tube from the throat (bronchus) may occur. The middle lobe bronchus is thus put under pressure, with collapse resulting in the blocked part of the lung. Treatment includes antituberculosis drugs, adrenal gland hormones, or surgical removal of the lobe.

Midrin, a trademark for a central nervous system drug. It contains a nerve impulse stimulant (isometheptene mucate), a tranquilizer (dichloralphenazone), and a painkiller (acetaminophen). It is used to treat migraine headaches.

midstream catch urine specimen, a urine specimen collected during the middle of a flow of urine. Some medical laboratories need the midstream catch urine for certain tests, rather than a urine sample containing the first or last part of the flow.

midwife, a person who assists women in childbirth. Among the responsibilities of the midwife are overseeing the woman's pregnancy, labor, delivery, and recovery after birth. The midwife may get the help of a physician when necessary or handle emergency measures as required.

migraine /mī′grān/, a throbbing headache, usually occurring on only one side of the head. There are severe pain, sensitivity to light, and other disturbances during the first phase. Attacks may last for hours or days. The disorder occurs more often in women than in men. Migraine may be inherited. The exact cause is not known. The head pain is related to widening of blood vessels, which may result from chemical changes that cause spasms of the vessels. Allergic reactions, excess carbohydrates, iodine-rich foods, alcohol, bright lights, or loud noises can begin attacks. Migraine may begin with sensations called auras. These may be seeing disturbances, as flashing lights or wavy lines, or a strange taste or odor. Other disturbances are tingling, dizziness, ringing in the ears, or a feeling that part of the body is distorted in size or shape. The first phase may also include nausea, vomiting, chills, excess urination, sweating, swollen face, irritability, and extreme tiredness. After an attack the patient often has dull head and neck pains and a great need for sleep. Aspirin seldom helps. Drugs that narrow arteries of the head can usually stop the headache from developing if taken early enough. **Migrainous cranial neuralgia,** also called **cluster headache,** is a variation of migraine. It features very painful, throbbing headaches. Other symptoms include sweating, tears, a runny nose, droopy eyelids, and swelling of the face. The headaches usually occur in groups within a few days or weeks. A long period without a headache may

M–N

follow. A usual attack begins suddenly with a burning sensation in an eye or temple. The resulting pain may last 1 or 2 hours. The pain may be helped by antihistamines.

migratory polyarthritis /mī'grətôr'ē/, arthritis of a number of joints, one after another, and finally settling in one or several. It occurs in patients with gonorrhea. Symptoms include a light fever and 1 to 5 days of pain in various joints, with signs of inflammation. Large joints are most affected. After the swelling goes down the skin over the joint may peel.

migratory thrombophlebitis, an abnormal condition in which blood clots in both deep veins and those near the skin. It may be linked to cancer, especially cancer of the pancreas. The disorder often shows up several months before other signs of cancer. See also **phlebitis.**

Mikulicz's syndrome /mik'yoolich'ēz/, an abnormal swelling of the saliva glands and tear glands. It is found in many diseases, including leukemia and tuberculosis.

mild, referring to gentleness, subtlety, or low intensity, as a mild infection.

miliaria /mil'ē·er'ē·ə/. See **heat rash.**

miliary /mil'ē·er'ē/, describing a condition with very small tumors, the size of millet seeds.

milium, *pl.* **milia,** a very small, white lump (cyst) of the skin. It is caused by a blockage of hair follicles and sweat glands. One kind is seen in newborn infants. It disappears within a few weeks. Another type is found mainly on the faces of middle-aged women. Milia may be treated with a harsh cleanser or by cutting and draining. Also called **whitehead.**

milk, a liquid released by the mammary glands of animals that suckle their young. It is a valuable nutrient for children and adults. It is nearly a complete food for infants, especially breast milk. Milk does not contain the necessary amount of iron. Its vitamin C content depends on the amount in the mother or the animal making the milk. Some persons show an allergic reaction to milk because of a lack of the enzyme lactase. See also **breast milk.**

milk baby, an infant with iron deficiency anemia. It is caused by drinking excess amounts of milk without adding iron-rich foods in the diet. Milk babies are overweight and have pale skin and poor muscle growth. They are likely to get infections. See also **anemia.**

milk-ejection reflex, a normal reflex in a nursing mother. It is caused by stimulation of the nipple, resulting in release of milk from the glands of the breast. Also called **let-down reflex.**

milker's nodule, a smooth, brownish-red tumor of the fingers or palm. The disease comes from tumors on the udder of a cow infected with cowpox virus. No treatment is needed.

milk fever, *nontechnical.* a fever that starts with the beginning of milk release (lactation) in the female breast. It means an infection is present.

milking, a way to release the contents of a duct or tube, to test for tenderness, or to get a sample for study. The examiner presses the structure with a finger and moves the finger firmly along the duct or tube to its opening. Also called **stripping.**

milk leg, inflammation with blood clotting in the vein of the upper leg (femoral), resulting in swelling and pain. It may occur after a severe illness with fever, or childbirth. Also called **phlegmasia alba dolens.**

milk of magnesia, a laxative and antacid containing magnesium hydroxide. It is given to relieve constipation and acid indigestion. Kidney disease, symptoms of appendicitis, or known allergy to this drug prohibits its use. Side effects include diarrhea and excess blood magnesium, usually occuring in patients who have kidney disease.

milk therapy, a food treatment for Curling's ulcer in patients who have been severely burned. Cool, homogenized milk is given in doses of 1 to 2 ounces (30 ml to 60 ml) every hour through a nose tube. As the milk is better absorbed and tolerated, feedings are increased. See also **ulcer.**

millicurie, a one-thousandth part of a curie (see **curie**) or 37 million disintegrations per second. Abbreviation: mCi.

milligram (mg), a metric unit of weight equal to one thousandth (10^{-3}) of a gram.

milliliter (ml), a metric unit of volume that is one thousandth (10^{-3}) of a liter.

millimeter (mm), a metric unit of length equal to one thousandth (10^{-3}) of a meter.

millirem, a one-thousandth part of a rem (see REM). Abbreviation: mrem.

milliroentgen, a one-thousandth part of a roentgen. Abbreviation: mR.

Milontin, a trademark for a drug used to treat convulsions (phensuximide).

Milpath, a trademark for a stomach drug. It contains a nerve drug (tridihexethyl chloride) and a drug to help the patient sleep (meprobamate).

Milprem, a trademark for a drug containing female sex hormones and a drug to help the patient sleep (meprobamate).

Miltown, a trademark for a drug to help the patient sleep (meprobamate).

Miltrate, a trademark for a heart drug. It contains a blood vessel widener (pentaerythritol tetranitrate) and a drug to help the patient sleep (meprobamate).

Milwaukee brace, a device that helps to keep the torso and the neck of a patient rigid. It is used to treat or correct spinal deformities. It is usually made of strong but light metal and fiberglass supports lined with rubber to protect against rubbing.

Minamata disease /min′əmä′tə/, a severe, wasting nerve disorder. It is caused by eating seed grain cooked with water containing mercury or of seafood taken from waters polluted with industrial mercury wastes. The term is taken from a tragedy involving Japanese who ate seafood from Minamata Bay. See also **mercury poisoning.**

mind, the part of the brain that is the seat of mental actions. It allows one to know, reason, understand, remember, think, feel, react, and adapt to all external and internal stimulations or surroundings.

mineral, 1. an inorganic substance occurring naturally in the earth's crust. It has a certain chemical makeup and, usually, a crystal-like structure. 2. a nutrient that is eaten in food as a compound, such as table salt (sodium chloride), rather than as a free element. Minerals are important in regulating many body functions.

mineral deficiency, the inability to use one or more of the mineral elements needed for human nutrition. Causes may be a birth defect, digestive disorder, or lack of that mineral in the diet. The symptoms vary, depending on the specific functions of the element in helping growth and keeping the body healthy. Minerals are part of all the body tissues and fluids. They act in nerve responses, muscle contractions, and the changes of nutrients in foods. They regulate electrolyte balance and the making of hormones. They strengthen skeletal structures. All mineral deficiencies are treated by adding the specific element to the diet, either as a pill or in the right foods. See also **electrolyte** and specific minerals.

mineralocorticoid, a hormone, released by the adrenal glands, that keeps blood volume normal. An excess of mineralocorticoid causes fluid to gather, high blood pressure, a lack of potassium, too much alkali, and a slight increase in salt in the blood. A lack of the hormone results in low blood pressure, collapse of the circulation, excess potassium, and heavy salt loss. Without the hormone an adult may lose as much as 25 g of salt a day. Injury and stress increase mineralocorticoid release.

mineral oil, a laxative, stool softener, skin softener, and solvent for dissolving substances for medicines. It is given to prevent and treat constipation. It is also given to prepare the bowel for surgery or examination. Symptoms of appendicitis, constipation, blockage or ulcer of the intestines, pregnancy, or known allergy to this drug prohibits its use. Side effects include laxative addiction, lack of vitamins, and stomach cramps.

Minerva cast, a body cast applied to the upper trunk and head, with spaces cut out for the face area and ears. The cast is used for keeping the head and part of the body rigid

in the treatment of neck and chest injuries and spinal infections in the neck. Also called **Minerva jacket.**

minimal care unit, a unit for the treatment of patients in a hospital who are able to move about and meet many of their own daily living needs but need some nursing care.

Minipress, a trademark for an anti-high-blood-pressure drug (prazosin hydrochloride).

Minocin, a trademark for an antibiotic (minocycline hydrochloride).

minocycline hydrochloride, an antibiotic given to treat many infections. Careful use is needed with kidney or liver disorders. Known allergy to this or similar antibiotics prohibits its use. Side effects include digestive disturbances, light sensitivity, loss of the sense of balance, and various allergic reactions. Use during pregnancy or in children under 8 years of age may result in discolored teeth.

minor surgery, any surgery procedure that does not need general anesthesia or breathing assistance.

minoxidil, a blood vessel widener. It is given to treat severe high blood pressure. Adrenal gland tumors or known allergy to this drug prohibits its use. The most serious side effects include rapid heart beat and other heart disorders, salt and water storing, excess hair growth, and digestive disturbances.

Mintezol, a trademark for a drug used to treat worm problems (thiabendazole).

Miochol, a trademark for a nerve blocking agent (acetylcholine chloride).

miosis /mī·ō′-/, 1. narrowing of the muscle of the iris, causing the pupil of the eye to become smaller. Certain drugs or an increase in light on the eye cause miosis. 2. an abnormal condition in which excess narrowing of the iris results in very small, pin-point pupils. Compare **mydriasis.**

Miostat, a trademark for a nerve signal stimulating drug (carbachol).

miotic /mī·ot′ik/, any substance or drug, as pilocarpine, that causes narrowing of the pupil of the eye. Such drugs are used to treat glaucoma.

Miradon, a trademark for a drug to prevent blood clots (anisindione).

miscarriage, an end of pregnancy before the twentieth week occurring by itself because of defects of the fetus or womb. More than 10% of pregnancies end as spontaneous abortions, almost all caused by defective eggs. **Inevitable abortion** refers to a condition in which sudden miscarriage cannot be prevented. There is bleeding, uterine cramping, widening of the cervix, and other symptoms. If heavy bleeding occurs, immediate emptying of the uterus may be required. A **threatened abortion** is a condition in pregnancy before the twentieth week of pregnancy. There is bleeding of the uterus and cramping sufficient to suggest

M–N

that miscarriage may result. It is generally managed with rest and observation. See also **abortion.**

missile fracture, a fracture caused by a fast-moving object, as a bullet or a piece of shrapnel.

mite, an insect with a flat, almost transparent body and four pairs of legs. Examples include chiggers and scabies mites. Some female mites burrow into the skin and lay eggs that hatch into larvae. The movements of the larvae cause heavy itching. See also **scabies.**

Mithracin, a trademark for an anticancer drug (plicamycin).

mitochondrion /mī′təkon′drē·on/, *pl.* **mitochondria,** a small, threadlike organ within the cytoplasm of a cell that controls cell life and breathing. Mitochondria are the main source of cell energy.

mitolactol /-lak′tôl/, an anticancer drug used for many cancers, including Hodgkin's disease.

mitomycin /-mī′sin/, an antibiotic given to treat certain cancers. Lack of clotting or other blood disorders or known allergy to this drug prohibits its use. Side effects include bone marrow disease, stomach and intestinal disturbances, hair loss, and skin reactions.

mitosis /mītō′-/, a type of cell division. It occurs in body cells and results in forming two identical cells, or daughter cells. Mitosis is the process by which the body makes new cells for both growth and repair of injured tissue. **Pathologic mitosis** refers to any cell division that is not typical and results in an unequal number of chromosomes. It usually causes a defect, as occurs in cancer and genetic disorders. Compare **meiosis.**

mitotane /mī′tətān/, an anticancer drug. It destroys normal and cancerous adrenal gland cells. It is given to treat cancer of the adrenal cortex. Known allergy to this drug prohibits its use. Side effects include stomach and intestinal symptoms, drowsiness, and hormone disorders.

mitral /mī′trəl/, referring to the mitral valve of the heart.

mitral regurgitation, a lesion of the mitral valve of the heart that causes the flow of blood back into the upper chamber (left atrium) from the lower chamber (left ventricle). Symptoms include breathing discomfort, fatigue, and irregular heart rate. The condition may result from a birth defect. Other causes are rheumatic fever, expansion of the left ventricle, and inflammation of the heart muscle. Congestive heart failure may eventually occur. Treatment depends on the cause. Surgery may be needed in cases of congestive heart failure. Also called **mitral insufficiency.** See also **valvular heart disease.**

mitral valve. See **heart valve.**

mitral valve prolapse (MVP), a failure of the mitral valve to close properly, causing a flow of blood back into the upper chamber of the heart (left atrium). It is caused by one or both small flaps (cusps) of the mitral valve sticking back into the atrium during narrowing of the lower chamber (ventricle). Most patients feel no symptoms. Some may have chest pain, an irregular heart rate, weakness, or breathing difficulty. The condition may lead to swelling of the left side of the heart. See also **valvular heart disease.**

mittelschmerz /mit′əlshmerts/, lower abdominal pain in the area of an ovary during ovulation. It usually occurs in the middle of the menstrual cycle. For many women, mittelschmerz is useful in identifying ovulation. Thus they know the time when pregnancy is most likely to occur.

mixed connective tissue disease (MCTD), a disorder with the combined symptoms of two or more diseases that affect connective tissue such as synovitis, myositis, and systemic lupus erythematosus. This condition may cause joint pain, inflammation of the muscles, arthritis, swollen hands, and breathing difficulty.

mixture, **1.** a substance made up of parts that are not chemically combined. **2.** a liquid drug containing one or more drugs. Compare **compound, solution.**

Moban, a trademark for a tranquilizer (molindone).

Mobidin, a trademark for a painkiller (magnesium salicylate).

mobilization center, an off-incident location at which emergency service personnel and equipment are temporarily located, pending assignment, release, or reassignment.

Möbius' syndrome /mē′bē·əs/, a disorder of body growth. It features paralysis on both sides of the face. It is usually linked to vision difficulties or other nervous system disorders, speech problems, and defects of the arms and legs. The condition is caused by a defect of nerves that control the muscles.

Moderil, a trademark for a high blood pressure drug (rescinnamine).

Modicon, a trademark for a birth control pill. It contains an estrogen (ethinyl estradiol) and a progestin (norethindrone).

modified milk, cow's milk in which the protein content has been reduced and the fat content increased to make it similar to human breast milk. See also **bottle feeding.**

molar, any of the 12 molar teeth, 6 in both the upper and lower dental arch. Each of the upper molars has three roots. The lower molars are larger than the upper and each has two roots.

molar pregnancy, pregnancy in which a tumorlike mass of cysts (called **hydatid mole**) instead of an embryo grows from the tissue of the early stage of the fertilized egg. It is more common in older and younger women than in those between 20 and 40 years of age. The cause of the disorder is not known. The signs of pregnancy are all heightened. The uterus grows more rapidly than is normal. Morning sickness is often severe and constant. Blood pressure is likely to be high. Blood levels of female hormones are very high. In most cases the mole is found when miscarriage is threatened or in progress. If the mole is not naturally aborted, it must be completely removed, because it may develop into a form of cancer.

mold, a fungus.

molding, the natural process by which a baby's head is shaped during labor as it is squeezed into and through the birth canal by the forces of labor. The head often becomes quite long. The bones of the skull may be caused to overlap slightly, without skull damage. Most of the changes caused by molding go back to normal during the first few days of life. There may also be a pooling of fluid between the scalp and skull of a newborn, called **caput succedaneum**. It is usually formed during labor as a result of the pressure of the cervix on the infant's head. The swelling begins to go down soon after birth.

molecule, the smallest unit of a substance that has the properties of an element or compound. See also **compound, element.**

molindone hydrochloride, a tranquilizer used to treat schizophrenia. Severe central nervous system disease or known allergy to this drug prohibits its use. Side effects include central nervous system reactions, falling blood pressure, and drowsiness.

molluscum /məlus′kəm/, any skin disease marked by soft, rounded masses or lumps. **Molluscum contagiosum** is a disease of the skin and mucous membranes caused by a virus. It features scattered white lumps and occurs most often in children. It is carried from person to person by direct or indirect contact. It lasts up to 3 years, although individual tumors last for only 6 to 8 weeks. Untreated, the tumors eventually disappear by themselves without scarring.

Mongolian spot, a harmless, bluish-black spot, occurring over the sacrum between the hipbones or the buttocks of some newborns. It is especially common in blacks, Native Americans, Southern Europeans, and Orientals. It usually disappears during early childhood.

mongolism. See **Down's syndrome.**

Monistat, a trademark for an antifungus drug (miconazole nitrate).

monitoring or monitoring survey, periodic or continuous determination of the amount of ionizing radiation or radioactive contamination present for purposes of health protection.

monitrice /mon′itris/, a childbirth coach who is specially trained in the Lamaze method of childbirth. See **Lamaze method.**

monoamine oxidase (MAO) /mon′ō·am′in/, an enzyme that makes nervous system hormones, as epinephrine, inactive.

monoamine oxidase (MAO) inhibitor, any of a group of drugs used to treat depression and anxiety. They are especially useful for anxiety linked to abnormal fears (phobias). MAO inhibitors are sometimes used to treat migraine headache and high blood pressure. The effects of the drugs vary greatly from patient to patient. Side effects include drowsiness, dry mouth, blood pressure that falls as one stands up, and constipation. MAO inhibitors interact with many drugs, one of which is ephedrine, which is in many common cold remedies. Patients taking MAO inhibitors are also given a list of foods to avoid, which can interact with the drug and cause severe high blood pressure. Among these foods are cheeses, red wine, smoked or pickled herring, beer, and yogurt.

monobenzone, a drug given to treat abnormal skin coloration (pigmentation), as vitiligo. It is not used for minor conditions, as freckles. Known allergy to this drug prohibits its use. Side effects include allergic reactions of the skin, and excess skin bleaching that can't be undone.

monoblast /mon′əblast/, a large, immature white blood cell. Some leukemias show by an excess amount of these cells in the marrow and an abnormal presence of them in blood circulation.

monocyte /-sīt/, the largest of the white blood cells. They have two to four times the diameter of a red blood cell.

monocytic leukemia /-sit′ik/, a cancer of blood-forming tissues in which the major cells are giant white blood cells (monocytes). Symptoms include discomfort, weakness, fever, loss of appetite, weight loss, a large spleen, bleeding gums, skin disorders, and anemia. There are two forms: **Schilling's leukemia** and the more common **Naegeli's leukemia.**

monocytosis /-sītō′-/, a large amount of giant white blood cells (monocytes) in the circulation.

monomphalus /mənom′fələs/, twins that are joined at the navel.

mononeuropathy /-nŏŏrop′əthē/, any disorder that affects a single nerve trunk. Some common causes are electric shock, radiation, and broken bones that may press or cut nerve fibers. Casts and bandages that are too tight may also damage a nerve by pressure. Accidental injection of penicillin and other drugs into the sciatic nerve can seriously injure the nerve. The nerve trunks beyond the spinal cord are especially open to pressure and damage. In a con-

M–N

dition called **multiple mononeuropathy** there is failure of several nerve trunks. It may be caused by various diseases, as uremia, diabetes mellitus, and some inflammatory disorders.

mononuclear cell /-nōō′klē·ər/, a white blood cell, including lymphocytes and monocytes, with a round or oval nucleus.

mononucleosis /-nōō′klē·ō′-/, an abnormal increase in the number of mononuclear white blood cells in the circulation. See also **infectious mononucleosis.**

monosaccharide /-sak′ərid/, a carbohydrate made up of one basic sugar unit.

monosomy /-sō′mē/, a birth defect with the lack of one chromosome from the normal set of 23 pairs. It usually involves the lack of one of the sex chromosomes, as occurs in the XO condition in Turner's syndrome.

monotropy /mənot′rəpē/, a condition in which a mother appears to be able to bond with only one infant at a time, such as one of a pair of twins.

monovulatory /mənōv′yələtôr′ē/, a normal condition in which the ovaries release one ovum during each menstrual cycle.

monozygotic (MZ) /-zīgot′ik/, referring to offspring grown from one fertilized egg (zygote), as occurs in identical twins. See also **twin.**

mons pubis, a pad of fatty tissue and rough skin that lies over the lower front bones of the female pelvis. After puberty, it is covered with pubic hair.

monster, a fetus that is badly disfigured and usually will not live.

Montgomery's gland, one of several oil glands on the areas (areolae) surrounding the nipples of the breasts. The glands normally get larger during pregnancy. The oily material that is released by the glands oils and protects the breast from infection and injury during breast feeding.

moon face, a condition in which a rounded, puffy face occurs in patients given large doses of steroid drugs, as those with rheumatoid arthritis or acute childhood leukemia. Features return to normal when the drug is stopped.

MOPP, an abbreviation for a drug combination used to treat cancer. It contains three antitumor drugs, Mustargen (mechlorethamine), Oncovin (vincristine sulfate), Matulane (procarbazine hydrochloride), and prednisone, an adrenal gland hormone. MOPP is given to treat Hodgkin's disease.

morbidity an illness or an abnormal condition or quality.

Morgagni's globule /môrgan′yēz/, a substance that may form from fluid clotting between the eye lens and the saclike capsule in which it is held, especially in cataract.

morning-after pill, *informal.* A large dose of an estrogen given by mouth to a woman within 24 to 72 hours after sexual intercourse. The purpose is to stop conception, most commonly in an emergency, as rape or incest. The woman is warned that the drug, taken over a short period of time, may cause serious problems if contraception fails. These include clots, severe nausea, and vomiting. Other problems are the risk of cancer-causing effects on the fetus or birth defects.

morning sickness, a common condition of early pregnancy. There may be frequent and long-lasting nausea, often in the morning, with vomiting, weight and appetite loss, general weakness, and discomfort. The cause is not known. It usually does not begin before the sixth week after the last menstrual period and ends by the twelfth to the fourteenth week of pregnancy. Eating frequent small, easily digested meals sometimes helps. Drugs may be given for severe cases. Nausea and vomiting after the sixteenth week is unusual. Severe vomiting of pregnancy means the patient must go to the hospital.

morphea /môr′fē·ə/, local hardening of the skin, with yellowish or ivory-colored, rigid, dry, smooth patches. It may lead to a hardness of tissue (sclerosis) elsewhere in the body. It is more common in women than men.

morphine sulfate, a narcotic given to reduce pain. Drug addiction or known allergy to this drug prohibits its use. Side effects include increased brain pressure, heart disturbances, breathing difficulties, and drug addiction.

mortality, 1. the condition of being subject to death. 2. the death rate, noted as the number of deaths per unit of population for a specific region, age group, disease, or other grouping.

Morton's plantar neuralgia, a severe throbbing pain that affects a branch of the nerves of the sole (plantar) of the foot.

morula /môr′ələ/, a solid ball of cells resulting from the cell divisions of the fertilized egg in the early stages of growth during pregnancy.

mosaicism /mōzā′isizm/, a condition in which an individual, developed from a single fertilized egg (zygote), has two or more cell populations that are different. Most commonly seen in humans is a variation in the number of chromosomes in the body cells. Normally, all body cells would have the same number of chromosomes.

mosquito bite, a bite of a bloodsucking insect of the subfamily Culicidae. It may result in a severe allergic reaction in an allergic person, an infection, or, most often, an itching sore. Mosquitoes are carriers of many infectious diseases. They are attracted by moisture, carbon dioxide, estrogens, sweat, or warmth.

motion sickness, a condition caused by uneven or rhythmic motions, as in a car, boat, or airplane. Severe cases feature nausea, vomiting, dizziness, and headache. With mild cases, there is headache and general discomfort. Antihistamines are used to stop the effect.

motor, **1.** referring to motion, as the body involved in movement, or the brain functions that direct body movements. **2.** referring to a muscle, nerve, or brain center that makes or takes part in motion.

motor apraxia, the inability to carry out certain planned movements or to handle small objects, although one knows the use of the object. The cause is a lesion in a part of the brain on the opposite side of the arm that cannot move. See also **apraxia.**

motor area, a part of the brain (cerebral cortex) that includes the centers that cause the voluntary muscles to contract. Removing the motor area from one of the brain's sides (hemispheres) causes paralysis of voluntary muscles. This happens especially to the opposite side of the body. Various parts of the motor area are linked to different body structures, as the lower arm, face, and hand.

motor neuron, one of various nerve cells that carry nerve signals from the brain or from the spinal cord to muscle or gland tissue. See also **nervous system.**

motor neuron paralysis, an injury to the spinal cord that causes damage to motor neurons. It results in various degrees of loss of movement, depending on where the damage is. **Lower motor neuron paralysis** involves an injury or lesion in the spinal cord. There is decreased muscle tone, weak or absent reflexes, local twitching of muscle groups, and progressive wasting of the muscles. **Upper motor neuron paralysis** involves an injury or lesion in the brain or spinal cord. Signs include increased muscle tone and spasticity of the muscles involved, hyperactive deep tendon reflexes, weak or absent superficial reflexes, and no local twitching of muscle groups.

Motrin, a trademark for an antiinflammatory drug (ibuprofen).

mouth, the open cavity at the upper end of the digestive tube. The opening, located in front of the teeth. It is surrounded externally by the lips and cheeks and internally by the gums and teeth. The mouth receives fluids from the salivary glands. The mouth cavity connects with the voicebox (pharynx) and is covered at the top by the hard and the soft palates. The tongue forms the large part of the floor of the cavity.

mouth-to-mouth resuscitation. See **resuscitation.**

moxalactam disodium, an antibiotic used to treat lower lung, stomach, urinary tract, bone and joint, and skin infections, and bacterial blood poisoning. Known allergy to this drug prohibits its use. It must be used carefully in patients allergic to the penicillins. Side effects include allergic reactions, blood disorders, and raised liver enzyme levels.

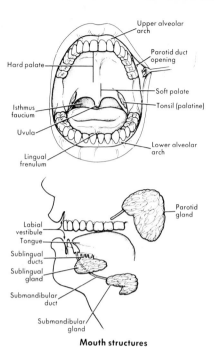

Mouth structures

Moxam, a trademark for an antibiotic (moxalactam).

moxibustion /mok′səbus′chən/, a method of relieving pain or changing the workings of a system of the body. A slow-burning substance is lit and held as near to the point on the skin as possible without causing pain or burning. It is sometimes used with acupuncture.

mucin /myoo′sin/, a carbohydrate that is the main part of mucus. It is present in most glands that release mucus. Mucin is the oily material that protects body surfaces from rubbing or wearing down.

mucinous carcinoma /-əs/, a tumor that is sticky because of the large amount of mucin released by its cells.

mucocutaneous /myoo′kōkyootā′nē·əs/, referring to the mucous membrane and the skin.

mucocutaneous lymph node syndrome (MLNS), a sudden illness with fever mainly of young children. Symptoms include inflamed mouth membranes, ''strawberry tongue,'' swollen lymph nodes in the neck, and redness and shedding of the skin on the arms and legs. Joint pain, diarrhea, ear disorders, pneumonia, and heart rhythm changes may also occur. The cause is unknown. Some people may inherit a condition that makes them unable to resist the disease. Treatment includes aspirin in large doses. It may be given over a long period of time. Also called **Kawasaki disease.**

mucoepidermoid carcinoma /-ep′idur′moid/, a cancer of gland tissues, especially the ducts of the salivary glands.

M–N

mucolytic /-lit′ik/, anything that dissolves or destroys the mucus.

mucopolysaccharidosis (MPS) /-pol′ēsak′əridō′-/, one of a group of inherited disorders of carbohydrate use. They feature greater than normal gatherings of substances making up sugars and mucins in the tissues. Symptoms include skeletal deformity, especially of the face, mental retardation, and slowed growth. There is a lowered life expectancy. The disorders may be found before birth by testing fetal cells present in amniotic fluid. After birth, a diagnosis is made through urine testing, x-ray films, and a family history. There is no successful treatment. **Hunter's syndrome (MPS II)** affects only males. Males born of women who carry the trait have a 50% chance of having the disorder. **Hurler's syndrome (MPS I)** causes severe mental retardation. Facial features of individuals affected by Hurler's syndrome include a low forehead and enlargement of the head, sometimes resulting from water on the brain. Hurler's syndrome usually results in death during childhood from heart or lung failures. **Morquio's disease (MPS IV)** results in abnormal muscle and bone growth in childhood. Dwarfism, hunchback, and knock-knees may occur. The disease may first show as the child, learning to walk, uses an abnormal, waddling gait.

mucoprotein /-prō′tēn/, a chemical compound present in all connective and supporting tissue that contains carbohydrates combined with protein.

mucopurulent /-pyo͞or′yələnt/, referring to a combination of mucus and pus.

mucous /myo͞o′kəs/, referring to mucus or the release of mucus.

mucous membrane, any of four major kinds of thin sheets of tissue cells that cover or line various parts of the body. Examples include linings of the mouth, digestive tube, breathing passages, and the genital and urinary tracts. It releases mucus and absorbs water, salts, and other substances. Compare **serous membrane, skin, synovial membrane.**

mucous plug, a collection of thick mucus in the cervix of the uterus. It is often released just before labor begins. The plug may be dry and firm. More often it is partly fluid and streaked with blood.

mucus /myo͞o′kəs/, the sticky, slippery material released by mucous membranes and glands. It has mucin, white blood cells, water, and cast-off tissue cells. **–mucoid,** *adj.,* **mucous,** *adj.*

Mudrane, a trademark for a lung drug. It contains a smooth muscle relaxing drug (theophylline), a stimulating drug (ephedrine hydrochloride), a drug to free up sputum (potassium iodide), and a drug to help the patient sleep (phenobarbital).

Müllerian duct, one of a pair of tubes in the human embryo that become the fallopian tubes, uterus, and vagina in females.

multiagency coordination system (MACS), the combination of facilities, equipment, personnel, procedures, and communications integrated into a common system with responsibility for coordination or assisting agency emergency operations.

multifactorial, referring to any condition or disease caused by two or more factors. Examples are diseases that involve inherited and environmental factors. Many disorders, as spina bifida, neural tube defects, and Hirschsprung's disease, are considered to be multifactorial.

multigravida /mul′tigrav′idə/, a woman who has been pregnant more than once.

multipara /multip′ərə/, *pl.* **multiparae,** a woman who has given birth to more than one living child.

multiple personality, an abnormal condition in which two or more personalities exist within the same individual. Awareness of the others among the various personalities may not occur. Each may take over at a particular time. Change from one to another is usually sudden and linked to stress. The condition is most often seen in young females. It may be treated with hypnosis, mind-altering drugs, or psychotherapy. Also called **split personality.**

multiple sclerosis (MS), a disease marked by loss of the protective myelin covering of the nerve fibers of the brain and spinal cord. It begins slowly, usually in young adulthood, and continues throughout life. There are cycles in which symptoms worsen or become milder. The first signs are numbness, or abnormal sensations in the arms and legs or on one side of the face. Other signs are muscle weakness, dizziness, and sight disturbances, as double vision and partial blindness. Later, there may be extremes in emotions, loss of muscle control, abnormal reflexes, and difficulty in urinating. As the disease continues, disability becomes greater. Because many other conditions cause similar symptoms, the diagnosis of MS is slow and difficult. There is no specific treatment for the disease. Drugs are used to treat the symptoms that occur. Physical therapy may help to delay or stop specific disabilities. The patient is told to live as normal and active a life as possible.

mummified fetus, a fetus that has died in the uterus and has dried up.

mumps, a viral disease with a swelling of the salivary glands near the neck. It is most likely to affect children between 5 and 15 years of age. In adulthood the infection may be severe. Antibodies from the mother usually prevents this disease in children under 1 year of age. Mumps is most contagious during the late winter and early spring. The mumps virus is carried in droplets or by direct contact. Symptoms include loss of appetite, headache, discomfort, and light fever, followed by earache, saliva gland swelling, and a temperature of 101° to 104° F (38.3° to 40° C). The patient feels pain when drinking sour liquids or when chewing. Although the patient must drink fluids to avoid dehydration, it may be difficult to swallow because of swollen saliva glands. Treatment includes keeping the patient isolated and drugs to reduce pain and fever. All cases of mumps are reported to health authorities. Vaccination within 24 hours of being exposed to the disease may halt the spread of the disease to others or may reduce its effects. Complications include arthritis, inflammation of the pancreas, heart muscle, ovary, testicles, and kidney. Also called **infectious parotitis.**

mumps live virus vaccine, an active drug given for vaccination against mumps. Halted immunity, use of steroid drugs, sudden infection, pregnancy, or known allergy to chicken proteins, neomycin, or this drug prohibits its use. Side effects include fever, inflamed saliva glands, and allergic reactions.

Mumpsvax, a trademark for a mumps live virus vaccine.

Munchausen's syndrome /munch'ousənz/, a condition in which a patient falsely claims to be sick or injured so as to receive medical treatment and hospitalization. The patient may imagine the symptoms and history of a real disease. The false symptoms will appear to get better with treatment. However, the patient may then seek treatment later for another imaginary disease.

murmur, a low pitched fluttering or humming sound in the body. See also **heart murmur.**

Murocoll, a trademark for an eye medicine.

muscle, a tissue made up of fibers that are able to contract, allowing movement of the parts and organs of the body. There are two basic kinds, striated muscle and smooth muscle. **Striated muscle,** also called voluntary muscle, includes all the muscles of the skeleton. It is made up of bundles of parallel, streaklike fibers under conscious control. It responds quickly to stimulation but is paralyzed by any pause in nerve supply. **Smooth muscle** is found in internal organs, such as the stomach and bowels. This kind of muscle is involuntary and reacts slowly to stimulation. It does not entirely lose its ability to contract if the nerves are damaged. The heart muscle (myocardium) is sometimes called a third (cardiac) kind of muscle. However, it is basically a striated muscle that does not contract as quickly as the skeletal muscles. Also, it is not completely paralyzed if it loses its nervous system stimulation.

muscle relaxant, a drug that reduces the ability of muscle fibers to contract. Such drugs are used to gain a lighter level of anesthesia during surgery and to control breathing of patients on ventilators. Other uses are to reduce muscle contractions in shock therapy and muscle spasms in con-

vulsions. The drugs are also used in the treatment of leg cramps at night.

muscular dystrophy, a group of diseases that feature weakness and wasting of skeletal muscles without the breakdown of nerve tissue. In all forms of muscular dystrophy there is a slow loss of strength with increasing disability and deformity. Each type of the disease differs in the muscles affected, the age at which it begins, and the rate of its progress. The basic cause is unknown. Diagnosis is based on examining a piece of muscle, muscle tests, and a family history. The disease is usually inherited and often affects both sexes. Family members who are carriers should be cautioned about the risk of transmitting this disease. No form of muscular dystrophy can be detected by examination of the amniotic fluid during pregnancy (amniocentesis). However, this procedure can determine the sex of the fetus. It is often recommended for carriers who are pregnant. **Duchenne's muscular dystrophy** occurs with progressive wasting of the muscles in the legs and pelvis and affects mostly males. It accounts for 50% of all muscular dystrophy diseases. It is a sex- (X-) linked inborn disease that appears gradually between the ages of 3 and 5 years. It spreads from the leg and pelvic muscles to the involuntary muscles. Linked muscle weakness produces a waddling walk and sway back. Muscles rapidly break down, and calf muscles become firm and large from fatty deposits. Affected children develop frozen flexed joints (contractures) and display winglike shoulder blades when they raise their arms. Such persons are usually confined to wheelchairs by the age of 12. Progressive weakening of heart muscle causes too rapid heart beats (tachycardia) and lung problems. **Fascioscapulohumeral dystrophy,** one of the main types, features wasting of the muscles of the face, shoulders, and upper arms. Early symptoms include not being able to pucker the lips, abnormal face movements when laughing or crying, face flattening, not being able to raise the arms over the head, and, in infants, not being able to suck. This disease is not usually fatal but spreads to all the voluntary muscles and commonly causes a thick lower lip. It is an inherited disease that may be carried to males and females. This form usually occurs before 10 years of age but may also start during adolescence. **Becker's muscular dystrophy** is a milder form and develops more slowly. It occurs in childhood between 8 and 20 years of age. **Distal muscular dystrophy** is a rare form that most often affects adults. It causes weakness and muscle wasting that begins in the arms and legs and then moves to the trunk and face. With **limb-girdle muscular dystrophy,** weakness and atrophy of the muscles begins in the shoulder or in the pelvis. The condition is progressive, spreading to other body areas, regardless of the area in which it begins. **Myotonic muscular dystrophy** occurs first in the hands and

M–N

feet, and later in the shoulders and hips. It features drooping eyelids, facial weakness, and speaking difficulties. **Pelvifemoral muscular dystrophy** is a form that begins in the hip. **Scapulohumeral muscular dystrophy** first affects the shoulder muscles and later often involves the pelvic muscles. No known treatment can halt the spread of this disease and the resulting muscle problems. However, exercises are used to relieve symptoms. The patient often becomes constipated because activity is increasingly limited. Some measures that may help keep the muscles working are physical therapy, surgery to reduce deformity, and the use of braces.

muscular system, all of the muscles of the body, namely, the smooth, cardiac, and striated muscles, considered as one structural group.

musculoskeletal /mus′kyəlōskel′ətəl/, referring to the muscles and the skeleton.

musculoskeletal system, all of the muscles, bones, joints, and related structures, as the tendons and connective tissue, that function in the movement of the parts and organs of the body.

musculoskeletal system assessment, an evaluation of the condition and functioning of the muscles, joints, and bones and of the body. The patient's general appearance, posture of the body, age, blood pressure, pulse, breathing, handgrip, skin conditions as bruises or rashes, and allergies are checked. Recent weight loss or gain are also checked. The physician asks about any pain or swelling in muscles, joints, and bones; weakness in arms and legs; limitations in movements; unsteadiness on the feet; or need for assistance. Also noted are any previous problems, as spinal surgery, partial paralysis, cerebral palsy, stroke, and bone diseases. The presence of muscle contractures and deformities, the range of motion of arms and legs, and the use of crutches or cane are noted. Diseases or conditions checked include injury to the spine, nerve damage, arthritis, bursitis, multiple sclerosis, and muscular dystrophy. Laboratory studies are important. Diagnosis may require x-ray films of bones, draining of joints, and tests of muscles.

mushroom poisoning, a condition caused by eating certain mushrooms, particularly two species of the genus *Amanita*. Muscarine, a substance in *Amanita muscaria,* causes poisoning in a few minutes to 2 hours. Symptoms include tears, excess saliva, sweating, vomiting, difficult breathing, stomach cramps, and diarrhea. In severe cases, convulsions, coma, and failure of the circulation may occur. Atropine is usually given in treatment. The more deadly but slower acting phalloidine, a substance in *A. phalloides* and *A. verna,* causes similar symptoms. It also causes liver damage, kidney failure, and death in 30% to 50% of the cases. Treatment includes emptying the stomach. This is followed by a saltwater enema. Intensive care

and removing the poison from the blood by cleansing the blood (hemodialysis) may prevent death.

Mustargen Hydrochloride, a trademark for an anticancer drug (mechlorethamine hydrochloride).

mutagen /myoo′təjən/, any chemical or physical agent that causes a gene change (mutation) or speeds up the rate of mutation. –**mutagenic,** *adj.,* **mutagenicity,** *n.*

Mutamycin, a trademark for an anticancer drug (mitomycin).

mutation, an unusual change in a person's genes that occurs by itself with or without the influence of a mutagen, as x-rays: The alteration changes the physical trait carried by the gene. Genes are stable units, but a mutation often is passed on to future generations.

mutism /myoo′tizm/, the inability or refusal to speak. The condition often results from an emotional conflict. It is most commonly seen in patients who are psychotic, neurotic, apathetic, or depressed. **Akinetic mutism** is a state in which a person is not able to or will not move or make sounds.

myalgia /mī·al′jə/, a muscle pain. It may be linked to many infectious diseases, as influenza, measles, and rheumatic fever. Muscle pain occurs in many disorders, as inflammation of connective and muscle tissue, excess release of parathyroid hormones, low blood sugar, and muscle tumors. Many drugs also may cause myalgia. – **myalgic,** *adj.*

Myambutol, a trademark for an antibiotic (ethambutol hydrochloride).

myasthenia /mī′əsthē′nē·ə/, abnormal weakness of a muscle or a group of muscles. –**myasthenic,** *adj.*

myasthenia gravis, an abnormal condition of long-term weakness of muscles. It occurs especially in the face and throat. It results from a defect in the movement of nerve signals between nerve fibers to muscles. Symptoms start with drooping upper eyelids, double vision, and weakness of facial muscles. The weakness may then extend to other muscles, as the breathing muscles. The disease occurs most often in young women and in men over 60 years of age. Restricted physical activity and bed rest are ordered. Drugs that stimulate nerve signals are usually given before meals. The patient's diet is changed if the ability to chew and swallow food is affected. A **myasthenia gravis crisis** is sudden increase in intensity of the disorder. Causes include infection, surgery, emotional stress, or a wrong size dose of a drug. Symptoms include breathing difficulty, extreme muscular weakness, swallowing and speaking difficulties, and fever. If the condition is caused by drugs, there may be loss of appetite, nausea, vomiting, and diarrhea. Excess saliva, sweating, blurred sight, dizziness, and muscle spasms may also occur. Emergency treatment includes getting oxygen into the lungs, as with special equipment. An opening into the throat (tracheostomy) may be made. If an eyelid is affected, the eye may be covered with a patch or eyedrops may be used. Range of motion exercises of arms and legs are done several times a day.

mycetoma /mī′sētō′mə/, a serious fungus infection involving skin, connective tissue, and bone. One kind is called **Madura foot,** a tropical fungal infection of the foot.

Mycitracin, a trademark for a combination of drugs containing three antibiotics (polymyxin B sulfate, bacitracin, and neomycin sulfate).

Mycolog, a trademark for a skin cream. It contains a hormone (triamcinolone acetonide), two antibiotics (neomycin sulfate and gramicidin), and an antifungus drug (nystatin).

mycophenolic acid /mī′kōfinō′lik/, an antibiotic that also stops the growth of fungi.

Mycoplasma /-plaz′mə/, microscopic organisms without rigid cell walls. They are considered to be the smallest of all free-living organisms. One species is a cause of walking (mycoplasma) pneumonia, pharyngitis, and other infections.

mycosis /mīkō′-/, any disease caused by a fungus. Some kinds of mycoses are athlete's foot and candidiasis. – **mycotic,** *adj.*

mycosis fungoides /fung·goi′dēz/, a skin cancer. Signs include a skin tumor, and tumors like those of Hodgkin's disease in lymph nodes and stomach and intestinal organs.

Mycostatin, a trademark for an antifungus drug (nystatin).

Mydriacyl, a trademark for an eye drug (tropicamide).

mydriasis /midrī′əsis/, widening of the pupil of the eye. It is caused by contraction of a muscle (dilator) of the iris, a covering of muscle fibers that moves out like the spokes of a wheel around the pupil. With a decrease in light or the action of certain drugs, the dilator pulls the iris outward. This makes the pupil larger.

mydriatic and cycloplegic agent /mid′rē·at′ik, sī′klōplē′jik/, any of several drugs that widen the pupil and paralyze the eye muscles. Such drugs are used in examination of the eye, and before and after many eye surgeries. They are also used in some tests for glaucoma. Blurred vision, thirst, flushing, fever, and rash may result from the drugs. In children and elderly patients more serious side effects may occur.

myelin /mī′əlin/, a fatty substance found in the coverings of various nerve fibers. The fat gives the normally gray fibers a white color. –**myelinic,** *adj.*

myelinolysis /-ol′-/, a disorder that dissolves the myelin sheaths around certain nerve fibers. It occurs in some alcoholic and undernourished patients.

myelin sheath, a fatty layer of myelin that wraps the signal-moving fibers (axons) of many nerve cells in the body. Some diseases, as multiple sclerosis, can destroy the myelin wrappings.

myelitis /mī′əlī′-/, an inflammation of the spinal cord with linked motor or sensory nerve problems. **Acute transverse myelitis** is the worst form and can develop quickly. Nerve problems often last after improvement. It may develop from many causes, such as multiple sclerosis, measles, pneumonia, and exposure to poisons. Some poisons can destroy a whole part of the spine. Pain and numbness below the spinal cord damage usually occurs. One or both legs may be unable to move. The severe spinal cord damage may cause shock with low blood pressure and low body heat. Loss of bowel control and reflexes are common. Chance of complete recovery is poor. See also **poliomyelitis.**

myeloblast /mī′əlōblast′/, a bone marrow cell from which a kind of white blood cell (granulocytic leukocyte) begins. –**myeloblastic,** *adj.*

myeloblastic leukemia, a cancer of blood-making tissues. It features many immature white blood cells (myeloblasts) in the circulating blood and tissues. **Rieder cell leukemia** is a form of this kind of cancer.

myelocele /mī′əlōsēl′/, a saclike bulge of the spinal cord through a defect in the spinal column, seen at birth. See also **myelomeningocele.**

myeloclast /-klast′/, a cell that breaks down the myelin sheaths of nerves of the central nervous system.

myelocystocele /-sis′təsēl/, a pouchlike (cystic) tumor of spinal cord substance that extends out through a defect in the spinal column. See also **myelomeningocele.**

myelocystomeningocele /-sis′təməning′gōsēl′/, a pouchlike (cystic) tumor. It contains both spinal cord substance and membrane (meninges) that extends out through a defect in the spinal column. See also **myelomeningocele.**

myelocyte /-sīt′/, an immature white blood cell. It is normally found in the bone marrow. These cells appear in the circulating blood only in certain forms of leukemia. – **myelocytic,** *adj.*

myelocytic leukemia /-sit′ik/. See **leukemia.**

myelodysplasia /-displā′zhə/, imperfect growth of any part of the spinal cord, especially of the lower part.

myelogram /-gram′/, **1.** an x-ray film of the spinal cord taken after the injection of a dye. It shows any distortions of the spinal cord, spinal nerve roots, and the surrounding space. **2.** a count of the different kinds of cells in a sample of bone marrow.

myeloid /mī′əloid/, **1.** referring to the bone marrow. **2.** referring to the spinal cord.

M–N

myeloid metaplasia, a disorder in which bone marrow tissue develops in abnormal sites. Signs include anemia, a large spleen, immature blood cells in the circulation, and blood cell formation in the liver and spleen. It may be linked to cancer, leukemia, or tuberculosis.

myeloma /mī'əlō'mə/, a bone-destroying tumor. It may develop at the same time in many sites and cause large areas of patchy destruction of bone. The tumor occurs most often in the ribs, vertebrae, pelvic bones, and flat bones of the skull. Intense pain and sudden fractures are common. An **endothelial myeloma** occurs most often in the long bones, especially the legs. Young people between 10 and 20 years of age are most often affected. Pain, fever, and increased numbers of white blood cells usually occur. Amputation is necessary for large tumors. X-ray therapy and chemotherapy are standard treatments. An **extramedullary myeloma** occurs outside of the bone marrow. It usually affects the abdominal organs or the nose, throat, and mouth. A **giant cell myeloma** is a tumor of very large cells in bone marrow. **Multiple myeloma** is a bone marrow cancer that destroys bone tissue, especially in flat bones. It causes pain, fractures, and bone deformities. A common effect is an abnormal curving of the spine. There also may be anemia, weight loss, breathing problems linked to rib fractures, and kidney failure.

myelomalacia /-məlā'shə/, abnormal softening of the spinal cord. It is caused mainly by a poor blood supply.

myelomeningocele /-məning'gōsēl'/, a central nervous system hernia. A sac containing the spinal cord, its membrane covering (meninges), and cerebrospinal fluid extends out through a break in the vertebral column. The condition is caused mainly by the failure of the nerve (neural) tube to close during pregnancy. It is obvious at birth. The hernia may be located at any point along the spinal column. It usually occurs in the lower back. The saclike structure may be covered with a thin layer of skin or with a fine membrane that can be easily broken. This makes the risk of infection greater. Usually the condition is linked to varying degrees of paralysis of the legs and to defects as clubfoot and joint deformities. Loss of anal and bladder control are also common. Hydrocephalus is the most common defect linked to myelomeningocele. See also **neural tube defect, spina bifida.**

myelopathy /mī'əlop'əthē/, any disease of the spinal cord.

myelopoiesis /-pō·ē'sis/, the formation and growth of the bone marrow. **Extramedullary myelopoiesis** is the growth of bone marrow (myeloid) tissue outside of the bone marrow.

myelosuppression, the halting of making blood cells and platelets in bone marrow.

myiasis /mī'yəsis/, infection or infestation of the body by the larvae of flies. They usually enter through a wound or an ulcer. They rarely come through the intact skin.

Myleran, a trademark for an anticancer drug (busulfan).

Mylicon, a trademark for an intestinal gas drug (simethicone).

mylohyoideus /mī'lōhī·oi'dē·əs/, one of a pair of flat triangular muscles that form the floor of the mouth. It acts to raise the tongue.

myocardial infarction (MI) /mī'ōkär'dē·əl/, a blockage of a heart artery. It is caused by hardening of the arteries (atherosclerosis) or a blood clot. This results in a dead tissue area in the heart muscle. Myocardial infarction often begins with a crushing, viselike chest pain that may move to the left arm, neck, or upper abdomen. It sometimes seems like indigestion or a gallbladder attack. The patient becomes ashen, clammy, and short of breath, may faint and may feel that death is near. Signs include rapid heart beat, a barely felt pulse, low blood pressure, above normal temperature, and heart beat irregularities. Emergency treatment of MI may require cardiopulmonary resuscitation (CPR) before the patient is taken to an intensive cardiac care unit of a hospital. In sudden MI, oxygen, heart drugs, and anticoagulants are usually given. Sleeping pills and painkillers are also given. The patient is usually given a low-sodium, low-cholesterol diet. Stool softeners and laxatives may be used to prevent straining.

myocardiopathy /-kär'dē·op'əthē/, any disease of the heart muscle. Also called **cardiomyopathy.**

myocarditis /-kärdī'-/, an inflammation of the heart muscle. It most often occurs as a sudden viral disease. It may also be caused by bacteria, fungus, or a chemical agent, or result from a connective tissue disease. It may lead to heart failure. Treatment includes painkillers, oxygen, antiinflammatory drugs, and rest to prevent shock or heart failure.

myocardium /-kär'dē·əm/, a thick layer of muscle cells that forms most of the heart wall. The myocardium contains few other tissues, except for blood vessels. It is covered inside by a smooth membrane (endocardium). The tissue of the myocardium that causes it to contract is made up of fibers like skeletal muscle tissue, but contains less connective tissue. Special fibers of myocardial muscle make up the contraction signal system of the heart. This includes the sinoatrial node, the atrioventricular node, the atrioventricular bundle, and the Purkinje fibers. Most of the myocardial fibers contract the heart. The heart uses free fatty acids as its main fuel, as well as important amounts of sugar and a small amount of amino acids. Oxygen, which affects the ability of muscle tissue to contract, is an important food for the myocardium. Without an oxygen supply, myocardial contractions decrease in a few minutes. The

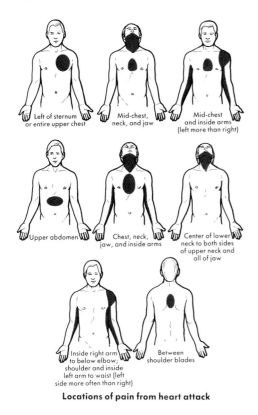

Left of sternum or entire upper chest

Mid-chest, neck, and jaw

Mid-chest and inside arms (left more than right)

Upper abdomen

Chest, neck, jaw, and inside arms

Center of lower neck to both sides of upper neck and all of jaw

Inside right arm to below elbow; shoulder and inside left arm to waist (left side more often than right)

Between shoulder blades

Locations of pain from heart attack

heart normally takes in about 70% of the oxygen reaching it by the coronary arteries. See also **epicardium, heart.** – **myocardial,** *adj.*

Myochrysine, a trademark for an antirheumatic drug (gold sodium thiomalate).

myoclonus /mī·ok′lənəs, mī′ōklō′nəs/, a spasm of a muscle or a group of muscles. –**myoclonic,** *adj.*

myodiastasis /-dī·as′təsis/, an abnormal condition in which there is separation of muscle bundles.

myogelosis /-jəlō′-/, a condition in which there are hardened areas or nodes within muscles, especially the gluteal muscles of the buttocks. There are no serious results of this condition. No treatment is necessary.

myoglobin /-glō′bin/, a form of hemoglobin found in muscle tissue. It is the cause of the red color of muscle and its ability to store oxygen. When found in the urine, the condition is called **myoglobinuria.**

myoma /mī·ō′mə/, a tumor of muscle. See also **fibroids, leiomyoma, rhabdomyoma.**

myometritis /-mətrī′-/, inflammation of the muscle wall (myometrium) of the uterus.

myometrium /-mē′trē·əm/, the muscular layer of the wall of the uterus.

myoneural /-no͞or′əl/, referring to a muscle and its nearby nerve, especially to nerve endings in muscles.

myopathy /mī·op′əthē/, a disorder of skeletal muscle that features weakness, wasting, and changes within muscle cells. Examples include any of the muscular dystrophies. A myopathy is different from a muscle disorder caused by nerve dysfunction. See also **muscular dystrophy.** – **myopathic,** *adj.*

myopia /mī·ō′pē·ə/, a condition of nearsightedness. Causes include lengthening of the eyeball or an error in deflecting rays so that parallel rays of light are focused in front of instead of on the retina. **Chromic myopia** is a kind of color blindness in which colors can be told apart only when the object is close to the eye. **Curvature myopia** is caused by an excess curve of the cornea in the eye. **Pathologic myopia** occurs with changes in the inside of the eyeball and bulging of the iris. Also called **nearsightedness, short sight.**

myorrhexis /mī′ôrek′sis/, a tearing or break in a muscle. –**myorrhectic,** *adj.*

myosarcoma /-särkō′mə/, a cancer of muscle tissue.

myosin /mī′əsin/, a protein that makes up nearly one half of the proteins in muscle tissue. An interaction between myosin and another protein, actin, makes muscle contraction possible.

myositis /-sī′-/, inflammation of muscle tissue, usually of the voluntary muscles. Causes of myositis include injury, infection, and invasion by parasites. **Dermatomyositis** is a disease of the connective tissues. Symptoms include itching, skin inflammation, and tenderness and weakness of the muscles. Muscle tissue is destroyed, often to the point where the person may not be able to walk or perform simple tasks. **Myositis fibrosa** occurs from an abnormal growth of connective tissue. **Myositis ossificans** is an inherited disease in which muscle tissue is replaced by bone. It begins in childhood with symptoms of stiffness in the neck and back. It continues to rigidity of the spine, body, arms, and legs. Some drugs may prevent the abnormal deposits of bone. There is no cure once it has occurred.

myotenotomy /-tənot′-/, division of a tendon done by surgery.

myotome /-tōm/, **1.** a group of muscles stimulated by a single spinal nerve segment. **2.** an instrument for cutting or dissecting a muscle.

myotomy /mī·ot′-/, the cutting of a muscle, done to get to tissues underneath. It is also used to relieve tightness in a circular band of muscles (sphincter), as in the esophagus or the pylorus of the stomach.

Myotonachol, a trademark for a nerve-stimulating drug (bethanechol chloride).

M–N

myotonia /-tō'nē·ə/, any condition in which muscles do not relax after contracting.

myotonic myopathy /-ton'ik/, any of a group of disorders with increased skeletal muscle contractions and decreased relaxation of muscles after contraction. **Myotonia congenita** is a mild form of skeletal muscle wasting seen in infants. The effects of the disorder are large, stiff muscles.

myringectomy /mir'injek'-/, surgical removal of the eardrum (tympanic membrane).

myringitis /-jī'-/, inflammation or infection of the eardrum. **Infectious myringitis** is a contagious condition with painful blisters on the eardrum.

myringomycosis /miring'gōmīkō'-/, a fungus infection of the eardrum.

myringoplasty /-plas'tē/, surgical repair of breaks in the eardrum with a tissue graft. It is done to correct hearing loss. Antibiotics are put on the area and a packing of absorbable sponge to hold the graft in place.

myringotomy /mir'ing·got'-/, surgical opening of the eardrum to relieve pressure or release pus from the middle ear. After the fluid is gently sucked out, ear drops may be used to improve drainage. If pain increases, it may have to be done again. Severe headache or confusion are possible side effects. Also called **tympanotomy.**

Mysoline, a trademark for a drug used to control convulsions (primidone).

mysophobia /mī'sə-/, an anxiety disorder. It features an abnormal fear of dirt, contamination, or getting dirty.

Mytelase Chloride, a trademark for a nerve-stimulating drug (ambenonium chloride).

myxedema /mik'sədē'mə/, the most severe form of decreased activity of the thryroid (hypothyroidism). Signs include swelling of the hands, face, feet, and tissues around the eye. The disease may lead to coma and death.

myxoma /miksō'mə/, a tumor of connective tissue. These tumors may grow to huge size. They are usually pale gray, soft, and jellylike. They may occur under the skin. They are also found in bones and in the genitals and urinary tract. **Atrial myxoma** is a benign tumor that grows in the wall dividing the upper chambers (atria) of the heart. It may cause irregular heart beats, nerve inflammation, nausea, weight loss, weakness, breathlessness, and fever. It may lead to fainting caused by a block in the flow of blood through the heart. **Cystic myxoma** is one that has had a saclike breakdown (cystic degeneration). An **enchondromatous myxoma** is one in which cartilage grows between the cells of connective tissue.

myxosarcoma /mik'səsärkō'mə/, a cancer that contains some jellylike (myxomatous) tissue.

myxovirus, any of a group of viruses usually carried by mucus. Some kinds of myxoviruses are the viruses that cause influenza, mumps, and croup.

N

Nabothian cyst /nābō′thē·ən/, a lump (cyst) formed in a small, mucus-releasing gland (nabothian) of the uterine cervix, commonly found in routine pelvic examination of women of reproductive age, especially in women who have had children. The pearly white, firm cyst seldom causes side effects.

nadolol, a nerve blocking drug given for chest pain (angina pectoris) and high blood pressure. Asthma, certain heart disorders, or known allergy to this drug prohibit its use. Side effects include spasms of the bronchial tubes, slow or irregular heart beat, heart failure, weakness, stomach and bowel problems, rashes, and other allergic reactions.

Naegeli's leukemia /nā′gəlēz/. See **monocytic leukemia.**

nafcillin sodium, an antibiotic used to treat infections caused by penicillin-immune staphylococci. Known allergy to this drug or to other penicillins prohibits its use. Side effects include allergic reactions, nausea, and vomiting.

nail, 1. a structure with a horny surface at the end of a finger or toe. Each nail has a root, body, and edge. The root fits into a groove in the skin. The nail ground substance (matrix) has long ridges, which are seen through the body of the nail. The matrix joins the body of the nail to the connecting tissue under the finger or toe. The whitish moon shape (lunula) near the root is less firmly joined to the connective tissue, which gives it a pale color. The cuticle is joined to the nail just ahead of the root. The nails grow longer when cells at the root divide. **2.** any of many metal nails used in bone and joint surgery to join bones or pieces of bone.

Naldecon, a trademark for a drug with two stimulants (phenylpropanolamine hydrochloride and phenylephrine hydrochloride) and two antihistamines (chlorpheniramine maleate and phenyltoloxamine citrate).

Nalfon, a trademark for an antiinflammatory drug used to relieve the pain of rheumatoid arthritis (fenoprofen calcium).

nalidixic acid, an antibiotic given to treat urinary tract infections. Kidney or liver disease, a history of seizures, or known allergy to this drug prohibits its use. Side effects include mild nervous system and stomach problems, seizures, and increased skull pressure.

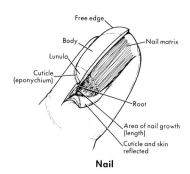

Nail

naloxone hydrochloride, a drug used to reverse narcotic depression or for sudden narcotic overdose. Known allergy to this drug prohibits its use. Side effects, when given to addicted patients, are those linked to narcotic withdrawal.

nandrolone decanoate /nan′drəlōn/, a male sex hormone given to treat a lack of testosterone, bone breakdown, female breast cancer, stimulation of growth, weight gain, and the making of red cells. Cancer of the male breast or prostate, liver disease, pregnancy, or known allergy to this drug prohibits its use. Side effects include hormone disturbances, excess hair growth, acne, and liver disorders.

nandrolone phenpropionate, a drug with male sex hormones given to treat bone breakdown, some anemias, and breast cancers of women. Cancer of the breast in males and some females, pregnancy, kidney disease, or known allergy to this drug prohibits its use. Side effects include excess hair growth, acne, various hormone effects, male features in females, liver disorders, and excess blood calcium in women with breast cancer.

nanism /nā′nizm/, an abnormal smallness or stunted growth; dwarfism.

nanocephalic dwarf /na′nōsəfal′ik/, a person affected with a birth defect (Seckel's syndrome). There is shortness, genital defects, mental retardation, a small head with very small jaws, large eyes, and a beaklike nose.

nanocormia /kôr′mē·ə/, an abnormal smallness of the body in relation to the head, arms, and legs. **–nanocormus,** *n.*

nanomelia /-mē′lyə/, abnormally small arms and legs in relation to the head and body.

nape, the back of the neck.

naphazoline hydrochloride /nəfaz′əlēn/, a drug that shrinks blood vessels, given to treat nasal congestion and some eye disorders. Glaucoma or known allergy to this drug or allergy to related drugs prohibits its use. Side effects include drowsiness, heart problems, and irritation to nasal mucous membranes.

naphthalene poisoning, a toxic condition caused by swallowing naphthalene or paradichlorobenzene. Symptoms include nausea, vomiting, headache, stomach pain, muscle spasm, and convulsions. Treatment includes making the patient vomit, flushing the stomach with water, a salt water laxative, and baking soda (sodium bicarbonate). Naphthalene and paradichlorobenzene are part of mothballs and moth crystals. Paradichlorobenzene is also used as an insecticide.

naphthol camphor, a blend of camphor and betanaphthol, used on the skin as an antiseptic.

napkin-ring tumor, a tumor that surrounds a tubelike structure of the body, as the intestine. It usually destroys the function of an organ and narrows its open area (lumen).

napping, periods of sleep, usually during the day. They may last from 15 to 60 minutes without reaching the level of deep sleep.

Naprosyn, a trademark for an antiinflammatory, antifever, and pain-relieving drug (naproxen).

naproxen, a nonsteroid drug given for the relief of inflammation of arthritis.

Naqua, a trademark for a diuretic and an anti-high-blood-pressure drug (trichlormethiazide).

Naquival, a trademark for a blood pressure drug containing a diuretic (trichlormethiazide) and a high blood pressure drug (reserpine).

Narcan, a trademark for a drug reversing the effects of narcotics (naloxone hydrochloride).

narcissism /när′sisizm/, an abnormal interest in oneself, especially in one's own body and sexual characteristics; self-love. Compare **egotism.**

narcissistic personality /-sis′-/, a personality with behavior and attitudes that show an abnormal love of the self. Such a person is self-centered and self-absorbed, is very unrealistic concerning abilities and goals, and, in general, assumes the right to more than is reasonable in relationships with others.

narcolepsy /när′kōlep′sē/, a disorder with sudden sleep attacks, sleep paralysis, and sight or hearing hallucinations at the onset of sleep. It begins in adolescence or young adulthood and lasts throughout life. Sleep periods may last from a few minutes to several hours. Temporary loss of muscle tone occurs during waking hours (cataplexy), or while the patient is asleep. Its cause is unknown, and no defects are found in the brain. Amphetamines and other stimulating drugs are used to stop the attacks. –**narcoleptic,** adj.

narcoleptic /-lep′-/, **1.** referring to a condition or substance that causes an uncontrollable desire for sleep. **2.** a patient with narcolepsy.

narcosis /närkō′-/, a state of stupor caused by narcotic drugs.

narcotic, 1. a substance that produces stupor. **2.** a narcotic drug. Narcotic painkillers (analgesics), made from opium or made artifically, change one's sense of pain. They also cause a heightened sense of well-being, mood changes, mental confusion, and deep sleep. They may slow breathing and coughing, narrow the pupils, cause muscle spasms, vomiting, and nausea, and reduce contractions of the intestines. Repeated use of narcotics may result in physical and psychologic addiction.

narcotic antagonist, a drug that is used mainly to work against the effects of narcotics.

Nardil, a trademark for an antidepressant drug (phenelzine sulfate).

nares /ner′ēz/, sing. **naris,** the openings in the nose that allow the passage of air to the throat (pharynx) and lungs during breathing. The **anterior nares** are the nostrils. A pair of openings in the back of the nasal cavity, called the **posterior nares,** connect with the upper throat. The **compressor naris** is the part of the nasal muscle that draws the nostril walls inward. The **dilatator naris** is the portion of the muscle covering the nose (nasalis) that widens the nostril.

nasal, referring to the nose and nasal cavity.

nasal cavity, the open area inside the nose that is divided into two chambers by the nasal wall (septum). Each chamber, called a **nasal fossa,** opens externally through the nostrils, and internally into the throat. Each fossa divides into a region (olfactory) for the sense of smell and one for breathing (respiratory). The olfactory section, containing special cells and nerves, is located in the top of the fossa. The respiratory area is lined with mucous membrane, many glands, nerves, and a group of widened veins and blood spaces. This area is easily irritated, causing the membrane to swell, blocking the breathing passages and the openings of sinuses.

nasal decongestant, a drug used for relief of symptoms in short- and long-term nasal problems and infected sinuses (sinusitis). Most are over-the-counter products made of a drug that shrinks blood vessels, as ephedrine or phenylephrine, and an antihistamine. A steroid drug may be added to reduce inflammation. Long-term use or a dose greater than usual may worsen the problem.

nasal glioma, a tumor made up of nerve tissue in the nasal opening (cavity).

nasal instillation of medication, putting (instilling) a drug into the nostrils by drops from a dropper or by a spray. Drops should be put in each nostril with the head tilted back. The mouth should remain open, and the head should stay in the tilted-back position for several minutes to let the drug spread through the nasal passages. A nasal spray can be used in a sitting position.

nasal sinus, any one of the many openings (cavities) in various bones of the skull. A sinus is lined with mucous membrane which lines the nasal cavity and is very sensitive. When irritated, the membrane may swell and block the sinuses. **Ethmoidal air cells** are many small, thin-walled cavities in the ethmoid bone of the skull. The **frontal sinuses** are two small cavities in the frontal bone of the skull. They connect to the nasal cavity. The frontal sinuses are lacking at birth, well developed between the seventh and eighth years, and reach their full size after puberty. The **maxillary sinuses** are a pair of large air cells forming a hole in the body of the upper jaw. The **sphenoidal sinuses** are a pair of cavities in the bone next to the nose under the eyes.

nasogastric feeding /nā′zōgas′-/, putting liquid food directly into the stomach using a tube that is inserted through the nose. Also called **tube feeding,** the process is used after mouth or stomach surgery, in severe burns, in paralysis or blockage of the food pipe (esophagus), in severe cases of a mental disorder causing severe weight loss (anorexia nervosa), and for unconscious patients or those unable to chew or swallow. See also **parenteral nutrition.**

nasogastric intubation, placing a tube through the nose into the stomach to remove gas or stomach contents; to give drugs, food, or fluids; or to get a sample for tests. After surgery and in any condition in which the patient can digest food but not eat it, the tube may be put in and left in place for tube feeding until the patient can eat normally. The tube is put in the nostril, where it is pushed forward and downward. The patient must bend the neck forward, take shallow, rapid breaths, and help move the tube into the stomach by swallowing. Resistance, gagging, and wincing may be lessened by a slow steady progress, and by proper lubrication of the tube. If left in place, the tube is attached with tape to the nose and to the cheek or jaw.

nasolabial reflex /-lā′bē·əl/, an infant's quick backward movement of the head, arching of the back, and stretching of the limbs in response to a light touch to the tip of the nose with an upward sweeping motion. The reflex disappears by about 5 months of age.

nasolacrimal /-lak′riməl/, referring to the nasal opening (cavity) and nearby tear (lacrimal) ducts. The **nasolacri-**

mal duct is a channel that carries tears from the lacrimal sac to the nasal cavity.

nasopharyngeal angiofibroma /-fe-rin′jē·əl/, a noncancerous tumor of the nose and throat. It is made of fiberlike connecting tissue with many blood vessel spaces. The tumor begins in puberty and is more common in boys than in girls. Typical signs are nose and eustachian tube blockage, muffled speech, and difficult swallowing.

nasopharyngeal cancer, a cancer of the throat area behind the nose (nasopharynx). Depending on the site of the tumor, there may be nasal blockage, middle ear inflammation (otitis media), hearing loss, sense or motor nerve damage, destruction of the skull bones, or disorders of the lymph nodes of the neck. Exposure to dusts of nickel, chromium, wood, and leather and to isopropyl oil increases the risk of this cancer.

nasopharyngoscopy /-fer′ing·gos′-kəpē/, a technique in physical examination in which the nose and throat are viewed using a number of devices, including a way to widen the nostrils, and a tubelike system with a lighting method.

natal, **1.** referring to birth. **2.** referring to the buttocks (nates).

nates /nā′tēz/. See **buttocks.**

National Eye Institute (NEI), a division of the National Institutes of Health, set up to support research in the normal workings of the human eye and seeing system.

National Health Service Corps (NHSC), a program of the United States Public Health Service (USPHS) in which health care persons work in areas that are underserved. Nurses, physicians, and dentists serve in rural and urban areas, usually in local health care agencies.

National Interagency Incident Management System (NIIMS), consists of five major subsystems that collectively provide a total systems approach to all-risk incident management. The subsystems are: the incident command system; training; qualifications and certification; supporting technologies; and publications management.

National Institute of Child Health and Human Development (N.I.C.H.H.D.), the part of the National Institutes of Health that is concerned with the growth, development, and health of the children of the United States.

National Institutes of Health (N.I.H.), an agency within the United States Public Health Service made up of several institutions and divisions, including the Bureau of Health Manpower Education, the National Library of Medicine, the National Cancer Institute, and several research institutes and divisions.

natriuresis /nā′trēyŏŏrē′-/, the release of more than normal amounts of salt (sodium) in the urine. It may be caused by diuretic drugs that help release sodium or from various

M–N

disorders of chemical and physical processes that take place in the body.

natural childbirth, labor and childbirth (parturition) done with little or no medicine. Some experts think it is safest for the baby and most satisfying for the mother. It needs a normal pregnancy, a large enough birth canal, strong interest by the mother, physical and emotional preparation, and constant, strong support of the mother during labor and birth. See also **Bradley method, Lamaze method, Read method.**

natural family planning method, any method of family planning that does not require a drug or a device to avoid pregnancy. Natural family planning methods need knowledge, the help and desire of the couple, plus correctly noting and recording the menstrual cycle information. The **basal body temperature method of family planning** relies on identifying the fertile period during a woman's menstrual cycle. The basal body temperature rises 0.5° to 1.0° F during ovulation. The increase varies somewhat from cycle to cycle in any one woman. Several cycles are observed, with records made of the temperature at the same time every morning before getting out of bed. Infection, stress, a bad night's sleep, medicine, or even room temperature can change the reading. If any of these factors are present, the woman notes them on her record. The fertile period is considered to continue until the temperature is above the baseline for 5 days. For birth control, the days following that period are considered "safe" unfertile days. Abstinence is required from 6 days before the earliest day that ovulation was noted to occur until the fifth day after the rise in temperature in the current cycle. The **ovulation method of family planning** depends on watching changes in the type and amount of cervical mucus as a means of telling the time of ovulation during the menstrual cycle. Certain hormones, especially estrogen, cause changes in the amount and type of cervical mucus. In the first days after menstruation, a small amount of thick mucus is released by the cervix. These "dry days" are "safe days," with ovulation several days away. The amount of mucus then increases; it is pearly-white and sticky, and gets clearer and less sticky as ovulation gets nearer; these "wet days" are "unsafe days." During and just after ovulation the mucus is clear, slippery, and elastic; it looks like the uncooked white of an egg. The day on which this sign is most clear is the "peak day," probably the day before ovulation. The 4 days following the "peak day" are "unsafe"; fertilization might occur. By the end of the 4 days, the mucus becomes pearly-white and sticky again and decreases in amount until menstruation occurs, which begins a new cycle. The **symptothermal method of family planning** uses both the ovulation and basal body temperature methods of family planning. It is safer than either

method used alone and requires fewer days of avoiding sexual intercourse, because it enables the fertile period of the menstrual cycle to be more exactly determined.

natural pacemaker. See **pacemaker.**

Naturetin, a trademark for a diuretic and blood pressure drug (bendroflumethiazide).

naturopathy /nā′chərop′əthē/, a system of disease treatment using natural foods, light, warmth, massage, fresh air, regular exercise, and the avoidance of drugs. Supporters believe that illness can be healed naturally by the body.

Nauheim bath /nou′hīm/, a bath taken in water through which carbon dioxide is bubbled. It is used with an exercise plan in the treatment of heart conditions.

nausea /nô′zē·ə, nô′zhə/, a sensation leading to the urge to vomit. Common causes are motion sicknesses, early pregnancy, intense pain, emotional stress, gallbladder disease, food poisoning, and various infections. –**nauseate,** v., **nauseous,** adj.

Navane, a trademark for a tranquilizer (thiothixene).

navel, the point on the abdomen at which the umbilical cord joined the fetal abdomen. In most adults it is a pushed-in space. In some it is a small lump of skin. It is located about halfway between the breastbone and the genital area. Also called **belly button, umbilicus.**

nearsightedness. See **myopia.**

Nebcin, a trademark for an antibacterial (tobramycin sulfate).

nebula /neb′yələ/, pl. **nebulae,** a slight eye (corneal) spot or scar that usually does not block sight and can be seen only by special lighting.

nebulization, a method of giving a drug by spraying it into the nose. The drug may be given with or without oxygen to help carry it into the lungs. **Heated nebulization** uses a heating device to make a spray with a higher water content than that of a cold atomizer. The mist may be given through a mask or in a tent. Croup in infancy is often treated with a heated nebulizer.

nebulizer, a device for making a fine spray. Nasal sprays are given by a nebulizer. Also called **atomizer.**

necatoriosis /ne′kətôr′e·ō′-/. See **hookworm infection.**

neck, a narrowed section, as the part of the body that connects the head with the body, or the neck of the upper leg bone (femur).

neck dissection, an operation to remove the lymph nodes of the neck to stop the spread of cancers of the head and neck. In a **radical neck dissection,** the tumor, nearby tissues, and lymph nodes on the affected side are removed in one mass from the angle of the jaw to the shoulder, forward to the middle, and back again to the angle of the jaw. A total removal of the voicebox (laryngectomy) may be done as part of the surgery.

neck righting reflex, an involuntary response in newborns. Turning the head to one side while the infant is lying face down causes the shoulders and body to turn in the same direction and allows the child to roll over. Lack of the reflex or its being present beyond about 10 months of age may mean there is central nervous system damage. See also **crawling reflex.**

necrobiosis lipoidica /nek′rōbī·ō′-/, a skin disease with thin, shiny, yellow to red spots (plaques) on the shins or forearms. These plaques may form crusts or ulcers. Usually linked to diabetes mellitus, it occurs most often in women. Treatment includes control of the diabetes and drugs.

necrosis /nekrō′-/, local tissue death that occurs in groups of cells because of disease or injury. In **coagulation necrosis,** blood clots block the flow of blood, keeping blood from nearby tissue. In **gangrenous necrosis,** lack of blood combined with bacterial decay causes rotting of tissue. See also **gangrene.**

necrotizing enteritis. See **food poisoning.**

necrotizing enterocolitis (NEC), a sudden inflammatory bowel disorder that occurs mainly in premature or low birth weight infants. The disease causes blood to move away from the stomach and intestinal tract. The result is tissue death with bacterial invasion of the intestinal wall. The stomach and intestinal lining are destroyed, which leads to a break in the bowel and poisoning of the intestinal area (peritonitis). Its cause is unknown. It may involve a lack of ability to fight normal intestinal bacteria rather than an infection from invading germs.

negative, the result of a laboratory test or physical examination that means a substance, condition, or disease is not present. This can mean that there is no medical problem.

negative feedback, a decrease in a body function in response to stimulation. For example, when the release of certain hormones reaches a certain level, a signal is given by another hormone to slow the release. Thus a constant level is kept.

negative pressure, less than standard atmospheric pressure, as in a vacuum or at an altitude above sea level. Some breathing assistance devices have a negative pressure that help a patient to breathe out.

negativism, a behavior attitude of resistance or refusal to cooperate with reasonable request. The response may be passive, as the stiff postures seen in catatonic schizophrenia, or active, as in a contrary act, like sitting down when asked to stand.

NegGram, a trademark for an antibiotic (nalidixic acid).

Nelson's syndrome, a hormone disorder that may follow removal of the adrenal gland. There is a large increase in the making of hormones by the pituitary gland. Treatment includes radiation to slow pituitary function and, sometimes, surgical removal of the pituitary.

nematocides /nem′ətōsīdz′/, chemicals used to kill nematode worms.

nematode /nem′ətōd/, a parasitic worm of the phylum Nematoda. All roundworms belong to this group.

Nembutal, a trademark for a barbiturate (pentobarbital), used as a sedative.

Neo-Cort-Dome, a trademark for a skin drug containing an adrenal hormone (hydrocortisone) and an antibiotic (neomycin sulfate).

neologism /nē·ol′əjizm/, a word made up by a psychiatric patient that has meaning only to the patient.

Neo-Medrol, a trademark for a skin drug containing an adrenal hormone (methylprednisolone) and an antibiotic (neomycin sulfate).

neomycin sulfate, an antibiotic given to treat infections of the intestine, sudden liver disorders, and skin infections. Kidney dysfunction, intestinal blockage, or known allergy to this drug or to any related drug prohibits its use. Side effects include nausea, vomiting, diarrhea, failure of the digestive system to absorb food, and allergic reactions.

Neonatal Behavior Assessment Scale, a scale for checking an infant's alertness, reactions irritability, and interaction with people. It is used to test the nervous system condition and the behavior of a newborn infant.

neonatal breathing /nē′ōnā′təl/, breathing in newborn infants that begins when fluid in the lungs is forced out by pressure of the chest during delivery or reabsorbed from the lungs into the bloodstream and lymph system. Air enters the lungs after birth, but forceful breathing is needed to keep the lungs full. These forces come from conditions such as temperature changes and certain reflexes. However, control of breathing rhythm is not fully developed at birth.

neonatal death. See **perinatal death.**

neonatal developmental profile, the growth status of a newborn infant based on three examinations: a chronologic age inventory, a brain and nerve examination, and a Neonatal Behavior Assessment score.

neonatal period, the period from birth to 28 days of age, a time of the greatest risk to the infant. About 65% of all deaths that occur in the first year of life happen in this 4-week period.

neonatal pustular melanosis, a skin disorder of the newborn. Blisters that appear at birth fill with pus. The sores disappear within 72 hours, leaving dark spots that gradually fade by about 3 months of age.

neonatal thermoregulation, the protection of body temperature of a newborn infant. To prevent the loss of body heat, the infant is dried with a warm towel immediately after birth and wrapped in a warm blanket. Placing the baby under a heater, on a warmed, padded surface, or skin-to-skin with the mother also reduces loss of heat. Infant bassinettes have high sides to prevent cross drafts. The surface area of the head of a newborn is quite large compared to the body, and heat loss from the head may be great; therefore, a cap or fold of blanket is placed around the head. The armpit (axillary) temperature of an infant is normally between 97.5° F (36.5° C) and 98.6° F (37° C), and the rectal temperature is normally 1° higher than the axillary temperature.

neonatal unit, a unit of a hospital that provides care and treatment for newborn infants through 28 days of age, or longer if needed.

neoplasm /-plazm/, any abnormal growth of new tissue that may be harmless (benign) or cancerous (malignant). A **benign neoplasm** is a tumor that has a fiber capsule and a regular shape. It does not grow very fast, become widespread, invade surrounding tissue, or spread to distant sites. It causes harm only by pressure and does not usually return after removal. A **histoid neoplasm** is a growth that resembles the tissues in which it originates. An **organoid neoplasm** is a tumor that looks like a body organ. A **malignant neoplasm** is a tumor that tends to grow, invade nearby tissues, and spread through the bloodstream. It usually has an irregular shape and is made up of imperfectly developed cells. Its harm varies with the kind of tumor and the condition of the patient. Also called **tumor.** See also **cancer. –neoplastic,** *adj.*

neoplastic fracture, a fracture resulting from bone tissue weakened by a tumor.

Neosporin, a trademark for a skin drug containing antibiotics (polymyxin B sulfate, neomycin sulfate, and bacitracin zinc).

neostigmine bromide, a nerve-stimulating drug given to treat myasthenia gravis. Bowel obstruction, urinary infection, or known allergy to this drug or to other bromides prohibits its use. Side effects include severe breathing problems, excess saliva, and intestinal cramps.

Neo-Synephrine Hydrochloride, a trademark for a blood vessel constricting drug (phenylephrine hydrochloride).

Neothylline, a trademark for a smooth muscle relaxant (dyphylline).

Neotrizine, a trademark for an antibiotic (trisulfapyrimidine).

nephrectomy /nefrek'-/, the surgical removal of a kidney. It is done to remove a tumor, drain a sore (abcess), or treat kidney bloating caused by urine pooling (hydronephrosis).

nephritis /nefrī'-/, any disease of the kidney with inflammation and abnormal function. **Interstitial nephritis** involves the structural connective tissue of the kidney. It may be acute or chronic. **Acute interstitial nephritis** is an allergic reaction to some drugs. Acute kidney failure, fever, and rash are common in this condition. Most people regain normal kidney function when the offending drug is stopped. **Chronic interstitial nephritis** is a disorder sometimes found with such conditions as blockage of the urinary tract, exposure of the kidney to toxin, or rejection of a transplant. Gradually, kidney failure, vomiting, weight loss, and anemia develop. If the cause is blockage of the urinary tract, rapid recovery may follow removal of the blockage; in other cases hemodialysis and kidney transplant may be needed. **Infective tubulointerstitial nephritis** is an acute kidney infection caused by certain germs. Symptoms include chills, fever, nausea and vomiting, and flank pain. The kidney may become enlarged, and part of it destroyed. **Lipomatous nephritis** is a rare condition in which the kidney filtration units are replaced by fatty tissue. Kidney failure may result. See also **glomerulonephritis.**

nephroangiosclerosis /nef'rō·an'jēōsklerō'-/, destruction of the small renal arteries, linked to high blood pressure. This condition is present in some patients between 30 and 50 years of age with high blood pressure. Early signs are headaches, blurred vision, and a diastolic blood pressure greater than 120 mm Hg. The heart is usually large. Proteins and red blood cells are found in the urine. Heart and kidney failure may occur if the disease is untreated. Treatment includes diet and high blood pressure drugs. Kidney dialysis is used when preventive measures fail. Also called **malignant hypertension.** See also **hypertension, kidney failure.**

nephrocalcinosis /-kal'sinō'-/, an abnormal condition of the kidneys in which deposits of calcium form in the filtering units. It usually occurs at the site of a previous inflammation or breakdown.

nephrogenic /-jen'ik/, beginning in the kidney.

nephrolith /-lith/, a stone formed in a kidney. **–nephrolithic,** *adj.*

nephrolithiasis /-lithī'əsis/, the presence of stones in the kidney. See also **kidney stone.**

nephron /nef'ron/, a filtering unit of the kidney, resembling a tiny funnel with a long stem and two twisted tubes. Each kidney contains about 1.25 million nephrons. See also **kidney.**

nephropathy /nefrop'əthē/, any inflammation or breakdown disorder of the kidney. See also **kidney disease.**

nephropexy /-pek'sē/, an operation to make stable a floating or drooping (ptotic) kidney.

nephroscope /-skōp/, an instrument used to break up and remove kidney stones. The nephroscope is inserted through the body wall, and the stones are found using x-rays. An ultrasonic probe giving off high-frequency sound waves breaks the stones into small pieces that are easily removed.

nephrotic syndrome /nefrot′ik/, a kidney disease marked by protein in the urine, abnormally low blood protein (albumin), and fluid gathering in the tissues. It may be caused by a problem in the kidney itself or result from other diseases, as diabetes mellitus and multiple myeloma. Treatment depends on the cause of disease. The disorder is usually successfully treated with adrenal gland hormones. Also called **nephrosis.**

nephrostomy /nefros′təmē/, a way in which a tube (catheter) is inserted into the kidney for drainage.

nephrotoxic /-tok′sik/, anything poisonous or destructive to a kidney.

nephrotoxin /-tok′sin/, a poison specifically destructive to the kidneys.

Neptazane, a trademark for a diuretic (methazolamide).

nerve, one or more bundles of signal-carrying fibers that connect the brain and the spinal cord with other parts of the body. Nerves carry inward (afferent) signals from receiving organs toward the brain and spinal cord, and outward (efferent) signals to the various organs and tissues. Each nerve consists of an outer sheath enclosing a bundle of nerve fibers. The sheath is made up of joining tissue. Single nerve fibers are wrapped in a membrane (neurilemma) in which some nerve fibers are also enclosed in a fatty insulating substance (myelin). See also **axon, dendrite, neuroglia, neuron.**

nerve accommodation, the ability of nerve tissue to adjust to a constant source and strength of stimulation so that some change in either strength or length of stimulation is needed to get its attention.

nerve compression, harmful pressure on one or more nerve branches, resulting in nerve damage and muscle weakness (atrophy). Any nerve that passes over a bony knob is at risk. The degree of damage depends on the amount and length of time of pressure. Activities in routine occupations, such as crossing the legs while seated, may put unnecessary pressure on some nerves.

nerve entrapment, nerve damage resulting from a trapped nerve. Nerves that pass over rigid knobs or through narrow bony and fiberlike tissue tunnels are particularly at risk. Signs of this disorder are pain or numbness and muscular weakness. Nerve damage occurs more often when joints are affected by swelling, as in rheumatoid arthritis. One of the most common types of entrapment is **carpal tunnel syndrome.**

nerve impulse, the electric and chemical processes by which messages are sent along the nerves.

nervous breakdown, *informal.* any mental condition that disrupts normal functioning.

nervous system, the arrangement of nerve cells that starts, oversees, and controls all of the functions of the body. It is divided into the central nervous system, made up of the brain and spinal cord, and the peripheral nervous system, which includes the cranial nerves and spinal nerves. These nerves combine and communicate to interact with all organs and tissues of the body with inward (afferent) and outward (efferent) nerve fibers. Afferent fibers carry sense signals, as pain and cold, to the central nervous system. Efferent fibers carry motor signals and movement commands from the central nervous system to the muscles and other organs. Somatic nerve fibers are linked to bones, muscles, and skin. Visceral nerve fibers are linked to the internal organs, blood vessels, and mucous membranes. The many functions of the nervous system are linked through a vast system of tiny structures, as neurons, axons, dendrites, and ganglia. See also **autonomic nervous system, central nervous system, peripheral nervous system.**

Nesacaine, a trademark for a local anesthetic (chloroprocaine).

Netromycin, a trademark for an antibiotic (netilmicin).

nettle rash, a fine, itching eruption resulting from skin contact with the stinging nettle. The common weed has leaves containing histamine. The stinging and itching lasts from a few minutes to several hours.

neural /nŏŏr′əl/, referring to nerve cells and their fibers.

neuralgia /nŏŏral′jə/, a painful condition caused by a variety of disorders that affect the nervous system. The term is usually linked to an affected body area, as facial neuralgia.

neural tube, the tube of tissue that lies along the central axis of the early embryo. It gives rise to the brain, the spinal cord, and other parts of the central nervous system.

neural tube defect, any defect of the brain and spinal cord caused by failure of the neural tube to close during growth during pregnancy. The defect often results from an abnormal increase in spinal fluid pressure on the neural tube during the first 3 months of pregnancy. It may occur at any point along the spinal column. The most severe defect is total lack of the skull and defective brain growth. Other serious defects, usually linked to severe mental and physical disorders, occur most often at the base of the skull. Most neural tube defects involve incomplete joining of one or more parts of the spinal column. There is constant risk of a break in the saclike lump of nerve tissues and a danger of infection. Immediate surgery is often necessary. Many

M–N

neural tube defects can be found during pregnancy by ultrasonic scanning of the fetus in the uterus. Such tests are done during the fourteenth to sixteenth week of pregnancy to allow abortion. See also **meningocele, myelomeningocele, spina bifida.**

neurasthenia /nŏŏr′əsthē′nē·ə/, **1.** a condition of nervous exhaustion and physical tiredness that often follows depression. **2.** a stage in the recovery from schizophrenia in which the patient is listless and seems unable to cope with routine activities and relationships. **–neurasthenic,** *adj.*

neurinoma /nŏŏr′inō′mə/, a tumor of the nerve covering (sheath). It is usually harmless but may become a cancer.

neuritis /nŏŏrī′-/, *pl.* **neuritides,** inflammation of a nerve. Some of the signs are nerve pain (neuralgia), sensitivity of the skin, loss of feeling, paralysis, muscular weakness, and slowed reflexes. With **multiple peripheral neuritis,** there is inflammation or breakdown of nerves of the arms and legs. Symptoms include numbness, tingling in the arms and legs, hot and cold sensations, and slight fever. There also may be pain, weakness, loss of reflexes, and in some cases paralysis. The disorder may be caused by poisons, such as arsenic, carbon monoxide, and lead, and drugs, such as for epilepsy, tuberculosis, and cancer. The condition may also occur in various diseases, such as diabetes and rheumatoid arthritis. Therapy consists of removal of the poison or treatment of the disease, rest, and drugs for pain.

neuroblastoma /nŏŏr′ōblastō′mə/, a cancer made up of cells that come from the tissues of life in the womb. The tumor may begin in any part of the nervous system, but it is most common in the adrenal glands of young children. The cancer spreads early and widely to lymph nodes, liver, lung, and bone. Symptoms may include an abdominal mass, breathing difficulty, and anemia. Active adrenal gland tumors cause irritability, flushing, sweating, high blood pressure, and fast heart beat. Early treatment with surgery, radiation, and chemicals is often successful. **Hutchison-type neuroblastoma** is one that has spread to the brain. A kind of neuroblastoma is **Pepper syndrome,** a cancer of the adrenal glands that spreads to the liver.

neuro check, *nontechnical.* a brief nerve test, usually done on coming to an emergency service of a hospital. The level of consciousness is noted as alert and aware, drowsy, listless, or in a coma. The movements of the arms and legs are noted to be voluntary or involuntary. The pupils of the eyes are checked for equal widening, reaction to light, and ability to focus. See also **neurologic assessment.**

neurocoele /-sēl/, a system of openings (cavities) in the brain and the central canal of the spinal cord. Also called **neural canal.**

neurodermatitis /-dur′mətī′-/, an itching skin disorder seen in anxious, nervous patients. Scratches and skin thickening are found on exposed areas of the body, as the forearms and forehead.

neurofibroma /-fībrō′mə/, a fiberlike growth of nerve tissue. Many growths of this type in the nervous system are often linked to defects in other tissues.

neurofibromatosis /-fī′brōmətō′-/, an inherited condition with many fiberlike growths (neurofibromas) of the nerves, skin, and other organs, and light brown (café au lait) spots on the skin. There may also be defects of the muscles, bones, and abdominal organs. Many large, stalklike soft tissue tumors may develop. An example is the famous case of the ''Elephant Man,'' in nineteenth-century England. Bone changes may result in skeletal defects, especially curving of the spine. The disorder is sometimes linked to meningocele, spina bifida, or epilepsy. Also called **multiple neuroma.**

neurogenic bladder /-jen′ik/, a urinary bladder disorder that can be caused by a tumor of the nervous system. To prevent infection and keep kidney functions, treatment aims at emptying the bladder completely and regularly. One example, called **flaccid bladder,** features continual filling and occasional overfilling of the bladder, lack of an urge to urinate, and inability to urinate at will. A **spastic bladder** is caused by a tumor of the spinal cord, injury, or multiple sclerosis. There is loss of bladder control and feeling, incontinence, and automatic, interrupted, incomplete emptying.

neurogenic fracture, a fracture linked to the destruction of the nerve supply to a bone.

neuroglia /nŏŏrog′lē·ə/, the supporting or connective tissue cells of the central nervous system. Compare **neuron.**

neurohormonal regulation /-hôr′mōnəl/, control of an organ or a gland by the combined effect of nervous system and hormone activity.

neurohypophyseal hormone /-hī′pōfiz′ē·əl/, a hormone released by the pituitary gland. Kinds of neurohypophyseal hormones are **oxytocin** and **vasopressin.** See also **pituitary gland.**

neurolepsis /-lep′-/, an altered state of consciousness with reduced physical movement, anxiety, and indifference to the surroundings. Sleep may occur, but usually the person can wake up and can respond to commands. Antipsychotic drugs usually cause neurolepsis.

neuroleptanalgesia /-lep′tanaljē′sē·ə/, a form of pain relief achieved by using a neuroleptic and a painkiller. Anxiety, physical movement, and sensitivity to pain are reduced. Sleep may or may not occur. The patient is conscious and can respond to commands.

neuroleptanesthesia /-anesthē′zhə/, a form of anesthesia achieved by giving a neuroleptic agent, a narcotic analgesic, and nitrous oxide in oxygen. The anesthesia is given slowly, but consciousness returns quickly after the patient stops breathing nitrous oxide.

neuroleptic /-lep′tik/, a drug that causes neurolepsis, as droperidol. See also **antipsychotic.**

neurologic assessment, an examination of a patient's nervous system. The physician will ask about weakness, numbness, headaches, pain, tremors, nervousness, irritability, or drowsiness. There will be questions about memory loss, periods of confusion, hallucinations, and loss of consciousness. The patient's general appearance, attention span, responses to stimulation, coordination, balance, and ability to follow commands are noted. Skin color and temperature, pupil size and reactions to light, breathing, and chest movements are observed. The pulse is checked. Strength of the handgrip and reflexes are tested. Speech is examined for slurring and ability to say certain words. The physician may ask about other diseases, as high blood pressure, cancer, and narrowing of the aorta, past illnesses linked to head injury, seizures, and motor sensory nerve, or emotional disturbances. There may be questions about sleep patterns, drugs, personality changes, and any family history of seizures, stroke, or mental illness. For a complete examination, laboratory tests may be needed, including spinal fluid analysis, x-ray films of the spinal cord (myelogram), and brain scan to locate possible tumors. See also **neuro check.**

neuroma /nŏŏrō′mə/, a noncancerous tumor made up mainly of nerve cells and nerve fibers. It may be soft or very hard and may vary in size up to 6 inches or more. Pain moves from the tumor to the ends of the affected nerve. It is not usually constant but may become continuous and severe. An **acoustic neuroma** is a benign tumor of the acoustic (eighth cranial) nerve that grows in the ear canal. Symptoms depend on the place and size of the tumor. They include ringing in the ear (tinnitus), loss of hearing, headache, facial numbness, swelling in the eye (papilledema), dizziness, and an unsteady walk. **Cystic neuroma** describes a tumor of nerve tissue that has broken down and become saclike. A **fascicular neuroma** is made up of covered (myelinated) nerve fibers. A **myelinic neuroma** is made up of myelinated nerve fibers. A **neuroma cutis** is a skin tumor that contains nerve tissue and may be very sensitive to pain. A **nevoid neuroma** contains many small blood vessels. A **traumatic neuroma** occurs after severe injury to a nerve. It is a tangled mass of nerve elements and fibrous tissue produced by the increase of nerve and connective tissue cells.

neuromuscular /-mus′kyələr/, referring to the nerves and the muscles.

neuromuscular blocking agent, a drug that interferes with the signals from motor nerves to skeletal muscles. Neuromuscular blocking agents are used to cause muscles to relax in anesthesia, to aid putting an airway tube into the throat, in electroshock therapy, and in treating tetanus, encephalitis, and poliomyelitis. Neuromuscular blocking drugs can cause spasm of the bronchial tubes, very high body temperature, falling blood pressure, or breathing paralysis. They must be used carefully, especially in patients with myasthenia gravis or with kidney, liver, or lung disorders, and in elderly and weak patients.

neuromyelitis /-mī′əlī′-/, an abnormal condition with inflammation of the spinal cord and nearby nerves.

neuron /nŏŏr′on/, the basic nerve cell of the nervous system. It contains a nucleus within a cell body with one or more fibers (axons or dendrites) extending from it. Some fibers are insulated by a fatty substance (myelin) and some fibers are uninsulated (unmyelinated). Some myelinated fibers carry signals of pressure, temperature, touch, and sharp pain. Others are linked to abdominal organs. Unmyelinated fibers carry signals of lengthy, burning sensations from the abdomen and outer body. Neurons are named according to the direction in which they carry signals and to the number of fibers they extend. Sensory neurons carry nerve signals toward the spinal cord and brain. Motor neurons carry nerve signals from the brain and spinal cord to muscles and gland tissue. Usually multipolar neurons have one axon to carry signals away from the cell body and several dendrites to carry signals toward the cell body. Most of the neurons in the brain and spinal cord are multipolar. Bipolar neurons, which are fewer than the other types, have only one axon and one dendrite. All neurons have at least one axon and one or more dendrites and are slightly gray in color when clustered, as in the brain and spinal cord.

neuronitis /-nī′-/, an inflammation of a nerve or nerve cell, especially of spinal nerves.

neuropathic joint disease /-path′ik/, a wasting disease of one or more joints. There is swelling, instability of the joint, bleeding, heat, and changes in bone tissue. Pain is usually less severe than would be expected for the damage to the joint. The disease results from an underlying disease, as syphilis, diabetes, leprosy, or a defect in pain sensation. Early guarding of the joint may prevent further damage. Surgery is seldom effective, and it may be necessary to cut off the limb.

neuropathy /nŏŏrop′əthē/, any abnormal condition with inflammation and wasting of the nerves, as that linked to lead poisoning. **Autonomic neuropathy** refers to nerve damage in the autonomic nervous system. This can cause extreme drops in blood pressure when standing up (orthostatic hypotension). **Compression neuropathy** is any dis-

M–N

order in which nerves are damaged by severe pressure or injury. The symptoms are numbness, weakness, or paralysis. **–neuropathic,** *adj.*

neuroplegia /-plē′jə/, nerve paralysis caused by disease, injury, or the effect of drugs given to achieve pain relief or anesthesia.

neurosarcoma /-särkō′mə/, a cancer made up of nerve tissue, connective tissue, and blood vessels. Also called **malignant neuroma.**

neurosis, any faulty way of handling worry or inner conflict. It usually involves using unconscious defense mechanisms that may lead to a neurotic disorder. This process, called **neurotic process,** in which an unconscious conflict, as a struggle between an idealized self-image and the real self, leads to feelings of anxiety. Defense mechanisms are used to avoid these uncomfortable feelings. Personality change and the symptoms of neurosis result. An example is anorexia nervosa, which may begin as an unconscious defense against facing sexual maturity and leads to a life-threatening disorder requiring forced feeding and psychotherapy. See also **neurotic disorder.**

neurosurgery, any surgery involving the brain, spinal cord, or nerves. Brain surgery is done to treat a wound, remove a growth or foreign body, relieve pressure on the brain, cut out an abscess, or treat other disorders. Kinds of brain surgery include craniotomy and lobotomy. Surgery of the spine is done to correct a defect, remove a growth, repair a herniated disk, or relieve pain. Kinds of spinal surgery include fusion and laminectomy. Surgery on nerves is done to remove a growth, relieve pain, or join a cut nerve. One kind of nerve surgery is sympathectomy.

neurosyphilis, infection of the central nervous system by syphilis organisms. If the brain is affected, partial paralysis may result. If the spinal cord is infected, wasting of the spinal cord (tabes dorsalis) with severe pains in the arms and legs may result. See also **syphilis, tabes dorsalis.** – **neurosyphilitic,** *adj.*

neurotic, 1. referring to neurosis or to a neurotic disorder. **2.** one who is afflicted with a neurosis. **3.** *informal.* an emotionally unstable person.

neurotic disorder, any mental disorder with symptoms that are distressing, unacceptable, and foreign to one's personality. Examples include severe anxiety, obsessions, and compulsive acts. The ability to function may be affected, but behavior generally stays within acceptable norms and sense of reality is not changed. There is no proof of a physical cause. The disorder is not simply a reaction to stress and may be long-lasting or come back if untreated. Kinds of neurotic disorders include **anxiety neurosis, obsessive-compulsive neurosis, psychosexual disorder, somatoform disorder.**

neurotoxic /-tok′sik/, anything having a poisonous effect on nerves and nerve cells, as the effect of lead on the brain and nerves.

neurotoxin /-tok′sin/, a poison that acts directly on the tissues of the central nervous system. It may move along the motor nerves to the brain, as the venom of certain snakes. Another example is the substance made by some bacteria, such as the botulism toxin.

neurotransmitter, any chemical that changes or results in the sending of nerve signals across spaces (synapses) separating nerve fibers. When a nerve signal reaches a knob at the end of a nerve fiber, the neurotransmitter chemical squirts into the gap (synaptic cleft) between fibers. It then binds to receptors on the nearby nerve fiber. This flow lets the signal move across to the next nerve fiber. Kinds of neurotransmitters include **acetylcholine, epinephrine, norepinephrine.**

neutral, a state exactly between two opposing values, qualities, or properties, as when a substance is neither acid nor alkaline. See also **acid, base.**

neutralization, the interaction between an acid and a base that makes a solution that is neither acidic nor basic. The usual products of neutralization are a salt and water.

neutralizing agents, those materials that can be used to neutralize the effects of a corrosive material.

neutral thermal environment, an artificial environment that keeps the body temperature normal to save oxygen and body energy. An incubator for a premature, sick, or low birth weight infant creates such an environment.

neutron, an elementary nuclear particle with a mass approximately the same as that of a hydrogen atom and carrying no electrical charge.

neutropenia /noo′trəpē′nē·ə/, an abnormal drop in the number of white blood cells (neutrophils) in the blood. Neutropenia is linked to leukemia, infections, rheumatoid arthritis, vitamin B_{12} deficiency, and a large spleen. Also called **granulocytopenia.**

neutrophil /-fil/, a grainlike white blood cell (leukocyte). Neutrophils are the circulating white blood cells necessary for removing or destroying bacteria, cell debris, and solid particles in the blood.

nevus /nē′vəs/, a colored skin spot that is usually harmless but may become cancerous. Any change in color, size, or texture or any bleeding or itching of a nevus should be checked. Also called **birthmark, mole.** See also **blue nevus, junction nevus.**

nevus flammeus. See **hemangioma.**

newborn, a recently born infant.

newborn intrapartal care, care of the newborn in the delivery area. During newborn intrapartal care, the throat and mouth of the infant are cleaned to remove excess mucus as the head is born. The baby is then put on the mother's stomach and covered with a warm, dry blanket or put by the nurse in an infant warmer. Apgar scores are given at 1 minute of age and at 5 minutes of age. Sometimes, another is given at 10 minutes of age. The baby is handled gently and quietly. Bright lights are often avoided, and contact with the mother is suggested. If a baby has good color, is alert, and can cry, suck, urinate, defecate, and respond to sound and light, the baby is almost always healthy and normal. If there are no problems, the nurse may put silver nitrate drops in the eyes, trim and clamp the umbilical cord, inject vitamin K, take footprints for identification, and diaper and wrap the baby. If abnormal function is seen, expert help may be called for as emergency measures are begun.

new drug, a drug for which the Food and Drug Administration needs proof of safety and effectiveness before its use is approved in the United States.

Nezelof's syndrome /nez′əlofs/, an abnormal condition with a lack of immune responses and little or no specific making of antibodies. The cause is not known. It affects both male and female brothers and sisters, pointing to a possible hereditary disorder. It causes increasingly severe, frequent, and finally fatal infections. Signs that often are seen in children up to 4 years of age include frequent pneumonia, middle ear infection, fungus infections, nose and throat infections, diarrhea, and a large spleen. The disease may make the lymph nodes and tonsils larger in some infants, but these structures may be totally lacking in others. Treatment includes monthly injections of gamma globulin or monthly infusions of fresh frozen blood plasma and the heavy use of antibiotics to fight infections. Immune function may be temporarily restored by a fetal thymus transplant. Repeated transplants are needed to keep the immunity.

NFPA, National Fire Protection Association.

niacin /nī′əsin/, a vitamin of the B complex group that dissolves in water, found in various plant and animal tissues. It acts in the breakdown and use of all major foods. It is necessary for healthy skin, normal working of the stomach and intestinal tract, caring for the nervous system, and production of the sex hormones. Rich sources of niacin are meats, poultry, fish, liver, kidney, eggs, nuts, peanut butter, brewer's yeast, and wheat germ. Symptoms of a lack include muscular weakness, general tiredness, loss of appetite, various skin spots, bad breath, inflammation of the mouth, lack of sleep, irritability, nausea, vomiting, frequent headaches, tender gums, tension, and depression. A severe lack leads to pellagra. The vitamin is not stored in the body, and any excess in the diet is released. Also called **nicotinic acid.** See also **pellagra.**

niacinamide /-am′īd/, a B complex vitamin. It is closely related to niacin but lacks blood vessel widening action. Also called **nicotinamide.**

nickel (Ni), a silvery-white metal element. Nickel causes more cases of allergic skin reaction (dermatitis) than all other metals combined.

nickel dermatitis, an allergic contact skin inflammation (dermatitis) caused by the metal, nickel. Exposure comes usually from jewelry, wristwatches, metal clasps, and coins. Sweating makes the rash worse. Treatment includes avoiding exposure to nickel and reducing sweating.

Niclocide, a trademark for a worming drug (niclosamide).

niclosamide, an antiworm (anthelmintic) drug given to treat beef tapeworm and fish tapeworm infestations. Known allergy to this drug prohibits its use. Its safety in pregnant or nursing mothers or small children has not been proven. Side effects include rectal bleeding, irregular heart rate, loss of hair, excess tissue fluid, nausea, and vomiting.

Nicobid, a trademark for two coenzymes (niacin and niacinamide) used as a vitamin supplement.

nicotine, a colorless, quick-acting poison in tobacco that is one of the major reasons for the ill effects of smoking. It is used to fight insects in farming and to fight parasites in veterinary medicine. Swallowing large amounts of nicotine causes excess saliva, nausea, vomiting, diarrhea, headache, dizziness, slowing of the heart beat, and, in severe cases, paralysis of breathing muscles. Treatment includes rinsing the stomach with a weak solution of potassium permanganate, followed by activated charcoal, and giving artificial respiration and oxygen, as needed. Pentobarbital is used to control seizures, ephedrine for low blood pressure, and nerve blocking agents to control abdominal symptoms.

nicotine poisoning, poisoning from swallowing nicotine. Excitement of the central and autonomic nervous systems is followed by depression of these systems. In fatal cases, death is from damaged function of the breathing center.

Niemann-Pick disease /nē′-/, an inherited disorder of fat use in which a substance (sphingomyelin) collects in the bone marrow, spleen, and lymph nodes. The disease, which in North America is most common among Jewish people, begins in infancy or childhood. Effects include a large liver and spleen, anemia, swelling of lymph nodes, and slow mental and physical breakdown. There is no effective treatment, and children with the disease usually die within a few years of the beginning of symptoms.

nifedipine, a coronary artery widening drug given to treat several types of chest pain (angina). Known allergy to this drug prohibits its use. Side effects include low blood pres-

M–N

sure, irregular heart rate, difficult breathing, nausea, dizziness, flushing, and headache.

night blindness, poor vision at night or in dim light from a lack of vitamin A, a birth defect, or other causes.

nightmare, a dream occurring during rapid eye movement (REM) sleep that brings out feelings of strong, inescapable fear, terror, distress, or extreme anxiety, usually awakening the sleeper. Compare **sleep terror disorder.**

night vision, an ability to see dimly lit objects. It stems from a condition linked to the rod cells of the retina. The rods contain a highly light-sensitive chemical, rhodopsin, or visual purple, which is necessary for being able to see in dim light. Night vision may be reduced by a lack of vitamin A, an important part of rhodopsin.

nikethamide, a central nervous system stimulating drug given to treat depression of the central nervous and respiratory systems. Known allergy to this drug prohibits its use. Side effects include rapid heart beat, high blood pressure, muscle spasms, and convulsions.

Nikolsky's sign, easy removal of the top layer (stratum corneum) of the skin from the bottom layer by rubbing apparently normal skin areas. It occurs in pemphigus and a few other blister-forming (bullous) diseases.

Nilstat, a trademark for an antifungus drug (nystatin).

NIOSH, (U.S.) National Institute for Occupational Safety and Health.

nipple, a small cylindric bump just below the center of each breast. The tip of the nipple has tiny openings to the milk (lactiferous) ducts, which carry milk from lobes where it is made. The nipple is surrounded by the areola. The color ranges from pink to brown, depending on the skin color of the individual. In pregnancy, the skin of the nipple darkens but lightens again when nursing of the infant ends. Stimulation of the nipple in men, as well as women, causes it to become erect. In women the nipple becomes larger and more sensitive after puberty.

nipple cancer, a cancer of the nipple and areola that is usually linked to a cancer in another part of the breast. It usually starts in the nipple and spreads to the areola. Also called **Paget's disease of the nipple.**

nipple discharge, a sudden release of fluid from the nipple. It may be normal, as colostrum in pregnancy, or a sign of disease.

nipple shield, a device to guard the nipples of a nursing mother. It is usually made of soft rubber and is used to let sore or cracked nipples heal while milk is still being made.

Nipride, a trademark for a blood vessel widening drug (sodium nitroprusside).

niridazole, a drug used to treat a liver fluke (schistosomal) infection. In the United States it is available from the Centers for Disease Control.

nit, the egg of a parasitic insect, as a louse. It may be found attached to human or animal hair or to clothing. See also **pediculosis.**

nitric acid /nī′trik/, a colorless, highly toxic acid that gives off suffocating brown fumes of nitrogen dioxide when exposed to air.

nitrite /nī′trīt/, a salt of nitrous acid used as a blood vessel widener and to fight spasms. Among the nitrites used in medicine are amyl, ethyl, potassium, and sodium nitrite.

nitrobenzene poisoning /nī′trōben′zēn/, poisoning from the absorption into the body of nitrobenzene, a pale yellow, oily liquid used in shoe dyes, soap, perfume, and artificial flavors. Exposure in industry occurs from breathing the fumes or absorbing it through the skin. Symptoms include headache, drowsiness, nausea, loss of muscle control, bluish skin color, and, in severe cases, breathing failure. Contaminated clothing is removed, and the skin is washed with vinegar, followed by soap and water. Oxygen, blood transfusion, and blood cleansing (hemodialysis) may be needed.

Nitrobid, a trademark for a coronary artery widening drug (nitroglycerin), used to treat chest pain (angina pectoris) caused by heart problems.

nitrofuran, one of a group of antimicrobial drugs used to treat infections caused by protozoa or by some bacteria. Nitrofurazone, one of the drugs, is used to treat skin wounds and infections, particularly burns. Furazolidone is used to treat bacterial and protozoal diarrhea and inflammation of the intestines (enteritis). Nitrofurantoin is used to treat urinary tract infections. Side effects include nausea, diarrhea, nerve disorders, allergic reactions, lung inflammation, and blood disorders.

nitrofurantoin, an antibiotic given to treat some urinary tract infections. Kidney disorders or known allergy to this drug prohibits its use. It is not given to children under 1 year of age or to pregnant or nursing women. Side effects include lung inflammation, nervous system disorders, anemia, stomach and bowel disturbances, and fever.

nitrofurazone, an antibiotic given to prevent and treat infection in second- and third-degree burns and to treat infections of the skin and mucous membranes. Known allergy to this drug prohibits its use. Side effects include severe allergic reactions and new infections.

nitrogen (N), an element that is a gas at normal temperatures. Nitrogen compounds, as nitroglycerin amyl nitrite, are often used to relieve symptoms of chest pain (angina pectoris). Nitrogen makes up about 78% of the atmosphere and is a part of all proteins and of most physical substances. In a 24-hour period the nitrogen released by a healthy person in the urine, feces, and sweat, together with nitrogen kept in skin and hair, equals the nitrogen taken in food and drink. The process of protein use explains this

nitrogen balance. Most of the body's nitrogen is blended into protein. Positive nitrogen balance occurs when the intake of nitrogen products for making tissue is greater than the nitrogen released. Negative nitrogen balance occurs when more nitrogen is released than is taken in, causing the waste or destruction of tissue.

nitroglycerin, a coronary artery widening drug (vasodilator) given for the prevention or relief of chest pain (angina pectoris). Known allergy to this drug prohibits its use. Side effects include falling blood pressure, flushing, headache, and fainting.

nitrosourea /-sōyŏŏr'ē·ə/, an anticancer drug used to treat brain tumors, bone tumors, Hodgkin's disease, gland cancers, liver tumors, long-term leukemias, and cancers of the breast and ovaries. Like other anticancer drugs, it can have severe side effects, including bone marrow disorders. Nausea and vomiting are common side effects. Carmustine and lomustine are typical examples of this group of drugs.

Nitrospan, a trademark for a coronary artery dilator (nitroglycerin).

Nitrostat, a trademark for a coronary artery widening drug (vasodilator) (nitroglycerin).

nitrous oxide (N₂O) /nī'trəs/, a gas used as an anesthetic in dentistry, surgery, and childbirth. It gives light anesthesia, delivered in various mixtures with oxygen. Nitrous oxide does not provide deep enough anesthesia to be used alone for major surgery. It is not given to patients with a lack of oxygen in the blood, lung disease, or intestinal blockage.

Nizoral, a trademark for an antifungus drug (ketoconazole).

NMR imaging, a way to make pictures of the internal structure and reactions of the body. Radio waves sent at the body form a signal called nuclear magnetic resonance (NMR). A computer uses the NMR signal to make an image of the internal body that is as good or better than x-ray films.

NOAA weather station, a mobile weather data collection and forecasting facility (including personnel) provided by the National Oceanic and Atmospheric Administration which can be used within the incident area.

nocardiosis /nōkär'dē·ō'-/, an infection with pneumonia and abscesses in the brain and tissues under the skin. The organism enters the breathing tract and spreads by the bloodstream. Surgical drainage of sores and sulfonamide therapy for 12 to 18 months may be necessary. Without treatment the disease is usually fatal.

no code, a note written in a patient record telling the staff members not to attempt to revive the patient in case of heart or lung failure. It is signed by a qualified, usually senior or attending, physician. This note is usually given only when a patient is so seriously ill that death is near and cannot be avoided. Also called **DNR.**

Noctec, a trademark for a strong sedative (chloral hydrate).

nocturia /noktŏŏr'ē·ə/, urination, especially excess urination, at night. It may be a symptom of prostate or kidney disease, or it may occur in persons who drink excess amounts of fluids, especially alcohol or coffee, before bedtime. Also called **nycturia.** Compare **enuresis.**

nocturnal /noktur'nəl/, **1.** referring to or occurring at night. **2.** describing an individual or animal that is active at night and sleeps during the day.

nocturnal emission, involuntary release of semen during sleep, usually linked to an erotic dream. Also called **wet dream.**

node, 1. a small, rounded mass. **2.** a lymph node.

nodular /nod'yələr/, referring to a small, firm, knotty structure or mass.

nodule /nod'yŏŏl/, a small node or nodelike structure.

Noludar, a trademark for a sedative (methyprylon).

Nolvadex, a trademark for a breast cancer drug (tamoxifen).

noma /nō'mə/, a sudden ulcer disease of the mucous membranes of the mouth or genitals. The condition is most often seen in children with poor nutrition and cleanliness. There is rapid and painless breakdown of bone and soft tissue along with a bad odor. Bacteria may be involved. Healing eventually occurs but often with disfiguring defects. Also called **gangrenous stomatitis.**

non-bulk packaging, packaging that has an internal volume of 119 gallons (450 liters) or less for liquids, a capacity of 882 pounds (400 kg) or less for solids, or a water capacity of 1000 pounds (453.6 kg) or less for gases. It may consist of single packaging (e.g., drum, carboy, cylinder) or combination packaging, which is one or more inner packagings inside an outer packaging (e.g., glass bottles inside a fiberboard box). Non-bulk packaging may be palletized or placed in overpacks for transport in vehicles, vessels, and freight containers. Examples include carboys, cylinders, and drums.

noncompliance, the failure of a patient to follow a physician's medical advice. The patient may have a health belief, a cultural or spiritual value, an economic difficulty, or a personal problem with the physician that results in missing appointments or not using drugs as ordered.

nondisjunction, failure of matching pairs of chromosomes to split properly during cell division (meiosis or mitosis). Nondisjunction causes many birth defects. Compare **disjunction.**

non-insulin-dependent diabetes mellitus (NIDDM). See **diabetes mellitus.**

M–N

noninvasive, referring to a test or treatment that does not require the skin to be broken or a cavity or organ of the body to be entered, as taking a blood pressure reading with a stethoscope and sphygmomanometer.

nonosteogenic fibroma /nonos'tēəjen'ik/, a common bone tumor, usually affecting the ends of the large long bones. It often does not cause symptoms and is only discovered during x-ray tests made for other reasons.

nonprotein nitrogen (NPN), the nitrogen in the blood that is not a part of protein. Examples include the nitrogen linked to urea and uric acid. Measurement of NPN is part of tests of kidney function.

non-rapid eye movement (NREM). See **sleep.**

nonspecific urethritis (NSU). See **urethritis.**

nontoxic, not poisonous. Also called **atoxic.**

nontropical sprue. See **sprue.**

Noonan's syndrome, a disorder in males, marked by short stature, low-set ears, webbing of the neck, and skeletal problems. Testicular function may be normal, but fertility is often decreased. The XY karyotype is normal. The cause is unknown.

norepinephrine /nôr'epinef'rin/, a hormone that increases blood pressure by blood vessel narrowing but does not affect the heart's output. It is released by the adrenal glands and is available also as a drug, levarterenol, given to maintain blood pressure in cases of severe low blood pressure.

norepinephrine bitartrate, a blood vessel narrowing drug given to treat heart and circulation disorders. Low blood volume, blood-clotting (coagulation) disorders, or known allergy to this drug prohibits its use. Side effects include local tissue death at the injection site, abnormally slow heart beat, headache, and high blood pressure.

norethindrone /nôreth'indrōn/, a hormone given to treat abnormal uterine bleeding and endometriosis. It is a part of birth control pills. Blood-clotting (coagulation) difficulties, liver disease, unusual vaginal bleeding, breast cancer, missed abortion, or known allergy to this drug prohibits its use. It should not be used during pregnancy. Side effects include breakthrough bleeding, lack of menstruation, stomach and intestinal problems, breast changes, and male features in a female fetus.

norethindrone acetate and ethinyl estradiol, a female sex hormone combination given for birth control, endometriosis, and excess menstrual bleeding. Blood-clotting (coagulation) disorders, heart disease, breast or reproductive organ cancer, unusual vaginal bleeding, gallbladder disease, liver tumor, or known allergy to this drug prohibits its use. It is not given to women over 40 years of age or during breast feeding, pregnancy, or suspected pregnancy. It is given carefully to women who smoke. Side effects

include blood clots, uterine tumors, porphyria, liver disease (jaundice), and stroke.

Norflex, a trademark for a skeletal muscle relaxant and antihistamine (orphenadrine citrate).

Norgesic Forte, a trademark for a drug containing a muscle relaxant (orphenadrine citrate) and APC (aspirin, phenacetin, and caffeine), used to relieve mild to moderate pain of short-term muscle and bone disorders.

norgestrel /nôrjes'trəl/, a hormone given alone or with estrogen as a birth control drug. Blood clotting, liver disorders, unusual vaginal bleeding, breast cancer, missed abortion, or known allergy to this drug prohibits its use. Side effects include lack of menstrual flow, abnormal uterine bleeding, breast changes, and male features in a female fetus.

Norinyl, a trademark for a birth control drug containing a progestin (norethindrone) and an estrogen (mestranol).

Norlac, a trademark for a food supplement containing multivitamins, calcium, and iron.

Norlestrin, a trademark for a birth control drug containing an estrogen (ethinyl estradiol) and a progestin (norethindrone acetate).

Norlutin, a trademark for a progestin (norethindrone).

normal, **1.** describing a usual, regular, or typical example of a set of objects or values. **2.** referring to persons in a nondiseased population.

normal-form radioactive materials, radionuclides in liquid, powder, gaseous, or other physical form, such that they might be dispersed if released from a shipping container.

normal human serum albumin, a solution made from proteins taken from healthy donors used to treat low blood protein, low blood volume, or shock.

normoblast /nôr'məblast/, an immature red blood cell that still has a nucleus. After the nucleus is released, the young red blood cell (erythrocyte) becomes known as a reticulocyte. Compare **erythrocyte.** See also **reticulocyte.** –**normoblastic,** *adj.*

normochromic /-krō'mik/, referring to a red blood cell of normal color, usually because it contains the right amount of hemoglobin.

Normosol-M, a trademark for a sugar solution with electrolytes.

normotensive, referring to normal blood pressure. –**normotension,** *n.*

Norpace, a trademark for a drug given to correct abnormal heart rates (disopyramide phosphate).

Norpramin, a trademark for an antidepressant (desipramine hydrochloride).

Nor-QD, a trademark for a birth control drug containing a progestin (norethindrone) but no estrogen.

nortriptyline hydrochloride, an antidepressant given to treat mental depression. Taking monoamine oxidase inhibitors at the same time, recent heart attack, or known allergy to this drug or to related drugs prohibits its use. It is used carefully in patients with a seizure disorder or a heart disease. Side effects includes drowsiness and stomach and intestinal, heart, and nervous system reactions. This drug interacts with many other drugs.

nose, a structure on the front of the skull that is a passageway for air to and from the lungs. The nose filters the air, warming, moistening, and checking it for foreign bodies that might irritate the lining of the breathing tract. The nose is the organ of smell and aids in speaking. The external portion, which grows out of the face, is much smaller than the internal portion, which lies over the roof of the mouth. The hollow interior portion is divided by a wall (septum) into a right and a left cavity. Each cavity is subdivided into a top, middle, and bottom opening by bony ridges (nasal conchae). The external nose has two nostrils, and the internal portion has two rear nostrils (posterior nares). Four pairs of sinuses drain into the nose. Mucous membrane with hairlike projections (cilia) lines the nose. See also **nasal cavity.**

nosebleed, bleeding from the nose. Causes include irritation of the soft lining of the nose, violent sneezing, fragile vessels in the nose, long-term infection, injury, high blood pressure, leukemia, or lack of enough vitamin K. Nosebleeds may cause breathing distress, dizziness, and nausea, and may lead to fainting. Emergency treatment includes seating the person upright with the head held forward to prevent swallowing blood. The person should breathe through the mouth and sit quietly. The bleeding may be stopped by pinching the nose firmly with the fingers. Pressing both thumbs directly under the nostril and above the lips may also block the blood supply to the nose. Cold compresses on the nose, lips, and the back of the head often help control bleeding. Continued bleeding needs treatment by a physician. Also called **epistaxis.**

nosecup, a device, inside a facepiece, that directs the wearer's exhalations away from the facepiece lens and thus prevents internal fogging (condensation) on the lens.

nosocomial infection /nō′sōkō′mē·əl/, an infection aquired during hospitalization. Also called **hospital-acquired infection.**

nostrils. See **nares.**

notch, a gap or a depression in a bone or other organ, as the sciatic notch, a groove in the hipbone.

notifiable, referring to conditions, diseases, and events that must, by law, be reported to a government agency. Examples include birth, death, smallpox, serious communicable diseases, and certain violations of public health regulations.

nourish, to furnish or supply the necessary foods for maintaining life.

nourishment, any substance that nourishes and supports the life and growth of a person.

Novahistine, a trademark for a drug containing an antihistamine (chlorpheniramine maleate) and a decongestant (phenylpropanolamine).

Novocain, a trademark for a local anesthetic (procaine hydrochloride).

NPH Iletin, a trademark for an insulin (isophane).

Nubain, a trademark for an artificial painkiller (nalbuphine hydrochloride) used with an anesthetic.

nuchal cord /noo′kəl/, a condition in which the umbilical cord is wrapped around the neck of the fetus in the uterus or as it is being born. Usually the cord is gently slipped over the infant's head. The shoulders may come through a single loose loop. The condition occurs in more than 25% of births, more often with long cords than with short ones.

nuclear family, a family unit made up of the biologic parents and their children. Breakup of a marriage results in breakup of the nuclear family.

nuclear magnetic resonance (NMR). See **NMR imaging.**

nuclear medicine, a branch of medicine that uses radioactive chemical elements (isotopes) in the diagnosis and treatment of disease.

nuclear radiation, particulate and electromagnetic radiation emitted from atomic nuclei in various nuclear processes. See also **alpha particle, beta particle, gamma ray, x ray,** and **neutron.**

nuclear scanning, a method of medical diagnosis. The size, shape, location, and function of various body parts is seen using radioactive material and a device that senses the radioactivity in the body. Also called **radionuclide organ imaging.**

nuclear weapon, a general name given to any weapon in which the explosion results from the energy released by reactions involving atomic nuclei — fission, fusion, or both.

nucleic acid /nookle′ik/, a chemical compound involved in making and storing energy, and carrying hereditary characteristics. A capsule-like protein coat (**nucleocapsid**) surrounds nucleic acid. Some viruses are made only of bare nucleocapsids. Kinds of nucleic acid are **deoxyribonucleic acid** and **ribonucleic acid.**

nucleocytoplasmic ratio /noo′klē·ōsī′təplaz′mik/, the balance between the nucleus and the cytoplasm of a cell. This balance is usually steady for a certain cell type. An increase in the nucleus is a sign of cancer.

nucleolus /nookle′ələs/, pl. **nucleoli,** any of the small, dense structures made up mostly of ribonucleic acid and located in the cytoplasm of cells. Nucleoli are needed to make cell proteins.

nucleon /noō′klē·on/,   a term applied to protons and neutrons within the nucleus.

nucleoplasm /-plazm′/,   the protoplasm of the nucleus, as opposed to the protoplasm of the cell outside of the nucleus. Compare **cytoplasm.**

nucleus /noō′klē·əs/,   **1.** the main controlling body in a living cell, usually surrounded by a membrane. It contains genetic codes for continuing life systems of the organism and for controlling growth and reproduction. **2.** a group of nerve cells of the central nervous system that have the same function, as supporting the sense of hearing or smell.

nucleus pulposus.   See **herniated disk.**

nuclide,   a general term referring to any nuclear species of the chemical elements. There are about 270 stable nuclides and about 1250 radioactive nuclides.

Nuhn's gland,   a gland in tissues on the bottom and near the tip of the tongue.

null cell,   a kind of white blood cell (lymphocyte) that grows in bone marrow. Stimulated by an antibody, these cells can apparently attack certain cells directly and are known as ''killer,'' or K, cells.

nullipara /nulip′ərə/,   a woman who has not given birth to a living infant. The term ''para 0'' also means nullipara. Compare **multipara, primipara.**

numbness,   a partial or total lack of feeling in a part of the body, because of anything that interrupts the sending of signals from sensory nerve fibers. Numbness is often seen with tingling.

nummular dermatitis /num′yələr/,   a skin disease with round blisters or eczema-like tumors on the forearms and front of the calves. The cause is unknown.

Numorphan Hydrochloride,   a trademark for a narcotic painkiller (oxymorphone hydrochloride).

Nupercainal,   a trademark for a local anesthetic (dibucaine hydrochloride).

nurse. See **registered nurse.**

nursery diarrhea,   diarrhea of the newborn. In nurseries, outbreaks of diarrhea from certain bacteria or viruses can be life-threatening to an infant. The newborn may be infected at birth by the mother's stool or infected later by the hands of hospital workers. Care includes restoring fluid and mineral balance and giving antibiotics.

nurse's aide,   a person who does basic nonmedical tasks in the care of a patient, as bathing and feeding, making beds, and moving patients.

nursing,   **1.** acting as a nurse, giving care that encourages and promotes the health of the patient being served. **2.** breast feeding an infant.

nursing-bottle caries,   tooth decay that occurs in children between 18 months and 3 years of age who are given a bottle at bedtime. It results in excess exposure of the teeth to milk or juice. Cavities (caries) form because pools of milk or juice may become food for acid-making bacteria. The acid destroys tooth enamel. Preventive measures include stopping the bedtime feeding or giving water instead of milk or juice in the nighttime bottle.

nursing home.   See **extended care facility.**

Nursoy,   a trademark for an allergy-free (hypoallergenic) food supplement for infants.

nutation,   nodding, especially involuntary nodding by some nervous system disorders.

Nutramigen,   a trademark for a milk substitute formula made from a soybean product and of milk sugar (lactose). It is given to infants or other patients who are unable to absorb a substance (lactose) in milk.

nutrient,   a substance that provides nourishment and aids in the growth and development of the body. **Essential nutrient** refers to the carbohydrates, proteins, fats, minerals, and vitamins necessary for growth and normal function. These substances are supplied by food, since some are not produced in the body in large enough amounts for normal health. **Secondary nutrient** refers to a substance that helps to digest food in the intestines.

nutrient artery of the humerus,   one of a pair of branches of the arteries near the middle of the arm.

nutrition,   **1.** nourishment. **2.** the sum of the steps involved in taking in nutrients and in their use by the body for proper functioning and health. The stages are ingestion, digestion, absorption, assimilation, and excretion. **3.** the study of food and drink as related to the growth and health of living organisms. A **nutritionist** is one who studies and puts into practice the rules and science of nutrition.

nutritional anemia,   a disorder with inadequate making of red blood cells caused by a lack of iron, folic acid, or vitamin B_{12}, or other food disorders. **Iron deficiency anemia** may be caused by too little dietary iron, poor absorption of iron, or chronic bleeding. Symptoms include pale skin, fatigue, and weakness. **Macrocytic anemia** features blocked blood cells and abnormal, large, fragile, red blood cells (macrocytes). Macrocytic anemia most often results from a lack of folic acid and vitamin B_{12}. **Megaloblastic anemia** is a blood disorder in which abnormal red blood cells (megaloblasts) are made and spread. These red blood cells are usually linked to a form of anemia (pernicious) in which there is a lack of vitamin B_{12} or folic acid. **Pernicious anemia** is a form of anemia that affects mainly older patients. It results from a lack of a substance (intrinsic factor) that is needed to process the vitamin B_{12} (cyanocobalamin) needed for red blood cells. The making of red blood cells in bone marrow is stopped. The condition is most often treated with injections of vitamin B$_{12}$, iron, and folic acid.

nutritional care, the ways involved in getting the proper foods, especially for the hospitalized patient. Depending on the patient's condition, food needs may be met by regular meals with menus selected from the ordered diet, by tube feeding, or by feeding through a vein (intravenous). Additional foods, when ordered by a physician, and fluids are offered between meals. Tooth cavities, loose teeth or dentures, gum problems, nausea, vomiting, diarrhea, or constipation may affect food care. Nutritional care will be needed for conditions of poor nutrition caused by an inability to swallow or to digest food or to absorb nutrients in the right amount for normal health. Symptoms include loss of weight, eating less food than is necessary, lack of interest in food, change in the taste of food, feelings of fullness right after eating small amounts, stomach pain, sores in the mouth, diarrhea, pale skin, weakness, and loss of hair. If indicated, as may be with overweight patients or those with disorders needing a highly restricted diet, the intake of food is limited.

nyctophobia /nik′tō-/, an obsessive, irrational fear of darkness.

Nydrazid, a trademark for an antibiotic (isoniazid).

nylidrin hydrochloride, a blood vessel widening drug given to treat circulation problems of the skin and inner ear. Sudden heart disease, rapid heart beat, Graves' dis

ease, chest pain (angina pectoris), or known allergy to this drug prohibits its use. Side effects include falling blood pressure, dizziness, rapid heart beat, nausea, and weakness.

Nylmerate, a trademark for an antimicrobial drug (phenylmercuric nitrate).

nymphomania, a disorder of women marked by an excessive desire for sexual satisfaction, often from an unconscious conflict, as a desire to disprove lesbianism or frigidity. See also **psychosexual disorder.**

nystagmus /nīstag′məs/, involuntary, rhythmic movements of the eyes side-to-side, up and down, around, or mixed. **Jerking nystagmus,** with faster movements in one direction than in the opposite direction, is the most common and occurs normally when a person watches a moving object. It may be a sign of barbiturate overdose or of another disorder. **Pendular nystagmus** has eye movements that are about equal in both directions. A disorder of the inner ear may cause rolling eye movements and is usually seen with dizziness and nausea. Other causes are various diseases of the retina of the eye and multiple sclerosis.

nystatin /nis′tətin/, an antifungus antibiotic given to treat fungal infections of the stomach and intestinal tract, vagina, and skin. Known allergy to this drug prohibits its use. Side effects include mild stomach distress and skin reactions.

O

O, symbol for **oxygen.**

oat cell carcinoma, a cancer that usually begins in the surface layer cells of one of the breathing tubes leading to the lungs. Tumors caused by these cells do not form areas of tissue but usually spread along the lymph system. One third of all cancers of the lung are of this type. Usually surgery cannot be done and chemotherapy and radiation do not work. Thus, the outlook is poor.

obesity, an abnormal increase in the amount of fat, mainly in the stomach and intestines, and in tissues beneath the skin. **Endogenous obesity** is caused by poor function of the hormone-making (endocrine) or chemical-processing (metabolic) systems. **Exogenous obesity** is overweight caused by greater calorie intake than the body needs. The characteristics of obesity include excess weight, low activity level, and bad eating habits, as eating when not hungry.

Obetrol, a trademark for a drug that has central nervous system stimulants (dextroamphetamine and amphetamine).

OB-Gyn, *informal.* abbreviation for **obstetrics and gynecology.**

objective, referring to a condition, as a health change, that is seen by others and is not subjective. An objective finding is often a physical sign, something that can be measured, as compared to a symptom, which is a subjective finding, as pain or nausea that another person cannot see or feel. **Objective data collection** refers to health information about a patient's problem gathered by a doctor or nurse through direct physical examination. This includes looking at the patient (observation); examining with the hands, as feeling for tissue masses (palpation); listening for sounds in the body (auscultation); laboratory tests; x-ray tests; and other tests.

oblique, referring to a slanting angle or any change from an up and down (vertical) or a sideways (horizontal) line. Some muscles have an oblique pattern. An **oblique fracture** is a bone break at a slanting angle.

oblique bandage, a bandage put on using spiraling circles in slanting turns, usually to an arm or leg.

obliquus externus abdominis /oblī'kwəs/, one of a pair of muscles of the abdomen. It helps to hold the contents of

this area and helps in urination, defecation, vomiting, childbirth, and forced breathing out. Both sides acting together flex the vertebral column. Also called **descending oblique muscle.**

obliquus internus abdominis, one of a pair of muscles of the abdomen. It helps to hold the contents of this area and helps in urination, defecation, vomiting, childbirth, and forced breathing out. Both sides acting together flex the vertebral column. Also called **ascending oblique muscle.**

observation, **1.** the act of watching carefully and closely. **2.** a report of what is seen or noticed.

obsession, a thought or idea with which the mind is always concerned and that usually deals with something irrational. The thought is not easily removed just by thinking or talking it through. It often leads to a compulsion, as an uncontrollable urge to clean a room that is not dirty. See also **compulsion.**

obsessional personality, a type of personality in which continuous, abnormal, uncontrollable, and unwanted thoughts lead to compulsive actions. The thoughts may be made up of simple ideas or desires or, more often, a group of ideas linked to past events or to events in the future. The person is orderly and neat and can be depended on, but is filled with feelings of not being good enough, and also is open to worry and not being able to make decisions.

obsessive-compulsive neurosis, a neurotic condition of being unable to resist or stop abnormal and uncontrollable urges, thoughts, or fears that are different from the person's judgments. The problem usually appears after the early teenage years resulting from fear, feelings of guilt, and worrying about punishment. Treatment may include psychotherapy to help the person tell the difference between real and unreal dangers.

obsessive-compulsive personality, a type of personality in which there is an uncontrollable need to do certain acts or rituals, as continous washing of hands or changing of clothes. When the acts or rituals become abnormal and more obvious, they can get in the way of everyday actions in society, becoming neurotic reactions.

obstetric anesthesia, any of various ways of giving a drug (anesthetic) to reduce pain during childbirth. It includes local anesthesia for a cut made to widen the opening of the birth canal (episiotomy), or regional anesthesia for labor or childbirth, as by nerve block. A nerve block or general anesthesia may be used for childbirth surgery (cesarean section). **Epidural anesthesia** numbs the pelvic, stomach, genital, or other area. A local anesthetic is injected into the epidural space of the spinal column. Epidural anesthesia is commonly used during labor and childbirth. **Pudendal block** is a form of regional anesthetic given to reduce the pain of the second stage of labor. It numbs the female genital region without affecting the contractions of the muscles of the uterus. See also **anesthesia.**

obstetrics, the branch of medicine dealing with pregnancy and childbirth. An **obstetrician** is a physician who specializes in obstetrics.

obstipation, a condition of serious and continuing constipation caused by a blockage in the intestines. See also **constipation.**

obstruction, 1. something that blocks or clogs an opening or passageway. **2.** the condition of being blocked or clogged. –**obstruct,** v., **obstructive,** adj.

obstructive airways disease, any blockage of the breathing tract that may be linked to symptoms of inflammation or unusual conditions in the bronchial tubes leading to the lungs, and a disorder caused by destructive changes in the tissues of these airways (emphysema). See also **asthma, cystic fibrosis, pulmonary disease.**

obstructive uropathy, any disease that blocks the flow of urine. The condition may lead to kidney disorders and a higher risk of urinary infection.

obtundation, the use of a drug that reduces pain by blocking feelings at some level of the central nervous system, as in use of anesthesia before surgery, use of narcotics to control pain, and use of a tranquilizer as a calming drug.

obturator /ob′tərā′tər/, a device used to block a passage or a canal or to fill in a space, as a device (prosthesis) placed in the mouth to bridge the gap in the roof of the mouth in a cleft palate.

obturator externus, the flat, triangle-shaped muscle covering the outer surface of the front wall of the pelvis. It rotates the thigh to the side.

obturator internus, a muscle that covers a large area of the lower part of the pelvis, where it surrounds a large opening on each side of the lower part of the hipbone (obturator foramen). It rotates the thigh to the side and pushes out and raises the thigh when it is flexed.

occipital artery /oksip′itəl/, one of a pair of branched arteries from the external carotid arteries that supplies blood to parts of the head and scalp.

occipital bone, the cuplike bone at the back of the skull that has a large opening (the foramen magnum) that links with the spinal canal.

occipital lobe. See **brain.**

occipitofrontalis /oksip′itōfrontā′lis/, one of a pair of thin, broad muscles covering the top of the skull. It is the muscle that pulls the scalp and raises the eyebrows and contains branches of the nerves for the face.

occiput /ok′sipət/, the back part of the head.

occlusal adjustment /oklōō′səl/, grinding the surfaces of the teeth to make the fit better between different parts of the mouth, including teeth, the bone beneath the gum, muscles used in chewing, and the joints between the upper and lower jaws (temporomandibular joints).

occlusal radiograph, an x-ray film made inside the mouth with the film placed between the facing (occlusal) tooth surfaces. A **bite-wing film** has a central tab or wing on which the teeth close to keep the film position rigid while x-ray films are taken.

occlusal trauma, an injury to a tooth and roots and bone beneath the gum resulting from accidents, problems at the corners of the jaws (temporomandibular joints), and teeth grinding.

occlusion, 1. a blockage in a canal, artery or vein, or passage of the body. **2.** any contact between the biting or chewing surfaces of the upper and lower teeth. **Balanced occlusion** is a closure of the teeth in which the upper and lower teeth on both sides make contact together. **Pathogenic occlusion** and **traumatic occlusion** both refer to an abnormal closure that may damage teeth, gums, and other parts of the mouth. **Working occlusion** refers to the closing contacts of teeth on the side of the jaw toward which the lower jaw (mandible) is moved.

occlusive, referring to something that causes a blockage or closing, as a taped bandage.

occult blood, blood that comes from an unknown place, with unclear signs and symptoms. Occult blood is usually in the stools of patients with stomach and intestinal diseases. It may be found by using a chemical test or by using a microscope to look closer at the blood.

occult carcinoma, a small cancer that does not cause serious symptoms. It may stay in one place and be found only at an autopsy following death from another cause, or it may spread (metastasize) through blood or lymph and be found in the results of tests done to look at the patient's disease. Also called **latent carcinoma.**

occult fracture, a broken bone that cannot be seen at first by using x-ray tests but may show up on x-ray films taken weeks later. It has the usual signs of pain and injury and may cause soft tissue swelling.

O–P

occupational accident, an injury caused by an accident to an employee that happens in the workplace. Accidents account for more than 95% of workplace injuries.

occupational disability, a condition in which a worker is unable to do a job properly because of an occupational disease or a workplace accident.

occupational disease, an illness that is caused by doing a certain job, usually from coming into contact with things that cause diseases, or from doing certain actions over and over again.

occupational health, the state of a worker being able to work well enough and hard enough to do the job well, not to miss work because of illness, to have few claims for disability payments, and to be able to work for a long time.

occupational history, a part of a health record in which questions are asked about the patient's job, source of income, effects of the work on health or the patient's health on the job, length of the job, and whether or not the patient is happy with the job. Certain side effects may be linked to a certain job or place of work. For example, a carpenter might be asked about muscle and bone problems. See also **health history.**

occupational medicine, a part of medicine that deals with preventing medical problems relating to work and especially to the health of workers in different kinds of workplaces and jobs.

occupational therapy, the training of patients with physical injury or illness, mental disease, or learning problems to work and live by themselves despite any health problem that keeps the patient from living a normal life. An **occupational therapist** is a person who is licensed to do this therapy.

ochronosis /ō'krənō'-/, a condition with deposits of brown-black color in connective tissue and cartilage. It is often caused by alkaptonuria or poisoning with phenol. Bluish spots may be seen on the whites of the eyes, fingers, ears, nose, genitals, mouth, and armpits. The urine may be dark colored. See also **alkaptonuria.**

ocular /ok'yələr/, **1.** referring to the eye. **2.** an eyepiece or system of lenses, as in a microscope.

ocular myopathy, a slow weakening of the muscles that move the eyeball. There may be drooping of the upper lid. The problem may affect one or both eyes and may be caused by damage to the nerve necessary for eye movement, a brain tumor, or a disease that affects nerves and muscles.

ocular spot, an unusual cloudiness in the eye. Red and black dots may be seen in the eye following bleeding in an eye vessel. Cloudiness in the lens is caused by cataracts. In one disease (asteroid hyalitis), often linked to diabetes, small white calcium deposits are found in the watery substance (vitreous humor) between the lens and retina.

oculocephalic reflex /ok'yəlōsefal'ik/, a test of the condition of the brainstem. When the patient's head is quickly moved to one side and then to the other, the eyes will usually take a moment to catch up with the head movement and then slowly move to the middle position. Failure of the eyes to do this properly means a brainstem tumor is on the opposite side of the head.

oculogyric crisis /-jī'rik/, condition in which the eyes are held in a fixed position, usually up and sideways, for minutes or several hours. It happens in patients who have recovered from sleeping sickness (encephalitis) but have signs of a nerve disorder (parkinsonism). In some cases the eyes are held down or sideways and there may be a sudden muscle movement (spasm) or closing of the lids.

oculomotor nerve, either of a pair of cranial nerves that control eye movements, supplying certain outside (extrinsic) and inside (intrinsic) eye muscles. Also called **third cranial nerve.**

Ocusert Pilo, a trademark for a nerve drug (pilocarpine).

odontectomy /ō'dontek'-/ the removal of a tooth.

odontitis, unusual growth of an immature (unerupted) tooth, usually caused by inflammation of the cells that make new teeth (odontoblasts). It may be caused by infection, tumor, or injury.

odontodysplasia /ōdon'tōdisplā'zhə/, an unusual condition in the growth of the teeth, resulting in a lack of the outer layers of the teeth (enamel and dentin). Also called **ghost teeth.**

odontoid process, the lump on the upper surface of the second cervical backbone (axis) in the neck. It is the place around which the first cervical backbone (atlas) turns, allowing the head to turn. Also called **dens.**

odontogenic fibroma /-jen'ik/, a tumor of the jaw that does not lead to cancer.

odontogenic fibrosarcoma, a cancer of the jaw.

odontogenic myxoma, a tumor of the jaw that does not lead to cancer.

odontoma /ō'dontō'mə/, a toothlike growth that looks like a hard tumor. It is made up of tooth tissues, as cementum and enamel, that may be in the form of teeth.

odor, a scent or smell. The sense of smell is set off when molecules in the air carry the odor to the nerve (olfactory) located inside the nose.

odynophagia /od'inōfā'jə/, a strong feeling of burning, squeezing pain while swallowing. It is caused by irritation of the mucous membranes or a muscle problem of the esophagus (gastroesophageal reflux), a germ or fungus infection, a tumor, or chemical irritation.

Oedipus complex /ed'əpəs, ē'də-/, a sexually excited feeling by a child for the parent of the opposite sex, usually with strong negative feelings for the parent of the same sex. Experts disagree on the cause, as the parents' supporting it, or its commonness, because it is not found in all countries.

Ogen, a trademark for a female sex hormone (estropipate).

oil, any of a large number of fatty liquid substances from animal, vegetable, or mineral matter that will not mix with water.

ointment, a creamlike medicine used on the skin and having one or more drugs. Various ointments are used as local painkillers, anesthetics, antiinfectives, astringents, irritants, or decoloring (depigmenting) and skin-softening (keratolytic) agents. Also called **salve, unction, unguent.**

olecranon /ōlek'rənon/, a bump on the lower arm bone (ulna) that forms the point of the elbow. It fits into the dent (olecranon fossa) of the upper arm bone (humerus) when the forearm is straightened out.

oleic acid /ōlē'ik/, a colorless, liquid fatty acid found in vegetable and animal fats. In store products, oleic acid is found in lotions, soaps, ointments, and food additives.

oleovitamin /ō'lē·ō-/, a mixture of fish liver oil or vegetable oil that contains one or more of the vitamins that are dissolved by fat or similar substances.

olfactory /olfak'tərē/, referring to the sense of smell. **–olfaction,** n.

olfactory center, the part of the brain responsible for being aware of odors.

olfactory nerve, one of a pair of nerves linked to the sense of smell. It is made up of many thin threads that spread through the mucous membrane of the smell-sensing area in the chamber behind the nose (nasal cavity). Passing into the skull, the fibers form links with the fibers of the cells in the olfactory bulb, a relay center between the nose and the brain. Also called **cranial nerve I.**

oligodactyly /ol'igōdak'tilē/, a birth defect that usually takes the form of the lack of one or more of the fingers or toes.

oligodendroglioma /-den'drōglī·ō'mə/, a brain tumor made up of cells that usually are part of the tissue around nerve cells. The tumor may grow to a large size. It grows in a number of different places of the brain.

oligodontia /-don'shə/, a dental problem that usually takes the form of having fewer than the normal number of teeth.

oligomeganephronia /-meg'ənefrō'nē·ə/, a type of inborn kidney problem with a lack of filtering units. It is linked with chronic kidney failure in children.

oligospermia /-spur'mē·ə/, lack of enough sperm in the semen.

oliguria /ol'igōōr'ē·ə/, a reduced ability to make and excrete urine, usually less than 500 ml (1 pint) a day. A result is that the waste products of the body's chemical processes (metabolism) cannot be released properly. It may be caused by body fluids and minerals that get out of balance, by kidney tumors, or by a urinary tract blockage. Compare **anuria.**

Ollier's dyschondroplasia /ōlyāz'/, a problem of bone growth in which the tissue necessary for bone growth spreads through the bones. It causes unusual and rough growth and, over time, badly formed bones. The long bones and the hipbone are the ones most often changed by this problem. Surgery to correct badly formed bones may be necessary and helpful, but the patient often becomes an invalid.

omentum /ōmen'təm/, an extension of the abdominal lining (peritoneum) that surrounds one or more nearby organs in the stomach and bowel area (abdomen). It divides into the greater omentum and lesser omentum. **–omental,** adj.

Omnipen, a trademark for an antigerm drug (ampicillin).

omphalitis /om'fəlī'-/, a disorder of the navel with redness, swelling, and pus in severe cases.

omphalocele /om'fəlōsēl'/, a hernia of intestinal organ material through a hole in the abdominal wall at the navel. The hole is usually closed surgically soon after birth.

onanism /ō'nənizm/. See **masturbation.**

onchocerciasis /on'kōsərsī'əsis/, a condition where worms multiply rapidly in the patient's body (filariasis), common in Latin America and Africa. It features bumps (nodules) under the skin, an itching rash, and eye tumors. The disease is carried by the bites of black flies that place their eggs under the skin. Eye problems may include inflammation and, rarely, blindness. Treatment includes drugs to kill the larvae and surgery to take out the nodules in order to remove adult worms. Protective clothing should be worn in black fly areas.

oncofetal protein /ong'kōfē'təl/, a protein made by or linked to a tumor cell, particularly a tumor from embryo tissue. An example of an oncofetal protein is alpha-feto-protein.

oncogene /-jēn/, a gene that may possibly cause cancer to grow. Normally, such genes play a role in the growth and spread of cells, but when changed in some way by a cancer-causing agent, as radiation, they may cause the cell to become cancerous.

oncogenic virus /-jen'ik/, a virus that is able to cause the growth of a cancer. Over 100 oncogenic viruses are known

O-P

to exist. Many "slow viruses," which may remain nonactive for years, are thought to cause cancer in humans.

oncology /ongkol′-/, the branch of medicine that deals with the study of tumors.

Oncovin, a trademark for an anticancer drug (vincristine sulfate).

oncovirus, a family of viruses linked to certain cancers (leukemia and sarcoma) in animals and, possibly, in humans.

Ondine's curse /ondēnz′/, a sudden inability to breathe, caused by loss of automatic control of breathing. (The term is taken from a fairy tale.) A problem in the breathing center's reaction to the buildup of carbon dioxide leaves the patient with too much carbon dioxide and lack of oxygen in the blood. There is no other problem with being able to breathe. This condition may be one cause of sudden infant death syndrome (SIDS). Causes of the disorder may be drug overdose, as with opiate narcotics; it may follow bulbar poliomyelitis or encephalitis; or it may occur after surgery that involves the brainstem or the higher parts of the spinal cord.

ontogeny /ontoj′ənē/, the life history of one living thing from a single-celled egg to the time of birth, including all phases of cell division and growth. Compare **phylogeny.**

onychia /onik′ē·ə/, inflammation of the finger under the nail (nail bed). Compare **paronychia.**

onychogryphosis /on′ikōgrifō′-/, a thickened, curved, clawlike overgrowth of fingernails or toenails.

onycholysis /on′ikol′isis/, the coming apart of a nail from its bed. It is linked to psoriasis, dermatitis of the hand, fungus infection, bacteria infection, and many other conditions.

ooblast /ō′əblast/, the female germ cell from which the egg grows.

oocyesis /ō′əsī·ē′sis/, a pregnancy with an embryo growing within the ovary instead of the uterus where it normally grows.

oogenesis /ō′əjen′əsis/, the growth of female eggs (ova). Growth actually begins during life in the womb when the very first germ cells in the fetal ovary make cells called **oogonia.** By the time of birth, the oogonia have multiplied and grown into primary **oocytes.** Each one has a layer of cells around it that form the primitive ovarian follicle. Every month, one, or sometimes two, of the primary oocytes break into a large secondary oocyte and a much smaller body that does not function. The second division begins at about the time of ovulation, resulting in one large mature egg, or **ootid,** and one or more smaller bodies that soon break apart. The mature egg has the haploid number of the mother's chromosomes that will join with the sperm during fertilization to form the zygote. If fertilization does not occur, the egg breaks apart and is released during men-

struation. A female baby is born with all the primary oocytes that will be used during her reproductive life.

oophorectomy /ō′əfôrek′-/, surgery to remove one or both ovaries. It may be done to take out a lump (cyst), a tumor, or an abscess, to treat endometriosis, or, in breast cancer, to take out the part of the body that makes the female sex hormone (estrogen), which helps to start some cancers. If both ovaries are removed, the patient will not be able to have children and menopause is started. In women who have not yet gone through menopause, one ovary or a part of one ovary may be left in place unless a cancer is present. The operation often is done with a removal of the uterus (hysterectomy). Unless a cancer is present, estrogen may be given to avoid the side effects of menopause. **Oophorosalpingectomy** is surgery to remove one or both ovaries and the fallopian tubes. The purpose, result, and treatment after surgery is like that of oophorectomy.

oophoritis /ō′əfôrī′-/, inflammation of one or both ovaries, usually occurring with inflammation of the fallopian tubes (salpingitis).

oosperm /ō′əspurm/, a fertilized egg; the cell caused by the joining of the sperm and the egg after fertilization occurs; a zygote.

opacity /ōpas′itē/, the condition of a thing that cannot be seen through (opaque or nontransparent), as a cataract opacity.

opaque /ōpāk′/, referring to a substance or surface that neither carries nor lets light come through.

open charting, a way to keep medical records in which the patient can look at his or her own chart.

open-circuit apparatus, breathing apparatus in which the wearer's exhalations are vented to the surrounding atmosphere.

operant conditioning. See **conditioning.**

operating microscope, a small microscope that is worn like glasses in front of each eye and is used in surgery where the things being operated on are very small, especially surgery of the eye or ear.

operating room (O.R.), a room or area in a hospital where patients are made ready for surgery, have surgery, and recover from the effects of the anesthetic needed for the surgery.

operation, any surgery, as an appendectomy or a hysterectomy.

operational period, the period of time scheduled for execution of a given set of operation actions as specified in the incident action plan.

Operations Coordination Center (OCC), the primary facility of the Multiagency Coordination System. It houses the staff and equipment necessary to perform the MACS functions.

operculum /ōpur′kyələm/, a covering, as the mucous plug that blocks the tube or channel of a uterus that has a fertilized egg in it.

Ophthaine, a trademark for a local anesthetic (proparacaine hydrochloride) liquid, used in eye (ophthalmic) procedures.

ophthalmia /ofthal′mē·ə/, inflammation of the outer surface (conjunctiva) or of the deeper parts of the eye. **Ophthalmia neonatorum** occurs in newborn babies. It is caused by the eyes coming into contact with chemicals, viruses, or germs. Irritation of the outer part of the eye caused by chemicals usually is the result of putting silver nitrate in the eyes of a newborn baby to keep a virus infection from starting. **Sympathetic ophthalmia** is an inflammation of parts of the eye that causes grainy, fiberlike bumps to form. It occurs in one eye (**sympathizing eye**) after the other has already been infected by an injury. Steroids may be helpful in treatment, but it may be necessary to remove the eye that was injured to save the other eye. See also **conjunctivitis.**

ophthalmic administration of medication, giving a drug by slowly dripping a liquid or creamy drug in the outer surface of the eye (conjunctiva). The patient should be lying back on a bed or sitting up with the neck leaned backwards. The loose tissue between the eyeball and the eyelid (conjunctival sac) is uncovered by a gentle pull on the tissue just below the lower eyelid. The eyedropper is not allowed to touch the eye, and the drug is not placed directly on the outer surface of the eye. The eyelid is slowly released, and the patient rolls the eye around a few times to spread the drug over the whole surface of the eye.

ophthalmology /-mol′-/, the branch of medicine that deals with the working, structures, and diseases of the eye, and finding their causes and treatments for them.

ophthalmoplegia /-mōplē′jə/, the loss of movement of the eye muscles. It may come about quickly in both eyes with serious myasthenia gravis, serious vitamin B_1 (thiamin) shortage, or botulism.

ophthalmoscope /ofthal′məskōp/, a tool for looking at the inside of the eye. It includes a light, a mirror with a hole through which the doctor may look, and a dial with lenses of different powers.

Ophthochlor, a trademark for an antibiotic (chloramphenicol) used to treat eye infections.

Ophthocort, a trademark for an eye drug that has an adrenal hormone (hydrocortisone acetate) and antibiotics (chloramphenicol and polymyxin B sulfate).

opiate /ō′pē·āt/, a narcotic drug that contains opium, drugs made from opium, or any of several partly artificial or artificial drugs that behave like opium. These drugs are used to cause sleep or help ease pain. Morphine and other opiates like it may cause unwanted side effects, as nausea, vomiting, dizziness, and constipation. Some patients may become more sensitive to pain after the opiate has worn off. Patients with low amounts of blood are more likely to have their blood pressure lowered because of morphine and drugs like it. Opiates should be used very carefully in overweight patients and in those with head injuries, or any problems linked to breathing. In patients with a large prostate, morphine may cause a serious buildup of urine, making it necessary to use a tube (catheter) in the urinary tract.

opisthorchiasis /ō′pisthôrkī′əsis/, infection with a kind of *Opisthorchis* liver worm commonly found in Asia, the Pacific Islands, and parts of Europe. Cancer of the bile ducts may be a late result. The disease is prevented by avoiding eating raw fish.

opisthotonos /ō′pisthot′ənəs/, a continuous severe spasm of the muscles causing the back to arch back, the head to bend back on the neck, the heels to bend back on the legs, and the arms and hands to flex rigidly at the joints.

opium, a dried or partly dried milky sap from the unripe capsules of the opium poppy (*Papaver somniferum* and *Papaver album*) producing nearly 10% or more of morphine. It is a narcotic painkiller and a drug that brings on sleep or hypnosis. Opium contains several alkaloids, including codeine, morphine, and papaverine.

opium alkaloid, any of several substances taken from the unripe seed pods of the opium poppy. Three of the alkaloids, codeine, papaverine, and morphine, are used in medicine for pain relief, but their use risks physical or psychologic addiction. Morphine is the basic, most common drug of its kind against which the painkiller effect of newer drugs for pain relief are tested. The opium alkaloids and the semiartificial drugs that are made from them, including heroin, act on the central nervous system, causing loss of pain, a change in mood, drowsiness, and mental slowness. In usual doses, the relief from pain is achieved without loss of consciousness.

opium tincture, a painkiller and antidiarrhea drug given to treat too much intestinal activity, cramping, and diarrhea. Drug addiction, the presence of poison in the bowel, or known allergy to this drug prohibits its use. Side effects include drug addiction, an enlarged colon, and central nervous system effects.

Oppenheim reflex, a sign of central nervous system disease. It is caused by firmly stroking downward on the front and inner surfaces of the lower leg, causing the great toe to straighten out and causing the fanning of other toes. See also **Babinski's reflex.**

Oppenheim's disease, an inborn disorder of infants, marked by flabby muscles, especially in the legs, and absent or very slow deep muscle reflexes. The infant seems unable to move during its first few months of life, and almost a third of the patients do not survive for 1 year.

opportunistic infection, an infection caused by a virus or by germs that are usually not harmful to normal persons. The patient becomes infected because the ability to fight off diseases has been reduced by a present disorder, such as diabetes mellitus, cancer, surgery, or a tube in the heart or urinary tract.

optic, referring to the eyes or to sight.

optic atrophy, wasting away of the optic disc in the innermost part of the eye (retina), caused by a breakdown of optic nerve fibers. In primary optic atrophy the disc is white with sharp outer edges and the central depression is large. In secondary atrophy the disc is gray, its outer edges are blurred, and the depression is filled in. Optic atrophy may be caused by a birth defect, inflammation, blockage of the central retinal artery or internal carotid artery, alcohol, or poisons. Breakdown of the disc may be seen with arteriosclerosis, diabetes, glaucoma, hydrocephalus, anemia, and different types of nervous system disorders.

optic disc, the small blind spot on the surface of the retina. It is the only part of the retina that is not sensitive to light. At its center is the entrance of the central artery of the retina. Also called (*informal*) **blind spot.**

optic glioma, a slow-growing tumor on the optic nerve made up of tissue from its supporting structure. It causes loss of sight, uneven eyes (strabismus), bulging eyeballs (exophthalmos), and eyes that cannot be moved.

optician, a person who grinds and fits eyeglasses and contact lenses by prescription.

optic nerve, one of a pair of cranial nerves made up mainly of fibers that start in the retina, travel through the thalamus at the base of the brain, and join with the visual cortex at the back of the brain. At a structure in the front part of the brain, called the optic chiasm, there is a crossing over of fibers from the inner half of the retina of one eye to the fibers of the other eye. The fibers left over from the outer half of each retina are uncrossed and pass to the visual cortex on the same side. The visual cortex works to sense light and shade and to sense objects by decoding nerve signals from the retina. Also called **cranial nerve II.**

optics, a field of study that deals with sight and the way that the workings of the eye and the brain are linked in order to sense shapes, patterns, movements, distance, and color. –**optic, optical,** *adj.*

optic system assessment, an eye checkup for current and past disorders or injuries that may result in problems in the patient's sight. The patient is tested to find if sight is blurred, double, reduced, lacking in one or both eyes, or reduced in darkness or in bright light. The physician asks if halos or lights are seen, if objects are seen when held too close or too far, if the eyes water, itch, feel tender, painful, or tired, and if an injury to the eye, face, or head has ever happened. Other observations include the kind of eyeglasses or contact lenses worn, the ability to blink, and the ability to focus. A report is made about eye inflammation, any discharge coming from the eye, bulging eyes, bleeding in the eye, and swelling, redness, or drooping of the eyelids. Also included are signs of aging, glaucoma, cataract, retinal detachment, or the presence of any disease, such as arteriosclerosis, diabetes mellitus, gonorrhea, or sinus problems. The patient's report of eye surgery or treatment earlier in life as well as a family history of glaucoma or diabetes is noted. The patient's job and hobbies are discussed to see if the patient is exposed to any possible dangers to the eyes. The use of alcohol and use of drugs, especially antibiotics, eye drugs, and certain drugs that increase the passing of urine (diuretics), are also noted. Other tests may include an x-ray film of the eyes and skull, a test for eyeball pressure (tonometry), and a brain scan.

Optimyd, a trademark for an eye drug that has an adrenal hormone (prednisolone sodium phosphate) and an antiinfection drug (sulfacetamide sodium).

optometry /optom′ətrē/, the practice of testing the eyes for the ability to focus and see, making corrective lenses, and suggesting eye exercises. See also **optician.**

oral administration of medication, giving a tablet, capsule, or solution or other liquid form of a drug by mouth. Water is usually given for swallowing with the drugs. Drugs with an unpleasant taste may be given with a flavoring to hide the taste. Drugs that are bad for the teeth should be given through a straw. Patients who have a hard time swallowing pills or capsules may find it easier to swallow the drug if they look up as they swallow. Giving a drug in the form of a tablet by placing it between the cheek and the teeth or gum until it dissolves is called **buccal administration.** Giving a drug, as nitroglycerin, usually in tablet form, by placing it beneath the tongue until the tablet dissolves is **sublingual administration.**

oral airway, a curved tube of rubber, plastic, or metal put in the throat while the patient is unconscious from general anesthesia during an operation. This tube helps to allow free passage of air and to keep the tongue from falling back over the windpipe.

oral cancer, a cancer on the lip or in the mouth. It usually occurs in patients around 60 years of age and is eight times more common in men than in women. Causes include alcoholism, heavy use of tobacco, poor mouth care, poorly fitting dentures, syphilis, and a low-iron disease (Plummer-Vinson syndrome). Leathery plaques, painless red patches, or a painless sore in the mouth area may be the first sign of oral cancer. Lymph glands are soon involved.

Local pain usually appears later. Treatment includes surgery and radiation.

oral contraceptive, an oral steroid drug for birth control. The two major steroids used are progestogen and a combination of progestogen and estrogen, both related to female sexuality. The steroids act by stopping the making of a hormone (gonadotropin releasing) by the hypothalamus. Therefore the pituitary gland does not get the signal to put out the hormones (gonadotropins) that usually cause the ovary to release an egg cell. This causes the endometrium lining of the uterus to become thin and the cervical mucus to become thick, thus stopping the sperm from getting through it. Before birth control pills are given, the woman should have a complete physical examination. While on the drug, she should be examined after 3 months and then once a year. Combination steroids are given for 3 weeks with no drug in the fourth week to allow for withdrawal bleeding (menstruation). Conditions that usually keep the patient from using birth control pills include diabetes mellitus, liver disease, high levels of blood fats, blood clotting problems, coronary heart disease, and sickle cell disease. Patients who are depressed or who have migraine headaches and those who are heavy cigarette smokers usually need more frequent medical checkups. An increased risk of circulation disorders occurs in women over 35 years of age who have used birth control pills for more than 5 years and who smoke cigarettes or who have other risk factors. A lack of menstrual flow may occur in women who stop taking birth control pills, particularly those who have a history of this condition. See also **contraception.**

oral hygiene, the practice of cleaning the teeth or mouth to take away bits of food, germs, and plaque. It includes massaging the gums, using dental floss or a water tool, or cleaning dentures and making sure of their proper fit to keep the gums healthy.

oral mucous membranes, the tissues lining the mouth that may be changed by different types of diseases, injuries, and treatments. Symptoms of damage include mouth pain or discomfort, a coated tongue, dry mouth, mouth tumors or ulcers, a lack of or decrease in saliva, bleeding gums, tooth cavities, and bad breath. Conditions that can cause changes in tissues of the mouth cavity include radiation to the head or neck, chemical or mechanical injury, bad mouth care, infection, poor nutrition, the effect of certain drugs, loss of water in the body, and breathing through the mouth.

oral poliovirus vaccine (OPV), a drug of changed live poliovirus that makes a patient immune to poliomyelitis. It is often given for a vaccination against poliomyelitis. Problems with the body's natural ability to resist infection and disease, using steroids at the same time, cancer, or severe infection prohibits its use. Side effects are uncommon. Also called **Sabin vaccine.**

oral stage, the first stage of psychosexual growth, occurring in the first 12 to 18 months of life when the feeding experience and other mouth-related activities are the main source of pleasure. To a great extent, experiences during this stage cause later feelings about food, love, being accepted and rejected, and other parts of the links between the patient and friends or family and the way people act.

Orasone, a trademark for an adrenal hormone (prednisone).

Ora-Testryl, a trademark for a male sex hormone used to treat sexual failure (impotence) (fluoxymesterone).

orbicularis oculi /ôrbik′yəler′is/, the muscular part of the eyelid made up of the palpebral, orbital, and lacrimal muscles. The palpebral muscle closes the eyelid gently; the orbital muscle closes it harder, as in winking.

orbicularis oris, the muscle that goes around the mouth, made up partly of fibers taken from other face muscles and partly of fibers that are in the lips. It closes and purses the lips.

orbit, one of a pair of bony, cup-shaped openings in the skull that contain the eyeballs and various eye muscles, nerves, and blood vessels that deal with the eyeballs.

orbital fat, a cushion of fat that lines the bony opening (orbit) in the skull that houses the eye. Loss of the fat causes the eye to look sunken. The fat may be replaced by tumor or other abnormal tissue in some diseases.

orbital pseudotumor, inflammation of the orbital tissues of the eye, marked by bulging eyes and swollen eyelids. The cause is not known.

orchidectomy /ôr′kidek′-/, an operation to take out one or both testicles. It may be done for serious disease or injury to the testicles or to control cancer of the prostate by taking out a source of male sex (androgenic) hormones. Also called **orchiectomy.**

orchiopexy /ôr′kē·ōpek′sē/, an operation to move an unlowered testicle into the sac that holds the testicles (scrotum), and attach it so that it will not move back into the intestinal area.

orchitis /ôrkī′-/, inflammation of one or both of the testicles, marked by pain. It is often caused by mumps, syphilis, or tuberculosis. Treatment includes supporting and raising the scrotum, cold packs, and painkillers.

Oretic, a trademark for a drug to increase the passing of urine (diuretic) (hydrochlorothiazide).

Oreticyl, a trademark for a blood pressure drug containing a diuretic (hydrochlorothiazide) and a high blood pressure drug (deserpidine).

Oreton Methyl, a trademark for a male sex hormone (methyltestosterone).

O–P

oreximania /ôrek′sē-/, a condition of extreme appetite and of too much eating. It often results from an unusual or unnatural fear of becoming thin when there is no great chance of that happening. Compare **anorexia.**

orf, a skin disease caused by a virus from sheep, in which painless blisters may become red, oozing bumps, finally crusting and healing. Treatment is not necessary. The condition heals by itself.

organ, a structural part of a system of the body made up of tissues and cells that allow it to do a certain job, as the liver, spleen, or heart. Each one of the organs that occur in pairs, as the lungs, can function by itself. The liver, pancreas, spleen, and brain may continue normal or near normal function with over 30% of its tissue damaged, destroyed, or taken out using surgery.

organic, **1.** referring to any chemical compound that has carbon in it. **2.** referring to an organ.

organic mental disorder, any mental or behavior problem caused by a physical problem of brain tissue. Causes may include cerebral arteriosclerosis, lead poisoning, or neurosyphilis. Also called **organic brain syndrome.**

organism, any individual living animal or plant able to live by using organs and bits of living substance found in most cells (organelles) in a way that each organ depends on the others.

organogenesis /ôr′gənōjen′əsis/. See **embryologic development.**

organoid, any structure that looks like an organ physically or by the way it works, especially an abnormal tumor mass.

organoid neoplasm. See **neoplasm.**

organotherapy, the treatment of disease by giving animal endocrine glands or the substance that comes from them. Whole glands are no longer put into patients, but substances taken from animal organs are widely used. Also called **Brown-Séquard's treatment.**

orgasm, the sexual climax, a series of strong muscle tightenings of the genitals over which there is no control. It is experienced as very pleasurable and is set off by intense sexual excitement. **–orgasmic,** *adj.*

orientation, being aware of where one is with regard to time, place, and knowing who the people around you are. Lack of orientation is usually a symptom of physical brain disease and most mental diseases.

orifice /ôr′ifis/, the entrance or outlet of any opening in the body, as the vaginal orifice.

Orimune, a trademark for a live poliovirus vaccine taken by mouth.

Orinase, a trademark for an antidiabetic drug (tolbutamide) taken by swallowing.

Ornade, a trademark for a drug that has a decongestant (phenylpropanolamine hydrochloride), an antihistamine (chlorpheniramine maleate), and a nerve signal blocker (isopropamide iodide), used for the relief of symptoms of upper breathing tract problems.

ornithine /ôr′nithin/, an amino acid that is not a part of proteins, but is a substance made while food is being made into energy by the body.

ornithine carbamoyl transferase, an enzyme in the blood that increases in patients with liver disease and other diseases.

Ornithodoros /ôr′nithod′ərəs/, a type of tick, some kinds of which carry the spirochetes of relapsing fevers.

orphan drug, any drug that is used by physicians and patients in other countries but is not sold in the United States. An orphan drug may not be for sale or use in the United States because the drug may not have been approved by the Bureau of Drugs of the Food and Drug Administration. The U.S. Orphan Drug Act of 1983 offers federal money to companies and research groups to make and sell drugs that before now have not been available in the United States.

orphenadrine citrate, a drug that relaxes skeletal muscles given to treat serious muscle strain. Myasthenia gravis, allergic reactions to similar drugs, or known allergy to this drug prohibits its use. Side effects include dry mouth, rapid heart beat, and allergic reactions.

orphenadrine hydrochloride, a nerve signal blocker and antihistaminic drug given to treat parkinsonism. Myasthenia gravis or other condition that keep doctors from using nerve signal blocking drugs or a known allergy to this drug prohibits its use. Side effects include nerve signal blocking problems and allergic reactions.

orthodontic appliance /ôr′thədon′tik/, any device used to change tooth position. A **fixed orthodontic appliance** is cemented to the teeth or attached by an adhesive. A **labiolingual fixed orthodontic appliance** has anchor bands attached to the first permanent molars of both jaws. An **extraoral orthodontic appliance** secures to a part of the face, the neck, or the back of the head to place traction on the teeth or jaws. An orthodontic device in the mouth to correct poor tooth contact is called an **intraoral orthodontic appliance.** A **removable orthodontic appliance** is placed inside the mouth and can be removed or replaced by the patient. A **Jackson crib** is a removable orthodontic appliance kept in position by crib-shaped wires. A **retaining orthodontic appliance** holds the teeth in place, after tooth movement, until the desired place is made stable.

orthodontics, a branch of dentistry that deals with crooked teeth (malocclusion) and problems of badly lined-up teeth.

orthomyxovirus /-mik′sō-/, a member of a family of viruses that includes several that cause the flu (human influenza).

Ortho-Novum, a trademark for a birth control pill that has a female sex hormone (mestranol) and a progestin (norethindrone).

orthopantogram /-pan′təgram/, an x-ray film showing a view of all of the teeth, jaw bones, and nearby structures on a single film.

orthopedics /-pē′diks/, the branch of medicine that deals with the skeleton, its joints, muscles, and other related structures.

orthopedic traction, a way to put a limb, bone, or group of muscles under tension by means of weights and pulleys. Traction is used mainly to change the position of bones and to keep broken bones rigid. It also is used to overcome muscle spasm, to stretch binding scar tissue (adhesions), to correct certain badly formed bones, and to help correct tightening of muscles (contractures) caused by arthritis. Skin or skeletal traction used on a leg allows the patient to move more easily in bed because the leg is balanced with weights and any slack in the ropes attached to the weights caused by the patient's movements is taken up by the traction device. A girdle that fits over the pelvis is used to stop low back pain and a halter is used to stop neck pain. Neck traction may also be used when a broken neck bone is thought to have occurred. **Skeletal traction** is one of the basic kinds of traction used to treat broken bones and to correct deformities of the skeleton. It is applied to the affected structure by a metal pin or wire put into the tissue of the structure and attached to traction ropes. It is often used when continuous traction is needed to allow a broken bone to heal properly. Infection of the pin may develop with skeletal traction, and a careful watch of pin sites is an important precaution. Another basic kind, called **skin traction,** may be used directly on the skin by attaching the rope-pulley-weight system in various ways. **Adhesive skin traction** is a method in which the weights are applied to the skin with sticky straps. With **nonadhesive skin traction,** foam-backed traction straps are used to attach traction weights, usually when only temporary traction is needed. The straps spread the traction pull over a wide area of the skin surface and decrease the risk of skin damage to the patient. **Balanced traction** is a system of suspension that supplements traction for treating fractures of the legs or after various operations on the lower parts of the body. A device used only with infants to keep legs rigid is called **Bryant's traction.** It treats a broken thigh (femur) or corrects an inborn dislocation of the hip. A frame supports weights, connected by ropes that run through pulleys to foot plates. One of the most common devices for leg disorders, **Buck's traction,** may be used on one or both legs. It is used to line up and keep rigid the legs in the treatment of broken bones and diseases of the hip and knee. The device is usually made up of a metal bar leading from a frame at the foot of the bed and supporting traction weights connected by a rope passing through a pulley to a cast or a splint around the legs. **Russell traction** combines suspension and traction to hold, position, and line up the lower legs. It is used to treat broken upper legs and to treat diseases or disorders of the hip and knee. A method called **90-90 traction** combines skeletal traction and suspension with a short-leg cast or a splint to keep still and position the leg in the treatment of a displaced broken thigh. It is especially used for children. A pin is inserted into bone in the knee area and attached to a riser running through a pulley and weight system. Use of 90-90 traction may also have a jacket restraint to help keep the patient rigid. One type of this traction is often used with adults to treat low back pain.

orthophoto maps, aerial photographs corrected to scale such that geographic measurements may be taken directly from the prints. They may contain graphically emphasized geographic features and may be provided with overlays of such features as water systems and important facility locations.

orthopnea /-pnē′ə, ôrthop′nē·ə/, an abnormal condition in which a patient must sit or stand to breathe deeply or comfortably. It occurs in many disorders of the heart and breathing systems, as asthma, emphysema, pneumonia, and chest pain (angina pectoris). See also **dyspnea.**

orthopsychiatry, the branch of psychiatry that studies mild mental and behavior disorders, especially in children, and tries to create new ways to help emotional growth.

orthoptic /ôrthop′tik/, referring to normal two-eyed (binocular) sight.

orthoptic examination, testing of the ability of the two eyes to work together correctly, resulting in a single image. If the patient has diplopia, two images are seen. If the patient has amblyopia only one picture may be seen by the working eye. Three-dimensional sight (stereoscopic) training may help in some conditions.

orthosis /ôrthō′-/, a system designed to control, correct, or make up for a badly shaped bone. Orthosis treatment often uses special braces. **Electric spinal orthosis** is an electric device that helps control curving of the spine (scoliosis) by stimulating the back muscles. The portable, battery-powered machine does not cure scoliosis, but it does stop the condition from getting worse.

orthotonos /ôrthot′ənəs/, a straight, rigid posture of the body caused by a muscle spasm. It may happen after being poisoned by strychnine or after a tetanus infection.

Ortolani's test /ôr′təlä′nēz/, a test of the stability of the hip joints in infants. The baby is placed on its back, with the hips and knees bent at right angles. The legs are pushed out until the outside of the knees touch the table. The examiner's fingers are stretched out along the outside of the thighs, with the thumbs holding the insides of the knees. The knees are turned to the inside and to the outside. A click or a popping feeling (Ortolani's sign) may be felt if the joint is not strong, because the end of the thigh bone (femur) moves out of the hip joint under pressure from the examiner's hands. See also **congenital dislocation of the hip.**

oscilloscope /osil′əskōp/,   a device that makes a picture of electric pulses by means of a TV-like screen. Oscilloscopes have many uses in medicine. For example, brain waves and heart beats can be displayed in order to watch and test their functions.

Osgood-Schlatter disease,   inflammation or partial coming apart of the point of attachment of the knee cap (patellar) ligament on the lower leg bone. Symptoms include swelling and tenderness near the top of a lower leg bone (tibia). It is caused by too much use of a thigh muscle (quadriceps). The condition is seen mainly in athletic adolescent boys. Exercise or any movement that straightens out the leg increases the problem. Treatment may require keeping the knee completely rigid in a cast. If the leg does not heal, surgery may be necessary.

OSHA,   U.S. Occupational Safety and Health Administration.

Osler's nodes,   tender, red bumps on the ends of fingers or toes. The condition is seen in an infection of the heart lining and valves (bacterial endocarditis) and usually lasts only 1 or 2 days.

Osler-Weber-Rendu syndrome /-randoo′/,   an inherited blood vessel disorder. It features bleeding from widened surface blood vessels (capillaries) in the skin and mucous membranes. Small red-to-violet sores are found on the lips, mouth and nasal mucous membranes, tongue, and tips of fingers and toes. Bleeding from the small sores is often heavy and may result in serious blood shortage (anemia). Blood replacement may be necessary for severe bleeding, and iron deficiency anemia may need continuous treatment.

osmosis /ozmō′-, os-/,   the movement of a fluid, as water, through a special tissue (semipermeable membrane) from a solution that has a lower amount of a dissolved substance to one that has a higher amount. Movement through the tissue happens until the levels of dissolved material in the solutions become equal.

osseous labyrinth /os′ē·əs/,   the bony part of the inside of the ear. It is made up of three cavities: the vestibule, the semicircular canals, and the cochlea, carrying sound vibrations from the middle ear to the acoustic nerve. All three cavities hold a fluid called perilymph.

ossicle /os′ikəl/,   a small bone, as the hammer (malleus), the anvil (incus), and the stirrup (stapes), the ossicles of the inner ear.   **–ossicular,** *adj.*

ossification,   the growth of bone. **Intramembranous ossification** is bone growth that has membrane growth go before it, as in the forming of the roof and the sides of the skull. **Intracartilaginous ossification** is bone growth that has the growth of rods of cartilage go before it, as that forming the bones of the arms and legs.

ossifying fibroma,   a slow-growing, noncancerous tumor of bone, seen most often in the jaws, especially the lower jaw. The tumor is made up of bone that grows within fiberlike connective tissue.

ostealgia /os′tē·al′jə/,   any pain that is linked to an abnormal condition within a bone, as osteomyelitis.

osteitis /os′tē·ī′-/,   an inflammation of bone, caused by infection, wasting away of bone, or injury. Symptoms include swelling, tenderness, dull, aching pain, and redness in the skin over the affected bone. **Osteitis fibrosa cystica** is a condition in which normal bone is replaced by cysts and fiberlike tissue. It is usually linked to excess production of thyroid hormone (hyperparathyroidism).

osteoarthritis /os′tē·ō·ärthrī′-/,   a common form of arthritis in which one or more joints have tissue changes. Symptoms include pain after exercise or use of the joint. Stiffness, tenderness to the touch, rubbing noises (crepitus), and a large joint develop. Lumps may form in bone tissue. Cartilage that normally cushions the joint becomes soft and breaks down. Small pieces of bone and cartilage may become loose and get caught inside the joint. Inflammation of the membrane lining the joint is common. Its cause is unknown but may include chemical, mechanical, inborn, metabolic, and endocrine factors. Also called **degenerative joint disease.** Compare **rheumatoid arthritis.**

osteoblast /-blast′/,   a cell that begins in the embryo and, during the early growth of the skeleton, works in forming bone tissue. Osteoblasts bring together the substances that form the bone and over time grow into osteocytes.

osteoblastoma /-blastō′mə/,   a small, noncancerous bone tumor that causes pain and loss of bone tissue. It occurs most often in the spine or bones of the legs or arms, usually in children and young adults. Treatment includes surgery.

osteochondroma /-kondrō′mə/,   a noncancerous tumor made of bone and cartilage.

osteochondrosis /-kondrō′-/,   a disease that affects the bone-forming centers in children. It begins by destroying and killing bone tissue, followed by regrowth of bone tissue. Kinds See also **Osgood-Schlatter disease, Perthes′ disease, Scheuermann's disease.**

osteoclasia /-klā′zhə/,   a condition in which bony tissue is destroyed and absorbed by large bone cells (osteoclasts). It may occur during growth or the healing of broken bones.

osteoclasis /os'tē·ok'ləsis/, an operation in which a surgeon breaks a bone on purpose that is badly shaped and reshapes it in a normal condition.

osteoclast /-klast'/, a large bone cell that works in periods of growth or repair. During healing of broken bones, or during some diseases, osteoclasts are set off by parathyroid hormone and also by a substance made by white blood cells (lymphocytes).

osteoclastoma /-klastō'mə/, a giant cell tumor of the bone that occurs most often at the end of a long bone. It often appears as a tissue mass that has a thin shell of new bone around it. The tumor may be harmless (benign) but is more often cancerous. It causes pain, loss of the ability of the bone to work correctly, and, in some cases, weakness followed by broken bones.

osteocyte /-sīt'/, a bone cell; a fully grown osteoblast that has become buried in the bone material (matrix). It connects with other osteoblasts to form a system of tiny canals within the bone substance.

osteodystrophy /-dis'trəfē/, any basic problem in bone growth. It is usually linked to problems in calcium and phosphorus use by the body and kidney disease, as in kidney osteodystrophy.

osteogenesis /-jen'əsis/, the beginning and growth of bone tissue. **Electrically stimulated osteogenesis** is a way to cause bone growth by putting in electrodes that send electric current to the bone. This is used for breaks that don't heal.

osteogenesis imperfecta, an inborn problem that causes poor growth of connective tissue. It features abnormally brittle and fragile bones that are easily broken by the slightest injury. In its worst form, the disease may be seen at birth (osteogenesis imperfecta congenita). The newborn baby has many broken bones and is usually badly deformed. Most infants with this condition die shortly after birth, although a few survive as badly deformed dwarfs with normal mental growth if no head injury has occurred. If the disease happens later (osteogenesis imperfecta tarda), it is usually less serious. Symptoms may appear when the child begins to walk, but they become less serious with age, and the high risk of having broken bones gets lower and often goes away after puberty. There is no known cure for the disease. Extreme care must be taken in handling patients. Treatment may include magnesium oxide to control symptoms linked to the condition. Also called **brittle bones.**

osteolysis /os'tē·ol'isis/, the destruction of bone tissue, caused by disease, infection, or poor blood supply. The condition often affects bones of the hands and feet. It is seen in disorders that affect blood vessels, as in Raynaud's disease, and systemic lupus erythematosus.

osteoma /os'tē·ō'mə/, a tumor of bone tissue.

osteomalacia /-məlā'shə/, an abnormal softening of the bone. There is a loss of calcium in the bone material, along with weakness, broken bones, pain, loss of desire to eat, and weight loss. The condition may be caused by not enough phosphorus and calcium in the blood to allow proper hardening of the bones. This lack of minerals may be caused by poor diet, a lack of vitamin D, or not getting enough sunlight, which the body needs to make use of vitamin D. Other causes are a disorder that disturbs the normal absorbtion of minerals and nutrients from the intestine. Treatment includes giving the necessary vitamins and minerals.

osteomyelitis /-mī'əlī'-/, an infection of bone and bone marrow. Symptoms include continuing and increasing bone pain, tenderness, local muscle spasm, and fever. It is usually caused by germs (often staphylococci) that enter the bone during an injury or surgery, or from a nearby infection, or through the bloodstream. The long bones in children and the spinal bones in adults are often places of infection caused by germs spreading through the bloodstream. Treatment includes bed rest and antiinfection drugs by injection for several weeks. Surgery may be necessary to take out dead bone and tissue, to fill holes, and to use artificial devices to keep the diseased bones and joints from moving. Long-term osteomyelitis may go on for years with periods of many or fewer symptoms in spite of treatment.

osteonecrosis /-nekrō'-/, the destruction and death of bone tissue, as caused by cancer, infection, injury, or not enough blood (ischemia).

osteopathy /os'tē·op'əthē/, the practice of medicine that uses all of the usual techniques of drugs, surgery, and radiation but looks more at the links between the organs and the muscle and skeletal system. Osteopathic physicians may correct structural problems by changing the position of bones in the treatment of health problems.

osteopetrosis /-pētrō'-/, an inborn disease with an increase in bone density. It usually results from a lack of large bone cells (osteoclasts). In its worst form, the bone marrow cavity is destroyed, causing severe low levels of blood (anemia), a badly shaped skull, and pressure on the skull nerves, which may cause deafness and blindness and lead to an early death. A milder form features short height, fragile bones that break easily, and a likelihood to develop a bone disease (osteomyelitis).

osteopoikilosis /-poi'kilō'-/, an inborn condition of the bones with many areas of dense calcium deposits all over the bone tissue. It causes a spotty look on x-ray film. Osteopoikilosis is usually harmless, most often without symptoms.

osteoporosis /-pôrō'-/, a loss of normal bone density with thinning of bone tissue and the growth of small holes in the

O–P

bone. The disorder may cause pain, especially in the lower back, frequent broken bones, loss of body height, and various badly formed parts of the body. It occurs most often in women who have gone through menopause, patients who are inactive or paralyzed, and patients taking steroid hormones. Estrogen, a female sex hormone, is often used to prevent postmenopausal osteoporosis.

osteosarcoma /-särkō′mə/, a type of cancer made up of bone cells.

osteosclerosis /-sklerō′-/, an abnormal increase in bone density. The condition occurs in different kinds of diseases and is often linked to poor blood circulation in the bone tissue, infection, and the forming of tumors.

osteotomy /os′te·ot′əmē/, the sawing or cutting of a bone. Kinds of osteotomy include block osteotomy, in which a section of bone is removed; cuneiform osteotomy to remove a bone wedge; and displacement osteotomy, in which a bone is rebuilt using surgery to change the way bones line up with each other on the areas of bones that carry most of the body's weight.

ostomy /os′təmē/, *informal.* using surgery to make an artificial opening in the body to allow the release of urine from the bladder or of feces from the bowel. A cut (stoma) in the wall of the abdomen is made using surgery. An ostomy may also be done to treat a blockage, infection, or injury of the urinary or intestinal tract. Each operation is named for the place of the ostomy in the body and its organs. For example, **cecocolostomy** connects the upper and lower part of the large intestine (the cecum and the colon); **cecoileostomy** connects the lower part of the small intestine with the upper part of the large intestine, the ileum to the cecum; **cecostomy** makes an opening from the abdomen into the cecum. It is done as a short-term measure to relieve blocked intestines in a patient who cannot have major surgery. In ostomy care, a long-term device is attached to the stoma as soon after surgery as possible. Each time the short-term or long-term device is changed, the skin around the stoma is washed with soap and water, rinsed carefully, and patted dry with a clean towel. If the skin is reddened or worn away, karaya powder, by itself or mixed with an ointment, is spread over the area before the device is put back in. A sticky substance may be used to keep a tight seal with the device, and deodorant drops or other odor controllers are added to the ostomy bag. The patient's diet must be planned according to the kind of ostomy. A patient with an ileostomy may need food high in sodium and potassium, as bananas, citrus juices, molasses, and cola. A diet of foods that the body can easily digest and absorb is best for most ostomy patients. How much fluid the patient drinks should also be closely watched. **Ostomy irrigation** refers to a way to clean, start, and control the release of an opening in the body made during surgery to allow better discharge of feces or urine. Fluids used to clean out the opening are often tap water and salt or drugs dissolved in a liquid. Various tools are needed, such as tubes (catheters), a container used during the cleaning of the device, and shields to keep leaking from occurring.

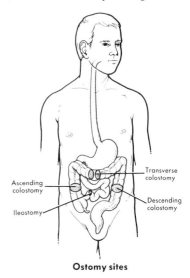

Ostomy sites

OTC. See **over the counter.**

otic /ō′tik/, referring to the ear.

otics, drugs used to treat inflammation of the outer ear canal or to take out excess ear wax (cerumen).

otitis /ōtī′-/, inflammation or infection of the ear. **Otitis externa** affects the outside canal of the ear or the larger part (auricle) outside the head. It is common in hot, humid weather. The main causes are allergy, germs, fungi, viruses, and injury. A patient may be allergic to nickel or chromium metal in earrings, to chemicals in hair sprays, to cosmetics, to hearing aids, and to certain drugs. Herpes simplex and herpes zoster viruses are often causes. Eczema, psoriasis, and seborrheic dermatitis also may affect the outer ear. Bruises of the ear canal may become infected. Swimming too much may wash out the ear wax that protects the ear and remove skin fats, leading to infection. **Otitis media** affects the middle ear, a common disease of childhood. Symptoms include a sense of fullness in the ear, with impaired hearing, pain, and fever. Germs, allergy, fungus, and several viruses also may be causes. An upper chest breathing infection often happens before the onset of otitis media. Germs and viruses get into the middle ear through the eustachian tube, which opens into the mouth and throat. Blockage of the eustachian tube and gathering of fluids may increase pressure within the middle ear, forcing infection into the porous mastoid bone next to the ear or breaking the eardrum (tympanic membrane). Usually only one ear gets this disorder. A tumorlike cyst may grow in the middle ear. Deafness may occur if many infections cause a broken eardrum. **Pneumococcal otitis media** may also spread to the membranes of the brain and spinal cord. Treatment for both forms includes aspirin or similar painkillers, careful cleaning, and antibiotics.

Otocort, a trademark for eardrops with a hormone (hydrocortisone), antiinfection drugs (neomycin sulfate and polymyxin B sulfate), and two painkillers (antipyrine, dibucaine).

otolaryngology /ō′tōler′ing·gol′-/, a branch of medicine that deals with diseases and disorders of the ears, nose, and throat, and nearby parts of the head and neck.

otolith righting reflex /ō′təlith/, a reflex in newborns. Tilting of the body when in an upright position causes the head to move back to the upright position. This movement allows the infant to raise the head. Not having this movement may mean there is something wrong with the baby's central nervous system.

otoplasty /-plas′tē/, plastic surgery to rebuild the outer ear. Some of the cartilage in the ears is removed in order to bring the outer ear closer to the head.

Otoreid-HC, a trademark for eardrops with a hormone (hydrocortisone) and antibiotics (neomycin sulfate and polymyxin B sulfate).

otorrhea /ō′tôrē′ə/, any substance discharged from the external ear. Otorrhea may contain blood, pus, or cerebrospinal fluid.

otosclerosis /-sklerō′-/, an inborn problem in which abnormal bone formation in the canal labyrinth of the inner ear causes noises in the ear, then deafness. The deafness may come between 11 and 30 years of age. Women get this condition twice as often as men. An operation to replace the stapes in the middle ear usually works to restore hearing.

otoscope /-skōp/, a tool used to look at the outer ear, the eardrum, and the tiny bones (ossicles) of the middle ear. It includes a light, a magnifying lens, and a device for blowing air into the ear (insufflation).

ototoxic /-tok′sik/, having a bad effect on the organs of hearing and balance or the eighth cranial (vestibulocochlear) nerve. Common ototoxic drugs include certain antibiotics, aspirin, and quinine.

Otrivin, a trademark for a drug that narrows blood vessels (xylometazoline hydrochloride), used as a nasal decongestant.

ounce (oz), a unit of weight equal to ¹⁄₁₆ of 1 pound avoirdupois.

outcome, the condition of a patient at the end of treatment or of a disease, including how well the patient is and the need for giving more care, drugs, support, or counseling.

outlet, an opening through which something can come out, as the pelvic outlet through which a baby comes during childbirth.

outlet contracture, an abnormally small pelvic outlet. It is important in childbirth because it may not let the baby come through the birth canal.

out-of-service resources, resources assigned to an incident but unable to respond for mechanical, rest, or personnel reasons.

outpatient, **1.** a patient, not staying in a hospital, who is being treated in an office, clinic, or other walk-in ambulatory care facility. **2.** referring to a health care facility for patients who do not need to be in a hospital. Compare **inpatient.**

ova and parasites test /ō′və/, a test using a microscope to look for parasites, as amebas or worms and their eggs (ova) in a patient's feces.

ovarian artery /ōver′ē·ən/, a slim branch of the abdominal aorta that takes blood to an ovary.

ovarian cancer, a cancer of the ovary. It occurs most often in women between 40 and 60 years of age and sometimes in adolescents.

ovarian carcinoma, a type of cancer of the ovaries that is not often found in the early stage. The tumor may have grown a great deal by the time it is found. Symptoms may include fluid buildup, swollen legs, and pain in the abdomen and backs of the legs. In women who have gone through menopause signs of the cancer may be swelling and pain in the intestine area, abnormal vaginal bleeding, weight loss, and changes in urination and bowel movement patterns. This cancer occurs often in the fifth decade of life and is the most common tumor of the reproductive system. The chance of getting the disease are increased by not being able to have children (infertility), having few or no children, having children later than normal, repeated miscarriage, endometriosis, Group A blood type, irradiation of pelvic organs, and exposure to chemicals that cause cancer, as asbestos and talc. Getting a pelvic examination each year after 40 years of age helps find the cancer at an early stage and helps the chances of recovery. A pap smear may show cancer cells if the tumor is far along. A test using high level sound waves (ultrasound examination) can show an ovarian tumor but does not show the difference between a harmless and cancerous tumor. A definite diagnosis requires surgery. The surgery that doctors suggest for ovarian cancer includes taking out the uterus, ovaries, fallopian tubes, and the connecting membranes (omentum). Radiation and chemotherapy are used after surgery. About one half of the tumors found to have cancer cannot be operated on.

ovarian cyst, a small globelike sac filled with fluid or semisolid material that grows in or on the ovary. It may

O–P

only stay there for a short time and can be harmless or dangerous. See also **dermoid cyst.**

ovarian varicocele, a varicose swelling of the veins of the broad ligament that helps support the ovaries. Also called **pelvic varicocele.**

ovarian vein, one of a pair of veins that come out from the broad ligament near the ovaries and the fallopian tubes.

ovary, one of the pair of female sexual reproduction organs (gonads) found on each side of the lower abdomen in a fold of the broad ligament, beside the uterus. Each ovary is normally firm, smooth, and like an almond in size and shape. At ovulation, an egg (ovum) is released from a small cavity (follicle) on the surface of the ovary. See also **ovulation.**

Ovcon, a trademark for a birth control pill containing a female sex hormone (ethinyl estradiol) and a progestin (norethindrone acetate).

overbite. See **bite.**

overclosure, an abnormal condition in which the lower jaw rises too far.

overcompensation, an extreme attempt to overcome a real or unreal physical or mental problem. The patient may or may not be aware of trying to solve the problem. See also **compensation.**

overhead personnel, personnel who are assigned to supervisory positions: incident commander, command staff, general staff, directors, supervisors, and unit leaders.

overjet, a side to side (horizontal) pushing out of upper teeth beyond the lower teeth.

overload, anything that pushes the body beyond normal limits and may harm health.

overoxygenation, an abnormal condition in which the amount of oxygen in the blood and other tissues of the body is greater than normal and the amount of carbon dioxide is less than normal. The condition features a fall in blood pressure, being less able to breathe, weakness, making errors in judgment, having numb hands and feet, nausea, and vomiting.

over the counter (OTC), referring to a drug that the consumer can buy without a prescription.

overweight, more than normal in body weight after taking into account height, body build, and age. See also **obesity.**

ovoflavin /ō'vəflā'vin/, a riboflavin (vitamin B_2) taken from the yolk of eggs.

ovoglobulin /-glob'yəlin/, a protein (globulin) taken from the white of eggs.

ovotestis /-tes'/, a sexual reproductive organ (gonad) that has tissue like that of both the ovary and testicles; a male and female (hermaphroditic) gonad. **–ovotesticular,** *adj.*

Ovral, a trademark for a birth control pill that has a progestin (norgestrel) and a female sex hormone (ethinyl estradiol).

Ovrette, a trademark for a birth control pill that has a progestin (norgestrel).

ovulation /ov'yəlā'shən/, releasing an egg (ovum) from the ovary after the breaking of a mature small cavity (follicle). Ovulation is brought on by the gonadotrophic hormones, follicle stimulating hormone (FSH), and luteinizing hormone (LH). The fully grown ovarian follicle also releases the hormones estrogen and progesterone. Ovulation usually occurs on the fourteenth day following the first day of the last menstrual period and often causes brief, sharp pain on the side of the ovulating ovary. **–ovulate,** *v.*

Ovulen, a trademark for a birth control pill that has a female sex hormone (mestranol) and a progestin (ethynodiol diacetate).

ovum /ō'vəm/, *pl.* **ova,** **1.** an egg. **2.** a female germ cell released from the ovary at ovulation.

oxacillin sodium, an antibiotic given to treat severe infections caused by penicillin-immune staphylococci. Known allergy to this drug or to any other penicillin prohibits its use. Side effects include severe allergic reactions, stomach and intestinal disturbances, and itching in the anal and genital areas.

Oxalid, a trademark for a drug (oxyphenbutazone) to treat inflammation and rheumatic disorders.

oxandrolone, a male sex hormone given to treat lack of testosterone, osteoporosis, and female breast cancer, and to start or increase growth, weight gain, and red blood cell production. Cancer of the male breast or prostate, liver disease, pregnancy, or known allergy to this drug prohibits its use. Side effects include excess hair growth (hirsutism), acne, liver disease, too many or too few minerals in the body, and hormone effects.

oxazepam, a mild tranquilizer given to help lower tension and nervousness.

oxidation, any process in which the amount of oxygen of a chemical compound is increased. **–oxidize,** *v.*

oxidizing agent, a chemical compound that easily gives up oxygen and attracts hydrogen from another compound.

Oxsoralen, a trademark for a skin-coloring drug (methoxsalen).

oxtriphylline, a bronchial tube widening drug given to treat bronchial asthma, bronchitis, and emphysema. Known allergy to this or a related drug prohibits its use. It is used carefully in patients with ulcers or with heart disease for whom making the heart beat faster might be harmful. Side effects include stomach and intestinal distress, irregular heart beat, nervousness, and not being able to sleep (insomnia).

oxybutynin chloride, a nerve drug given to treat a bladder that is not working correctly (neurogenic). Glaucoma, problems of the stomach and intestinal or urinary tract, or known allergy to this drug or to other drugs like it prohibits its use. Side effects include reduced sweating, urinary bloating, blurred sight, rapid heart beat, and severe allergic reactions.

oxycephaly /ok′sēsef′əlē/, a birth defect of the skull in which premature closing of the joints or seams (sutures) of the skull results in increased upward growth of the head, giving it a long, narrow look with the top pointed or cone-shaped. –**oxycephalus,** *n.,* **oxycephalous,** *adj.*

oxycodone hydrochloride, a narcotic painkiller used to treat moderate to severe pain. It is used carefully in many conditions, including head injuries, asthma, kidney or liver disease, or unstable heart condition. Known allergy to this drug prohibits its use. Side effects include sleepiness, dizziness, nausea, constipation, breathing and circulation problems, and drug addiction.

oxygen (O), a gas that is necessary for human life and has no taste, odor, or color. In breathing therapy, oxygen is given to increase the amount of oxygen and thus to lower the amount of other gases in the blood. In anesthesia, oxygen is a carrier gas for the delivery of anesthetic drugs to the tissues of the body. See also **oxygen toxicity.**

oxygenation, the process of combining or treating with oxygen. –**oxygenate,** *v.*

oxygen consumption, the amount of oxygen in milliliters per minute necessary for normal body functions.

oxygen mask, a device used to give oxygen. It is shaped to fit snugly over the mouth and nose and may be held in place with a strap or with the hand.

oxygen therapy, any method used to give oxygen to relieve oxygen shortage (hypoxia). If the hypoxia results from heart disease, a high level of oxygen may be given by a mask. Humidity and drugs in aerosol form may be given with oxygen. Oxygen therapy may help relieve low blood pressure, heart rhythm disorders, rapid heart beat, headache, confusion, and nausea.

oxygen toxicity, a condition of oxygen overdose that can cause dangerous tissue changes, as a form of blindness (retrolental fibroplasia) or a type of emphysema (bronchopulmonary dysplasia).

oxygen transport, the way oxygen is absorbed in the lungs by the hemoglobin in red blood cells and carried to tissue cells all over the body. This process is possible because hemoglobin is able to combine with large amounts of oxygen when it is at high levels, as in the lungs, and to release this oxygen when the oxygen level is low, as in the body tissues. See also **hemoglobin.**

oxymetazoline hydrochloride, a decongestant given to treat nasal congestion. Hyperthyroidism, diabetes, use of a monoamine oxidase inhibitor within 14 days, or known allergy to this drug prohibits its use. Side effects include central nervous system activity, and, in children, a severe disorder with coma, falling blood pressure, and slow heart beat.

oxymetholone, a male sex hormone given to treat a lack of testosterone, an abnormal bone disease (osteoporosis), and female breast cancer, and to increase the rate of growth, weight gain, and the making of red blood cells. Cancer of the male breast or prostate, liver disease, pregnancy or suspected pregnancy, or known allergy to this drug prohibits its use. Side effects include excess hair growth (hirsutism), acne, liver disease, having too much or too little minerals in the body, and hormone effects.

oxymorphone hydrochloride, a narcotic painkiller given to reduce moderate to severe pain, as a drug before surgery, and during anesthesia. Drug addiction or known allergy to this drug prohibits its use. Side effects include drug addiction, urinary bloating, and breathing or circulation problems.

oxyopia /ok′sē·ō′pē·ə/, unusually good sight. A patient with normal (20/20) vision when standing 20 feet from the standard Snellen eye chart can read the seventh line of letters, each of which is ⅛ inch high. A patient with oxyopia can read smaller letters at that distance.

oxyphenbutazone, a nonsteroid antiinflammatory drug given to treat arthritis, bursitis, gout, and other conditions with inflammation.

oxyphenonium bromide, a nerve drug given to treat peptic ulcer. Glaucoma, disorders of the stomach or intestinal or urinary tract, or known allergy to this or a related drug prohibits its use. Side effects include lower level of sweating, urinary bloating, rapid heart beat, blurred sight, and severe allergic reactions.

oxytetracycline, an antibiotic given to treat germ and rickettsial infections. Pregnancy, early childhood, or known allergy to this or to other tetracyclines prohibits its use. The drug is used carefully in patients who have kidney or liver disease. Side effects include stomach and intestinal ailments, being sensitive to light, possible new and serious infections, and different kinds of allergic reactions. The teeth of children exposed to the drug in the uterus or before 8 years of age may become badly discolored.

oxytocic /-tō′sik/, any one of many drugs that start the smooth muscle of the uterus to pull in (contract). An oxytocic can cause and increase rhythmic contractions in the uterus at any time, but high doses are needed for such responses in early pregnancy. These drugs are often used to start labor at the end of pregnancy. They are also used to control bleeding and correct uterine muscle tone after

O–P

childbirth, to cause uterine contractions after cesarean section or other uterine surgery, and to cause an abortion. The U.S. Food and Drug Administration has ruled that oxytocin should be used to end a pregnancy only in cases where continued pregnancy is seen as a greater risk to the mother or to the fetus than the risk of causing labor by drugs. These drugs are used very carefully in pregnant women with certain problems, such as severe blood pressure disorders. The risk of using these drugs is much higher in mothers who have just had uterine surgery or who have had a recent disease or injury. The most serious side effect is continued contractions of the uterus that may cause death of the fetus or a break in the uterus.

oxytocin /-tō′sin/, a hormone produced by the pituitary gland that starts uterine contractions in bringing on or increasing labor and release of milk from the breast. It also refers to a substance or drug that is like the hormone. See also **oxytocic.**

oxytocin challenge test, a test to see if the fetus is able to tolerate continuation of pregnancy or the likely stress of labor and childbirth. Other tests to check the well-being of the fetus may be done before physicians decide on an emergency childbirth by surgical opening (cesarean section) or causing labor. See also **stress test.**

ozena /ōzē′nə/, a condition of a decrease in the bony ridges and mucous membranes inside the nose. Symptoms include crusting of nasal fluids, discharge, and a very bad smell. Ozena may occur after long-term inflammation of the nasal mucosa.

ozone shield, the layer of ozone, a form of oxygen, that hangs in the atmosphere from 20 to 40 miles above the surface of the earth. It protects the earth from excess ultraviolet radiation.

ozone sickness, an abnormal condition caused by the breathing of ozone that may get into jet aircraft at altitudes over 40,000 feet. Symptoms include headaches, chest pains, itchy eyes, and sleepiness. Exactly why and how ozone causes this condition is not known. It is more common early in the year and occurs more often in flights over the Pacific Ocean.

P

PABA, abbreviation for **paraaminobenzoic acid.**

Pabanol, a trademark for a sunscreen (paraaminobenzoic acid).

pabulum /pab′yələm/, any substance that is a food or nutrient.

pacemaker, 1. a group of special nervous tissue at the junction of a great vein (superior vena cava) and the right chamber (atrium) of the heart. It causes the heart to contract. The right and left chambers (atria) then carry the signal on to another area (atrioventricular node), which causes the lower chamber of the heart to contract. 2. an artificial device for keeping a normal rhythm of heart contraction through electric signals to the heart muscle. A pacemaker may be permanent, sending the stimulus at a constant and fixed rate. It may also fire only on demand, as when the heart does not contract at a certain rate. Also called **cardiac pacemaker.**

pachyderma /pak′ēdur′mə/, thick skin.

pachyonychia congenita /-ōnik′ē·ə/, a birth defect with thick nails on the fingers and the toes, and with thick skin on the palms of the hands and soles of the feet.

pacifier, 1. something that soothes or comforts. 2. a nipple-shaped object used by infants and children for sucking. Pacifiers can be dangerous if they are too small or made poorly. The object can be swallowed or get stuck in the throat and block the air passage. The safest pacifiers are made in one piece, so that only the nipple fits into the mouth, with an easy-to-hold handle.

Pacini's corpuscles /päsē′nēz/, special pressure sense organs that look like tiny white onions, each joined to the end of one nerve fiber in the skin. They are found in the palm of the hand, sole of the foot, genitals, and joints.

pack, 1. a treatment in which all or part of the body is wrapped in hot or cold, wet or dry towels, or in ice for many reasons. Cold packs are used to bring down high temperatures and swellings or to lower body temperatures (hypothermia) during heart surgery or organ transplants. 2. a dressing to cover a wound or to fill the space left after removing a tooth.

package, an assembly consisting of the external structure and the internal container for transporting radioactive material.

packed cells, blood cells taken from the liquid portion (plasma) of the blood. They are given in severe anemia to restore normal levels of hemoglobin and red cells without overloading the bloodstream with excess fluids. See also **bank blood.**

pad, 1. a mass of soft material used to cushion shock, prevent wear, or soak up wetness. Abdominal pads are used to soak up fluids or to keep organs apart during surgery. 2. a mass of fat that cushions many structures, as the fat pad of the knee cap.

Paget's disease /paj′əts/, a bone disease of unknown cause, usually affecting older people. Most cases are mild and without symptoms. However, bone pain may be the first symptom. Bowed lower leg bones (saber shins), forward curve of the spine (kyphosis), and broken bones are caused by the soft, abnormal bone. The skull gets bigger. Headaches and warmth over the places affected are caused by more blood flowing through them. No treatment is needed for mild cases. Also called **osteitis deformans.**

Paget's disease of the nipple. See **nipple cancer.**

Pagitane Hydrochloride, a trademark for a nerve drug (cycrimine hydrochloride).

pagophagia /pā′gōfā′jə/, an abnormal condition with a craving to eat large amounts of ice. It is linked to a lack of iron in the diet.

pain, an unpleasant sense caused by signals from some sense nerve endings. It is a basic symptom of inflammation and is an important clue to the cause of many disorders. Pain may be mild or severe, chronic, acute, cutting, burning, dull, or sharp, exactly or poorly located, or referred. **Acute pain** describes severe pain, as may follow surgery or injury, occur with heart attacks, or occur with other diseases. Serious pain in patients with skeletal problems is caused by the covering over the bones (periosteum), the joint surfaces, and the artery walls. Muscle pain after bone surgery results from lack of blood to the muscle. Serious belly pain often causes the patient to lie on one side and draw up the legs in the fetal position. **Chronic pain** refers to pain that continues or returns over a long period. It can be caused by a number of diseases or abnormal conditions, as rheumatoid arthritis. Chronic pain is often less severe than acute pain. The patient with chronic pain usually does

O–P

329

not have increased pulse and rapid breathing because these nervous system reactions to pain cannot be sustained for a long time. Scarring, continuing psychologic stress, and the frequent need for drugs can slow treament of patients with chronic pain. **Referred pain** is felt at a place different from that of an injured or diseased organ or part of the body. The pain of heart vessel disease (angina) may be felt in the left shoulder, arm, or jaw. In disease of the gallbladder, pain may be felt in the right shoulder or chest. See also **abdominal pain, chest pain, ischemic pain, low back pain, parietal pain.**

pain assessment, an examination of the things that make a patient's pain worse or better. It is used to diagnose and treat disease or injury. Reactions to pain vary widely among different people and depend on many different physical and mental factors. Patients also express their feelings of pain in different ways. A physician may ask a patient to describe the cause of the pain, if known, how strong it is, its location, and when it started. The patient should note anything that happened before the pain started, and how the pain is treated or handled. Severe pain causes pale skin, cold sweat, "goose bumps," wide pupils, and higher levels of the pulse, breathing rate, blood pressure, and muscle tension. The length of pain is noted in terms of hours, days, weeks, months, or years. Pain patterns are linked to many sensations, as burning, sticking, aching, or rhythmic throbbing.

pain intervention, relieving pain caused by disease and injury. Useful pain intervention depends on the type of pain, the physical and mental sources of the pain, and the patterns linked to different kinds of pain. The most common method of pain intervention is to give narcotic painkillers, as morphine. Many believe that using painkillers without taking into account mental help is not useful. Nearly everyone has a mental and emotional, as well as physical, effect of pain. For that reason, pain intervention often uses methods that combine both mental and physical measures. Short-term pain in the first 24 to 48 hours after surgery is often hard to relieve, even with narcotics. The type of pain intervention also depends on how the patient describes the pain. Mild pain is sometimes relieved by having the patient watch television, have visitors, or read. Moderate pain may be relieved by a mixture of these actions and giving drugs. Intervention to relieve severe pain often includes giving narcotics, working with the patient and family or hospital workers. In relieving all types of pain, removing anything that makes pain worse is a goal. Pain often gets worse in a cold room because the patient's muscles tend to contract. But putting on something cold, as an ice pack, often relieves pain by bringing down swelling. Dealing with pain gets harder as the patient gets more tired. Tranquilizers may make pain worse,

because they block otherwise useful ways of reducing pain. Overactivity may cause tiredness and fear, thus making the pain worse. Religious beliefs may help the patient to lessen pain or raise the ability to deal with it. Religious beliefs, however, may make pain worse if the patient sees the pain as punishment. Repeated daily use of any opiate drug will lessen the effect of the drug, so the dose will have to be made larger over time. The narcotic painkillers act on the central nervous system, but the nonnarcotic drugs (as the salicylates) act on where the pain is. Some nonnarcotic drugs can reduce inflammation and fever, as aspirin, indomethacin, or ibuprofen. In patients who are allergic to or are unable to take aspirin, acetaminophen may be used. Nerve block may be done by injecting alcohol. A nerve may also be cut to reduce pain. Other techniques include acupuncture and hypnosis. Newly identified painkillers made by the body are the enkephalins and the endorphins. Some studies show that the enkephalins are ten times as strong as morphine in lowering pain. See also **pain assessment.**

pain mechanism, the group of nerves that carry unpleasant senses and feelings of pain through the body. Two ideas about how pain happens are the gate control theory and the pattern theory. The gate control theory says that pain signals in the nervous system excite a group of small nerve cells that form a "pain pool." These nerve cells become overactive until they reach a level where a "gate" opens up and allows the pain signals to go to higher brain centers. The pattern theory says that the strength of a signal causes a pattern, which the brain senses as pain. This pain feeling is controlled by the strength and amount of activity of nervous system end organs. Some believe that two chemical substances made by the body (bradykinin and histamine) cause pain. The fear of pain is second only to the fear of death for most people. It is known that fear and worry often make pain worse.

pain receptor, any of the many free nerve endings in the body that warn of possible harmful changes, as excess pressure or temperature. The free nerve endings making up most of the pain receptors are found mainly in the skin and in some mucous membranes. They also appear in the eye (cornea), in the hair roots, and around sweat (sudoriferous) glands. Any kind of activity, if it is strong enough, can act on the pain receptors in the skin and the mucosa, but only major changes in pressure and some chemicals can act on the pain receptors in the inner organs. Referred pain results only from acting on the pain receptors in deep structures, as the organs in the abdomen, the joints, and the skeletal muscles, but never from pain receptors in the skin.

paint, 1. to apply a drug solution to the skin. 2. a drug solution that is used in this way. Kinds of paint include **antiseptic, germicide,** and **sporicide drugs.**

pain threshold, the point at which a stimulus, usually one linked to pressure or temperature, starts pain receptors working and causes a feeling of pain.

palate /pal′it/, the roof of the mouth. It is divided into the hard palate and the soft palate. –**palatal, palatine,** *adj.*

palatine bone /pal′ətin/, one of a pair of bones of the skull, forming the back part of the hard palate, and part of the nasal space.

palladium (Pd) /pəlā′dē·əm/, a hard, silvery metal element used in high-grade surgery instruments and in dental devices.

palliate /pal′ē·āt/, to soothe or relieve. –**palliation,** *n.,* **palliative** /pal′i·ətiv/, *adj.*

pallor, an abnormal paleness or lack of color in the skin.

palm, the lower side of the hand, between the wrist and bases of the fingers, when the hand is held stretched out with the thumb toward the body's middle. –**palmar,** *adj.*

palmar aponeurosis /pä′mər/, connective tissue (fascia) that surrounds the muscles of the palm. Also called **palmar fascia.**

palmar erythema, redness from inflammation of the palms of the hands.

palmaris longus /palmer′is/, a long, slender muscle of the forearm. It flexes the hand.

palmar reflex, a reflex that curls the fingers when the palm of the hand is tickled.

palmomental reflex /pal′mōmen′təl/, an abnormal nerve effect caused in some people by scratching the palm of the hand at the base of the thumb. The muscles of the chin and corner of the mouth on the same side of the body as the scratching contract. Also called **palm-chin reflex.**

palpation, a technique used in physical examination in which the examiner checks the texture, size, feel, and location of parts of the body with the hands. **Cardiac palpation** is a way to examine the heart by feeling the vibrations through the chest at certain spots between the ribs near the breastbone.

palpebra /pal′pəbrə/. See eyelid.

palpebral fissure /pal′pəbrəl/, the opening between the the upper and lower eyelids.

palpitate, to flutter or throb rapidly, as in the very fast beating of the heart under conditions of stress and in some heart problems.

palpitation, a pounding or racing of the heart. It is linked to normal emotion responses or with some heart disorders. Some people may complain of pounding hearts and show no sign of heart disease.

palsy /pôl′zē/, a loss of control of some muscles, or a form of paralysis. For example, **acute radial nerve palsy** refers to damage to the radial nerve of the arm, causing a weakening of the muscles of the forearm. It may be caused by too much pressure on the radial nerve. Some kinds of palsy are **Bell's palsy, cerebral palsy, Erb's palsy.**

Pamine, a trademark for a nerve drug (methscopolamine bromide).

panacea /pan′əsē′ə/, **1.** a remedy. **2.** an ancient name for an herb or a potion with the ability to heal.

Panafil, a trademark for a skin drug with an enzyme (papain).

panarthritis /pan′-/, inflammation of many joints of the body. –**panarthritic,** *adj.*

pancake kidney, a birth defect in which the left and right kidneys are joined into a single mass in the pelvis.

pancarditis /-kärdī′-/, inflammation of the whole heart.

Pancoast's syndrome, 1. a lung tumor condition. The signs are pain in the arm, an x-ray shadow at the top of the lung, and weakening of the muscles of the arm and the hand. The signs are caused by the damaging effects of the tumor on the nerve in the neck (brachial plexus). **2.** an abnormal condition caused by bone destruction in one or more ribs, and sometimes the spine.

pancreas /pan′krē·əs/, a fish-shaped, grayish-pink gland about 5 inches long that stretches across the back of the abdomen, behind the stomach. It releases insulin, glucagon, and some enzymes of digestion. Small ducts from the releasing cells empty into the main duct that runs the length of the organ. The main duct empties into the intestine at the same spot as the exit of the common bile duct. About 1 million cell units (islands of Langerhans) are in the pancreas. Beta cells release insulin, which helps control the body's use of carbohydrate. Alpha cells release glucagon, which counters the action of insulin. Other units of the pancreas release enzymes that help digest fats and proteins.

pancreatectomy /pan′krē·ətek′-/, the removal of all or part of the pancreas. It is done to remove a cyst or tumor, treat inflammation of the pancreas, or repair an injury. If the whole pancreas is removed, a type of diabetes develops that needs strict control of both diet and insulin dose.

pancreatic cancer /pan′krē·at′ik/, a cancer of the pancreas. Symptoms are loss of appetite, gas in the intestines, weakness, a large weight loss, stomach or back pain, liver disease (jaundice), itching, and signs of diabetes. The patient may pass clay-colored stools. Insulin-releasing tumors cause low blood sugar (hypoglycemia), especially in the morning. Symptoms of peptic ulcer may be felt. In some cases, there may be diarrhea, low blood potassium, and a lack of stomach acid.

pancreatic dornase, an enzyme from beef pancreas and used to treat lung diseases.

O–P

pancreatic duct, the main releasing channel of the pancreas. The **accessory pancreatic duct** is a small opening into the pancreatic duct or the first section of the small intestine (duodenum).

pancreatic enzyme, any one of the digestion enzymes released by the pancreas. See also **chymotrypsin, pancreatic juice.**

pancreatic hormone, any one of several hormones released by the pancreas. Major hormones are insulin and glucagon. See also **glucagon, insulin.**

pancreatic insufficiency, any condition with not enough release of pancreatic hormones or enzymes. Loss of appetite, failure of the body to absorb food, stomach pain, discomfort, and heavy weight loss often occur. Alcohol-caused pancreatitis is the most common form of the condition.

pancreatic juice, the fluids released by the pancreas. They are made as a reaction to the arrival of food in the first part of the intestine (duodenum). Pancreatic juice contains water, protein, salts, and many enzymes. The juice is needed to break down proteins into amino acids, to turn fats in the diet to fatty acids, and to change starch to simple sugars.

pancreatin /pan′krē·ətin′/, pancreas enzymes from swine or cattle given to aid digestion to replace natural human pancreas enzymes in cystic fibrosis and after surgery to remove the pancreas. Known allergy to this drug or to pork or beef protein prohibits its use. Large doses may cause nausea or diarrhea.

pancreatitis /-tī′-/, inflammation of the pancreas. **Acute pancreatitis** is often the result of damage to the gallbladder (biliary tract) by alcohol, injury, infection, or drugs. Symptoms are severe abdominal pain moving to the back, fever, loss of appetite, nausea, and vomiting. There may be yellowing of the skin (jaundice). Acute pancreatitis is often fatal. The causes of **chronic pancreatitis** are like those of the acute form. When the cause is alcohol abuse, there may be calcium deposits and scars in the smaller ducts of the pancreas. There is stomach pain, nausea, and vomiting, as well as undigested fat and protein in the feces. Insulin levels may go down. Some patients get diabetes mellitus.

pancreatoduodenectomy /pan′krē-ətōdoo′ədənek′-/, surgery in which the head of the pancreas and the loop of intestine (duodenum) that surrounds it are removed.

pancreatolith /pan′krē·at′ōlith/, a stone in the pancreas.

pancytopenia /pan′sītəpē′nē·ə/, a marked reduction in the number of red and white blood cells and platelets. See also **anemia.**

pandemic /pandem′ik/, a disease that occurs throughout a population, as a large influenza epidemic.

panencephalitis /pan′ensef′əlī′-/, inflammation of the whole brain. It is often caused by a virus. **Rubella panencephalitis** is a disease of adolescents and linked to the rubella virus. It is a long-term disease affecting motor nerves. **Subacute sclerosing panencephalitis** is caused by the measles virus. Symptoms include widespread brain inflammation, personality change, seizures, blindness, fever, and death. The condition occurs in children and in adolescents who have had measles at a very early age. No useful treatment is known.

panesthesia /pan′esthē′zhə/, the total of all feelings. Compare **cenesthesia.**

panhypopituitarism /panhī′pōpitoo′itərizm/, general faulty working of the pituitary gland. **Postpubertal panhypopituitarism** may be caused by the death of pituitary gland tissue from blood clots during or after giving birth. Symptoms are weakness, not being able to make breast milk, loss of menstrual flow and body hair, and loss of sex drive. Other effects include slow heart beat and wasting away (atrophy) of the thyroid and adrenal glands. **Prepubertal panhypopituitarism** occurs with a brain growth (cyst) or tumor in childhood. It causes the body to stay very small (dwarfism) with normal body shape, below normal sexual development, low levels of hormone functions, and yellow, wrinkled skin. Diabetes insipidus may be present, and there may be sight problems or even total blindness.

panic, a strong, sudden fear or feeling of worry that causes terror that may result in being unable to move or in senseless, uncontrolled behavior.

Panmycin Hydrochloride, a trademark for an antibacteria and antiprotozoa drug (tetracycline hydrochloride).

panniculus /panik′yələs/, *pl.* **panniculi,** a membrane made of many sheets of fiberlike tissue (fascia) covering a structure in the body.

pannus /pan′əs/, an abnormal condition of the eye (cornea) in which it becomes filled with blood vessels and grainy tissue just under the surface.

panophthalmitis /pan′ofthalmī′-/, inflammation of the whole eye, usually caused by a bacteria infection. Symptoms are pain, fever, headache, drowsiness, and swelling. The iris may appear muddy and gray.

Panoxyl, a trademark for an acne drug (benzoyl peroxide).

Panteric, a trademark for an enzyme (pancreatin).

pantothenic acid /pan′təthen′ik/, a member of the vitamin B complex, and an important element in food.

Panwarfin, a trademark for a drug used to stop blood clotting (warfarin sodium).

papain /pəpā′ēn/, an enzyme of the papaya used to clean wounds and help in healing.

Papanicolaou test /pap′ənik′ōlā′ō/, a simple method of examining tissue cells shed by a body organ. It is used most often to detect cancers of the cervix, but it may be used for tissue samples from any organ. A smear is usually taken by collecting a few loose cells in the vagina. The technique allows early diagnosis of cancer and has helped lower the death rate from cervical cancer. Also called (informal) **Pap test.** See also **Pap smear.**

papaverine hydrochloride, a smooth muscle relaxing drug given to treat heart or abdomen organ spasms. Complete heart block or known allergy to this drug prohibits its use. Side effects include liver disease (jaundice), high blood pressure, and irregular heart rate.

papilla /pəpil′ə/, pl. **papillae, 1.** a small pimple or nipple-shaped bump, as the cone-shaped (conoid) papillae on the surface of the tongue. **2.** the optic papilla, a tiny white disc in the retina of the eye. It is known as the "blind spot."

papillary adenoma /pap′iler′ē/, a noncancer tumor in which the membrane lining of glands forms bumps that grow into or out of a surface.

papillary carcinoma, a cancer with many fingerlike bumps. It is the most common type of thyroid tumor.

papillary muscle, any of the muscles joined to the tendons (chordae tendineae) in the chambers (ventricles) of the heart. The papillary muscles help to open and close the heart valves.

papilledema /pap′iladē′mə/, swelling of the optic disc caused by pressure in the skull.

papillitis /pap′ili′-/ an abnormal condition with inflammation of a papilla.

papilloma /pap′ilō′mə/, a noncancer tumor with a branching or stalk. An **intracanicular papilloma** is a benign warty growth in some glands, especially the breast. An **intracystic papilloma** is a formed gland tissue tumor (cystic adenoma).

papillomatosis /-mətō′-/, a condition in which there is widespread growth of abnormal nipplelike bumps.

papillomavirus, the virus that causes warts in humans.

papovavirus /pap′ə-/, one of a group of small viruses that may cause cancer.

pappus, the first growth of beard with downy hairs.

Pap smear, informal. a sample of tissue (epithelial) cells and cervical mucus collected during a pelvic examination for a cancer test using the Papanicolaou system. See also **Papanicolaou test.**

Pap test, informal. Papanicolaou test.

papular scaling disease /pap′yələr/, a skin disorder in which there are raised, dry, scalelike bumps. An example is **psoriasis.**

papule /pap′yōōl/, a small, solid, raised pimplelike skin bump, as of acne. Compare **macula.** **–papular,** adj.

-para, a combining form meaning a "woman who has given birth to children in a number of pregnancies."

paraaminobenzoic acid (PABA), a substance often linked to the vitamin B complex, found in cereals, eggs, milk, and meat. It is used as a sunscreen and may also be useful in treating some skin diseases.

paraaminosalicylic acid (PAS, PASA), a drug given to treat tuberculosis. Known allergy to the drug prohibits its use. It may interact with other drugs. Side effects include nausea, vomiting, diarrhea, and stomach pain.

parabiotic syndrome /per′əbī·ot′ik/, a condition that can occur between identical twin fetuses so that one gets more placental blood than the other. One twin may become anemic and the other have an excess of blood.

paracentesis /-sentē′-/, a way in which fluid is taken from a space of the body.

paracetamol. See **acetaminophen.**

paracoccidioidomycosis /-koksid′ēoi′dōmīkō′-/, a long-term, sometimes fatal, fungus infection. It causes ulcers of the mouth, voicebox (larynx), and nose. The disease occurs in Mexico and South America.

Paradione, a trademark for a drug used to fight seizures (paramethadione).

paradoxic agitation, a period of unexpected excitement that sometimes follows the use of a sleeping pill or tranquilizer.

paradoxic breathing, a condition in which part of the lung empties when breathing in and fills when breathing out. It may be caused by an open chest wound or rib cage damage.

paraffin bath /per′əfin/, placing heat on a surface of the body using melted paraffin. It is effective for heating injured or swollen areas, and used for patients with arthritis and rheumatism or any joint problem. Also called **wax bath.**

Paraflex, a trademark for a skeletal muscle relaxing drug (chlorzoxazone).

Parafon Forte, a trademark for a drug with a painkiller (acetaminophen) and a skeletal muscle relaxing drug (chlorzoxazone). It is used to relieve painful muscle and bone conditions.

paragonimiasis /per′əgon′imī′əsis/, an infection with a lung fluke (Paragonimus kellicotti). It occurs most often in North American minks and can be carried to humans. The disease may also be caused by eating fluke cysts in infected freshwater crabs or crayfish. Cooking shellfish properly prevents the disease.

parainfluenza virus /-in′flōō·en′zə/, a virus that causes lung infections in infants and young children and, less commonly, in adults. There are four types of the virus. Types 1 and 2 parainfluenza viruses may cause a form of bronchitis or croup. Type 3 is a cause of croup, bronchitis, and bronchopneumonia in children. Types 1, 3, and 4 are

O–P

linked to throat inflammation (pharyngitis) and the common cold. Compare **influenza, rhinovirus.**

Paral, a trademark for a sleeping pill and tranquilizer (paraldehyde).

paraldehyde /peral'dəhīd/, a clear, colorless, strong-smelling liquid used as a lotion. It may be given to cause sleep.

paralysis /pəral'əsis/, *pl.* **paralyses,** the loss of muscle use or the loss of feeling, or both. It may be caused by many problems, ranging from injury to disease and poisoning. Paralyses may be named for the cause, the effects on muscle tone and their spread, or the part of the body affected. **Flaccid paralysis** features the weakening or the loss of muscle tone. **Spastic paralysis** is the uncontrolled tightening of one or more muscles with related loss of muscular function. –**paralytic,** *adj.*

paralysis agitans /aj'itəns/. See **Parkinson's disease.**

paralytic ileus /pêr'əlit'ik/, a lowering in or lack of intestine activity that may come after surgery, injury to the wall of the abdomen, or in severe kidney disease. It may also be linked to a broken backbone or broken ribs, heart attack, severe ulcers, heavy metal poisoning, or any severe disease. Paralytic ileus is the most common cause of blocked intestines. The symptoms are a tender and bloated abdomen, lack of bowel sounds, lack of gas, nausea, and vomiting. Fluids are given through the veins, and drugs to make the digestive tract contract (peristalsis) are given. Also called **adynamic ileus.**

paramedical personnel, health care workers other than physicians, dentists, foot doctors, and nurses who have special training in health care. Kinds of paramedical personnel include Emergency Medical Technicians, audiologists, and x-ray technologists. Also called **allied health personnel.**

paramethadione, an antiseizure drug given to prevent seizures in petit mal epilepsy. Blood disorders, severe kidney or liver damage, or known allergy to this drug prohibits its use. Side effects include skin reactions, blood disorders, and liver disease (hepatitis). Drowsiness and day blindness may occur.

parametritis /-mētrī'-/, an inflammation of the structures around the uterus. See also **pelvic inflammatory disease.**

paramnesia /per'amnē'zhə/, a memory defect in which one believes one remembers events that never happened. Compare **déjà vu.**

paramyxovirus /-mik'sō-/, a member of a family of viruses that includes the viruses that cause mumps and some lung infections.

paranasal /-nā'zəl/, near or alongside the nose.

paranasal sinus, one of the spaces in many bones around the nose, as the frontal sinus in the forehead.

paranoia, a mental disorder marked by a complex system of thinking. Delusions of persecution and grandeur usually center on one major theme, as a job situation or an unfaithful spouse. Symptoms include being wary of others, unwilling to change habits, being resentful, being hostile, being very angry, and demanding unrealistic things of others. **Acute hallucinatory paranoia** is a disorder in which one sees and hears things that are not there and believes things that are not true. **Querulous paranoia** features very strong discontent and habitual complaining, usually about imagined slights by others.

paranoiac /per'ənoi'ak/, a person with symptoms of paranoia.

paranoid, 1. a person with a paranoid disorder. **2.** *informal.* a person who is too suspicious or who feels overly persecuted.

paranoid disorder, any of a large group of mental disorders marked by a damaged sense of reality and continuing delusions. An **acute paranoid disorder** is a condition that begins and develops quickly, and usually lasts less than 6 months. It is most commonly seen in persons who have had big changes in their environment, such as immigrants, refugees, prisoners, military inductees, and, in a less severe form, those leaving home for the first time. A **shared paranoid disorder** is one in which two close or related patients have exactly the same symptoms. See also **paranoia.**

paranoid personality disorder, a behavior with extreme distrust of others. The person's own mistakes and failures are blamed on others. Symptoms include hostility, stubborness, envy, exaggerated self-importance, tenseness, and lack of passive or tender feelings. The condition is seen more commonly in men than in women. The breakdown of the personality in this condition is less severe than in paranoid schizophrenia.

paranoid reaction, a behavior associated with aging and with the gradual formation of delusions, usually of a persecution, and often accompanied by hallucinations. Other signs of senilty, such as memory loss and confusion, do not usually accompany the reaction, and the person stays aware of time, place, and self.

paranoid schizophrenia, a form of schizophrenia marked by preoccupation with absurd and changeable delusions, usually of persecution or jealousy, accompanied by hallucinations. Symptoms include extreme anxiety, exaggerated suspiciousness, anger, and violence. The condition occurs most often during middle age. See also **schizophrenia.**

parapertussis /-pərtus'is/, an acute bacterial infection with symptoms closely resembling those of whooping cough (pertussis). It is usually milder, although it can be fatal. It is possible to have both infections at the same time.

parapharyngeal abscess /-ferin′jē·əl/, a pus-forming infection of tissues next to the throat, usually as a complication of acute inflammation or tonsillitis. Infection may spread to the jugular vein where it may cause infected blood clots. Antibiotics and surgical drainage may be required.

paraphimosis /-fīmō′-/, an inability of the penis foreskin to return to its normal position after it has been retracted. Caused by narrowing or inflammation, the condition may lead to gangrene. Compare **phimosis.**

paraplegia /-plē′jə/, an abnormal condition of motor nerve or sensory loss in the legs, resulting from damage to the spinal cord. This condition may also involve the back and abdominal muscles and cause degrees of paralysis. Such injuries commonly occur in automobile, motorcycle, and sporting accidents, falls, and gunshot wounds. Less common causes are disease conditions, such as scoliosis and spine bifida. Signs of paraplegia often develop immediately after injury and include loss of sensation, motion, and reflexes below the level of spinal damage. Depending on the completeness of damage to the spinal cord, the person may lose bladder and bowel control and develop lack of sexual functions. An incomplete spinal cord injury does not usually stop sensation or control in the anal region, or toe movement. A complete spinal cord injury destroys sensation and voluntary muscle control and usually causes the permanent loss of muscle function beyond the injury. Treatment seeks to stabilize the injured spinal area, restore any damaged nerve structures, and rehabilitate the person as quickly as possible. At the accident scene, when spinal cord injury is suspected, the person must not be moved until strapped on a board.

parapsoriasis /-sərī′əsis/, a group of chronic skin diseases resembling psoriasis, with reddish skin and scaly lesions but no symptoms involving other parts of the body.

parapsychology, a branch of psychology concerned with the study of alleged psychic phenomena, like clairvoyance, extrasensory perception, and telepathy.

paraquat poisoning /per′əkwət/, a condition caused by swallowing a highly poisonous pesticide (paraquat dichloride). Fibrous growths in the lungs and damage to the esophagus, kidneys, and liver develop several days after exposure. Most often, poisoning results from accidental exposure on the job.

parasite /-sīt/, an organism living in or on and obtaining nourishment from another organism. A **facultative parasite** may live on a host but is capable of living independently. An **obligate parasite** is one that depends entirely on its host for survival.

parasitemia /-ē′mē·ə/, the presence of parasites in the blood.

parasympathetic /-sim′pəthet′ik/, referring to a part of the autonomic nervous system. The actions of the parasympathetic part are begun by the release of a chemical (acetylcholine), and affect body resources. Parasympathetic nerve fibers slow the heart and cause intestine activity (peristalsis). They also help release fluids from tear, saliva, and digestion glands. They begin the release of bile and insulin, widen some blood vessels, and narrow the pupils, esophagus, and tubes in the lung (bronchioles). They also relax muscles during urination and defecation. See also **autonomic nervous system.**

parasympatholytic /-sim′pəthōlit′ik/. See **anticholinergic.**

parasympathomimetic /-mimet′ik/, referring to a substance causing effects like those caused by acting on a parasympathetic nerve. The parasympathomimetic drugs include those used to treat urine buildup and to counter the action of some muscle-relaxing drugs. Also called **cholinergic.**

parathion poisoning /per′əthī′on/, a harmful condition caused by swallowing, breathing in, or taking in through the skin a chemical used to kill insects (parathion). Symptoms include nausea, vomiting, stomach and bowel cramps, confusion, headache, lack of muscle control, seizures, and breathing difficulty. Emergency treatment is needed.

parathyroid gland /-thī′roid/, one of many small structures, usually four, joined to the thyroid gland. The parathyroid glands release a hormone that helps to keep the level of blood calcium normal.

parathyroid hormone (PH), a hormone released by the parathyroid glands that acts to keep a constant level of calcium in body tissues. The hormone controls the movement of calcium in the body and controls its passing out of the body. Loss of the parathyroid glands results in low blood calcium, leading to muscle spasms, seizures, and death if the hormone is not replaced. See also **hypoparathyroidism.**

paratrooper fracture, a break of the end of the lower leg bone and the ankle. It often occurs when a person jumps from a high platform and lands feet first on the ground, putting a high force on the ankles.

paratyphoid fever /-tī′foid/, a bacteria infection, caused by *Salmonella*. Symptoms look like typhoid fever, although milder. See also **salmonellosis, typhoid fever.**

Paredrine, a trademark for a nerve drug (hydroxyamphetamine hydrobromide).

paregoric /-gôr′ik/, a mixture of opium, camphor, and other items given to treat diarrhea and as a painkiller. Known allergy to this or a similar drug prohibits its use. It

O-P

should not be used when diarrhea is caused by a poison. There are usually no side effects.

parenchyma /pəreng'kimə/, the working tissue of an organ as opposed to supporting or connective tissue.

parent, a mother or father; one who has offspring. **–parental,** *adj.*

parenteral /pəren'tərəl/, not in or through digestion, as in taking a drug by injection instead of by mouth. **–parenterally,** *adv.*

parenteral absorption, taking up substances into the body other than by the digestive tract.

parenteral nutrition, food given by a vein, usually in fluids that contain salt (saline) with glucose, amino acids, minerals (electrolytes), vitamins, and drugs. They are not a total diet but keep fluids and minerals balanced after surgery and in other conditions. **Total parenteral nutrition (TPN),** is a way to give full nutrition when needed for a long time. A catheter is placed in the vein that drains into the right upper chamber of the heart (superior vena cava). The method is used for conditions in which feeding by mouth cannot be done or give enough of the essential nutrients. Examples include a long coma, severe uncontrolled malabsorption, or extensive burns. In infants and children it is used when feeding by way of the stomach and intestinal tract is a serious problem, as in long-term intestinal blockage, a too short gut length, or severe diarrhea. A strict infection-free environment must be kept because infection is a grave and ever present danger of this treatment.

parent figure, a parent or someone else who cares for a child. The parent figure gives physical, social, and emotional support needed for normal growth.

parent image, a concept that a child forms concerning the roles and traits of the mother and father.

paresis /pərē'-, per'əsis/, **1.** less than total paralysis related in some cases to nerve inflammation. **2.** a late sign of the third stage of syphilis (neurosyphilis) with paralysis, tremors, seizures, and mental decline, caused by damage to brain nerve cells. Also called **general paresis. –paretic,** *adj.*

paresthesia /per'esthē'zhə/, a sensation sometimes described as numbness, tingling, or a "pins and needles" feeling. Some factors, as posture, activity, rest, swelling, congestion, or disease may change the feeling.

pargyline hydrochloride, a monoamine oxidase (MAO) inhibitor used to treat moderate to severe high blood pressure.

parietal /pərī'ətəl/, **1.** referring to the outer wall of a space or organ. **2.** referring to the parietal bone of the skull, or the parietal lobe of the brain.

parietal lobe. See **brain.**

parietal pain, a sharp feeling of distress in the membrane lining the chest. The pain is made worse by breathing and chest movements. Causes include pneumonia, tuberculosis, cancer, or fluid building up from heart, liver, or kidney disease. See also **chest pain, pain.**

Parinaud's conjunctivitis /per'inōz/, an eye membrane (conjunctiva) disorder that most often affects only one side and is followed by swollen and tender nearby lymph nodes. The condition is linked to many infections, as rabbit fever (tularemia) and cat-scratch fever.

parity /per'itē/, a system for labeling a woman by the number of live and dead children she has given birth to at more than 28 weeks of pregnancy. The total number of pregnancies is noted by the letter "P" or the word "para." A para 4 (P4) gravida 5 (G5) has had 4 births after 28 weeks out of 5 pregnancies and 1 abortion or miscarriage before 28 weeks.

parkinsonism /pär'-/, a nerve system disorder caused by damage to nerves in the brain. Symptoms include rigid muscles, mild paralysis, slow shuffling gait, tremor, and difficulty in chewing, swallowing, and speaking. Signs of parkinsonism look like those of Parkinson's disease and may result from brain disease, syphilis, malaria, polio, or carbon monoxide poisoning. Parkinsonism often occurs in patients given tranquilizers. See also **Parkinson's disease.**

Parkinson's disease, a slowly growing disorder caused by damage to brain cells. Symptoms include tremors that occur while at rest, "pill rolling" movements of the fingers, and a masklike face. Other symptoms are a shuffling gait, a slightly bent-over posture, rigid muscles, and weakness. It is usually a disease of unknown cause (idiopathic) affecting persons over 60 years of age. However, it may occur in younger persons, especially following brain inflammation (encephalitis) or poisoning by carbon monoxide, metals, or some drugs. Parkinson's disease patients may drool, have a heavy appetite, be unable to stand heat, have oily skin, be emotionally unstable, and have judgment problems. The symptoms are made worse by tiredness, excitement, and frustration. It rarely damages the ability to think and reason. Treatment is to correct the imbalance in some brain substances (dopamine, acetylcholine). Also called **paralysis agitans.**

Parlodel, a trademark for a parkinsonism drug (bromocriptine).

Parnate, a trademark for an antidepressant drug (tranylcypromine sulfate).

paronychia /per'ənik'ē·ə/, an infection of the fold of skin at the edge of a nail.

parosmia /pəroz'mē·ə/, any disorder of the sense of smell.

parotitis /per'ətī'-/. See **mumps.**

paroxysm /per'əksizm/, **1.** a marked rise in symptoms. **2.** a fit, seizure, or spasm. –**paroxysmal**, *adj.*

paroxysmal hemoglobinuria /per'oksiz'məl/, the sudden passage of a blood substance (hemoglobin) in urine. It can occur following exposure to low temperatures. See also **Marchiafava-Micheli disease.**

paroxysmal nocturnal dyspnea (PND), a disorder with sudden attacks of breathing problems, most often occurring after several hours of sleep lying down. It is most often caused by fluid in the lungs linked to a heart disease (congestive heart failure). There is also coughing, a feeling of not being able to breathe, cold sweat, and rapid heart beat. Sleeping with the head propped up on pillows may help breathing at night.

paroxysmal nocturnal hemoglobinuria (PNH), a disorder in which red blood cells are destroyed, resulting in bloody urine, especially at night. A basic membrane defect in the red blood cells is involved. The cause is unknown, but it is linked to abnormal bone marrow. Occurring mainly in adults between 25 and 45 years of age, it has symptoms of stomach and bowel pain, back pain, and headache. Treatment includes giving blood, iron, and drugs to halt blood clotting.

Parsidol, a trademark for an antiparkinsonian drug (ethopropazine hydrochloride).

parthenogenesis /pär'thənōjen'əsis/, a type of reproduction in which a living thing grows from an unfertilized egg (ovum).

partial hospitalization program, a health care service that provides treatment to patients who use only day or night hospital services, rather than stay in the hospital 24 hours a day.

parturition /pär'tyərish'ən/, the process of giving birth.

passive-aggressive personality, a behavior in which strong actions or opinions are given in an indirect, nonviolent manner, as pouting or being difficult, stubborn, and forgetful.

passive-dependent personality, a behavior marked by helplessness, being unable to make a decision, and often clinging to and seeking support from others.

passive lingual arch, a dental device that helps keep the tooth space and dental arch length normal when the baby teeth are lost too early.

passive smoking, the breathing in by nonsmokers of the smoke from other people's smoking. Especially patients with long-term heart and lung diseases and allergies can be harmed.

Pasteurella /pas'tərel'ə/, a group of bacteria, including species that cause disease in humans. *Pasteurella* infections may be carried by animal bites.

pasteurized milk /pas'chərīzd/, milk that has been treated by heat to destroy disease bacteria. By law, pasteurization needs a temperature of 145° F to 150° F for not less than 30 minutes. This is followed by a temperature of 161° F for 15 seconds and then rapid cooling.

patch, a small, flat spot on skin that differs from the nearby area in color or texture. Also called **macule.**

patch test. See **allergy testing.**

patella /pətel'ə/. See **kneecap.**

patellar ligament, a ligament that stretches from the tendon above the knee across the kneecap (patella). It joins a bone of the lower leg (tibia).

patellar reflex. See **deep tendon reflex.**

patent ductus arteriosus (PDA), an abnormal opening between two arteries (pulmonary artery, aorta) caused by the fetal blood vessel (ductus arteriosus) failing to close after birth. See also **congenital heart disease.**

Paterson-Kelly syndrome, a digestive system disorder linked to a lack of iron (iron deficiency anemia). Webs of tissue grow in the upper part of the tube to the stomach (esophagus), making swallowing solids difficult.

Pathibamate, a trademark for a stomach and bowel drug with a nerve drug (tridihexethyl chloride) and a tranquilizer (meprobamate).

-pathic, 1. a combining form referring to an illness or affected part of the body. **2.** a combining form referring to a form or system of treatment.

Pathilon, a trademark for a nerve signal blocker (tridihexethyl chloride).

pathogen /path'əjən/, any microorganism able to cause a disease. –**pathogenic**, *adj.*

pathologic retraction ring, a ridge that may form around the uterus between the upper and lower parts during the second stage of a blocked labor. The lower part becomes bloated and thin, and the upper part becomes too thick. Also called **Bandl's ring.** Compare **constriction ring, physiologic retraction ring.**

pathology /pathol'-/, the study of the traits, causes, and effects of disease, as seen in the structure and workings of the body. In **autopsy pathology,** a disease is studied in a body after death. This includes looking at tissues under a microscope and doing laboratory tests. **Clinical pathology** is the laboratory study of disease by a pathologist. It includes the study of blood (hematology), microorganisms (bacteriology), chemistry, and immune systems (serology). –**pathologic**, *adj.*

pathway, a group of nerve cells (neurons) that make a route for nerve signals between any part of the body and the spinal cord or the brain.

patient, someone who receives health care.

patient interview, a step-by-step interview of a patient, to get information that can be used to develop a care plan.

patient record, a group of papers that is a record of each time a patient had treatment and medical care. The record

O–P

is private and is most often held by the hospital or other health care service. Data in the record are given only to the patient, or with written permission. Also called *(informal)* **chart.**

Patient's Bill of Rights, a list of patient's rights set up by the American Hospital Association. It offers some guides for protection of patients by stating the duties that a hospital and its staff have toward patients and their families during a stay in the hospital.

patrol unit, any light, mobile unit, having limited pumping and water capacity.

Pauwel's fracture /pou'əlz/, a break of the neck of the upper leg bone (femur), near the socket of the hipbone.

Pavabid, a trademark for a smooth muscle relaxing drug (papaverine hydrochloride).

Pavacap, a trademark for a smooth muscle relaxing drug (papaverine hydrochloride).

Pavulon, a trademark for a nerve and muscle drug (pancuronium bromide) used during anesthesia.

PCB, abbreviation for **polychlorinated biphenyls.**

peak level, the highest amount, usually in the blood, that a substance reaches during a certain time. An example is

A Patient's Bill of Rights

The American Hospital Association Board of Trustees' Committee on Health Care for the Disadvantaged, which has been a consistent advocate on behalf of consumers of health care services, developed this bill of rights, which was approved by the AHA House of Delegates February 6, 1973. The following rights are affirmed:

1. The patient has the right to considerate and respectful care.

2. The patient has the right to obtain from his physician complete current information concerning his diagnosis, treatment, and prognosis in terms the patient can be reasonably expected to understand. When it is not medically advisable to give such information to the patient, the information should be made available to an appropriate person in his behalf. He has the right to know, by name, the physician responsible for coordinating his care.

3. The patient has the right to receive from his physician information necessary to give informed consent prior to the start of any procedure and/or treatment. Except in emergencies, such information for informed consent should include but not necessarily be limited to the specific procedure and/or treatment, the medically significant risks involved, and the probable duration of incapacitation. Where medically significant alternatives for care or treatment exist, or when the patient requests information concerning medical alternatives, the patient has the right to such information. The patient also has the right to know the name of the person responsible for the procedures and/or treatment.

4. The patient has the right to refuse treatment to the extent permitted by law, and to be informed of the medical consequences of his action.

5. The patient has the right to every consideration of his privacy concerning his own medical care program. Case discussion, consultation, examination, and treatment are confidential and should be conducted discreetly. Those not directly involved in his care must have the permission of the patient to be present.

6. The patient has the right to expect that all communications and records pertaining to his care should be treated as confidential.

7. The patient has the right to expect that within its capacity a hospital must make reasonable response to the request of a patient for services. The hospital must provide evaluation, service, and/or referral as indicated by the urgency of the case. When medically permissible a patient may be transferred to another facility only after he has received complete information and explanation concerning the needs for and alternatives to such a transfer. The institution to which the patient is to be transferred must first have accepted the patient for transfer.

8. The patient has the right to obtain information as to any relationship of his hospital to other health care and educational institutions insofar as his care is concerned. The patient has the right to obtain information as to the existence of any professional relationships among individuals, by name, who are treating him.

9. The patient has the right to be advised if the hospital proposes to engage in or perform human experimentation affecting his care or treatment. The patient has the right to refuse to participate in such research projects.

10. The patient has the right to expect reasonable continuity of care. He has the right to know in advance what appointment times and physicians are available and where. The patient has the right to expect that the hospital will provide a mechanism whereby he is informed by his physician or a delegate of the physician of the patient's continuing health care requirements following discharge.

11. The patient has the right to examine and receive an explanation of his bill regardless of source of payment.

12. The patient has the right to know what hospital rules and regulations apply to his conduct as a patient.

the highest blood glucose level reached during a glucose tolerance test.

pectin, a substance found in fruits and vegetables. It adds bulk to the diet. See also **dietary fiber.**

pectineus /pektin′ē·əs/, one of the thigh (femoral) muscles. It moves the thigh and turns it toward the middle of the body.

pectoralis major /pek′tərā′lis/, a large fan-shaped muscle of the upper chest wall. It flexes and rotates the arm in the shoulder joint.

pectoralis minor, a thin, triangle-shaped muscle under the muscle of the upper chest wall (pectoralis major). It rotates the shoulder blade (scapula), draws it down and forward, and raises the upper ribs in forced breathing.

Pediaflor, a trademark for a dental drug (sodium fluoride). It is used to prevent cavities in children.

Pedialyte, a trademark for a balanced mixture of electrolytes.

Pediamycin, a trademark for an antibiotic (erythromycin ethylsuccinate).

pediatric dose /pē′dē·at′-/, the correct amount, times of giving the dose, and total number of doses of a drug to be given to a child or infant based on the age, weight, body surface area, and the action of the drug in the child. Many formulas have been made to figure the pediatric dosage from a standard adult dose. **Clark's rule** is one way to calculate the correct dose of a drug for a child. The formula is: weight in pounds/150 × adult dose. A second way, called **Cowling's rule,** uses this formula: (age at next birthday/24) × adult dose. **Young's rule** is a method used to calculate the dose of a drug for a child 2 years of age or more. The formula is: (age in years) ÷ (age + 12) × adult dose.

pediatric hospitalization, keeping a child or infant in a hospital for testing or treatment. No matter what the age or the degree of illness or injury, being in a hospital is a major crisis in a child's life, and may cause behavior reactions. Some hospitals tell parents to take part in the care of the child through rooming-in or visiting often.

pediatric nutrition, having the right foods and enough calories to be correct for the many stages of a child's growth. Diet needs vary with age and activity of the child. During infancy the need for protein is important because of the rapid change in height and weight. Through the preschool and middle childhood years, growth is uneven and occurs in spurts, with a changing appetite and calorie use. The growth phase during adolescence needs more calories and vitamins, but food habits are often changed by emotional factors, peer pressure, and fad diets. A special problem is overfeeding in the early childhood years.

pediatrics, a branch of medicine concerned with the growth and care of children. Its special focus is on the diseases of children and their treatment and prevention. – **pediatric,** adj.

pediatric surgery, the special care of the child having surgery for injuries, defects, or diseases. In addition to the usual fears and emotional problems of illness and being in the hospital, the child is often worried about being put to sleep for the surgery. The child fears the operation itself, possible death, the loss of control while asleep, and any change in the body or damage to body parts. See also **pediatric hospitalization.**

pediculosis /pədik′yəlō′-/, an infestation with bloodsucking lice. Lice cause severe itching, often resulting in infection from scratching the skin. Body lice lay eggs in the seams of clothing; crab and head lice attach their eggs to hairs. Lice are spread by direct contact with bedding, with people, or from borrowed combs and clothing. Body lice may carry some diseases. These include returning fevers, typhus, and trench fever. See also **crab louse, louse bite.**

pedigree, 1. line of descent. **2.** a chart that shows the genetic makeup of a person's ancestors with those affected by a disease or trait, and those who are carriers of inherited diseases.

pedophilia /ped′əfil′ə/, **1.** an abnormal interest in children. **2.** a disorder in which sexual activity with children is the desired way to get sexual pleasure. –**pedophilic,** adj.

peduncle /pədung′kəl/, a stalk or stemlike connecting part of a growth or tissue.

Peeping Tom. See **voyeurism.**

Peganone, a trademark for an antiseizure drug (ethotoin).

pellagra /pəlag′rə, pəlā′grə/, a disease resulting from a lack of a B complex vitamin (niacin) or an amino acid (tryptophan). Persons with diets made up of foods lacking in tryptophan, as cornmeal and porkfat, are at risk. Symptoms include scaly sores, especially on skin exposed to the sun, inflammation of the mucous membranes, diarrhea, and mental problems. **Pellagra sine pellagra** is a form in which skin symptoms are absent.**Typhoid pellagra** is a form in which the symptoms also include continued high temperatures. Treatment and prevention include a well-balanced diet rich in liver, eggs, milk, and meat.

pelvic, referring to the pelvis.

pelvic brim, the curved top of the bones of the hips. Below the brim is the pelvis.

pelvic cellulitis, a bacterial infection of the tissues (parametrium) around the cervix. It may occur after childbirth or an abortion. It may have spread from a first

O–P

infection in the genitals. Symptoms include fever, chills, and sweats, stomach pain that spreads, or the uterus failing to return to its nonpregnant size.

pelvic congestion syndrome, a condition marked by long-term low back pain, urinary difficulty, menstrual disorders, vague lower bowel pain, vaginal discharge, and discomfort during sexual intercourse.

pelvic diaphragm, a group of pelvic muscles stretched like a hammock across the pelvic space. The muscles hold the contents of the abdomen and support the pelvic organs.

pelvic examination. See **female reproductive system assessment.**

pelvic floor, the muscles and tissues surrounding the bottom of the pelvis.

pelvic inflammatory disease (PID), a disease of the female pelvic organs, usually caused by bacteria. Symptoms include fever, foul-smelling vaginal discharge, pain in the lower abdomen, abnormal bleeding, and painful sexual intercourse. There may also be soreness or pain in the uterus, an ovary, or a fallopian tube. Severe PID may need a hysterectomy to avoid fatal blood poisoning. If the cause is infection by a sexually carried disease, the woman's sexual partners are also treated with antibiotics. PID is most often very painful. The woman may have to stay in bed and need narcotic painkillers. PID often results in scars, blocked fallopian tubes, and the inability to have children. See also **endometritis.**

pelvic inlet, the inlet to the true female pelvis surrounded by the sacral and pubic bones. An infant must pass through the inlet to enter the true pelvis and be born through the vagina. The size of the inlet is an important measurement to be made in examining the pelvis in pregnancy.

pelvic minilaparotomy, an operation in which the lower abdomen is entered through a small cut. It is done most often to sterilize the tubes, but it is also done for diagnosis and to treat a pregnancy outside of the uterus, an ovarian lump (cyst), displaced tissue from the uterine lining (endometriosis), and an inability to have children. It is often done in the physician's office, although some women may need to stay in the hospital for a short time. See also **sterilization.**

pelvic outlet, the space surrounded by the bones at the bottom of the true pelvis, through which the fetus must pass during childbirth. It is bounded by the tip of the tailbone (coccyx), ligaments, and a joint of the pelvis (pubic symphysis). In women, the shape and size of the pelvic outlet are not standard and are important in childbirth. See also **pelvic inlet.**

pelvic rotation, a walking pattern with the movement of the pelvis to the right and the left. It is used to diagnose many diseases and abnormal conditions of bones and joints.

pelvifemoral /pel′vifem′ərəl/, referring to the structures of the hip joint. Included are the muscles and the space around the bony pelvis and the head of the upper leg bone (femur).

pelvimetry /pelvim′ətrē/, measurement of the bony birth canal. In **clinical pelvimetry** the size of the birth canal is determined by feeling specific bony landmarks in the pelvis and estimating the distances between them. This is usually done during the first vaginal examination of a pregnant woman. With **x-ray pelvimetry,** a radiographic examination is made. The diameter of the baby's head is also determined when there is doubt that the head can pass safely through the pelvis in labor.

pelvis, *pl.* **pelves,** the lower part of the trunk of the body. It is made up of four bones: the two hip (innominate) bones on the front and sides, and the lower backbone (sacrum) and tailbone (coccyx) at the bottom of the spinal column. It divides into the greater (false) pelvis and the lesser (true) pelvis. The greater pelvis is the larger part of the space above a bony rim that divides the two parts. The lesser pelvis is below the rim. Its bony walls are more complete than those of the greater pelvis. A **pelvic classification** is a system of measuring the bones of the female pelvis to find if they are suited for vaginal birth. Categories include android, anthropoid, gynecoid, and platypelloid. An **android pelvis** has a structure that is typical of a male. The bones are thick and heavy. The opening is heart-shaped. In a female, childbirth may be hard unless the android pelvis is large and the baby is small. An **anthropoid pelvis** has an oval opening; the front-to-back diameter is much greater than the side-to-side. If the pelvis is large, normal childbirth is possible. This type of pelvis is present in 40% of nonwhite women and in more than 25% of white women. A **gynecoid pelvis** has an opening between the two pelvic bones that is nearly round. The lowest bone of the spine (sacrum) is parallel to the back of the joint between the pelvic bones, the sidewalls are straight, and the spines of the hip bones do not slant in. It is the ideal pelvic type for childbirth. A **platypelloid pelvis** has a round inlet, but the back section is made shorter by its flat and heavy border. Vaginal birth is not often possible in women who have platypelloid pelves.

pemoline, a nervous system stimulant. It is given to treat minimal brain defects and attention deficit disorders in children. Known allergy to this drug prohibits its use. Side effects include inability to sleep, seizures, and hallucinations.

pemphigoid /pem′figoid/, a skin disease marked by blisters (bullae) and red patches or an itching rash. The skin effects may be linked to an inner cancer.

pemphigus /pem′figəs/, a disease of the skin and mucous membranes. It is marked by thin-walled blisters (bullae) on the skin or the mucous membrane. The bullae break open easily. The patient loses weight, becomes weak, and is at risk for infections.

penetration, the flow of a hazardous liquid chemical through zippers, stitched seams, and pinholes or other imperfections in the material. Chemical protective clothing can be penetrated at several locations, including the face piece and exhalation valve, suit exhaust valves, and suit fasteners. The potential for penetration generally increases at excessively hot or cold temperatures.

penicillamine (D-penicillamine) /pen′isilam′in/, a drug given to bind with and remove metals from the blood. It is used to treat lead poisoning. It is also given to relieve symptoms of rheumatoid arthritis when other drugs have failed. Known allergy to this drug or a form of anemia prohibits its use. It is not given during pregnancy or to patients with kidney disorders. Side effects include fever, rashes, and blood disorders. Severe bone marrow disease is linked to long-term use of this drug.

penicillin /pen′isil′in/, any of a group of antibiotics taken from cultures of the fungus *Penicillium* or made in a laboratory. Many penicillins are given by mouth or injection to treat bacteria infections. Allergic reactions are common in patients who get penicillin. Side effects may appear even when the drug has not been used before. The reason for this may be an unnoticed use of a food or other substance with traces of the antibiotic. The most common allergic reactions to penicillin are rash and fever. Some patients have a severe skin inflammation.

penicillinase /-ās/, an enzyme made by some bacteria, including staphylococci, that stops the action of penicillin. This causes resistance to the antibiotic. It is used to treat the side effects of penicillin. Also called **beta-lactamase.**

penicillin G, an antibiotic given to treat many infections. Known allergy to this drug or any penicillin prohibits its use. Side effects include allergic reactions, nausea, and diarrhea.

penicillin G benzathine, a long-acting form of penicillin used to treat some streptococcal and other infections. It is given by slow, deep injection over 12 hours to several days. Allergy to this drug or to other penicillins prohibits its use. Side effects include allergic shock (anaphylaxis).

penicillin V, an antibiotic given to treat infections. Known allergy to this drug or to any penicillin prohibits its use. Side effects include allergic shock (anaphylaxis).

penile cancer /pē′nīl/, a cancer of the penis that occurs mainly in men whose foreskin has not been removed. It is linked to genital herpesvirus infection and poor personal washing. Treatment involves part or total removal of the penis and removal of lymph nodes in the groin.

penis, the outer reproductive organ of a male. The penis is made up of three tubular masses of spongy tissue covered with skin. Two of them (corpora cavernosa) partly surround a third one (corpus spongiosum). The corpus spongiosum contains the tube (urethra) that drains the bladder.

penniform, referring to the shape of a feather, especially in muscle fibers.

pentaerythritol tetranitrate, a heart blood vessel widening drug given to relieve chest pain (angina pectoris). Known allergy to this drug prohibits its use. It is not given in severe anemia, brain bleeding, or head injury. Side effects include low blood pressure, allergic reactions, headaches, and flushing.

Pentids, a trademark for an antibiotic (penicillin G potassium).

pentobarbital, a tranquilizer and sedative given before surgery, to treat an inability to sleep, and to control seizures.

pentose, a sugar made by the body and also found in some fruits, as plums and cherries.

pentosuria /pen′təsoo̅r′ē·ə/, a condition in which a sugar (pentose) is in the urine. Pentosuria may be caused by an inherited defect.

Pentothal, a trademark for a barbiturate drug (thiopental sodium), used as an anesthetic and to aid anesthesia.

pep pills, *slang.* amphetamines.

pepsin, an enzyme released in the stomach that speeds up the breakdown of protein. Pepsin from pork and beef stomachs is sometimes used to aid digestion. See also **enzyme.**

peptic ulcer, an area of loss of mucous membrane of the stomach or any other part of the digestive system coming into contact with juices that have stomach acid and pepsin. A **duodenal ulcer,** one in the first part of the small intestine (duodenum), is the most common type of peptic ulcer. A **channel ulcer** is a rare type of peptic ulcer found in the pyloric canal, which is between the stomach and the first segment of the intestine (duodenum). Acute ulcers are almost always shallow and occur in groups. They may be without symptoms and heal without scars. Chronic ulcers are true ulcers. They are deep and single and cause symptoms. The muscle coat of the wall of the tract is permanently damaged. A scar forms, and the mucous membrane may heal, but not the muscle under it. Peptic ulcers are caused by many factors. They include an excess amount of stomach acid, loss of covering of the mucous membrane, stress, inherited defects, and using some drugs. Chronic ulcers cause a gnawing pain in the upper stomach. The pain is not affected by a change in body position. Antacids and many, small bland meals may help. The cause is treated if known. Treatment includes drugs to lower the acid and spasms of the stomach and to relieve stress. If a break and bleeding occur, surgery may be necessary. In most cases, ulcers heal completely and pain may be controlled simply, often with the correct use of antacids and other drugs. Also called **gastric ulcer.** See also **ulcer.**

peptide /pep′tīd/, a molecule chain of two or more amino acids. See also **amino acid, polypeptide, protein.**

perception, noting and sensing nerve signals from the sense organs. The ability to judge depth or the distance between objects is called **depth per- ception.** Vision from both eyes is essential to this ability. **Facial perception** refers to the ability to judge the distance and direction of objects through a feeling in the skin of the face. It is commonly felt by those who are blind. **Stereognostic perception** refers to the ability to recognize objects by the sense of touch.

perceptual defect, any of a broad group of disorders of the nervous system that slow down the conscious sensing of nerve signals.

perceptual deprivation, the lack of or reduced important signals. It may result from constant background noise or constant poor lighting.

Percodan, a trademark for a nervous system drug with two narcotic painkillers (oxycodone hydrochloride and oxycodone terephthalate).

Percogesic, a trademark for a lung drug with an antihistamine (phenyltoloxamine citrate) and a painkiller (acetaminophen).

Percorten Acetate, a trademark for an adrenal gland hormone drug (desoxycorticosterone acetate).

percussion, a tapping in medical tests used to guess the size, borders, and texture of some chest organs and organs in the abdomen. It is also used to detect the presence and amount of fluid in a body space. **Immediate** or **direct percussion** refers to tapping (percussion) done by striking the fingers on the surface of the chest or abdomen. **Indirect, mediate,** or **finger percussion** is striking a finger of one hand on a finger of the other hand as it is placed over an organ. **Palpatory percussion** is done using light pressure with the flat of the hand.

percutaneous /pur′kyo͞otā′nē·əs/, a medical procedure done through the skin, as a biopsy or fluid taken out from below the skin using a needle.

percutaneous catheter placement, placing a tube (catheter) into a blood vessel (artery) through the skin, and moving it to a tissue or an organ to be studied.

percutaneous transluminal coronary angioplasty (PTCA), a technique to treat heart disease and chest pain (angina pectoris). Fatty material (plaques) in the blood vessels (arteries) of the heart are flattened against the vessel walls. It makes the blood flow better. A tube (catheter) is put into the vessel through the skin. A small balloon at the tip of the catheter is filled up and emptied many times to flatten the plaques.

Perez reflex, the normal response of an infant when on its back with a finger pressed along the spine from the lower back (sacrum) to the neck. This includes crying, moving the arms and legs, and holding up the head and hips. If the reflex still occurs after 6 months of age, it may mean there is brain damage.

perforate, to make a hole. –**perforation,** *n.*

perforating fracture, an open broken bone caused by an object, as a bullet, making a small surface wound.

perforation of the uterus, an accidental break in the uterus, as may occur during an abortion or by a birth control device (IUD).

perfusion, 1. fluid passing through an organ or a part of the body. **2.** a method for giving a drug meant for a remote part of the body by sending it through the blood.

Pergonal, a trademark for a hormone drug used to treat an inability to have children.

Periactin Hydrochloride, a trademark for an antihistamine used to relieve itching (cyproheptadine hydrochloride).

perianal abscess /per′ē·ā′nəl/, a pus-making infection beneath the skin around the anus. See also **abscess.**

periapical /per′ē·ap′ikəl/, referring to the tissues around the root of a tooth, including the gums and bones.

periapical abscess, an infection around the root of a tooth, usually spread from tooth cavities. The abscess may go into nearby bone or, more often, to soft tissues.

periarteritis /per′ē·är′tərī′-/, an inflammation of the outer coat of a blood vessel (artery) and the tissue around the vessel.

periarteritis nodosa, a disease of the connective tissue with many large bumps (nodules) in groups along blood vessels (arteries). This causes blockage of the blood vessels, resulting lack of blood in some places (ischemia), bleeding, tissue death, and pain. The early signs of the disease are rapid heart beat, fever, weight loss, and stomach pain.

pericarditis /-kärdī′-/, an inflammation of the membrane (pericardium) covering the heart. It is linked to injury, cancer, heart attack, and other diseases. The first stage is marked by fever, chest pain that moves to the shoulder or neck, breathing difficulty, and a dry cough. During the second stage, fluid gathers in the heart membrane, slowing down heart movement. Heart sounds become soft, weak, and distant. A bulge is seen on the chest over the heart. If the fluid has pus in it, a high fever, sweat, chills, and physical collapse also occur. **Adhesive pericarditis** refers to scar tissue that binds the layers of the heart membrane or the membrane (pericardium) and the partition between the lungs (mediastinum), diaphragm, or chest wall. It may interfere with the normal movements of the heart. Surgery may be needed to remove fluid or to find the cause of the disease.

pericardium /-kär′dē·əm/, *pl.* **pericardia,** a double-layered sac of membranes around the heart. The inner part (serous pericardium) divides into a membrane that sticks to the heart's surface. The other lines the inside of the outer part (fibrous pericardium) of the sac. Between the two layers is the pericardial space. It contains fluid that oils tissue surfaces, allowing the heart to move easily while contracting. –**pericardial,** *adj.*

pericholangitis /-kō′lanjī′-/, inflammation of the tissues around bile ducts in the liver. It is caused by a disease of the intestines (ulcerative colitis) and is marked by fever, chills, and yellow skin (jaundice). See also **colitis.**

perilymph /-limf/, a clear fluid in the inner ear.

perinatal /-nā′təl/, referring to the time and process of giving birth or being born.

perinatal death, 1. the death of a fetus weighing more than 1000 g at 28 or more weeks of pregnancy. **2.** the death of an infant between birth and 28 days after birth. Also called **neonatal death.**

perinatology /-tol′-/, a branch of medicine that studies the anatomy and physiology of the mother and her infant during pregnancy, childbirth, and the 28 days after birth.

perineum /-nē′əm/, the part of the body between the inner thighs on either side, with the buttocks to the rear and the sex organs at the front. –**perineal,** *adj.*

period, *nontechnical.* menses.

periodic, happening again and again.

periodic apnea of the newborn. See **apnea.**

periodontal /per′ē·ōdon′təl/, referring to the space around a tooth.

periodontal cyst, a fluid-filled sac that occurs most often at the bottom of a tooth root.

periodontal disease, disease of the tissues around a tooth.

periodontal ligament (PDL), the fiberlike tissue that joins the teeth to the sockets (alveoli). It is made up of many bundles of connective tissue in groups and linked up with blood vessels, lymph vessels, and nerves.

periodontitis /-ōdontī′-/, inflammation of the tissue that joins the teeth and gums. **Juvenile periodontitis** is an abnormal state that may affect children and adolescents. There is severe pocketing and bone loss.

periosteum /per′ē·os′tē·əm/, a fiberlike covering of the bones, except at their ends. It has an outer layer of connective tissue with some fat cells and an inner layer of fine stretchy fibers. Periosteum has the nerves and blood vessels that supply the bones.

periostitis /-ostī′-/, inflammation of the fiberlike coverings of bones (periosteum). Infection or injury causes tenderness and swelling around the bone, pain, fever, and chills.

peripheral /pərif′ərəl/, referring to the outer parts of an organ or body.

peripheral acrocyanosis of the newborn, a normal, temporary condition of the newborn. It is marked by pale bluish skin on the hands and feet, especially the fingers and toes. The blueness fades as the baby begins to breathe easily but returns if the baby becomes chilled.

peripheral nervous system, the motor and sense nerves outside of the brain and spinal cord. The system has 12 pairs of skull nerves, 31 pairs of spinal nerves, and their many branches in body organs. Sense nerves carry signals to the brain and spinal cord (central nervous system). Motor nerves carry signals from the brain to other parts of the body. The sense and motor nerves travel together but divide at the spinal cord level. Some nerves (somatic) act on the body wall; others (visceral) supply internal organs. The autonomic nervous system is a part of the peripheral system. See also **autonomic nervous system.**

peripheral neuropathy, any disorder of the motor and sense nerves outside of the brain and spinal cord (peripheral nervous system). An example is numbness or tingling feelings (paresthesia).

peripheral resistance, a resistance to the flow of blood outside the major blood vessels.

peripheral vascular disease, any abnormal condition that affects the blood vessels outside of the heart and the major vessels. Symptoms include numbness, pain, paleness, high blood pressure, and damaged pulses. Causes include being overweight, cigarette smoking, stress, and lack of activity. When linked to an infection of the heart (bacterial endocarditis), blood clots may form in tiny blood vessels (arterioles) causing tissue death (gangrene) in many parts of the body, as the tip of the nose, fingers, or toes. Some kinds of peripheral vascular disease are **arteriosclerosis** and **atherosclerosis.**

peripheral vision, an ability to see objects that are to the side of the body, rather than straight ahead.

O-P

peristalsis /per′istôl-/, the wavelike, rhythmic contraction of smooth muscle. It forces food through the digestive tract, bile through the bile duct, and urine through the ureters.

peritoneal cavity /per′itōnē′əl/, a space between the outer (parietal) and the inner (visceral) layers of the membrane lining the abdomen (peritoneum).

peritoneal dialysis. See **dialysis.**

peritoneum /-tōnē′əm/, a large oiled membrane that covers the entire wall of the abdomen and is folded over the inner organs (viscera). It is divided into an outer (parietal) membrane and an inner (visceral) one. The **parietal peritoneum** is the part that lines the wall of the abdomen. The **visceral peritoneum** is the largest membrane in the body that covers the viscera. The free surface of the peritoneum is oiled by fluid that permits the organs to glide against the wall and against one another. A part (mesentery) of the peritoneum fans out from the main membrane to hold the small intestine. –**peritoneal,** *adj.*

peritonitis /-tōnī′-/, a painful inflammation of the membrane that covers the wall of the abdomen (peritoneum). It is caused by bacteria or substances in the space in the abdomen because of a wound or an abnormal hole (perforation) in an organ. Peritonitis is caused most often by a break in the appendix. When the condition is caused by scar tissue between two surfaces, it is called **adhesive peritonitis.** Symptoms of peritonitis include swelling of the abdomen, pain, nausea, vomiting, rapid heart beat, chills and fever, and rapid breathing. Shock and heart failure may follow. See also **appendectomy, appendicitis.**

Peritrate, a trademark for a blood vessel widening drug (pentaerythritol tetranitrate).

permanent tooth. See **dentition, tooth.**

Permapen, a trademark for an antibiotic (penicillin G benzathine).

permeable /pur′mē·əbəl/, allowing fluids and other substances to pass through. See also **osmosis.**

permeation, the process by which a hazardous liquid chemical moves through a given material on the molecular level. This process is significant in PPE contamination and decontamination.

Permissible Exposure Limit (PEL) or **Recommended Exposure Limit (REL),** the maximum time-weighted concentration at which 95% of exposed, healthy adults suffer no adverse effects over a 40-hour work week. It is an 8-hour, time-weighted average concentration, unless otherwise noted. PELs are expressed in either ppm or mg/cu meter. They are commonly used by OSHA in evaluating work place exposures and can be found in the NIOSH *Pocket Guide to Chemical Hazards.*

Permitil, a trademark for a tranquilizer (fluphenazine hydrochloride).

pernicious anemia /pərnish′əs/. See **nutritional anemia.**

peroneal /per′ənē′əl/, referring to the outer part of the leg.

peroneal muscular atrophy, an abnormal, inherited condition. It involves weakening or wasting of the foot and ankle muscles, and hammertoes. Affected people often have high arches and an awkward walk, caused by weak ankle muscles.

perphenazine, an antipsychotic drug given to treat psychotic disorders and to control severe nausea and vomiting in adults.

PERRLA, abbreviation for *pupils equal, round, react to light, accommodation.* It notes the condition of the eyes, the size and shape of the pupils, their reaction to light, and their ability to focus as normal. It is used to note results of an eye test.

Persa-Gel, a trademark for an acne drug (benzoyl peroxide).

Persantine, a trademark for a heart vessel widening drug (dipyridamole).

Persistin, a trademark for a nervous system drug with painkillers (aspirin and salicylsalicylic acid).

persona, *pl.* **personae,** the role that a person takes and presents to the world to satisfy the demands of society or as part of some mental conflict. The persona masks the person's inner being or unconscious self.

personal care services, the services done by health care workers to help patients in meeting the demands of daily living.

personality, the pattern of behavior each person develops as a means of dealing with the surroundings and their cultural, ethnic, and other standards.

perspiration. See **sweat.**

Perthes' disease /per′tās/, abnormal changes in the growth of the bone substance in the upper leg bone (femur) in children. It may begin with death and the breakdown of bone forming tissues, followed by regrowth or rehardening of the bone.

Pertofrane, a trademark for an antidepressant (desipramine hydrochloride).

pertussis /pərtus′is/. See **whooping cough.**

pertussis immune globulin, a passive vaccinating drug used against whooping cough. Known allergy to this drug prohibits its use. A side effect can be allergic shock.

pertussis vaccine, an active vaccinating drug given to fight whooping cough (pertussis) when combined diphtheria, pertussis, and tetanus vaccine cannot be used. A lack of blood platelets (thrombocytopenia) or known allergy to the vaccine prohibits its use. Side effects include severe allergic reactions, pain at the injection site, and fever.

perversion, 1. any varying from what is considered normal or natural behavior. 2. *informal.* any of a number of sexual acts that vary from what is considered normal adult behavior.

pes /pēz/, the foot or a footlike structure.

pes cavus, a defect of the foot with a very high arch and very long toes. The condition may be present at birth or appear later because the muscles of the foot contract or become unbalanced, as in nerve or muscle diseases. Surgery is needed in severe cases, especially in children. In milder forms the pain can be relieved by special shoes. Also called **clawfoot.**

pessary /pes'ərē/, a device placed in the vagina to treat a falling uterus (prolapse), or other problems of the vaginal space. It is used to treat women whose older age or poor general condition prevents surgery. Pessaries are also used in younger women in checking for a backward bending of the uterus (retroversion). The pessary is sometimes used in pregnancy to hold the uterus in a forward position. A pessary must be removed, usually daily, for cleaning.

pesticide poisoning, a condition caused by swallowing or breathing a substance used for pest control. See also **malathion poisoning, parathion poisoning, rodenticide poisoning.**

petechiae /pētē'kē·ē/, *sing.* **petechia** /-ē·ə/, tiny purple or red spots that appear on the skin because of small spots of bleeding under the skin. Petechiae range from pinpoint to pinhead size and are even with the skin surface. Compare **ecchymosis.** –**petechial,** *adj.*

petit mal seizure /pətē'mäl', pet'emäl'/. See **epilepsy.**

Petrogalar, a trademark for a laxative (mineral oil).

petrolatum, a soft, purified substance obtained from petroleum and used in ointments. Also called **petroleum jelly.**

petroleum distillate poisoning, a harmful condition caused by swallowing or breathing a petroleum product, as gasoline, kerosene, fuel oil, or model airplane cement, and some solvents. Nausea, vomiting, chest pain, dizziness, and severe depression of the nervous system are symptoms. Severe or fatal lung problems may occur. Vomiting should be avoided.

Peyer's patches /pī'ərz/, groups of lymph nodes in the end of the small intestine (terminal ileum) near where it joins with the large intestine (colon).

peyote /pā·ō'tē/, a cactus from which a hallucinogenic drug, mescaline, is made.

Peyronie's disease /pārōnēz'/, a growth of fiberlike tissue on the erection tissue (corpora cavernosa) of the penis. The main symptom of Peyronie's disease is a painful erection.

Pfizerpen, a trademark for an antibiotic (penicillin G potassium).

pH, a scale showing the levels of acid or alkaline in a solution. A value of 7.0 is neutral. Below 7.0 is acid. Above 7.0 is alkaline. See also **acid, acid-base balance.**

phagocyte /fag'əsīt/, a cell that is able to surround, eat, and digest small living things, as bacteria. **Fixed phagocytes** do not move in the blood. They include fixed cells and some connective tissue cells. **Free phagocytes** move in the blood and include white blood cells (leukocytes) and free cells.

phagocytosis /-sītō'-/, the process by which some cells of the body, as cells that help the body fight bacteria, eat and get rid of small living things and cell wastes.

phakomatosis /fak'ōmətō'-/, *pl.* **phakomatoses,** a group of inherited diseases marked by noncancerous tumorlike bumps (nodules) of the eye, skin, and brain. See also **cerebroretinal angiomatosis, neurofibromatosis, tuberous sclerosis.**

phalanx /fālan'gks/, *pl.* **phalanges** /fālan'jēz/, any one of the narrowing bones making up the fingers of each hand and the toes of each foot. Each hand or foot has 14 phalanges.

phallic stage, the period in mental and sexual growth between 3 and 6 years of age when awareness and playing with the genitals is the main source of pleasure. See also **psychosexual development.**

phantom limb syndrome, a sense nerve feeling common after the removal of a limb. The patient has feeling in the missing limb. See also **pseudesthesia.**

pharmaceutic /fär'məsoo'-/, referring to pharmacy or medical drugs.

pharmacokinetics /fär'məkōkinet'-/, the study of the action of drugs in the body.

pharmacology /-kol'-/, the study of the making, ingredients, uses, and actions of drugs.

pharmacy, a place for making and giving out drugs.

pharyngeal reflex /ferin'jē·əl/. See **gag reflex.**

pharyngeal tonsil. See **adenoid.**

pharyngitis /'fer'injī'-/, inflammation or infection of the throat (pharynx), usually causing symptoms of a sore throat. Symptoms may be relieved by painkillers, drinking warm or cold liquids, or salt water gargles. See also **strep throat.**

pharynx /fer'ingks/, the throat, a tubelike structure that is a passage for both the breathing and digestive tracts. It also works in speech as it changes shape to allow one to form vowel sounds. The pharynx is made of muscle and is lined with mucous membrane. It contains the openings of the hearing (eustachian) tubes, nasal space (posterior nares), voice box (larynx), gullet (esophagus), and the tonsils. It is divided into three regions. The **nasopharynx** is behind the nose from the back of the nasal opening to the soft palate.

O-P

The **oropharynx** extends from the soft palate in the back of the mouth to the level of the hyoid bone below the lower jaw. The **laryngopharynx** extends from the hyoid bone at the base of the tongue to the esophagus. Also called **throat.** See also **larynx.**

phenacemide, an antiseizure drug given to treat severe epilepsy. It is used for mixed seizures that do not respond to other drugs. Pregnancy, behavior problems, or known allergy to this drug prohibits its use. Side effects include anemia, mental problems, and kidney and liver inflammation.

phenacetin, a painkiller given to relieve pain and to lower fever. Known allergy to this drug prohibits its use. Repeated use should be avoided in anemia, heart, lung, liver, or kidney disease. Side effects include liver disease, fever, and skin rash.

Phenaphen, a trademark for a painkiller, antifever drug (acetaminophen).

phenazopyridine hydrochloride, a urinary tract painkiller for bladder inflammation (cystitis) or other urinary tract infections. Kidney problems or known allergy to this drug prohibits its use. Side effects include headache and stomach and bowel problems.

phendimetrazine tartrate, a drug given to lower the appetite in treating problems of being overweight caused by eating too much. Heart disease, high blood pressure, an overactive thyroid, sight problems (glaucoma), a history of drug abuse, use of nervous system stimulating drugs or monoamine oxidase inhibitors, or known allergy to this drug prohibits its use. Side effects include nervous system excitement, high blood pressure, an inability to sleep, dry mouth, and addiction.

phenelzine sulfate, a monoamine oxidase (MAO) inhibitor given to treat depression.

phenindione, a drug to stop blood clotting given to prevent and treat many different kinds of blood clots.

pheniramine maleate, an antihistamine given to treat many allergic reactions, including runny nose and skin rash. Asthma or known allergy to this drug prohibits its use. It is not given to newborn infants or nursing mothers. Side effects include drowsiness, skin rash, allergic reactions, dry mouth, and rapid heart beat.

phenmetrazine hydrochloride, a drug given to lower the appetite. It is used to treat being overweight caused by eating too much. Heart disease, high blood pressure, an overactive thyroid, sight problems (glaucoma), history of drug abuse, use of a nervous system stimulating drug or a monoamine oxidase (MAO) inhibitor, or known allergy to this or other drugs like it prohibits its use. It is not used for children under 12 years of age. Side effects include nervous system excitement, high blood pressure, an inability to sleep, and dry mouth.

phenobarbital, a barbiturate, antiseizure, and tranquilizing drug given to treat many seizure disorders and as a long-acting sleeping pill.

phenocopy /fē′nōkop′ē/, a physical trait or condition that is caused by outside things, but looks like a trait that is inherited. Conditions as deafness, mental retardation, and eye clouding (cataracts) can be inherited, but they can also result from infections or other causes.

phenol /fē′nôl/, a highly poisonous, harsh chemical taken from coal or plant tar or made in a laboratory. It has a strong odor and is a strong cleaning fluid (carbolic acid).

Phenolax, a trademark for a laxative (phenolphthalein).

phenol camphor, an oily mixture of camphor and phenol, used to sterilize things and to relieve toothache.

phenolphthalein laxative, a laxative that acts on the wall of the bowel. It is given to treat long-term constipation and to prevent straining. It is given to patients recovering from surgery and those with heart disease or high blood pressure.

phenol poisoning, harsh poisoning caused by swallowing compounds with phenol, as carbolic acid, creosote, and naphthol. Phenol poisoning causes burns of the mouth, seizures, and failure of all major systems. The skin around the mouth and nose should be washed, as well as any burns on the skin. Narrowing (stricture) of the esophagus can happen because of a high level of tissue damage.

phenomenon /finom′ənon/, a sign that is often linked to an illness or condition and is important in diagnosing something.

phenothiazine tranquilizers, any of a group of drugs used to treat mental problems, as an antihistamine to control vomiting and to put a patient to sleep before surgery. The most widely used drugs are chlorpromazine and prochlorperazine. These drugs are not used in pregnancy.

phenotype /fē′nōtīp/, **1.** the traits of an individual or group one can see. They are caused by the interactions of heredity and the environment. **2.** a group of organisms that look like each other. Compare **genotype.** **–phenotypic,** *adj.*

phenoxybenzamine hydrochloride, a blood pressure drug given to control high blood pressure and sweating when a patient has adrenal tumors (pheochromocytoma). Low blood pressure or known allergy to this drug prohibits its use. Side effects include very low blood pressure and rapid heart beats.

phensuximide, an antiseizure drug given to prevent and treat seizures in petit mal epilepsy. Known allergy to this or a related drug prohibits its use. Side effects include blood disorders and kidney damage with blood in the urine.

phentermine hydrochloride, a drug given to lower the appetite to treat being overweight caused by eating too much. Hardening of the arteries, heart disease, high blood pressure, sight problems (glaucoma), overactive thyroid, or known allergy to this or other drugs like it prohibits its use. Side effects include an inability to sleep, rapid heart beat, and high blood pressure.

phenylalanine (Phe), an amino acid needed for the normal growth of infants and children. It is also needed for normal protein use all through life. It is found in large amounts in milk, eggs, and other foods. See also **amino acid, phenylketonuria, protein.**

phenylbutazone, an antiinflammatory drug given to treat severe symptoms of arthritis, bursitis, and other conditions with inflammation.

phenylephrine hydrochloride, a nervous system drug given to keep the blood pressure at a set level. It is also used in the nose and eyes to narrow blood vessels. Sight problems (narrow-angle glaucoma), use of monoamine oxidase inhibitors, or known allergy to this drug prohibits its use. Side effects include heart problems, a high rise in blood pressure, and allergic reactions.

phenylketonuria (PKU) /fe′nəlkē′tōnŏŏr′ē·ə/, a birth defect in which an enzyme needed to change an amino acid (phenylalanine) in the body into another substance (tyrosine) is lacking. Buildup of phenylalanine is poisonous to brain tissue. Signs include skin rashes (eczema), a mousy odor of the urine and skin, and mental retardation. Treatment is a diet free of phenylalanine. See also **Guthrie test.** –**phenylketonuric,** *adj.*

phenylpropanolamine hydrochloride, a blood vessel narrowing drug given to relieve a stuffy nose and other cold symptoms. High blood pressure, heart artery disease, use of monoamine oxidase inhibitors at the same time, or known allergy to this drug prohibits its use. Side effects include nervousness, an inability to sleep, loss of appetite, and high blood pressure.

phenytoin, an antiseizure drug given to treat grand mal and motor seizures and to control the heart rhythm. Known allergy to this drug or to related drugs prohibits its use. It is used with caution in patients with liver or blood problems and some heart disorders. Side effects include loss of muscle control, uncontrolled eye movements, and allergic reactions. This drug interacts with many other drugs.

pheochromocytoma /fē′ōkrō′mōsītō′mə/, a tumor of the adrenal gland that causes too much release of two hormones (epinephrine and norepinephrine). Signs include high blood pressure, headache, sweating, excess blood sugar, nausea, vomiting, and fainting spells.

phimosis /fīmō′-/, tightness of the foreskin (prepuce) of the penis that will not allow the foreskin to be pulled back. It may be the result of infection.

phimosis vaginalis /vaj′inā′lis/, an inherited narrowness of the opening of the vagina.

phi phenomenon /fī/, a feeling of motion that is caused by lights that flash on and off at a certain rate. Also called **stroboscopic illusion.**

pHisoHex, a trademark for a cleanser with an antiinfective drug (hexachlorophene) used mainly before surgery. It should not be used for bathing infants.

phlebitis /flebī′-/, inflammation of a vein, often along with formation of a clot. It occurs most commonly as the result of injury to the vessel wall, abnormal increased clotting of the blood, infection, and chemical irritation. Less blood flow after surgery, prolonged bedrest, sitting, or standing, or a long period of vein catheterization are other causes. The vessel feels hard and thready or cordlike and is extremely sensitive to pressure. The surrounding area may be red and warm to the touch. The entire limb may be pale, cold, and swollen. Deep vein phlebitis features aching or cramping pain, especially in the calf when the patient walks or bends the foot backward. Treatment may include anticlotting therapy and moist heat applied to the affected area. As swelling becomes less, an exercise program is started. Also called **thrombophlebitis.**

phlebothrombosis /fleb′ōthrombō′-/, an abnormal blood problem in which a clot forms in a vein. It is most often caused by poor blood flow, a blocked vein, or blood that clots faster than normal. In contrast to phlebitis, the wall of the vein is not inflamed. See also **phlebitis.**

phlebotomus fever /flēbot′əməs/, a mild infection, caused by a virus carried to humans by the bite of an infected sandfly. Symptoms include fever, headache, eye pain and inflammation, muscle pain, and a rash.

phlebotomy /flebot′-/, entry into a vein to release blood, as in getting blood from a donor. It is done to treat an excess of red blood cells (polycythemia vera). Also called **venesection.**

phlegm /flem/, thick mucus released by the tissues lining the breathing passages.

phobia, an anxiety problem with an overwhelming and irrational fear. In a **simple phobia,** the fear centers on specific things, as animals, dirt, light, or darkness. In a **social phobia,** there is a strong wish to avoid, and an unreasonable fear of, situations in which the patient may be closely watched and judged by others, as speaking, eating, or performing in public, or using public toilets or transportation. The patient may faint, have a racing heart rate, sweat, and have nausea and feelings of panic. The fear, which is not realistic, often results from something unpleasant from the past. The strong need to avoid the feared object or situation can alter regular behavior, which can result in changes in life patterns and interactions with others. Although the cause may be known, the patient feels

O–P

unable to overcome the fear. Treatment is behavior treatment to reduce the anxiety. See also specific entry.

phocomelia /fō′kōmē′ly·ə/, a birth defect in which the feet or hands or both are joined to the body by short, distorted stumps. It is seen as a side effect of a drug (thalidomide) taken during early pregnancy. Also called **seal limbs.**

phocomelic dwarf /-mē′lik/, a dwarf in whom the long bones of any or all of the arms and legs are very short.

phonic /fon′ik, fō′-/, referring to voice, sounds, or speech.

phosphatase /fos′fətāz/, an enzyme that starts chemical reactions with phosphorus. See also **catalyst, enzyme, phosphorus.**

phosphate /fos′fāt/, a substance that is very important in living cells in storing and using energy. It also helps carry genetic data within a cell and from one cell to another.

Phospholine Iodide, a trademark for an eye drug (echothiophate iodide).

phospholipid /fos′fōlip′id/, one of a class of chemical compounds, widely found in living cells. It contains phosphoric acid, fatty acids, and nitrogen. Two kinds of phospholipids are **lecithin, sphingomyelin.**

phosphoric acid, a clear, odorless liquid that is irritating to the skin and eyes and poisonous if swallowed.

phosphorus (P) /fos′fərəs/, a nonmetal chemical element. It is needed to digest protein, calcium compounds, and glucose. The body uses phosphorus from milk, cheese, meat, egg yolk, whole grains, peas, and nuts. A lack of phosphorus can cause weight loss, anemia, and abnormal growth.

phosphorus poisoning, a condition caused by swallowing white or yellow phosphorus, sometimes found in rat poisons, fertilizers, and fireworks. Symptoms include nausea, throat and stomach pain, vomiting, diarrhea, and an odor of garlic on the breath.

photoallergic contact dermatitis, a skin reaction that occurs 24 to 48 hours after being exposed to light in a person who is put at risk by a substance (photosensitizer) that builds up in the skin. It is changed to active allergic material by light. Avoiding both the substance and sunlight at the same time prevents the reaction. See also **photosensitizer.**

photochemotherapy, a kind of chemical treatment in which the effect of a drug is made stronger by exposing the patient to light. See also **chemotherapy.**

photon, energy emitted or absorbed in the form of electromagnetic radiation. Gamma rays are examples of photons.

photophobia, 1. abnormal reaction to light, as by the eyes. It occurs in albinos and many diseases that affect the eye membrane (conjunctiva) and cornea, as measles.

2. an anxiety disorder marked by an unreal fear of light with a need to avoid light places.

photosensitive, referring to a strong reaction of skin to sunlight often caused by certain drugs. A brief exposure to sunlight or to an ultraviolet lamp may cause swelling, pimples, hives, or acute burns in patients who are photosensitive. See also **photosensitizer, phototoxic.**

photosensitizer, anything that may cause an allergic reaction, as in the skin, when combined with light. Common photosensitizers are antibiotics (sulfanilamide), antiseptics (hexachlorophene), some birth control pills, tranquilizers (phenothiazene), and a substance (psoralen) found in many plants, as carrots and mustard.

photosynthesis /-sin′thəsis/, a process by which plants with green coloring (chlorophyll) make carbohydrates from carbon dioxide and water. They use sunlight for energy and release oxygen.

phototherapy, treatment of disorders by using light, as ultraviolet light. Ultraviolet light may be used to treat acne, bed sores, and other skin disorders. **Phototherapy in the newborn** is a treatment for a bile-coloring disorder (hyperbilirubinemia) that causes yellowing (jaundice) in the skin of a newborn. The infant's bare skin, with eyes and sex organs covered, is exposed to a strong fluorescent light. The bluish light speeds up the release of the bile coloring (bilirubin) in the skin.

phototoxic, showing a quickly growing reaction of the skin when it is exposed to a substance that causes the reaction (photosensitizer) and light. See also **photosensitive, photosensitizer.**

phrenic nerve /fren′ik/, one of a pair of branches of the fourth neck (cervical) nerve. It is a motor nerve to the diaphragm that helps to move it in breathing. The **accessory phrenic nerve** joins the phrenic nerve at the base of the neck or in the chest.

phycomycosis /fī′kōmīkō′-/, a fungus infection. Severe infection in the lungs sometimes occurs with late diabetes mellitus that is untreated or out of control. See also **zygomycosis.**

phylogeny /filoj′ənē/, the growth of the structure of a species as it changed from simpler forms of life. Compare **ontogeny.**

physical abuse, one or more times of forceful behavior that result in physical injury.

physical or **chemical hazard statement,** a statement displayed on a side panel, as necessary. It will list special flammability, explosion, or chemical hazards posed by the product.

physical examination, a test of the body to find out its state of health, using any or all of the means of testing. The physical examination, medical history, and first laboratory tests are the basis on which a diagnosis is made and on which treatment is decided on.

physical fitness, the ability to carry out daily tasks normally, without becoming too tired, and with enough energy left to meet emergencies or to enjoy leisure activities.

physical medicine, using physical therapy to return diseased or injured patients to a useful life. See also **rehabilitation.**

physical therapy, the treatment of disorders with physical agents and methods. Some types are massage, moving muscles and bones, exercises, cold, heat, and light. Also called **physiotherapy.**

physician, 1. a health care worker who has earned a degree of Doctor of Medicine (MD) after an approved course of study at an approved medical school. An MD most often enters a hospital internship program for 1 year of training after getting the degree before beginning practice or further training in a specialty. To practice medicine, an MD has to get a license from the state in which the services will be done. **2.** a health care worker who has earned a degree of Doctor of Osteopathy (D.O.) by completing a course of study at an approved college of osteopathy. Osteopathic physicians and medical physicians follow nearly the same courses of training and practice. Osteopathic medicine places special stress on the physical defects of tissues as a cause of illness and on treatment that is moving body structures.

physician extender, a health care worker who is not a physician but who does certain medical actions also done by a physician.

physician's assistant (PA), a person trained to assist a physician. A physician directs and oversees the physician's assistant. Also called **physician's associate.**

physiologic retraction ring, a ridge around the inside of the uterus that forms during the second stage of normal labor. Compare **constriction ring, pathologic retraction ring.**

physiology /fiz′ē·ol′-/, the study of the processes and workings of the human body.

physostigmine salicylate, a drug given to treat nervous system side effects caused by drugs able to block normal nerve signals. Asthma, gangrene, diabetes, heart and blood vessel disease, or blocked intestines or urinary tract prohibits its use. It is not given to patients taking some nerve muscle blocking drugs. Side effects include excess saliva, slow heart beat, seizures, and high blood pressure.

phytohemagglutinin test /fī′tōhem′əglōō′tinin/, a test to find persons who are carriers of cystic fibrosis. It is done by exposing blood cells to a plant antibody (phytohemag-

glutinin). A normal reaction makes more cell protein. See also **cystic fibrosis.**

pia mater /pī′ə mā′tər, pē′ə/, the most inner of the three membranes (meninges) covering the brain and the spinal cord. It carries a rich supply of blood vessels, which serve the nervous tissue. Compare **arachnoid, dura mater.**

pica /pī′kə/, a craving to eat things that are not foods, as dirt, clay, chalk, glue, ice, starch, or hair. It may occur with poor diet, with pregnancy, and in some forms of mental illness.

Pick's disease, a mental disorder that occurs in middle age. Affecting mainly the front part of the brain, it causes neurotic behavior, slow changes in personality, emotions, reasoning, and judgment. See also **dementia.**

pickwickian syndrome, an abnormal condition with being overweight, breathing difficulty, tiredness, and excess red blood cells.

picornavirus /pīkôr′nə-/, one of a group of small viruses (RNA) that cause polio, throat infections, brain inflammation (meningitis), and other diseases. See also **virus.**

picrotoxin, a powerful nervous system stimulating drug taken from the seeds of a Southeast Asian fruit, (*Anamirta cocculus*).

PID, abbreviation for **pelvic inflammatory disease.**

piebald /pī′bôld/, having patches of white hair or skin because of a lack of color-forming of pigment cells (melanocytes) in those areas. It is inherited. Compare **albinism, vitiligo.**

Pierre Robin's syndrome, a group of birth defects occurring together that includes a small lower jaw, cleft lip and cleft palate, and defects of the eyes and ears. Intelligence is most often normal. Plastic surgery may repair the defects, but speech or dental treatments and counseling are often needed.

pigeon breast, a birth defect with a breastbone that pushes out. It may cause heart and lung problems that sometimes need surgery. **–pigeon-breasted,** *adj.*

pigeon breeder's lung, a breathing disorder caused by allergic material in bird droppings.

pigment, any organic coloring material made by the body tissues, as melanin. **–pigmentary, pigmented,** *adj.*, **pigmentation,** *n.*

piles /pīlz/. See **hemorrhoids.**

pill, a rounded or oval-shaped drug to be swallowed whole.

Pilocar, a trademark for a nerve drug (pilocarpine hydrochloride).

pilomotor reflex /pī′lō-/, erection of the hairs of the skin in response to cold, emotion, or irritation of the skin. Also called **gooseflesh.**

pilonidal cyst /-nī′dəl/, a hairy lump (cyst) that often grows in the skin of the lower back. The cysts may be

O–P

noted at birth by a pushed-in space, sometimes a hairy dimple, in the middle of the back. If a cyst becomes infected, it is removed, and the space is closed after the infection has been treated.

pilonidal fistula, a cystlike channel (fistula) close to the tip of the tailbone (coccyx). Also called **pilonidal sinus.**

pilosebaceous /-sibā′shəs/, referring to a hair sac (follicle) and its oil gland.

pilus /pē′ləs, pī′-/, *pl.* **pili,** a hairlike structure.

Pima, a trademark for a cough syrup (potassium iodide).

pimple, a small swelling of the skin, often an infection of a pore. See also **acne, furuncle, papule, pustule.**

pin, 1. to secure and hold fragments of bone with a nail in surgery. **2.** a small metal rod or peg, used by dentists as a support in rebuilding a tooth.

pineal gland /pin′ī·əl/, a cone-shaped structure in the brain. No one knows exactly what it does. It may release a hormone (melatonin), which appears to stop the release of another (luteinizing) hormone. Also called **pineal body.**

pinealoma /pin′ē·əlō′mə/, a tumor of the pineal gland in the brain.

pindolol, a drug given alone or with a fluid-releasing (diuretic) drug to treat high blood pressure. Asthma or heart disorders prohibits its use. It must be used with caution in patients with diabetes. Side effects include slow or rapid heart beat, low blood pressure, fainting, and stomach and bowel problems.

pine tar, a common part of creams, soaps, and lotions used to treat long-term skin conditions, as eczema or psoriasis.

ping-ponging, *slang.* an illegal practice in which a patient is passed from one physician to another so that a health program or service can charge for many unneeded tests.

pinocytosis /pī′nōsītō′-/, the process by which fluid is taken into a cell. The cell membrane develops a pouchlike space, fills with fluid from outside the cell, then closes around it, forming a tiny pond of fluid in the cell.

pinta /pēn′tə/, a skin infection carried by flies or other insects in Latin America.

pin track infection, a condition in which infections may develop at the sites where traction pins are inserted into a body part. Signs of infection are redness at the sites, pus draining and odor, pins slipping, high body temperature, and pain. Treatment is with antibiotics.

pinworm infection, an infection by the common pinworm *(Enterobius vermicularis),* which looks like a small white thread. The worms infect the large intestine. The females deposit eggs in the anal area, causing itching and insomnia. It is possible for an entire family to become infected by contact with bedclothes or hands of the patient. Treatment for the whole family may be necessary. Treatment with

drugs usually completely rids the body of pinworms. Also called **enterobiasis.**

piperacetazine, a tranquilizer given to treat psychotic and behavior disorders in mentally retarded patients. Parkinson's disease, use of nervous system depressing drugs, liver or kidney disease, low blood pressure, or known allergy to this or drugs like it prohibits its use. Side effects include low blood pressure, liver disease, blood disorders, allergic reactions, and many nervous system reactions.

piperazine citrate, a worming (anthelmintic) drug given to treat infestation by pinworms or roundworms. Liver or kidney damage, seizures, or known allergy to this drug prohibits its use. Side effects include, most often because of an overdose, stomach cramps, diarrhea, dizziness, sight problems, and fever.

Pipracel, a trademark for an antibiotic (piperacillin).

piriformis /pir′ifôr′mis/, a flat, triangular muscle that moves the thigh and helps to extend it.

Pirquet test /pērkā′/. See **tuberculin test.**

Pitocin, a trademark for a uterus-stimulating drug (oxytocin).

Pitressin, a trademark for a fluid-gathering hormone drug (vasopressin).

pitting, 1. small, puncturelike dents in fingernails or toenails, often a result of a skin disorder (psoriasis). **2.** a pushed-in space that remains for a short time after pressing fluid-swollen skin with a finger.

pituitary dwarf /pitoo′iter′ē/, a dwarf whose slowed growth is caused by a lack of growth hormone. It results from a defect of part of the pituitary gland. The body is normally shaped, with no face or skeleton defects, and there is normal mental and sexual growth. It is usually found in childhood. Also called **hypophyseal dwarf.**

pituitary gland, the small gland joined to another gland (hypothalamus) at the base of the brain. It supplies many hormones that control many needed processes of the body. The pituitary is divided into two lobes. The **adenohypophysis** is the front (anterior) lobe. It gives off many hormones, including growth hormone. These hormones control the thyroid, gonads, adrenal cortex, breast, and other endocrine glands. Hormones from the hypothalamus gland control the adenohypophysis. The **neurohypophysis** is the back (posterior) lobe of the pituitary gland. It is the source of antidiuretic hormone (ADH) and oxytocin. ADH hormone causes cells in the kidney to reabsorb more water, thereby reducing the amount of urine. Oxytocin causes strong contractions of the pregnant uterus and causes milk to flow from breasts. The pituitary gland is larger in a woman than in a man and becomes larger during pregnancy. Also called **hypophysis cerebri.**

Pituitrin, a trademark for something taken from the fluid-gathering and labor-causing hormone of the pituitary gland.

pit viper, any one of a family of poisonous snakes. Except for coral snakes, all poisonous snakes naturally found in the United States are pit vipers. See also **snakebite.**

pityriasis alba /pit′ərī′əsis/, a common skin disease marked by round or oval, finely scaling patches without skin color (pigment), usually on the cheeks. The itching sores are easy to spot and occur mostly in children and adolescents. Treatment includes special creams.

pityriasis rosea, a skin disease in which a slightly scaling, pink rash spreads over unexposed parts of the body. The **herald patch,** a large, more scaly sore, appears before the pink rash by several days. The smaller sores tend to follow the normal crease lines of the skin.

pivot joint, a joint in which movement is limited by the joint to moving back and forth. The elbow is a pivot joint. See also **synovial joint.**

PKU, abbreviation for **phenylketonuria.**

placard. See **vehicle warning placard.**

placebo /pləse′bō/, an inactive substance given as if it were a real dose of a needed drug. The substance may be a saltwater solution, distilled water, or sugar. Placebos are used in drug studies to compare the effects of the inactive substance with those of an experimental drug. They are also given to patients who cannot be given a real or potent drug. The benefit to the patient of a placebo may sometimes outweigh the ethical, moral, and legal problems raised by giving it.

placebo effect, a physical or emotional change occurring after a placebo is taken. The change may be for the better, meeting the results the patient expects.

placenta /pləsen′tə/, a temporary blood-rich structure in the uterus through which the fetus takes in oxygen, food, and other substances and gets rid of carbon dioxide and other wastes. The placenta begins to form on about the eighth day of pregnancy when the forming embryo (blastocyst) invades the wall of the uterus and becomes joined to it. The embryo cell layer invades the mother's tissues with fingerlike bumps (chorionic villi). Separating the villi are lakes of blood in the wall of the uterus. The mother's blood flows into the lakes surrounding the villi, allowing food, gases, and other substances to pass into the fetal blood flow. The mother's surface has a dark red, rough, liverlike look. The fetal surface is smooth and shiny. **Placenta accreta** refers to a placenta that invades the uterine muscle, making separation from the muscle difficult. **Placenta battledore** is a condition in which the umbilical cord is in the margin or edge of the placenta, instead of near the center.

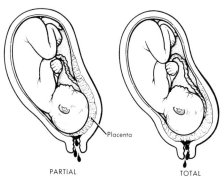

Placenta previa

placental insufficiency, an abnormal condition of pregnancy, marked by slowed growth of the fetus and uterus. Also called **placental dysfunction.** See also **intrauterine growth retardation.**

placenta previa /prē′vē·ə/, a condition in which the placenta is buried abnormally in the uterus so that it partly or completely covers the opening of the cervix. It is the most common cause of painless bleeding in the third 3 months of pregnancy. Its cause is unknown. As the cervix opens during labor, the placenta is slowly separated from the blood vessels in the lining of the uterus. This results in bleeding that usually begins slowly, is painless, and continues to heavy bleeding that is life-threatening to the mother and the baby. The condition may be discovered before bleeding begins by ultrasound or by vaginal examination in the normal course of prenatal care. If severe bleeding occurs, immediate cesarean section is most often needed to stop the bleeding and save the mother's life, regardless of the stage of the fetus' growth. If the placenta is next to or near, rather than touching or covering, the opening of the cervix, labor and birth through the vagina may be attempted. **Central placenta previa** is a problem in which the placenta is implanted in the lower part of the uterus so that it completely covers the narrow lower end of the uterus (cervix). With **marginal placenta previa,** the placenta becomes stuck in the lower part of the uterus. Its edges touch or spread to some degree over the opening of the uterine cervix. Bleeding may be so light as to pose no serious problem. **Partial placenta previa** is a condition in which the placenta partly covers the opening of the cervix. As the cervix widens in labor, the part of the placenta that lies over it breaks apart, causing bleeding.

Placidyl, a trademark for a tranquilizer (ethchlorvynol).

plagiocephaly /plā′jē·ōsef′əlē/, a defect of the skull in which early or irregular closing of the borders of the skull results in the unequal growth of the head, making it look unbalanced. Also called **plagiocephalism.** See also **craniostenosis.** –**plagiocephalic, plagiocephalous,** *adj.*

O–P

plague /plāg/, an infectious disease carried by the bite of a flea from a rodent infected with the bacillus *Yersinia pestis*. Plague is mainly an infectious disease of rats or other rodents. The rat fleas feed on humans when their normal hosts have been killed by the plague. Widespread human infections may follow. **Bubonic plague** is the most common form of plague. **Black Death** usually refers to the epidemic of bubonic plague in the fourteenth century that killed over 25,000,000 people in Europe. Symptoms include painful swollen lymph nodes (buboes) in the armpit, groin, or neck, fever as high as 106° F, exhaustion with a high thready heart rate, low blood pressure, confusion, and bleeding into the skin from the surface blood vessels. **Septicemic plague** is a form of bubonic plague in which blood poisoning (septicemia) and inflammation of the membranes covering the brain and spinal cord occurs. **Sylvatic plague** is a native disease of wild rodents that may be carried to humans by the bite of an infected flea. It is found on every continent except Australia. **Pneumonic plague** is a rapidly fatal form of plague with pneumonia. There are two forms: **primary pneumonic plague** results from the lungs being infected during bubonic plague; **secondary pneumonic plague** is caused by breathing infected bits of sputum from a patient with pneumonic plague. Vaccination with plague vaccine gives partial immunity; infection with the disease gives lifetime immunity. Treatment includes antibiotics and draining the buboes. See also **bubo.**

plague vaccine, an active vaccinating drug made with killed plague bacilli. It is given to vaccinate against plague after a possible exposure or to protect travelers in high risk areas. An inability to fight infections or strong infection prohibits its use. Side effects include allergic reactions, inflammation at the injection site, headache, and general discomfort.

planning meeting, a meeting, held as needed throughout the duration of an incident, to select specific strategies and tactics for incident control operations and for service and support planning.

plantago seed /plantā′gō/, a bulk-forming laxative taken from *Plantago psyllium* seeds. It is given to treat constipation and diarrhea.

plantar, referring to the sole of the foot. Also called **volar.**

plantaris /plantär′is/, one of the muscles at the back of the leg. It flexes the foot and the leg. Compare **gastrocnemius, soleus.**

plantar reflex, the normal response of flexing the toes when the outer surface of the sole is firmly stroked from the heel to the toes. Compare **Babinski's reflex.**

plantar wart. See **wart.**

plantigrade /plan′tigrād/, referring to the human pattern of walking on the sole of the foot with the heel touching the ground.

plaque /plak/, **1.** a flat, often raised patch on the skin or any other organ of the body. **2.** a patch of fatty buildup (atherosclerosis) on the lining of a blood vessel (artery). **3.** also called **dental plaque.** a thin film on the teeth made up of material in saliva and containing bacteria.

Plaquenil Sulfate, a trademark for an antimalaria, antiarthritis, and lupus-suppressing drug (hydroxychloroquine sulfate).

plasma /plaz′mə/, the watery, colorless fluid in lymph and blood in which the white and red blood cells and platelets float. It is made up of water, electrolytes, proteins, sugar (glucose), fats, bile coloring (bilirubin), and gases. Plasma is needed to carry the many parts of the blood through the bloodstream and keep the acid-base balance of the body. Plasma makes up about 50% of the total volume of blood. **Blood plasma** contains glucose, proteins, amino acids, and other foods, urea and other waste products, as well as hormones, enzymes, vitamins, and minerals. Compare **serum.**

plasma cell, a cell found in the bone marrow, connective tissue, and, sometimes, the blood. Plasma cells are used in the body's fight against disease and are formed in large numbers in bone marrow cancer.

plasma cell leukemia, an abnormal tumor of blood-forming tissues in which most of the cells in the blood are plasma cells. In most cases plasma cell leukemia is fatal, but some patients respond to treatment with anticancer and hormone drugs.

plasmapheresis /-fərē′-/, removing plasma from blood taken from a patient. It is also a mixture made from the cell parts of the plasma, and putting this mixture back into the patient. It is used to treat some diseases. Compare **leukapheresis, plateletpharesis.**

plasma protein, any of the proteins in blood plasma. These substances (as albumin, fibrinogen, prothrombin, and the gammaglobulins) help to keep water balance and blood pressure normal. Fibrinogen and prothrombin are needed for blood clotting.

plasma volume, the total amount of plasma in the body. It rises in diseases of the liver and spleen and in a lack of vitamin C. It lowers in an adrenal gland disorder (Addison's disease), loss of fluids, and shock.

plaster, **1.** any material made of a liquid and a powder that hardens when it dries. It can be used in shaping a cast to keep a broken bone aligned, as plaster of paris. **2.** a home treatment made of a semisolid mixture placed on a part of the body, as a mustard plaster.

plastic surgery, the change, replacement, or rebuilding of the outer parts of the body. It is done to correct a structural plate   353   plexus

or cosmetic defect. In corrective plastic surgery, the surgeon may use tissue from the patient or from another person or artificial material. The artificial tissue must not be irritating. It must have a texture that is right for the body part. It must also be able to hold its shape and form for a long time. Implants are often used in making breasts larger (mammoplasty). Skin grafts are common in plastic surgery. Simpler techniques (Z-plasty, Y-plasty) are often done instead of a graft in parts of the body covered by loose, stretchy skin, as the neck and throat. A coloring may be added to the skin of a graft to change the color of the graft to make it look like the skin around it. See also specific entry.

plate, a flat structure or layer, as a thin bone.

platelet /plāt′lit/, the smallest of the cells in the blood. Platelets are disk-shaped and have no hemoglobin. They are needed for blood clotting. Compare **erythrocyte, leucocyte.** See also **hemoglobin.**

plateletpheresis /-fərē′-/, the removal of platelets from blood. The rest of the blood is put back into the patient. Compare **leukapheresis, plasmapheresis.**

Platinol, a trademark for an anticancer drug (cisplatin).

platinum (Pt), a silvery-white, soft metallic element. It is used in dentistry and to make chemicals that must be able to stand high temperatures.

Platyhelminthes, a group of parasitic flatworms that includes tapeworms and flukes,

platysma /plətiz′mə/, one of a pair of wide muscles at the side of the neck. The platysma draws down the lower lip and the corner of the mouth.

play, any action that is fun, entertaining, amusing, or diverting. It is important in childhood for normal personality growth and as a means for growing physically, mentally, and socially. With **active play,** the child is doing, not watching. In **associative play,** a group of children do similar or identical activities without a definite goal. The children may borrow or lend toys and may do like others in the group. However, each child acts independently, as on a playground or among a group riding bicycles. **Cooperative play** refers to any organized play among a group of children. Activities are planned to achieve some goal. This usually takes place among older children.

play therapy, a form of mental treatment in which a child plays in a safe and guided place with games and toys set up by a health care worker. This person watches the behavior, affect, and speech of the child to gain data for the child's thoughts, feelings, and daydreams.

pledget /plej′ət/, a small, flat compress made of cotton gauze, a piece of cotton, or material like it. It is used to wipe the skin, soak up fluids, or clean a small surface.

-plegia, a combining form meaning a paralysis in a certain area.

Plegine, a trademark for a drug used to lower the appetite (phendimetrazine tartrate).

plethora /pleth′ərə/, a term given to the beefy red color of a newborn.

plethysmograph /pləthiz′məgraf/, an instrument for listing changes in the size of hands, feet, and organs by measuring changes in the amount of blood.

pleura /ploor′ə/, pl. **pleurae,** a two-layered membrane surrounding the lung. The visceral pleura covers the surface of the lung, dipping into spaces between the lobes. The parietal pleura lines the chest wall. The two parts of the pleura are separated from each other by an oily fluid. –**pleural,** adj.

pleural cavity, the space within the chest (thorax) that holds the lungs.

pleural effusion, an abnormal buildup of fluid in the lungs. Symptoms are fever, chest pain, breathing difficulty, and a dry cough. The fluid comes from swollen lung surfaces.

pleurisy /ploor′əsē/, inflammation of the linings of the chest. Symptoms include breathlessness and stabbing pain. It stops normal breathing with spasms on the affected side of the chest. Pleurisy without fluid buildup is called dry (fibrinous). **Adhesive pleurisy** refers to a fusion of the layers of the pleura. The main symptom is pain when breathing in or moving. Causes include lung cancer, pneumonia, a blood clot in the lung, and tuberculosis.

pleurodynia /ploor′ədin′ē·ə/, inflammation of the muscles (intercostal) between the ribs and those that attach the diaphragm to the chest wall. Symptoms are sudden severe pain and tenderness, fever, headache, and loss of appetite. The pain is made worse by movement and breathing. The lungs are not affected. **Epidemic pleurodynia** is an infection caused by a virus that mainly affects children. Symptoms include severe pain in the stomach or lower chest, fever, headache, sore throat, fatigue, and extreme muscle aches. The symptoms may continue for weeks or stop after a few days and recur weeks later. There is no specific treatment. Complete recovery is usual. Also called **devil's grip.**

pleuropneumonia, a combination of lung lining inflammation (pleurisy) and pneumonia.

pleurothotonos /-thot′ənəs/, an uncontrolled, severe, long-term contraction of the muscles of one side of the body. It results in a twisting of the body to that side and is usually linked to tetanus infection or strychnine poisoning. –**pleurothotonic,** adj.

plexiform neuroma, a tumor made of twisted bundles of nerve fibers. Also called **Verneuil's neuroma.**

plexus, pl. **plexuses,** a group of joined nerves, blood vessels, or lymph vessels. The body has many plexuses, as the cardiac plexus and the solar plexus.

O–P

plica /plī′kə/, *pl.* **plicae** /plī′sē/, a fold of tissue in the body, as the circular folds (plicae circulares) of the small intestine. –**plical,** *adj.*

plicamycin, an anticancer drug given to treat cancer of the testicles, and excess blood calcium linked to cancer. Blood disorders, kidney or liver disease, bone marrow defect, or known allergy to this drug prohibits its use. Side effects include blood defects, nausea, and mouth inflammation.

plug, a mass of tissue cells, mucus, or other matter that blocks a normal opening or passage of the body, as a cervical plug.

Plummer's disease, a thyroid growth (goiter) with a harmful condition from an overactive thyroid or tumor. Also called **toxic nodular goiter.**

Plummer-Vinson syndrome, a disorder with iron deficiency anemia and webs of tissue in the gullet (esophagus) that cause swallowing difficulty. Also called **sideropenic dysphagia.**

PMT, abbreviation for **premenstrual tension.**

PND, abbreviation for **postnasal drip.**

pneumococcal vaccine /nōō′mōkok′əl/, an active vaccination drug with foreign bodies (antigens) of the 14 types of *Pneumococcus* linked to 80% of the cases of pneumococcal pneumonia. It is given to patients over 2 years of age who are at high risk of getting severe pneumococcal pneumonia. Pregnancy, early childhood (under 2 years of age), or known allergy to the vaccine prohibits its use. Side effects include inflammation at the site of injection, fever, and allergic reactions.

pneumococcus /-kok′əs/, *pl.* **pneumococci** /-kok′sī/, a bacterium (*Diplococcus pneumoniae*), the most common cause of bacterial pneumonia. More than 85 subtypes are known. See also **pneumonia.**

pneumoconiosis /-kō′ne·ō-/, any disease of the lung caused by the long-term breathing of dust, most often mineral dusts. See also **anthracosis, asbestosis, silicosis.**

pneumocystosis /-sistō′-/, a lung infection from a parasite (**Pneumocystis carinii**) commonly seen in patients who are weak or at high risk because of loss of resistance to infections. Symptoms include fever, cough, rapid breathing, and bluish skin (cyanosis). The death rate is near 100% in untreated patients. Also called **interstitial plasma cell pneumonia,** *Pneumocystis carinii* **pneumonia.** See also **acquired immune deficiency syndrome (AIDS).**

pneumomediastinum /-mē′de·əstī′nəm/, the presence of air or gas in the space between the lung lining (pleural) sacs of the chest.

pneumonectomy /-nek′-/, the removal of all or part of a lung.

pneumonia /nōōmō′ne·ə/, inflammation of the lungs, commonly caused by bacteria (*Diplococcus pneumoniae*). Parts of the lungs become plugged with a fiberlike fluid.

Symptoms include severe chills, a high fever (which may reach 105° F), headache, cough, and chest pain. Red blood cells leaking into the air sacs of the lungs cause a rust-colored sputum. As the disease continues, sputum may become thicker and have pus. The patient may have painful attacks of coughing. Breathing often becomes painful, shallow, and rapid. The pulse rate goes up, often over 120 beats a minute. Other signs may be heavy sweating and bluish skin. Viruses, rickettsiae, and fungi may also cause pneumonia. **Aspiration pneumonia** is caused by taking foreign material or vomit into the lungs. It can occur when a patient vomits during or after surgery. It also occurs when a patient is intoxicated or otherwise unconscious and vomits. Treatment includes suctioning the vomit from the lungs and giving oxygen. **Eosinophilic pneumonia** features lung inflammation with a buildup of white blood cells (eosinophils) in the lungs. The disease may be caused by an allergy to fungus, plant fibers, wood dust, bird droppings, or other foreign substance. **Hypostatic pneumonia** occurs in elderly or weak persons who remain in the same position for long periods. Gravity tends to speed up fluid congestion in one area of the lungs, increasing the likelihood of infection. **Interstitial pneumonia** is a diffuse, chronic inflammation of the lungs. Symptoms include clubbing of the fingers, bluish skin, and fever. The cause may be an allergy to certain drugs or an autoimmune reaction. X-ray films of the lungs show patchy shadows and mottling. Heart or respiratory failure may cause death. **Lobar pneumonia** is a severe infection of one or more of the lobes of the lungs. *Streptococcus pneumoniae* bacteria usually cause the disease but other bacteria can also produce it. With an early diagnosis, appropriate antibiotic therapy is highly successful. Complications include lung abscess, lung collapse, pus accumulation, and inflammation of the membrane surrounding the heart (pericarditis). Precautions against spread of the contagious disease are important. Because the fatality rate in the elderly and those with other diseases is high, a preventive injection of pneumococcal vaccine is recommended for them. **Mycoplasma pneumonia,** also called walking pneumonia, is a contagious disease of children and young adults. Symptoms include dry cough, fever, harsh or reduced breath sounds and fine bubbling or crackling noises on breathing in. There may be complications of sinus problems, chest pain (pleurisy), nerve inflammation, or heart disorders. In untreated adults, long-term cough, weakness, and discomfort are common. Treatment of pneumonia includes bed rest, fluids, antibiotics, painkillers, and, if needed, oxygen. Ice packs or cold, wet compresses may be needed to lower the fever. Fever, loss of fluids, and breathing through the mouth result in a need for special care of the mouth and nose. Mild pneumonia is often treated at home. See also **bronchopneumonia.**

pneumonitis /-nī′-/, *pl.* **pneumonitides,** an inflammation of the lung. It may be caused by a virus or be a reaction to chemicals or organic dusts, as bird droppings or molds. Dry cough is a common symptom.

pneumothorax /-thôr′aks/, a collection of air or gas in the chest (pleural space) causing the lung to collapse. It may be the result of an open chest wound that permits air to enter, the break of an air-filled blister (vesicle) on the lung's surface, or a severe bout of coughing. Pneumothorax may begin with a sudden, sharp chest pain, followed by difficult, rapid breathing. The patient must learn how to turn, cough, breathe deeply, and do passive exercises without making the condition worse.

pocket face mask, a device to aid in mouth-to-mouth resuscitation to prevent contact with the patient's mouth. It may be used with supplemental oxygen when fitted with an oxygen inlet.

podalic /pōdal′ik/, referring to the feet.

podiatry /pōdī′ətrē/, the diagnosis and treatment of diseases and other disorders of the feet.

poikiloderma of Civatte /poi′kilōdur′mə/, a common skin inflammation with red patches on the face and neck that become dry and scaly. The patient often has skin reactions to sunlight. Also called **reticulated pigmented poikiloderma.** See also **photosensitive.**

poison, any substance that damages health or destroys life when swallowed, breathed in, or soaked up by the body in small amounts. Most doctors agree that, depending on the size of the dose, any substance can be harmful. There are few workable antidotes. Treatment for poisoning is based mainly on getting the poison out the body before it can be absorbed. Poisons that injure the nervous system often cause permanent damage because parts of the brain cannot regrow. The harmful effects of chemicals may be divided into local and system effects. Local effects, as those from swallowing harmful substances, involve the site of the first contact between the body and the poison. System effects depend on the soaking up and spread of the poison. System poisoning most often affects the nervous system but may also affect the blood flow, blood and blood-forming tissues, skin, and liver, kidneys, and lungs. Muscles and bones are less often affected. See also **poisoning treatment,** and specific types of poisoning. –**poisonous,** *adj.*

poison control center, one of a nearly worldwide group of services that offer data about all aspects of poisoning, keep records of their rate, and refer patients to treatment centers.

poisoning treatment, the care given a patient who has been exposed to or who has taken a harmful drug or chem-

ical. In the case of poisoning by mouth, the first thing to do is to remove the poison quickly. If vomiting does not occur, it should be started after first finding out what the poison is, if possible. However, if the poison is gasoline, kerosene, or a harsh or burning substance, vomiting should *not* be started. Before attempting to start vomiting, the victim, if conscious, should be given one or two glasses of milk or water. A carbonated beverage should never be given for poisoning by mouth. Because of the danger of high levels of salt (sodium) in the blood, the victim, especially a child, should not be given water with salt or mustard. Syrup of ipecac can be given, if handy, to start vomiting, and the dose can be repeated one time. But if the ipecac does not cause vomiting, working on the victim's gag reflex at the back of the throat may help. Ipecac should not remain in the stomach or be given with milk or charcoal, both of which can affect its action. As in other emergencies, a physician should be called to take charge of the case. If one is not available, the nearest poison control center should be called for help.

poison ivy, any of several species of climbing vine (*Rhus*), with shiny, three-pointed leaves. Common in North America, it causes severe allergic reactions in many people. Blisters with itching and burning result that may be treated with lotions, cold compresses, or hormone lotions or creams. People who are extremely allergic to poison ivy may be given preventive treatment with a *Rhus* antigen after contact, before symptoms begin. Careful washing of the exposed skin after suspected contact may prevent the reaction. Also common in North America, and of the *Rhus* group, are **poison oak,** a vine, and **poison sumac,** a shrub. Symptoms of contact with these plants and treatment are like those for poison ivy. See also **rhus dermatitis, urushiol.**

poker spine. See **bamboo spine.**

Polaramine, a trademark for an antihistamine (dexchlorpheniramine maleate).

polarity /pōler′itē/, the existence or display of opposing qualities, or emotions, as pleasure and pain, love and hate, or strength and weakness. It is important for mental well-being.

polarity therapy, a type of massage based on the idea that the body has positive and negative energy patterns that must be balanced to keep the body healthy.

polio /pō′lē·ō/, *informal.* poliomyelitis.

polioencephalitis /-ensef′əlī′-/, inflammation of the gray matter of the brain caused by a virus (poliovirus). **Polioencephalomyelitis** includes the spinal cord.

poliomyelitis /-mī′əlī′-/, a disease caused by a virus. There are mild forms of the disease and others that cause paralysis. The disease is carried from person to person. Stress increases the chance of getting the virus. Older peo-

O–P

ple and pregnant women are more likely to get the serious form. The mild form lasts only a few hours with fever, headache, nausea, and vomiting. A longer lasting form also includes irritation of brain membranes (meninges) with pain and stiffness in the back. See also **poliovirus.**

poliomyelitis vaccine. See **poliovirus vaccine.**

poliosis /pō′lē·ō′-/, loss of hair coloring. It may be an inborn problem and can occur over the whole body. It may also be seen only in patches.

poliovirus, the virus that causes poliomyelitis. There are three different types of this very small virus. Getting infected by or vaccinated with one type does not keep the patient from getting the others.

poliovirus vaccine, a vaccine made from poliovirus to keep a person from getting the disease. TOPV (trivalent live oral vaccine), or Sabin vaccine, should be given to children under 18 years of age. IPV (inactivated poliovirus vaccine), or Salk vaccine, should be given to infants and children who have not formed a defense against the disease and for adults who have not been vaccinated.

pollutant, an unwanted substance in the environment, usually with unhealthy effects. Pollutants can be in the atmosphere as gases or dust that irritate lungs, eyes, and skin, and as substances in water, foods or beverages.

polyarteritis nodosa /pol′ē·är′təri′-/, a serious blood vessel disease in which small and medium-sized arteries become swollen and damaged. This causes the death of the tissues they supply with blood. Any organ or organ system may be affected. The disease attacks men and women between 20 and 50 years of age. Symptoms are high temperatures, pain in the abdomen, weight loss, and nerve damage. If the kidneys are affected, high blood pressure, fluid gain (edema), and a poison (urea) in the blood result.

polychlorinated biphenyls (PCB), a group of chemical compounds used to make plastics, insulation, and chemicals to slow the spread of flames. All can be poisonous and cancer-causing. Mild contact with PCBs may cause a skin disorder (chloracne); serious contact may cause liver damage.

Polycillin, a trademark for an antibiotic (ampicillin).

polyclonal /-klō′nəl/, referring to a group of cells or living things that are exactly alike and come from cells that are exactly alike.

Polycose, a trademark for a food supplement that has carbohydrates from cornstarch.

polycystic kidney disease (PKD) /-sis′-/, an abnormal condition of kidneys that have become too big and have lumps (cysts). There are three forms of the disease. **Childhood polycystic disease (CPD)** may cause death within a few years because the liver and kidney stop working. **Adult polycystic disease (APD)** may be present at birth, and may affect one kidney or both. There is pain in the outer side of the hip, thigh, and buttock (flank) and high blood pressure. The kidneys stop working, causing poisons in the blood (uremia) and death. **Congenital polycystic disease (CPD)** is a birth defect that affects all or only a small part of one or both kidneys.

polycystic ovary syndrome, a disorder with a failure to ovulate or menstruate in a woman, an abnormal growth of body hair (hirsutism), and not being able to become pregnant. It is caused by the endocrine gland getting out of balance with higher levels of some hormones (testosterone, estrogen, and luteinizing) and lower levels of others.

polycythemia /-sīthē′mē·ə/, an abnormal increase in the number of red blood cells. It may occur with lung or heart disease, or being in high altitudes for a long time. Also called **Osler's disease.** See also **altitude sickness, erythrocytosis.**

Actions in selected situations with a conscious victim who has ingested poison

Corrosive or caustic substances

Do not attempt to neutralize the substance.
Do not induce vomiting.
Offer the victim a glass of milk or water.

Noncorrosive substances

The decision on whether to induce vomiting depends on the substance ingested, the amount ingested, and the victim's condition. In general, when pure petroleum distillates are ingested, vomiting is *not* indicated.
For other materials, vomiting may be induced. The Regional Poison Center can help in this evaluation.

Methods of inducing vomiting

1. Give 1 tbsp (15 ml) syrup of Ipecac followed by 1 glass of water. (Dose can be repeated once only if vomiting does not occur within 15 to 20 minutes.) Do not allow emetic to remain in stomach.
2. Physician's order: Apomorphine hydrochloride 0.03 mg/lb subcutaneously. (Contraindicated if respiratory depression is present or patient is comatose.) Apomorphine is rarely used. Can be reversed by the administration of naloxene.

Information supplied by the American Association of Poison Control Centers, University of California Medical Center, San Diego.

polydactyly /-dak′-tile/, a birth defect with more than the normal number of fingers or toes. The defect can often be corrected by surgery shortly after birth. Also called **hyperdactyly, polydactylism.**

polydipsia /-dip′sē·ə/, having too much thirst. Some conditions increase urination, which leads to low blood volume and thirst. These include diabetes and some kidney disorders. **Compulsive polydipsia** is a neurotic, compelling urge to drink large amounts of liquid. The condition is emotional. It is not caused by any physical disorder or lack. Extreme cases can result in death.

polyestradiol phosphate, an anticancer drug given for cancer of the prostate and breast cancer. Male breast cancer, a blood clotting disorder (thrombophlebitis), or known allergy to this drug prohibits its use. Side effects include loss of sex drive, not being able to have sex, and growth of breasts in males.

polygene /-jēn/, any of a group of genes that alone have a small effect but work together to form a trait. Examples include genes that affect size, weight, or intelligence.

polyleptic /-lep′-/, any disease or condition that has many phases of high and low levels of seriousness of symptoms.

polymer /-mər/, a chemical compound formed by linking a number of small molecules (monomers).

polymerization, a reaction during which a monomer is induced to polymerize by the addition of a catalyst or other unintentional influences, such as excessive heat, friction, contamination. If the reaction is not controlled, it is possible to have an excessive amount of energy released.

polymorphous /-môr′fəs/, referring to things that exist in many different forms, possibly changing in structure at different stages.

polymorphous light eruption, a common reaction to sunlight or ultraviolet light in patients who are sensitive to sunlight. Small, red pimples and blisters appear on otherwise normal skin, then disappear within 2 weeks.

Polymox, a trademark for an antibiotic (amoxicillin).

polymyalgia rheumatica /-mī·al′jə/, a disease of the large arteries that may appear in people over 60 years of age. Two disorders are thought to be involved in the same disease with slightly different symptoms. One form (polymyalgia rheumatica) affects the muscles, with pain and stiffness of the back, shoulder, or neck, usually becoming more severe when the patient gets up in the morning. There may also be a headache. The other disorder (cranial arteritis) affects the arteries at the side and back of the head, causing a severe, throbbing headache. See also **temporal arteritis.**

polymyxin, an antibiotic used to treat some bacterial infections. Allergies to this drug prohibit its use. It is used very carefully in patients with kidney problems. Side effects include kidney damage, nerve disorders, pain or irritation at the place of shots, and allergic reactions of the skin or mucous membranes.

polymyxin B sulfate, an antibiotic given for infections of the urinary tract, blood, and eye. Known allergy to this drug prohibits its use. Extreme care is necessary when it is given to people with kidney problems. Side effects include kidney and nervous system disorders, drug fever, and allergies when used on the skin.

polyopia /-ō′pē·ə/, a sight problem in which something is seen as many images; multiple vision. The condition can occur in one or both eyes. See also **diplopia.**

polyp, a small tumorlike growth that comes from a mucous membrane surface.

polypeptide /-pep′tīd/, a chain of amino acids that is usually smaller than a protein. See also **amino acid, peptide.**

polypharmacy, the use of a number of different drugs by a patient with one or several health problems.

polyploid /-ploid/. See **euploid.**

polyposis /-po′-/, an abnormal condition with many tumors or growths (polyps) on an organ or tissue. **Familial polyposis** is a disorder with polyps in the colon and rectum. The disease, which has high cancer potential, is inherited. A kind of familial polyposis is **Gardner's syndrome,** a disorder that includes a fiberlike change of bone tissue in the skull, extra teeth, tumors, and cysts.

polysaccharide /-sak′ərīd/, a carbohydrate that contains three or more molecules of simple carbohydrates. Starch is an example.

Polysporin, a trademark for an eye and skin drug that has antibiotics (polymyxin B sulfate and bacitracin).

Polytar Bath, a trademark for a drug that has two drugs for helping with itching, scaling skin (antieczema) (coal tar and pine tar).

polythiazide, a drug given to treat high blood pressure and edema.

polyuria /-yo͝or′ē·ə/, the release of abnormally large amounts of urine. Some causes are diabetes (insipidus or mellitus), use of drugs that increase the passage of urine (diuretics), and too much fluid intake.

Poly-Vi-Flor, a trademark for a children's drug given by mouth that has several vitamins and sodium fluoride.

polyvinyl chloride (PVC), a common plastic material that releases hydrochloric acid when burned. It may be a cause of cancer.

POMP, an acronym for a drug combination, used in the treatment of cancer, that has three anticancer drugs, Purinethol (mercaptopurine), Oncovin (vincristine sulfate), methotrexate, and adrenal hormone (prednisone).

Pompe's disease. See **glycogen storage disease.**

O–P

Pondimin, a trademark for a drug to reduce appetite (fenfluramine hydrochloride).

pons /ponz/, *pl.* **pontes** /pon'tēz/, any bridge of tissue that connects two parts of a structure or an organ of the body. See also **brain.**

Ponstel, a trademark for an antiinflammatory and pain-killing drug (mefenamic acid).

Pontocaine Hydrochloride, a trademark for a local anesthetic (tetracaine hydrochloride).

pooled plasma, a thin, colorless, or slightly yellow liquid part of whole blood for use when whole blood cannot be gotten. See also **bank blood.**

popliteal artery /poplit'ē·əl, pop'litē'əl/, a part of the femoral artery of the upper leg that continues below the knee. It brings blood to muscles of the thigh, leg, and foot.

population, any group that is marked by a certain trait or situation.

population at risk, a group of people who share a trait that causes each member to be at risk to a disease, as cigarette smokers who work with asbestos.

pork tapeworm infection. See **tapeworm infection.**

porphyria /pôrfir'ē·ə/, a group of inborn disorders in which there is an abnormal increase in the body of substances called porphyrins. There are two major kinds of porphyria. **Erythropoietic porphyria,** in which large amounts of porphyrins are made in bone marrow, and **hepatic porphyria,** in which large amounts are made in the liver. Signs common to both are being sensitive to light, pain in the abdomen, and nerve damage. **Acute intermittent porphyria (AIP)** involves sudden attacks of pain from the nerves. Women are affected more often, and attacks often are started by hormone changes of menstruation, pregnancy, and during puberty. Other factors are starvation or crash dieting, infections, and a wide range of drugs. Any part of the nervous system can be affected. A common effect is belly pain. Other effects can include nerve damage, seizures, coma, hallucinations, and difficult breathing. A high-carbohydrate diet may reduce the attacks.

Portagen, a trademark for a substance added to food that has protein, carbohydrate, and fat.

portal hypertension, an increased blood pressure in the portal system caused by blockage in the liver's blood supply. Also called **renovascular hypertension.**

portal system, the network of veins that drains the blood from the stomach and intestinal portion of the digestive tract, spleen, pancreas, and gallbladder and carries blood from these organs to the liver.

portoenterostomy /pôr'tō·en'təros'-/, surgery to open the bile duct. A part of the intestine is sewed to an opening in the liver. This lets bile flow directly into the intestine.

port-wine stain. See **hemangioma.**

position, any one of many postures of the body, as the anatomical, prone, or supine positions. See specific entry.

positive, **1.** referring to a laboratory test showing that a substance or a reaction is present. **2.** referring to physical examination showing that there is a disease change.

positive-pressure apparatus, also known as pressure-demand apparatus, breathing apparatus with a regulator that supplies air when the wearer inhales and also allows a small constant flow to the facepiece. This constant airflow creates an air pressure in the facepiece greater than that of the surrounding atmosphere.

positive-pressure resuscitation, delivering oxygen to the non-breathing patient using an oxygen-powered, manually triggered ventilating device.

postconcussional syndrome, a condition that follows a head injury. Symptoms include dizziness, being unable to focus one's thoughts, headache, being sensitive to noise and other signals, and nervousness. Also called **posttraumatic syndrome.**

posterior, referring to or placed in the back part of a structure. Compare **anterior.**

posterior costotransverse ligament, one of the five ligaments of each joint in the spine.

posterior longitudinal ligament, a thick, strong ligament attached to the back of each backbone and running from the base of the skull to the tailbone (coccyx).

posterior palatal-seal area, the area of soft tissues between the hard and soft palates. It is use by dentists to locate the proper place for a denture.

posterior tibial artery, one of the parts of the popliteal artery of the leg.

postictal /postik'təl/, referring to the time after serious muscle contractions that the patient cannot control (convulsion). –**postictus,** *n.*

postinfectious, occurring after an infection.

postmastectomy exercises /-mastek'-/, exercises that help keep muscles from tightening up and freezing the joints following breast removal (mastectomy). The patient should flex and straighten out the fingers of the arm on the side where the breast was removed as well as the forearm as soon as she returns to her room after recovery from anesthesia and surgery. On the first day after surgery she squeezes a rubber ball in her hand. Brushing the teeth and hair are useful exercises. Other exercises include four that are called climbing the wall, arm swinging, rope pulling, and elbow spreading. They are done as follows:
★Climbing the wall: The patient stands facing a wall, toes close to the wall. The elbows are bent, and the palms of the hands are placed on the wall at shoulder height. The hands are moved up the wall together until the patient feels pain

or pulling on the place where the cut was made in surgery, then returned to the starting position.

★Arm swinging: While standing, the patient bends forward from the waist, letting both arms relax and hang normally. The arms are swung together from the shoulders from left to right and then in circles straight out over the floor, swinging clockwise and counterclockwise. She straightens up slowly.

★Rope pulling: A rope is looped over a shower rod or a hook. Each end of the rope is held and the patient pulls one end of the rope then the other, raising one arm after the other to the height at which pain is felt at the surgical cut or pulling can be felt. The rope is shortened until the arm on the side where the breast was removed is raised almost directly overhead.

★Elbow spreading: The hands are clasped behind the neck and the elbows are slowly raised to chin level while holding the head straight. Slowly, the elbows are spread apart to the point at which pain or pulling is felt. With proper exercise, full range of motion returns, and both arms can be extended fully and equally high over the head. Many activities of daily life give the patient good exercise, as reaching for things on high shelves and gardening.

postmature,   overly developed or matured. See also **dysmaturity.**   –**postmaturity,** n.

postmature infant,   an infant born after the end of the forty-second week of pregnancy, usually with signs of the placenta becoming weak. The baby may have dry, peeling skin, long fingernails and toenails, and folds of skin on the thighs and, sometimes, on the arms and buttocks. Low blood sugar and potassium are common. To avoid the problem, labor may be brought on before the term of pregnancy reaches 42 weeks.

postmenopausal,   referring to the period of life following menopause.

postmortem,   examination after death. Also called **autopsy, necropsy, postmortem examination.**

postmyocardial infarction syndrome /-mī′əkär′dī·əl/,   a condition that may occur days or weeks after a serious heart attack. Symptoms include fever, inflamed heart with a friction rub, pleurisy, fluid buildup, and joint pain.

postnasal drip (PND),   a drop-by-drop release of nasal mucus into the back of the throat, often with a bad taste, and bad breath. Causes are the nose being irritated, sinusitis, or too much fluid being released by the nasal mucosa.

postoperative,   referring to the period of time following surgery. It begins with getting over the effects of anesthesia and goes through the time needed for the effects of the anesthetic or surgery to end.

postpartal care /-pär′təl/,   care of the mother and her newborn baby during the first few days after childbirth (puerperium). Changes that may have occured while the baby was in the uterus are watched. The uterus pulls in after childbirth and causes bleeding to slow. The liquids released from the uterus (lochia) change color during the first few days. A red liquid is released for up to a week, then turns yellow, and, finally, becomes clear and sticky. The muscles around the stomach and intestinal area are soft, but muscle tone comes back with time and exercise. On the third day, the milk usually begins to fill the breasts. The bond between the mother and baby may become closer by contact between the mother and baby. Breast feeding, bottle feeding, nutrition, care of the navel and diaper areas, baby baths, safety, and exercises are taught to new mothers. Being tired, enlarged breasts, sadness, and minor blood clots (thrombophlebitis) are common, but not usual.

postpartum /-pär′təm/,   after childbirth.

postpartum depression,   an abnormal condition that may follow childbirth. Symptoms range from mild ''blues'' to a severe, suicidal mental state where the patient loses touch with reality (psychosis). Severe depression occurs about once in every 2000 to 3000 pregnancies. The cause is not known.

postpericardiotomy syndrome /-per′ēkär′dē·ot′-/,   a condition that sometimes occurs after surgery on the heart membrane (pericardium). Symptoms include pain and the patient finding it hard to breathe, often with no fever. See also **pericarditis.**

postprandial /-pran′dē·əl/,   after a meal.

postsynaptic /-sinap′-/,   **1.** located after a gap between nerves (synapse). **2.** occurring after a synapse has been crossed by a nerve signal (impulse). See also **synapse.**

posttraumatic stress disorder.   See **stress reaction.**

postural drainage /pos′chərəl/.   See **drainage.**

posture,   the position of the body with respect to the space around it. A posture is made by the muscles that move the limbs, by feeling in muscles and joints (proprioception), and by the sense of balance.

potassium (K),   an alkali-metal element needed by all plants and animals to live. Potassium in the body helps to control the nerves and muscles. Foods that have potassium are whole grains, meat, beans (legumes), fruit, and vegetables. Increased kidney release may be caused by chemicals or drugs that increase passage of urine (diuretics) and other drugs, or by kidney disorders. Loss of potassium can also occur through vomiting, diarrhea, surgical drainage, or the long-term use of laxatives.

potassium chloride (KCl),   a drug to treat low blood potassium and digitalis intoxication. Too much blood potassium, use of certain drugs (spironolactone or triamterene), or known allergy to this drug prohibits its use. Side

O–P

effects include high blood levels of potassium, and open sores (ulcers) in the small bowel.

potassium iodide, a drug to treat inflammation of the breathing tubes (bronchitis), asthma, and other disorders. Serious bronchitis, pregnancy, or known allergy to this or drugs like it prohibits its use. Side effects include allergy, goiter, low levels of thyroid (myxedema), bowel problems, and skin sores.

potentiation /pōten'shē·ā'shən/, a condition in which the effect of two drugs given together is greater than the effect of the drugs given each by themselves.

Pott's fracture, a break of the lower leg bone (fibula) near the ankle, often with tearing of a ligament. Also called **Dupuytren's fracture.**

poultice /pōl'tis/, a soft, moist, substance spread between layers of gauze or cloth and placed hot onto a body surface. It may help blood flow and reduce pain.

Povan, a trademark for a drug to treat patients with worms (pyrvinium pamoate).

povidone-iodine, an antigerm chemical used to disinfect wounds. It is also used to treat infections and burns. Known allergy to this drug or to iodine prohibits its use. Side effects include itching of the skin, redness, and swelling.

Powassan virus infection, a form of brain inflammation (encephalitis) caused by a virus carried by ticks found in eastern Canada and the northern United States.

powder bed, a treatment used to keep large areas of the body in contact with a powdered drug. It is usually repeated three times a day. The powder is spread on the sheet from a shaker. The patient lies on the powdered sheet. The powdered sheet is then wrapped around the body in order to keep the powder touching the body. The treatment may be used for skin disorders, such as bedsores.

pox, **1.** any of several skin disorders marked by a rash of pimples, small blisters, or pus-filled sores. **2.** the pitlike scars of smallpox.

poxvirus, one of a group of like (family) viruses that includes the living things that cause smallpox and vaccinia.

ppm, abbreviation for *parts per million.*

practitioner, a person with the training and skills to practice in a special medical field.

Prader-Willi syndrome, a disorder with an inborn lack of muscle tone, too much appetite, being overweight, and mental slowness (retardation). When diabetes mellitus occurs with these other symptoms, the condition is called Royer's syndrome.

pralidoxime chloride, a drug used to reverse the effect (antidote) of poisoning from insect and rodent poisons and to treat drug overdosage in myasthenia gravis. Known allergy to this drug prohibits its use. It should not be used in poisoning by carbamate insect poisons. Side effects include dizziness, fast heart beat and breathing, and weak muscles.

Pramosone, a trademark for a skin balm that has a hormone (hydrocortisone acetate) and a local anesthetic (pramoxine hydrochloride).

pramoxine hydrochloride, a local anesthetic to take away pain and itching in skin disorders, hemorrhoids, anal fissure, and minor burns.

prandial /pran'dē·əl/, referring to a meal; it is used in relation to timing, as after eating (postprandial) or before eating (preprandial). –**prandiality,** *n.*

precipitate /prəsip'itāt/, **1.** to cause a substance to separate or to settle out of a liquid in which it is dissolved. **2.** an event that occurs quickly or without being expected.

Precision, a trademark for a food supplement that has no lactose, cholesterol, and gluten.

precision rest, a stiff denture support. It is made up of two tightly fitting parts. One part rests firmly against the gums.

precocious, referring to the early, often premature, physical or mental traits.

precordial /prēkôr'dē·əl/, referring to the precordium, which is the part of the chest over the heart.

precordial movement, any motion of the front wall of the chest in the area over the heart.

precordial thump, a method to restore the heartbeat of a person whose heart has stopped (cardiac arrest). The person doing it raises one fist 8 to 12 inches above the person's chest and brings it down quickly in one blow. If the heart does not start beating, chest compression and mouth-to-mouth breathing (CPR) are started.

prednisolone /prednis'əlōn/, a hormone (glucocortocoid) used to treat inflammation of the skin and eyes, and to stop the body from having a reaction to an allergic substance.

prednisone /pred'nisōn/, a hormone (glucocorticoid) used to treat severe inflammation and to stop the body from having a reaction to an allergic substance.

preeclampsia /prē'iklamp'sē·ə/, an abnormal condition with very high blood pressure after the sixth month of pregnancy. Other symptoms of preeclampsia are protein in the urine and swollen ankles (edema). It occurs in 5% to 7% of pregnancies, and most often in the first pregnancy. The risk gets higher the more the patient weighs, having a tumorlike mass (hydatid mole) in the uterus or too much amniotic fluid (hydramnios). A type of kidney injury (glomeruloendotheliosis) is a common sign of preeclampsia. After the pregnancy, the signs and symptoms of the disease go away and the kidney disorder heals. Preeclampsia causes the level of nitrogen to get out of balance, the patient becomes irritable, the reflexes react too strongly, there are kidney disorders, and the body's mineral gets out of balance. Further problems include placenta coming away from the uterus, blood cell destruction, bleeding in the brain, eye damage, fluid in the lungs, and lower birth weight of the fetus. The most serious problem is a condition of coma or seizures (eclampsia), which can result in the death of the mother and fetus. Treatment includes rest, use of a calming drug, magnesium sulfate, and high blood pressure drugs. If eclampsia is about to occur, forced childbirth or childbirth by surgical opening (cesarean section) may be necessary. See also **eclampsia.** Also called **toxemia of pregnancy.**

preexcitation /prē·ek′sītā′shən/,   early contraction of part of the heart muscle.

Pregestimil, a trademark for a food supplement for infants.

pregnancy,   the process of growth and development within a woman's reproductive organs of a new individual. It goes from the time of conception through the phases where the embryo grows and the baby develops as the fetus to birth. Pregnancy lasts about 266 days (38 weeks) from the day the egg is fertilized by the sperm, but it may last 280 days (40 weeks; 10 lunar months; $9\frac{1}{3}$ calendar months) from the first day of the last menstrual period (LMP). The date of childbirth, or expected date of confinement (EDC) is based on the LMP even if a woman's periods are not regular. If a woman is certain that sexual intercourse occurred only once during the month of conception, the EDC may be figured as 266 days from that date. There are three **positive signs of pregnancy:** heart tones of the fetus, heard through a stethoscope; fetal skeleton, seen on x-ray film or with other methods (ultrasound); and parts of the fetus felt by pressing gently on the abdomen (palpation). Pregnancy begins after sexual intercourse at or near the time of the egg being released (ovulation). This is usually about 14 days before a woman's next expected menstrual period. Of the millions of sperm cells in the vagina during sexual intercourse, thousands may reach the female egg (ovum) in the fallopian tube. But only one is able to enter the egg for union of the male and female germ cells, which causes conception. The fertilized egg (zygote) is the original body cell of the new individual. Its cells begin to divide as it moves to the uterus where it implants itself in the wall. Parts of the uterus and the embryo combine to form the placenta, which provides the fetus with nutrients from the woman's body and remove waste made by the fetus. However, the blood of the fetus and the woman's body do not normally mix. The embryo (conceptus) is, in some ways, like an animal that lives off another animal (parasite) within the mother. An **ectopic pregnancy** is one in which the fetus develops outside of the uterus. This can occur because of a defect in the fallopian tube or uterus. A **cornual pregnancy** is a type of ectopic pregnancy. The

fertilized egg stays in the part of the fallopian tube that is within the top of the uterus. An **ovarian pregnancy** is one in which the embryo grows in the ovary rather than in the womb. Ectopic pregnancy is rare. Diagnosis is made by ultrasound or x-ray films. The placenta and fetus must be removed. See also **molar pregnancy, tubal pregnancy.**

★PSYCHOLOGIC CHANGES: The effects of pregnancy on the woman's feelings are normal and healthy. A pregnant woman becomes very aware of the fast and unavoidable changes her body is going through. She finds new interest in herself. Her concern for the perfection of her baby, her looking ahead to labor, and her thoughts about the new role of motherhood improve her emotions.

★CARDIOVASCULAR CHANGES: The heart must pump 30% to 50% more blood during pregnancy. The increase begins at about the sixth week and reaches a peak about the sixteenth week. The pulse rate rises during pregnancy to about 80 to 90 beats per minute. Blood pressure may drop slightly after the twelfth week of pregnancy. The circulation of blood to the uterus near the end of pregnancy (term) is about one liter per minute, using about 20% of the total heart output.

★PULMONARY CHANGES: Though the breathing level (vital capacity) remains the same in pregnancy, the breathing rate and other factors increase.

★KIDNEY CHANGES: The rate of blood being filtered by the kidneys increases from between 30% to 50% during pregnancy. The urinary tract expands greatly (hydronephrosis of pregnancy). It is caused by pressure on the ureters from the uterus getting bigger.

★GASTROINTESTINAL CHANGES: Hormone effects that increase during pregnancy cause some smooth muscles to relax in the stomach and intestines. Heartburn may result. Lower bowel activity and pressure on the bowel from the uterus getting bigger may result in constipation. Nausea and vomiting may occur, usually early in pregnancy, probably caused by the effect of a hormone (human chorionic gonadotropin).

★ENDOCRINE CHANGES: The way the thyroid gland works changes in a way that looks like a disorder of too much thyroid secretion. Adrenal gland hormone levels get higher and may be the cause of streaks on the skin in the intestinal area. Sugar processing by the body is changed, and the need for insulin is increased. The placenta makes hormones that supply the lining (decidua) of the uterus, start the growth of the breast milk sacs (acini), and help breast tissue get ready for making milk (lactation). The breasts become firm and more painful early in pregnancy. As the breasts get larger and softer, the tenderness disappears. The circular area (areola) around the nipple becomes more deeply colored, and its glands become larger. A clear or whitish watery substance (colostrum) begins to come

O-P

out from the nipple. Sweating increases. Redness of the skin can be easily seen. Hair growth may be started. Pinpoint bleeding in the skin is very common. Streaks (stria) over the intestinal area, breasts, and buttocks appear in some women. More skin pigment (melanin) causes freckles to get darker. The dark line (linea nigra) in the midline of the lower intestinal area becomes darker and longer. The skin over the nose and above the eyebrows may get darker. This is called chloasma, or the "mask of pregnancy." Normal weight gain is different for each woman, within wide limits. Average weight gain is 20 to 25 pounds, but greater increases are common. The body's need for iron, protein, and calcium increase more than the body's needed overall increase in intake of calories and other nutrients.

pregnancy test. See **HCG radioreceptor assay.**

preload, the first stretch of heart muscle (myocardia) fiber as blood begins to flow into the lower heart chambers (ventricles). The amount of stretch affects the force and rate of movement (velocity) of the next contraction of heart muscles.

Preludin, a trademark for a drug to lower the desire for eating (phenmetrazine hydrochloride).

premalignant fibroepithelioma /prē′məlig′nənt/, a raised "flesh"-colored tumor formed out of ribbons of tissue on a stalk. The tumor occurs most often on the lower trunk of older people. It may become a basal cell cancer.

Premarin, a trademark for sex hormone drug (estrogen).

Premarin with Methyltestosterone, a trademark for a hormone drug that has Premarin and a male sex hormone (androgen) (methyltestosterone).

premature, 1. not fully grown or mature. **2.** occurring before the usual time. –**prematurity,** *n.*

premature contraction, any drawing together of the heart chambers that occurs too soon with respect to the normal heart rhythm. See also **arrhythmia.**

premature ejaculation, an uncontrolled, untimely spurting (ejaculation) of semen. It is often caused by worry during sexual intercourse. See also **ejaculation, nocturnal emission.**

premature infant, any infant, no matter what birth weight, born before 37 weeks of pregnancy. Since exact age of the fetus is often hard to know, low birth weight is an easy way to tell if the infant is premature. Prematurity may be caused by blood disorders, long-term disease, serious infection, or multiple births. The premature infant may appear small and scrawny, with a large head in relation to body size, and a weight of less than 2500 grams (5.5 pounds). The skin is bright pink, smooth, and shiny, and the blood vessels can be seen easily. The arms and legs are straight, not flexed, as in babies born full-term. There is

little skin fat, little hair, few creases on the soles of the feet and palms, and poorly developed ear cartilage. Problems of premature babies include chilling, breathing problems, poor sucking and swallowing reflexes, and small stomachs. Other problems may include kidney, liver, and intestinal breakdown. With treatment in a care unit for young babies, survival rates get better each year. Many very small babies now grow normally, and those who do not have seizures or breathing problems in the first few days after birth will not have serious damage. Also called **preterm infant.** Compare **postmature infant.**

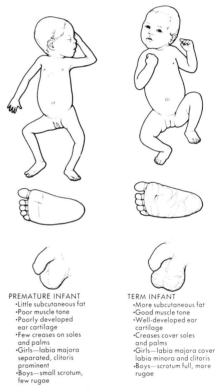

PREMATURE INFANT
·Little subcutaneous fat
·Poor muscle tone
·Poorly developed
 ear cartilage
·Few creases on soles
 and palms
·Girls—labia majora
 separated, clitoris
 prominent
·Boys—small scrotum,
 few rugae

TERM INFANT
·More subcutaneous fat
·Good muscle tone
·Well-developed ear
 cartilage
·Creases cover soles
 and palms
·Girls—labia majora cover
 labia minora and clitoris
·Boys—scrotum full, more
 rugae

Comparison of premature and term infants

premature labor. See **labor.**

premedication, any calming drug or other drug given before anesthesia or a test.

premenopausal, referring to the time of life before the menopause.

premenstrual tension (PMT), nervous tension, irritability, weight gain, fluid buildup, headache, and sore breasts that occur each month in the days just before the start of menstruation.

premolar /prēmō′lər/, one of eight teeth, four in the upper jaw and four in the lower jaw, found on the side and behind the canine teeth. The premolars appear during childhood and normally stay until old age. Also called **bicuspid.**

prenatal /prēnā′təl/,   occurring before birth.

prenatal development, the entire process of growth that occurs between conception and birth. When an egg (ovum) is fertilized, it begins the process of fetal growth and birth. During the first 14 days the first cell formed by the union of sperm and egg (zygote) divides several times. It becomes a ball of cells that is ready to be attached to the wall of the uterus. A very simple placenta appears, and the cell mass becomes a three-layered disk. Next, the basic structures of the body begin to form. A nerve tube grows as the first stage of a central nervous system. Simple blood vessels and blood cells, a heart tube, and umbilical cord vessels form and begin to work. Arm and leg buds may be seen, and the gut, lungs, and kidneys start to form. By the fifth week, the brain has begun to grow quickly, the heart tube splits into chambers, the roof (palate) of the mouth and the upper lip are formed, and the urinary and genital system develops. By the end of the seventh week, all basic body systems are present. The period of time from the eighth week to birth is called the fetal stage. Between the seventeenth and the twentieth weeks of pregnancy, the mother often first feels the baby move. The fetus looks like a very small baby at this time. It has eyebrows and tiny nipples. The fetus has been seen at this age sucking its thumb and holding its own umbilical cord. At 28 weeks fat begins to develop under the skin, fingernails and toenails are present, the eyelids have split and the eyes may open, and the scalp hair has grown a lot. In a modern young baby (neonatal) intensive care unit, more than 80% of the babies born at 28 weeks will live. As the fetus reaches term, between 38 and 42 weeks, the fatty coating on the body starts to go away. In males, the testes are in the scrotum; in females, the labia majora meet in the midline and cover the labia minora and the clitoris. At 40 weeks, the average fetus weighs 7¼ pounds and is between 19 and 22 inches long. Prenatal growth may be affected by several things. Between 2 and 14 weeks of pregnancy, x-rays or other radiation and some drugs may have serious effects on body structures and workings. Various viruses, poor eating, injury, or disease in the mother may also affect a quickly growing structure or organ. After 14 weeks when all the organs, systems, and parts of the body have formed, harmful things may affect the workings of the fetus, but serious damage to the structures of the fetus is not likely to occur.

prenatal diagnosis, examining the developing fetus to find any inborn disorder or other problem. X-ray examination and tests using sound waves (ultrasound scanning) can show growth of the fetus and find certain defects. Through using a needle placed into the amniotic sac to withdraw fluids (amniocentesis), fetal cells may be obtained from the amniotic fluid to find inborn disorders and other inborn problems. Use of a device to see into the fetus (fetoscopy) allows fetal blood to be taken out from a blood vessel of the placenta and looked at for disorders, as thalassemia, sickle cell anemia, and Duchenne's muscular dystrophy. Also called **antenatal diagnosis.** See also **amniocentesis, fetoscope, genetic counseling, genetic screening.**

preoperative care, the care given a patient before surgery. The person's nutritional and health condition, medical and surgical history, allergies, physical handicaps, signs of infection, drugs being used, and waste elimination habits are noted and recorded. The signed informed consent statement, the physician's orders for care before surgery, and the patient's I.D. bands are checked by a nurse. Blood pressure, temperature, pulse, and breathing are taken. Before bedtime, the patient showers, using an antigerm soap; nothing is given by mouth after dinner unless ordered by a physician. Before leaving for the operating room, the patient urinates, and any dentures, contact lenses, and valuables are removed for safekeeping.

prepayment, paying in advance for health care services by holders of a health insurance plan, as Blue Cross/Blue Shield.

preprandial /prēpran′dē·əl/,   before a meal.

prepuce /prē′pyo͞os/,   a layer of skin that forms a cover that folds back, as the foreskin of the penis.

presbycardia /prez′bikär′dē·ə/,   an abnormal heart condition, that affects mainly older persons. It is marked by the heart muscle losing its stretchiness and changes in the fibers of the heart valves.

presbycusis /-kyo͞o′-/,   the normal loss of good hearing that goes with aging.

presbyopia /-ō′pē·ə/,   farsightedness caused by a loss of stretching of the lens of the eye. The condition often occurs with old age. Compare **accommodation.** –**presbyopic,** adj.

prescribe, 1. to write an order for a drug, treatment, or process. **2.** to suggest a certain way to treat a patient for a disorder.

prescription, an order for drugs, treatment, or a device given by someone who has authority to do so, usually a doctor. The order is given to a person, such as a pharmacist, who has the power to fill the order. The prescription is usually in written form and has the name and address of the patient, the date, the ℞ symbol (superscription), the drug prescribed (inscription), directions to the pharmacist or other person who will fill the order (subscription), directions to the patient that must appear on the label, the prescriber's signature, and, usually, a code number that is needed to refill the original prescription.

prescription drug, a drug that can be given to the public only with a doctor's prescription. Only the Food and Drug

Administration can classify a drug as a prescription drug.

presenile dementia /prēsē′nīl/. See **Alzheimer's disease.**

presenting part, the part of the fetus that is closest to the opening of the cervix, just before or during labor.

pressor, a substance that often causes blood pressure to go up.

pressure, a force, or stress, put against a surface by a fluid or an object.

pressure acupuncture, one kind of acupuncture in which pressure, as from the tip of a finger, is put on certain points of the body. See also **acupuncture.**

pressure bandage, a bandage put on to stop bleeding, stop swelling, or give support for varicose veins.

pressure edema, 1. swelling of the legs caused by a pregnant uterus pushing against the large veins of the lower abdomen. **2.** a swelling of the scalp of the fetus after of the head has come out of the mother's body.

pressure point, a point over an artery where the pulse may be felt. Pressure on the point often helps to stop the flow of blood from a wound past that point.

pressure regulator, a device connected to an oxygen cylinder to reduce the cylinder pressure to a safe working level.

presumptive signs, signs of a pregnancy that may not mean the woman is actually pregnant. They include missing a menstrual period and morning sickness. See also **Chadwick's sign.**

presynaptic /prē′sinap′-/, **1.** located near or before a nerve gap (synapse). **2.** occurring in a nerve before a synapse is crossed.

pretibial fever /prētib′ē·əl/, an infection in which one of the signs is a rash on the front of the legs. Other symptoms are headache, chills, fever, and muscle pain. Also called **Fort Bragg fever.**

prevention, any action taken to prevent illness and help make for good health. **Secondary prevention** is a level of preventive medicine that aims to detect disease early, send the patient to the right doctor, and start the right treatment as soon as possible.

preventive, referring to things that slow, stop, or break up the path of an illness or to lower the risk of a disease.

preventive care, medical care that focuses on preventing disease and on keeping people in good health. Getting vaccine shots (immunization) is an example of preventive care.

priapism /prī′əpizm/, a problem with the penis remaining erect too long. This is often painful and is not often linked to being sexually excited. It may be caused by urinary stone (calculi) or a sore inside the penis or the central nervous system. It sometimes occurs in men who have sickle cell anemia or severe leukemia. Treatment may include surgery.

priapitis /prī′əpī′-/, inflammation of the penis.

prickly heat. See **heat rash.**

prilocaine hydrochloride, a local anesthetic used to block the nerves and for regional anesthesia.

primaquine phosphate, a drug used to treat malaria and keep it from coming back during recovery from the disease. Arthritis, use of bone marrow depressants or related drugs, or known allergy to this drug prohibits its use. Side effects include blood disorders and pain in the abdomen.

primary, first in order of time, place, development, or importance.

primary care, the first contact with a doctor for treatment of illness, that leads to a decision on a way to treat a health problem.

prime mover, a muscle that acts directly to bring about a movement. Most body movements need the combined action of many muscles.

primidone, a drug to control muscle spasms (anticonvulsant) used to treat seizure disorders, including grand mal, psychomotor, and focal epilepsy-like seizures. Porphyria or known allergy to this or similar drugs prohibits its use. Side effects include anemia, dizziness, and loss of control of certain muscles.

primigravida /prim′igrav′idə/, a woman pregnant for the first time, shown by the term ''gravida I'' on the woman's medical records. Compare **multigravida, primapara.** –**primigravid,** *adj.*

primipara /primip′ərə/, *pl.* **primiparae,** a woman who has given birth to one healthy infant, shown by the term ''para 1'' on the woman's medical records. Compare **multipara, nullipara, primagravida.**

primitive, formed early in the course of growing; existing in an early or simple form.

primordial dwarf /prīmôr′dē·əl/, a person who is very short but is otherwise normal. The person has normally shaped body parts and normal mental and sexual development. The condition may be inborn, with failure of the body to use growth hormones.

Principen, a trademark for an antibiotic (ampicillin).

Priscoline Hydrochloride, a trademark for a drug that enlarges blood vessels located away from the center of the body (tolazoline hydrochloride).

privileges, rights given to a physician or dentist by a hospital governing board to give care to the hospital's patients. Clinical privileges are limited to the doctor's license, experience, and skill. Emergency privileges may be given by a hospital in an emergency without regard to the physician or dentist's normal standing. Temporary privileges may be given to a physician or dentist to give health care to patients for a limited period or to a certain patient.

Privine Hydrochloride, a trademark for a drug that increases the activity of nerves (naphazoline hydrochloride).

p.r.n., (in prescriptions) abbreviation for a Latin phrase *(pro re nata)* meaning ''as needed.''

probable signs, medical signs of a strong chance of pregnancy. Examples include enlargement of the abdomen, softening of the cervix (Goodell's sign), muscle contractions in the uterus (Braxton Hick's sign), and hormone test results that show pregnancy is likely. Compare **presumptive signs.**

Pro-Banthine, a trademark for an ulcer drug (propantheline bromide).

probenecid, a uric acid and antibiotic drug used to treat an inborn form of arthritis (gout). It is also used to prolong the action of other drugs used to treat some infections, as gonorrhea. Kidney stones, blood disorders, or known allergy to this drug prohibits its use. It is not started during serious attack of gout. It is not given to children under 2 years of age. Use of drugs, such as aspirin, lowers the effect of probenecid. Side effects include low levels of red blood cells in the blood (anemia), headache, urinating often, and minor allergic reactions. It reacts with many other drugs.

procainamide hydrochloride, a drug used to treat various heart disorders. Myasthenia gravis, heart block, or known allergy to this or drugs like it prohibits its use. Side effects include stomach and intestinal problems, allergic reactions, and white blood cell disorders.

procaine hydrochloride, a local anesthetic given by injection, such as Novocain. Side effects include nerve and heart reactions if too quickly absorbed.

procarbazine hydrochloride, an anticancer drug used to treat various cancers, including Hodgkin's disease and lymphomas.

Procardia, a trademark for a calcium channel blocker (nifedipine).

procerus /prōsir′əs/, one of three muscles of the nose. It pulls down the eyebrows and wrinkles the nose.

process, 1. a series of linked events that follow one after another from a given state or condition. **2.** a natural growth that comes out from a bone or other body part.

prochlorperazine, a drug used to combat mental disorders (antipsychotic) and control vomiting and nausea (antiemetic).

procidentia /prō′siden′shə/, the falling or dropping down of an organ, such as the uterus.

procreation, the process of producing offspring. **–procreate,** *v.,* **procreative,** *adj.*

proctitis /proktī′-/, inflammation of the rectum and anus caused by infection, injury, drugs, allergy, or radiation injury. Symptoms include minor pain and the urge to def-

ecate without being able to do so. Pus, blood, or mucus may be present in the stools, and straining (tenesmus) may occur. Also called **rectitis.**

Proctocort, a trademark for an adrenal hormone (hydrocortisone).

proctology /proktol′-/, the branch of medicine that deals with treating disorders of the colon, rectum, and anus.

proctoscope /prok′təskōp/, an instrument used to look at the rectum and the lower end of the colon. It is made up of a light mounted on a tube. Compare **sigmoidoscope.**

prodrome /prō′drōm/, an early sign of a health disorder or disease. **–prodromal,** *adj.*

product name, brand or trade name printed on front panel of a hazardous material container. If the product name includes the term ''technical,'' as in Parathion-Technical, it generally indicates a highly concentrated pesticide with 70% to 99% active ingredients.

Professional Standards Review Organization (PSRO), an organization formed under the Social Security Act Amendments of 1972 to look at the services given under Medicare, Medicaid, and Maternal Child Health programs.

progeny /proj′ənē/, **1.** offspring; an individual that comes from a mating. **2.** the descendants of a known or common ancestor.

progeria /prōjir′ē·ə/, an abnormal condition marked by early aging. It commonly begins with the appearance in childhood of gray hair, wrinkled skin, and small size. There may be the posture and body build of an aged person and a lack of pubic and facial hair. Death usually occurs before 20 years of age. Compare **infantilism.**

Progestasert, a trademark for a female sex hormone (progesterone).

progestational /prō′jestā′shənəl/, referring to a drug with effects like those of progesterone, the female sex hormone. Natural and synthetic kinds of progesterone are used to treat menstrual disorders.

progesterone /prōjes′tərōn/, a natural progestational hormone used to treat various menstrual disorders or inability to become pregnant. Blood clotting, liver problems, breast cancer, missed abortion, or allergy to this drug prohibits its use. Side effects include pain at the place of injection, and problems in the body's chemical processes.

progestin /projes′tin/, **1.** progesterone. **2.** any of a group of hormones, natural or synthetic, released by the corpus luteum, placenta, or adrenal cortex with progesterone-like effects on the uterus.

progestogen /projes′təjən/, any natural or synthetic female sex (progestational) hormone. Also called **progestin.**

O–P

prognathism /prog'nəthizm/,   a condition in which the face looks abnormal because one or both jaws project forward.

prognosis /prognō'-/,   predicting the likely outcome of a disease based on the condition of the patient and the usual action of the disease.

progressive,   referring to the process of the signs and symptoms of a disease or condition becoming more obvious and severe as it develops.

progressive patient care,   a system of care in which patients are placed in units on the basis of their needs for care. The needs are based on the degree of illness and include intensive care, intermediate care, and minimal care.

progressive relaxation,   a way to combat tension and worry by tensing and relaxing groups of muscles in sequence.

projection,   1. anything that thrusts or juts outward, as from a bone. **2.** a subconscious way to defend oneself by attributing traits, ideas, or actions that one cannot accept in oneself on another person.

projectile vomiting,   vomiting that is very forceful.

projective test,   a mental test that uses inkblots, a series of pictures, or unfinished sentences to bring out responses that show the patient's true personality. See also **Rorschach test.**

Proketazine Maleate,   a trademark for a calming drug (carphenazine maleate).

prolactin (PRL) /prōlak'tin/,   a hormone that is made and released into the bloodstream by the pituitary gland. Prolactin, acting with other hormones, starts the growth of the mammary glands. After childbirth, it helps to start and maintain the making of breast milk. This occurs in response to suckling by the infant. When suckling stops, prolactin slows and the breasts stop making milk. Also called **lactogenic hormone, luteotropin.**

prolapse /prō'laps/,   the falling, sinking, or sliding of an organ from its normal position or place in the body, as a prolapsed uterus.

proliferation /prōlif'ərā'shən/,   the rapid spread of like forms of tissues. The term often refers to increases of lumps (cysts) or bacteria.

proline (Pro) /prō'lin/,   an important amino acid found in many proteins of the body, especially collagen. See also **amino acid, protein.**

Proloid,   a trademark for a thyroid hormone drug (thyroglobulin).

prolonged release,   the trait or quality of a drug that is released over a long period of time. The most common form is a drug in a soft capsule that dissolves and has tiny pellets of the drug for release at different rates in the intestine.

Proloprim,   a trademark for an antibiotic (trimethoprim).

promethazine hydrochloride,   an antihistamine and calming drug used to treat motion sickness, nausea, irritation of the mucus in the nose (rhinitis), itching, and skin rash.

pronation /prōnā'shən/,   **1.** a lying-flat position, in which the body faces downward. **2.** the turning of the forearm so that the palm of the hand faces downward and backward. –**pronate,** *v.,* **prone,** *adj.*

pronator teres,   a muscle of the forearm. It turns the hand downward or backward (pronates).

prone,   referring to the position of the body when lying face downward. Compare **supine.**

Pronemia,   a trademark for a body-building drug containing iron, vitamin B_{12}, a chemical to allow vitamin B_{12} to be absorbed (intrinsic factor concentrate), vitamin C, and folic acid.

Pronestyl,   a trademark for a drug that slows the heart rate (procainamide hydrochloride).

propantheline bromide,   a drug used to treat peptic ulcer.

proparacaine hydrochloride,   a fast-acting, local anesthetic used for various eye (ophthalmologic) procedures, including taking out foreign objects from the eye. One drop gives 15 minutes of eye anesthesia. Also called **proxymetacaine.**

prophase /prō'fāz/,   the first phase of nuclear division of tissue cells (mitosis) and of germ cells (meiosis).

prophylactic /prō'filak'-/,   something that keeps a disease from spreading. See also **condom.**

prophylaxis /prō'filak'sis/,   prevention of or protection against disease. It may mean using a biological, chemical substance or a mechanical device to destroy germs or viruses or keep them from entering the body.

Propine,   a trademark for an eye drug (dipivefrin hydrochloride).

Propionibacterium,   a kind of bacteria found on the skin of humans, in the gut of humans and animals, and in dairy products. One species (P. acne) is common in acne blisters.

propionicacidemia /prō'pē·on'ikas'idē'mē·ə/,   an inborn defect in which the body is not able to use certain amino acids (threonine, isoleucine, and methionone). It causes mental and physical retardation.

Proplex,   a trademark for human clotting factor IX.

propoxyphene,   a mild narcotic painkiller used to relieve mild to moderate pain. Use of calming or antidepressant drugs, current alcohol or drug abuse, or known allergy to aspirin prohibits use of this drug. It should be not used by people who are suicidal, those who may tend toward alcohol or drug addiction, or pregnant women. Side effects include liver problems, severe slowing of the central nervous system from a drug overdose or reaction with another drug, nausea, dizziness, sleepiness, or vomiting.

propranolol hydrochloride, a nerve blocking agent used to treat chest pain (angina pectoris), irregular heart rhythm, and high blood pressure. Asthma, irregular heart rhythms, heart failure, use of monamine oxidase (MAO) inhibitors, or known allergy to this drug prohibits its use. Side effects include heart failure, heart block, breathing difficulty, stomach and intestine problems, and allergic reactions. Withdrawal symptoms may occur in some patients.

proprietary, referring to an institution or a product, as a drug or device, run or made for profit.

proprietary hospital, a hospital run as a profit-making organization.

proprietary medicine, any drug that is protected from competition because the chemicals it is made out of or the way it is made are protected by trademark or copyright.

proprioception /prō′prē·əsep′shən/, feeling linked to cues from within the body that help one to know the positions of body parts and the motions of the muscles and joints.

proptosis /proptō′-/, bulging, pushing out or out of place of a body organ or area.

proscribe, to forbid. **–proscriptive,** *adj.*

prosencephalon /pros′ensef′əlon/, the part of the brain that has the thalamus and hypothalamus. It controls important body functions and affects thinking, appetite, and feelings. Also called **forebrain.** Compare **mesencephalon.** **–prosencephalic,** *adj.*

Pro Sobee, a trademark for a milk-substitute formula that is made from soy beans and has no milk in it. It is given to infants with a milk processing disorder (galactosemia) and patients who cannot drink milk without a harmful reaction. See also **galactosemia, lactose intolerance.**

prostacyclin (PGI₂) /pros′təsī′klin/, a prostaglandin. It is formed mainly in human blood vessel walls and slows blood platelet clumping.

prostaglandin (PG) /-glan′din/, one of several strong hormonelike fatty acids that act in small amounts on certain organs. They are used to end pregnancy and to treat asthma and too much stomach acid.

Prostaphlin, a trademark for an antibiotic (oxacillin sodium).

prostate /pros′tāt/, a gland in men that surrounds the neck of the bladder and the urethra. It releases a substance that makes semen into a liquid. It is a firm structure about the size of a chestnut, and is made up of muscle and gland tissue. The substance released by the prostate gland is made up of alkaline phosphatase, citric acid, and various enzymes. **–prostatic,** *adj.*

prostatectomy /pros′tətek′-/, surgical removal of part of the prostate gland. It may be done for an enlarged prostate (benign prostatic hypertrophy). If the gland is cancerous, total removal may be necessary. The most common way (transurethral) uses an instrument put in through the urethra. Shavings of tissue from the prostate gland are cut off at the bladder opening. An opening between the scrotum and anus is used to remove tissue for examination when early cancer is suspected or when stones (calculi) are removed.

prostatic /prostat′ik/, referring to the prostate gland.

prostatitis /pros′tətī′-/, inflammation of the prostate gland. It is usually caused by infection. The patient feels urgent needs to urinate frequently and has a burning sensation during urination.

prosthesis /prosthē′-/, *pl.* **prostheses, 1.** a device designed to replace a missing part of the body, such as an artificial limb. Two examples are artificial heart valves: the **caged-ball prosthesis** made up of a plastic ball in a metal cage, and the **caged-lens prosthesis** made up of a plastic disk in a metal cage. A **maxillofacial prosthesis** replaces part, or all, of the upper jaw, nose, or cheek. It is applied when plastic surgery using normal body tissue is not adequate. **2.** a device designed and applied to make a part of the body work better, as a hearing aid or denture.

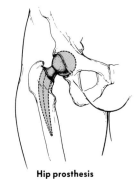

Hip prosthesis

prosthodontics /pros′thədon′-/, a branch of dentistry that deals with making artificial devices that take the place of missing teeth.

prostration, a condition of being severely worn out and unable to exert oneself further, as from heat or stress.

protamine sulfate, a drug produced from fish sperm used to lower or reverse the effect of an overdose from a drug used to block blood clot
ting (heparin). Pregnancy, allergy to fish, or known allergy to this drug prohibits its use. Side effects include low blood pressure, troubled breathing, and slow heart beat.

protease /prō′tē·ās/, an enzyme that helps the breakdown of protein. See also **proteolytic.**

O–P

protection factor, the ratio of contaminants in the atmosphere outside the facepiece to the contaminants inside the facepiece.

protein /prō'tēn, -tē·in/, any of a large group of complex, organic nitrogen compounds. Each is made up of linked amino acids that have the elements carbon, hydrogen, nitrogen, and oxygen. Some proteins also have sulfur, phosphorus, iron, iodine, or other necessary elements of living cells. Twenty-two amino acids are necessary for body growth, development, and health. The body can make 14 of these amino acids, called nonessential, while the other eight must be obtained from food. Protein is the main building material for muscles, blood, skin, hair, nails, and the inside organs. It is also needed to form hormones, enzymes, and antibodies. It is necessary for proper release of body wastes. Foods high in protein are meat, poultry, fish, eggs, milk, and cheese.

protein-bound iodine (PBI), iodine that is attached (bound) to protein in blood serum. The measurement of PBI shows the level of a thyroid gland hormone (thyroxine) in the blood. Low PBI is a sign of too low a thyroid level. A PBI of more than the normal values shows too much thyroid.

protein metabolism, the ways by which protein in foods is used by the body for energy and to make other proteins. Food proteins are first broken down into amino acids, then absorbed into the bloodstream and used in body cells to form new proteins. Excess amino acids may be changed by liver enzymes for use as sources of energy. They may also be changed into glucose or fat to be stored. Urea, a waste from the body's use of protein, is released in urine and sweat.

proteinuria /-ŏŏr'ē·ə/, having large amounts of protein in the urine, such as albumin. Proteinuria is often a sign of kidney disease, but it can also be caused by heavy exercise or fever. **Orthostatic proteinuria** is the presence of protein in the urine of some people who have been standing. It disappears when they lie down and is not medically important. It usually occurs in teenagers. Also called **albuminuria.**

proteolipid /prō'tē·ōlip'id/, a compound of protein and fat (lipid) in which lipid forms more than half of the molecule.

proteolysis /prō'tē·ol'isis/, a process in which water added to the bonds that link protein units causes the protein molecule to break down. Many enzymes may cause this effect.

proteolytic /-lit'ik/, referring to any substance that helps the breakdown of protein.

Proteus /prō'tē·əs/, a type of bacteria often linked to hospital (nosocomial) infections. It is normally found in feces, water, and soil. It may cause wound infections, bacteria in the blood, and shock. *Proteus vulgaris* is often the cause of urinary tract infections. *Proteus morgani* causes diarrhea in infants.

prothrombin /prōthrom'bin/, a blood plasma protein that forms thrombin, the first step in blood clotting. It is made in the liver if the body has enough vitamin K. Also called **factor II.**

prothrombin time (PT), a test for blood clotting defects. A clotting substance (thromboplastin) and calcium are added to a sample of the patient's blood plasma and, at the same time, to a sample of normal blood plasma. The length of time needed to clot in both samples is compared. See also **blood clotting.**

proton, an elementary nuclear particle with a positive electric charge equal numerically to the charge of the electron and having a mass about equal to that of a hydrogen atom.

protoplasm /prō'tōplazm/, the living substance of a cell, usually made up of water, minerals, and animal and vegetable compounds.

protoporphyria /-pôrfir'ē·ə/, higher levels of protoporphyrin in the blood and feces.

protoporphyrin /-pôr'firin/, a kind of coloring (porphyrin) that mixes with iron and protein to make many important body chemicals, such as hemoglobin and myoglobin. See also **heme.**

protozoa /-zō'ə/, *sing.* **protozoon,** single-celled tiny living things that are the lowest form of animal life. About 30 kinds of protozoa cause diseases in humans.

protozoal infection /-zō'əl/, any disease caused by protozoa. Some kinds of protozoal infections are **amebic dysentery, malaria, trichomonas vaginitis.**

proud flesh. See **granulation tissue.**

Proventil, a trademark for a drug to expand the breathing tubes (albuterol).

Provera, a trademark for a hormone (medroxyprogesterone acetate).

provider, a hospital, clinic, or health care professional, or group of health care professionals, who give a service to patients.

provitamin, a substance found in certain foods that the body may convert into a vitamin. Also called **previtamin.**

proximal, a body part that is nearer to a point, such as the trunk of the body, than other parts of the body.

proximity suits, suits designed for short duration, close proximity exposures to flame and radiant heat, such as in aircraft crash, fire, and rescue (CFR) operations. The outer shell is a highly reflective, aluminized fabric over an inner shell of a flame-retardant fabric. These ensembles are not designed to offer any substantial chemical protection.

prurigo /prŏŏrī′gō/, inflammation of the skin. It features severe itching and many small pimples capped by tiny blisters. Later, because of repeated scratching, crusting and skin thickening may occur. Treatment depends on the cause.

pruritus /prŏŏrī′təs/, the symptom of itching. Scratching often causes secondary infection. Some causes are allergy, infection, liver disease (jaundice), or a tumor. Some relief may come from using antihistamines, starch baths, hormone creams, or cool water. **Pruritus ani** is an itching of the skin around the anus. Some causes are contact dermatitis, hemorrhoids, pinworms, psoriasis, and fungus. **Pruritus vulvae** is itching of the outer genitals of a female. Some causes are skin disorders (dermatitis) and fungus (candidiasis).

psammoma /samō′mə/, a tumor that has small hard grains (psammoma bodies). It occurs in the brain tissues, pineal body, and ovaries. Also called **sand tumor.**

pseudochylous ascites /sŏŏ′dōkī′ləs/, the abnormal buildup in the peritoneal cavity of a milky fluid that is like chyle. It is a sign of a tumor or infection in the intestinal area. See also **ascites, chyle.**

pseudocyesis /-sī·ē′sis/, a condition in which a woman thinks she is pregnant when she is not. Some signs and symptoms look like pregnancy, such as failure to menstruate, although no egg has been fertilized. Also called **false pregnancy, pseudopregnancy.**

pseudocyst /-sist/, a cavity without a lining that has gas or liquid. Draining by surgery is the usual treatment.

pseudoephedrine hydrochloride, a drug that affects the nervous system, used to reduce congestion in the nose and the eustachian tube. Known allergy to this drug or similar drugs prohibits its use. It may interact with drugs to control mental depression (MAO inhibitors) or high blood pressure. It is given with caution to patients who have high blood pressure, glaucoma, heart disease, diabetes, or urinary problems. Side effects include an increase in the activity of the central nervous system, headache, and rapid heart beat.

pseudogout. See **chondrocalcinosis.**

pseudohermaphroditism /-hərmaf′rōditizm′/, a condition in which a person has either male testicles or female ovaries but the body features of the opposite sex. See also **feminization, hermaphroditism.**

pseudojaundice /-jôn′dis/, a yellow skin color caused by eating too much carotene-rich food, such as carrots.

Pseudomonas /sŏŏdom′ənas/, a kind of bacteria often found in wounds, burns, and infections of the urinary tract.

pseudopregnancy. See **pseudocyesis.**

pseudotumor, a false tumor.

psilocybin /sī′lōsī′bin/, a psychedelic drug that produces mood changes and may cause people to see things that are not there.

psittacosis /sit′əkō′-/, a pneumonia-like illness caused by a bacterium (*Chlamydia psittaci*). It is given to humans by infected birds, especially parrots. The symptoms include fever, cough, and severe headache. Also called **parrot fever.**

psoas major /sō′əs/, a long muscle in the lower (lumbar) area of the back. It moves the thigh in circles and bends the spine.

psoas minor, a long, slim muscle of the pelvis. It flexes the spine.

psoralen, a chemical that makes things sensitive to light. After being exposed to ultraviolet light, psoralens react to increase the coloring (melanin) in the skin. Natural psoralens are found in buttercups, carrot greens, celery, clover, dill, figs, limes, and parsley. Some psoralen-type chemicals are used in drugs to help skin tanning. They are also used to treat skin diseases, as psoriasis and vitiligo. Such drugs should be applied carefully to keep the skin from becoming too sensitive to light.

psoriasis /sərī′əsis/, an inborn skin disorder in which there are red patches with thick, dry, silvery scales. It is caused by the body making too many skin cells. Sores may be anywhere on the body but are more common on arms, scalp, ears, and the pubic area. A type of arthritis may go along with the skin disease. **Guttate psoriasis** is a form with scaly patches all over the body. A lung infection may cause this reaction. **Pustular psoriasis** is a form in which groups of sores occur every few days in cycles that repeat for weeks or months. Hospital treatment for this type may be needed to replace fluids in the body, and provide drugs and sedation. Treatment for less severe forms includes hormone creams, ultraviolet light, tar soap baths, creams and shampoos.

psychedelic /sī′kədel′ik/, describing a mental state of altered senses in which a person may see things that are not there (hallucination). The person may feel very happy or fearful. It is caused by the use of drugs or other substances that affect the brain.

psychiatric emergency service, a hospital service that treats patients with severe mental problems on a 24-hour-a-day basis.

psychiatric foster care /sīkē·at′-/, a service for mental patients who have been released from a hospital and get care in a foster home.

psychiatric home care, a service for mental patients who get care in their home.

psychiatric inpatient unit, a hospital ward or like area used for the treatment of persons admitted to a hospital (inpatients) who need mental care around the clock.

O–P

psychiatry /sīkī′ətrē/, the branch of medical science that deals with the causes, treatment, and prevention of mental, emotion, and behavior disorders. **Biologic psychiatry** is a branch that stresses the physical, chemical, and nervous system as the causes of and treatments for mental and emotional disorders. **Existential psychiatry** emphasizes an analytical, total approach in which mental disorders are problems within the total structure of a person's existence and not caused by biological or cultural factors. **–psychiatric,** *adj.*

psychic trauma, an emotional shock or injury that leaves lasting effect on the subconscious mind. Causes of psychic trauma are abuse in childhood, rape, and loss of a loved one.

psychoanalysis /sī′kō·ɔnal′isis/, a branch of psychiatry founded by Sigmund Freud that deals with the study of the mental aspects of human development and behavior. It is a system of mental treatment that seeks to use the power of the unconscious mind. The theory uses such techniques as having patients rapidly say what a word or idea makes them think about, and analyzing dreams.

psychoanalyst /-an′əlist/, a physician who works with mental treatment, usually a psychiatrist, who has had special training in analyzing the mind (psychoanalysis) and who uses psychoanalytic techniques.

psychobiology, the study of behavior in terms of the way the body and the mind work together.

psychodrama, a form of group therapy in which people act out their emotional problems in order to find new solutions (role playing).

psychogenic /-jen′ik/, starting in the mind. See also **psychosomatic.**

psychogenic pain disorder, a disorder of continuing and severe pain for which there seems to be no physical cause. See also **somatoform disorder.**

psychologic test, any of a group of standard tests designed to measure traits as intelligence, the desire or lack of desire to undertake activities, values, worries and fears.

psychologist, a person who specializes in the study of the structure and function of the brain and related mental processes. A clinical psychologist is one who is qualified to test and counsel patients with mental and emotional disorders. See also **psychotherapist.**

psychology, the study of behavior and the functions and processes of the mind. **Applied psychology** is a practical use of psychology. See also **psychologist.**

psychomotor, referring to self-controlled muscle movements linked with the nervous system.

psychomotor development, the skills developed by a child that use both the mind and muscles. These include being able to turn over, sit, or crawl at will in infancy; and

later to walk, talk, control urination and defecation, and begin to solve problems.

psychomotor seizure. See **epilepsy.**

psychopath /-path/, a person with a personality disorder whose behavior goes against normal social ways (antisocial). Also called **sociopath.**

psychopathy /sīkop′əthē/, any disease of the mind, inborn or one that develops. it may or may not involve lower than normal intelligence. Also called **psychopathia.**

psychopharmacology /-fär′məkol′-/, the study of the effects of drugs on behavior and mental functions.

psychophysical preparation for childbirth, a program that prepares women for childbirth. They learn about the childbirth process, ways to exercise and improve muscle tone and strength, and ways to breathe and relax for comfort during labor. Different methods may be taught, as the Bradley, Lamaze, or Read methods.

psychophysiologic disorder /-fiz′ē-əloj′ik/, any of a large group of mental disorders that involve an organ or organ system controlled by the autonomic nervous system. For example, a peptic ulcer may be caused or made worse by feelings. Also called **psychosomatic illness, psychosomatic reaction.**

psychosexual, referring to the mental and emotional aspects of sex. See also **psychosexual development, psychosexual disorder. –psychosexuality,** *n.*

psychosexual development, the growth of the personality through a series of stages from infancy to adulthood. Each stage is usually a certain period of childhood and is linked to a way of getting pleasure from various bodily urges. Solving the conflicts of each of the stages should lead to normal development. The stages of development are oral, anal, phallic, latency, and genital. Also called **libidinal development.**

psychosexual disorder, any condition of abnormal sexual feelings, desires, or activities with mental causes. See also **gender identity disorder, psychosexual dysfunction.**

psychosexual dysfunction, any problem of sexual adjusting or disorder, such as sexual failure (impotence) or lack of sexual excitement (frigidity), caused by a mental problem.

psychosis /sīkō′-/, *pl.* **psychoses,** any major mental disorder with a physical or emotional source. The personality may not be able to function smoothly. Often there is also severe depression, excitement, and mistaken beliefs (illusions). There may be those who hold false beliefs (delusion) and see things that are not there (hallucination). These disturbances may prevent the patient from functioning normally. Care in a hospital is often needed. With **acute psychosis,** the ability to process facts is lessened. It sometimes has a known physical cause. Delirium and acute brain syndrome are associated with known physical disorders of the brain. These cause disorientation, loss of memory, and lapses in consciousness. With **functional psychosis,** there are personality changes and the loss of ability to function in reality. However, there is no sign that the disorder is related to brain functions. See also **bipolar disorder, organic mental disorder, paranoia, schizophrenia.**

psychosocial assessment, a review of a patient's mental health, social position, and ability to function with other people. The patient's physical status, appearance, and behavior are reviewed for factors that may show emotional problems or mental illness.

psychosomatic /-sōmat′ik/, the display of an emotional problem through physical disorders. See also **psychogenic, psychophysiologic disorder.**

psychosomatic medicine, the branch of medicine that deals with the links between mental and emotional reactions and the processes of the body. It is based on the idea that the body and mind cannot be divided and that both physical and mental methods should be used in the study and treatment of illness.

psychosurgery, surgery that cuts certain nerve pathways in the brain. It is done to treat some cases of long-term anxiety, overexcitement (agitation), or disorders in which the patient is uncontrollably absorbed by a certain idea or action (obsessional neuroses). The surgery is performed only when the condition is severe and other treatments do not work. A limited section of the front lobe of the brain may be removed (prefrontal lobotomy), and connecting fibers in the frontal lobe may be cut. A marked change in personality is a result. Modern drugs are used instead of psychosurgery in many cases.

psychotherapist, one who practices psychotherapy. The ways psychotherapy is defined and licenses are awarded differ from state to state. Compare **psychoanalyst.**

psychotherapy, any of a number of ways to treat mental and emotional disorders by mental techniques instead of physical means. **Brief psychotherapy** refers to treatment that usually focuses on a specific problem and is limited to a specified number of sessions with the therapist. It is aimed at solving personality or behavior problems rather than trying to analyze the unconscious. **Directive therapy** uses an approach in which the therapist asks questions and offers interpretations. In **nondirective therapy** the therapist does not give advice or interpret. Instead, the patient is helped to identify conflicts and to understand his or her own feelings and values.

psychotic /sīkot′ik/, **1.** referring to psychosis. **2.** a patient who shows the symptoms of a psychosis.

psychotic insight, a stage in the development of a psychosis where the patient develops an idea that justifies a system of false beliefs. With the new insight, the factors that were confusing before become a part of the pattern of the delusion.

psychotropic drugs /-trop′ik/, drugs that affect the mental functions or behavior of a person.

pterygoideus lateralis /ter′igoi′dē·əs/, one of the jaw muscles used to chew food.

ptomaine /tō′mān/, a group of nitrogen compounds found in decaying proteins. Because injection of the substances causes side effects, the compounds were at one time viewed as poisonous.

ptosis /tō′sis/, the dropping down (prolapse) of an organ or part. An example is the drooping of one or both upper eyelids. It is caused by weakness of the muscle that raises the eyelid, or failure of a nerve that controls the muscle.

ptotic kidney /tō′tik/, a kidney that is abnormally located in the pelvis.

ptyalin /tī′əlin/, an enzyme in saliva that helps to digest starch. Also called **amylase.**

pubarche /pyoobär′kē/, the start of sexual maturity (puberty). It is marked by the first signs of adult sexual traits.

puberty /pyoo′bərtē/, the period of life at which both males and females are first able to reproduce. **Prepuberty** is the period just before puberty, lasting about 2 years. During the period there are important body changes, such as quick growth and the first signs of pubic hair and other signs of sexual maturity. **Postpuberty** is a period of about 1 to 2 years following the time when the person is able to create offspring.

pubic symphysis /pyoo′bik sim′fi-/, the slightly movable joint of the front of the pelvis.

pubis /pyoo′bis/, *pl.* **pubes,** one of the bones that help form the hip. Compare **ilium, ischium.**

public health, a field of medicine that deals with the general health of the community. It is active in such areas as water supply, waste disposal, air pollution, and food safety.

pubococcygeus exercises /pyoo′bōkoksij′ē·əs/. See **Kegel exercises.**

pudendal nerve /pyooden′təl/, one of the branches of a nerve network that carry nerve signals to the rectum and genital areas, and the penis or clitoris.

pudendum /pyooden′dəm/, the outer genitals, especially of women. See also **vulva.**

puerperal /pyoo·ur′pərəl/, referring to the time right after childbirth or to a woman who has just given birth.

puerperal fever, a bacterial infection and blood poisoning that sometimes follows childbirth. It may be caused by using pregnancy and childbirth methods that are not free from germs. The symptoms include fever, fast heart beat, swollen uterus, and bloody discharge (lochia). If not

O–P

treated, kidney failure, shock, and death may occur. The germ causing the disease is most often one of the bacteria (streptococci) known to destroy blood. Also called **child-bed fever, puerperal sepsis.**

puerperal sepsis. See **puerperal fever.**

puerperium /pyoo̅'ərpir'ē·əm/, the period of 6 weeks following childbirth.

Pulex /pyoo̅'leks/, a type of flea that carries certain infections, such as plague and typhus.

pulmonary /pool̅'məner'ē/, referring to the lungs or the breathing system. Also **pulmonic** /pool̅mon'ik/.

pulmonary disease, a disorder with cough, chest pain, shortness of breath, bloody sputum, abnormal breathing noises, and wheezing. Less common symptoms may be arm and shoulder pain, slight pain in the calf of the leg, swelling of the face, headache, hoarseness, pain in the joints, and drowsiness. Pulmonary diseases are of either a blocking (obstructive) or tightening (restrictive) nature. Obstructive breathing diseases are caused by an obstacle in the airway. Such blockages may be swelling of the membranes lining the breathing tubes, or thick substances released by them. **Chronic obstructive pulmonary disease (COPD)** is an incurable condition in which lungs are able to take in less and less air over a period of time. Symptoms include problems in breathing while exercising or in breathing in or out deeply, and sometimes a long-term cough. Causes include chronic bronchitis, emphysema, and asthma. It is made worse by cigarette smoking and air pollution.**pulmonary edema,** fluid in lung tissues. It is often caused by congestive heart failure, but also occurs as a side effect of drugs, infections, inflammation of the pancreas, or kidney failure. Pulmonary edema also may follow a stroke, skull fracture, near drowning, the breathing in of poisonous gases, the rapid flow of whole blood, or fluids in the veins. In congestive heart disease, fluid from the blood is pushed through walls of tiny blood vessels (capillaries) in the lungs into open spaces of the lungs. The patient with pulmonary edema breathes quickly, shallowly, and with difficulty. The patient may be restless and hoarse and have pale or bluish skin. He or she may cough up frothy, pink sputum. The veins of the neck, arms, and legs are usually swollen. Severe pulmonary edema is an emergency. Treatment includes bedrest in a sitting position, narcotic painkillers, a heart tonic, a drug that acts quickly to increase the passing of urine (diuretic), and a drug to enlarge the breathing tubes. Mechanical breathing help may be ordered by the doctor.

pulmonary function test (PFT), a test of the ability of the lungs to exchange oxygen and carbon dioxide during normal breathing.

pulmonary stenosis. See **stenosis.**

pulmonary trunk, a short, wide blood vessel that carries blood from the right lower heart chamber (ventricle) to the lungs.

pulmonary valve. See **heart valve.**

pulmonary vein, one of a pair of large blood vessels that return blood from the lungs to the left upper heart chamber (atrium). Compare **pulmonary trunk.**

pulp, any soft, spongy tissue, as that in the spleen or the pulp chamber of a tooth.

pulp canal. See **root canal.**

pulp cavity, the space in a tooth that has the dental pulp.

pulpitis /pulpī'-/, infection of the dental pulp.

pulsatile /pul'sətīl/, referring to a rhythmic pulsing.

pulse, the effect on an artery caused by the movement of blood from the heart as it contracts. The pulse matches each beat of the heart. The normal number of pulse beats per minute in the average adult is from 60 to 100. The average pulse rate for a newborn baby is 120 beats per minute. It slows throughout childhood and adolescence. Girls, beginning about 12 years of age, and women have higher rates than boys and men. A **bigeminal pulse** is an abnormal pulse in which two beats in close succession are followed by a pause during which no pulse is felt. A **bounding pulse** feels full and springlike when touched. It occurs because of increased force of the heart contraction or an increased amount of blood in the veins. A **thready pulse** is an abnormal pulse that is weak and often fairly rapid. The artery does not feel full, and the rate may be difficult to count. It is a sign of a loss of circulating fluid (hypovolemia), as occurs with severe bleeding. A **trigeminal pulse** is an abnormal pulse in which every third beat is absent. A **quadrigeminal pulse** is one in which a pause occurs after every fourth beat. Differences may be caused by exercise, injury, illness, and emotions. For example, **Corrigan's pulse** is a throbbing pulse that occurs during great excitment, in various heart disorders, and as a result of hardening of the arteries (arteriosclerosis). A **wiry pulse** is an abnormal pulse that is strong but small.

pulse point, any one of the places on the surface of the body where the pulse can be easily felt. The most commonly used pulse point is over the radial artery on the thumb side of the wrist. Other pulse points are over the temporal artery in front of the ear and over the common carotid artery under the chin at the throat. An **abdominal pulse** is in the large artery (abdominal aorta) that carries blood to the organs and legs. An **apical pulse** is heard with a stethoscope placed over the top (apex), or pointed lower part, of the heart. A **brachial pulse** can be felt in the space in front of the elbow. A **carotid pulse** can be felt by gently pressing a finger in the groove between the voice box (larynx) and the muscle in the neck. A **dorsalis pedis pulse** is felt between the first and second metatarsal bones on the top of the foot. A **femoral pulse** is felt in the groin from the femoral artery. The **popliteal pulse** can be felt behind the knee in the popliteal artery. A **posterior tibialis pulse** is felt on the ankle, just behind to the bulge of the ankle bone (talus). A **venous pulse** is usually felt over the inner or outer or jugular veins in the neck. The pulse in the jugular vein is taken to read the pressure of the pulse and the form of the pressure wave, especially in a patient with a cardiac conduction defect or cardiac arrhythmia.

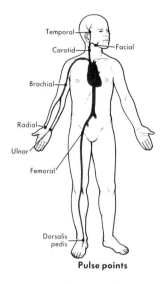

Pulse points

pulvule /pul'vyool/,   a gelatin capsule that has a dose of a drug in powder form.

pump,   a device used to move liquids or gases by suction or pressure, as a stomach pump.

punctum lacrimale /lak'rimā'lē/,   a tiny opening in the edge of each eyelid that is linked to the tear (lacrimal) duct.

puncture wound,   an injury caused by a cut of the skin by a narrow object, as a knife, nail, glass, or other material. In such an injury to the eye, a lung, or other organ, the object should not be taken out until the person has been taken to a medical facility. Minor puncture wounds are treated with thorough cleansing. A tetanus booster shot is usually given for such wounds.

pupil,   an opening in the form of a circle in the iris of the eye. The pupil lies behind the cornea and in front of the lens. The pupil is the window of the eye through which light passes to the lens and the retina. Its size changes as the eye responds to changes in light, emotions, and other signals. See also **dilatator pupillae. –pupillary,** *adj.*

purgative /pur'gətiv/,   a strong drug usually given by mouth, to bring about bowel movements.

purge,   1. to empty the bowels, as with a laxative or drug given to cause vomiting (cathartic). **2.** to make free of an unwanted substance or an emotional problem.

purine /pyoor'ēn/,   any one of a large group of nitrogen compounds. They may be end products of digestion of proteins in the diet. Purines are in many drugs and other substances, including caffeine. Too much blood uric acid may occur in people who are not able to use up purines. Foods that are high in purines include anchovies and sardines, liver, kidneys, legumes, and poultry.

Purinethol,   a trademark for an anticancer drug (mercaptopurine).

Purkinje fibers /pərkin'jə/,   heart muscle fibers that help carry the electric signals that control heart contractions.

Purodigin,   a trademark for a heart drug (digitoxin).

purpura /pur'pyərə/,   a disorder with bleeding beneath the skin or mucous membranes. It causes black and blue spots (ecchymoses) or pinpoint bleeding.

purulent /pyoor'oōlənt/,   making or having pus.

pus,   a creamy, thick, pale yellow or yellow-green fluid that comes from dead tissue. Its main substance is white blood cells. Its most common cause is infection by bacteria.

pustule /pus'chool/,   a small blister that usually has pus. **–pustular,** *adj.*

putrefaction /pyoo'trəfak'shən/,   the decay of animal or plant tissue, especially proteins. It makes foul-smelling compounds, as ammonia.

putromaine /pyootrō'mān/,   any poisonous substance made by the decay of food within a living body.

PVC,   abbreviation for **polyvinyl chloride.**

P.V. Carpine,   a trademark for a drug to increase the activity of nerves (pilocarpine nitrate).

pyelogram /pī'əlōgram'/,   an x-ray picture of the kidneys and tubes that carry urine from the kidneys to the bladder (ureters) taken after a dye has been injected. Also called **urogram.**

pyelolithotomy /-lithot'-/,   surgery in which kidney stones are taken out of the tube that carries urine from the kidney to the bladder (ureter).

pyelonephritis /-nəfrī'-/,   a pus-forming infection of the kidney. **Acute pyelonephritis** is usually caused by an infection that moves upward from the lower urinary tract to the kidney. In females, it is often caused by bacteria in the opening of the urethra (meatus). The disorder comes on fast, with fever, chills, pain, nausea, and a frequent need to urinate. Antibiotics are given for 10 days to 2 weeks. **Chronic pyelonephritis** develops slowly after a infection of the kidney caused by bacteria. It may get worse and lead to kidney failure. Most cases are linked to some form of blockage, as a stone in the ureter.

O–P

pygmy /pig′mē/, a very small person with normal body shape; an undeveloped dwarf. Also spelled **pigmy.**

pyknic /pik′nik/. See **somatotype.**

pyloric sphincter /pīlôr′ik/, a thick muscular ring in the pylorus, separating the stomach from the first part of the small intestine (duodenum). Also called **pyloric valve.**

pyloric stenosis. See **stenosis.**

pyloroplasty /pīlôr′əplas′tē/, surgery done to relieve pyloric stenosis. In the treatment of an ulcer of the first part of the small intestine (duodenal), the operation allows the alkaline substances released by the duodenum to flow back into the stomach.

pylorospasm /-spazm/, a spasm of the pyloric sphincter of the stomach.

pylorus /pīlôr′əs/, a tube-shaped part of the stomach that angles toward the first segment of the intestine (duodenum).

Pyocidin Otic, a trademark for a drug used to treat ear infections (otic) that has a hormone (hydrocortisone) and an antibiotic (polymyxin B sulfate).

pyoderma /pī′ōdur′mə/, any pus-forming skin disease, as impetigo.

pyogenic /-jen′ik/, pus-making.

Pyopen, a trademark for an antibiotic (carbenicillin disodium).

pyorrhea /pī′ôrē′ə/, **1.** a releasing of pus. **2.** a pus-forming inflammation of the gums. **–pyorrheal,** *adj.*

pyramidal tract /pīram′idəl/, a nervous system pathway made up of nerve fibers with nerve cell bodies in the brain that direct the muscles that can be controlled at will.

Pyribenzamine Hydrochloride, a trademark for an antihistamine (tripelennamine hydrochloride).

Pyridium, a trademark for a painkiller (phenazopyridine hydrochloride).

pyridostigmine bromide, a drug that increases the activity of the nerves used to treat myasthenia gravis. Blockage of the intestines or urinary tract, slow heart beat, low blood pressure, or known allergy to this or like drugs prohibits its use. Side effects include nausea, diarrhea, cramps in the stomach and intestines, muscle cramps, and weakness.

pyridoxine /pir′idok′sin/, a vitamin that is part of the B complex group of vitamins. It helps to build and break down amino acids. Foods high in pyridoxine are meats, especially organ meats, whole-grain cereals, soybeans, peanuts, wheat germ, and brewer's yeast. Common symptoms of shortage are an acnelike skin disorder about the eyes, nose, and mouth and behind the ears, cracked lips, nervousness, sadness, nerve irritation, and blood disorders. Also called **vitamin B₆.**

pyrilamine maleate, an antihistamine used to treat different reactions, such as runny nose and skin rash. Asthma or known allergy to this drug prohibits its use. It is not given to newborn infants or nursing mothers. Side effects include drowsiness, skin rash, dry mouth, and fast heart beat.

pyrogen /pī′rəjən/, any drug or substance that causes a rise in body temperature. See also **fever.** **–pyrogenic,** *adj.*

pyromania /pī′rō-/, an uncontrollable urge to set fires. The condition is found mainly in men. Someone with the condition (called a **pyromaniac**) feels great tension before setting the fire and much pleasure while watching it burn. **–pyromaniacal,** *adj.*

piromaniac. See **pyromania.**

pyrophoric materials, materials that ignite spontaneously in air without an ignition source.

pyrosis /pīrō′-/. See **heartburn.**

Pyrroxate, a trademark for a drug that has a substance to stop muscle spasms (methoxyphenamine hydrochloride), an antihistamine (chlorpheniramine maleate), two painkillers (aspirin and phenacetin), and a stimulant (caffeine).

pyrvinium pamoate, a drug used to treat worms, especially pinworms. Pregnancy or known allergy to this drug prohibits its use. Side effects include nausea, cramping, and diarrhea. Stools and vomit will be stained bright red by the drug.

pyuria /pīyo͞or′ē·ə/, white blood cells in the urine. It is a sign of infection of the urinary tract. Pyuria conditions that have no bacteria may be caused by an infection from viruses of the bladder and urethra. See also **bacteriuria.**

Q

q.d., in prescriptions, abbreviation for *quaque die,* a Latin phrase meaning "every day." Also called **quotid.**

Q fever, a sudden feverish illness, usually involving the respiratory system, caused by the *Rickettsia burnetii.* The disease is spread through contact with infected animals. This happens by breathing in the rickettsiae from their hides or other tissues, or drinking infected raw milk. A high fever may persist for 3 weeks or more. Treatment with antibiotics usually works within 36 to 48 hours. People who are regularly exposed to domestic animals should be vaccinated against Q fever.

q.h., in prescriptions, abbreviation for *quaque hora,* a Latin phrase meaning "every hour."

q.2h., in prescriptions, abbreviation for *quaque secunda hora,* a Latin phrase meaning "every 2 hours."

q.3h., in prescriptions, abbreviation for *quaque tertia hora,* a Latin phrase meaning "every 3 hours."

q.i.d., in prescriptions, abbreviation for *quater in die,* a Latin phrase meaning "4 times a day."

q.s., in prescriptions, abbreviation for *quantum sufficit,* a Latin phrase meaning "quantity required."

quack, a totally unqualified person posing as an expert, as a person pretending to be a physician. Also called **charlatan.**

quadriceps femoris /kwod′riseps fem′əris/, a group of four muscles of the thigh that function to extend the leg.

quadrigeminal /-jem′inəl/, **1.** in four parts. **2.** a fourfold increase in size or frequency.

Quadrinal, a trademark for a respiratory drug. It contains a smooth muscle relaxant (theophylline calcium salicylate), a nerve stimulant (ephedrine hydrochloride), an expectorant (potassium iodide), and a sedative-hypnotic (phenobarbital).

quadriplegia /-plē′jə/, paralysis of the arms, the legs, and the body below the level of an injury to the spinal cord. This disorder is often the result of a spinal cord injury in the area of the fifth to the seventh vertebrae. Automobile accidents and sporting mishaps are common causes. Compare **hemiplegia, paraplegia.**

quadruplet /kwod′rooplit, kwodrup′lit/, any one of four offspring born at the same time during a single pregnancy.

qualified, referring to a health professional or health facility that is recognized by an appropriate agency or organization as meeting good standards of performance. The standards relate to the professional ability of an individual or the eligibility of an institution to offer an approved health care program.

qualitative test /kwol′ita′tiv/, a test that shows the presence or lack of a substance.

quality factor, referring to the biologic damage that radiation can produce. The same doses of different types of radiation can cause differing levels of damage.

quantitative test /kwon′titā′tiv/, a test that determines the amount of a substance per unit volume or unit weight.

quarantine /kwôr′əntēn/, **1.** the isolation of patients with a communicable disease or of those exposed to a communicable disease during the contagious period. The purpose is to prevent spread of the illness. **2.** the practice of holding travelers or ships, trucks, or airplanes coming from places of epidemic disease for the purpose of inspection or disinfection.

quartan /kwôr′tən/, happening again on the fourth day, or at about 72-hour intervals.

Quelidrine, a trademark for a respiratory drug. It contains two nerve stimulants (phenylephrine hydrochloride and ephedrine hydrochloride), an antihistamine (chlorpheniramine maleate), a cough drug (dextromethorphan hydrobromide), and a drug that releases sputum (ammonium chloride).

Quengle cast /kweng′gəl/, a two-section, hinged plaster cast. It keeps rigid the lower leg from the foot or ankle to below the knee and upper thigh to just above the knee. The two parts of the cast are connected by special hinges at knee level. The cast is used for the gradual correction of broken kneejoints.

quercetin /kwur′sitin/, a yellow dye. It is found in oak bark, the juice of lemons, asparagus, and other plants. It is used to reduce abnormal small blood vessel (capillary) weakness.

Questran, a trademark for a cholesterol control drug (cholestyramine resin).

Quibron, a trademark for a respiratory drug. It contains a smooth muscle relaxant (theophylline) and a drug that releases sputum (guaifenesin).

quick connect, a plastic or similar connecting device that is attached to or implanted in a patient who will be joined to an electromechanical apparatus, as an artificial heart.

quickening, the first feeling by a pregnant woman of movement of the baby in her uterus. It usually occurs between 16 and 20 weeks of pregnancy.

quinacrine hydrochloride, an antiworm (anthelmintic) and an antimalarial drug. It is given to treat protozoa and tapeworm infestations, and to treat and suppress malaria. Pregnancy, use of primaquine at the same time, or known allergy to this drug prohibits its use. Side effects include severe psoriasis, anemia, severe liver destruction, nausea, vomiting, and liver disease (jaundice).

Quinaglute, a trademark for a heart rhythm control drug (quinidine gluconate).

Quincke's pulse /kwing'kēz/, an abnormal alternate paleness and reddening of the skin seen by pressing the front edge of the fingernail and watching the blood in the nail bed disappear and return. This pulsation is commonly seen in major blood vessel (aortic) problems and other abnormal conditions. It may also occur in otherwise normal individuals. Also called **capillary pulse.**

quinethazone, a diuretic and high blood pressure drug. It is given to treat high blood pressure (hypertension) and fluid pooling (edema).

Quinidex, a trademark for a heart rhythm control drug (quinidine sulfate).

quinidine /kwin'idin/, an antiarrhythmic drug. It is given to treat heart rhythm irregularities. Known allergy to this drug prohibits its use. It should not be used in patients with heart block. Side effects include heart rhythm problems, high blood pressure, and cinchona alkaloid overdose. Rare, but possibly fatal, allergic reactions may occur.

quinine /kwī'nīn/, a white, bitter crystal-like alkaloid. It is made from cinchona bark. It is used in antimalaria drugs.

quinine sulfate, an antimalaria drug with antifever, pain relief, and muscle-relaxant activity. It is given to treat malaria, particularly malaria caused by *Plasmodium falciparum,* and to treat night leg cramps. An inherited disorder (glucose-6-phosphate dehydrogenase deficiency) or certain heart disorders prohibit its use. Side effects include symptoms of cinchona drug overdose, ringing in the ears (tinnitus), headache, and visual, hearing, and stomach and bowel problems.

Quinora, a trademark for a heart rhythm drug (quinidine sulfate).

quintan /kwin'tən/, happening again on the fifth day, or at about 96-hour intervals.

quintuplet /kwin'tŏŏplit, kwintup'lit/, any one of five offspring born at the same time during a single pregnancy.

R

rabbit fever. See **tularemia.**

rabies /rā′bēz/, an often fatal virus disease of the nervous system. The virus is found mainly in wild animals, such as skunks and raccoons. Contact with an infected animal carries the virus to an unvaccinated dog or cat. Humans most often get the virus from a bite or exposure of a mucous membrane or break in the skin to the saliva of an infected animal. The virus moves along nerves to the brain, and then to other organs. A dormant period ranges from 10 days to 1 year. Symptoms include fever, headache, numbness, and muscle ache. After many days, severe brain inflamation, confusion, very painful muscle spasms, seizures, paralysis, coma, and death result. There have been few nonfatal cases. Survival has been the result of extreme medical care. There is no treatment once the virus has reached the nervous system tissue. Immediate treatment of bites from rabid animals may prevent the disease. The wound should be cleaned with soap, water, and a disinfectant. A deep wound may be burned out, and a vaccination drug (rabies immune globulin) may be injected directly into the base of the wound. For active vaccination, a series of injections into muscles with another vaccine (human diploid cell rabies vaccine) or duck embryo vaccine is begun. If the first is used, injections are given on the day of exposure and on days 3, 7, 14, 28, and 90. Great effort is made to find and examine the animal that is supposed rabid. It is first isolated and carefully watched. If the animal is well in 10 days, there is little danger of rabies being caused from the bite. Also called *(obsolete)* **hydrophobia.** –**rabid** /rab′id/, *adj.*

rabies immune globulin (RIG), a mixture of a vaccine (antirabies immune globulin) used with rabies duck embryo vaccine for possible treatment in patients who may have been exposed to rabies. Prior use of this drug or known allergy to it, to gamma globulin, or to thimerosal (Merthiolate) prohibits its use. Side effects include soreness at the site of injection, fever, and allergic reactions.

rabies vaccine, a sterile mixture of killed rabies virus made from duck embryo. It is used to vaccinate and prevent rabies after exposure. Allergy to chicken or duck eggs or to protein prohibits its use. Side effects include severe allergic reactions and pain and inflammation at the site of injection.

race, a vague, unscientific term for a group of genetically related people who share some physical traits.

racemose /ras′əmōs′/, describing a structure in which many branches end in forms like a bunch of grapes, as the air sacs (alveoli) of the lungs.

Racet, a trademark for a skin cream with a hormone (hydrocortisone) and an antiinfection drug (iodochlorhydroxyquin).

rachischisis /rəkis′kisis/, a groove or cleft (fissure) in one or more backbones at birth. A fissure of the entire spinal column and spinal cord (**complete rachischisis**) is a rare birth defect. See also **neural tube defect, spina bifida.**

rachitic /rəkit′ik/, referring to rickets.

rachitis /rəkī′tis/, **1.** rickets. **2.** an inflammatory disease of the spine.

rad /rad/, abbreviation for *radiation absorbed dose;* the basic unit of a taken-in dose of ionizing radiation.

radarkymography /rā′därkīmog′rəfē/, a method for showing the size and outline of the heart. Using a radar tracking device, it shows images made by electric signals passed over the chest surface on a screen.

radial artery /rā′dē·əl/, a blood vessel (artery) in the forearm. It divides into 12 branches to the forearm, wrist, and hand.

radial keratotomy, an operation in which a series of tiny shallow cuts are made on the cornea of the eye. The cuts cause the cornea to bulge slightly. This most often corrects the eye for mild to moderate nearsightedness (myopia).

radial nerve, the largest branch of a group of nerves (brachial plexus) that supplies the skin of the arm and some of the muscles.

radial reflex, a normal reflex in which flexing of the forearm is caused by tapping at the wrist. Flexing of the fingers may also occur if the reflex is very active.

radiant energy, the energy given off by radiation, as radio waves, visible light, and x-rays.

radiate, to move or spread from a common point.

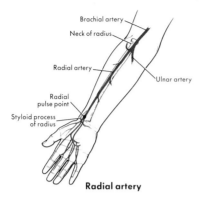

Brachial artery
Neck of radius
Radial artery
Ulnar artery
Radial pulse point
Styloid process of radius

Radial artery

radiate ligament, a ligament that connects a rib with a backbone and a linked disk.

radiation, 1. the giving off of energy, rays, or waves. **Electromagnetic radiation** refers to every kind of electrical and magnetic radiation. It is thought of as a whole range of energy. It includes energy with the shortest wavelength, as gamma rays, to that with the longest wavelength, as long radio waves. **Gamma radiation** refers to rays from radioactive elements that come from nuclear decay or nuclear reactions. Gamma radiation can injure, distort, or destroy body cells and tissue, especially cell nuclei, but controlled radiation is used to diagnose and treat various diseases. **Ionizing radiation** refers to electromagnetic rays such as x-rays and others that break substances in their paths into ions. Ionizing radiation kills cells or slows their growth. It causes gene changes and chromosome breaks. **Nonionizing radiation** does not change the electric charge of atoms in tissue. **Natural radiation** is radioactivity in the soil and rocks or that reaches the earth from space as radiation from the sun and particles from beyond the solar system. 2. the use of a radioactive substance to diagnose or treat a disease.

radiation caries, tooth decay (caries) caused by radiation. This form of caries is often a side effect of radiation treatment for cancer of the mouth and jaw. See also **dental caries.**

radiation detector, a device used to detect the presence and amount of radiation, which cannot be seen, felt, or otherwise noted by the human senses. A Geiger counter (Geiger-Müller detector) is an example of a radiation detector.

radiation hazard, a condition under which persons might receive radiation in excess of the maximum permissible dose. There are both internal and external radiation hazards. See **external exposure** and **internal exposure.**

radiation hygiene, the method of protecting human beings from injury by radiation damage. Measures to lessen exposure to outside radiation include using protective barriers of radiation-absorbing material, ensuring safe distances between people and radiation sources, and lowering exposure times.

radiation oncology, treatment of cancer through radiation.

radiation sickness, a condition resulting from exposure of the body to radiation. The seriousness of the condition depends on the amount of radiation, length of time of exposure, and the part of the body affected. Moderate exposure may cause headache, nausea, vomiting, loss of appetite, and diarrhea. Long-term exposure may cause an inability to have children (sterility), damage to the fetus in pregnant women, leukemia or other forms of cancer, loss of hair, and eye clouding (cataracts).

radical dissection, the removal of tissue in a large area surrounding a surgery site. Most often it is done to find and remove all possible cancer tissue to lower the chance of the cancer returning.

radical mastectomy. See **mastectomy.**

radical therapy, 1. a treatment meant to cure, not only relieve symptoms. 2. an extreme treatment; not conservative, as radical mastectomy rather than simple or partial mastectomy.

radicular cyst /rədik′yələr/, a sac (cyst) that is joined to the tip of the root of a tooth.

radio cache, a cache may consist of a number of portable radios, a base station, and in some cases, a repeater stored in a predetermined location for dispatch to incidents.

radioactive, giving off radiation as the result of the decay of the nucleus of an atom.

radioactive contamination, the unwanted buildup of radioactive material in the body or the area around the body, as clothing or tools. Any article found to be contaminated by a radioactive source in treating a patient must be gotten rid of following hospital or federal standards for removing radioactive waste.

radioactive element, a chemical element subject to decay of its nucleus with the release of alpha or beta particles or gamma rays. All elements with atomic numbers greater than 83 are radioactive. Many radioactive elements not found in nature have been made in laboratories. Some kinds of radioactive elements are radium and uranium.

radioactive iodine. See **radioiodine**

radioactive iodine excretion test, a method of checking thyroid gland action by measuring the amount of radioactive iodine in the urine. The patient is given an oral tracer dose of radioactive iodine (^{131}I). Normally, 5% to 35% of the dose is taken up by the thyroid. Absorption is higher in an overactive gland (hyperthyroidism) and lower in an underactive gland (hypothyroidism).

radioactivity, the release of radiation (particles or waves) as a result of nuclear decay. Radioactivity is part of all chemical elements with an atomic number greater than 83.

radioactivity hazards, the ability of a material to emit any form of radioactive energy.

radiobiology, the branch of science dealing with the effects of radiation on body systems.

radiograph, an x-ray picture.

radiography /rā′dē·og′rəfē/, the use of radiation, as x-rays, to make images on photographic film. **Digital radiography (DR)** is an x-ray test that uses a computer to create the image.

radioimmunoassay (RIA) /-im′yənōas′ā/, a method used to find the amount of a protein in the blood. A radioactive substance known to react in a certain way with the suspected protein is injected and any allergic reaction is noted.

radioiodine /-ī′ədīn/, a radioactive isotope of iodine. It is used to treat some thyroid conditions. It is also used in many methods of diagnosis.

radioisotope /-ī′sətōp/, a radioactive isotope of an element.

radioisotope scan, an image of the gamma rays released by a radioactive isotope, showing its level in a body site, as the thyroid gland, brain, or kidney. Radioactive isotopes used in scanning may be given by mouth or injected in a vein.

radiological survey. See **monitoring.**

radiology /-ol′-/, the branch of medicine that deals with radioactive substances, as in diagnosing and treating a disease. A **radiologist** is a physician who studies and practices radiology.

radionuclide /-noo′klīd/, any of the radioactive isotopes of cobalt, iodine, and other elements, used in nuclear medicine to treat tumors and cancers. They are also used for nuclear images of inner parts of the body. See also **nuclear scanning.**

radiopaque /-pāk′/, referring to anything that stops the passage of x-rays or other radiant energy. Bones are mostly radiopaque. They show as white areas on an x-ray film. Lead is very radiopaque. It is widely used to shield x-ray equipment and atomic power sources. A **radiopaque dye** is a chemical that blocks the passage of x-rays. Radiopaque iodine mixtures are used to outline the inside of hollow organs, as heart chambers, blood vessels, and the bile ducts in an x-ray film.

radiopharmaceutic /-fär′məsoo′tik/, a radioactive drug. A **diagnostic radiopharmaceutic** is one that allows images of body organs or structures to be obtained. In this way it is possible to tell if structures or functions are normal. The drug is given to the patient. It then emits radiation which can be detected by a special machine. This process is used for diagnosis. A **research radiopharmaceutic** is one in which a small amount of a radioactive element is given to study its spread in the body. It may later be used without a radioactive element. A **therapeutic radiopharmaceutic** is given to a patient to get radiation to the inner body tissues, as iodide 131 or cesium 137.

radioresistance, the ability of cells, tissues, or organs to resist the effects of radiation. –**radioresistant,** *adj.*

radiosensitivity, the lack of ability of cells, tissues, or organs to resist the effects of radiation. Cells of the intestine are the most radiosensitive of the body. Cells that divide regularly but mature between divisions, as sperm cells, are next. Long-lived cells that most often do not divide (mitosis) unless there is a good starting agent include the liver, kidney, and thyroid cells. Least sensitive are cells that have lost the ability to divide, as nerve cells.

radiosensitizers, drugs that raise the killing effect of radiation on cells.

radiotherapy, a treatment for cancer by using x-rays or gamma rays. It is painless, but the possible side effects include redness or darkening of the skin, shedding of skin cells, itching or skin pain, and hair loss. There is also possible fluid buildup, nausea, vomiting, headache, loss of ability to fight infection, and other problems. **Interstitial therapy** is a form of radiotherapy in which needles or wires that contain radioactive material are put in tumor areas. **Intracavitary therapy** is a form in which radioactive sources are put in a body cavity to irradiate the walls of the cavity or nearby tissues. The patient lies on a table from which it is possible to talk to the radiotherapist in a nearby booth. After a dose of radiation, the patient is placed in a noninfecting room or, if needed, in isolation. Skin care is given after irradiation. Antivomiting drugs and vitamins are given as needed. Feedings through the veins may be needed if the person's appetite declines. Before leaving the hospital, the patient learns to follow hospital practices for skin care, tooth brushing and mouthwashes, fluid intake, and a high-protein, well-balanced diet. Eating just before and after irradiation should not be done. The patient must avoid tight clothing, high or low temperatures, exposure to sunlight, tub baths, or showers until allowed by a doctor. Persons with infections must also be avoided. Any problems, as signs of infection, an inability to eat, severe diarrhea, headache, or pain at the site of the therapy must be

Q–R

reported. Radiotherapy can control or stop many forms of cancers from growing and can relieve some tumors that cannot be operated on.

radium (Ra), a radioactive metal element. Radium salts have been used as radiation sources to treat cancer but are now being replaced by cobalt and cesium. **Radium insertion** refers to putting the metal radium (Ra) into the body, as the uterus, to treat cancer.

radius /rā′dē·əs/, *pl.* **radii,** one of the bones of the forearm. Its upper end is small and forms a part of the elbow joint. The lower end is large and forms a part of the wrist joint.

radon (Rn), a radioactive, gaseous element. Radon is a decay product of radium and is used in radiation cancer therapy. A **radon seed** is a small sealed tube of glass or gold with a decay product of radium (radon) put into body tissues to treat cancers.

rale /rāl, räl/, an abnormal breath sound heard in the chest with a stethoscope. Fine rales have a crackling sound caused by air entering the lower air sacs (alveoli) of the lungs that have a buildup of fluids. It is heard in congestive heart failure, pneumonia, or early tuberculosis. Coarse rales start in the larger bronchial tubes or windpipe (trachea) and have a lower pitch. An **atelectatic rale** gives an abnormal intermittent crackling sound. It usually disappears after the patient being examined coughs or breathes deeply several times. A **bubbling rale** is a feature of moisture moving in the lungs. An abnormal hollow, metal-like sound heard in the chest is a **cavernous rale.** It is caused by the movement of a diseased lobe of a lung while breathing. A **dry rale** occurs when air passes through a narrowed bronchial tube in the lungs. A **gurgling rale** gives an abnormal coarse sound heard especially over large hollows or over a windpipe nearly filled with fluids. An abnormal whistling sound, called a **sibilant rale,** may be made by a person with a lung or breathing disease. It is caused by air passing through clogged mucus. A **sonorous rale** is a snoring sound that may be made by the vibration of a mass of thick released matter lodged in a tube leading from the lung to the throat. This sound is linked with various lung or breathing disorders.

Ramsay Hunt's syndrome. See **herpes zoster oticus.**

ramus /rā′məs/, *pl.* **rami,** a small, branchlike structure extending from a larger one, as a branch of a nerve or blood vessel (artery).

range of motion exercise. See **exercise.**

ranitidine, a histamine H₂ that slows stomach acid release used to treat small intestine (duodenal) and stomach ulcers and excess stomach acid conditions. Known allergy to this drug prohibits its use. The drug should be used in pregnancy only if clearly needed. Side effects include headaches and rashes.

ranula /ran′yələ/, *pl.* **ranulae,** a large saclike swelling in the floor of the mouth, most often caused by a blockage of the ducts of the saliva glands.

rape, a sexual attack, heterosexual or homosexual. The legal definitions vary from state to state. Rape is a crime of violence or one done under the threat of violence. Its victims are treated for medical and mental injury. The victim is often frightened and feels at risk, degraded, and abused. General physical tests may reveal cuts, bruises, and other injuries. Pelvic or sex organ examinations may show injury to the inner or outer sex organs or anus. A careful physical examination is done and a detailed medical record is drawn up. Samples are gotten for laboratory tests and evidence. In the case of a woman who has been raped by a man, a pregnancy test is done and injuries are treated. If the test is positive, birth control pills may be given. Antibiotics are often given to prevent a venereal disease. Privacy for the medical record and examination and police interview is given. The police must be informed in every case. The victim must sign a special form to allow samples to be released to a law enforcement agency. In general, it is the role of medical staff members to examine, treat, and collect samples as needed, not to decide that rape has occurred. In law, **statutory rape** means sexual intercourse with a female below the age of consent, which varies from state to state.

rape counseling, counseling by a trained person given to a victim of rape. Rape counseling ideally begins at the time the crime is first reported, as in an emergency room. The counselor offers support for the victim by accepting the person in a noncritical way. Counseling workers may be a link between the victim and medical, legal, and law-enforcement workers. This involves staying with the victim during medical tests, police or district attorney's questioning, and throughout the criminal justice process.

rape trauma syndrome, a phase of mental and emotional confusion and a longer phase of regrouping in the victim's life. The cause of the disorder is the shock of the rape. The signs of rape shock are emotional and physical reactions. These are feelings of anger, guilt, embarrassment, fear of violence and death, humiliation, and a wish for revenge. There are many physical problems, as digestive problems, discomfort in the sex organs and urinary system, tension, and disturbed patterns of sleep, activity, and rest. The long-term phase of rape shock features changes in the usual patterns of daily life, nightmares and irrational fears (phobias), and a need for support from friends and family. A silent reaction sometimes occurs. Signs are a rise in fear during the interview about the rape, denying the rape happened, or refusing to discuss it, a sudden change in the victim's usual sexual relations, a marked change in sexual behavior, an increase in nightmares, and the sudden appearance of phobic reactions.

Rape preventive measures

Prevention of attack

Set house lights to go on and off by timer.
Keep light on at all entrances.
Place safety locks on windows and doors.
Have key ready before reaching door of house or car.
Look in car before entering.
Insist on identification before letting a stranger in house; check identification with agency if suspicious.
Do not list first name on mailbox or in telephone directory.
Make arrangements with neighbor for needed assistance.
Be alert when walking in street; walk in lighted areas.
Walk down center of street if possible.
Avoid lonely or enclosed areas.

If attacked

Run toward a lighted house; yell ''Fire.''
Spit in rapist's face; act bizarre; vomit.
Rip off rapist's glasses.
Step hard on his foot (instep).
Aim at eyes—try to gouge eyes, scrape face.
Hit throat at Adam's apple (larynx).
Use fighting and screaming with caution; this may scare some rapists, encourage others.
Try talking to avoid rape.
If powerless, make close observations about rapist, car, location.

---

raphe /rā′fē/, a line that marks the joining of the halves of many similar parts of the body, as the raphe penis, which appears as a narrow, dark streak on the bottom of the penis.

rapid eye movement (REM). See **sleep.**

rapid relief, ranges from several seconds to several minutes, depending on the size of the opening, type of container, and the nature of its contents. Responders may often have time to reach a safe location or develop tactical counter measures. This behavior is associated with releases from containers under pressure, through relief valve actuations, broken or damaged valves, punctures, splits, tears, or broken piping.

rapport /rapôr′/, a sense of understanding, harmony,

accord, confidence, and respect in a relation between two persons, as rapport between a therapist and patient in mental therapy.

raptus, any sudden or violent state of excitement, seizure, or attack. **Raptus haemorrhagicus** is a sudden, heavy bleeding. **Raptus maniacus** is a sudden, violent attack of mania. **Raptus melancholicus** is an attack of very high excitement or frenzy that occurs during the course of depression. **Raptus nervorum** is a sudden, violent attack of nervousness that may be marked by cramps.

rash, a skin inflammation. Kinds of rashes include butterfly rash, diaper rash, and heat rash.

Rashkind procedure /-rash′kind/, making larger an opening in the heart wall (cardiac septum) between the right and left chambers (atria). It is done to relieve congestive heart failure in newborns by allowing better mixing between blood with oxygen in it from the lungs and blood from the rest of the body. An empty balloon is passed through a vein to an opening (foramen ovale) into the left chamber of the heart. The balloon is then filled and pulled through the opening, making it larger. Also called **balloon septostomy.**

ratbite fever, an infection carried to humans by the bite of a rat or mouse. Symptoms include fever, headache, nausea, vomiting, a rash on palms and soles, and painful joints. It lasts an average of 2 weeks. Treatment with antibiotics is effective.

ratio, the relation of one quantity to one or more other quantities shown as a relation of one to the others, and written either as a fraction (8/3) or linearly (8:3).

rational, **1.** referring to a treatment based on an understanding of the cause and processes of a specific disease and the possible effects of the drugs or methods used in treating the disorder. **2.** sane; able to reason or act normally.

rationale /rash′ənal′/, a system of reasoning or a statement of the reasons used in explaining data or happenings.

rationalization, a way of making believable reasons to explain a behavior.

rattle, an abnormal sound heard in the lungs in some forms of lung disease. It is a coarse vibration caused by the movement of moisture and the division of the walls of small air passages during breathing.

rattlesnake bite. See **snakebite.**

Raudixin, a trademark for a blood pressure drug (purified *Rauwolfia serpentina*).

Q-R

Rauwiloid, a trademark for a blood pressure drug (alseroxylon).

rauwolfia serpentina, the dried root from *Rauwolfia serpentina,* used as the source of a drug given to treat high blood pressure. Mental depression, peptic ulcer, ulcerative colitis, electroshock, or known allergy to this drug prohibits its use. It can interact adversely with MAO inhibitors. Side effects include symptoms like parkinsonism, sight problems (glaucoma), heart rhythm irregularities, and stomach and bowel bleeding.

Rauzide, a trademark for a heart drug with a fluid-releasing action (bendroflumethiazide) and a blood pressure drug (*Rauwolfia serpentina*).

ray, a beam of radiation, as heat or light, moving away from a source.

Raynaud's phenomenon /rānōz′/, attacks of blood flow interruptions (ischemia) of the fingers, toes, ears, and nose. The effect is caused by exposure to cold or by emotional stimulations. Symptoms include severe paling of the affected area, followed by bluish skin, then redness. There is also numbness, tingling, burning, and often pain. The attacks are often linked to other health conditions, as rheumatoid arthritis, shoulder girdle nerve compression, drug poisoning, some protein defects, high lung vessel pressure, and injury. It is called **Raynaud's disease** if the symptoms have occurred for at least 2 years and there is no evidence of another cause. Treatment depends on finding and treating any other disease. It may be controlled by protecting the body from the cold and by the use of mild tranquilizers and blood vessel widening drugs.

Raynaud's sign. See **acrocyanosis.**

RBC, abbreviation for *red blood cell.* See **erythrocyte.**

RDA, abbreviation for **recommended daily allowance.**

Reach to Recovery, a national volunteer service that offers counseling and support to women who have breast cancer.

reaction, a response to a substance, treatment, or other stimulation, as an antigen-antibody reaction in immunology, or an allergic reaction.

reaction formation, a mental defense mechanism in which a patient avoids anxiety through behavior and attitudes that are the opposite of ignored impulses and drives. The false behavior conceals these feelings.

reactivity, the ability of a material to undergo a chemical reaction with the release of energy. It could be initiated by mixing or reacting with other materials, application of heat, physical shock, etc.

Read method, a method preparing "natural childbirth" set up by Dr. Grantly Dick-Read. Read held that childbirth is a normal, physical process and that the pain of labor and birth is mental from fear and tension. To help the mother relax and to function well in labor and recovery after birth, he set up a group of exercises to be done often in classes. They could also be done at home. During the early and midfirst stage of labor, contractions are 2 to 5 minutes apart. The mother lies on her back with her knees bent. Stomach breathing is used during contractions. Her hands are placed over her lower stomach, fingers touching. She breathes deeply and slowly — in through her nose and out through her mouth. The stomach wall rises with each breath in, which she can feel with her hands. During the late part of the first stage of labor, contractions are 1½ to 2 minutes apart. Rib cage (costal) breathing is used during contractions. Her hands are placed on her sides, over the ribs. She breathes in less deeply, feeling her ribs move sideways against her hands. Each breath is drawn in through her nose and breathed out through her mouth. The stomach wall does not rise and fall with this kind of breathing. At the end of the first stage of labor, near full widening, contractions may be very strong, occurring every 1½ to 2 minutes. The mother lies on her back with her knees bent. Panting breaths are then used during the contractions. The mother holds one of her hands on her breastbone (sternum). It rises and falls as she pants lightly and rapidly through her mouth. Panting helps the woman not to push. During the second (expulsive) stage of labor after full widening of the cervix, the contractions occur every 1½ to 2 minutes. The woman has an urge to bear down and push. The woman lies back, head and shoulders held in a partly sitting position. She is helped to draw her legs up, holding them with her hands behind the lower thighs, thighs on her stomach and spread apart. As each contraction begins, she raises her head, takes a deep breath, tucks her chin on her chest, blocks the flow of air from her lungs, and bears down. During each contraction she may need to blow the air out, refill her lungs, and push again two or three times. Many who support using some parts of the Read method strongly say that a woman in labor should not lie on her back. Falling blood pressure may result in this position, because the uterus can fall back onto the body's main blood vein (vena cava). This results in a lack of oxygen for the fetus. Today, the woman using the Read method spends most of labor lying on her side or in a partly sitting position with her knees, back, and head supported. Compare **Bradley method, Lamaze method.** See also **natural childbirth.**

reagent /rē·ā′jənt/, a chemical substance known to react in a specific way. A reagent is used to find or make another substance in a chemical reaction.

reagin-mediated disorder /rē′ājin-/, an allergic reaction, as hay fever or an allergic response to an insect sting. It is caused by foreign bodies (antibodies), called **reagins.** The antibodies start the release of histamine and other substances that cause symptoms. Reactions range from a simple rash (wheal and flare) on the skin to near fatal allergic shock. Allergens that commonly cause these reactions are plant spores, pollens, animal danders, stings, blood proteins, foods, and some drugs. See also **allergy, anaphylaxis, hay fever.**

reality orientation, an action that helps confused or deluded persons toward a sense of reality, as by repeating the hour, day, month, and weather.

reapproximate /rē′əprok′simāt/, to rejoin tissues divided by surgery or an accident. It is done to restore their proper places.

reasonable care, the degree of skill and knowledge used by an able health care worker in treating and caring for the sick and injured.

reasonably prudent person doctrine, a concept that a person with common sense will use standard care and skill in meeting the health care needs of a patient.

rebase /rēbās′/, a process of refitting a denture by replacing its base material without changing its relation with the other teeth.

rebound, 1. recovery from illness. 2. a sudden muscle cramp after a time of relaxing. It is often seen in conditions in which some reflexes are lost.

rebound tenderness, a sign of inflammation of the lining of the stomach and intestine wall (peritoneum) in which pain is caused by the sudden release of a hand that had been pressing on the stomach space. See also **appendicitis, peritonitis.**

rebreathing bag, a flexible bag joined to a face mask. The rebreathing bag may store gases used for anesthesia during surgery or for oxygen while trying to revive a non-breathing patient. It may be squeezed to pump the gas or air into the lungs.

recannulate /rēkan′yəlāt/, to make a new opening through an organ or tissue, as opening a passage through a blocked blood vessel.

receptor, a sense nerve ending that responds to specific kinds of action.

recessive gene. See **gene.**

reciprocal inhibition /risip′rəkəl/, a notion in behavior treatment that if something causing worry (anxiety) occurs at the same time as a response that lowers anxiety, it may cause less anxiety. An example is the use of deep chest or stomach breathing and relaxing the deep muscles seem to lower anxiety and pain in birth.

Recklinghausen's tumor, a noncancerous smooth muscle tumor with connective tissue and other elements. It occurs in the wall of the fallopian tube or uterus. Also called **adenomyosis of the uterus.**

reclining, leaning backward. –**recline,** *v.*

recombinant /rēkom′binənt/, referring to a cell or organism that results from the rejoining (recombination) of genes in the DNA molecule. The cause may be natural or artificial.

recombinant DNA, a DNA molecule that has been broken into pieces that are then put back together in a new form. Parts of DNA material from another organism of the same or a different species may also be placed into the molecule.

recommended daily allowances, the amount of foods, such as vitamins, suggested as the needed part of one's daily food intake to stay healthy.

reconstitution, the repair of tissue damage.

recovery room, an area next to the operating room to which surgery patients are taken while still asleep, before being returned to their rooms. Life signs, as breathing, are carefully watched as the patient wakes up. The recovery room has machines and a special trained nursing staff.

recreational therapy, a form of mental treatment in which games or other group actions are used as a means of changing unwanted behavior, making the patient have social interests, or making speaking to others easier in depressed, withdrawn patients.

recrudescence /rē′krōōdes′əns/, a return of symptoms of a disease during a time of getting better.

rectal instillation of medication, putting (instilling) a drug pill, cream, or gel into the rectum. Some conditions treated by it are constipation and hemorrhoids. The pill may be self-oiled, or it may need to be oiled. The pill is gently placed past the anal muscle (sphincter). Sometimes a drug may be given in an enema. See also **enema.**

Rectal Medicone, a trademark for a rectal drug with a local anesthetic (benzocaine), an antiseptic (oxyquinoline sulfate), a drug that causes contractions, (zinc oxide), and a protective drug (Peruvian balsam).

rectal reflex, the normal response (defecation) to feces in the rectum. Also called **defecation reflex.**

rectocele /rek′təsēl/, a sticking out of the rectum and the back wall of the vagina into the vagina. The condition occurs after the muscles of the vagina and pelvic floor have been weakened by childbirth, old age, or surgery. It may mean an inborn weakness in the wall and may, if severe, cause painful sexual intercourse and difficulty in emptying the bowel. Surgery to rebuild the wall is often helpful and is joined with any other needed pelvic or vaginal repair. Also called **proctocele.** Compare **cystocele.**

rectosigmoid /-sig′moid/, a part of the body that includes the lower part of the large intestine (sigmoid colon) and the upper part of the rectum.

rectum /rek′təm/, the part of the large intestine, about 12 cm long, that is parallel to the lower part of the large intestine (descending sigmoid colon), just before the anal canal. It follows the curve of the end of the backbone.

Q–R

rectus muscle, any of many muscles of the body with a somewhat straight form. The **rectus abdominis** is one of a pair of muscles of the stomach and intestines, reaching the whole length of the front of the stomach and intestines. It flexes the spinal column, tenses the stomach and intestine walls, and helps to press the contents of the stomach and intestines. The **rectus femoris** is a muscle of the thigh and one of the four parts of another leg muscle (quadriceps femoris muscle). It flexes the leg.

recumbent /rikum'bənt/, lying down or leaning backward. See also **reclining.** –**recumbency,** n.

recurrent bandage, a bandage that is wrapped many times around itself. It is most often used for the head or the end of a limb that has been cut off.

recurvatum /rē'kərvā'təm/, backward-bending, as of the knee when caused by weakness of a leg muscle or a joint disorder.

red blood cell count (RBC). See **blood count.**

red blood cell, red cell. See **erythrocyte.**

red cell indices, a series of signs noted in a red blood cell sample. They include size, hemoglobin content, and hemoglobin amount. Red cell indices are useful in making diagnoses of many kinds of anemia.

Red Cross. See **American Red Cross.**

red infarct, a disorder in brain tissue that has become oxygen-starved (ischemic) by lack of blood. With slowed blood flow, red blood cells leak into the working tissue of the brain. A well-formed pool of blood (hematoma) does not occur, only a buildup of red blood cells (erythrocytes).

red marrow. See **bone marrow.**

reduce, 1. to restore a body part to its usual place after it has been moved. To reduce a broken bone, the ends or pieces are brought back into line. A rupture (hernia) may be reduced by returning the bowel to its normal place. If done by outside movement alone, it is said to be closed. If surgery is needed, it is said to be open. **2.** to decrease the amount, size, extent, or number of something, as of body weight.

reduction diet, a diet that is low in calories. It is used to lose weight. The diet should have fewer calories than the body uses each day while also having all foods needed to stay healthy. A diet of this type may allow 1200 calories per day from the basic food groups. Meats are most often broiled, roasted, stewed, or lightly fried. Vegetables are steamed or eaten raw. Starches and fats are limited, and fresh fruits are eaten instead of desserts. Foods not to be eaten are sugar-sweetened soft drinks, fried foods, pastries, and most snack foods. A lack of vitamins and minerals may result if such a diet is not carefully planned. Also called **low-caloric diet, reducing diet.**

Reed-Sternberg cell, one of a number of large, abnormal cells in the lymph system in a cancer (Hodgkin's disease). The number and size found are the reason for the diagnosis of the specific type of Hodgkin's disease.

reentry, a common cause of heart rhythm problems in which the heart muscle tissue reacts more than once to the same nerve signal.

referral /rifur'əl/, a process in which a patient or the patient's family is given more medical help. For example, a doctor may help a patient find a community health nurse after the patient leaves a hospital.

referred pain /rifurd'/. See **pain.**

reflex action, the unwilled working or movement of any organ or part of the body in response to a specific action. The reflex action occurs at once, without using the will or conscious thinking. An **attitudinal reflex** is any reflex triggered by a change in position of the head. A **chain reflex** is a series of reflexes, each aroused by the preceding one. A **conditioned reflex** is one that is developed by linking a behavior with a specific, repeated stimulus. An example is an experiment (Pavlov's) in which a dog drooled at the ringing of a bell, if the bell was rung before every feeding. A **coordinated reflex** is a series of muscular actions with a purposeful, set progression. An example is the act of swallowing.

reflexology, a system of treating some disorders by massaging the soles of the feet, using methods like those of acupuncture.

reflux /rē'fluks/, an abnormal backward or return flow of a fluid. For example, **gastroesophageal reflux** is a backflow of contents of the stomach into the esophagus. It often results from a failure of a band of muscle (esophageal sphincter) to close. Gastric juices are acid and produce burning pain in the esophagus, called heartburn. Repeated returns of reflux may cause inflammation, ulcers, or narrowing of the esophagus. See also **hepatojugular reflux, vesicoureteral reflux.**

refraction, 1. a test to find and to correct light-focusing errors of the eye. **2.** the change of direction of energy as it passes from one place to another of a different makeup.

refractometer /rē'frektom'ətər/, a device for finding what lenses may be needed to correct a sight defect in a patient's eyes.

refractory /rifrak'tərē/, referring to a disorder that resists treatment.

refractory period, the time after the excitement of a nerve cell or the pulling in of a muscle during which the cell membrane recharges.

Refsum's syndrome /ref'soomz/, a birth defect of fat processing in which a substance (phytanic acid) cannot be broken down. Symptoms include unsteadiness, defects of the bones and skin, nerve inflammation, and an eye disorder (retinitis pigmentosa). Foods with animal fat and milk products should not be eaten. Also called **phytanic acid storage disease.**

regimen /rej′əmen/, a strictly controlled treatment, as a diet or exercise schedule.

regional anesthesia, anesthesia of a part of the body by giving a numbing medication to block a group of sensory nerve fibers. **Brachial plexus anesthesia** is an anesthetic block of the region supplied by the brachial plexus nerves. **Conduction** or **nerve block anesthesia** is done by injecting a local anesthetic into a nerve. This blocks the nerve signals from moving up and down the nerve. A nerve block put in a neck nerve, called **cervical plexus anesthesia,** is used for operations on the area between the jaw and collarbone. Complications may include vertebral artery bleeding, phrenic nerve block or paralysis (the phrenic nerve controls the diaphragm), or nerve block of the voice box manifested by sudden hoarseness. **Continuous anesthesia** is a way of blocking nerve signals to an area below the naval. It is used for operations or labor. A small tube is inserted into the back near the base of the spine and a small amount of an anesthetic solution is given at intervals. **Subarachnoid block anesthesia** is a form of spinal anesthesia involving the injection of an anesthetic into the space at the base of the brain. See also **anesthesia.**

regional control, the control of cancer in body parts that are the first stages of spread of the disease from the first site.

registered nurse (RN), a professional nurse who has completed a course of study at an approved school of nursing and who has taken and passed an examination. A registered nurse may use the initials RN after the signature.

Regitine Hydrochloride, a trademark for a nerve-blocking drug (phentolamine hydrochloride).

Reglan, a trademark for a digestive system stimulating drug (metoclopramide hydrochloride).

regression, 1. a backward movement (retreat) in conditions, signs, or symptoms. **2.** a return to an early form of behavior.

Regroton, a trademark for a heart and blood vessel drug with a fluid-releasing drug (chlorthalidone) and a high blood pressure drug (reserpine).

regular diet, a full, well-balanced diet with all of the foods needed for growth, repair of tissues, and normal working of the organs. It contains foods with proteins, carbohydrates, fats, minerals, and vitamins in amounts that meet the specific caloric needs of the person. Also called **full diet, normal diet.**

Regular Iletin II, a trademark for insulin injection (crystalline zinc insulin).

regulator, a device, between the air cylinder and the facepiece, that reduces the pressure of the air coming from the cylinder.

regulator gauge, a gauge, connected to the regulator, that indicates the pressure of the air reaching the regulator; used as an indication of the air pressure in the air cylinder.

regurgitation /rigur′jitā′shən/, **1.** the return of swallowed food into the mouth. **2.** the backward flow of blood through a defect in a heart valve, named for the affected valve. See also **reflux.**

rehabilitation /rē′habil′itā′shən/, restoring a patient or a body part to normal or near normal after a disease or injury.

rehabilitation center, a center giving treatment and training for returning to normal (rehabilitation). The center may offer job training, physical treatment, and special training, as speech therapy.

Reifenstein's syndrome /rī′fənstīnz/, an inherited form of male sexual dysfunction. It features not being able to make sperm, testicles that have not lowered into the scrotum, femalelike breasts, and a lack of the male sex hormone (testosterone).

reimbursement, a method of payment, commonly by a third party payer. It could be a health insurance agency paying for medical treatment or hospital costs.

reinforced attack, those resources requested in addition to the initial attack.

reinforcement, a mental process in which a response is made stronger by the fear of punishment or the hope of reward.

Reiter's syndrome /rī′tərz/, an arthritic disorder of adult males that may result from a virus or fungus infection. It most often affects the ankles, feet, and lower back joints. It is linked to a disease of eye membranes (conjunctivitis) and one of the bladder tube (urethritis). Symptoms include diarrhea, mild fever, conjunctivitis, and ulcers on the palms and the soles. Arthritis often lasts after the first problems go away. Treatment includes antibiotics and drugs to relieve pain and inflammation.

rejection, 1. an immune system response to bodies or substances that the body tissues see as foreign, as grafts or transplants. **2.** the act of keeping out or denying affection to another person.

Rela, a trademark for a skeleton muscle relaxing drug (carisoprodol).

relapse, the return of a disease after the patient seems to have recovered.

relapsing fever, any of many infections marked by times of fever and caused by *Borrelia* bacteria. The disease is carried by both lice and ticks and is often seen during wars and famines. It has occurred in the western United States but is more common in South America, Asia, and Africa.

The first symptoms include a sudden high fever (104° to 105° F), chills, headache, muscle pains, nausea, and a rash. Yellow skin (jaundice) is common during the later stages. Each attack lasts 2 or 3 days and peaks with high fever, heavy sweating, and a rise in heart and breathing rate. Victims often relapse after 7 to 10 days of normal temperature and recover over time. Treatment is with antibiotics, but they can cause a side effect, so treatment may be stopped during a high fever. Bed rest, sponge baths, and aspirin ease the symptoms. Clothing and bedding must be cleaned to destroy any lice or ticks.

relapsing polychondritis, an inflammation and breakdown of cartilage. Most often the ears and noses of middle-aged persons are affected. The disease results in floppy ears, a collapsed nose, hearing loss, or hoarseness and airway blockage because of damage in the voice box (larynx) and windpipe (trachea). Steroid hormone drugs are used.

relative biologic effectiveness (RBE), a measure of the ability of a specific radiation to kill cells, as for cancers. It is compared with a specific level of x-rays.

relaxation, 1. a lowering of tension, as when a muscle relaxes between contractions. **2.** a lowering of pain.

relaxation therapy, treatment in which patients are taught to do breathing and relaxing exercises and to think about something good when a harmful action is done. The Lamaze method of childbirth uses relaxation therapy. Many yoga exercises and mental (biofeedback) methods may be used. Some patients learn to relax stiff muscles, to stop migraine attacks, or to lower their blood pressure.

releasing hormone (RH), one of many substances made by a part of the brain (hypothalamus) and released into the pituitary gland through a blood vein. Each of the releasing hormones acts on the pituitary to release a certain hormone. For example, the releasing hormone for growth hormone is a ''message'' sent to the pituitary to release growth hormone. Also called **releasing factor.**

REM, 1. abbreviation for **rapid eye movement.** See also **sleep. 2.** A unit of biological radiation dose such that the number of rems of radiation is equal to the number of rads absorbed multiplied by the quality factor of the given radiation (for a specified effect). See **RAD, quality factor.**

remission, the partial or complete lack of symptoms of a long-term disease. Remission may be natural or the result of treatment. If the remission lasts for many years, the disease is said to be cured. Compare **cure.**

remittent fever /rimit′ənt/, daily changes of a fever with increases and lack of symptoms (remissions) but never a return to normal.

remote afterloading, a radiation therapy method in which a device is placed in or on the patient and then loaded from a remote safe source with a strong radioisotope. Remote afterloading is used to treat head, neck, vaginal, and cervical tumors.

remotivation group, a group of mental patients that is set up to raise the interest, awareness, and speech among others of the withdrawn and inpatient members of the group.

Remsed, a trademark for an antivomiting and antihistamine drug (promethazine hydrochloride).

renal /rē′nəl/, referring to the kidney.

renal artery, one of a pair of large branches of the the major artery (abdominal aorta) serving the kidneys, adrenal glands, and ureters. The left renal artery is somewhat higher than the right. Before reaching the kidney, each artery divides into four branches.

renal biopsy, the removal of a sample of kidney tissue (biopsy) for a microscope test. It is done to find the cause of a kidney disorder, to help find the stage of the disease, and to find the right treatment. An open biopsy requires a cut through the body wall, offers a better view of the kidney, and carries a lower risk of bleeding. A closed biopsy is done by drawing a piece of tissue through a hollow needle. The needle is quickly taken out and a pressure bandage is put on.

renal calyx, the first unit in the system of funnel-like tubes (ducts) in the kidney. Each unit divides into two parts. It then joins others to form the opening (renal pelvis) to the outside of the kidney. Urine is then emptied through the ureters.

renal cell carcinoma, a cancer of the kidney. The tumor may grow in any part of the kidney. It becomes a large mass that may grow into the branches of the kidney vein. Blood in the urine and pain are commonly present. Spread of the cancer, as to the lungs and bones, may occur early in the disease. Treatment includes surgery and radiation. Also called **clear cell carcinoma of the kidney.** See also **Wilms' tumor.**

renal cortex, the soft, grainy, outer layer of the kidney. It has about 1.25 million tiny tubes. They remove body wastes from the blood in the form of urine. A **renal corpuscle** is one of the small, round, deep red bodies in the cortex of the kidney. The corpuscles are thought to be part of a filter system through which nonprotein substances in blood plasma enter small tubes (tubules) in the kidney for urination.

renal diet, a diet given for long-term kidney failure. It controls the intake of protein, potassium, sodium, phosphorus, and fluids. Protein is limited. Some vegetables and fruits may be eaten. Special flours and breads that have no protein and are low in potassium and sodium may be used. The low potassium level of the diet also makes it useful in conditions of excess blood potassium. Since this diet is not complete, vitamins and some minerals are needed.

renal dwarf, a dwarf whose slowed growth is caused by kidney failure.

renal failure. See **kidney failure.**

renal osteodystrophy, uneven bone growth and loss of minerals caused by long-term kidney failure.

renal scan, an outline, or scan, of the kidneys made to find their size, shape, and exact place. It is used to help diagnose a tumor or other defects. See also **scanning.**

Renese, a trademark for a fluid-releasing drug (diuretic) and a high blood pressure drug (polythiazide).

renin /rē′nin/, an enzyme, made by and stored in a kidney area that surrounds each blood vessel as it enters a filter (glomerulus). The enzyme affects the blood pressure.

rennin /ren′in/, a milk-curdling enzyme that occurs in the stomach juices of infants and is also in the substance (rennet) made in the stomach of cattle.

Renoquid, a trademark for an antibiotic (sulfacytine).

reovirus /rē′ō-/, a type of virus found in the breathing and digestive tracts in relatively healthy people. Some disorders, as upper breathing tract disease, may be caused by this virus.

Repen-VK, a trademark for an antibiotic (penicillin V potassium).

replacement, the substitution of a missing part or substance with a like part or substance, as to replace lost blood with donor blood.

replication, 1. a means of reproducing, or copying; a folding back of a part to form a double. 2. the process by which chromosome material is doubled in the cell.

reporting locations, any one of six facilities/locations where incident assigned resources may check in. The locations are: incident command post—resources unit (RESTAT). Base, camp, staging area, helibase, or division supervisor for direct line assignments. (Check in at one location only.)

repression, 1. the act of holding back or down. 2. a mental defense mechanism in which unwanted thoughts, feelings, or desires are pushed from the conscious into the unconscious mind. Because of the painful feeling of guilt or unpleasant content, the thoughts may remain hidden in the mind. They may, however, continue to affect behavior and may lead to other disorders.

reproduction, 1. the way animals and plants make offspring. In humans, the germ cells, the male sperm and the female egg, join during fertilization to form the new person. 2. creating a like structure, situation, or factor. 3. remembering an early thought, sense, or lesson.

reproductive system, the male and female sex glands, nearby ducts and glands, and the outer sex organs. They create offspring. In women these include the ovaries, fallopian tubes, uterus, vagina, clitoris, and vulva. In men these include the testicles, epididymis, vas deferens, seminal vesicles, ejaculatory duct, prostate, and penis. Also called **genital tract.**

rescinnamine, a drug used to treat mild high blood pressure that affects the heart, nervous system, or both. Mental depression, use of electroshock, or known allergy to this drug prohibits its use. Side effects include digestive, heart, and central nervous system problems.

rescue medical, any manned ground vehicle capable of providing emergency medical services.

resect /risekt′/, to remove tissue or an organ from the body by surgery. Resection of an organ may be part or complete.

reserpine, a drug used to treat high blood pressure and some nerve disorders.

reserve, a possible ability of the body to keep life processes normal by changing to meet a need, as heart (cardiac) reserve or lung (pulmonary) reserve. See also **homeostasis.**

reservoir of infection, a constant source of infectious disease. People, animals, and plants may be reservoirs of infection.

resident, a doctor in training after an internship.

resident bacteria, bacteria living in a certain area of the body.

residential care facility, a health care center, as a nursing home. It gives nonmedical care to patients who, because of physical, mental, or emotional disorders, are not able to live by themselves.

residual /rizij′oo·əl/, referring to the part of a substance that stays after much of it has been removed. An example is residual urine that stays in the bladder after urination.

residual volume, the air that stays in the lungs after breathing out as much as possible.

resistance, fighting a force, as the body fighting infection.

resonance, an echo or other sound made in the body by tapping (percussion) the skin over a body organ or space during a physical test. —**resonant,** *adj.*

resorcinated camphor /rizôr′sinā′tid/, a mixture of a mild irritant (camphor) and and antiseptic (resorcinol), used to treat lice infestations and itching.

resorcinol, an antiseptic used as a skin-peeling drug in skin diseases.

resorption, the loss of tissue, as bone, by the breakdown of the tissue. An example is the reduced size of the dental ridge of a jaw after a tooth has been taken out.

resources, all personnel and major items of equipment available, or potentially available, for assignment to incident tasks on which status is maintained.

Resource Conservation and Recovery Act (RCRA), establishes framework for the proper management and disposal of all hazardous wastes, including treatment, storage, and disposal. Also establishes installation and notification requirements for underground storage tanks.

Respid, a trademark for a smooth muscle relaxing drug (theophylline).

respiration, the give and take of oxygen and carbon dioxide in the body's tissues, from the lungs to the level of the cells. The rate changes with the age and condition of the person.

respirator, a machine used to aid or act as the breathing stimulant of patients with respiratory failure. See also **respiratory therapy.**

respiratory /res'pərətôr'ē, rispī'rə-/, referring to breathing (respiration).

respiratory acidosis. See **acidosis.**

respiratory alkalosis. See **alkalosis.**

respiratory assessment, a checkup of a patient's breathing system. The patient is asked about coughs, wheezes, shortness of breath, becoming tired easily, having chest or stomach pain, chills, fever, heavy sweating, dizziness, or swelling of the feet and hands. Signs of confusion, wide nostrils, bluish lips or nails, swelling (clubbing) of the fingers, fever, and loss of appetite are noted. The patient's breathing is closely watched for slow, rapid, irregular, shallow, or waxing and waning (Cheyne-Stokes) breathing. Rapid, slow, or abnormal heart beats, or signs of congestive heart failure, as abnormal breathing sounds, fluid buildup, swollen spleen and liver, bloated stomach, or pain are recorded. Tapping the chest (percussion) is done to check for drumlike sounds, dull or flat sounds, wheezing, friction rubs, or the carrying of spoken words through the chest wall. Also checked are prior breathing disorders and operations, long-term conditions, current drugs, smoking habits, and the family history of breathing disorders. Laboratory tests include chest x-ray films, complete blood count, a heart rate test (electrocardiogram), and lung tests.

respiratory center, a group of nerve cells in the brain that control the rhythm of breathing in response to changes in levels of oxygen and carbon dioxide in the blood and cerebrospinal fluid. Change in the amount of oxygen and carbon dioxide or hydrogen levels start nerve cells that send signals to the respiratory center, raising or lowering the breathing rate. This is needed for normal breathing. The respiratory center is harmed by barbiturates, anesthetics, tranquilizers and morphine.

respiratory distress syndrome of the newborn (RDS), a lung disease of the newborn. It features airless air sacs (alveoli), rigid lungs, more than 60 breaths a minute, a widened nose, cramps of rib cage muscles, grunting on breathing out, and fluid buildup in the arms and legs. The condition occurs most often in premature babies and in babies of mothers with diabetes. Causes include overfilled

air sacs and, at times, a growth of a fiberlike (hyaline) membrane, bleeding in the lungs, lowered heart output, and very low blood oxygen. The infant either completely recovers with no aftereffects or dies in a few days. Treatment includes correcting shock and lack of oxygen. Also called **hyaline membrane disease.**

respiratory exchange ratio (R), the amount of carbon dioxide breathed out compared to the amount of oxygen breathed in.

respiratory failure, the inability of the heart and lung systems to keep enough of a transfer of oxygen and carbon dioxide in the lungs. Respiratory failure may be caused by lack of oxygen (hypoxemic failure) or a transfer of gases problem (ventilatory failure). A sign of hypoxemic failure is excess breathing (hyperventilation). This occurs in diseases such as emphysema, fungus infections, leukemia, pneumonia, lung cancer, or tuberculosis. Ventilatory failure occurs in conditions such as bronchitis, emphysema, brain diseases, injury, or tumors of the nerve and muscle system or the chest. Respiratory failure in long-term lung diseases may be caused by added stress, as heart failure, surgery, anesthesia, or upper breathing tract infections. Treatment of respiratory failure includes clearing the airways by suction, giving lung drugs (bronchodilators), or making an airway (tracheostomy).

respiratory rate, the normal rate of breathing at rest, about 12 to 16 breaths per minute. The rate may be more rapid in fever, lung infection, gas gangrene, left-sided heart failure, and other disorders. **Bradypnea** is an abnormally slow rate of breathing. Slower breathing rates may result from head injury, coma, or narcotic overdose. **Hyperpnea** is a deep, rapid, or labored breathing. It occurs normally with exercise, and abnormally with pain, fever, hysteria, or any condition in which the supply of oxygen is inadequate, as heart disease and lung disease. **Hypopnea** is shallow or slow breathing. In well-conditioned athletes it is normal and is accompanied by a slow pulse. It is serious when it occurs in damage to the brainstem, accompanied by a rapid, weak pulse. **Tachypnea** is an abnormally rapid rate of breathing, as seen with too high body temperature (hyperpyrexia). See also **apnea, dyspnea, orthopnea.**

respiratory rhythm, a regular cycle of breathing in and out, controlled by nerve signals carried between muscles in the chest and breathing centers in the brain. The normal cycle may be changed by a long breathing-out phase in diseases of the airway, as asthma, bronchitis, and emphysema, or by Cheyne-Stokes breathing in patients with raised brain pressure or heart failure.

respiratory syncytial virus (RS virus), a member of a subgroup of viruses (myxoviruses) that cause epidemics of bronchitis, pneumonia, and the common cold. Symptoms include fever, cough, and severe tiredness. Treatment includes rest, aspirin, and nasal drugs.

respiratory therapy (RT), any treatment that maintains or improves the function of the respiratory tract. See also **continuous positive airway pressure, intermittent mandatory ventilation, IPPB.**

respiratory tract, the system of organs and structures that transfers oxygen and carbon dioxide between the air outside and the blood flowing through the lungs. It also warms the air passing into the body. The speech function is helped by air for the throat (larynx) and the vocal cords. The respiratory tract is divided into two parts. The **lower respiratory tract** includes the left and the right bronchi and the alveoli where the exchange of oxygen and carbon dioxide occurs during the breathing cycle. The bronchi, which are branches of the windpipe (trachea), divide into smaller bronchioles in the lung tissue; the bronchioles divide into alveolar ducts; the ducts into alveolar sacs; and the sacs into alveoli. The lower respiratory tract is a common site of infections, obstructive conditions, and lung cancer. The **upper respiratory tract** consists of the nose, the nasal cavity, the ethmoidal air cells, the frontal sinuses, the sphenoidal sinuses, the maxillary sinus, the larynx, and the trachea. The upper tract moves air to and from the lungs and filters, moistens, and warms the air. Infection and irritation of the upper tract are common and often spread to the lower respiratory tract, where they may cause serious complications. See also **larynx, lung, nose, trachea.** Also called **respiratory system.**

RESTAT, an acronym for resource unit. A unit within the planning section.

restless legs syndrome, an irritating feeling of uneasiness, tiredness, and itching deep in the muscles of the leg. This occurs often in the lower part of the leg. There may also be twitching and sometimes pain. The only relief is walking or moving the legs. The condition may be linked to many nervous system disorders.

restoration, any tooth filling, inlay, crown, denture, or other dental device that restores or replaces lost tooth structure, teeth, or mouth tissues. **Faulty restoration** refers to any dental work that contains flaws, as overhanging or incomplete tooth fillings. Such faults may cause inflammatory diseases of the teeth and mouth. Also called **prosthetic restoration.**

Restoril, a trademark for a sedative (temazepam).

restraint, any of many devices used to prevent the movement of patients to protect them from injury. A **diaper restraint** is often used to treat children with orthopedic disorders. It provides traction of the legs when other methods do not work. It fits over the pelvic area like a diaper, with rings attached at the four corners. A strap is threaded through the rings and attached to the top of the bed. A

jacket restraint is used to hold the patient's trunk still in traction and to keep the patient from sitting up in bed. The restraint is attached to both sides of the bed frame by buckled webbing straps. A **sling restraint** may be put over the pelvic area or the abdominal area to keep patients rigid in traction. Restraints often cause emotional problems for the patient and should be carefully used. Restraints that are too tight may cause skin irritation. Any that fit too loosely do not serve their purpose. Restraints are most often removed every 4 hours to check the skin condition and to give skin care.

resuscitation /risus'itā'shən/, the process of keeping a patient in lung or heart failure alive. Resuscitation uses methods of artificial breathing and chest compression and treats the cause of the failure. **Mouth-to-mouth resuscitation** is done most often with chest compressions. The victim's nose is sealed by pinching the nostrils closed. The head is tilted back. Air is breathed by the rescuer through the mouth into the lungs. With **mouth-to-nose resuscitation,** the mouth of the victim is covered and held closed. Air is breathed through the victim's nose. See also **cardiopulmonary resuscitation.** –resuscitate, *v.*

resuscitator /-tər/, a device for pumping air into the lungs. It is made of a mask that fits snugly over the mouth and nose, a storage place for air, and a pump.

retainer, the part of a dental device that connects a tooth with part of a bridge. It may be an inlay or a crown. It also may be any clasp, attachment, or device for fixing or keeping rigid a dental fixture. For example, an **extracoronal retainer** is one that lies largely outside the crown (coronal) part of a tooth, or a direct clasp that fastens on a tooth on its outer surface. An **intracoronal retainer** is one that lies largely within the tooth crown, as an inlay, or a direct retainer used in making removable partial dentures. A **radicular retainer** is one that lies in the body of a tooth, most often in the root.

retarded, very slow. –retard, *v.*, retardation, *n.*

retch, a strong attempt to vomit without bringing anything up.

retention, 1. resisting movement or being moved. 2. the ability of the digestive system to hold food and fluid. 3. the inability to urinate or defecate. 4. the ability of the mind to remember data. 5. the ability of a dental device or filling to stay in place without moving under stress. 6. temporary containment of the material in an area where it can be absorbed, neutralized, or vacuumed for proper disposal. Retention tactics are intended to be more permanent and may require resources such as portable basins, bladder bag, or other special construction.

retention procedure, a method set up by state laws or mental health codes for putting a patient in a mental hos-

Q–R

pital. Most states name four types of retention: emergency, informal, involuntary, and voluntary.

Retet, a trademark for an antibiotic (tetracycline).

reticular /ritik′yələr/, having a netlike pattern or structure of veins.

reticular activating system (RAS), a working system in the brain needed for the level of consciousness, from sleep to full attention. A group of nerve fibers in many parts of the brain (thalamus, hypothalamus, brainstem, and cerebral cortex) are part of the system.

reticular formation, a small, thick cluster of nerve cells in the brainstem. It controls breathing, heart beat, blood pressure, and other vital functions of the body. The state of the body is constantly checked through joinings with the sense and motor nerve tracts.

reticulocyte /ritik′yələsīt′/, immature red blood cells that usually make up less than 1% of the flowing red blood cells. A greater amount shows a higher rate of red cell making.

reticuloendothelial system (RES) /-en′dōthē′lē·əl/, a working system of the body mainly used to defend against infection and to dispose of the products of the breakdown of cells. It is made up of large cells (macrophages), the cells of the liver (Kuppfer cells), and the cells (reticulum) of the lungs, bone marrow, spleen, and lymph nodes.

reticuloendotheliosis /-lē·ō′-/, an abnormal condition with increased growth and spread of the cells of a defense system of the body (reticuloendothelial system).

retina /ret′inə/, a 10-layered, nervous tissue membrane of the eye, continuous with the optic nerve. It receives images of objects outside the eye and carries signals through the optic nerve to the brain. The retina contains visual purple (rhodopsin), a substance that adapts the eye to changes in light. The retina becomes clouded if exposed to direct sunlight. The outer surface of the retina is in contact with the coating of the eye (choroid); the inner surface with the watery part of the eye (vitreous body). There is a thin spot in the exact center of the back surface where focus is best. See also **eye.**

Retin-A, a trademark for an acne drug (tretinoin).

retinaculum /ret′inak′yələm/, *pl.* **retinacula,** a structure that holds an organ or tissue in place.

retinal /ret′inəl/, **1.** the active form of vitamin A needed for night, day, and color vision. See also **retinene, vitamin A. 2.** referring to the retina of the eye.

retinal detachment, a separation of the retina of the eye from the covering (choroid) in the back of the eye. The first symptom is often the sudden appearance of many spots seen floating loosely in the affected eye. There may also be flashing lights seen as the eye is moved. The patient may not seek help, because the number of spots tends to decrease during the days and weeks after the detachment.

Because the retina does not contain sense nerves that relay feelings of pain, the condition is painless. The condition most often results from a hole in the retina that allows the watery substance (vitreous humor) to leak between the choroid and the retina. Severe injury to the eye, as a bruise or penetrating wound, may be the cause, but in most cases retinal detachment is the result of internal changes in the vitreous chamber linked to aging or, less often, to inflammation inside the eye. Detachment often begins at the thin outer edge of the retina and reaches gradually under the thicker, more central areas. When the center becomes affected, the eyesight is distorted, wavy, and unfocused. If the detachment is not halted, total blindness of the eye will result. Surgery is often needed to repair the hole and prevent the leak of vitreous humor. If the condition is found early, when the hole is small and the amount of vitreous humor lost is not large, the retinal hole may be closed by causing a scar to form on the choroid and to join to the retina around the hole. The scar may be caused by heat, electric current, or cold.

retinene /ret′inin/, either of the two yellow colorings (carotenoid pigments) found in the rods of the retina that are sources of vitamin A and are set into motion by light. See also **retinal, retinol.**

retinoblastoma /ret′inōblastō′mə/, an inherited tumor growing from eye (retinal) germ cells. Signs are lessened sight, unfocused eyes, a detached retina, and an abnormal pupil reflex. The rapidly growing tumor may invade the brain and spread to distant sites. Treatment includes removal of the eye and as much of the optic nerve as possible, followed by radiation and chemical treatments. It occurs in both eyes in about 30% of cases. Because it is an inherited condition, genetic counseling is urged.

retinol /ret′inôl/, a form of vitamin A. It is found in the retinas of the eyes of mammals. Also called **vitamin A₁.**

retinopathy /ret′inop′əthē/, an eye disorder without inflammation that results from changes in the eye (retinal) blood vessels.

retraction, 1. the moving of tissues to expose a part or structure of the body. **2.** a backward movement of the teeth.

retraction of the chest, the visible sinking-in of the soft tissues of the chest between the ribs, as occurs with increased breathing effort. In infants, breastbone retraction also occurs with only a slight increase in breathing effort.

retroflexion, an abnormal placement of an organ in which the organ is tilted back and folded over on itself.

retrograde, 1. moving backward; moving in the opposite direction to that which is thought to be normal. **2.** breaking down; going back to an earlier state or worse condition.

retrograde cystoscopy, a method in radiology for testing the bladder in which a tube (catheter) is put through the urethra into the bladder, allowing the urine in the bladder to pass through the catheter. A dye is put in to fill the bladder. The shape of the bladder is looked at, using many x-ray films or fluoroscopy, as the bladder is emptied. See also **cystoscopy.**

retrolental fibroplasia /ret'rōlen'təl/, a disorder caused by giving excess amounts of oxygen to premature infants. A fiberlike tissue forms behind the lens of the eye, resulting in blindness.

retroperitoneal /-per'itōnē'əl/, referring to organs closely attached to the stomach and intestine walls and partly covered by the lining (peritoneum), rather than held up by that lining.

retroperitoneal fibrosis, a long-term inflammation in which fiberlike tissue surrounds the large blood vessels in the lower back. It often causes a narrowing of the middle of the bladder tubes (ureters). Symptoms include low back and stomach pain, weakness, weight loss, fever, and, with urinary tract involvement, excess urination and other urinary problems. Sometimes it spreads up to involve the small intestine (duodenum), bile ducts, and the large blood vessel of the abdomen (superior vena cava). Methysergide, a drug taken to prevent migraine headaches, is one known cause of this condition. Treatment includes stopping the use of methysergide and surgery.

retroperitoneal lymph node dissection, removal of lymph nodes behind the linings of the abdomen (peritoneum), most often done in an attempt to get rid of sites of lymph gland cancer or the spread of cancers that start in pelvic organs or the sex organs.

retropharyngeal abscess /-ferin'jē·əl/, a buildup of pus in the tissues behind the throat (pharynx) causing difficulty in swallowing, fever, and pain. Treatment includes giving antibiotics and draining.

retrouterine /ret'rōyōo'tərin/, behind the uterus.

retroversion /-vur'zhən/, **1.** a common condition in which an organ is tipped backward, often without bending or other twisting. The uterus may be retroverted in as many as 25% of normal women. Uterine retroversion is measured as first, second, or third degree, depending on the angle of tilt with respect to the vagina. No treatment is needed. **2.** an abnormal condition in which the teeth or other jaw structures are behind their normal places. –**retrovert,** *v.*

revascularization, restoring through surgery the blood flow to an organ or a tissue being replaced, as in bypass surgery.

reversed bandage, a roller bandage that is turned on itself with a half twist so that it lies smoothly, conforming to the contour of the arm or leg. See also **roller bandage.**

review of systems (ROS), a system-by-system review of the person's health history of the body. It is begun during the first interview with the patient and completed during the physical examination, as physical findings prompt further questions. One outline of the systems and some of the signs and symptoms that might be noted or reported are as follows.

★SKIN: bruising, discoloration, itching, birthmarks, moles, ulcers, and changes in the hair or nails.

★BLOOD: abrupt or heavy bleeding, fatigue, swollen or tender lymph nodes, paleness, and a history of anemia.

★HEAD AND FACE: pain, injury, and difficulty in seeing.

★EARS: ringing in the ears, change in hearing, discharge from the ears, deafness, and dizziness.

★EYES: change in sight, pain, inflammation, infections, double vision, sight defects, blurring, and tearing.

★MOUTH AND THROAT: dental problems, hoarseness, difficulty in swallowing, bleeding gums, sore throat, ulcers, and sores in the mouth.

★NOSE AND SINUSES: discharge, nosebleed, sinus pain, and blockage.

★BREASTS: pain, change in shape or skin color, lumps, and discharge from the nipple.

★BREATHING TRACT: cough, sputum, change in sputum, night sweats, shortness of breath, and wheezing.

★HEART AND BLOOD VESSEL SYSTEM: chest pain, difficulty in breathing, rapid heart beat, weakness, intolerance of exercise, varicose veins, swelling of hands and feet, known heart murmur, high blood pressure, and heart attack.

★DIGESTIVE SYSTEM: nausea, vomiting, diarrhea, constipation, quality of appetite, change in appetite, difficulty in swallowing, gas, heartburn, change in bowel habits, and the use of laxatives or other drugs to alter the function of the digestive tract.

★URINARY TRACT: lack of urine, change in color of urine, change in times of urination, pain with a desire to urinate, not being able to urinate, and fluid buildup.

★GENITAL TRACT (female): menstrual history, use of birth control pills and devices, discharge, pain or discomfort, itching, and a history of venereal disease.

★GENITAL TRACT (male): penis discharge, pain or discomfort, itching, sores, blood in the urine, and a history of venereal disease.

★SKELETAL SYSTEM: heat, redness, swelling, limited movement, deformity, and pain in a joint or a limb, the neck, or back, especially with movement.

Q–R

★NERVOUS SYSTEM: dizziness, tremor, irregular muscle movements, difficulty in speaking, change in speech, paralysis, loss of sensation, seizures, and fainting.

★ENDOCRINE SYSTEM: tremor, rapid heart beat, intolerance of heat or cold, too much urine, an excess thirst, excess speech, seizures, and goiter.

★MENTAL STATUS: nervousness, instability, depression, unreal fears, sexual problems, criminal behavior, lack of sleep, night terrors, mania, memory loss, and confusion.

Reye's syndrome /rāz/, a combination of brain disease and fatty invasion of the inner organs that may come after a virus infection. Symptoms include a rash, vomiting, and confusion about 1 week after the beginning of the illness. In the late stage, there may be extreme confusion followed by coma, seizures, and stopped breathing. It often affects patients under 18 years of age. A liver test shows fatty breakdown and confirms the diagnosis. The death rate ranges from 20% to 80%, depending on the severity of symptoms. The cause of Reye's syndrome is unknown. It has been linked to influenza B, chickenpox (varicella), the enteroviruses, and the Epstein-Barr virus. There is no specific treatment. Prompt correction of any imbalance in vital functions is very important for the outcome.

rhabdomyoma /rab′dōmī·ō′mə/, a tumor of muscle that may occur in the uterus, vagina, throat, or tongue, and may or may not be a cancer. A related disorder (congenital tumor nodules) occurs in the heart.

rhabdomyosarcoma /-mī′ōsärkō′mə/, a cancer that occurs most often in the head and neck. It is also found in the sex organs and urinary tract, legs and arms, body wall, and abdomen. In some cases, the disease comes after an injury. The first symptoms depend on the site of the tumor. They are related to tissue or organ damage, as swallowing difficulty, vaginal bleeding, bloody urine, or a block in the flow of urine. Removal is rarely possible because the tumor tends to spread. Removing an affected leg or arm may help. Radiation and chemical treatments with anticancer drugs may lengthen the life of the patient.

rhabdovirus, a member of a family of viruses that includes the one that causes rabies.

rhagades /rag′ədēz/, cracks or breaks in the skin that has lost its stretching ability. It is very common around the mouth.

Rh₀(D) immune globulin, a vaccinating drug used to prevent Rh allergy after abortion, miscarriage, childbirth, or pregnancy outside of the uterus (ectopic). It is not given to those already vaccinated. The most serious side effect is allergic shock.

Rheomacrodex, a trademark for a blood plasma expander (dextran 40).

rheumatic aortitis /rŏŏmat′ik/, an inflammatory condition of the major blood vessel (aorta) in the body. It occurs in rheumatic fever and results in damage to the aorta wall that may develop into patches of scarlike tissue (fibrosis). A similar condition linked to rheumatic fever, called **rheumatic arteritis,** may occur in other blood vessels (arteries and arterioles).

rheumatic fever, a disease that may develop within 1 to 5 weeks after recovery from a sore (strep) throat or from scarlet fever. It most often occurs in young children and may affect the brain, heart, joints, and skin. Early symptoms include fever, joint pains, nose bleeds, stomach pain, and vomiting. The major effects of this disease are a form of arthritis in many joints. It also causes heart problems, as chest pain, and, in severe cases, symptoms of heart failure. Another disorder (Sydenham's chorea) may develop and is commonly the only, late sign of rheumatic fever. This may at first appear as an increased awkwardness and a habit of dropping objects. Irregular body movements may worsen, and sometimes the tongue and the face muscles are affected. Other problems may be skin disorders, a rise in the number of white blood cells, anemia, and protein in the urine. There is no specific test for rheumatic fever. A return of rheumatic fever is common. Except for heart inflammation, all effects of this disease often go away without any permanent problems. Treatment includes bed rest and drugs, as penicillin, steroid drugs, or aspirin.

rheumatic heart disease, damage to heart muscle and heart valves caused by attacks of rheumatic fever. The heart damage may be found during the disease, or it may be discovered long after the disease has gone away. Heart murmurs, abnormal pulse rate and rhythm, heart block, and congestive heart failure often result. Deaths are often caused by heart failure or infection in the heart. Long-term rheumatic heart disease may require no treatment except for close watching. If signs of poor heart action occur, heart drugs, fluid-releasing drugs (diuretics), and a low-sodium diet are often given. It may be necessary to correct or replace the valves. Patients with a history of rheumatic fever or signs of rheumatic heart disease may get daily doses of penicillin by mouth or monthly injections to protect against streptococcal infections.

rheumatism, *nontechnical.* any of many conditions with inflammation of the bursae, joints, ligaments, or muscles. Symptoms include pain, limited movement, and tissue damage. –**rheumatic, rheumatoid,** *adj.*

rheumatoid arthritis, a long-term, destructive connective tissue disease that results from the body rejecting its own tissue cells (autoimmune reaction). There is inflammation of the membranes (synovial) lining the joints and increased release of synovial fluid. This leads to thickening of the synovial membrane and swelling of the joint. The adult form of rheumatoid arthritis first appears in early middle age, between 36 and 50 years of age, most often in women. First symptoms include fatigue, weakness, and poor appetite. Other early signs are mild fever, anemia, and red blood cells changes. The symptoms listed by the American Rheumatism Association are morning stiffness, joint pain or tenderness, swelling of at least two joints, arthritic nodes found at pressure points (as the elbows), changes in the joint seen on x-ray films, a positive rheumatoid factor blood test, and changes in the content of synovial fluid. The diagnosis is done by x-ray studies and blood tests. Aspirin-type drugs are given. Steroids are given with caution because of side effects. Other treatments, as diathermy, ultrasound, warm paraffin applications, and exercise under water are sometimes used.

rheumatoid factor (RF), a type of antibody often found in the blood of patients with rheumatoid arthritis. Rheumatoid factors are present in about 70% of such cases. They may also be found in other diseases, as tuberculosis, parasitic infections, and leukemia.

Rh factor, a substance (antigen) in the red blood cells of most people. A person with the factor is Rh+ (Rh positive). A person lacking the factor is Rh− (Rh negative). If an Rh− person receives Rh+ blood, red blood cell are destroyed and anemia occurs. An Rh+ fetus may be exposed to antibodies to the factor made in the Rh− mother's blood. Red cell destruction occurs and, if untreated, a fatal condition (erythroblastosis fetalis) results. Transfusion, blood typing, and crossmatching depend on Rh+ and ABO blood group labeling. The Rh factor was first found in the blood of a species of the rhesus (Rh) monkey. It is in the red cells of 85% of people. See also **blood group, erythroblastosis fetalis.**

rhinencephalon /rī′nensef′əlon/, *pl.* **rhinencephala,** a part of each brain side (cerebral hemisphere) that contains the limbic system, which is linked to the emotions. See also **limbic system.**

rhinitis /rīnī′-/, inflammation of the mucous membranes of the nose, with a nasal discharge. It may be seen with a sinus infection.

rhinopathy /rīnop′əthē/, any disease or defect of the nose.

rhinoplasty /ri′nōplas′tē/. See **cosmetic surgery.**

rhinorrhea /rī′nôrē′ə/, **1.** the free release of mucus from the nose. **2.** the flow of spinal fluid from the nose following an injury to the head.

rhinoscopy /rīnos′kəpē/, the examination of the nasal passages to inspect the mucosa, and to detect inflammation or defects, such as a crooked nose. The nasal passages may be looked at from the front, by putting a device in the nostrils. They can also be looked at from behind, by putting a device in through the back of the throat.

rhinosporidiosis /rī′nōsporid′ē·ō′-/, an infection caused by a fungus. There are fleshy red growths (polyps) on the mucous membranes of nose, the lining of the eye (conjunctiva), the back of the throat (nasopharynx), and the soft palate. The most effective treatment is to burn off the growths (electrocautery).

rhinotomy /rīnot′-/, an operation in which a cut is made along one side of the nose. It is done to drain pus from a sore or a sinus infection.

rhinovirus, any of about 100 distinct, small RNA viruses that cause about 40% of breathing illnesses. The infection features a dry, scratchy throat, stuffy nose, tiredness, and headache. There is little fever. The fluids from the nose last 2 or 3 days. Children may also get a cough. The treatment is general and may include rest, painkillers, antihistamines, and decongestants. See also **cold.**

rhitidosis /rit′idō′-/, a wrinkling, as of the cornea of the eye.

Rh negative. See **Rh factor.**

rhodopsin /rōdop′sin/. See **rod.**

RhoGAM, a trademark for a vaccinating drug (Rh₀(D) immune globulin).

rhomboideus major /romboi′dē·əs/, a muscle of the upper back. It draws the shoulder blade toward the backbone while holding it up and drawing it slightly upward.

rhonchi /rong′kī/, *sing.* **rhonchus,** abnormal sounds heard in an airway blocked by thick fluids, muscle spasms, tumors, or outside pressure. The constant rumbling sounds are lower when the patient breathes out, and they clear on coughing. Sibilant rhonchi are high pitched and are heard in the small tubes (bronchi), as in asthma. Sonorous rhonchi are lower pitched and are heard in the large bronchi, as in tracheobronchitis. Dry rales are called rhonchi. Compare **rale.**

rhotacism /rō′təsizm/, a speech disorder marked by a defective pronunciation of words with the sound /r/, by the excess use of the sound /r/, or by using another sound for /r/.

Rh positive. See **Rh factor.**

rhus dermatitis /ro͞os/, a skin rash resulting from contact with a plant of the genus *Rhus,* as poison ivy, poison oak, or poison sumac. See also **contact dermatitis.**

rhythm, the relation of one signal to nearby signals as measured in time, movement, or regular action.

rhythm method. See **natural family planning method.**

rhytidoplasty /ritid′ōplas′tē/. See **cosmetic surgery.**

rib, one of the 12 pairs of elastic arches of bone forming a large part of the chest (thoracic) skeleton. The first seven ribs on each side are called **true ribs** because they join to the breastbone (sternum) and the backbones (vertebrae). The other five ribs are called **false ribs.** The first three join

Q–R

the ribs above. The last two are free at their ends and are called **floating ribs.**

rib fracture, a break in a bone of the chest caused by a blow or crushing injury or by violent coughing or sneezing. The ribs most commonly broken are the fourth to eighth. If the bone is shattered or the break is displaced, sharp pieces may pierce the lung. Symptoms include pain, especially on taking a deep breath, and quick, shallow breathing. The site of the break may be very tender to the touch. The crackling of bone pieces rubbing together may be heard. Breath sounds may show other signs of damage. The location and nature of the break are found by chest x-ray films. Blood or air in the chest, collapsed lung, pneumonia, and other problems may occur. Broken ribs may be splinted with an elastic belt, an Ace bandage, or adhesive tape. The patient must learn how to breathe deeply, cough, and do exercises while wrapped in tape. If taping and painkilling drugs fail to relieve pain, a regional nerve block may be done.

riboflavin /rī′bōflā′vin/, a part of the B vitamin complex. It is important in preventing some sight disorders, as cataracts. Small amounts of riboflavin are found in the liver and kidneys. It is not stored in any large amount in the body and must come from the diet. Common sources are organ meats, milk, cheese, eggs, green leafy vegetables, meat, whole grains, and peas. A lack of riboflavin causes skin tumors, sensitivity to light and other eye disorders, trembling, sluggishness, dizziness, fluid buildup, inability to urinate, and vaginal itching. Also called **vitamin B$_2$.**

ribonucleic acid (RNA) /-nōōklē′ik/, a nucleic acid, found in both the nucleus and cytoplasm of cells. It carries gene data from the nucleus to the cytoplasm. In the cytoplasm, RNA puts together proteins. **Messenger RNA** is a part of RNA that sends information from DNA (deoxyribonucleic acid) to the protein-making ribosomes of cells. See also **deoxyribonucleic acid.**

ribosome /-sōm/, a tiny organ (organelle) in the cytoplasm of cells. Ribosomes act with messenger RNA and transfer RNA to join together amino acid units into a larger protein molecule according to a series of reactions by a genetic code.

rice diet, a diet made up only of rice, fruit, fruit juices, and sugar. Vitamins and iron are given. (Salt is not used.) It is sometimes given to treat high blood pressure, long-term kidney disease, and overweight. The diet is somewhat changed after the blood pressure is lowered and other symptoms are eased. It should not be followed for any length of time, because it may lead to nutrition problems. Also called **Duke diet, Kempner rice-fruit diet.**

rickets, a condition caused by the lack of vitamin D, calcium, and phosphorus. It is seen most often in infancy and childhood. It features abnormal bone growth. Symptoms include soft bones causing defects, as bowlegs and knock-knees, swellings on the ends and sides of the bones, muscle pain, chest defects, a curved spine, swollen liver and spleen, heavy sweating, and general tenderness of the body when touched. Prevention and treatment are a diet rich in calcium, phosphorus, and vitamin D and enough exposure to sunlight.

rickettsia /riket′sē·ə/, *pl.* **rickettsiae,** any organism of the genus *Rickettsia*. Rickettsiae are small, round, or rod-shaped, special bacteria. They live inside the cells of lice, fleas, ticks, and mites. They are carried to humans by bites from these insects. Rickettsial diseases have caused many of history's worst epidemics. The many species are told apart on the basis of the diseases they cause. The spotted fever group is Rocky Mountain spotted fever, rickettsialpox, and others. Another group causes different forms of typhus. Treatment often includes antibiotics.

rickettsialpox /riket′sē·əlpoks′/, a mild infectious disease caused by *Rickettsia akari*. It is carried from mice to humans by mites. Symptoms include a crusted sore, chills, fever, headache, tiredness, muscle pain, and a rash that looks like chickenpox. About 1 week after the symptoms begin, small pimples appear. These become dry and form scabs. The scabs fall off, leaving no scars. Antibiotics help recovery.

rider's bone, a bony deposit that sometimes grows in horseback riders on the inner side of the lower end of the tendon of a thigh muscle.

Rieder cell leukemia /rē′dər/. See **myeloblastic leukemia.**

Rifadin, a trademark for an antibiotic (rifampin).

rifampin, an antibiotic used to treat or prevent tuberculosis, meningitis, and leprosy. Liver disorders or known allergy to this or like drugs prohibits its use. Side effects include liver disorders, stomach upset, aches and cramps, and discolored urine, saliva, and sweat. This drug interacts with many other drugs.

Riga-Fede disease, a tumor of the tongue (lingual frenum) in some infants. It is caused by early teeth rubbing on it.

right-handedness. See **handedness.**

right lymphatic duct, a vessel that carries lymph from the right upper area of the body into the blood. The duct joins two veins (right internal jugular and right subclavian) in the neck. At its opening are two valves that prevent blood from flowing back into the lymph system. See also **lymphatic system.**

right pulmonary artery, the longer, slightly larger of the two blood vessels (arteries) carrying blood from the heart to the lungs. It begins at the right lower heart chamber (ventricle) from a short blood vessel (pulmonary trunk), bends to the right, and divides into two branches at the root of the right lung.

right-sided heart failure. See **heart failure.**

rigidity, a condition of hardness or stiffness. **–rigid,** *adj.*

rigor /rig′ər, rī′gər/, **1.** a rigid condition of the tissues of the body, as in rigor mortis. **2.** a violent attack of shivering that may come with chills and fever.

rigor mortis /môr′tis/, the rigid stiffening of the muscles shortly after death.

Rimactane, a trademark for an antibiotic (rifampin).

ringworm, a contagious fungal disease. It features circular, bald patches of from 1 to 6 cm in diameter with slight redness of the skin (erythema), scaling, and crusting. Treatment is made up of 3 to 6 weeks of griseofulvin given by mouth. Also called **tinea capitis.** See also **tinea.**

Rinne tuning fork test /rin′ē/, a method of testing the ability to hear sounds of some frequencies. While each ear is tested, the other is covered. The stem of a vibrating fork is placed first outside of the ear, then on the bone behind the ear. It is held until the sound is no longer heard at each of these positions. The person with normal hearing senses the sound for a longer time when conduction is by air outside of the ear, instead of by bone. In conductive hearing loss, the sound is heard for a longer time when conducted by bone than by air. In hearing loss from a sense nerve disorder, the sound is heard longer when conducted by air, but hearing by both air and bone conduction is lowered.

Riopan, a trademark for an antiacid (magaldrate).

risk factor, a factor that causes a person or a group of people to be at risk to an unwanted or unhealthful event. **Relative risk** is the chance that a disease or side effect will occur given certain conditions or factors. It is compared with what would be expected. An example is the relative risk of lung cancer in someone who smokes cigarettes as compared with the risk in someone who does not smoke.

risorius /risôr′ē·əs/, one of the 12 muscles of the mouth. It retracts the angles of the mouth, as in a smile.

Risser cast, a fiberglass or plaster cast that surrounds the body and reaches over the neck as far as the chin. The cast prevents movement of the body. It is used to treat a spine disorder (scoliosis).

Ritalin Hydrochloride, a trademark for a nervous system stimulating drug (methylphenidate hydrochloride).

ritodrine hydrochloride, a nerve drug used in pregnancy to stop the uterus from contracting in labor that begins too soon. It is not given before the twentieth week of pregnancy. Known allergy to this drug prohibits its use. Side effects include rapid heart beat, headache, nausea, and changes in blood pressure.

Ritter's disease, an infection of newborns that begins with red spots about the mouth and chin. The rash spreads over the entire body. General shedding of skin follows. Blisters and yellow crusts may also be present. Ritter's disease is often fatal unless treated with antibiotics.

RN, abbreviation for **registered nurse.**

RNA, abbreviation for **ribonucleic acid.**

Robaxin, a trademark for a skeletal muscle relaxing drug (methocarbamol).

Robicillin VK, a trademark for an antibiotic (penicillin V potassium).

Ro-Bile, a trademark for a drug with many digestive enzymes.

Robimycin, a trademark for an antibiotic (erythromycin).

Robinul, a trademark for a peptic ulcer drug (glycopyrrolate).

Robitet, a trademark for an antibiotic (tetracycline or tetracycline hydrochloride).

Robitussin, a trademark for a cough syrup (guaifenesin). It is used in many cough drugs, and with an antihistamine it is used to stop coughing or to ease breathing.

Rocaltrol, a trademark for a calcium-controlling drug (calcitriol).

Rocky Mountain spotted fever (RMSF), an infectious disease carried by ticks in the warm zones of North and South America. It is caused by bacteria (*Rickettsia*). Symptoms include chills, fever, severe headache, muscle pain, mental confusion, and rash. Bleeding sores, constipation, and upset stomach are common. Early treatment with antibiotics is important. More than 20% of untreated patients die from shock and kidney failure. Prevention includes using insect repellents and wearing protective clothing. Inspecting the body for ticks and careful removal of any found is needed. Care must be taken not to crush ticks, because infection may be gotten through breaks in the skin. Vaccination with killed vaccine is suggested for those often exposed to ticks. See also **typhus.**

rod, one of of the tiny nerve cells shaped like a cylinder on the surface of the retina of the eye. Rods have a chemical (rhodopsin) that allows the eye to detect dim light. Rhodopsin is the purple-colored part in the rods. It forms from a protein (opsin) and a part of vitamin A (retinal). It breaks down when struck by light. It starts the sending of nerve signals. Short times of darkness allow the opsin and the retinal to remake the rhodopsin. Closing the eyes is a natural reflex that allows the remaking of rhodopsin. Compare **cone.**

rodenticide poisoning, a harmful condition caused by swallowing a substance used to kill rats, mice, or other rodents. See also **phosphorus poisoning, thallium poisoning, warfarin poisoning.**

Q–R

roentgen (R) /rent'gən, ren'jən/, an amount of x-rays or gamma rays. In radiology, it is the unit of the emitted dose. See **x-ray.**

role playing, a method in which a person acts out a real or imagined situation as a means of understanding mental conflicts.

Rolfing. See **structural integration.**

roller bandage, a long, tightly wound strip of fabric that may vary in width. It is used as a circular bandage.

Romberg sign, a sign of loss of the sense of position in which the patient loses balance when standing erect, feet together, and eyes closed. Also called **Romberg test.**

Rondec-DM, a trademark for a drug with an antihistamine (carbinoxamine maleate), an antitussive (dextromethorphan hydrobromide), and a nasal and lung drug (pseudoephedrine hydrochloride).

Rondomycin, a trademark for an antibiotic (methacycline hydrochloride).

rooming-in, a practice that allows mothers and new babies to remain together in the hospital as they would at home rather than being separated.

root, the part of an organ or a structure that is firmly joined to something, as the root of the tooth.

root canal, the space that has the pulp in the root of a tooth. An **accessory root canal** branches to the side of the pulp canal in a tooth. A **collateral pulp canal** comes out of the root of a tooth at a place other than the tip. Also called **pulp canal.**

root curettage, the scraping of the root surface of a tooth to remove plaque and help healthy gum tissues grow.

rooting reflex, a normal response in newborns when the cheek is touched or stroked along the side of the mouth. The infant turns the head toward the touched side and begins to suck. The reflex goes away by 3 to 4 months of age but it may last until 12 months of age.

root retention, a method to remove the crown of a root canal treated tooth and keep enough of the root and gums to hold a removable dental device (prosthesis).

Rorschach test /rôr'shäk, -shäkh/, a mental test set up by the Swiss psychiatrist Hermann Rorschach. It is made up of 10 pictures of inkblots. The person studies the cards and responds by telling what images and emotions each design suggests. Replies are judged according to whether the response is to the entire image or only a part of it, and whether color, shading, shape, or location of certain picture parts are important. Other factors are whether movement is seen and the complexity of each response.

rosacea /rōzā'shē·ə/, a long-term form of acne seen in adults. It is linked to widened blood vessels of the nose, forehead, and cheeks. **Rhinophyma** is a form of rosacea. There is overgrowth of tissue, redness, prominent blood vessels, swelling, and defects of the skin of the nose.

Treatment is scouring or surgery. Also called **acne rosacea.**

roseola infantum /rōzē'ələ/, an illness of infants and young children. There is an abrupt, high fever, mildly sore throat, and swollen lymph nodes. Seizures may occur. After 4 or 5 days the fever drops to normal and a faint, pink, pimplelike rash appears on the neck, body, and thighs. The rash may last a few hours to 2 days. There is no specific treatment or vaccine. Aspirin or acetaminophen are often used to try to control fever. Antiseizure drugs may be needed.

rotation, **1.** a turning around an axis. **External rotation** is a turning outward or away from the midline of the body. For example, a leg is turned out when the toes point away from the body's midline. **Lateral rotation** is a turning away from the midline of the body, as when twisting to the left or right. **Medial rotation** is a turning toward the middle of the body. **Neutral rotation** is the placement of a leg or arm that is turned neither toward nor away from the body's middle. When lying on the back with the leg neutrally rotated, the toes should point straight up. **2.** one of the basic kinds of motion allowed by many joints, as the rotation of the head on its central axis, the bones of the neck. **3.** the turning of a baby's head to go through the pelvis.

Rotor syndrome, an inherited condition of the liver, with a mild yellowing of the skin (jaundice) but without other symptoms. The gallbladder works normally.

roughage /ruf'ij/. See **dietary fiber.**

roundworm, any worm of the class Nematoda, which includes the hookworm and the pinworm.

route of administration, any one of the ways in which a drug may be given. Examples are into a muscle (intramuscularly), into the nose (intranasally), into a vein (intravenously), into the mouth (orally), into the rectum (rectally), under the skin (subcutaneously), under the tongue (sublingually), on the skin surface (topically), or into the vagina (vaginally). Some drugs can be given only by one route. Taking the medication by the prescribed route allows for peak effectiveness. Taking the medication by another route may be damaging.

rubber, *informal.* a **condom.**

rubber dam, a thin sheet of latex rubber for separating one or more teeth during dental work.

rubbing alcohol, a disinfectant for skin and devices. It has 70% ethyl alcohol by volume. The rest is made up mainly of water. It may cause dryness of the skin. Rubbing alcohol is for outer use only and is flammable.

rubefacient /roo'bəfā'shənt/, something that increases the reddish color of the skin.

rubella /roobel'ə/, a contagious virus disease (German measles). Symptoms include those of a mild upper breathing tract infection, fever, swollen lymph nodes, joint pain, and a fine, red rash. The virus is spread by droplets from coughs or sneezes. The dormant time is from 12 to 23 days. The symptoms usually last only 2 or 3 days except for the joint pain, which may last longer or return. One attack gives lifelong immunity. If a woman gets rubella in the first 3 months of pregnancy, birth defects may result, such as heart disorders, cataracts, deafness, and mental retardation. An infant exposed to the virus in the uterus at any time during pregnancy may carry the virus for up to 30 months after birth. A vaccine is used for all children to lower the chances of an epidemic and thus to protect pregnant women. Spread of the virus from a recently vaccinated person rarely occurs. The illness itself is mild and needs no special treatment.

rubella and mumps virus vaccine,   a live viruses vaccine used for vaccination against rubella and mumps. Infection or known allergy to this drug prohibits its use. It is not given to a patient whose immune function is slowed or to a pregnant woman. Pregnancy is avoided for 3 months after vaccination. Side effects include allergic reactions.

rubella embryopathy,   any birth defect in an infant caused by German measles (rubella) in the mother in the early stages of pregnancy.

rubella virus vaccine,   a live virus vaccine used to vaccinate against German measles (rubella). Fever, infection, untreated tuberculosis, or allergy to certain animal proteins prohibits its use. It is not given to pregnant women. Pregnancy should be avoided for 3 months after vaccination. Side effects include allergic reactions and pain.

rubeola /roōbē′ələ/.   See **measles.**

rubescent /roōbes′ənt/,   reddening.

Rubin's test,   a test of female infertility by checking the opening of the fallopian tubes. Carbon dioxide gas (CO_2) is sent under pressure through a tube (cannula) put into the cervix. The CO_2 is passed through from a needle connected to a pressure gauge. If the tubes are open, the gas passes from the uterus and enters the stomach space. The recorded pressure then falls. There may be shoulder pain from irritation of the diaphragm. If the tubes are blocked, gas can-

not escape from the tubes into the stomach space and the pressure remains high. After the test, the patient rests for 3 hours. Crampy pain, dizziness, nausea, and vomiting may occur. A position with the pelvis higher than the head allows the gas to stay in the pelvis and gives some relief.

rubivirus /roō′bē-/,   a member of the virus family, as rubella virus.

rubor /roō′bôr/,   redness, especially when there is swelling.

Rubramin PC,   a trademark for vitamin B_{12} (cyanocobalamin).

rudiment /roō′dəmənt/,   an organ or tissue that is incompletely grown or does not work.   –**rudimentary,** *adj.*

ruga /roō′gə/, *pl.* **rugae,**   a ridge or fold, as the rugae of the stomach, which form large folds in the mucous membrane of that organ.

rule of nines,   a way of estimating the amount of body surface covered by burns. It is done by giving 9% to the head and each arm, twice 9% (18%) to each leg and the front and back of the body and 1% to the space between the anus and the urethral opening (perineum). This is changed in infants and children because of the different body size.

rumination /roō′minā′shən/,   the spitting up (regurgitation) of small amounts of undigested food with little force after every feeding. It is commonly seen in infants. It may be a symptom of overfeeding, of eating too fast, or of swallowing air. See also **vomit.**

rupture /rup′chər/,   a tear or break in an organ or body tissue. It includes those instances when other tissues break through the opening. See also **hernia.**

Russell dwarf,   a patient with Russell's syndrome. It is an inherited disorder in which there is short height with many defects of the head, face, and skeleton. Patients also show many degrees of mental retardation.

rutin /roō′tin/,   a substance (bioflavonoid) taken from buckwheat and used to treat weak small blood vessels (capillaries).

Q–R

S

Sabin-Feldman dye test, a test for toxoplasmosis.

Sabin Vaccine. See **oral poliovirus vaccine.**

sac, a pouch or a baglike organ.

saccharide /sak′ərīd/, any of a large group of carbohydrates, including all sugars and starches. Almost all carbohydrates are saccharides. See also **carbohydrate, sugar.**

saccharin /sak′ərin/ a white, crystal-like artificial sweetener, sweeter than table sugar (sucrose). Saccharin is often used as a substitute for sugar.

Saccharomyces /sak′ərōmī′sēz/, a genus of yeast fungi, including brewer's and baker's yeast, as well as some harmful fungi, that cause such diseases as bronchitis, candidiasis, and pharyngitis.

saccharomycosis /-mīkō′-/, infection with yeast fungi, as the genera *Candida* or *Cryptococcus.*

saccule /sak′yool/, a small bag or sac, as the air saccules of the lungs. –**saccular,** *adj.*

sacral /sā′krəl, sak′rəl/, referring to the sacrum.

sacral foramen, one of a number of openings between the vertebrae in the pelvic area through which the nerves pass.

sacral plexus, a network of nerves that control motion and feeling. It lies against the inner back wall of the pelvis. It becomes the sciatic nerve and serves the upper legs and pelvic area.

sacroiliac /sak′rō·il′ē·ak/, referring to the part of the skeleton that includes the sacrum and the ilium bones of the pelvis.

sacrospinalis /-spīnā′lis/, a large muscle of the back. It straightens and supports the vertebral column and the head, and it pulls the ribs downward.

sacrum /sā′krəm/. See **vertebra.**

saddle joint, a kind of joint, as the wrist and thumb. Compare **pivot joint.**

sadism /sā′dizm, sad′izm/, **1.** abnormal pleasure from causing physical or mental pain or abuse to others; cruelty. **2.** a mental and sexual disorder marked by the wish to hurt or destroy the self-respect of another person, either a willing or unwilling partner, to get sexual satisfaction. The condition is usually long-term, is usually found in men, may be caused by conscious or unconscious desires, and,

in serious cases, can lead to rape, torture, and murder. Compare **masochism.** –**sadistic,** *adj.*

sadist, a person who suffers from or practices sadism.

sagittal suture /saj′itəl/, the saw-toothed line in the top of the skull that is formed where two bones (parietal) of the skull come together.

salicylate /səlis′ilāt/, any of several widely used drugs that are made from salicylic acid.

salicylate poisoning, a poisonous condition caused by eating salicylate, most often in aspirin or oil of wintergreen. It features rapid breathing, vomiting, headache, irritability, low blood sugar, and, in severe cases, convulsions and breathing failure. Treatment usually includes a quick cleaning out of the stomach, the use of vitamin K if there is bleeding, and proper steps to treat loss of water, glucose, and potassium. Sodium bicarbonate should not be taken by mouth.

salicylic acid /sal′isil′ik/, a drug used to treat warts and other growths on the skin and to help fight infections caused by a fungus. Diabetes, poor circulation, or known allergy to this drug prohibits its use. Side effects include skin inflammation, nausea, and ringing in the ears.

saline cathartic /sā′lin/, one of a large group of laxatives used to empty the bowel. It usually takes effect withing 3 to 4 hours.

saline solution, a solution containing salt (sodium chloride). A **saline infusion** is the injection of a mild salt solution into a vein. **Saline irrigation** is the washing out of a body space or wound with a salt solution.

saliva, the clear, viscous fluid secreted by glands in the mouth. Saliva contains water, mucin, organic salts, and the enzyme ptyalin that helps digest food. It keeps the mouth wet, starts to digest starches, and helps in chewing and swallowing food.

salivary /sal′iver′ē/, relating to saliva or to the forming of saliva.

salivary duct, any one of the tubes that carry saliva.

salivary fistula, an abnormal hole between a salivary gland or duct and the mouth or the skin of the face or neck.

salivary gland, one of the three pairs of glands that make the mouth wet, thus aiding in digesting food. The **parotid**

glands are the largest pair of salivary glands. They lie inside the cheek just below and in front of the outer ear. The **sublingual glands** are a pair of small salivary glands found under the mucous membrane of the floor of the mouth beneath the tongue. They are narrow, almond-shaped structures. The **submandibular glands** are a pair of round, walnut-sized salivary glands found below the jaw in the front of the neck.

salivary gland cancer, a cancer of a salivary gland, found most often in a parotid gland. About 75% of tumors that develop in the salivary glands are harmless, slow-growing, and painless rubbery bumps. On the other hand, cancerous tumors are fast-growing, hard, lumpy, and often very sore. Pain and facial muscle tightening and palsy may occur. Treatment includes surgery, x-rays, and chemotherapy.

salivation, the secreting of saliva by the salivary glands.

Salk Vaccine. See **poliovirus vaccine.**

Salmonella /sal′mənel′ə/, a genus of moving rod-shaped bacteria that includes species causing typhoid fever, paratyphoid fever, and some forms of infection of the digestive tract (gastroenteritis).

salmonellosis /sal′mənelō′-/, infection of the digestive tract caused by eating food contaminated with a species of *Salmonella.* Symptoms include sudden, sharp pain in the stomach or bowels, fever, and bloody, watery diarrhea that occur 6 to 48 hours after eating. Nausea and vomiting are common. Symptoms usually last from 2 to 5 days, but may persist for up to 2 weeks. Dangerous loss of water may occur. There is no special cure. Cooking food long enough, keeping food in the refrigerator, and careful hand-washing may help prevent the disease. See also **food poisoning.**

salol camphor /sal′ôl/, a clear, oily mixture of camphor and phenyl salicylate, used to kill germs on contact.

salpingectomy /sal′pinjek′-/, removal of one or both fallopian tubes, done to remove a cyst or tumor, to cut out an abscess, or, if both tubes are removed, to sterilize. Often the operation is done with removal of the uterus or ovaries.

salpingitis /-jī′-/, inflammation or infection of the fallopian tube. See also **pelvic inflammatory disease.**

salpingostomy /sal′ping·gos′-/, an operation in which a new opening is made in a fallopian tube. This is done to clear a tube that has been closed by infection, by long-term inflammation, or to drain an abscess. A device may be put in to keep the fallopian tube open.

salt, **1.** a substance made by mixing together an acid and a base. **2.** sodium chloride (common table salt). **3.** a substance, as magnesium sulfate (Epsom salt), used as a purgative.

salt depletion, the loss of salt from the body through too much sweating, diarrhea, vomiting, or urination, without replacing what was lost. See also **heat exhaustion.**

salt-free diet. See **low-sodium diet.**

Saluron, a trademark for a drug used to treat high blood pressure and to make the patient urinate more (hydroflumethiazide).

salve /sav, säv/. See **ointment.**

Sandhoff's disease, a type of Tay-Sachs disease that includes defects in two enzymes (hexosaminidase A and B). It features a more rapid course and is found in the general population, not restricted, as is Tay-Sachs disease. See also **Tay-Sachs disease.**

sanguineous /sang·gwin′ē·əs/, relating to blood.

Sanorex, a trademark for an appetite-controlling drug (mazindol).

Sansert, a trademark for a vasoconstrictor (methysergide maleate).

Santyl, a trademark for an enzyme (collagenase).

saphenous nerve /səfē′nəs/, the largest and longest branch of the femoral nerve that goes along the inner side of the leg. One branch of the saphenous nerve below the knee goes to the ankle. Another branch below the knee goes to the inner side of the foot.

SAR, search and rescue.

sarcoidosis /sär′koidō′-/, a long-term disease of unknown cause. Small, round bumps form in the tissue around many organs of the body, including the lungs, spleen, liver, and skin. The sores usually go away after a period of some months or years, but lead to widespread grainy inflammation and fibrous tissue. With **sarcoidosis cordis,** grainy growths develop in the heart. The number and the size of the growths vary. Mild cases with few growths are without symptoms. In severe cases the heart may have many growths, and heart failure may follow.

sarcoma /särkō′mə/, a cancer of the soft tissues usually appearing at first as a painless swelling. About 40% of sarcomas occur in the legs and feet, 20% in the hands and arms, 20% in the trunk, and the rest in the head or neck. The growth tends to spread very quickly. It is usually not caused by an injury, but it can grow in burn scars. Treatment includes surgery, x-rays, and chemotherapy. See specific sarcomas.

sarcoma botryoides /bot′rē·oi′dēz/, a tumor that can grow in muscle cells, found most often in young children and marked by a painful, grapelike mass in the upper vagina or on the cervix or the neck of the bladder.

sarcoplasmic reticulum /sär′kōplaz′mik/, a network of little tubes and sacs in muscles attached to the skeleton that plays an important part in tensing and relaxing the muscles.

S

sartorius /särtôr′ē·əs/, the longest muscle in the body, stretching from the pelvis to the calf of the leg. It is a narrow muscle that runs across the top of the thigh at an angle from the outside of the pelvis to the inside of the knee. It causes the thigh to move up and out and causes the leg to move in.

saturated, having absorbed or dissolved the largest possible amount of a given substance, and unable to absorb any more.

saturated fatty acid. See **fatty acid.**

satyriasis /sat′irī′əsis/, excessive or uncontrollable sexual desire in the male. Also called **satyromania.** Compare **nymphomania.**

sauna bath, a bath in which steam is used to induce sweating, followed by rubbing of the body, and ending with a cold shower.

Sayre's jacket /serz/, a cast used for support in treating injuries to and defects of the spinal column.

scabicide /skab′isīd/, any one of a large group of drugs that destroy the itch mite, *Sarcoptes scabiei.* These drugs are applied to the skin as a lotion or a cream. All are possibly poisonous and may irritate the skin. They are used with caution in treating children.

scabies /skā′bēz/, a contagious disease caused by the itch mite. There is intense itching of the skin and damage to the skin from scratching. A rash often occurs on the fingers, wrists, and thighs. The mite, passed by close contact with infected humans or domestic animals, burrows into the layers of the skin where the female lays eggs. Two to 4 months later, the eggs hatch and the itching begins. Treatment includes drugs and lotions.

scalp, the skin that covers the top of the head. The face and ears are not included.

scalp medication, a cream, ointment, lotion, or shampoo used to treat skin disorders of the scalp. A shampoo is usually used first. The hair is dried, combed, and parted in the middle, and the medication is spread with the fingertips. After treatment, the medication may need to be washed off the scalp and hair with an alkaline shampoo.

scanning, carefully looking at a part of the body, an organ, or a system of the body by making a picture of the area. Sometimes a substance is injected to make a certain area or body part stand out on the x-ray film. The liver, brain, and thyroid can be looked at, tumors can be found, and function may be studied by various scanning methods. –**scan,** *n., v.*

scanography /skanog′rəfē/, a special method of making an x-ray of an organ of the body. It is used mainly for making x-ray tests of the long bones.

scaphocephaly /skaf′ōsef′əlē/, a defect of the skull present at birth in which the skull has an unusually long narrow shape. It is often linked with mental retardation.

scaphoid bone /skaf′oid/, either of two similar bones of the hand and the foot. Also called **navicular bone.**

scapula /skap′yələ/. See **shoulder blade.**

scapulohumeral /skap′yəlōhyoo′mərəl/, referring to the muscles and the area around the shoulder blade (scapula) and long bone of the upper arm (humerus) that make up the shoulder.

scapulohumeral reflex, a normal response to tapping the side of the scapula nearest the spine, causing the arm to jerk. If the arm does not move, it may be a sign of damage to the spine.

scar. See **cicatrix.**

scarify /sker′əfī/, to make a number of light cuts into the skin; to scratch. Vaccination for smallpox is done by scarifying the skin under a drop of vaccine.

scarlet fever, a very easily spread disease of childhood caused by a type of *Streptococcus.* The infection features sore throat, fever, enlarged lymph nodes in the neck, weakness, and a widespread bright red rash. Also called **scarlatina.**

SCF, standard cubic foot.

SCFM, standard cubic feet per minute.

Scheuermann's disease /shoi′ərmunz/, an abnormal disease of the skeleton that leaves the patient a hunchback. Its cause is not known. It occurs most often in children between 12 and 16 years of age, and more often in girls than boys. It begins very slowly and is often linked with a history of unusual physical activity or participation in sports. Symptoms include poor posture with tiredness, stiffness, and pain in the back. If the disease is discovered early, the posture may be cured. Otherwise, the posture becomes fixed within a period of 6 to 9 months. This disease may be treated by putting the body in a cast for 10 or 12 months. After the cast is taken off, the patient must do a special set of exercises. In adults, continuous pain in the middle and lower back may be a sign of a milder form, and an operation may be needed. See also **spinal curvature.**

Schick test, a skin test to find out if the person can catch diphtheria. A small amount of a substance that fights diphtheria germs is injected into the skin. Redness and swelling at the site of injection is a positive reaction, showing that the patient can get diphtheria. A negative reaction has no skin signs and shows that the patient cannot get diphtheria.

Schilder's disease /shil′dərz/, a group of serious nerve diseases that begin in childhood. These diseases attack parts of the brain, and many of the symptoms are like those of multiple sclerosis. There is no known treatment. The cause may be viral or genetic.

Schiller's test /shil′ərz/, a test used to choose sections of the skin in the vagina or cervix for further tests in looking for possible cancers.

Schilling's leukemia /shil'ingz/.   See **monocytic leukemia.**

Schilling test,   a test used to find a blood disease (pernicious anemia). The patient swallows a small amount of cobalt, then waits for 24 hours. The urine is then tested.

schistosomiasis /shis'tōsōmī'əsis/,   an infection caused by a parasite *(Schistosoma)* in humans by contact with freshwater fouled with human waste (feces). One worm may live in one part of the body, laying eggs often, for up to 20 years. The eggs attack the mucous membrane, causing it to become thick and to develop small growths. Symptoms depend on the part of the body infected. *Schistosoma* may be found in the bladder, rectum, liver, lungs, spleen, intestines, and some veins. It may cause pain, blockage, damage to the infected organ, and anemia. Treatment includes drugs called schistosomacides that kill the worms. Schistosomiasis most often occurs in the tropics and in the Orient.

schizoaffective disorder /skit'sō-afek'tiv/,   a condition that has some of the same symptoms as schizophrenia and bipolar disorder or other major emotional disorders.

schizoid /skit'soid, skiz'oid/,   **1.** typical of or resembling schizophrenia; schizophrenic. **2.** a person, not necessarily a schizophrenic, who shows the traits of a schizoid personality.

schizoid personality disorder,   a state marked by the lack of the ability to make friends. Other symptoms are a lack of feelings, the wish to be alone all the time, and no concern for the opinions and feelings of others. The person is not able to show anger or any hostile feelings and does not seem to react to disturbing experiences. It may lead to schizophrenia.

schizophasia /skit'səfā'zhə, skiz'ə-/,   the rambling babble typical of some types of schizophrenia.

schizophrenia /-frē'nē·ə/,   any of a large group of mental disorders in which the patient loses touch with reality and in which the person is no longer able to think or act normally. It can be mild or serious, with a need to spend some time in a hospital. Treatment includes tranquilizers and other drugs, counseling, and group therapy. **Acute schizophrenia** is the sudden onset of identity crisis. Symptoms include confusion, emotional turmoil, fear, depression, and strange behavior. **Catatonic schizophrenia** is a form in which times of extreme withdrawal are followed by times of extreme excitement. Symptoms while in the withdrawal stage include not speaking, stupor, and rigid muscles. While in the stage of excitement, the person's aimless, constant actions may range from mild agitation to violence. **Childhood schizophrenia** begins before puberty. It may be caused by either organic brain damage or environmental conditions. It features withdrawal into fantasy and obsessions, and failure to communicate verbally.

Repetitive gestures, a lack of emotions, and a severely blocked sense of identity also occur. **Disorganized schizophrenia** is a form that begins at a young age, usually at puberty. A more severe decay of the personality occurs than in other forms of the disease. Symptoms include inappropriate laughter and silliness, odd mannerisms, talking and gesturing to oneself; bizarre and often obscene behavior and extreme social withdrawal. There are often hallucinations and delusions, which are most often of a sexual, religious, or paranoid nature. Another form, called **latent schizophrenia,** shows mild symptoms of the disease in a person with no previous history of psychotic behavior. **Process schizophrenia** is a form caused by tissue changes in the brain rather than by outside causes. It usually begins slowly and moves to a mental state that cannot be reversed. A form caused by outside factors rather than by physical changes in the brain is called **reactive schizophrenia.** It often begins rapidly. Symptoms last a short time and the patient appears well both before and following the episode. **Residue schizophrenia** is a form in which the patient has had at least one psychotic episode, often with delusions and hallucinations. Signs of the illness, as withdrawal and strange behavior, may last. A slow, gradual form, called **simple schizophrenia,** features a lack of feeling, a lack of concern for others, and no energy or wish to be around other people.

schizophrenic /-fren'ik/,   **1.** relating to schizophrenia. **2.** a person with schizophrenia.

schizophreniform disorder /-fren'iform/,   a condition exhibiting the same symptoms as schizophrenia but marked by a sudden beginning with resolution in 2 weeks to 6 months.

schizotypal personality disorder /-tī'pəl/,   a condition marked by odd thinking, talking, and acting that is not serious enough to be schizophrenia. See also **schizoid personality disorder, schizophrenia.**

Schneiderian carcinoma /shnīdir'ē·ən/, a skin cancer of the mucous membranes in the nose and sinuses.

school phobia,   a fear of going to school, found mainly in young children. It usually goes away as the child grows older; if it does not go away, counseling may be needed.

schwannoma /shwänō'mə/,   a harmless, single, self-contained tumor arising in the coverings of certain nerves. Also called **neurilemoma, Schwann cell tumor.**

sciatic /sī·at'ik/,   near the hip, as the sciatic nerve or the sciatic vein.

sciatica /sī·at'ikə/,   inflammation of the sciatic nerve, usually with pain and soreness along the thigh and leg. It may lead to a wasting of the muscles of the lower leg.

sciatic nerve,   a long nerve stretching through the muscles of the thigh, leg, and foot, with many branches.

S

science, a system that attempts to organize facts learned by study and to explain how the world and everything in it works. **Pure science** is concerned with learning new facts only for the sake of gaining new knowledge. **Applied science** is the practical use of scientific theory and laws.

scirrhous carcinoma /skir'əs/, a hard, fiberlike, very fast-spreading cancer in which the cancer cells occur one at a time or in groups. It is the most common form of breast cancer. See also **breast cancer.**

sclera /sklir'ə/, the tough, hard, dense membrane covering most of the back of the eyeball. It helps the eyeball hold its shape. The muscles that move the eyeball are attached to the sclera. It is the white visible portion of the eyeball.

scleredema /sklir'ədē'mə/, a skin disease without a known cause. It may follow a strep infection. It features hard areas of tissue that spread from the face or neck to the rest of the body, except for the hands and feet. It will go away by itself, but often comes back. There is no specific treatment.

sclerodactyly /skler'ōdak'tilē/, a deforming of the muscles and skeleton affecting the hands of patients with scleroderma. The fingers are frozen in a half-bent position, and the fingertips are pointed and have sores.

scleroderma /-dur'mə/, a fairly rare disease affecting the blood vessels and connective tissue. It features fibrous breakdown of tissue in the skin, lungs, and other internal organs. There are symptoms like rheumatoid arthritis. It occurs most often in middle-aged women. Steroid drugs are used in treatment, but there is no cure.

scleromalacia perforans /-məlā'shə/, a condition of the eyes in which the sclera is attacked as a complication of rheumatoid arthritis, causing parts of the eye to be exposed. Glaucoma, cataracts, and a detached retina may result.

sclerose /sklerōz'/, to harden or to cause hardening. –**sclerotic,** *adj.*

sclerosing solution, a liquid that causes inflammation in tissues. It may be used in burning out ulcers, in stopping bleeding, and in treating hemangiomas.

sclerosis /sklerō'-/, a condition with hardening of tissue resulting from any of several causes, including inflammation, the deposit of mineral salts, and damaged connective tissue fibers. –**sclerotic,** *adj.*

scoliosis /skō'lē·ō'-/. See **spinal curvature.**

scopolamine hydrobromide, a drug used to treat nausea and vomiting, as a sedative, and in eye operations. Some kinds of glaucoma, asthma, blocking of the intestines, severe ulcerative colitis, or known allergy to this drug prohibits its use. Side effects include blurred vision, central nervous system effects, a fast heart beat, dry mouth, decreased sweating, and allergic reactions.

scopophilia /skō'pəfil'yə/, **1.** sexual pleasure from looking at sexually exciting scenes or at another person's genitals; voyeurism. **2.** an unhealthy desire to be seen; exhibitionism.

scopophobia, an unhealthy fear of being seen or stared at by others. The condition is common in schizophrenia. See also **phobia.**

scorpion sting, a painful wound of a scorpion, a member of the spider family with a hollow stinger in its tail. The stings of many species are only slightly poisonous, but the sting of certain scorpions may lead to death, especially in small children. The first pain is followed within several hours by numbness, nausea, muscle spasm, shortness of breath, and convulsion. It is treated by putting ice on the wound. Severe cases require a doctor's care. An antivenin is available in some areas.

screening, 1. a beginning step, as a test or examination, to detect the most obvious sign of illness before further testing. **2.** testing a very large number of patients to find a certain disease, as high blood pressure.

scrotal cancer /skrō'təl/, a cancer of the scrotum. It begins as a small sore that may become an ulcer. The sore occurs most often in elderly men who have been exposed to soot, pitch, crude oil, mineral oils, or arsenic fumes from copper smelting. Treatment involves cutting out the tumor.

scrotum /skrō'təm/, the bag of skin that holds the testicles. In older men, in sick men, and in warm weather, the scrotum becomes long and floppy. The left side of the scrotum usually hangs lower than the right. See also **testis.** –**scrotal,** *adj.*

scurvy, a disease that is caused by a lack of vitamin C in the diet. Symptoms include weakness, anemia, edema, spongy gums, often with open sores in the mouth and loosening of the teeth, bleeding in the mucous membranes, and hard bumps of the muscles of the legs. **Infantile scurvy** most commonly occurs because cow's milk, unfortified with vitamin C, is the principal food in an infant's diet. Families are counseled to use a formula supplemented with this vitamin. A **scorbutic pose** is the typical posture of a child with scurvy, with thighs and legs half-bent and hips turned outward. The child usually lies still without moving the hands or feet because of the pain that any movement causes. Scurvy is treated and prevented by taking vitamin C and eating fresh vegetables and fruits.

seal limbs. See **phocomelia.**

sealed source, a radioactive source sealed in an impervious container that has sufficient mechanical strength to prevent contact with and dispersion of the radioactive material under the conditions of use and wear for which it was designed. Many sealed sources do not meet DOT special-form test criteria.

seasickness.   See **motion sickness.**

sea urchin sting,   an injury from any sea urchin in which the skin is pierced and, in some species, venom released. A poisonous sting features pain, muscular weakness, numbness around the mouth, and shortness of breath. The spines must be taken out at once, and a doctor's care may be needed. In all cases the broken spines cause local pain and irritation. Infection may result. See also **stingray.**

seawater bath,   a bath taken in warm seawater or in saline solution.

sebaceous /sibā′shəs/,   fatty, oily, or greasy, usually referring to the oil-secreting glands of the skin or to their secretions.

sebaceous cyst.   See **wen.**

sebaceous gland,   one of the many small saclike organs in the skin. They are found all through the body near all types of body hair but are especially in the scalp, the face, the anus, the nose, the mouth, and the external ear. They are not found in the palms of the hands and the soles of the feet.

seborrhea /seb′ôrē′ə/,   any of several common skin conditions in which there is too much grease (sebum) made that causes very oily skin or dry scales.

seborrheic dermatitis /-rē′ik/,   a common, long-term, inflammatory skin disease with dry or moist greasy scales and yellowish crusts. Common sites are the scalp, eyelids, face, outer surfaces of the ears, armpits, breasts, and groin. An example is **cradle cap,** a common condition of the head and face of infants. It consists of thick, yellow, greasy scales on the scalp. **Seborrheic blepharitis** is a form in which the eyelids are abnormally red and the edges are covered with a grainy crust. Seborrheic dermatitis is treated with special shampoos, creams, lotions, and drugs. See also **dandruff.**

sebum /sē′bəm/,   the oily secretion of the sebaceous glands of the skin, composed of keratin, fat, and cellular debris. Mixed with sweat, sebum forms a moist, oily, acidic film that is mildly harmful to bacteria and fungus and protects the skin against drying.

secobarbital,   a drug that is used to calm and put a patient to sleep.

Seconal,   a trademark for a drug used to calm and put a patient to sleep (secobarbital).

second opinion,   the patient's right to ask to be seen by another doctor so that the patient will get more knowledge about his or her health. It is most often used when the first doctor wants to operate on the patient's body.

secondary,   less important, second in order, or less well-developed.

secondary occlusal traumatism,   a strain caused by biting down so hard that it injures an already weak part of the gums that hold the teeth. The strain may not be too much for normal tissues but can be harmful to weakened areas.

secondary sex characteristic,   any of the visible bodily features of sexual maturity that develop as the patient grows older. These features include the growth of body hair and the development of the penis or breasts and the labia.

secondary survey,   patient interview, vital signs, and the physical examination performed after the primary survey.

secrete,   to release a substance into a cavity, vessel, or organ or onto the surface of the skin, as a gland.   −**secretion,** n.

secretin /sikrē′tin/,   a hormone made by the lining of the intestines that helps digest food. It also helps to make bile.

secretin test,   a test of the pancreas using the hormone, secretin. It is used to test for certain cancers and diseases of the pancreas.

section,   that organizational level having functional responsibility for primary segments of incident operations such as: operations, planning, logistics, finance. The section level is organizationally between branch and incident commander.

sector officers,   those individuals assigned by the incident commander to manage specific geographical areas or specific functions. They include the hazard sector officer and the safety officer.

secundigravida /səkun′dəgrav′idə/,   a woman who is pregnant for the second time. Also called **gravida 2.**   −**secundigravid,** adj.

secundipara /sek′əndip′ərə/,   a woman who has borne two live children in separate pregnancies.

security seal,   a seal or device, provided on a hazardous materials package, that enables one to easily determine whether the package has been opened.

sedation,   a drug-caused state of quiet, calmness, or sleep, as by means of a sedative or sleeping pill.

sedative,   a drug that slows down or calms the patient. Some sedatives affect the whole body and some affect one or two parts at a time. Barbiturates and nonbarbiturate sedatives, as chloral hydrate, and various minor tranquilizers, are used to bring sleep, ease pain, aid the giving of anesthesia, and treat convulsions, nervous attacks, and irritable bowel syndrome. See also **sedative-hypnotic.**

sedative bath,   putting the body in water for a very long time, used especially to calm excited patients.

sedative-hypnotic,   a drug that temporarily slows down the central nervous system, used mostly to bring sleep and to calm nervousness. It is used to treat a lack of sleep, nervous attacks, and convulsions and to help activate anes-

S

thesia. These drugs should be used carefully because they can become habit-forming. See also **barbiturate.**

segmental fracture, a bone break in which several large pieces of bone break away from the broken bone. If the ends of these pieces come through the skin, it is called an open fracture; if they stay inside of the skin, it is called a closed fracture.

segmental resection, an operation in which a part of an organ, gland, or other part of the body is cut out.

segmentation method, a method for filling tooth root canals in which a cone is cut into sections and the tip section sealed into the tip of a root. The other sections are usually warmed and pressed against the first piece with a plugger. More cone segments are then added until the canal is filled.

seizure. See **convulsion.**

seizure threshold, the amount of stimulus necessary to cause a seizure. All humans can have seizures if the stimulus is strong enough. Those who have sudden seizures for no apparent reason are said to have a ''low seizure threshold.''

selective inattention, ignoring something unpleasant on purpose.

selenium (Se), a metal-like element related to sulfur. It is found in very small amounts in food. Eating a very large amount over a long period of time may be harmful. It is used, in small amounts and mixed with other drugs, to treat dandruff and some other scalp diseases.

selenium sulfide, a drug used to kill fungus and to treat certain scalp diseases. Sudden inflammation of the scalp or known allergy to this drug prohibits its use. Side effects include dermatitis after long skin contact or keratitis after getting it in the eyes accidentally.

self-catheterization, a method done by a person to empty the bladder and prevent it from becoming overfilled with urine. The person who cannot empty the bladder completely but can retain urine for 2 to 4 hours at a time can usually be taught self-catheterization.

self-diagnosis, forming an opinion about one's own health or sickness without asking a doctor.

self-help group, a group of people who meet to talk together about health matters. Usually these groups are not led by a doctor or nurse. Compare **group therapy.**

self-limited, (of a disease or condition) tending to resolve without treatment.

Selsun, a trademark for a drug used to kill fungus and to treat certain scalp diseases (selenium sulfide), used as a shampoo.

semen /sē′mən/, the thick, whitish fluid released by the male sex organs that carries the sperm. Also called **seminal fluid, sperm.** –**seminal,** *adj.*

semicircular canal, any of three bony, fluid-filled loops inside the inner ear, involved in the sense of balance. See also **ear.**

semilunar valve, 1. a valve with half-moon-shaped cusps, as the aortic valve and the pulmonary valve. **2.** any one of the cusps forming such a valve. See also **heart valve.**

semimembranosus /sem′ēmem′brəno̅′səs/, one of three muscles at the back and inside of the thigh. It helps to bend the leg.

seminal duct /sem′inəl/, any tube through which semen passes, as the vas deferens or the ejaculatory duct.

seminal fluid test, any of several tests of semen to detect defects in the male sexual system and to determine fertility. Normal values in some of these tests are sperm count, 60 million to 150 million/ml of seminal fluid; pH, more than 7 (7.7 average); ejaculation volume, 1.5 to 5.0 ml; motility, 60% of sperm.

seminal vesicle, either of the paired, saclike glands that lie behind the bladder in the male and act as part of the reproductive system. The seminal vesicles release a fluid that forms part of semen.

semination, the introduction of semen into the female genital tract.

seminiferous /sem′inif′ərəs/, carrying or releasing semen, as the tubules of the testicles.

seminoma /-no̅′mə/, the most common cancer of the testicles. See also **testicular cancer.**

semipermeable membrane /-pur′mē·əbəl/, a membrane that allows certain substances to pass through, but does not allow others, depending on the size of the atoms.

semitendinosus /-ten′dino̅′səs/, one of three muscles on the back of the thigh that help to move the leg.

senescent /sines′ənt/, aging or growing old. See also **senile.** –**senescence,** *n.*

Sengstaken-Blakemore tube, a thick catheter with three tubes and two balloons, used to stop bleeding in the throat. Attached to a tube, one balloon is blown up in the stomach and exerts pressure against the upper opening. Similarly attached, another longer and narrower balloon exerts pressure on the walls of the throat. The third tube is used for removing the contents of the stomach.

senile, relating to or characteristic of old age or the process of aging, especially the wasting of the mind and body that come with aging. See also **aging.**

senile involution, a pattern of steady shrinking and breakdown in tissues and organs that come in old age.

senile psychosis, a mental disorder of the aged that is caused by a shrinking of the brain. It is not known why this happens. Symptoms include loss of memory, not being able to think clearly, and periods of confusion and irritability, all of which may be more or less serious. It is more common in women than men. There is no known cure.

senopia /senō′pē·ə/, an eye condition in which the hardening of the lenses causes the eyes to focus better on things nearby. It is linked with a disorder (lenticular nuclear sclerosis) that commonly leads to the development of cataracts.

sensation, 1. a feeling, impression, or awareness of a bodily state or condition that occurs whenever a nerve is excited and sends a signal to the brain. A **deep sensation** is the awareness of pain, pressure, or tension in the deep layers of the skin, muscles, or joints. These sensations are carried to the brain by way of the spinal cord. A **delayed sensation** is not felt until sometime after the cause has stopped. An **epigastric sensation** is a weak, sinking feeling of unclear cause. It is most often centered in the pit of the stomach but may occur elsewhere in the belly. A **primary sensation** comes directly from something (stimulus) that causes the sensation. A **referred sensation** is felt at a place other than where the action occurs. A **subjective sensation** is a feeling that is not linked with or is not directly caused by something outside of the body. **Superficial sensation** refers to what is felt in the surface layers of the skin in response to touch, pressure, temperature, and pain. 2. a feeling of a mental or emotional state, which may or may not be caused by something outside of the body.

sense, 1. the ability or structure that allows events both inside and outside of the body to be felt and understood. The major senses are sight, hearing, smell, taste, touch, and pressure. Other senses include hunger, thirst, pain, temperature, ability to feel the muscles move, space, time, and being able to tell when the stomach, bladder, and bowel are full or empty. 2. the ability to feel; a sensation. 3. normal mental ability. 4. to perceive through a sense organ.

sensitivity, 1. ability to feel, transmit, or react to a stimulus. 2. allergy to a substance, as a drug or an antigen. See also **allergy, hypersensitivity.** –**sensitive,** *adj.*

sensitization, an acquired reaction in which specific antibodies develop in response to an antigen. This is done on purpose in vaccination by injecting a disease-causing organism that has been changed so that it is no longer infectious. It remains able to cause the making of antibodies to fight the disease. Allergic reactions are sensitization reactions that result from excess sensitization to a foreign protein.

sensitized, referring to tissues that have been made susceptible to antigenic substances. See also **allergy.**

sensory deprivation, an unwilling loss of bodily awareness caused by being shut off from outside for a very long time. It can cause panic, confusion, depression, and hallu-

cinations. It may be linked with various handicaps and conditions, as blindness, heavy sedation, and long isolation.

sensory nerve, a nerve that carries sense signals from the parts of the body to the brain or spinal chord. Compare **motor nerve.**

sensory-perceptual overload, a state in which the loudness and strength of numerous sensations go beyond the ability of the patient to sort them out.

separator, a tool used to hold teeth apart when the dentist needs to work between two teeth.

sepsis /sep′sis/, infection. –**septic,** *adj.*

septal defect /sep′təl/, an abnormal defect usually present at birth in the wall (septum) separating two chambers of the heart. **Atrial septal defect (ASD)** is a birth defect with a hole in the septum between the two upper heart chambers (atria). The severity of the condition depends on the size and location of the hole. Atrial septal defects cause an increased flow of blood containing oxygen into the right side of the heart. Surgery can close the hole in most cases. Unless the defect is severe it is usually not done until later childhood to prevent problems. A **ventricular septal defect (VSD)** is a hole in the septum separating the ventricles, permitting blood to flow from the left ventricle to the right ventricle and to recirculate through the pulmonary artery and lungs. It is the most common heart defect, present at birth. Treatment consists of surgical repair of the defect, preferably in early childhood.

septate /sep′tāt/, relating to a structure divided by a septum.

septicemia /sep′tisē′mē·ə/. See **blood poisoning.**

septic shock. See **shock.**

septostomy /septos′-/, an operation to make a hole in a septum.

Septra, a trademark for a drug used to kill bacteria.

septum /sep′təm/, *pl.* **septa,** a dividing wall, as found separating the chambers of the heart. The **nasal septum** is the wall dividing the nostrils. It is made up of bone and cartilage covered by mucous membrane.

sequester /sikwes′tər/, to keep apart, or away from others, as a patient sequestered to prevent the spread of an infection.

sequestrum /sikwes′trəm/, *pl.* **sequestra,** a fragment of dead bone that is partly or totally broken free from the nearby healthy bone. **Primary sequestrum** refers to a piece of dead bone that totally breaks free. **Secondary sequestrum** refers to a piece that partly comes away from healthy bone in the course of some diseases, but can be pushed back into place.

sequoiasis /sikwoi′əsis/, a type of pneumonia common among workers in redwood sawmills. It is caused by a fungus in the sawdust. Symptoms include chills, fever,

S

cough, shortness of breath, loss of appetite, nausea, and vomiting.

Ser-Ap-Es, a trademark for drug used to treat high blood pressure.

Serax, a trademark for a tranquilizer (oxazepam).

Serentil, a trademark for a phenothiazine tranquilizer (mesoridazine).

serial extraction, the pulling out of certain baby teeth over a number of years, to prevent crowding when the permanent teeth grow in.

serine (Ser) /ser′ēn/, an amino acid found in many proteins in the body.

Seromycin, a trademark for a drug to treat tuberculosis (cycloserine).

serotonin /ser′ətō′nin, sir′-/, a substance found naturally in the brain and intestines. Serotonin is released from certain cells when the blood vessel walls are damaged. It acts as a strong vessel-narrowing substance.

serous fluid /sir′əs/, a thin watery liquid.

serous membrane, one of the many thin sheets of tissue that line certain areas inside the body, as the sac that surrounds the heart. Between the inner layer of serous membrane covering various organs and the outer layer of the organ itself is a space kept wet by serous fluid. The fluid allows the covered organ to move easily, as the lungs, which move in breathing. Compare **mucous membrane, skin, synovial membrane.**

Serpasil, a trademark for a high blood pressure drug (reserpine).

Serpasil-Apresoline, a trademark for a drug containing two high blood pressure medicines (reserpine and hydralazine hydrochloride).

Serpasil-Esidrix, a trademark for a high blood pressure drug containing a diuretic (hydrochlorothiazide) and an antihypertensive (reserpine).

serratus anterior /serā′təs/, a thin muscle of the chest wall stretching from the ribs under the arm to the shoulder blade. It moves to raise the shoulder and arm.

serum /sir′əm/, **1.** also called **blood serum.** any thin, watery fluid, especially one that keeps serous membranes wet. **2.** any clear, watery fluid that has been separated from its more solid elements, as the liquid from a blister. **3.** the clear, thin, and sticky liquid part of the blood that remains after clotting. **4.** a vaccine made from the serum of a patient who has had some disease and used to protect another patient against that same infection or poison.

serum albumin, an important substance found in the blood. It is needed to help control blood pressure. See also **normal human serum albumin.**

serum glutamic oxaloacetic transaminase (SGOT), an enzyme found in various parts of the body, especially the heart, liver, and muscle tissue. The body makes more of it when there has been some cell damage.

serum glutamic pyruvic transaminase (SGPT), an enzyme normally found in large amounts in the liver. Having much more of it than normal in the blood is a sign of liver damage.

serum sickness, a sickness that may occur 2 to 3 weeks after being given an antiserum. It is caused by a reaction to the donor serum. Symptoms include fever, a swollen spleen, swollen lymph nodes, skin rash, and joint pain. Treatment may include the use of steroids. See also **antiserum.**

sesamoid bone /ses′əmoid/, any one of numerous small, round bones buried in certain tendons that go through much stress and strain. The largest is the kneecap.

severe combined immunodeficiency disease (SCID), an illness marked by the total or partial lack of certain cells in the body fluids that fight infection. It is a disease of the genes. It is usually fatal. Its cause is not yet known.

sex, 1. a division of male or female based on many features, as body parts and genetic differences. Compare **gender. 2.** sexual intercourse.

sex chromosome, a chromosome that is responsible for the sex determination of offspring; it carries genes that transmit sex-linked traits and conditions. In humans and mammals there are two distinct sex chromosomes, the X and the Y chromosomes, which are unequally paired and appear in females in the XX combination and in males as XY. Compare **autosome.**

sex-linked disorder, any disease or abnormal condition that is caused by a defect in the genes.

sexual abuse, taking advantage of another person by fondling, rape, or forcing another to take part in unnatural sex acts or other perverted behavior. When children are victims, they tend to get a harmful feeling of loss of control of themselves.

sexual dysfunction, a sex-related difficulty. It may be a physical or mental problem. **Female sexual dysfunction** is an inability of a woman to have or enjoy satisfactory sexual intercourse and orgasm. Symptoms include pain, spasms, a complete inability to reach orgasm, and being unable to be aroused sexually. Causes include anxiety, fear, and negative feelings about sexual arousal and intercourse. **Male sexual dysfunction** is an inability of a man to carry on his sex life to his own satisfaction. Symptoms include difficulties in starting and maintaining an erection, ejaculating too soon, inability to ejaculate, and loss of desire. Men are often ashamed of the problem and ask the physician to treat a ''prostate problem.'' See also **impotence, premature ejaculation.**

sexual harassment, any bothersome act of a sexual nature, including sexual talk, committed by someone in power, as a boss or supervisor. Sexual harassment on the job is against the law. Sexual harassment may involve a man and a woman, two men, or two women.

sexual history, (in a patient record) the part of the patient's personal history concerned with sexual activity. A sexual history is very important for deciding the proper treatment of a disease of the reproduction system or sexual difficulties, or for contraception, abortion, or sterilization. The extent of the history varies with the patient's age, condition, and the reason for securing the history.

sexual intercourse. See **coitus.**

sexuality, 1. all of the physical, functional, and mental traits that are shown by one's sex identity and sex behavior. **2.** the genital organs that tell apart males from females.

sexually deviant personality, a sexual behavior that differs a great amount from what is considered normal for a society.

sexually transmitted disease (STD), a contagious disease usually caught by sexual intercourse or genital contact. These diseases are quite common. Some kinds are gonorrhea, syphilis, scabies, herpes genitalis, trichomoniasis, genital candidiasis, chlamydial infections, and AIDS. Also called **venereal disease.** See also specific entry.

sexual psychopath, an individual whose sexual behavior is openly perverted, antisocial, and criminal. See also **antisocial personality disorder.**

sexual reassignment, a sex change.

shallow breathing, a kind of breathing that is slow, shallow, and usually not very useful. It is usually caused by drugs.

sheath, a tubelike structure that surrounds an organ or any other part of the body, as the sheath of the rectus abdominis muscle or the sheath of Schwann, which covers various nerve fibers.

Sheehan's syndrome, a condition occurring after giving birth in which the pituitary gland is damaged. It is caused by a lessening of blood circulation after bleeding of the womb.

sheep cell test, a method that mixes human blood cells with the red blood cells of sheep. It is used to diagnose several diseases, as DiGeorge's syndrome.

sheet bath, applying of wet sheets to the body, used mainly to treat burns.

shellfish poisoning, an illness caused by eating clams, oysters, or mussels that are tainted with the parasite known as the "red tide." The symptoms appear within a few minutes and include nausea, lightheadedness, vomiting, and tingling or numbness around the mouth, followed by paralysis of the hands and feet and, possibly, the inability to breathe. The poison is not destroyed by cooking; however, the illness is less serious if the water used in cooking

is not eaten or drunk. It is treated with drugs after breathing has been restored. **Vibrio parahaemolyticus** is a species of microorganism of the genus *Vibrio,* the cause of food poisoning linked with the eating of uncooked or undercooked shellfish, especially crabs and shrimp. Thorough cooking of seafood prevents the infection linked with *Vibrio,* which causes watery diarrhea, stomach cramps, vomiting, headache, chills, and fever.

shell shock. See **stress reaction.**

shell teeth, a type of tooth disease in which the teeth are not formed properly.

shield, anything used to prevent or reduce the passage of radiation. A shield may be a mound of earth, a vehicle, a building, etc. Generally dense materials such as lead, steel, or concrete make the best shields.

shigellosis /shig′əlō′-/, a serious infection of the bowel marked by diarrhea, stomach pain, and fever, that is carried by hand-to-mouth contact with the feces of infected individuals. The disease occurs only rarely in the United States but is native to underdeveloped areas of the world. It is treated with drugs. Shigellosis infections must be reported to the public health department. Also called **bacillary dysentery.**

shin bone. See **tibia.**

shingles. See **herpes zoster.**

shin splints, a painful condition of the lower leg caused by strain after very hard exercise, as running. It often results from a lack of proper training. Treatment usually involves rest and exercise therapy. Surgery is sometimes necessary.

shipping name, the proper shipping name or other common name for a hazardous material; also any synonyms for the hazardous material.

shipping package warning label, a special label affixed to a package of hazardous material to identify the package contents. DOT regulations **shipping papers** or **documents,** forms containing a description of the materials being transported. These papers must accompany all shipments of radioactive material.

Shirodkar's operation /shir′odkärz′/, an operation done to repair a damaged or defective cervix. It allows a pregnancy to develop normally.

shock, a serious state of collapse that occurs when not enough blood flows through the body causing very low blood pressure, a lack of urine, and dangerous cell disorders. The signs and symptoms of different kinds of shock are very much alike. The pulse and breathing become faster. The person may appear to be very nervous, with weakness, low body temperature, pale skin, and cold sweat. Shock may be caused by a heart problem, changes in the blood vessels, or an injury. Other causes are bleeding, vomiting, diarrhea, not drinking enough liquid, or improp-

S

er action of the kidneys. **Primary shock** is a state of physical collapse very like fainting. It may be caused by pain or fright. Primary shock is often mild, and will go away by itself in a short time. Severe injury may make the shock last longer and merge primary shock with secondary shock. **Secondary shock** is caused by many types of serious injury or disease. Blood pressure drops and death may occur in a fairly short time unless proper treatment is given. Secondary shock is often linked with heatstroke, crushing injuries, heart attacks, poisoning, very serious infections, burns, and other life-threatening conditions. **Hemorrhagic shock** often occurs with secondary shock from a sudden, rapid loss of large amounts of blood. Severe injuries often cause such blood losses, which, in turn, produce low blood pressure. **Hypovolemic shock** is caused by massive blood loss, circulatory failure, and too little blood to the tissues. The loss of about one fifth of total blood volume in the affected person can produce this condition. Disorders that may cause hypovolemic shock are fluid loss from too much sweat, severe diarrhea, long-term vomiting, intestinal blockage, inflammations in the belly, and severe burns. Severe kidney or brain damage may result. Treatment includes replacing blood and fluid volumes, and the control of bleeding. Death occurs within a relatively short time unless treatment is quickly given to restore normal blood volume. A form of shock caused when the heart fails to supply enough blood to the body is called **cardiogenic shock.** It is linked with heart attack (myocardial infarction) and heart failure. Cardiogenic shock is an emergency that needs quick treatment. It is deadly about 80% of the time. Treatment may include giving fluids in the vein, or drugs. Devices, as pacing catheters, are also used. **Septic shock** occurs in blood poisoning (septicemia). Symptoms include fever, rapid heart beat, fast breathing, and confusion or coma. Septic shock usually follows signs of severe infection, often in the urinary system or in the intestines. **Speed shock** is a side effect to shots or drugs that are given too quickly. Signs include a flushed face, headache, a tight feeling in the chest, uneven pulse, loss of consciousness, and heart attack. **Spinal shock** is linked with serious injury to the spinal cord. **Neurogenic shock** is a form of shock from blood vessels widening in the arms and legs as a result of damage in the nervous system. **Vasogenic shock** results from blood vessels widening from factors that directly affect them, such as poisons. See also **anaphylactic shock, electric shock, insulin shock.**

shock trousers, a pair of trousers that can be filled with air that put pressure on the legs to treat shock and very low blood pressure.

short-acting, referring to a drug that begins to take effect very soon after being taken by the patient.

shoulder, the place where the collarbone and the shoulder blade meet and where the arm attaches to the trunk of the body.

shoulder blade, one of the pair of large, flat, three-sided bones that form the back of the shoulder. Also called **scapula.**

shoulder-hand syndrome, a disorder of the nerves and bones that occurs most commonly after a heart attack but may be linked with other problems. Symptoms include pain and stiffness in the shoulder and arm, limited joint motion, swelling of the hand, muscle wasting, and a loss of calcium from the underlying bones.

shoulder joint, the ball and socket joint of the humerus and the shoulder blade. Also called **humeral articulation.**

shreds, very shiny little threads of mucus in the urine, showing an infection in the urinary tract. Also called **mucous shreds.**

shunt, 1. to reroute the flow of a body fluid from one place to another. **2.** a tube or device put into the body to redirect a body fluid from one place to another. An **external shunt** is a tube or series of containers that passes over the surface of the body. Various shunts are put in to drain excess cerebrospinal fluid from the brain in hydrocephalus. A **ventriculoatrial shunt** is put in between the brain (cerebral ventricle) and the right atrium of the heart. A **ventriculoperitoneal shunt** is placed between a cerebral ventricle and the abdomen. A **ventriculopleural shunt** diverts spinal fluid from enlarged ventricles into the chest, usually in the newborn.

Shy-Drager syndrome, a rare, gradual nerve disorder of young and middle-aged adults. Symptoms include very low blood pressure, no bladder or bowel control, trembling, stiffness, lack of coordination, and muscle wasting. Treatment includes drugs to control the muscles and blood pressure.

sialogogue /sī·al′əgog/, anything that causes saliva to be released.

sialography /sī′·əlog′rəfē/, a method in making x-ray pictures in which a salivary gland is filmed after a dye is injected into its duct.

sialolith /sī·al′əlith/, a small stone formed in a salivary gland or duct.

sialorrhea /sī·al′ôrē′ə/, a flow of too much saliva that may be linked with a number of conditions, as acute inflammation of the mouth, mental retardation, mercury poisoning, pregnancy, teething, alcoholism, or malnutrition. Also called **hypersalivation, ptyalism.**

Siamese twins. See **twin.**

Siblin, a trademark for a bulk laxative containing psyllium seed.

sickle cell, an abnormal, crescent-shaped red blood cell typical of sickle cell anemia.

sickle cell anemia, a serious, long-term, incurable blood disease. It attacks the red blood cells and results in joint pain, blood clots, fever, and long-term anemia, with enlargement of the spleen, lack of energy, and weakness. A **sickle cell crisis** is a serious, short attack that occurs in children with sickle cell anemia. The most common form is a painful closing of the blood vessels. It is linked with an infection in the lungs or throat or in the intestines. Typical symptoms are acute stomach pain, painful swelling of the soft tissue of the hands and feet (hand-foot syndrome), and joint pain, often so severe that movement of the joint is limited. Persistent headache, dizziness, convulsions, visual or auditory disturbances, facial nerve palsies, coughing, shortness of breath, and rapid breathing may occur if the central nervous system or lungs are affected. A common problem of young children with sickle cell anemia is the high risk of infection that may be greatly increased during periods of crisis. **Sickle cell trait** is a form without anemia. People who have the trait are told of it and advised of the possibility of having an infant with sickle cell disease if both parents have the trait.

sickle cell thalassemia, a blood disorder in which the genes for sickle cell and for thalassemia are both inherited. See also **thalassemia.**

sick sinus syndrome, a group of disorders linked with problems in a part (sinus node) of the heart. The condition may be caused by several types of heart disease. The most common symptoms are weakness, lightheadedness, dizziness, and episodes of near fainting to actual loss of consciousness. At present the only treatment is by implanting a pacemaker.

side effect, any reaction that results from a medication or therapy. Usually, although not necessarily, the effect is not wanted. Such reactions may be nausea, dry mouth, dizziness, blood disorders, blurred vision, discolored urine, or a ringing or roaring in the ears.

sideroblastic anemia /sid′ərōblas′-/, any one of a group of long-term blood disorders. It affects the red blood cells. The cause of the disease is not known. Treatment may include extract of liver, pyridoxine, folic acid, and blood transfusion. See also **anemia.**

siderosis /sid′ərō′-/, **1.** a type of lung disease caused by the inhalation of iron dust or particles. **2.** an increase in the amounts of iron in the blood.

sight, 1. the sense of vision. It is the major function of the eye. **2.** that which is seen.

sigmoid /sig′moid/, **1.** relating to an **S** shape. **2.** the sigmoid colon. See also **colon.**

sigmoidectomy /sig′moidek′-/, cutting out the sigmoid bend of the colon, most commonly done to remove a can-cerous tumor. Most cancers of the lower bowel occur in the sigmoid colon.

sigmoid mesocolon, a fold of membrane that connects the sigmoid colon to the pelvic wall.

sigmoidoscope /-dos′kəpē/, an instrument used to examine the sigmoid colon. It consists of a tube and a light, allowing the mucous membrane lining the colon to be looked at.

sign, something seen by an examiner, as a fever, a rash, or the sound heard in the chest in lung disease. Many signs go along with symptoms, as bumps and rashes are often seen when a patient complains of itching. See also **symptom.**

silicosis /sil′ikō′-/, a lung disorder caused by inhaling silicon dioxide over a long period of time. Silicon dioxide is found in sands, quartzes, flints, and many other stones. Small fiberlike growths develop in the lungs. In advanced cases, there may be severe shortness of breath. Silicosis occurs among industrial workers exposed to silica powder in manufacturing processes.

Silvadene, a trademark for a drug that kills bacteria (sulfadiazine silver).

silver (Ag), a whitish precious metal used in certain medications and, blended together with other metals, to fill teeth.

silver cone method, a method for filling tooth root canals. A small silver cone is sealed into the tip of a root canal, and any canal space that is left is filled with another sealer.

Silver dwarf, a person who has **Silver's syndrome,** a disorder present at birth in which short stature is linked with each side of the body being a different size, numerous deformities of the head, face, and skeleton, and early puberty.

Silverman-Anderson score, a system for rating the amount of difficulty in breathing.

silver salts poisoning, a poisonous condition caused by swallowing silver nitrate. Symptoms include discoloration of the lips, vomiting, stomach pain, dizziness, and convulsions. Treatment includes rinsing the stomach with salt water, followed by soothing fluids. Treatment of convulsions and low blood pressure may also be needed.

silver sulfadiazine, a drug used on the skin to prevent or treat infection in second- and third-degree burns. Known allergy to this drug, to silver, or to sulfonamides prohibits its use. It is not given in the last weeks of pregnancy or to newborn or premature infants. Side effects include rashes, fungal infections, and some blood disorders.

simethicone, a drug used to prevent the patient from passing gas. It is used to reduce excess gas in the stomach and intestines. Side effects include belching and rectal flatus.

simian crease /sim′ē·ən/, a single crease across the palm from the joining of the front and back creases of the palm,

S

seen in birth defects, as Down's syndrome. Also called **simian line.**

Similac preparations, a trademark for a group of commercial milk products that are prepared especially for infant feeding. The formulas are packaged in both powder and liquid form.

sinciput /sin′sipət/, the upper half of the head.

Sinemet, a trademark for a central nervous system drug.

Sinequan, a trademark for an antidepression drug (doxepin hydrochloride).

sinew, the tendon of a muscle. See also **tendon.**

sinoatrial block /sī′nō·ā′trē·əl/. See **heart block.**

sinoatrial (SA) node, a cluster of hundreds of cells in the heart. It generates nerve signals that cause the heart to beat. Implanting an artificial pacemaker is a common operation for individuals suffering from a defective sinoatrial node. More than 150,000 persons are leading active lives with permanently implanted devices.

sinus /sī′nəs/. See **nasal sinus.**

sinusitis /sī′nəsī′-/, inflammation of one or more nasal sinuses. It may be a complication of an upper respiratory infection, dental infection, allergy, a change in atmosphere, as in air travel or underwater swimming, or a defect of the nose. With swelling of nasal mucous membranes the openings from sinuses to the nose may be blocked, causing pressure, pain, headache, fever, and local tenderness. Complications include spread of infection to bone, brain, or meninges. Treatment includes steam inhalations, nasal decongestants, analgesics, and, if infection is present, antibiotics. Surgery to improve drainage may be done to treat chronic sinusitis.

sinus node, an area of special heart tissue that generates the cardiac electric impulse and is in turn controlled by the autonomic nervous system. Also called **sinus pacemaker.**

Sippy diet, a very limited diet for peptic ulcer patients. It consists of hourly servings of milk and cream for several days, with the gradual addition of eggs, refined cereals, pureéd vegetables, crackers, and other simple foods until the regular bland diet is reached. Because the diet limits all fresh vegetables and fruits, additional iron and vitamins should be used to prevent deficiency.

sirenomelia /sī′rənomē′lyə/, a birth defect in which both legs have grown together and there are no feet.

Sister Kenny's treatment, a polio treatment in which the patient's limbs and back are wrapped in warm, moist woolen cloths and, after the pain goes away, the patient is taught to exercise affected muscles, especially by swimming. Equally important is passive movement of affected limbs while massaging the muscles at the same time, carried out after hot packs.

SITSTAT, an acronym for the situation unit. A unit within the planning section.

situs /sī′təs/, the normal position or location of an organ or part of the body.

sitz bath /sits/, literally (German) "seat" bath, a bath in which only the hips and buttocks are soaked in water or saline solution. The procedure is used for patients who have had surgery in the area of the rectum. Also called **hip bath.**

SI units, the international units of physical amounts. Examples of these units are the volume of a liter, the length of a meter, or the precise amount of time in a minute. A group of scientists (Comité International des Poids et Mesures) meets regularly to define the units.

Sjögren-Larsson syndrome /shō′grenlär′sən/, a condition present at birth, marked by dry, scaly skin, mental deficiency, and spastic paralysis.

SK-Ampicillin, a trademark for an antibacterial drug (ampicillin).

SK-Bamate, a trademark for a sedative (meprobamate).

skeletal fixation, any method of holding together the fragments of a broken bone by the attaching of wires, screws, plates, or nails. See also **external pin fixation.**

skeletal system, all of the bones and cartilage of the body that provide the framework for the muscles and organs.

skeleton, the supporting frame for the body. It has 206 bones that protect delicate structures, provide attachments for muscles, allow body movement, serve as major reservoirs of blood, and produce red blood cells. See also **bone.**

Skene's glands /skēnz/, the largest of the glands that open into the urethra of women.

skilled nursing facility (SNF), an institution or part of an institution that meets guidelines for accreditation set by the sections of the Social Security Act that determine the basis for Medicaid and Medicare payments for skilled nursing care, including rehabilitation and various medical and nursing procedures. It is required by law that the care of every patient be under the supervision of a physician, that a physician be available on an emergency basis, that records be kept regarding the condition and care of every patient, that nursing service be available 24 hours a day, and that at least one full-time registered nurse be employed.

Skillern's fracture, an open fracture of the thumb (distal radius) linked with a greenstick break.

skimmed milk, milk from which the fat has been removed. Most of the vitamin A is removed with the cream, although all other nutrients remain. It appears as fluid skimmed milk, fortified skimmed milk, nonfat dry milk, and a form of buttermilk. Also called **nonfat milk, skim milk.**

skin, the tough, supple membrane that covers the entire surface of the body. It is the largest organ of the body and is composed of five layers of cells. Each layer is named for its unique function, texture, or position. The deepest layer is the **stratum basale.** It anchors the more superficial layers to the underlying tissues, and it provides new cells to replace the cells lost by abrasion from the outermost layer. The cells of each layer move upward as they mature. Above the stratum basale lies the **stratum spinosum.** The cells in this layer have tiny spines on their surfaces. As the cells move to the next layer, the **stratum granulosum,** they become flat, lying parallel with the surface of the skin. Over this layer lies a clear, thin band of tissue called the **stratum lucidum.** The boundaries of the cells are not visible in this layer. The outermost layer, the **stratum corneum,** is made up of scaly plaques of dead cells that contain keratin. This horny layer is thick over areas of the body subject to abrasion, as the palms of the hands, and thin over other more protected areas. The color of the skin varies according to the amount of melanin in the epidermis. Genetic differences determine the amount of melanin. The skin helps to cool the body when the temperature rises by radiating the heat flow in widened blood vessels and by providing a surface for the evaporation of sweat. When the temperature drops, the blood vessels narrow, and the production of sweat lessens. Also called **cutaneous membrane, integument.**

skin absorption, the introduction of a chemical or toxic product into the body by way of the skin. Skin absorption can occur with no sensation to the skin itself. Pain or irritation are not always present as warning signs of absorption. Some poisons are so concentrated that a few drops placed on the skin may result in death. Skin absorption is enhanced by abrasions, cuts, heat, and moisture. This can create critical problems when working at incidents involving biological and etiological agents. Anyone with open cuts or abrasions should be absolutely prohibited from working in areas where they may be exposed.

skin cancer, a cancer of the skin caused by contact with various chemical substances or by too much exposure to the sun or other sources of ultraviolet light. Skin cancers, the most common and most curable cancers, are also the most frequent secondary lesions in patients with cancer in other sites. Risk factors are a fair complexion, xeroderma pigmentosa, vitiligo, senile and seborrheic keratitis, Bowen's disease, radiation dermatitis, and hereditary basal cell nevus syndrome. The most common skin cancers are basal cell carcinomas and squamous cell carcinomas. A certain diagnosis may be made by cutting the cancer out, which may be the only treatment needed for small lesions. Surgery is usually used if the lesion is large, if bone or cartilage is invaded, or if lymph nodes are involved. Radiother-

apy may also be used. Despite the curability of skin cancer it causes many deaths because people fail to obtain treatment.

skinfold calipers, an instrument used to measure the width of a fold of skin, usually on the back of the upper arm or over the lower ribs of the chest.

skin graft, a portion of skin implanted to cover areas where skin has been lost through burns or injury or by surgical removal of diseased tissue. To prevent tissue rejection of permanent grafts, the graft is taken from the patient's own body or from the body of an identical twin. Skin from another person or animal can be used as a short-term cover for large burned areas to lessen fluid loss.

skin prep, a method of cleaning the skin with an antiseptic before surgery or injecting a fluid into a vein. Skin preps are done to kill bacteria and germs and to reduce the risk of infection. Various skin prep devices may be used.

skin tag, a small brown or "flesh"-colored loose lump of skin, occurring most often on the neck of an older person. Also called **cutaneous papilloma.**

skin test, a test to determine the reaction of the body to a substance by watching what happens when a certain substance is injected into the skin or is wiped on the skin. Skin tests are used to detect allergies and to diagnose disease. Kinds of skin tests include **Schick test** and **tuberculin test.** See also **allergy testing.**

SK-Penicillin VK, a trademark for an antibacteria drug (penicillin V potassium).

SK-Pramine, a trademark for an antidepression drug (imipramine hydrochloride).

SK-65 Compound, a trademark for a drug containing painkillers (propoxyphene hydrochloride, aspirin, and phenacetin) and a stimulant (caffeine).

SK-Tetracycline, a trademark for an antibiotic (tetracycline).

skull, the bony structure of the head, consisting of the skull (cranium) and the skeleton of the face. The cranium, which holds and protects the brain, consists of eight bones. The skeleton of the face has 14 bones. The base of the skull is the floor of the skull to which the spine attaches. The **calvaria** is the skull cap or upper, domelike part of the skull.

sleep, a state marked by lessened consciousness, lessened movement of the skeletal muscles, and slowed-down metabolism. People normally sleep in patterns that follow four definite, gradual stages. These four stages make up three fourths of a period of typical sleep and are called, as a group, **non-rapid eye movement (NREM)** sleep. The remaining time is usually occupied with **rapid eye movement (REM)** sleep. The REM sleep periods, lasting from a few minutes to half an hour, alternate with the NREM peri-

S

ods. Dreaming occurs during REM time. Individual sleep patterns change throughout life because daily needs for sleep gradually diminish from as much as 20 hours a day in infancy to as little as 6 hours a day in old age. Infants tend to begin a sleep period with REM sleep, whereas REM activity usually follows the four stages of NREM sleep in adults.

sleeping pill, 1. a sedative taken for insomnia or for sedation after an operation. **2.** an over-the-counter pill, sold as an aid to sleeping. Any drugs that slow down the central nervous system should not be used by pregnant or breast feeding women or by patients with asthma or glaucoma.

sleep terror disorder, a condition occurring during sleep that features repeated episodes of waking up suddenly, usually with a panicky scream, accompanied by intense fear, confusion, agitation, jerking arms or legs, and total amnesia concerning the event. The disorder is usually seen in children, is more common in boys than in girls, and is not at all regular but is more likely to occur if the individual is very tired or under stress or has been given a tricyclic antidepressant or neuroleptic at bedtime. When the condition occurs during a daytime nap, it is called **pavor diurnus. Pavor nocturnus** occurs in children during night sleep. See also **nightmare.**

sleepwalking, a condition occurring during sleep that features moving parts of the body, usually ending up by leaving the bed and walking about, with no memory of the event upon waking up. The episodes, which usually last from several minutes to half an hour or longer, are seen mostly in children, more often in boys than in girls, and are more likely to occur if the person is very tired or under stress or has taken a sedative at bedtime. Seizure disorders, central nervous system infections, and injury may be part of the cause, but the condition is more often related to fear and nervousness. In adults, the condition is less common. Also called **somnambulism.**

sling, a bandage or device used to hold an injured part of the body.

slipped disk. See **herniated disk.**

Slo-Phyllin, a trademark for a bronchodilator (theophylline).

slough /sluf/, **1.** to shed or cast off dead tissue cells of the uterus, which are shed during menstruation. **2.** the tissue that has been shed.

Slow-K, a trademark for a slow-release tablet of an electrolyte replacement (potassium chloride).

slow virus, a virus that remains inactive in the body after first infection. Years may go by before symptoms occur. Several wasting diseases of the central nervous system are believed to be caused by slow viruses.

SMA, a trademark for a food supplement for infants.

small cardiac vein, one of five tiny veins within the heart. Also called **right coronary vein.**

small intestine. See **intestine.**

smallpox, a highly contagious virus-caused disease marked by fever, prostation, and a blisterlike rash. It is caused by one of two species of poxvirus, variola major or variola minor (**alastrim**). Alastrim is a mild form of smallpox. Because human beings are the only carrier for the virus, worldwide vaccination with vaccinia, a related poxvirus, has been effective in wiping out smallpox. For several years no natural case of the disease has been known to occur. Also called **variola.**

smegma /smeg′mə/, a substance released by sebaceous glands, especially the cheesy, foul-smelling secretion often found under the foreskin of the penis and at the base of the labia minora near the glans clitoris.

smell, 1. the special sense that allows odors to be perceived. **2.** any odor, pleasant or unpleasant.

Smith fracture, a broken wrist; a reverse Colles' fracture.

smoke diver, highly trained user of an SCBA.

smoke inhalation, the breathing in of noxious fumes or irritating dust that may cause severe lung damage. Lung disease, suffocation, and serious injury to the lungs and throat may occur. Symptoms include irritation of the throat and lungs, singed nasal hairs, shortness of breath, a lack of oxygen, dusty gray spittle, wheezing, noisy breathing, restlessness, nervousness, cough, and hoarseness. Fluid in the lungs may develop up to 48 hours after exposure.

smooth muscle. See **muscle.**

snakebite, a wound resulting from piercing of the flesh by the fangs of a snake. Bites by snakes known to be nonpoisonous are treated as puncture wounds; those produced by an unknown or poisonous snake need immediate attention.

sneeze, a sudden, forceful, involuntary burst of air through the nose and mouth occurring as a result of irritation to the mucous membranes of the throat, as by dust, pollen, or virus infection.

Snellen test, a vision test using a **Snellen chart.** Letters, numbers, or symbols are arranged on the chart, large on top and getting smaller toward the bottom. The person being tested stands 20 feet from the chart and reads as many of the symbols as possible, reading each line and proceeding downward from the top. A score is assigned. A person who can read what the average person can read at 20 feet has 20/20 vision.

snout reflex, an abnormal response caused by tapping the nose, resulting in a marked facial grimace. It usually indicates the presence of a brain tumor.

social readjustment scale, a checklist that can be used to measure the amount of stress in a person's life. It is thought

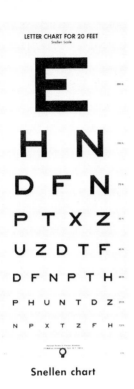

LETTER CHART FOR 20 FEET
Snellen Scale

Snellen chart

that a person with a very stressful life is more likely to get sick.

Social Security Act, a federal law that provides for a national system of old age assistance, survivors' and old age insurance benefits, unemployment insurance and payments, and other public welfare programs, including Medicare and Medicaid.

soda, a compound of sodium, particularly sodium bicarbonate, sodium carbonate, or sodium hydroxide.

sodium (Na), a soft, grayish and metallic element, needed in small amounts for health. It is eaten in the form of salt. It is also used in many forms to make various medicines. Sodium salts, as sodium bicarbonate, are widely used in medications.

sodium arsenite poisoning, a poisonous condition caused by eating sodium arsenite, an insect poison and weed-killer. The typical symptoms of arsenite poisoning are similar to those of arsenic poisoning, as is the treatment. See also **arsenic poisoning.**

sodium bicarbonate, a substance used to control excess acid in the stomach and to treat stomach ulcers and indigestion. Pyloric blockage, kidney disease, heart disease, or bleeding ulcer prohibits its use. Side effects include stomach bloating, acid rebound, alkalosis, and excess potassium and sodium in the blood.

sodium chloride, common table salt, used for many medical procedures.

sodium nitroprusside (SNP), a vessel-widening drug. It is used in the emergency treatment of high blood pressure and in heart failure. Certain forms of high blood pressure or known allergy to the drug prohibits its use. Side effects include muscle spasms, a rapid fall in blood pressure, or symptoms of cyanide poisoning.

sodium phosphate, a salt-based laxative. It is used to achieve prompt, thorough evacuation of the bowel and, in lower dosage, for laxative effect. Congestive heart failure, stomach pain, collection of fluids, enlargement of the colon, low blood volume, salt-restricted diet, or allergy to this drug prohibits its use. Side effects include loss of water, low blood volume, and stomach cramps.

sodium-restricted diet. See **low sodium diet.**

sodium salicylate, a drug used to treat pain and fever.

sodium sulfate, a salt-based drug used to treat constipation by causing a bowel movement. Heart disease, low blood volume, or allergy to this drug prohibits its use. It should not be used very often. Side effects include loss of water, low blood volume, and chemical imbalances in the body.

sodomy /sod'əmē/, **1.** anal intercourse. **2.** intercourse with an animal. **3.** a vague term for "unnatural" sexual intercourse.

soft diet, a diet that is soft in texture, low in residue, easily digested, and well tolerated. It provides the essential nutrients in the form of liquids and semisolid foods, as milk, fruit juices, eggs, cheese, custards, tapioca and puddings, strained soups and vegetables, rice, ground beef and lamb, fowl, fish, mashed, boiled, or baked potatoes, wheat, corn, or rice cereals, and breads. Left out are raw fruits and vegetables, coarse breads and cereals, rich desserts, strong spices, all fried foods, veal, pork, nuts, and raisins. It is commonly recommended for people who have disorders of the stomach or intestines, or serious infections, or for anyone unable to eat a normal diet.

soft palate, the structure composed of mucous membrane, muscular fibers, and mucous glands, hanging from the back of the hard palate forming the roof of the mouth. When the soft palate rises, as in swallowing and in sucking, it closes off the nose and sinuses from the throat and mouth. The back edge of the soft palate hangs like a curtain between the mouth and the voice box. The uvula is the small, round piece of flesh hanging from the back of the soft palate. Compare **hard palate.**

solar plexus, a network of nerves found behind the stomach in the middle of the body. It is one of the most important nerve centers in the body. It is sometimes called "the pit of the stomach."

S

solar radiation, the ultraviolet rays from the sun. Overexposure may result in sunburn, scaly skin, skin cancer, or sores linked with a sensitivity to light.

Solatene, a trademark for a sunscreen (beta-carotene), used to treat certain skin diseases.

soleus /sō′lē·əs/, one of three muscles found at the back of the calf. It is a broad flat muscle that moves the foot.

Solfoton, a trademark for a drug used to prevent convulsions and as a sleeping pill (phenobarbital).

Solganal, a trademark for a drug used to treat rheumatism (aurothioglucose).

solid, a dense body, structure, or substance that has length, width, and thickness, is not a liquid or gas, contains no significant hollowness, and has no openings on its surface.

solubility, the ability of a solid, liquid, gas, or vapor to dissolve in water. The ability of one material to blend uniformly with another, as in a solid in liquid, liquid in liquid, gas in liquid, or gas in gas.

Solu-Cortef, a trademark for a steroid (hydrocortisone sodium succinate).

Solu-Medrol, a trademark for a steroid (methylprednisolone sodium succinate).

solution, a mixture of one or more substances dissolved in another substance. A solution may be a gas, a liquid, or a solid.

solvent, 1. any liquid in which another substance can be dissolved. **2.** a liquid, as benzene, carbon tetrachloride, and certain oil-based liquids that when breathed in can be poisonous, and can do damage to mucous membranes of the nose and throat and the tissues of the kidney, liver, and brain. Repeated exposure over a very long time can add to addiction, brain damage, blindness, and other serious results, some of them fatal. See also **benzene poisoning, carbon tetrachloride, petroleum distillate poisoning.**

Soma, a trademark for a skeletal muscle relaxing drug (carisoprodol).

somatoform disorder /sō′mətōfôrm′, sōmat′ō-/, any of a group of nervous disorders with symptoms that look like a physical illness or disease, for which there is no real disease. The symptoms are usually caused by some mental conflict within the patient's mind. Kinds of somatoform disorders are **conversion disorder, hypochondria, psychogenic pain disorder.**

somatomegaly /-meg′əlē/, a condition in which the body is abnormally large because of hormonal imbalance within the body.

somatosplanchnic /sōmat′ōsplangk′nik/, relating to the trunk of the body and the internal organs of the lower body, as the stomach and intestines.

somatostatin /-stat′in/, hormone that controls growth and helps to control the release of certain other hormones.

somatotropic hormone, somatotropin. See **growth hormone.**

somatotype /-tīp/, **1.** body build or physique. **2.** the classification of body types based on certain physical traits. An **ectomorph** is a body type that is slender and fragile and with most distinct parts grown from the ectoderm. An **endomorph** has a soft, round body build with a large trunk and thighs, tapering limbs, and fat throughout the body. A **mesomorph** is a body type made up mainly of muscle, bone, and connective tissue, structures that develop from the middle (mesodermal) tissue cell layer of the embryo. **Asthenic habitus** refers to a slender body build with long limbs, an angular profile, and prominent muscles or bones. An **athletic habitus** is a well-proportioned, muscular body with broad shoulders, thick neck, deep chest, and flat stomach. **Pyknic** describes a stocky body structure with short, round limbs, a full face, a short neck, and a tendency to become fat.

somnambulism /somnam′byəlizm/. See **sleepwalking.**

somnolent /som′nələnt/, **1.** sleepy or drowsy. **2.** tending to cause sleepiness. **–somnolence,** *n.*

Somophyllin, a trademark for a bronchodilator (theophylline).

soporific /sop′ərif′ik/, referring to a substance, condition, or method that causes sleep. See also **hypnotic, sedative.**

Sorbitrate, a trademark for a drug used to treat angina (isosorbide dinitrate).

sordes /sôr′dēz/, *pl.* **sordes,** dirt or waste matter, especially the crusts consisting of food, germs, and cells that collect on teeth and lips during a fever illness or one in which the patient takes nothing by mouth. Sordes gastricae is undigested food and mucus in the stomach.

sore, 1. a wound, ulcer, or lesion. **2.** tender or painful.

Sorrin's operation, an operation to treat an abscess of the gums.

s.o.s., (in prescriptions) abbreviation for *si opus sit,* a Latin phrase meaning "if necessary."

space maintainer, a fixed or movable device for holding open the space formed by the early loss of one or more teeth. A **space obtainer** is a device used to widen the space between two teeth next to one another. A **space regainer** is used to move a displaced permanent tooth into its normal position.

span-of-control the supervisory ratio of from three to seven individuals with five being established as a general rule of thumb.

sparganosis /spär′gənō′-/, an infection with larvae of the fish tapeworm, marked by painful swellings under the skin or swelling and destruction of the eye. It is caught by drinking contaminated water or in undercooked, infected frog flesh. Treatment includes surgery and local injection of ethyl alcohol to kill the larvae. See also **tapeworm infection.**

Sparine, a trademark for a phenothiazine antipsychotic and antivomiting drug (promazine hydrochloride).

spasm, 1. a sudden unconscious muscle tightening, as habit spasms, hiccups, stuttering, or a tic. **2.** a convulsion or seizure. **3.** a sudden, brief tightening of a blood vessel, bronchus, esophagus, pylorus, ureter, or other hollow organ. Compare **stricture.**

spastic, of or relating to spasms or other uncontrolled tightenings of the skeletal muscles. See also **cerebral palsy. –spasticity,** *n.*

spastic bladder. See **neurogenic bladder.**

spastic colon. See **irritable bowel syndrome.**

spatial dance /spā′shəl/, body shifts or movements used by individuals as they try to adjust the distance between them. See also **spatial zones.**

spatial zones, the areas of personal space in which most people function. Four basic spatial zones are the intimate zone, in which distance between individuals is less than 18 inches; the personal zone, between 18 inches and 4 feet; the social zone, extending between 4 and 12 feet; and the public zone, beyond 12 feet.

special care unit, a hospital unit with the necessary special equipment and personnel for handling critically ill or injured patients, as an intensive care unit, burn unit, or cardiac care unit.

special sense, the sense of sight, smell, taste, touch, or hearing.

special-form radioactive materials, materials that are encapsulated or are in a solid form or matrix such that, if released from a package, they would maintain their integrity. Such materials might present a direct radiation exposure problem, but there would be little possibility of loose contamination and/or dispersal.

specialist, a health care professional who makes a detailed study of one part of the body and the related diseases, or of a particular type of disease. A specialist usually has advanced training.

species (Sp) /spē′sēz, spē′shēz/, *pl.* **species (sp., spp)** /spē′sēz, spē′shēz/, the category of living things below genus in rank. A species includes individuals of the same genus who are similar in structure and chemical composition and who can interbreed. See also **genus.**

specific activity, the total activity of a given radionuclide per unit mass. Units are generally curies per gram.

specific gamma-ray constant, for a nuclide emitting gamma radiation, the exposure rate at a meter from a unit point source of a gamma-emitting nuclide.

specific gravity, the weight of a material as compared with the weight of an equal volume of water. If the specific gravity is less than one, the material is lighter than water and will float. If the specific gravity is greater than one, the material is heavier than water and will sink.

specific immune globulin, a special substance made from human blood that is used to protect against a specific disease, as varicella zoster immune globulin.

specification packages (DOT), shipping packages meeting the design and construction standards prescribed in the Code of Federal Regulations, 49 CFR Part 178.

specimen /spes′imən/, a small sample of something, tested to show the nature of the whole, as a urine specimen.

Spectazole, a trademark for a fungus-killing drug (econazole nitrate).

spectinomycin hydrochloride, an antibiotic. It is used to treat gonorrhea and certain infections in patients who are allergic to penicillin. Known allergy to this drug prohibits its use. Side effects include lessened urine, rash, chills, fever, dizziness, and nausea.

Spectrobid, a trademark for a certain kind of penicillin (bacampicillin).

Spectrocin, a trademark for a drug used to kill bacteria infections on the skin (neomycin sulfate and gramicidin).

speculum /spek′yələm/, a tool used to hold open a body space to make examination possible, as an ear speculum, an eye speculum, or a vaginal speculum.

speech, the making of definite vocal sounds that form words to express one's thoughts or ideas. It involves the complex coordination of the muscles and nerves of the organs involved in making sound. Any nerve or muscle injury or defect involving these organs results in various speech defects or disorders.

speech dysfunction, a condition which in some way affects the ability to speak. It may be caused by lack of blood to the brain, brain tumor, tube in the throat, or removal of the voice box. It may also be caused by a physical defect, as a cleft palate, or a psychosis. It may even apply to language barriers. Symptoms include slurring, stuttering, and problems in forming words or in expressing thoughts. Disorientation may also occur. **Anarthria** results from the loss of control of the muscles of speech. The patient is unable to say words. The defect is usually caused by damage to a nerve. **Aphonic speech** is a defect in which everything is whispered. With **ataxic speech,** there is faulty formation of the sounds. The cause is a disorder of the nerves to the muscles. Abnormal speech caused by diseases of a part of the brain (cerebellum) is called **cerebellar speech.** There is slow, jerky, and slurred pronunciation of words. The tone may be intermittent and explosive or monotonous and unvaried in pitch. **Explosive speech** is slow, jerky speech alternating with sudden loud words. This is often seen in brain disorders. **Mirror**

S

speech has the order of syllables in a word reversed. With **scamping speech,** consonants or whole syllables are left out of words because of the person's inability to shape the sounds. With **scanning speech,** words are clipped and broken because the person stops between syllables. With **slurred speech,** words are not spoken clearly or completely but are run together or only partly said. The condition may be caused by weakness of the muscles of the lips, tongue, and mouth, damage to a motor nerve, brain disease, drug usage, or carelessness.

speech pathology,   **1.** the study of defects of speech or of the organs of speech. **2.** the diagnosis and treatment of defects of speech as practiced by a speech pathologist or a speech therapist.

sperm.   See **semen, spermatozoon.**

spermatic cord /spərmat′ik/,   a structure by which each testicle is attached to the body. The left spermatic cord is usually longer than the right, thus the left testis usually hangs lower than the right. Each cord is made up of arteries, veins, lymphatics, nerves, and the excretory duct of the testicles.

spermatic duct.   See **vas deferens.**

spermatic fistula,   an abnormal passage leading to or away from a testicle or a seminal duct.

spermatocele /spur′mətōsēl′/,   a cystlike swelling, that contains sperm. It lies above, behind, and separate from the testis; it is usually painless and requires no therapy.

spermatocide /-sīd′/,   a chemical substance that kills spermatozoa. Also called **spermicide.**

spermatozoon /-zō′ən/, *pl.* **spermatozoa** /-zō′ə/,   the male seed, contained in semen, that fertilizes the female egg in the womb in order to create a fetus. It looks like a tiny tadpole, with a head, a neck, and a tail that propels it.

sphenoid bone /sfē′noid/,   the bone at the base of the skull. It looks like a bat with its wings spread.

sphenomandibular ligament /sfē′nōmandib′yələr/,   one of a pair of flat, thin ligaments that connect the top of the jaw bone to the skull.

spherocytic anemia /sfir′osit′ik/,   an inherited blood disorder with misshaped red blood cells. Attacks of stomach pain, fever, jaundice, and enlargement of the spleen occur. Because repeated transfusions are often needed to treat the anemia, too much iron in the blood may develop. Removal of the spleen may then be necessary.

spherocytosis /-sītō′-/,   the abnormal presence of diseased red blood cells in the blood.

sphincter /sfingk′tər/,   a circular band of muscle fibers that narrows a passage or closes a natural opening in the body, as the outer anal sphincter, which closes the anus.

sphingolipid /sfing′gōlip′id/,   a substance found in large amounts in the brain and other tissues of the nervous system, especially membranes.

sphingomyelin /-mī′əlin/,   any of a group of sphingolipids containing phosphorus. It occurs mainly in the tissue of the nervous system, generally in membranes, and in the fats (lipids) in the blood.

sphingomyelin lipidosis,   any of a group of diseases marked by an abnormality in the ability of the body to store sphingolipids. An example is **Niemann-Pick disease.** See also **lipidosis.**

sphygmograph /sfig′məgraf/,   an instrument that records the force of the arterial pulse on a graph called a sphygmogram. It may be useful in determining the health of the heart.

sphygmomanometer /-mənom′ətər/,   a device for measuring the blood pressure. It consists of an arm or leg cuff with an air bag attached to a tube and a bulb for pumping air into the bag, and a gauge for showing the amount of air pressure being pressed against the artery. See also **blood pressure.**

spica bandage /spī′kə/,   a figure-of-eight bandage in which each turn usually overlaps the next to form a succession of **V**-like designs. It may be used to give support, to apply pressure, or to hold a dressing in place on the chest, limbs, thighs, or pelvis.

spica cast,   a cast applied to hold in place part or all of the trunk of the body and part or all of one or more arms or legs. It is used to treat various fractures, as of the hip and the thigh, and in correcting hip deformities. A **bilateral long-leg spica cast** encases the trunk as far as the nipples and both legs as far as the toes. A horizontal crossbar connects the cast at ankle level. A **shoulder spica cast** uses a diagonal shoulder support between the hip and arm parts. It is used to treat shoulder dislocations and injuries, and to put into place and keep rigid the shoulder after surgery. A **one-and-a-half spica cast** is used to keep the body rigid from the nipple line, one leg as far as the toes, and the other leg as far as the knee. A slanted crossbar joins the parts of the cast covering the legs. This type of cast is used during recovery of surgery to repair the hip or a broken upper leg and for repairing hips that are badly formed. A **unilateral long-leg spica cast** is one that holds rigid one leg and the trunk of the body as far as the nipple line. It is used to treat a broken thigh or to correct or maintain a correction of a hip deformity.

spider antivenin.   See **black widow spider antivenin.**

spider bite,   a puncture wound made by the bite of a spider. Fewer than 100 of some 30,000 species of spiders are known to bite. Two of them, the black widow spider and the brown recluse spider, found in the United States, are poisonous.

spina bifida /spī′nə bif′ədə, bī′fədə/,   a nerve tube defect present at birth that results in a gap in the bone that surrounds the spinal cord. Spina bifida is relatively common, occurring about 10 to 20 times per 1000 births. The gap may be very small, a condition that only rarely needs treatment, or it may be large enough to allow parts of the spinal cord to come through, in which case surgery may be needed. Direct symptoms are rarely noted in spina bifida, which is often diagnosed accidentally during x-ray examinations needed for other reasons. **Spina bifida anterior** refers to a gap along the front surface of the spinal column. The defect is often linked with growth defects of the organs of the lower body. **Spina bifida cystica** is a growth defect of the central nervous system in which a cyst containing meninges (meningocele), spinal cord (myelocele), or both (myelomeningocele) sticks out through a gap in the spine. The sac can easily break, causing the leakage of fluid and a higher risk of infection. **Spina bifida occulta** refers to a gap in the spine in the lower back without hernia of the spinal cord. The defect, which is quite common, occurs in about 5% of the population and is identified from outside by a dimple, dark tufts of hair, certain blood vessel disorders, or soft tumors beneath the skin. There is usually no nerve damage linked with the defect. However, certain disorders may occur, as problems with gait and foot weakness and with the bowel and bladder sphincters.

spinal canal /spī′nəl/,   the space within the bones of the spinal column.

spinal column,   the flexible group of backbones. It is made up of 33 vertebrae that are separated by spongy disks. The spine is made stronger by several curves. The spinal column also protects the spinal cord that runs inside of it. Also called **spine, vertebral column.** See also **vertebra.**

spinal cord,   a long, almost round structure found in the spinal canal and reaching from the base of the skull to the upper part of the lower back. A major part of the central nervous system, the adult cord is about 1 cm in diameter with an average length of 42 to 45 cm and a weight of 30 g. The cord carries sense and movement signals to and from the brain and controls many reflexes. The **central canal** of the spinal cord is a tunnel that runs the entire length of the spinal cord. It carries the fluid of the brain and spinal cord. This fluid flows into the canal from a space in the brain. See also **spinal nerves.**

spinal cord compression,   an abnormal and often serious condition caused by pressure on the spinal cord. Symptoms range from temporary numbness of an arm or leg to permanent paralysis, depending on the cause, severity, and location of the pressure. Causes include spinal fracture, vertebral dislocation, tumor, bleeding, and edema linked with a crushing or bruising injury with contusion. See also **herniated disk.**

spinal cord injury,   any of the severe injuries to the spinal cord, often linked with widespread effects on the muscles and skeleton. Common spinal cord injuries are spinal fractures and dislocations, as those commonly suffered by individuals involved in car accidents, airplane crashes, or other violent impacts. Such injuries may cause varying degrees of paralysis. Spinal cord injuries produce a state of spinal shock, with paralysis and complete loss of skin feeling at the time of the injury. Within a few weeks, the muscles affected may become spastic, and the skin feeling may return to a slight degree. The motor and the sensory losses that continue a few weeks after the injury are usually permanent. Treatment varies a great deal and involves many different methods, such as special exercises.

spinal cord tumor,   a growth on the spinal cord. Symptoms usually develop slowly and may progress from prickling skin on one side of the body to stabbing pain, weakness in one or both legs, abnormal deep tendon reflexes, and, in advanced cases, some type of paralysis. Function of the nervous system is sometimes disturbed, causing areas of dry, cold, bluish-pink skin or profuse sweating of the legs and feet. Tumors of the spinal cord may arise at any age but appear most often in the third decade of life and are one fourth as common as brain cancers.

spinal curvature,   any continuous, abnormal change of shape of the vertebral column from its normal position. **Kyphosis** is a forward, humplike curvature of the spine. Kyphosis may be caused by rickets or tuberculosis of the spine. If the curvature progresses, there may be moderate back pain. **Kyphoscoliosis** is a forward and to the side, humplike curvature of the spine, often associated with a heart disorder (cor pulmonale). **Lordosis** is an abnormal, increased degree of forward curvature of any part of the spine. **Scoliosis** is a sideways curve of the spine that results in an **S** shape of the back, a common defect in childhood. **Congenital scoliosis** refers to a defect that is present at birth. It increases with growth and age. The degree of deformity varies greatly. **Idiopathic scoliosis** is the most common type of scoliosis, evident in 70% of all patients with scoliosis and up to 80% of those with structural scoliosis. It may occur at any age, but three types mostly occur in certain age groups. The infantile type affects 1- to 3-year-olds. The juvenile type affects 3- to 10-year-olds. The adolescent type affects preadolescents and adolescents. The most common type is the adolescent type. The signs of scoliosis include unlevel shoulders, a prominent shoulder blade, a prominent breast, a prominent flank area, an unlevel or a prominent hip, poor posture, and obvious curvature. Other signs include occasional pain, fatigue, and decreased lung function. Nerve defects are commonly

S

linked with severe curvature and vary according to how much the curvature has pushed on the spinal cord. Spinal curvature is usually diagnosed with the use of x-ray tests. Early discovery and treatment may prevent it from getting worse. Treatment includes braces, casts, exercises, and corrective surgery.

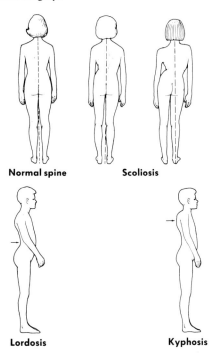

Normal spine   **Scoliosis**

Lordosis   **Kyphosis**

Spinal curvatures

spinal fluid. See **cerebrospinal fluid.**

spinal fusion, the joining of an unstable part of the spine, done by skeletal traction or keeping the patient rigid in a body cast but most often by surgery.

spinal manipulation, the forced passive movement of spinal bones. It may be done to treat sprains, breaks, and dislocations.

spinal nerves, the 31 pairs of nerves that are connected to the spinal cord. They are without special names and are numbered according to the level where they leave the cord. See also **spinal cord.**

spinal puncture. See **lumbar puncture.**

spinal tract, any one of the pathways for nerve signals that are found in the white matter of the spinal cord.

spindle cell carcinoma, a rapidly growing tumor.

spine. See **spinal column.**

spinnbarkeit /spin'bärkīt', shpin'-/, the clear, slippery texture of an uncooked egg white, typical of cervical mucus during ovulation. It is a valuable sign of the most

fertile period in a woman's menstrual cycle. Observation of spinnbarkeit is useful in natural methods of family planning, in the evaluation of infertility, and in finding the best time for artificial insemination.

spinocerebellar disorder /spī'nōser'əbel'ər/, an inherited disorder with a gradual wasting of the spinal cord and brain, often involving other parts of the nervous system as well. These disorders tend to occur within families. They usually attack early, during childhood or adolescence. No treatment is known. Some kinds of spinocerebellar wasting are **ataxia telangiectasia, Charcot-Marie-Tooth atrophy, Dejerine-Sottas disease, Friedreich's ataxia, Refsum's syndrome.**

spiral fracture, a bone break in which the break of bone tissue is in a corkscrew fashion following the long axis of the broken bone.

spirograph /spī'rəgraf/, a device for recording breathing movements.

spirometry /spīrom'ətrē/, laboratory test of the lungs by means of a spirometer, a machine that measures and records the amount of inhaled and exhaled air. Information is recorded on a chart, called a spirogram.

spironolactone, a drug that controls a certain hormone (aldosterone). It is used to treat primary hyperaldosteronism, edema of heart failure, cirrhosis of the liver with edema, kidney damage, high blood pressure, and a lack of potassium in the blood. Certain kinds of kidney disorder or too much potassium in the blood prohibits its use. Side effects include too much potassium in the blood, the growth of male breasts, mental confusion, loss of coordination, impotence, lack of menstruation, hairiness, and a patchy rash.

splanchnocele /splangk'nōsēl/, hernia of any internal organ of the lower body.

spleen, a soft, blood-vessel-filled, egg-shaped organ found between the stomach and the diaphragm on the left half of the body. It is considered part of the lymphatic system. It has a dark purple color. The exact function of the spleen is not known, but it helps keep the blood healthy. The size of the spleen becomes larger during and after digestion and often during illness. See also **lymphatic system.**

spleen scan, an x-ray test of the spleen done to find a tumor, damage, or other problem.

splenectomy /splēnek'-/, the removal by surgery of the spleen.

splenic flexure syndrome /splen'ik/, a pain coming back time after time and a bloating in the area of the stomach caused by a pocket of gas trapped in the large intestine below the spleen. The symptoms are eased by a bowel movement or by breaking wind.

splenomegaly /splē'nōmeg'əlē/, an abnormal enlargement of the spleen linked with certain types of high blood pressure and anemia, Niemann-Pick disease, or malaria.

splint, **1.** a device for holding in place any part of the body. It may be stiff (of metal, plaster, or wood) or flexible (of felt or leather). A **caliper splint** is a leg splint made of two metal rods extending from a band around the thigh or the pelvis. The lower ends of the rods are attached to a metal plate under the shoe. **2.** (in dentistry) a device for anchoring the teeth or changing the bite. Compare **brace, cast.**

splinter fracture, a crushing break resulting in thin, sharp bone chips.

splinter hemorrhage, bleeding that looks like a splinter under a finger- or toenail. It is seen after injury and in patients with bacterial endocarditis.

spondylitis /spon'dilī'-/, inflammation of any of the spinal vertebrae, usually marked by stiffness and pain. The condition may follow injury to the spine, or it may be the result of infection or rheumatoid disease. See also **ankylosing spondylitis.**

spondylosis /spon'dilō'-/, a condition of the spine marked by stiffness of a vertebral joint.

sponge bath, the method of washing the patient with a damp washcloth or sponge, used when a full bath is not needed or as a method of reducing body temperature.

spongioblastoma /spon'jē·ōblastō'mə/, a tumor made up of cells from the embryo that remain and later affect the spinal cord canal. An example is **spongioblastoma unipolare,** a rare growth occurring in the spinal cord or brain.

spontaneous evolution, the unassisted birth of a fetus in the crosswise (transverse) position. **Denman's spontaneous evolution** refers to an unaided turning of the fetus just before birth from a crossway position to a bottom-down position (breech).

sporadic, (of a number of events) occurring at scattered, interrupted, and seemingly random intervals.

spore, a form taken by some bacteria that is resistant to heat, drying, and chemicals. Under proper conditions the spore may change back into the active form of the bacterium. Diseases caused by spore-forming bacteria include anthrax, botulism, gas gangrene, and tetanus.

sporicide /spôr'isid/, any substance used to kill spores.

sporotrichosis /spôr'ōtrikō'-/, a common, long-term, fungus-caused infection usually with skin ulcers and little bumps under the skin. It rarely spreads to bones, lungs, joints, or muscles. The fungus is found in soil and rotting vegetation and usually enters the skin by accidental injury. Treatment may include amphotericin B.

sprain, an injury to the tendons, muscles, or ligaments around a joint, marked by pain, swelling, and discoloration of the skin over the joint. The length of time and seriousness of the symptoms vary with the amount of damage to the tissues. Treatment requires support, rest, and alternating cold and heat. X-ray pictures are often used to be certain that no break has occurred.

sprain fracture, a break that results from the separation of a tendon or ligament linked with the separation of a bone.

sprinter's fracture, a break of a certain part of the pelvis caused by a fragment of bone being pulled by a very strong muscle spasm.

sprue, a long-term disorder caused by poor absorption of nutrients in the small intestine. Symptoms include diarrhea, weakness, weight loss, poor appetite, pale skin, muscle cramps, bone pain, ulcers of the mucous membrane lining the digestive tract, and a smooth, shiny tongue. It occurs in both tropic and nontropic forms and affects both children and adults. **Nontropical sprue** is a condition due to an inborn inability to digest foods that contain gluten. **Tropical sprue** is of unknown cause and occurs in the tropics and subtropics. Symptoms include diarrhea, loss of appetite, and weight loss. Treatment includes use of antibiotics, folic acid, iron, calcium, and vitamins, as well as a balanced diet high in protein and normal in fat content. See also **celiac disease, malabsorption syndrome.**

SPRX, a trademark for a drug used to lessen appetite (phendimetrazine tartrate).

sputum /spyoo'təm/, material coughed up from the lungs and spit out through the mouth. It contains mucus, cellular debris, or microorganisms, and it may also contain blood or pus. The amount, color, and contents of the sputum are important in the diagnosis of many illnesses, including tuberculosis, pneumonia, and cancer of the lung.

squamous cell /skwā'məs/, a flat, scaly cell.

squamous cell carcinoma, a slow-growing cancer often found in the lungs and skin and occurring also in the anus, cervix, larynx, nose, bladder, and other sites. The typical tumor, a firm, red, horny, painless little bump, often results from overexposure to the sun.

squeeze dynamometer, an instrument for measuring the strength of the grip of the hand.

squint. See **strabismus.**

SSKI, a trademark for a drug used to clear mucus and other matter from the mouth and throat (potassium iodide).

stabilization, **1.** the physical process of becoming stable. **2.** the seating of a fixed or removable denture so that it will not tilt or be moved under pressure. **3.** the control of induced stress loads and the development of measures to counteract such forces so that the movement of the teeth or of a device does not irritate nearby tissues.

Stadol, a trademark for a painkilling drug (butorphanol tartrate) used as an aid to anesthesia.

stages of dying, the five emotional and behavioral stages that have been identified as occurring after a patient first

S

learns of approaching death. A period of denial, followed by anger, bargaining, depression, and, finally, acceptance are the stages the dying patient goes through. The family often goes through like stages. Sensitive care and support through all stages of dying may help the patient accept death more quickly and easily. When the patient denies the truth and will not follow directions, one neither argues nor agrees with the person. During the stage of anger, the patient is encouraged to express the anger. In the period in which the patient tries to make bargains, as ''If I could live until . . . ,'' it may help to discuss the importance of events and people in earlier life. When depression sets in, efforts to cheer the patient or stop the crying should not be made. The patient may want only the most beloved person to be present. In the final stage of acceptance, the patient may feel less pain and discomfort, become peaceful and accept care from people who are close.

staging area, that location where incident personnel and equipment are assigned on a three (3) minute available status.

standard cubic foot, the amount of air in a cubic foot at sea level and at 70° F.

standard of care, the minimum accepted level of emergency care to be provided as set forth by law, administrative orders, guidelines published by emergency care organizations and societies, local protocols and practice, and what has been accepted in the past (precedent).

stanozolol /stənō′zəlôl/, a male hormone steroid. It is used to treat aplastic anemia and osteoporosis. Cancer of the breast or prostate, nephrosis, pregnancy, or known allergy to this drug prohibits its use. Side effects include various hormone disorders in males and females, allergic reactions, and disorders of the stomach and bowels.

stapedectomy /stā′pədek′-/, removal of the stapes of the middle ear and replacing it with a small plastic tube of stainless steel wire, done to restore hearing in the treatment of otosclerosis. Possible complications include infection of the ear, rejection of the replacement, and leaking of fluid, with ringing in the ear and dizziness.

stapes /stā′pēz/, one of the three small bones in the middle ear, resembling a tiny stirrup. It carries sound vibrations to the inner ear. See also **ear.**

Staphage Lysat (SPL), a trademark for an active immunizing drug (staphylococcal antigen phage lysed) used in staphylococcal infection.

Staphcillin, a trademark for a bacteria-killing drug (methicillin sodium).

staphylococcal infection /staf′ilōkok′əl/, an infection caused by any one of several disease-causing types of *Staphylococcus.* It commonly results in the formation of abscesses on the skin or other organs. Staphylococcal infections of the skin include carbuncles, folliculitis, and furuncles. Presence of the germ in the blood may result in endocarditis, meningitis, or osteomyelitis. Staphylococcal pneumonia often follows influenza or other viral disease and may be linked with long-term or weakening illness. Acute infection of the digestive tract may result from a poison made by certain species of staphylococci in tainted food. Treatment usually includes bed rest and pain-killing and other drugs. Surgical drainage, especially of deep abscesses, is often necessary.

staphylococcal scalded skin syndrome (SSSS), an abnormal skin condition, with reddening, peeling, and scabs, that gives the skin a scalded look. It is caused by infections. SSSS is more common in the newborn infant because of undeveloped immunity and kidney systems. It is treated with antibiotics.

Staphylococcus /-kok′əs/, a type of bacteria. Some kinds are normally found on the skin and in the throat; certain kinds cause severe, pus-forming infections or produce a poison, which may cause nausea, vomiting, and diarrhea. See also **staphylococcal infection.**

startle reflex, a normal reflex in an infant caused by a sudden loud noise. It results in drawing up the legs, an embracing position of the arms, and usually a short cry.

starvation, **1.** a condition caused by the lack of proper food over a long period of time and marked by numerous disorders of the body and metabolism. **2.** the act or state of starving or being starved. See also **malnutrition.**

stasis /stā′sis, stas′is/, **1.** a disorder in which the normal flow of a fluid through a vessel of the body is slowed or stopped. **2.** stillness.

stasis dermatitis, a condition, caused by too little circulation in the legs. Symptoms include a swelling of the ankles, a tan-colored skin, patchy reddening, tiny, round, purplish-red spots, and hardening of the skin. It can lead to shrinking of the skin and tissues. Treatment includes correcting the underlying vein problem, antibiotics, and steroids.

statement of practical treatment, located near the signal word on the front panel of a hazardous materials container, it is also referred to as the ''first aid statement'' or ''note to physician.'' It may have precautionary information as well as emergency procedures for exposures. Antidote and treatment information may also be added.

static, without motion, at rest, in balance.

Statobex, a trademark for a drug used to control appetite (phendimetrazine tartrate).

status, **1.** a specified state or condition, as emotional status. **2.** a continuing state or condition, as a long-lasting asthma attack (status asthmaticus).

status asthmaticus /azmat′ikəs/. See **asthma.**

status epilepticus /ep′ilep′tikəs/, a medical emergency marked by continual attacks of convulsive seizures occurring without intervals of consciousness. Unless convulsions are stopped, permanent brain damage results. The cause may be the sudden withdrawal of anticonvulsant drugs, low blood sugar, a brain tumor, a head injury, a high fever, or poisoning. Therapy includes anticonvulsant drugs, nutrients, and electrolytes, preferably given in an intensive care unit.

STCC number, the Standard Transportation Commodity Code number used in the rail industry; a seven-digit number assigned to a specific hazardous material or group of materials & used in determination of rates. For hazardous material, the STCC number will begin with the digits ''49.''

Stearns' alcoholic amentia /sturnz/, a form of insanity brought on by alcohol. There is an emotional disturbance of a less severe nature than that of delirium tremens but longer lasting and with greater mental clouding and amnesia.

steatorrhea /stē'ətorē'ə/, greater than normal amounts of fat in the feces, marked by frothy, foul-smelling fecal matter that floats, as in celiac disease, some malabsorption syndromes, and any condition in which fats are poorly absorbed by the small intestine.

Steele-Richardson-Olszewski syndrome, a rare nerve disorder of unknown cause, occurring in middle age, more often in men. It features paralysis of eye muscles, loss of coordination, neck and trunk rigidity, and other signs like those of Parkinson's disease.

Stelazine, a trademark for a tranquilizer (trifluoperazine).

stellate fracture /stel'āt/, a bone break in the form of a star.

stem cell leukemia, a cancerous growth on a blood-making organ. The disease is extremely acute and has a rapid, relentless course. See also **leukemia.**

stenosis /stinō'-/, an abnormal condition marked by the tightening or narrowing of an opening or passageway in a body structure. **Cicatricial stenosis** refers to the narrowing of a duct or tube caused by scar tissue. **Valvular stenosis** is a defect in valves of the heart. The condition may be present at birth, or it may be caused by some disease, such as rheumatic fever. One kind, **aortic stenosis,** is a defect of the aortic valve in the heart. The flow of blood is blocked at the left bottom chamber (ventricle) into the aorta. This causes a lower output of blood from the heart and lung congestion. Symptoms include chest pain, a heart murmur, and a faint pulse. Left heart failure may occur. **Mitral valve stenosis** is a defect in the left upper chamber (atrium) of the heart. Reduced blood pumping causes weakness, breathing difficulty, and bluish skin color. Right heart failure may result. Diagnosis and treatment are similar for both of these valve defects. Chest x-rays are

made, a tube is put into the heart (cardiac catheterization), and sounds of the heart are graphed (echocardiography). Surgery is often done to correct the defect. An artificial heart valve may be put in. **Pulmonary stenosis** is most often a birth defect, marked by enlargement of the right lower heart chamber (ventricle). There is little increase in the amount of blood pumped between contractions. Early diagnosis and surgery may prevent heart failure. **Pyloric stenosis** is a narrowing of a band of muscle (pyloric sphincter) at the outlet of the stomach. It can block the flow of partly digested food into the small intestine. The condition may occur as a birth defect, but can also develop in adults as a result of ulcers. Forceful vomiting is a sign of the disorder in infants. Surgery is needed to widen the stomach outlet.

Sterapred, a trademark for a nerve-blocking drug (prednisone).

stereotypy /ster'ē·ətī'pē, stir'-/, the continuous, improper repetition of actions, body postures, or speech patterns, usually occurring with a lack of variation in thought. It is often seen in patients with schizophrenia.

sterile /ster'il/, **1.** barren; unable to produce children because of a physical abnormality, often the lack of sperm in a man or blockage of the fallopian tubes in a woman. Compare **impotence. 2.** aseptic. –**sterility,** *n.*

sterilization, 1. a process or act that makes a person unable to produce children. See also **hysterectomy, tubal ligation, vasectomy. 2.** a technique for destroying microorganisms using heat, water, chemicals, or gases. – **sterilize,** *v.*

sternal node /stur'nəl/, a lymph gland in one of the three groups in the front of the rib cage. They drain the lymph from the breast, the surface of the liver, and the deep stomach wall. See also **lymphatic system.**

sternoclavicular articulation /stur'nōkləvik'yələr/, the double joint between the breastbone (sternum) and the collar bone (clavicle). It is at the center and top of the rib cage.

sternocostal articulation /-kos'təl/, the flexible joint of the cartilage of each true rib and the sternum. Each sternocostal articulation also has five ligaments.

sternohyoideus /-hī·oi'dē·əs/, one of the four muscles in the front of the neck that stretch from near the collar bone up to the voice box (larynx). It is used in swallowing and speaking.

sternothyroideus /-thīroi'dē·əs/, one of the four muscles in the front of the throat that stretch from near the collar bone up to the voice box (larynx). It is used in swallowing and speaking.

sternum /stur'nəm/, the long, flat bone in the middle of the front of the ribcage. It is sometimes called the ''breastbone''. The sternum is longer in men than in women.

S

sterognosis /ster'ognō'-/,   **1.** the sense of feeling and understanding the form and nature of objects by the sense of touch. **2.** perception by the senses of the solidity of objects.

steroid /stir'oid/.   See **corticosteroid.**

stertorous /stur'tərəs/,   relating to an act of breathing that is labored or struggling; having a snoring sound.

stethoscope /steth'əskōp/,   an instrument consisting of two earpieces connected by means of flexible tubing to a diaphragm, which is placed against the skin of the patient's chest or back to hear heart and lung sounds.

Stevens-Johnson syndrome,   a serious, sometimes fatal inflammatory disease affecting children and young adults. It features fever, blisters on the skin, and open sores on the mucous membranes of the lips, eyes, mouth, nasal passage, and genitals. Pneumonia, pain in the joints, and weakness are common. The disorder may be an allergic reaction to drugs, or it may follow pregnancy, herpesvirus I, or another infection. Treatment includes bed rest, antibiotics, and other drugs.

stibogluconate sodium,   a drug used to fight leishmaniasis available from the Center for Disease Control.

Stieda's fracture /stē'dəz/,   a fracture of the end of the thigh bone (femur).

stigma /stig'mə/,   **1.** a moral or physical blemish. **2.** a physical trait that serves to identify a disease or a condition.

stillbirth,   the birth of a fetus that died before or during delivery.

stillborn,   referring to an infant that was born dead.

Stilphostrol,   a trademark for a female hormone (diethylstilbestrol diphosphate).

stimulant,   any substance that speeds up a body system.

stimulus, *pl.* **stimuli,**   anything that excites an organism or part to function, become active, or respond. –**stimulate,** *v.*

sting,   an injury caused by a sharp, painful puncture of the skin, often accompanied by irritating chemicals or the poison of an insect or other animal. In cases of allergy, a highly poisonous sting, or numerous stings, shock may occur. Kinds of stings include bee, jellyfish, scorpion, sea urchin, and shellfish stings.

stingray,   a flat, long-tailed fish that has barbed spines on its back that are connected to sacs of venom. Spasm of the skeletal muscles, severe local pain, seizures, and shortness of breath may occur if the skin is broken by the spines. The wound is washed with cold salt water, and the injured limb is placed in very hot water for 30 to 60 minutes; an antiseptic is applied and tetanus protection is given.

stoma,   **1.** a pore or opening on a surface. **2.** an artificial opening from an internal organ to the surface of the body, created surgically, as for a colostomy, ileostomy, or tra-

cheostomy. **3.** a new opening created surgically, between two body structures, as for a gastroenterostomy.

stomach,   the main organ of digestion, which is divided into a body and a pylorus. It receives and partly digests food and drink funneled from the mouth through the throat and moves material into the intestines. The shape of the stomach is changed by the amount of contents, stage of digestion, development of the muscles, and condition of the intestines. It is lined with mucous membranes that have many blood vessels and nerves, and contains several important glands.

stomach pump,   a pump for removing the contents of the stomach through a tube passed through the mouth or nose into the stomach.

stomatitis /stō'mətī'-/,   any inflammatory condition of the mouth. It may result from infection by bacteria, viruses, or fungi, from exposure to certain chemicals or drugs, from vitamin deficiency, or from some diseases. **Angular stomatitis** refers to soreness and redness at the corner of the mouth. **Aphthous stomatitis** a condition in which painful canker sores in the mouth return again and again. The cause is unknown, but it may be an immune response. **Pseudomembranous stomatitis** is a severe mouth inflammation with a fluid release. It may result from bacteria or chemicals. Symptoms include problems in swallowing, pain, fever, and swelling of the lymph glands.

stomatognathic system /stō'mətōnath'ik/,   the combination of organs, structures, and nerves involved in speech and reception, chewing, and swallowing of food. This system is composed of the teeth, jaws, tongue, lips, and surrounding tissues, muscles, and nerves that control these structures.

stool.   See **feces.**

strabismus /strəbiz'məs/,   an abnormal condition in which the eyes do not move together or are "crossed." An inward deviation of one eye in relation to the other eye is called convergent or internal strabismus or **esotropia.** The outward deviation of one eye in relation to the other is called divergent or external strabismus or **exotropia.** Also called **squint.**

straight sinus,   one of the six vein passages on the top and front of the brain, draining blood from the brain into the jugular vein. It has no valves.

strain,   **1.** damage, usually muscular, that results from excessive physical effort. **2.** an emotional state reflecting mental pressure or fatigue.

straitjacket,   a coat of canvas with long sleeves that can be tied behind the wearer's back to prevent movement of the arms. It is used to restrain violent or uncontrollable people.

strangulation,   the tightening or closing of a tubular structure of the body, as the throat, a section of bowel, or the blood vessels of a limb, that prevents function or slows circulation. See also **intestinal strangulation.**

strap, 1. a band, as that made of adhesive plaster, that is used to hold dressings in place or to attach one thing to another. **2.** to bind securely.

strapping, putting overlapping strips of adhesive tape to an arm, leg, or other parts of the body or body area to exert pressure and hold a structure in place, done to treat strains, sprains, dislocations, and some fractures.

stratum /strā′təm, strat′əm/, *pl.* **strata,** an even, thick sheet or layer, usually linked with other layers, as the stratum basale of the skin.

strawberry mark. See **hemangioma.**

strawberry tongue, a symptom of scarlet fever, marked by a strawberry-like color of the tongue.

strep throat, *informal.* an infection of the throat and tonsils caused by a germ *(Streptococcus).* Symptoms include sore throat, chills, fever, swollen lymph glands in the neck, and, sometimes, nausea and vomiting. The symptoms usually begin suddenly a few days after exposure to the germs in airborne droplets or after direct contact with an infected person.

streptococcal infection /strep′təkok′əl/, an infection caused by disease-causing bacteria of one of several types of *Streptococcus* or their poisons. Almost any organ of the body may be involved. The infections occur in many forms, including endocarditis, erysipelas, impetigo, meningitis, pneumonia, scarlet fever, tonsillitis, and urinary tract infection. See also **strep throat.**

Streptococcus /-kok′əs/, a type of bacteria, causing many diseases in humans. **Beta-hemolytic streptococci** cause most of the acute streptococcal infections seen in humans, including rheumatic fever and many cases of pneumonia and septicemia. Penicillin is usually prescribed to treat these infections.

streptomycin sulfate /-mī′sin/, an antibiotic. It is used to treat tuberculosis, endocarditis, and certain other infections. Labyrinthitis or known allergy to this drug prohibits its use. It must be used with caution in damaged kidney function and in the elderly. Side effects include damage to the ears and hearing, kidney damage, muscle weakness, and allergic reactions.

stress, any emotional, physical, social, economic, or other factor that requires a response or change, as severe loss of fluid, which can cause a rise in body temperature, or a separation from parents, which can cause a young child to cry. See also **general adaptation syndrome.**

stress fracture, a bone break, especially of one or more of the foot bones, caused by repeated, long-term, or abnormal stress.

Stress-producing life events in ranked order

1. Death of spouse
2. Divorce
3. Marital separation
4. Jail term
5. Death of close family member
6. Personal injury or illness
7. Marriage
8. Fired at work
9. Marital reconciliation
10. Retirement
11. Change in health of family member
12. Pregnancy
13. Sex difficulties
14. Gain of new family member
15. Business readjustment
16. Change in financial state
17. Death of close friend
18. Change to different line of work
19. Change in number of arguments with spouse
20. Mortgage or loan major purchase (home, etc.)
21. Foreclosure of mortgage or loan
22. Change in responsibilities at work
23. Son or daughter leaving home
24. Trouble with in-laws
25. Outstanding personal achievement
26. Spouse begins or stops work
27. Begin or end school
28. Change in living conditions
29. Revision of personal habits
30. Trouble with boss
31. Change in work hours or conditions
32. Change in residence
33. Change in schools
34. Change in recreation
35. Change in church activities
36. Change in social activities
37. Mortgage or loan for lesser purchase (car, TV, etc.)
38. Change in sleeping habits
39. Change in number of family get-togethers
40. Change in eating habits
41. Vacation
42. Christmas
43. Minor violations of the law

Reprinted with permission from Holmes, T.H., and Rahe, R.H.: J. Psychosom. Res. 11:213-218, 1967, Pergamon Press, Ltd.

stressor, anything that causes wear and tear on the body's physical or mental resources. See also **general adaptation syndrome.**

stress reaction, a response to extreme anxiety. Also called **posttraumatic stress disorder,** it is caused by a shocking or tragic event, such as a natural disaster, an airplane crash, or physical torture. Symptoms include going over memories or nightmares again and again, having no interest in daily life, having bad, restless sleep, and having headaches. One form is **combat fatigue,** which results from the physical and mental stress of warfare. It is usually temporary but sometimes leads to permanent neurosis. **Shell shock,** also caused by the stress of combat, may be any of a number of mental disorders, ranging from extreme fear to dementia. Treatment for a stress reaction includes the use of drugs to calm the patient and help for the patient's mental state (psychotherapy). See also **general adaptation syndrome.**

stress test,   a test that measures a system of the body when subjected to carefully controlled stress. This kind of test is often used to test the heart and lungs, and the health of the fetus in pregnant women. An **exercise electrocardiogram (exercise ECG)** is used in a stress test to diagnose disease of the arteries of the heart. It is recorded while a person walks on a treadmill or pedals a stationary bicycle. Abnormal changes in heart function may appear during exercise. Some abnormalities will not show on ECG during rest. See also **oxytocin challenge test.**

stria /strī′ə/, *pl.* **striae,**   a streak or a narrow furrow in the skin that often results from a stretching of the skin, as seen on the stomach after pregnancy. Purplish striae are one of the classic findings in a disorder of the pituitary gland (Cushing's syndrome). Also called **stretch mark.**

striated muscle /strī′ātid/.   See **muscle.**

stricture /strik′chər/,   an abnormal narrowing of the tube of a hollow organ, as the throat, pylorus of the stomach, ureter, or urethra, because of inflammation, pressure from outside the body, or scarring. Treatment depends on the cause. Compare **spasm.**

stridor /strī′dər/,   an abnormal, high-pitched breath sound, caused by a blockage in the throat or larynx. It is usually heard when breathing in. Stridor may indicate a tumor or inflammation. Compare **rales, rhonchi.**

strike team,   specified combinations of the same kind and type of resources, with common communication and a leader.

string carcinoma,   a cancer of the large intestine, usually of the colon that, in an x-ray photo, causes the intestine to appear to be tied in segments like a string of large beads.

stripping,   **1.** an operation for the removal of the long and the short saphenous veins of the legs. With **subcutaneous stripping,** a varicosed saphenous vein is removed by inserting an acorn-tipped rod, tying the vein to the rod, and drawing it out. **2.** the removal of a very small amount

of enamel from the top and sides of teeth to ease crowding.

stroke,   a blood clot (embolus) or bleeding in the brain. This results in lack of oxygen to the brain tissues that are normally supplied by the vessels. The after-effects of a stroke depend on the location and extent of damage. Paralysis, weakness, speech defect, inability to understand language, or death may occur. Symptoms usually go away somewhat after the first few days as brain swelling subsides. Physical therapy and speech therapy may restore much lost function. Also called **cerebrovascular accident.**

stroke prone profile,   a list of risk factors that show whether a person may be likely to have a stroke. The factors include advanced age, high blood pressure, previous attacks of poor circulation, cigarette smoking, heart disorders, embolism, family history of strokes, use of birth control pills, diabetes mellitus, lack of exercise, overweight, and high cholesterol.

stroma /strō′mə/, *pl.* **stromata,**   the supporting tissue for an organ. An example is the vitreous stroma, which encloses the vitreous humor of the eye.

strongyloidiasis /stron′jəloidī′əsis/.   See **threadworm infection.**

structural integration,   a method of deep massage intended to help by realigning the body by changing the length and tone of certain tissues. It is believed by some that improper posture and mental and bodily injuries may have a bad effect on a person's energy level, self-image, muscular efficiency, perceptions, and general health. Also called **Rolfing.** See also **massage.**

structure,   a part of the body, as the heart, a bone, a gland, a cell, or a limb.

Stryker wedge frame,   a special bed that allows the patient to be turned over as needed. It is used to treat patients with certain disorders of the spine or with very bad burns.

Stuartnatal 1+1,   a trademark for a drug given by mouth to pregnant women, containing vitamins and minerals.

stump,   the part of a limb that is left after amputation. A **stump hallucination** is the feeling of the continued presence of an amputated limb. See also **phantom limb syndrome.**

stupor,   a condition in which a person seems unaware of the surroundings or is almost unconscious. The condition occurs in nerve and mental disorders. With **anergic stupor,** the person is quiet, listless, and nonresistant. A **benign stupor,** a state of apathy or lethargy, occurs in severe depression. A **delusion stupor,** seen in catatonic schizophrenia, is a state in which a patient is unresponsive.

An **epileptic stupor** is the state of being unaware or unresponsive directly after an epileptic seizure.

Sturge-Weber syndrome, a disease of the nerves of the skin marked by a port-wine-colored noncancerous tumor on the face. It may be linked with certain kinds of brain damage, certain eye disorders, and seizures. There is no known cure. Drugs may be given to control convulsions.

stuttering, a speech defect marked by halting speech, involving many hesitations, stumbling, repeating the same syllables, and holding some sounds for a long time. The condition may result from a brain or nerve disorder or an injury to the organs of speech, but in most cases the cause is emotional and mental. Hesitancy in speech are normal traits of language development during the preschool years. If too much emphasis or stress is placed on this pattern, the child becomes conscious of the difficulties and may develop a fear of speaking. Stuttering can usually be cured until about 7 years of age. If stuttering continues, treatment by a speech therapist may be necessary.

sty, a pus-forming infection on the edge of the eyelid formed in the root of an eyelash. Treatment includes compresses and antibiotic eye medicines; it occasionally requires opening and drainage. Compare **chalazion.** Also called **hordeolum.**

stylohyoideus /stī'lōhī·oi'dē·əs/, one of the neck muscles.

stylohyoid ligament /-hī'oid/, the ligament attached to the side of the head that runs to the throat.

stylomandibular ligament /stī'lōmandib'yələr/, one of a pair of special fibrous bands of tissue that forms part of the jaw joint (temporomandibular).

styptic /stip'tik/, **1.** a substance used to control bleeding. **2.** acting as an agent to control bleeding.

subacromial bursa /subəkrō'mē·əl/, the small fluid-filled sac in the shoulder joint.

subacute /-əkyoot'/, relating to a disease or other abnormal condition present in a patient who appears to be well. The condition may be identified or discovered by means of a laboratory test or by x-ray test.

subarachnoid hemorrhage /-ərak'noid/, a bleeding into a fluid-filled space between the layers of membranes at the base of the brain near the spine. The cause may be an injury or breaking of an aneurysm. The first symptom is a sudden painful headache that begins in one area and then spreads, becoming dull and throbbing. Other symptoms include dizziness, stiffness of the neck, vomiting, drowsiness, sweating and chills, stupor, and loss of consciousness. It may result in continued unconsciousness, coma, and death.

subcapital fracture, a break just below the head of a bone that pivots in a ball and socket joint.

subcapsular cataract /-kap'syələr/, a condition marked by cloudiness beneath the capsule of the lens of the eye.

subclavian /-klā'vē·ən/, situated under the clavicle, or collarbone, as the subclavian artery.

subclavian artery, one of a pair of arteries that rise in the neck and supply blood to the vertebral column, spinal cord, ear, and brain.

subclavian steal syndrome, a disorder caused by a blockage in the subclavian artery near the beginning of the vertebral artery. The block causes a change in blood pressure and blood flow. Symptoms include attacks of paralysis of the arm and pain behind the ear and in the back of the skull. Very different blood pressure readings from the arms are sometimes symptoms of the condition.

subclavius /-klā'vē·əs/, a short muscle of the chest wall. It moves the shoulder down and forward.

subclinical, relating to a disease or abnormal condition that is so mild it produces no symptoms.

subcutaneous /sub'kyoota'nē·əs/, beneath the skin.

subcutaneous nodule, a small, solid bump beneath the skin that can be detected by touch.

suberosis /soo'bərō'-/, a lung disease caused by an allergic reaction to cork dust.

subgingival calculus /-jin'jivəl/, a small stone, made up of collected minerals, bits of food, and other matter found in the mouth, which occurs on the teeth or in the gum next to the teeth.

subgingival curettage, a method of removing some growths on or within the gums. It is used to reduce swelling and to restore the health of the gums.

subinvolution, a condition that occurs when the womb does not return to normal after the birth of a child. It features longer and heavier bleeding after childbirth and, on pelvic examination, a larger and softer uterus than would be expected at that time.

Sublimaze Citrate, a trademark for a powerful painkilling drug (fentanyl citrate).

sublingual /-ling'gwəl/, beneath the tongue.

subluxation /-luksā'shən/, a partial dislocation. For example, a **shoulder subluxation** is an injury to the tissues around the shoulder joint.

submandibular duct /-mandib'yələr/, a tube through which a submandibular gland releases saliva. Also called **submaxillary duct.**

submucous /-myoo'kəs/, beneath a mucous membrane.

subperiosteal fracture /-per'ē·os'tēəl/, a break in a bone beneath the membrane that covers each bone.

subphrenic /-fren'ik/, referring to the area beneath or under the diaphragm.

substance abuse, the overuse of and addiction to a stimulant, depressant, or other chemical substance, leading to effects that are harmful to the patient's health, or the welfare of others.

S

substance P, a nerve-carrying substance that is made by the body. Its uses include widening of the vessels, tightening of the intestines and other smooth muscles, a part in the release of saliva and urine, and in the function of the nervous systems.

substratum /-strā′təm/, any underlying layer; a foundation.

subthalamus /-thal′əməs/, a portion of the brain that serves as a center for signals from the eye and eye spaces. –**subthalamic,** *adj.*

subtle, not severe and having no serious results, as a mild infection.

subungual hematoma /-ung′gwəl/, a pool of blood beneath a nail, usually resulting from injury. The pain accompanying this condition may be quickly eased by burning or drilling a small hole through the nail to release the blood.

succus /suk′əs/, *pl.* **succi** /suk′sī/, a juice or fluid, usually one released by an organ.

succussion splash /səkush′ən/, a sound heard in the body of a patient who has free fluid and air or gas in a hollow organ or body space. This sound may be heard over a normal stomach but may also be heard with hernias or blockages.

sucking blisters, the pale, soft pads on the upper and lower lips of a baby that look like blisters but are not. They form as soon as the baby begins to suck well, at the breast or on a bottle.

suckle, 1. to provide nourishment, specifically to breast-feed. 2. to take in as nourishment, especially by feeding from the breast.

Sucostrin, a trademark for a drug used in anesthesia (succinylcholine).

sucrose /soo′krōs/, sugar derived from sugar cane, sugar beets, and sorghum.

sucrose polyester (SPE), an artificial fat that, when added to the diet, lowers blood cholesterol levels by increasing the excretion of cholesterol in the feces. It is made to have the texture and taste of margarine or vegetable oil and adds no calories to the diet.

suction curettage, a method of removing material from the womb by suction. The cervix is widened, a tube is inserted into the womb, and suction is applied. Also called **vacuum aspiration.** Compare **dilatation and curettage.**

suction device, a vacuum-, air-, or oxygen-powered device that is used to remove blood, secretions, or other fluids from a patient's mouth, throat, or stoma. Electrical, oxygen, and manually powered units are available.

Sudafed, a trademark for a vessel-narrowing drug (pseudoephedrine hydrochloride), used as a decongestant and bronchodilator.

sudden infant death syndrome (SIDS), the unexpected and sudden death of a seemingly normal and healthy infant that occurs during sleep and with no physical evidence of disease. It is the most common cause of death in children between 2 weeks and 1 year of age. The origin is unknown. Also called **crib death.**

Characteristics of SIDS

Factors	Occurrence
Incidence	1.5 to 2 per 1000 live births
Peak age	2 to 4 months; 90% occur by 6 months
Sex	Higher percentage of males affected
Time of death	Usually during nighttime
Time of year	Increased incidence in winter
Birth	Higher incidence in:
	Premature infants
	Multiple births
	Neonates with low Apgar scores
	Infants with central nervous system disturbances
Feeding habits	Not significant; breast feeding does not prevent SIDS
Siblings	Ten times greater incidence
Possible causes	CNS anomaly
	Cardiovascular anomaly
	Airway anomaly
	Infection
	Chronic hypoxia

sudoriferous gland /soo′dôrif′ərəs/. See **sweat gland.**

sudorific /soo′dôrif′ik/, referring to a drug, substance, or condition, as heat or emotional tension, that causes sweating. Also called **diaphoretic.**

suicide, the intentional taking of one's own life. Early signs of suicidal intent include depression; expressions of guilt, tension, and nervousness; insomnia; loss of weight and appetite; neglect of personal appearance; and direct or indirect threats to commit suicide.

sulcus /sul′kəs/, a depression or furrow on an organ or as in the chest cavity that holds up part of the lung.

sulfacetamide, an antibacteria drug used to protect against infection after eye injury and to treat some eye diseases. It is also used to treat infections of the urinary system. Known allergy to the drug or to other sulfonamides or kidney damage prohibits its use. Side effects include local pain, growth of other bacteria, and an allergic reaction to the drug.

Sulfacet-R, a trademark for a drug containing a substance to prevent scabies (sulfur), an antibacteria drug (sulfacetamide sodium), and an antiseptic and cell-tightening substance (zinc oxide).

sulfacytine, an antibacteria drug. It is used to treat infection of the urinary tract. Porphyria, urinary tract blockages, or known allergy to sulfonamides prohibits its use. Side effects include sensitivity to light, severe allergic reactions, and blood disorders.

sulfamethizole, an antibacteria drug used to treat infection, mainly of the kidney and urinary tract. Porphyria, urinary tract blockages, or known allergy to sulfonamides prohibits its use. Side effects include sensitivity to light, blood disorders, and severe allergic reactions.

sulfamethoxazole, an antibacteria drug used to treat otitis media, bronchitis, and some urinary tract infections. It is not given during the last 3 months of pregnancy, during breast feeding, or to children under 2 months of age. Known allergy to sulfonamides prohibits its use. Side effects include rash, fever, and other allergic reactions.

sulfamethoxazole and trimethoprim, an antibacteria drug used to treat urinary tract infections, otitis media, and a bowel infection (shigellosis). It is used with caution in patients with kidney and liver damage, or with known allergy to either drug or to sulfonamides. It is not for use in infants under 2 months of age or in the last 3 months of pregnancy. Side effects include rashes, fever, and other allergic reactions.

Sulfamylon, a trademark for an antiinfection drug (mafenide acetate).

sulfasalazine, a sulfonamide drug used to treat mild to moderate ulcerative colitis and as therapy in severe cases. Urinary blockage or known allergy to sulfonamides or to salicylates prohibits its use. It is not given during the last 3 months of pregnancy. Side effects include urine and digestive problems, loss of appetite, blood diseases, and severe allergic reactions.

sulfhemoglobin, a form of hemoglobin containing a bound sulfur molecule that stops normal oxygen binding. It is present in the blood in small amounts.

sulfinpyrazone, a drug used to aid in excreting uric acid in the urine. It is used to treat gout and gouty arthritis. Peptic ulcer, ulcerative colitis, kidney failure, or known allergy to this drug or to phenylbutazone prohibits its use. Side effects include ulcers in the stomach and intestines, blood disorders, and dermatitis.

sulfisoxazole, an antibacteria drug used to treat conjunctivitis and urinary tract infections. Porphyria, urinary tract blockage, or known allergy to this drug or to sulfonamide drugs prohibits its use. It is not given during the last 3 months of pregnancy or to children under 2 months of age. Side effects include blood disorders and severe allergy reactions.

sulfiting agents, food preservatives used in processing of various foods and by restaurants to impart a ''fresh'' appearance to salad fruits and vegetables. The chemicals can cause a severe reaction in persons who are allergic to sulfites. The reactions include flushing, faintness, hives, headache, distress in the stomach and intestines, breathing difficulty, and, in extreme cases, loss of consciousness and death.

sulfonamide /səlfon′əmīd/, one of a large group of artificial drugs that are effective in treating infections.

Sulfoxyl, a trademark for a drug containing a disinfectant (benzoyl peroxide) and a substance to prevent scabies (sulfur).

sulfur (S) /sul′fər/, a tasteless, odorless chemical element that is used to make sulfuric acid and used commercially in many industrial processes. Sulfur has been used to treat gout, rheumatism, and bronchitis and as a mild laxative. The sulfonamides, or sulfa drugs, are used to treat various bacteria infections.

sulfuric acid /sulfyoor′ik/, a clear, colorless, oily, highly dangerous liquid that creates great heat when mixed with water. A very poisonous substance, sulfuric acid causes severe skin burns, blindness on contact with the eyes, serious lung damage if the vapors are breathed in, and death if it is eaten or drunk. It is used in various ways in industry, such as in the making of fertilizers. Weak solutions of sulfuric acid are used to treat gastric hypoacidity and serious diarrhea.

sulindac, an antiinflammatory drug. It is used to treat osteoarthritis, rheumatoid arthritis, and ankylosing spondylitis.

Sulkowitch's test, a test of the urine for calcium. Also called **S's test.** See also **hypercalciuria.**

Sultrin, a trademark for a vaginal drug containing antibacterials (sulfathiazole, sulfacetamide, and sulfabenzamide).

Sumycin, a trademark for an antibiotic (tetracycline hydrochloride).

sundowning, a condition in which elderly patients tend to become confused at the end of the day. Many of them have trouble seeing and varying degrees of hearing loss. With less light, they lose visual cues that help them to make up for their sensory losses.

sunstroke. See **heatstroke.**

Supen, a trademark for an antibacteria drug (ampicillin).

superfecundation /soo′pərfe′kəndā′shən/, the fertilization of two or more eggs released during one menstrual cycle by sperm from the same or different males during separate acts of sexual intercourse.

superfetation /-fētā′shən/, the fertilization of a second egg after the onset of pregnancy, resulting in the presence of two fetuses of different degrees of maturity developing within the uterus at the same time. Also called **superimpregnation.**

superficial, **1.** relating to the skin or another surface. **2.** not grave or dangerous.

superficial inguinal node, a lymph gland in one of the two groups in the upper thigh that supply the skin of the penis, scrotum, perineum, buttocks, and abdominal wall below the level of the navel.

superficial reflex, any nerve reflex begun by stimulation of the skin. The **abdominal reflex** is caused by firmly stroking the skin of the belly. The muscles contract, and the navel moves toward the side stroked. An **anal reflex** is caused by stroking the skin around the anus. This results in a contraction of the anal muscle (sphincter). This reflex may be lost in a nerve (neurologic) disease. The **cremasteric reflex** is triggered by stroking the skin of the upper inner thigh in a male. This normally causes the testicle to draw up toward the body. The reflex is lost in certain nervous system diseases. Compare **deep tendon reflex.**

superficial vein, one of the many veins between the layers of tissue just under the skin. Compare **deep vein.**

superinfection, an infection that occurs while treating another infection. It often results from change in the normal tissue favoring growth of some organisms by lowering the vitality and then the number of competing organisms, as yeast microbes thrive during penicillin therapy used to cure a bacterial infection.

superior, found above or higher, as the head is superior to the torso. Compare **inferior.**

superior costotransverse ligament, one of five ligaments that help connect each rib to the spine.

superior mesenteric artery, a large artery in the lower body that supplies blood to the small intestine and parts of the colon.

superior mesenteric vein, a branch of the vein that drains the blood from the small intestine, the cecum, and the colon.

superior radioulnar joint, the pivot joint of the elbow. The joint lets the lower arm move in circles. Also called **proximal radioulnar articulation.**

superior sagittal sinus, one of six vein paths in the back of the membrane covering the brain (dura mater) that drains blood from the brain.

superior subscapular nerve /subskap'yələr/, one of two small nerves on opposite sides of the body that supply the top part of the muscle in the front of the shoulder.

superior thyroid artery, one of a pair of arteries in the neck that supply the thyroid gland and several muscles in the head.

superior ulnar collateral artery, a long, slender division of the main artery of the upper arm.

supernumerary nipples, a larger than normal number of nipples, which are usually not linked with glands underneath. They may vary in size from small pink dots to that of normal nipples.

supination /soo'pinā'shən/, one of the kinds of turning allowed by certain joints, as the elbow and the wrist joints, which allow the palm of the hand to turn up. See also **supine.** Compare **pronation.** –**supinate,** v.

supine /səpīn', soo'pīn/, lying flat on the back, face up. Compare **prone.** See also **body position.**

supporting area, any of the areas of the upper or lower jaw that are considered best able to bear the force of chewing with false teeth.

suppository /səpoz'itôr'ē/, an easily melted cone or cylinder of material mixed with a drug for placing in the rectum, urethra, or vagina. Drugs given in this way are absorbed into the system. This route is especially useful in babies, in patients who won't cooperate, and in cases of vomiting or certain digestive disorders.

suppurate /sup'yərāt/, to make pus.

supraclavicular /soo'prəkləvik'yələr/, the area of the body above the collarbone (clavicle).

supraclavicular nerve, one of a pair of nerves that run along the collarbone from the neck to the shoulder.

supracondylar fracture /-kon'dilər/, a break between the bulges (condyles) at the big end of an arm or thigh bone.

supragingival calculus /-jin'jivəl/, a stony deposit, made up of various minerals, bits of food, and other matter found in the mouth, that forms on the teeth.

suprascapular nerve /-skap'yələr/, one of a pair of nerves that run from the neck to the shoulder and shoulderblade.

Surfacaine, a trademark for a local anesthetic (cyclomethycaine sulfate).

surface therapy, a form of x-ray treatment given by placing a radioactive substance on or near a part of the skin.

Surfadil, a trademark for a drug containing a substance to treat an allergy or a cold (methapyrilene hydrochloride) and an anesthetic (cyclomethycaine sulfate).

Surfak, a trademark for a drug used to soften feces (docusate calcium).

surfer's nodules, small bumps on the skin of the knees, ankles, feet, or toes of a surfer caused by repeated contact of the skin with a gritty, sandy surfboard. They get smaller and go away if surfing is stopped. Treatment includes injection of steroids.

surgery, a branch of medicine concerned with diseases and injury needing an operation. –**surgical,** adj.

surgical ligature, an operation in which the gum is opened to allow a metal band to be placed around a tooth that has not come through. Tiny chains fastened to the band are attached to a device that forces the tooth out.

surgical sectioning, a dental operation in which a tooth is broken into several pieces in order to make it easier to remove it.

Surital Sodium, a trademark for a barbiturate (thiamylal sodium), used with an anesthetic.

Surmontil, a trademark for an antidepression drug (trimipramine maleate).

survey instrument, a portable instrument used for detecting and measuring radiation under varied physical conditions. The term covers a wide range of devices such as the CD V-700 Geiger counter, the CD V-715 ionization chamber, and many other similar instruments.

susceptibility /səsep′təbil′itē/, the condition of being more than normally likely to fall ill to a disease or disorder. –**susceptible,** *adj.*

suspension, a treatment that uses traction equipment, including metal frames, ropes, and pulleys, to relieve the weight on various parts of the body. One use is for disorders of the spine and consists of hanging the patient by the chin and shoulders. **Balanced suspension** is a system for suspending the legs. It is used as an aid to healing of fractures or after surgical operations. **Hyperextension suspension** is used to position hip muscles after an operation. This relieves the weight of the lower limbs and properly positions the muscles of the hip, without applying traction to the lower limbs involved. **Lower extremity suspension** is used to treat bone fractures and correct abnormalities of the legs. **Upper extremity suspension** treats bone fractures and corrects abnormalities of the upper limbs. It relieves the weight of the upper limb involved rather than exerting traction.

sutilains /soo′tilānz/, an enzyme used to treat certain wounds, ulcers, and second- and third-degree burns. Wounds opening into major body spaces or containing exposed major nerves or nervous tissue, or certain types of ulcer prohibits its use. It is not given during pregnancy. Side effects include bleeding, numbness (paresthesias), and dermatitis.

sutura /sootoor′ə/, *pl.* **suturae,** an immovable, fiberlike joint in which certain bones of the skull are connected by a thin layer of tissue. They form a connection in various ways. For example, one kind has toothlike processes that interlock along the margins of connecting bones. Another has curved and jagged edges that overlap.

suture /soo′chər/, **1.** a border or a joint, as between the bones of the cranium. **2.** to stitch together cut or torn edges of tissue with suture material. **3.** a surgical stitch taken to repair a cut, tear, or wound. A **button suture** is a means of passing the suture material through buttons on the surface of the skin and knotting. It is used to prevent the suture from cutting through the skin. **4.** material used for surgical stitches, as absorbable or nonabsorbable silk, catgut, wire, or synthetic material.

swab, a stick or clamp for holding absorbent gauze or cotton, used for washing, cleansing, or drying a body surface, for collecting a specimen for laboratory tests, or for applying a topical medication.

swanneck deformity, a defect of the kidney tubules linked with rickets.

sweat, the fluid or the release of fluid by the sweat glands through pores in the skin. Also called **perspiration,** it is made up of water with salt (sodium chloride), phosphate, urea, ammonia, and other waste products. A small amount of perspiration is continually released by the sweat glands in the skin. It helps control body temperature. The loss of fluid from the body by evaporation, as normally occurs during breathing, is called **insensible perspiration.** The portion that evaporates before it may be observed also contributes to insensible perspiration.

sweat bath, a bath given to induce sweating.

sweat duct, any one of the tiny tubes carrying sweat to the surface of the skin from the sweat glands throughout the body. The sweat ducts in the armpits and in the groin are larger than in other parts of the body.

sweat gland, one of about 3 million tiny structures within the skin that make sweat. The average quantity of sweat secreted in 24 hours varies from 700 to 900 g. The number of glands per square centimeter of skin varies in different parts of the body. They are found in great numbers on the palms of the hands and on the soles of the feet and fewest in the neck and the back. They are completely absent in the deeper parts of the ear canal, the prepuce, and the glans penis. Also called **sudoriferous gland.** Compare **sebaceous gland.**

sweating. See **diaphoresis.**

sweat test, a method for measuring sodium and chloride released from the sweat glands, often the first test performed to detect cystic fibrosis. The sweat glands are made to work with a drug, and the sweat that results is tested. The test is very trustworthy, and although it may be useful at any age, it is usually done on infants from 2 weeks to 1 year of age. See also **cystic fibrosis.**

Sweet localization method, a type of x-ray test used to find a foreign body in the eye by making two x-ray films of the eye while the patient's head is held still.

swimmer's ear, infection of the ear carried in the water of a swimming pool.

S

swimmer's itch, an allergic skin condition caused by sensitivity to tiny wormlike organisms (schistosome cercarias) that die under the skin, leading to reddening of the skin and the appearance of a rash lasting 1 or 2 days. Treatment includes skin lotions and drugs to relieve itching.

swimming pool conjunctivitis, a virus infection with symptoms of fever, sore throat, and red eyes (conjunctivitis). The disease spreads quickly in warm weather. Infected water in lakes and swimming pools is a common cause of the infection. Also called **pharyngoconjunctival fever.**

Sydenham's chorea /sid′ənhamz/. See **chorea.**

symmelia /simē′lyə/, a defect of the fetus marked by the growing together of the lower limbs with or without feet.

Symmetrel, a trademark for an antivirus drug (amantadine hydrochloride).

symmetrical, (of the body or parts of the body) equal in size or shape; very similar in placement about an axis. Compare **asymmetrical.** –**symmetry,** *n.*

symmetric tonic neck reflex. See **crawling reflex.**

sympathectomy /sim′pəthek′-/, an operation done to ease pain in some vessel diseases, as arteriosclerosis, claudication, and Buerger's disease, and to increase the blood flow through a graft area. The sheath around an artery carries the sympathetic nerve fibers that control tightening of the vessel. Removing part of the sheath causes the vessel to relax and expand and allows more blood to pass through it.

sympathetic amine /sim′pəthet′ik/, a drug that causes effects that look like those made normally by the sympathetic nervous system.

sympathetic nervous system. See **autonomic nervous system.**

sympathetic trunk, one of a pair of chains of nerves that lie along the side of the spine from the base of the skull to the tailbone. Each trunk is part of the sympathetic nervous system.

sympathizing eye. See **ophthalmia.**

sympatholytic /sim′pəthōlit′ik/. See **antiadrenergic.**

sympathomimetic /-mimet′ik/, a drug that causes effects that look like those from the sympathetic nervous system. They are used as decongestants, to treat lung diseases, and to treat low blood pressure and shock. Side effects include nervousness, headache, anxiety, vertigo, nausea, vomiting, widened pupils, and some urine disorders. See also **adrenergic.**

symphalangia /sim′fəlan′jē·ə/, a birth defect in which webbing of the fingers or toes occurs in varying degrees, often along with other defects of the hands or feet. See also **syndactyly.**

symphocephalus /sim′fəsef′ələs/, twin fetuses joined at the head. The term is often used as a general term for fetuses with varying degrees of the defect.

symphyseal angle /simfiz′ē·əl/, (in dentistry) the angle of the chin, which may be striking out, straight, or receding, according to type.

symphysis /sim′fisis/, *pl.* **symphyses** /-ēz/, a joint made of cartilage in which bony surfaces lying next to one another are firmly united by fiberlike cartilage. Also called **fibrocartilaginous joint.**

sympodia /simpō′dē·ə/, a birth defect marked by fusion of the lower limbs.

symptom, something felt or noticed by the patient that can help to detect a disease or disorder. See also **sign.**

symptothermal method of family planning /simp′təthur′məl/. See **natural family planning method.**

sympus /sim′pəs/, a deformed fetus in which the legs are completely grown together or twisted and the pelvis and genitals are defective.

Synalar, a trademark for a nerve blocking drug (fluocinolone acetonide).

synapse /sin′aps/, **1.** the point where one nerve signal jumps from one nerve cell to another. Normally, nerve signals only travel in one direction; they are also subject to fatigue, oxygen deficiency, anesthetics, and other chemical agents. **2.** to form a synapse or connection between nerve cells. –**synaptic,** *adj.*

synchilia /singkē′lyə/, a birth defect in which the lips are partly or totally grown together.

syncope /sing′kəpē/, a fainting spell. It usually follows a feeling of lightheadedness and may often be prevented by lying down or by sitting with the head between the knees. It may be caused by many different factors, including emotional stress, pooling of blood in the legs, heavy sweating, or sudden change in room temperature or body position. Many patients, especially men, suffer such attacks during violent coughing spells because of rapid changes in blood pressure. Syncope may also result from any of a number of heart and lung disorders.

syndactyly /sindak′tilē/, a birth defect marked by the growing together of the fingers or toes. It varies in degree of severity from partial webbing of the skin of two digits to complete union of the fingers or toes and the growing together of the bones and nails.

syndrome, a group of signs and symptoms that occur together and are typical of a particular disorder or disease.

syndrome of inappropriate antidiuretic hormone secretion (SIADH), an abnormal condition with a release of too much of a certain hormone that creates an imbalance in the body. It is linked with some lung cancers. Symptoms include weight gain despite loss of appetite, vomiting, nausea, muscle weakness, and irritability. There may be coma and convulsions.

synechia /sinek′ē·ə/, *pl.* **synechiae,** a scarring together (adhesion) of the iris to the cornea or lens of the eye. It may develop from glaucoma, cataracts, or keratitis or as a complication of surgery or injury to the eye. Blindness may develop. Treatment includes widening the pupils with a drug, followed by treatment of the cause.

Synemol, a trademark for a nerve-blocking drugs (fluocinolone acetonide).

Synkayvite, a trademark for an artificial form of vitamin K (menadiol sodium diphosphate).

Synophylate, a trademark for a bronchodilator (theophylline sodium glycinate).

synotia /sīnō′shə/, a birth defect marked by the drawing together of the ears in front of the neck, often with the absence of the lower jaw.

synovectomy /sin′ōvek′-/, the cutting out of a synovial membrane of a joint.

synovia /sinō′vē·ə/, a clear, sticky fluid, resembling the white of an egg, released by synovial membranes and acting as a lubricant for many joints, bursae, and tendons. It contains mucin, albumin, fat, and mineral salts. Also called **synovial fluid.** –**synovial,** *adj.*

synovial membrane /sinō′vē·əl/, the inner layer of a capsule surrounding a freely movable joint. The synovial membrane secretes into the joint a thick fluid that normally oils the joint but that may collect in painful amounts when the joint is injured.

synovial sarcoma, a cancer that begins as a soft swelling and often spreads through the bloodstream to the lung before it is discovered.

synovitis /sin′əvī′-/, inflammation of the synovial membrane of a joint that results from a wound or an injury, such as a sprain or severe strain of the knee. Fluid collects, the joint is swollen, tender, and painful, and motion is limited. In most cases, the fluid is absorbed without medical or surgical treatment.

synthetic, relating to a substance that is artificial instead of natural.

Synthroid, a trademark for a thyroid hormone (levothyroxine sodium).

Syntocinon, a trademark for a drug used to speed up childbirth (oxytocin).

syphilis, a sexually carried disease caused by a type of bacteria *(Treponema pallidum),* marked by three clear stages over a period of years. Any organ system may become involved. The bacteria are able to pass into a fetus in the womb, causing syphilis in the newborn at birth. In the first stage **(primary syphilis),** a small, painless, red pus-forming bump appears on the skin or mucous membrane between 10 and 90 days after exposure. The sore may appear anywhere on the body where contact with a sore on an infected person has occurred, but is seen most often in the pelvic region. It quickly forms a painless, bloodless ulcer, called a chancre, releasing a fluid that swarms with bacteria. The chancre may not be noticed by the patient, and many people may become infected. It heals by itself within 10 to 40 days, often giving the mistaken impression that the sore was not serious. The second stage **(secondary syphilis)** occurs about 2 months later, after the bacteria have spread throughout the body. Symptoms include loss of appetite, nausea, fever, headache, hair loss, bone and joint pain, a rash that does not itch, flat white sores in the mouth and throat, or pimples on the moist areas of the skin. The disease remains highly contagious at this stage. The symptoms usually continue for up to 3 months but may recur over 2 years. The third stage **(tertiary syphilis)** may not develop for 3 to 15 or more years. Soft, rubbery tumors, called gummas, appear that fester and heal by scarring. Gummas may develop anywhere on the surface of the body and in the eye, liver, lungs, stomach, or sexual organs. Tertiary syphilis may be painless, unnoticed except for gummas, or there may be deep, burrowing pain. The ulceration of the gummas may result in punched-out areas of the mouth, nose, and throat. Various parts of the body, including the nervous system and the heart, may be damaged or destroyed, leading to mental or physical disorders and premature death. **Syphilitic aortitis,** an inflammation of the large artery (aorta), may occur in tertiary syphilis. Widespread widening with plaques containing calcium on the inner coat and scars on the outer coat results. There may be damage to the valves, and the formation of blood clots, such as in the brain. Symptoms include pain in the middle of the chest, shortness of breath, bounding pulse, and high blood pressure. **Syphilitic periarteritis** is inflammation of the outer coat of one or more arteries occurring in tertiary syphilis. **Congenital syphilis** caused by infection in the womb may result in the birth of a deformed or blind infant. The infant may appear to be well until, at several weeks of age, snuffles, sometimes with a bloodstained discharge, and skin sores are observed, particularly on the palms and soles or in the genital region.

S

Visual or hearing defects, early old age (progeria), or poor health may develop. The clouding of the cornea, notched teeth, and deafness characteristic of inborn syphilis is called **Hutchinson's triad.** Syphilis is sometimes detected from blood tests, but often only the patient's report of exposure is evidence. Treatment includes antibiotics in the first and second stages. Any sexual partners who have been exposed to syphilis should be reported so that they can be treated. In many states, active cases of syphilis must, by law, be reported to the Department of Health.

syringe /sir'inj/, a device for withdrawing, injecting, or instilling fluids. An example is the **bulb syringe,** blunt-tipped and of flexible rubber or plastic, used mainly for flushing out openings, as the ear.

syringomyelocele /siring'gōmī'əlōsēl'/, a condition in which a section of the spinal cord sticks out through a hole, present at birth, in the spinal column. It forms a fluid-filled sac. See also **spina bifida.**

system, a collection of parts that make a whole. Systems of the body, as the cardiovascular or reproductive systems, are made up of structures specially adapted to perform functions necessary for life.

systemic /sistem'ik/, of or relating to the whole body rather than to a single area or part of the body.

systemic lupus erythematosus (SLE). See **lupus erythematosus.**

systemic remedy, a substance that is given by mouth, or placed in the intestines or rectum to be absorbed into the bloodstream for treatment of a health problem. Drugs given systemically may have various local effects, but the intent is to treat the whole body.

systole /sis'təlē/, the tightening of the heart, driving blood into the aorta and lung arteries. The systole is heard as the first heart beat and felt as the pulse. An **aborted systole** is a heart beat that is too early and may be so weak that a pulse is not felt in the wrist — **systolic** /sistol'ik/, *adj.*

T

tabes dorsalis /tā′bēz dôrsā′lis/, an abnormal condition marked by the slow breakdown of all or part of the body and the progressive loss of reflexes at the outer part of the body. This disease involves the spinal cord. It destroys the large joints of affected limbs in some individuals. Some surveys have indicated that about 40% of patients with neurosyphilis have tabes dorsalis.

tablet, a small, solid dose form of a drug. It may be pressed or molded in its manufacture. It may be of almost any size, shape, weight, and color. Most tablets are meant to be swallowed whole. However, some may be dissolved in the mouth, chewed, or dissolved in liquid before swallowing.

Tacaryl, a trademark for an antihistamine (methdilazine).

TACE, a trademark for female hormone (chlorotrianisene).

tachycardia /tak′ikär′dē·ə/, an abnormal condition in which the heart wall contracts regularly but at a rate greater than 100 beats per minute. The heart rate normally speeds up in response to fever, exercise, or nervous excitement. Tachycardia also occurs with lack of oxygen (anoxia), as caused by anemia, congestive heart failure, bleeding, or shock. Tachycardia acts to increase the amount of oxygen given to the cells of the body by increasing the amount of blood circulated through the vessels. **Double tachycardia** is the firing of two rapid heart contraction impulses that occur on their own, but at the same time. One impulse controls the upper chambers (atria) and one the lower chambers (ventricles). **Junctional tachycardia** is an automatic heart rhythm of greater than 100 beats per minute. It is often caused by digitalis toxicity. **Ventricular tachycardia** refers to a fast heart beat that usually begins in the ventricular system.

tachyphylaxis /-filak′sis/, an event in which the repeated use of some drugs results in a marked decrease in effectiveness.

tachypnea /-pnē′ə/. See **respiratory rate.**

tactile /tak′təl/, referring to the sense of touch.

tactile anesthesia, the absence or lack of the sense of touch in the fingers. It can possibly result from injury or disease. This condition can be inborn or acquired. It may cause the patient to get severe burns, serious cuts, bruises, or scraped areas.

tactile corpuscle, any one of many small, oval end organs linked to the sense of touch. They are widely distributed throughout the body in outer areas, as the hand and foot, front of the forehead, skin of the lips, mucous membrane of the tongue, eyelid, and skin of the nipples of the breasts. Also called **Meissner's corpuscle.**

tactile image, a mental concept of an object as perceived through the sense of touch. See also **image.**

Tagamet, a trademark for a histamine H_2 receptor antagonist (cimetidine).

talbutal, a barbiturate sedative-hypnotic. It is given as a sleeping drug (hypnotic) to treat the inability to sleep (insomnia). Previous addiction to sedative-hypnotics, porphyria, blocked liver function, or known allergy to this drug or to other barbiturates prohibits its use. Side effects include lowered breathing, drug hangover, allergic reactions, porphyria, and physical dependence.

talipes /tal′ipēz/, a deformity of the foot. It is usually inherited. The foot is twisted and relatively fixed in an abnormal position. Talipes refers to deformities that involve the foot and ankle. Pes refers only to a deformity of the foot.

talus /tā′ləs/. See **ankle bone.**

Talwin, a trademark for a painkiller (pentazocine).

tamoxifen, a cancer drug that counters the effects of a female hormone (estrogen). It is used to relieve advanced breast cancer in women whose tumors are estrogen-dependent.

tampon, a pack of cotton, a sponge, or other material. Its purpose is to check bleeding or absorb fluids in cavities or canals or hold displaced organs in position.

tamponade /tam′pənād′/, stoppage of the flow of blood to an organ or a part of the body by pressure, as by a tampon or a pressure dressing applied to stop a bleeding.

Tangier disease /tan′jir/, a rare lack of high-density lipoproteins. It runs in families. It features low blood cholesterol and an abnormal orange or yellow color of the tonsils and throat. There may also be large lymph nodes, liver, and spleen, muscle wasting, and disorders of the nervous system (peripheral neuropathy). No specific treatment is known.

tannin, any of a group of substances that cause contractions. It comes from plants. Tannic acid, a mixture of tannins, is used in the treatment of burns.

tanning, a process in which the color of the skin deepens as a result of exposure to ultraviolet light. Skin cells with dark pigment (melanin) darken immediately. New melanin is formed within 2 to 3 days. It moves upward rapidly. This allows the darkening process to continue.

tantrum, a sudden outburst or violent display of rage, frustration, and bad temper. It usually occurs in a poorly adjusted child and certain emotionally disturbed persons. It is used mainly as an attempt to control others and the surroundings. Also called **temper tantrum.**

TAO, a trademark for an antibacterial (troleandomycin).

Tapazole, a trademark for a thyroid inhibitor (methimazole).

tapeworm infection, an intestinal infection by one of several species of parasitic worms called tapeworms or cestodes. The tapeworm species that most often infects humans is *Taenia saginata*. It is in the tissues of cattle during its larval stage. It infects the intestine of humans in its adult form and may grow to a length of between 12 and 25 feet. Symptoms of intestinal infection with adult worms are usually mild or absent. However, diarrhea, stomach pain, and weight loss may occur. Diagnosis is made when eggs or portions of the adult worm are passed in the stool. The drugs niclosamide and quinacrine are used to loosen and dissolve the worm so that it may be released. **Pork tapeworm infection** is caused by the pork tapeworm (*Taenia solium*). This tapeworm can use humans as both a place for its young to grow and for the adult worm. Humans are usually infected with the adult worm after eating undercooked pork that has tapeworms in it. **Fish tapeworm infection** is carried to humans when they eat raw or undercooked freshwater fish infected by a tapeworm (*Diphyllobothrium latum*). It is common in warm areas throughout the world and is found in the Great Lakes area of the United States.

Taractan, a trademark for a tranquilizer (chlorprothixene).

Tarbonis, a trademark for a drug that relieves eczema. It contains coal tar.

Tarcortin, a trademark for a drug that raises the concentration of liver glycogen and blood sugar (hydrocortisone) and relieves eczema (crude coal tar).

tardive dyskinesia, an abnormal condition with involuntary, repetitive movements of the muscles of the face, the limbs, and the trunk. This disorder most commonly affects older people who have been treated for extended periods with phenothiazine drugs to relieve the symptoms of parkinsonism. The involuntary movements may slacken or disappear after weeks or months. See also **antiparkinsonian.**

tardy peroneal nerve palsy, an abnormal condition in which the peroneal nerve is compressed where it crosses the smaller leg bone. Such compression may occur when a person falls asleep with the legs crossed.

tardy ulnar nerve palsy, an abnormal condition that features wasting of the hand muscles and difficulty in movement. It may be caused by injury of the ulnar nerve at the elbow. Symptoms include numbness of the small finger, of part of the ring finger, and of the elbow border of the hand. Treatment includes the use of a doughnut cushion for the elbow to relieve the pressure on the ulnar nerve. Severe cases of this disorder may be corrected by surgery.

target cell, 1. an abnormal red blood cell (leptocyte) marked, when stained and examined under a microscope, by a dark center surrounded by a pale ring circled by a dark, irregular band. Target cells occur in the blood after the removal of the spleen (splenectomy) and in blood diseases (anemias, hemoglobin C disease). **2.** any cell having a specific receptor that reacts with a specific hormone, antigen, antibody, antibiotic, sensitized tumor cell, or other substance.

target organ, 1. (in radiotherapy) an organ that receives a therapeutic dose of irradiation, as for the treatment of a tumor. **2.** (in endocrinology) an organ most affected by a specific hormone, as the thyroid gland, which is the target organ of thyroid-stimulating hormone released by the pituitary gland.

Tarpaste, a trademark for a drug used against eczema (tar distillate) in a paste.

tarsal /tär′səl/, referring to the tarsus (ankle bone) or to the eyelid.

tarsal bone, any one of seven bones comprising the ankle, made up of the talus, calcaneus, cuboid, navicular, and the three cuneiforms.

tarsal gland, one of numerous oil glands on the inner surfaces of the eyelids. Bacterial infection of a tarsal gland causes a sty. Compare **ciliary gland.**

tarsal tunnel syndrome, an abnormal condition marked by pain and numbness in the sole of the foot. This disorder may be caused by a broken ankle that presses the posterior tibial nerve. It may be corrected by orthopedic therapy or by surgery.

tarsometatarsal /tär′sōmet′ətär′səl/, referring to the bones of the foot between toes and ankle (metatarsus) bones and the ankle of the foot.

tarsus /tär′səs/, *pl.* **tarsi,**   **1.** the area between the foot and the leg (the ankle). **2.** a plate of cartilage (also called **tarsal plate**) that forms each eyelid.

tartar /tär′tär/,   a hard, gritty deposit. It is made of organic matter, phosphates, and carbonates that collect on the teeth and gums. An excess of tartar may cause gum disease and other dental problems. See also **gingivitis, pyorrhea.**

tartaric acid /-ter′ik/,   a colorless or white powder found in various plants and prepared commercially for use in baking powder, some beverages, and a drug causing vomiting (tartar emetic).

task force,   a group of resources with common communications and a leader temporarily assembled for a specific mission.

taste,   the sense of perceiving different flavors in soluble substances that contact the tongue and send nerve impulses to special taste centers in the cortex and the thalamus of the brain. The sense of taste is linked with the sense of smell. The four basic taste sensations are sweet, sour, bitter, and salty. All other tastes are combinations of these four basic flavors. The front of the tongue is most sensitive to salty and sweet substances. The sides of the tongue are most sensitive to sour substances. The back of the tongue is most sensitive to bitter substances. The middle of the tongue produces virtually no taste sensation.

taste bud,   any one of many outer taste organs distributed over the tongue and the roof of the mouth. Adults have about 9000 taste buds. Each taste bud rests in a spheric pocket. Taste (gustatory) cells and supporting cells form each bud. Also called **gustatory organ.**

tattoo,   permanent color put into the skin by the introduction of foreign color. A tattoo may accidentally occur when a bit of graphite from a broken pencil point is embedded in the skin. Small tattoos can be removed by surgery. Mechanical abrasion (dermabrasion) of the skin is preferred for removal of large areas of pigment.

Tavist,   a trademark for an antihistamine (clemastine).

taxonomy /takson′əmē/,   a system for classifying organisms on the basis of natural relationships and giving them appropriate names.   **–taxonomic,** *adj.*

Taylor brace,   a padded steel brace used to support the spine.

Tay-Sachs disease /tā-saks′/,   an inherited nerve breakdown disorder of fat processing. It is caused by a lack of an enzyme that results in the pooling of fats in the brain. It occurs foremost in families of Eastern European Jewish origin, specifically Ashkenazic Jews. It features progressive mental and physical retardation and early death. Symptoms first appear by 6 months of age. After this age, no new skills are learned, and there is loss of those skills already learned. Convulsions, blindness, loss of control of muscles, mental breakdown, and paralysis occur. Most children die between 2 and 4 years of age. There is no specific treatment for the condition. Intervention is merely to take care of symptoms and to offer some relief. The disease can be diagnosed before birth through amniocentesis. See also **lipidosis, Sandhoff's disease.**

TB,   abbreviation for **tuberculosis.**

T bandage,   a bandage in the shape of the letter T. It is used for the pelvic floor (perineum) and sometimes for the head.

T cell,   a small circulating white blood cell (lymphocyte) made in the bone marrow. It matures in the thymus gland or as a result of exposure to a hormone (thymosin) released by the thymus. T cells live for years. They have several functions but mainly involve immune responses, such as graft rejection and delayed allergy. One kind of T cell, the **helper cell,** affects the production of antibodies by B cells; a **suppressor T cell** suppresses B cell activity. Compare **B cell.** See also **antibody, immune response.**

teaching hospital,   a hospital with recognized programs in medical, nursing, or related health personnel education.

team practice,   professional practice by a group of professionals that may include physicians, nurses, and others, as a social worker, nutritionist, or physical therapist. They organize the care of a specified number of patients as a team, usually in an outpatient setting.

teardrop fracture,   a tear-shaped break of one of the short bones, as a vertebra.

tear duct,   any duct that carries tears, including the ducts in the eyelids and nose, and the ducts of the tear glands.

tearing,   watering of the eye. It it usually caused by excess tear production from strong emotion, infection, or irritation by a foreign body. Tearing occurs when more tears are made than are drained by the ducts and sacs of the eyes.

technetium (Tc),   a radioactive, metallic element. Isotopes of technetium are used in radioisotope scanning methods of internal organs, as the liver and spleen.

technical information specialist,   those individuals who provide specific expertise, concerning a hazardous material to the incident commander either in person, by telephone, or through other electronic means. They may represent the manufacturer or shipper or be otherwise familiar with the chemicals or problems involved. CHEMTREC and CHEMNET often provide an excellent way to reach information sources in any given area of expertise.

technical specialists,   personnel with special skills who are activated only when needed. Technical specialists may be needed in the areas of fire behavior, water resources, environmental concerns, resource use, and training areas.

technique,   the method and details followed in performing a procedure, as those used in conducting a laboratory test,

T–Z

a physical examination, a psychiatric interview, or a surgical operation.

Tedral, a trademark for a drug to help breathing. It is made up of a bronchi widener (theophylline), a stimulation (adrenergic) drug (ephedrine hydrochloride), and a sleeping and relaxation (sedative-hypnotic) drug (phenobarbital).

teether, an object, as a teething ring, on which an infant can bite or chew during the teething process.

teething, the process of the eruption of the first (deciduous or baby) teeth through the gums. The structure found in the mouth of the infant before the coming out of the baby teeth is called **predeciduous dentition.** Teething normally begins between the sixth and eighth months of life and continues until the complete set of 20 teeth has appeared at about 30 months. Discomfort and inflammation result from the pressure against the tissue supporting the teeth as the crown of the tooth breaks through the membranes. General signs of teething include excess drooling, biting on hard objects, irritability, difficulty in sleeping, and refusal of food. Fever or diarrhea often occurs during teething. However, it points to illness rather than to teething. The pain and inflammation may usually be soothed by cold, as with a frozen teething ring, cold metal spoon, or ice wrapped in a washcloth. Use of teething powders and procedures, as rubbing or cutting the gums, are discouraged because of the possibility of infection or problems from swallowing the drug.

teething ring, a circular device, usually made of plastic or rubber, on which an infant may chew or bite during the teething process.

Teflon, a trademark for a substance (polytetrafluorethylene) used for the construction of surgical implants.

Tegopen, a trademark for an antibacterial (cloxacillin sodium).

Tegretol, a trademark for a painkiller and a drug that prevents convulsions (carbamazepine).

telangiectasia /təlan′jē·ektā′zhə/, permanent widening of groups of capillaries and small veins (venules). Common causes are damage from excess sunlight, some skin diseases, as rosacea, too high levels of female hormone, and collagen blood vessel diseases.

telangiectatic epulis /-tat′ik/, a harmless, red tumor of the gum. It contains visible blood vessels. Low-grade or long-term irritation usually occurs. The tumor is easily injured.

telangiectatic glioma, a tumor made up of nerve (glial) cells and a network of blood vessels. This gives the mass a vivid pink appearance.

telangiectatic nevus, a common skin condition of newborn infants. It features flat, deep-pink localized areas of capillary widening. They occur foremost on the back of the

neck, lower back part of the head, upper eyelids, upper lip, and bridge of the nose. The areas go away by about 2 years of age.

telepathist /təlep′əthist/, a person who believes in telepathy.

telepathy /-thē/, the unproved communication of thought from one person to another by means other than the physical senses. –**telepathic,** adj., **telepathize,** v.

teletherapy /tel′ē-/, radiation therapy given by a machine that is positioned at some distance from the patient. Typically, a teletherapy unit can turn around a patient and thus allow use of beams that intersect at the tumor. This lowers the dose to surrounding normal tissue.

telophase /tel′əfāz/, the final of the four stages of nuclear division in certain cell divisions (mitosis and meiosis). See also **anaphase, interphase, meiosis, mitosis, prophase.**

Temaril, a trademark for an antihistamine (trimeprazine tartrate).

temazepam, a sleeping drug. It is given for the occasional sleeping problems (insomnia). Pregnancy or breast feeding prohibits its use. It is not advised for patients under 18 years of age. Side effects include confusion, loss of appetite, lack of muscular coordination (ataxia), palpitations, hallucinations, and involuntary rapid movements of the eyeball (nystagmus).

temperature, a relative measure of heat or cold. See also **body temperature, fever.**

template /tem′plit/, (in genetics) the strand of DNA that acts as a mold for the synthesis of messenger RNA. This messenger RNA has the same sequence of nucleic acids as the DNA strand. It carries the code to the ribosomes for the synthesis of proteins.

temporal arteritis /tem′pərəl/. See **arteritis.**

temporal artery, any one of three arteries on each side of the head: the superficial temporal artery, the middle temporal artery, and the deep temporal artery.

temporal bone, one of a pair of large bones forming part of the skull. It has many cavities and small empty spaces linked to the ear, as the tympanic cavity and the auditory tube. Each temporal bone consists of four portions: the mastoid, the squama, the petrous, and the tympanic.

temporal bone fracture, a break of the temporal bone of the skull. It is sometimes marked by bleeding from the ear. Diminished hearing or facial paralysis may occur.

temporalis /tem′pôrā′lis/, one of the four muscles of food chewing. The temporalis closes the jaws. Also called **temporal muscle.**

temporal lobe. See **brain.**

temporomandibular joint /-mandib′yələr/, one of two joints connecting the lower jaw bone to the temporal bone of the skull. It is a combined hinge and gliding joint.

temporomandibular joint syndrome (TMJ), an abnormal condition with facial pain and poor function of the lower jaw. It is apparently caused by a defective or dislocated temporomandibular joint. Some common signs are the clicking of the joint when the jaws move, limitation of jaw movement, and partial dislocation.

temporoparietalis /-pərī′ətā′lis/, one of a pair of broad, thin muscles of the scalp. It acts to wrinkle the forehead, to widen the eyes, and to raise the ears.

tenacious /tənā′shəs/, referring to fluids that are sticky or adhesive or otherwise tend to hold together, as mucus and sputum.

tenaculum /tənak′yələm/, *pl.* **tenacula,** a clip or clamp with long handles used to grasp and hold an organ or a piece of tissue. Kinds of tenacula include the **abdominal tenaculum,** which has long arms and small hooks, the **forceps tenaculum,** which has long hooks and is used in gynecologic surgery, and the **uterine** or **cervical tenaculum,** which has short hooks or open, eye-shaped clamps used to hold the the lower narrow end of the uterus (cervix).

tendon, one of many white, glistening fibrous bands of tissue that attach muscle to bone. Except at points of attachment, tendons are tubular shaped in delicate fibroelastic connective tissue. Larger tendons have a thin inner dividing wall (septum), a few blood vessels, and specialized sterognostic nerves. Tendons are extremely strong and flexible and inelastic and occur in various lengths and thicknesses. Compare **ligament.** –**tendinous,** *adj.*

tendonitis /ten′dənī′-/, inflammation of a tendon. It usually results from strain. Treatment may include rest, corticosteroid injections, and support.

tenesmus /tənez′məs/, persistent, ineffectual spasms of the rectum or bladder. It goes along with the urge to empty the bowel or bladder.

tennis elbow, a painful and sometimes disabling inflammation of the muscle and tissues of the elbow. It is caused by repeated strain on the forearm. Also called **epicondylitis.**

Tenormin, a trademark for a beta-blocker (atenolol).

tenosynovitis /ten′ōsin′ōvī′-/, inflammation of a tendon sheath usually caused by calcium deposits, repeated strain, or injury. In some instances, movement yields a crackling noise over the tendon.

tenotomy /tənot′-/, the total or partial severing of a tendon. It is done to correct a muscle imbalance, as in the correction of squint (strabismus) of the eye or in clubfoot.

Tensilon a trademark for a nerve drug (edrophonium). It is used as an antitoxic drug and as a diagnostic aid in muscle weakness (myasthenia gravis).

tension, 1. the act of pulling or straining until strained. **2.** the condition of being tense, or under pressure. It is marked physically by a general increase in muscle tonus, heart rate, breathing rate, and alertness. See also **stress.**

tension headache. See **headache.**

tensor, any one of the muscles of the body that tenses a structure. An example is the **tensor fasciae latae,** a muscle of the buttocks region that acts to flex the thigh and rotate it slightly toward the middle. Compare **abductor, adductor, depressor, sphincter.**

tent, 1. a transparent cover, usually of plastic, supported over the upper part of a patient by a frame. It is used to treat breathing conditions. It gives a controlled environment into which steam, oxygen, vaporized drugs, or droplets of cool water may be sprayed, as an oxygen tent. **2.** a cone made of various materials put into a cavity (or its entrance or outlet) of the body to widen its opening. **3.** a pack placed in a wound to hold it open. This ensures that healing goes from the base of the wound upward to the skin.

tentorial herniation /tentôr′e·əl/, a bulging out of brain tissue. It is caused by increased pressure in the brain. It results from edema, bleeding, or a tumor. Symptoms include severe headache, fever, flushing, sweating, abnormal reflex of the pupils, drowsiness, low blood pressure, and loss of consciousness.

tentorium /tentôr′ē·əm/, *pl.* **tentoria,** any part of the body that looks like a tent.

Tenuate, a trademark for a drug that lessens the appetite (diethylpropion hydrochloride).

Tepanil, a trademark for a drug that lessens the appetite (diethylpropion hydrochloride).

tepid, moderately warm to the touch.

teramorphous /ter′əmôr′fəs/, of the nature of or characteristic of a monster.

teras /ter′əs/, *pl.* **terata,** a severely deformed fetus; a monster. –**teratic,** *adj.*

teratism /ter′ətizm/, any inborn or developmental anomaly that is produced by inherited or environmental factors, or by a combination of the two. It can be any condition in which a severely defective fetus is produced. Examples include: **atresic teratism,** in which any of the normal openings of the body, as the mouth, nostrils, anus, or vagina, fail to form; **ceasmic teratism,** in which parts of the body that should be fused are not, as in cleft palate; **hypergenetic teratism,** in which there is excessive growth of a part or organ or the entire body, as in gigantism; and **symphysic teratism,** in which there is a fusion of normally separated parts or organs, as a horseshoe kidney, or in which parts close prematurely, as the skull bones in craniostenosis.

teratogen /ter′ətəjen/, any substance, agent, or process that blocks normal growth of the fetus, causing one or

T–Z

more developmental abnormalities in the fetus. Teratogens act directly on the developing organism or indirectly, affecting such structures as the placenta. The type and extent of the defect are determined by the specific kind of teratogen and its mode of action. It also depends on the embryonic process affected, and the stage of development at the time the exposure occurred. Compare **mutagen.** – **teratogenic,** *adj.*

teratogenesis /ter'ətōjen'əsis/, the development of physical defects in the embryo.

teratoma /ter'ətō'mə/, a tumor made up of different kinds of tissue, none of which normally occur together or at the site of the tumor. Teratomas are most common in the ovaries or testes.

terbutaline sulfate, a beta-adrenergic stimulant. It is given as a bronchial widener to treat asthma, bronchitis, and emphysema and as a uterine relaxant to treat premature labor. Irregular heart beat (cardiac arrhythmias) or known allergy to this drug prohibits its use. Side effects include dizziness, irregular heart rate, nervousness, and trembling.

teres /tir'ēz/, *pl.* **teretes** /ter'ətēz/, a long, cylindric muscle. The **teres major,** a shoulder muscle, acts to pull forward, extend, and rotate the arm to the middle. The **teres minor,** also a shoulder muscle, acts to rotate the arm outwards, pull up the arm, and to strengthen the shoulder joint.

terminal, (of a structure or process) near or approaching its end, as a terminal bronchiole or a terminal disease. – **terminate,** *v.,* **terminus,** *n.*

terminal drop, a rapid decline in mental function and coping ability that occurs 1 to 5 years before death.

terminal sulcus of right atrium, a shallow channel on the outer surface of the right heart chamber (atrium) between the upper and lower venae cavae veins.

term infant, any newborn, regardless of birth weight, born after the end of the thirty-seventh and before the beginning of the forty-third week of gestation. Infants born at term usually measure from 48 to 53 cm from head to heel. They weigh between 2700 and 4000 g.

terpin hydrate and codeine elixir, a preparation of the drug terpin hydrate. It promotes coughing up (expectorant). It is made of sweet orange peel tincture, benzaldehyde, glycerin, alcohol, syrup, water, and the cough-suppressing narcotic codeine. Terpin hydrate reduces secretions and promotes healing of the mucous membrane. Codeine depresses the cough center in the medulla oblongata. Prolonged use may lead to addiction.

Terra-Cortril, a trademark for a drug with a glucocorticoid (hydrocortisone) and an antibiotic (oxytetracycline).

Terramycin, a trademark for an antibiotic (oxytetracycline).

Terrastatin, a trademark for a drug with an antifungal (nystatin) and an antibiotic (oxytetracycline).

tertian /tur'shən/, occurring every 48 hours or 3 days, including the first day of occurrence, as tertian malaria, in which fever occurs every third day. Compare **quartan.** See also **malaria.**

tertiary /tur'shē·er'ē/, tursh'ərē/, third in frequency or in order of use; belonging to the third level of a system, as a tertiary health care facility.

tertiary health care, a specialized level of health care. It includes diagnosis and treatment of disease and disability in large hospitals with specialized intensive care units, advanced diagnostic support services, and highly specialized personnel. It offers a highly centralized care to the population of a large region; in some cases, to the world.

tertiary prevention, a level of health care that deals with the return of a patient to a state of greatest usefulness with the least risk of renewed physical or mental disorders.

Teslac, a trademark for a drug that blocks the growth of tumors (testolactone).

Tessalon, a trademark for a local anesthetic agent (benzonatate).

test, 1. an examination or trial intended to establish a principle or determine a value. 2. a chemical reaction or reagent that has clinical importance. 3. to detect, identify, or conduct a trial. See also **laboratory test.**

testicle. See **testis.**

testicular /testik'yələr/, referring to the testicle.

testicular artery, one of a pair of long, slender branches of the abdominal aorta, arising backwards to the kidney arteries and supplying the testicles.

testicular cancer, a malignant disease of the testicles. It occurs most often in men between 20 and 35 years of age. An undescended testicle is often involved. In many cases the cancer is detected after an injury. However, injury is not thought to be a cause. Patients with early testicular cancer often have no symptoms. Cancer cells may have moved to the lymph nodes, the lungs, and liver before the original tumor can be felt. Radiation, surgical removal, and chemotherapy are recommended for treatment. Chemotherapeutic agents, used in various combinations, are increasing the survival of patients with testicular cancer.

testicular duct. See **vas deferens.**

testicular vein, one of a pair of blood veins that arises from networks of veins (venous plexuses) that drain blood from the testicles.

testis /tes'tis/, *pl.* **testes,** one of the pair of male gonads that produce semen. The adult testes are suspended in the scrotum by the spermatic cords. In early fetal life they are within the abdominal cavity behind the lining (peritoneum). Before birth they normally lower into the scrotum.

Each testis is an oval body about 4 cm long, 2.5 cm wide. It weighs about 12 g. The ducts in which the sperm is stored (epididymis) are located on the back of the testis. A man with both testes undescended is sterile but may not be impotent. **Aberratio testis** refers to a testicle that does not move down correctly. See also **scrotum.**

testolactone, a drug that counteracts tumor growth. It is given to treat postmenopausal breast cancer and to premenopausal women whose ovarian function has been ended. Pregnancy, breast feeding, or known allergy to this drug prohibits its use. It is not given to men. Side effects include excess calcium in the blood (hypercalcemia) and numbness or tingling.

testosterone /testos′tərōn/, a naturally occurring hormone that stimulates the growth of male characteristics (androgen). It is given for androgen lack, female breast cancer, stimulation of growth, weight gain, and red blood cell production. Cancer of the male breast or prostate, liver disease, pregnancy or suspected pregnancy, or known allergy to this drug prohibits its use. Side effects include fluid buildup, masculinization, acne, and a blood disease (erythrocythemia).

testosterone propionate, a drug that stimulates the growth of male characteristics.

test tube, a tube made of clear material having one open end. It is used in many laboratory functions. See also **tube.**

tetanus /tet′ənəs/, a sudden, potentially deadly infection of the central nervous system. It is caused by a bacteria-formed poison (exotoxin) produced by an anaerobic bacillus, *Clostridium tetani.* Symptoms include irritability, headache, fever, and painful spasms of the muscles resulting in lockjaw. More than 50,000 people a year die of tetanus infection worldwide. The toxin is a nerve poison and is one of the most lethal poisons known. *C. tetani* infects only wounds that contain dead tissue. The bacillus is commonly found in the top layers of the soil. It is a normal inhabitant of the intestinal tracts of cows and horses. Therefore, barnyards and fields fertilized with manure are heavily contaminated. The bacillus may come into the body through a puncture wound, abrasion, cut, or burn. It also may come into the body via the uterus in abortion, through afterbirth contamination (sepsis), or through the stump of the umbilical cord of the newborn. The infection occurs in two forms. The first one shows a sudden beginning, high mortality, and a short incubation period (3 to 21 days); the second one shows less severe symptoms, a lower mortality, and a longer incubation period (4 to 5 weeks). Wounds of the face, head, and neck are the ones most likely to result in fatal infection, because the bacillus may travel rapidly to the brain. Prompt and thorough cleansing and removal of foreign bodies from the wound are neces-

sary for prevention. A booster shot of tetanus toxoid is given to previously vaccinated people. Tetanus-immune globulin and a series of three injections of tetanus toxoid are given to those not vaccinated. People who are known to have been adequately immunized within 5 years do not usually need vaccination. Also called **lockjaw.**

tetanus and diphtheria toxoids (Td), an active vaccination drug with detoxified tetanus and diphtheria toxoids that slowly makes antibodies to the diseases. It is a vaccination against tetanus and diphtheria in children under 7 years of age when whooping cough vaccine present in the usual diphtheria, pertussis, and tetanus trivalent vaccine is prohibited. Lessened resistance (immunosupression), use of corticosteroids at the same time, or serious infection prohibits its use. Side effects include allergic reactions and stinging at the site of injection.

tetanus antitoxin (TAT), a tetanus immune serum that neutralizes exotoxins in tetanus infection. It is given for short-term vaccination against tetanus after possible exposure to the organism and in tetanus treatment. It is not given if the more effective tetanus immune globulin is available or if there is a known allergy to equine serum. Side effects include allergic reactions and pain and inflammation at the site of injection.

tetanus immune globulin (TIG), an injectable solution prepared from the globulin of an immune human. It is effective and much safer than tetanus antitoxin. It is given for short-term vaccination against tetanus after possible exposure to the organism and tetanus treatment. Known allergy to this drug prohibits its use. It should not be substituted for tetanus toxoid. Side effects include an overreaction (anaphylaxis), fever, pain, and inflammation at the site of injection.

tetanus toxoid, an active immunizing agent prepared from detoxified tetanus toxin that makes antibodies in the body. This gives permanent immunity to tetanus infection. It is given for primary active immunization against tetanus. Lessened resistance (immunosuppression) or immunoglobulin abnormalities, serious infection, or illness prohibits its use. Side effects include an allergic reaction, pain, and inflammation at the site of injection.

tetany /tet′ənē/, a condition with cramps, convulsions, twitching of the muscles, and sharp bending of the wrist and ankle joints. These symptoms are sometimes linked with attacks of harsh breathing sounds (stridor). Tetany is a sign of an abnormality in calcium processing.

Tetrachel, a trademark for an antibiotic (tetracycline hydrochloride).

tetracycline /tet′rəsī′klēn/, an antibiotic with many uses. It is given to treat many bacterial and rickettsial infections. Blocked liver or kidney function or known allergy to this drug prohibits its use. Because it may cause permanent

T–Z

discoloration of the teeth, its use is prohibited in the last half of pregnancy and during a child's first 8 years of life. Side effects include poisoning of the kidneys and liver, disorders of the stomach and intestines, inflammation of the small intestine and colon (enterocolitis), lesions with growth of fungus in the anogenital area, blood diseases, and rashes.

tetracycline hydrochloride, a tetracycline antibiotic. It is given to treat a variety of infections. Known allergy to this drug or to other tetracyclines prohibits its use. Use during pregnancy or in children under 8 years of age may result in discoloration of the child's teeth. It is to be given carefully with kidney or liver problems. Side effects include potentially serious secondary infections, various allergic reactions, toxic reactions due to light exposure (phototoxicity), and disorders of the stomach and intestines.

Tetracyn, a trademark for an antibiotic (tetracycline hydrochloride).

tetrahydrocannabinol (THC), the active substance of marijuana, hashish, bhang, and ganja. THC increases pulse rate, causes eye reddening, gives a feeling of great excitement, and has variable effects on blood pressure, breathing rate, and pupil size. The drug affects memory, cognition, and the senses. It decreases motor coordination, and increases appetite. See also **cannabis.**

tetrahydrozoline hydrochloride, an adrenergic constrictor of vessels. It is given to treat nose and nose-throat (nasopharangeal) congestion and as an eye vasoconstrictor. Glaucoma or known allergy to this drug or to other vasoconstrictors prohibits its use. It is used carefully in patients who have heart disease. Side effects include irritation to mucosa, rebound nasal congestion, and effects linked with systemic absorption, including sedation and alterations in heart function.

tetralogy of Fallot /tetral'-, falō'/, an inborn heart problem that is made up of four defects: lung narrowing (pulmonic stenosis), a defect in the dividing wall of the lower chamber of the heart (ventricular septal defect), malposition of the aorta so that it arises from the septal defect or the right ventricle, and enlargement of the right ventricle. The main symptoms in the infant are bluish skin from too little hemoglobin (cyanosis) and lack of oxygen (hypoxia), usually during crying, difficulty in feeding, failure to gain weight, and poor development. In older children a typical squatting position and clubbing of the fingers and toes are evident. **Trilogy of Fallot** is a variation with three defects: a heart wall defect and a wasting of both lower heart chambers. Treatment includes supportive measures and surgery. Also called **Fallot's syndrome.** See also **blue baby.**

tetraploid /tet'rəploid/. See **euploid.**

Tetrastatin, a trademark for an antiinfective drug with an antifungal (nystatin) and an antibiotic (tetracycline hydrochloride).

Tetrex, a trademark for an antibiotic (tetracycline phosphate complex).

Texacort, a trademark for a skin drug with a glucocorticoid (hydrocortisone).

T fracture, a break in the rounded end of a bone (condyle) in which the fracture lines are T-shaped.

thalamus /thal'əməs/, *pl.* **thalami,** one of a pair of large, oval organs forming part of the brain. It is made up mainly of gray substance. It translates impulses from receptors for pain, temperature, and touch. It also joins in associating sensory impulses with pleasant and unpleasant feelings, in the arousal mechanisms of the body, and in the mechanisms that produce reflex movements. Compare **epithalamus, hypothalamus, subthalamus.** –**thalamic,** *adj.*

thalassemia /thal'əsē'mē·ə/, a disease marked by abnormal and short-lived red blood cells. People of Mediterranean origin are more often affected than others. It is a genetically carried disease occurring in two forms. **Thalassemia major (Cooley's anemia),** a form evident in infancy, is recognized by anemia, fever, failure to thrive, and too large spleen (splenomegaly). Frequent transfusions are needed to keep up oxygen-carrying capacity of the blood. Red cells are rapidly destroyed, releasing large amounts of iron to be deposited in the skin, which becomes bronzed and freckled. The iron is also deposited in the heart, liver, and pancreas, which become fibrous and function poorly. The spleen may become so large that breathing movement is blocked and the other organs are crowded. Headache, stomach pain, weakness, and loss of appetite often occur. **Thalassemia minor,** the other form, is marked only by a mild anemia and minimal red blood cell changes. Thalassemia minima is a form that lacks clinical symptoms although patients show some evidence of the disease. Education and counseling about the disease, and referral for genetic counseling are needed.

thalidomide /thalid'əmīd/, a sleeping pill. It is withdrawn from general use because of its potential for creating defects in the growing fetus, particularly defects of limbs, hands, and feet (phocomelia), when taken during pregnancy. It is sometimes given to treat leprosy.

thallium poisoning, a toxic condition caused by swallowing or the absorption through the skin of thallium salts, especially thallium sulfate. Symptoms include stomach pain, vomiting, bloody diarrhea, trembling, delirium, and baldness (alopecia). Thallium has been used in insect and rodent poisons, fireworks, and some cosmetic hair removers. However, this very toxic and cumulative poison was banned for use in household products in 1965.

Tham, a trademark for a buffering agent (tromethamine), used to treat acid-base disturbances.

thanatophoric dwarf /than'ətōfôr'ik/, an infant with severe shortness or smallness of the limbs (micromelia). The limbs usually extend straight out from the trunk. There are also an extremely narrow chest and defects of the spine. Death usually occurs from breathing problems shortly after birth.

Thanatos /than'ətəs/, a freudian term for the death instinct.

the Blues, *informal.* referring to Blue Cross (an insurance system that pays the costs of treatment by a hospital or clinic) and Blue Shield (an insurance system that pays the costs of treatment by a professional).

theca /thē'kə/, *pl.* **thecae** /thē'sē/, a sheath or capsule.

theca cell tumor, an uncommon, harmless fibroid tumor of the ovary. The tumors are typically solid masses with yellow, fatty streaks. They are often linked to excess female hormone production.

Theden's bandage /tā'dənz/, a roller bandage applied below the injury and continued upward over a compress. It is used to stop bleeding.

thelarche /thelär'kē/, the beginning of female pubertal breast growth that normally occurs before puberty at the beginning of the phase of fast growth between 9 and 13 years of age. **Premature thelarche** is breast growth in a female without other evidence of sexual maturation. Compare **menarche.**

thenar /thē'när/, **1.** the ball of the thumb. **2.** referring to the thumb side of the palm.

Theobid, a trademark for a smooth muscle relaxant (theophylline).

Theo-Dur, a trademark for a bronchial widener (theophylline).

Theolair, a trademark for a bronchial widener (theophylline). It is used for the relief of sudden bronchial asthma.

Theophyl, a trademark for a smooth muscle relaxant (theophylline).

theophylline, a bronchial widener. It is given to relax the smooth muscle of the bronchial passages in the treatment of bronchospasm in bronchial asthma, bronchitis, and emphysema. High blood pressure, heart disease, liver disease, kidney disease, or treatment at the same time with other xanthines prohibits its use. Side effects include allergy, bleeding in the stomach and intestines, palpitations, and seizures.

theoretic effectiveness, (of a contraceptive method) the effectiveness of a drug, device, or method in preventing pregnancy if used consistently and exactly as intended, without error. Compare **use effectiveness.**

Theovent, a trademark for a smooth muscle relaxant (theophylline).

therapeutic, 1. beneficial. **2.** referring to a treatment.

therapeutic equivalent, a drug that has in essence the same effect in the treatment of a disease or condition as one or more other drugs. A drug that is a therapeutic equivalent may or may not be chemically or bioequivalent. See also **bioequivalent, chemical equivalent, generic equivalent.**

therapeutic recreation specialist, a person who helps patients in their recovery or rehabilitation after physical or emotional illness or disability. This specialist plans and supervises recreation programs.

therapeutic temperature, treatment through increased body temperature (hyperthermia), temperatures between 42° and 45° C (107° and 113° F).

therapist, a person with special skills, gained through education and experience, in one or more areas of health care.

therapy, the treatment of any disease or abnormal condition. For example, breathing therapy gives some drugs for patients suffering from diseases of the breathing tract.

thermal /thur'məl/, referring to the production, application, or upkeep of heat.

thermal stress, hazardous material container stress that generally indicates temperature extremes, both hot or cold. Examples include fire, sparks, friction or electricity, and ambient temperature changes. Extreme or intense cold, such as that found with cryogenic materials may also act as a stressor. Clues of thermal stress include the operation of safety relief valves or the bulging of a container.

thermogenesis /thur'mōjen'əsis/, mak- ing of heat, especially by the cells of the body. –**thermogenetic,** *adj.*

thermography /thurmog'rəfē/, a method for sensing and recording on film hot and cold areas of the body by means of an infrared detector that reacts to blood flow. Disease states that have increased or decreased blood flow show patterns of heat changes that can be distinguished from those of normal areas. –**thermographic,** *adj.*

thermolabile /-lā'bil/, easily destroyed or changed by heat. Also called **heat labile.**

thermometer, an instrument for measuring temperature. It is usually made of a sealed glass tube, marked in degrees of Celsius or Fahrenheit. It has a liquid, as mercury or alcohol. The liquid rises or falls as it expands or contracts according to changes in temperature. An **air thermometer** is one that uses air instead of mercury. An **electronic thermometer** gives temperature quickly by electronic means. **Invasive thermometry** measures tissue temperature using probes directly in the tissue. A **surface thermometer** shows the temperature of the skin of any part of the body.

T–Z

A **thermistor** is a kind of thermometer for measuring very small changes in temperature.

thermoneutral environment, 1. an environment that keeps body temperature at an optimum point at which the least amount of oxygen is consumed. **2.** an environment that enables a newborn to keep a body temperature of 36.5° C (97.7° F) with a minimal requirement of energy and oxygen.

thermopenetration, the use of heating techniques to make warmth within the body tissues for therapeutic purposes. Also called **transthermia.**

thermoregulation, the control of heat production and heat loss; keeping the body temperature normal through physical mechanisms set off by the hypothalamus.

thermostat, a device for the automatic control of a heating or cooling system.

thermotaxis, 1. the normal adjustment and control of body temperature. **2.** the movement of an organism in response to heat, either toward the stimulus (positive thermotaxis) or away from the stimulus (negative thermotaxis). Also called **thermotropism.**

thermotherapy, the treatment of disease by the application of heat. It may be given as dry heat with heat lamps, heating (diathermy) machines, or electric pads. Hot water bottles or moist heat with warm compresses or immersion in warm water are other methods. Warm soaks or compresses may be used to treat local infections, to relax muscles, and to relieve pain in patients with motor problems. It also helps to promote circulation in outer blood vessel (peripheral vascular) disorders, as thrombophlebitis. –**thermotherapeutic,** *adj.*

theta wave. See **brain waves.**

thiabendazole, a drug that destroys worms (anthelmintic). It is given to treat a variety of worm infestations, including hookworms, roundworms, and pinworms. Some skin diseases or known allergy to this drug prohibits its use. Side effects include loss of appetite, central nervous system effects, severe disturbances of the stomach and intestines, dizziness, and low blood pressure.

thiamine /thī′əmin/, a water-soluble, crystalline compound of the B complex vitamin group. It is necessary for normal processing and for the health of the heart and nervous systems. Thiamine joins with pyruvic acid to form a coenzyme necessary for the breakdown of carbohydrates into glucose. Rich sources of thiamine are pork, organ meats, green leafy vegetables, legumes, sweet corn, egg yolk, and corn meal. Brown rice, yeast, the germ and husks of grains, berries, and nuts are other rich sources. It is not stored in the body and must be supplied daily. A lack of thiamine affects chiefly the nervous system, the circulation, and the stomach and intestines. Symptoms include irritability, emotional disturbances, loss of appetite, nerve

inflammation, increased pulse rate, difficult breathing (dyspnea), lessened intestinal ability to move spontaneously (mobility), and heart irregularities. Severe lack causes beriberi. Also called **vitamin B$_1$.**

thiethylperazine maleate, a drug that relieves nausea and vomiting (antiemetic). Parkinson's disease, central nervous system disorders, liver or kidney dysfunction, severe low blood pressure, or known allergy to this type of drug prohibits its use. Side effects include low blood pressure, liver toxicity, uncontrolled movements, blood disease, and allergic reactions.

thigh, the section of the lower limb between the hip and the knee.

thigh bone. See **femur.**

thimerosal, an antiinfective. It is given as an eye antiseptic. It is also given as a skin disinfectant after and before operations. Use of permanganates at the same time, strong acids, salts of heavy metals, or known allergy to this drug or to compounds with mercury prohibits its use. Side effects include eruptions at the site of application. Mercury poisoning has been reported when large doses of this drug are given.

thinking, the mental process of forming images or concepts, and problem-solving through the sorting, organizing, and classification of facts. **Concrete thinking** is a stage reached in a child between 7 and 11 years of age in which thought becomes more logical. Problem solving is based on what is seen. The literal meaning of words is still present. It is preceded by the ability to combine different beliefs (syncretic thinking). **Abstract thinking** is the last stage in the growth of the thought processes. This type of thinking appears from about 12 to 15 years of age.

thioamide derivative, one of a group of antithyroid drugs given to treat excess thyroid gland activity (hyperthyroidism). Thioamide drugs act by blocking the making of thyroid hormone.

thioguanine, an antitumor drug. It is given to treat some cancerous tumor diseases, including the serious leukemias. Known allergy or resistance to this drug prohibits its use. It is not given to pregnant women. Side effects include bone marrow depression, distress of the stomach and intestines, and inflammation of the mouth.

Thiomerin, a trademark for a mercurial drug that promotes the release of urine (mercaptomerin sodium).

thiopental sodium, a potent, short-acting drug to aid sleep and relaxation. It is used as a general anesthetic for surgical procedures that are expected to require 15 minutes or less. It is also used as an induction agent for other general anesthetics.

thioridazine hydrochloride, a antipsychotic. It is given for childhood behavioral disorders, mental disorders of the elderly, depression, and alcohol withdrawal. Parkinson's disease, use at the same time of central nervous system depressants, liver or kidney dysfunction, severe low blood pressure, or known allergy to this or similar drugs prohibits its use. Side effects include low blood pressure, poisoning of the liver, uncontrolled movements, blood disease, and allergic reactions.

Thiosulfil, a trademark for a sulfonamide antibacterial (sulfamethizole).

thiotepa, an antitumor alkylating drug. It is given to treat some cancerous diseases, including cancer of the breast and ovary, and urinary bladder cancers. Bone marrow depression, pregnancy, liver or kidney dysfunction, or known allergy to this drug prohibits its use. Side effects include bone marrow depression, loss of appetite, nausea, and headache.

thiothixene, a thioxanthene antipsychotic. It is given to treat sudden agitation and mild to severe psychotic disorders. Parkinson's disease, use at the same time of central nervous system depressants, liver and kidney dysfunction, severe low blood pressure, known allergy to this drug or to phenothiazine drugs prohibits its use. It is not advised for children under 12 years of age. Side effects include low blood pressure, poisoning of the liver, uncontrolled movements, blood diseases, and allergic reactions.

thioxanthine derivative, any one of a group of antipsychotic drugs, each of which is similar to the phenothiazenes in indication, action, and side effects.

thiphenamil hydrochloride, a nerve-blocking drug. It is given to treat stomach and intestine pain caused by excess movements (hypermotility) and spasms. Narrow-angle glaucoma, asthma, obstruction of the urine, genital, or digestive tracts, severe inflammation of the lower bowel (ulcerative colitis), or known allergy to this drug prohibits its use. Side effects include blurred vision, central nervous system effects, rapid heart beat (tachycardia), dry mouth, decreased sweating, and allergic reactions.

thirst, a perceived desire for water or other fluid. The sensation of thirst is usually referred to the mouth and throat.

Thiuretic, a trademark for a drug that stimulates urine release (hydrochlorothiazide).

Thomas' splint, 1. a rigid splint made of steel bars that are curved to fit the involved limb and held in place by a cast or a rigid bandage. It is used to treat long-term joint diseases. **2.** also called **Thomas' ring splint.** a rigid metal splint that extends from a ring at the hip to beyond the foot. It is used to treat a broken leg. It is used together with many traction and suspension devices to immobilize and position a fractured thigh of the patient after and before surgery.

thoracic /thôras´ik/, referring to the chest (thorax).

thoracic duct, a common trunk of many lymphatic vessels in the body. It begins high in the abdomen, directed toward the second lumbar backbone, enters the chest through the diaphragm, and goes up into the neck. See also **lymphatic system.**

thoracic fistula, an abnormal opening in the chest wall that ends blindly or that communicates with the chest cavity.

thoracic medicine, the branch of medicine concerned with the diagnosis and treatment of disorders of the structures and organs of the chest, especially the lungs.

thoracic nerves, the 12 spinal nerves on each side of the thorax, including 11 intercostal nerves and one subcostal nerve. They are distributed mainly to the walls of the chest and stomach. See also **autonomic nervous system.**

thoracic outlet syndrome, a type of nerve disorder. It features an abnormal sensation of the fingers. It may be caused by nerve root pressure from a neck disk or by pressure of the middle nerve in the carpal tunnel (carpal tunnel syndrome).

thoracic parietal node, one of the lymph glands in the chest. See also **lymphatic system, lymph node.**

thoracic vertebra. See **vertebra.**

thoracic visceral node, one of the lymph glands connected to the part of the lymphatic system that serves certain structures within the chest, as the thymus, heart sac, esophagus, windpipe, lungs, and bronchi. See also **lymphatic system, lymph node.**

thoracocentesis /thôr´əkōsentē´-/, surgery to enter the chest wall with a needle for the removal of fluid for diagnostic study or treatment. It may also be done for the removal of a specimen for biopsy. It is usually done using local anesthesia. The patient is seated leaning forward over a table that is chest-high. Puncture of the chest wall may be used to treat cancer of the lung (bronchogenic carcinoma). Fluid samples may be examined for red and white blood cell counts, protein, glucose, enzymes, and microorganisms that may be present. Also called **thoracentesis.**

thoracostomy /-kos´-/, a cut made into the chest wall to provide an opening for draining.

thoracotomy /-kot´-/, a surgical opening into the chest cavity.

thorax, the chest area, with the bone and cartilage containing the principal organs of respiration and circulation and covering part of the abdominal organs. The chest (thorax) of women has less capacity, a flat bone forming the front wall of the chest (sternum), and more movable upper ribs than that of men. Also called **chest.**

Thorazine, a trademark for a phenothiazine (chlorpromazine). It is used as a drug that prevents or relieves nausea and vomiting, and as a tranquilizer.

T–Z

thorium (Th), a heavy, grayish, radioactive, metallic element. Thorium is used in in radiation therapy.

threadworm infection, a disorder of the small intestine caused by the worm *Strongyloides stercoralis,* acquired when larvae from the soil penetrate intact skin, causing an itching rash. The larvae pass to the lungs by way of the bloodstream, sometimes causing pneumonia. Larvae then move up the air passages to the throat, are swallowed, and develop into adult worms in the small intestine. Bloody diarrhea and disorders of the intestines may result. Treatment often includes giving a drug, thiabendazole. Also called **strongyloidiasis.**

three-day measles. See **rubella.**

threonine (Thr) /thrē′ōnin/, an essential amino acid needed for proper growth in infants and for keeping the nitrogen balance in adults. See also **amino acid, protein.**

threshold, the point at which a stimulus is great enough to make an effect. For example, a pain threshold is the point at which a person first becomes aware of pain.

threshold limit value (TLV), the maximum concentration of a chemical to which workers can be exposed for a fixed period, as 8 hours per day, without developing a health problem.

threshold limit value/ceiling (TLV/C), the maximum concentration that should not be exceeded, even instantaneously.

threshold limit value/short term exposure limit (TLV/ STEL), minute time-weighted average exposure that should not be exceeded at any time, nor repeatedly more than four times daily with a 60-minute rest period required between each STEL exposure. These short-term exposures can be tolerated without suffering from irritation, chronic or irreversible tissue damage, or narcosis of a sufficient degree to increase the likelihood of accidental injury, impairing self-rescue, or reducing worker efficiency. TLV/ STELs are expressed in ppm and mg/cu meter.

threshold limit value/time weighted average (TLV/ TWA), the maximum airborne concentration of a material to which an average, healthy person may be exposed repeatedly for 8 hours each day, 40 hours per week without suffering adverse effects. They are based upon currently available data and are adjusted on an annual basis by organizations such as the American Council of Governmental Industrial Hygienists (ACGIH). Because TLVs involve and 8-hour exposure, they are difficult to adapt for emergency response operations. TLV/TWAs are expressed in ppm and mg/cu meter. (The lower the concentration, the more toxic the substance.)

thrill, a fine vibration, felt by an examiner's hand on the body of a patient over the site of a bulging of an artery wall (aneurysm) or on the region over the heart and lower chest (precordium). Compare **bruit, murmur.**

throat. See **pharynx.**

throb, a deep, pulsating kind of discomfort or pain. –**throbbing,** *adj., n.*

thrombectomy /thrombek′-/, the removal of a solid mass (thrombus) from a blood vessel. It is done as emergency surgery to restore circulation to the affected part. Before surgery, anticlotting therapy is begun. An x-ray of the arteries is done to locate the clot. Using general anesthesia, a lengthwise incision is made into the blood vessel and the clot is removed. Compare **embolectomy.**

thrombin /throm′bin/, an enzyme formed in blood during the clotting process from prothrombin, calcium, and thromboplastin. Thrombin causes fibrinogen to change to fibrin, essential in the formation of a clot. See also **blood clot, thrombus.**

thromboangiitis obliterans /throm′bō·an′jē·ī′tis oblit′ ərənz/. See **Buerger's disease.**

thrombocytopenia /-sī′təpē′nē·ə/, an abnormal blood condition in which the number of platelets is reduced. It is usually caused by breakdown of tissue in bone marrow linked to certain tumor diseases or an immune response to a drug. Thrombocytopenia is the most common cause of bleeding disorders. All drugs are stopped because nearly any drug may cause the condition. Transfusion may be necessary.

thrombocytopenic purpura, a bleeding disorder marked by a decrease in the number of platelets. This results in many bruises, red blood spots (petechiae), and bleeding into the tissues. It may occur secondary to a number of causes, including infection and drug allergy and poisoning. It is considered to be an immune response against one's own body tissues (autoimmunity). The acute form usually but not always occurs in children between 2 and 6 years of age. It is harmless. Complete recovery usually is apparent within 6 weeks. The long-term form usually occurs in adults between 20 and 50 years of age. Recovery is rarely spontaneous. It often requires removal of the spleen (splenectomy). **Thrombotic thrombocytopenic purpura (TTP)** is a form with blood and nerve abnormalities. It is seen in a long-term form and in a sudden intense form that may lead to death in weeks. Therapy includes steroids and removal of the spleen.

thrombocytosis /-sītō′-/, an abnormal increase in the number of platelets in the blood. **Benign thrombocytosis,** or **secondary thrombocytosis,** has no specific symptoms. It usually occurs after removal of the spleen (splenectomy), a blood disease (hemolytic anemia), bleeding, or a lack of iron, as a response to exercise, or after treatment with an antitumor drug (vincristine). It may also occur in advanced cancer or Hodgkin's disease or in other lymph cancers. **Essential thrombocythemia** features periods of spontaneous bleeding alternating with blood-clotting episodes. Compare **thrombocytopenia.**

thromboembolism /-em′bōlizm/,   a condition in which a blood vessel is blocked by a clot (embolus) carried in the bloodstream from the site of formation of the clot. The area supplied by a blocked artery may tingle and become cold, numb, and bluish colored (cyanotic). Treatment includes quiet bed rest, warm wet packs, and anticlotting drugs to prevent the formation of additional clots. Removal of clots by surgery (embolectomy) may be needed. A clot in the lungs causes a sudden, sharp, chest or upper stomach pain, breathing difficulty (dyspnea), a violent cough, fever, and spilling of blood (hemoptysis).

thrombophlebitis /-fləbī′-/,   See **phlebitis.**

thromboplastin,   a complex substance that starts the clotting process by changing prothrombin to thrombin in the presence of calcium. It is found in most tissue cells and, in somewhat different form, in red and white blood cells. See also **blood clotting.**

thrombosis /thrombō′-/, *pl.* **thromboses,**   an abnormal blood condition in which a clot develops within a blood vessel of the body. **Cerebral thrombosis** refers to a clotting of blood in any brain blood vessel. A **coronary thrombosis** blocks a coronary artery. It often causes heart attack and death. With **venous thrombosis,** there is a clot in a vein in which pain, inflammation, and swelling may follow if the vein is closed. See also **blood clotting, cavernous sinus syndrome.**

thrombus /throm′bəs/, *pl.* **thrombi,**   a cluster of platelets, fibrin, clotting factors, and other cell elements of the blood usually attached to the interior wall of a vein or artery. It can block a blood vessel. An **agonal thrombus** forms in the heart in the process of dying. A **ball thrombus** is a relatively round blood clot. A **hyaline thrombus** is a clear, colorless mass consisting of broken down red blood cells. A **laminated thrombus** is arranged in layers apparently formed at different times. A **white thrombus** is a clot of blood elements with chiefly white blood cells and with few or no red blood cells. Also called **blood clot.** Compare **embolus.**

thrush,   infection of the tissues of the mouth from a fungus.

thumb,   the first and shortest finger (digit) of the hand. It is classified by some anatomists as one of the fingers. Other anatomists classify the thumb separately, regarding it as composed of one metacarpal bone and only two phalanges, while the fingers have three phalanges.

thumbsucking,   the habit of sucking the thumb for oral satisfaction. It is normal in infants and young children as a pleasure-seeking or comforting device, especially when the child is hungry or tired. The habit reaches its peak when the child is between 18 and 20 months of age. It normally goes away as the child grows and becomes older. Thumbsucking beyond 4 to 6 years of age may lead to teeth that do not properly close. It may also lead to an abnormality of the bony tissue of the thumb.

thymic /thī′mik/,   referring to the thymus gland.

thymol /thī′môl/,   a synthetic or natural thyme oil. It is a part of some over-the-counter drugs used to treat hemorrhoids, a skin disease (acne), and athlete's foot (tinea pedis).

thymoma /thīmō′mə/,   a usually benign tumor of the thymus gland. It may be linked to muscle disease (myasthenia gravis) or an immune deficiency disorder.

thymosin /thī′məsin/,   **1.** a naturally occurring hormone released by the thymus gland. It is present in greatest amounts in young children and lessens in amount throughout life. **2.** an experimental drug derived from bovine thymus extracts. It is given as a drug that changes resistance to certain diseases.

thymus /thī′məs/,   a single, unpaired gland that is located in the upper chest cavity extending upwards into the neck to the lower edge of the thyroid gland. Research has established that the thymus is the primary central gland of the lymphatic system. The endocrine activity of the thymus is believed to depend on the hormone thymosin. This hormone is critical to the immune system. The size of the organ relative to the rest of the body is largest when the individual is about 2 years of age. The thymus usually attains its greatest absolute size at puberty. After puberty, the organ shrivels as fatty tissue replaces the receding thymic tissue. With aging, the gland may change in color from pinkish-gray to yellow. In the elderly individual it may appear as small islands of thymic tissue covered with fat. Compare **spleen.**

Thypinone,   a trademark for the synthetic thyrotropin-releasing hormone (protirelin). It is used to help in the diagnostic assessment of thyroid function. Thyrotropin is naturally released by the pituitary gland and stimulates the thyroid gland.

Thyrar,   a trademark for thyroid hormone.

thyrocervical trunk /thī′rōsur′vikəl/,   one of a pair of short, thick arteries supplying many muscles and bones in the head, neck, and back.

thyroglobulin /-glob′yəlin/,   a purified extract of pork thyroid. It is given to treat diseases caused by a lack of thyroid release. Heart disease, abnormal pituitary gland function, or known allergy to this drug prohibits its use. Side effects when given in excess doses include trembling, nervousness, irregular and too rapid heart rate (tachycardia), and abnormal heart beats. See also **thyroid hormone.**

thyroid.   See **thyroid gland, thyroid hormone.**

T–Z

thyroid cancer, a cancer of the thyroid gland. It is usually features slow growth. There is a high rate of thyroid cancer in survivors of exposure to atomic bomb explosions and in patients who have been treated with radiation for a large thymus in infancy or for acne or other skin disorders in adolescence. Large soft thyroid glands and tumors in the sacs of the thyroid gland (follicular adenomas) may be a beginning of cancerous thyroid tumors. The first sign of cancer may be an increase in size of the thyroid gland, a lump that can be felt by hand, hoarseness, difficult swallowing (dysphagia), breathing problems (dyspnea), or pain on pressure. Total or partial removal of the thyroid gland and related lymph nodes is usually recommended. Radioactive iodine may be given after the operation. High doses of thyroid are often used to suppress thyroid-stimulating hormone (TSH) in an effort to cause the disappearance of remaining tumor dependent on TSH. Cancer of the thyroid is twice as common in women as in men. Although it is diagnosed most frequently in patients between 30 and 50 years of age, it may occur in children and the elderly.

thyroid cartilage, the largest cartilage of the larynx. It is made up of two thin flat plates fused together at an acute angle in the middle line of the neck to form the Adam's apple.

thyroidectomy /thī′roidek′-/, the surgical removal of the thyroid gland. It is done for large soft thyroid glands, tumors, or excess thyroid gland activity (hyperthyroidism) that does not respond to iodine therapy and antithyroid drugs. All but 5% to 10% of the gland is removed. Regrowth usually begins shortly after surgery. The thyroid function may return to normal. For cancer of the thyroid, the entire gland is removed, along with surrounding structures from neck to collarbone.

thyroid function test, any of several laboratory tests done to evaluate the function of the thyroid gland. Often several of the tests are done at the same time.

thyroid gland, an organ at the front of the neck. It is made up of lobes connected in the middle. The thyroid gland is slightly heavier in women than in men. It becomes bigger during pregnancy. The thyroid gland releases the hormone thyroxin directly into the blood. It is essential to normal body growth in infancy and childhood. Its removal may cause lowered bodily activity. The thyroid needs iodine to make thyroxine. Compare **parathyroid gland.**

thyroid hormone, an iodine-containing compound released by the thyroid gland, mainly as thyroxine (T_4) and in smaller amounts the four times more potent triiodothyronine (T_3). These hormones affect body temperature, regulate protein, fat, and carbohydrate catabolism in all cells. They keep up growth hormone release, skeletal maturation, and the heart rate, force, and output. They promote central nervous system growth, stimulate the making of many enzymes, and are necessary for muscle tone and vigor. The production of thyroid hormones is too great in excess thyroid gland activity (hyperthyroidism) and related diseases. A too small or absent production (hypothyroidism) causes serious disorders, such as myxedema or cretinism. Thyroid hormones gotten from animal glands and synthetic compounds are used as replacement therapy in patients with hypothyroidism. Overdosage or a rapid increase in the dosage may result in signs of excess thyroid gland activity, as nervousness, tremor, rapid heart beat (tachycardia), irregular heart beat (cardiac arrhythmia), and menstrual irregularity.

thyroiditis /thī′roidī′-/, inflammation of the thyroid gland. Infections may cause sudden thyroiditis with pus and abscess formation. **Fibrous thyroiditis** (Riedel's struma) is a disorder in which dense fiberlike tissue replaces normal thyroid tissue. It usually occurs in one lobe of the gland but sometimes in both lobes, the windpipe, and surrounding muscles, nerves, and blood vessels. The disease occurs more often in women than in men and usually shows up after 40 years of age. Symptoms include a sense of choking, breathlessness, and swallowing problems. **Lymphocytic thyroiditis** (Hashimoto's disease) is a disorder of the immune system that attacks the thyroid gland. The disease seems to be inherited, but it is 20 times more common in women than in men. It occurs most often between 30 and 50 years of age but may arise in young children. The thyroid develops a goiter which can cause difficult swallowing and a feeling of local pressure. Treatment includes thyroid hormone. **Radiation thyroiditis** occasionally occurs 7 to 10 days after the treatment of hyperthyroidism with radioactive iodine 131. With **subacute thyroiditis** (de Quervain's thyroiditis), there is inflammation of the thyroid. Symptoms include tenderness of the gland, fever, difficult swallowing, fatigue, and severe pain in the neck, ears, and jaw. It often occurs after a viral infection of the lungs. Treatment includes drugs to fight inflammation, as aspirin. Steroids are given for prolonged or severe cases.

thyroid storm, a crisis in uncontrolled excess thyroid gland activity (hyperthyroidism). It is caused by the release into the bloodstream of increased amounts of thyroid hormones. Symptoms include fever that may reach 106° F, a rapid pulse, sudden breathing problems, fear, restlessness, irritability, and extreme exhaustion. The patient may become delirious, fall into a coma, and die of heart failure.

thyroid-stimulating hormone (TSH), a substance released by the front lobe of the pituitary gland. It controls the release of thyroid hormone and is necessary for the growth and function of the thyroid gland. Also called **thyrotropin.** See also **thyroid hormone.**

Thyrolar, a trademark for a thyroid hormone (liotrix).

thyronine. See **thyroid hormone.**

thyrotropin (systemic), a preparation of beef thyroid stimulating hormone. It increases the uptake of radioactive iodine in the thyroid and the release of thyroxine by the thyroid. It is given in diagnostic tests and in the treatment of thyroid cancer. Clotting of the heart arteries or known allergy to this drug prohibits its use. It should not be given in untreated low adrenal function (Addison's disease) or after heart attack. Side effects include excess thyroid gland activity, allergic reactions, low blood pressure, and irregular heart beats.

thyrotropin-releasing hormone, a substance of the hypothalamus that stimulates the release of thyrotropin (thyroid-stimulating hormone) from the front pituitary gland.

Thytropar, a trademark for bovine thyroid stimulating hormone (thyrotropin).

tibia /tib′ē·ə/, the second longest bone of the skeleton. It is located in the middle of the lower leg. It joins with the fibula and the femur, forming part of the knee joint. Also called **shin bone.**

tibialis anterior /tib′ē·ā′lis/, one of the outside muscles of the lower leg.

tibial torsion, a twisting rotation of the tibia on its longitudinal axis.

tic, unwilled movements of a small muscle group, as of the face. The movements are often caused by emotions rather than any physical disorder. A tic may be made worse by stress or anxiety. It is generally brought under control quickly. Multiple grimacing and blinking spasms occur in Gilles de la Tourette's syndrome.

Ticar, a trademark for an antibiotic (ticarcillin).

tic douloureux /tēk do͞olo͞oro͝e′/. See **trigeminal neuralgia.**

tick bite, a puncture wound produced by the toothed beak of a bloodsucking tick. Ticks carry several diseases to humans. Nervousness, loss of appetite, and tingling and headache followed by muscle pain may occur. Symptoms often disappear when the attached tick is carefully removed with forceps. Placing a drop of alcohol on the tick or coating it with petrolatum or nail polish makes removal easier. See also **Lyme arthritis.**

tick paralysis, a disorder caused by several species of ticks that release a poison. Symptoms include weakness, loss of muscle coordination, and paralysis. The tick must feed on the host for several days before the symptoms appear. Because breathing, lip, tongue, throat, and vocal cord paralysis can cause death, it is important to search for ticks. They are often hidden in scalp hair on a patient with the symptoms.

t.i.d., (in prescriptions) abbreviation for *ter in die,* a Latin phrase meaning "three times a day."

tidal volume (TV), the amount of air inhaled and exhaled during normal breathing. See also **pulmonary function test.**

tide, a change, increase or decrease, in the concentration of a particular component of body fluids, as acid tide, fat tide. –**tidal,** *adj.*

Tietze's syndrome /tē′tsēz/, a disorder marked by swellings without pus of one or more rib cartilages causing pain that may radiate to the neck, shoulder, or arm and feel like the pain of heart artery disease. The syndrome may go along with breathing infections.

Tigan, a trademark for a drug used against nausea and vomiting (trimethobenzamide hydrochloride).

timed release. See **prolonged release.**

timolol maleate, a beta-adrenergic receptor blocking drug. It is given for lowering eye pressure in long-term open-angle and secondary glaucoma. Bronchial asthma, COPD, slow heart beat (sinus bradycardia), or known allergy to this drug prohibits its use. It is used carefully in patients who are sensitive to beta-adrenergic receptor blocking drugs. Side effects include blurring of vision and mild eye irritation.

Timoptic, a trademark for a beta-adrenergic receptor blocking agent (timolol maleate).

Tinactin, a trademark for an antifungal (tolnaftate).

Tindal Maleate, a trademark for a phenothiazine (acetophenazine maleate), used as a tranquilizer.

tinea /tin′ē·ə/, a group of fungal skin diseases. They are caused by several kinds of parasitical fungi. They are marked by itching, scaling, and, sometimes, painful sores. Tinea is a general term that refers to infections of various causes, which are seen on several sites. The specific type is usually designated by a modifying term. Diagnosis is made by demonstrating fungus on smear or by culture. See also **athlete's foot, jock itch, ringworm.**

tine test. See **tuberculin test.**

tingling, a prickly sensation in the skin or a part of the body. It goes along with less sensitivity to stimulation of the sensory nerves. It is felt by a patient as the area is numbed by local anesthetic or by exposure to the cold, or as it "goes to sleep" from pressure on a nerve.

tinnitus /tinī′təs/, tinkling or ringing heard in one or both ears. It may be a sign of hearing injury.

T-Ionate-P.A., a trademark for a drug that stimulates male characteristics (testosterone cypionate).

tissue, a collection of similar cells that act together in doing a particular function.

tissue plasminogen activator (TPA), a clot-dissolving substance produced naturally by cells in the walls of blood

T–Z

vessels. It has been used to remove blood clots blocking heart arteries.

tissue response, any reaction or change in living cell tissue when it is acted on by disease, toxin, or other outer stimulus. Some kinds of tissue responses are **immune response, inflammation, necrosis.**

tissue typing, a series of tests to evaluate whether tissues of a donor and a recipient fit with each other. It is done before a transplant. It is done by identifying and comparing a large series of human leukocyte antigens (HLA) in the cells of the body. See also **human leukocyte antigen, immune system, transplant.**

titanium (Ti), a grayish, brittle metallic element. Titanium dioxide is the active part in a number of skin ointments and lotions.

titer /tī'tər/, **1.** a measurement of the concentration of a substance in a solution. **2.** the quantity of a substance needed to get a reaction with another substance.

Title III, Superfund Amendments and Reauthorization Act of 1986 (SARA-Title III), the emergency planning and community Right-To-Know act requires notification of both local emergency planning committee and the state emergency response commission of hazardous substances that exceed reportable planning quantities. Also, certain chemical manufacturing facilities are required to notify the EPA of ''normal'' toxic chemical releases annually.

titubation /tich'əbā'shən/, unsteady posture with a staggering or stumbling style of walking. It also features a swaying head or trunk while sitting. It may be caused by a brain disease. Compare **ataxia.**

TMJ. See **temporomandibular joint syndrome.**

toadstool poisoning, a toxic condition. It is caused by eating certain varieties of poisonous mushrooms. See **mushroom poisoning.**

tobacco, a plant whose leaves are dried and used for smoking and chewing, and in snuff. See also **nicotine.**

tobacco withdrawal syndrome, a change in mood or performance linked to stopped or lessened exposure to nicotine. Symptoms may range from lack of concentration to anxiety and temper outbursts.

tobramycin sulfate, an aminoglycoside antibiotic. It is used to treat outer eye infections, blood poisoning (septicemia), and lower breathing tract and central nervous system infections. Kidney problems, use of strong drugs that stimulate urine release, or known allergy to this or other aminoglycosides prohibits its use. Side effects include harm to nerves, hearing, and balance (ototoxicity), and harm to the kidney cells (nephrotoxicity).

Tobruk plaster /tō'brook/, a plaster cast splint with tapes for skin traction coming through openings in the plaster and connected with Thomas' splint. It covers and immobilizes the leg from foot to groin.

tocanide hydrochloride, a drug taken by mouth to treat irregular heart beats (cardiac arrhythmias).

tocodynamometer /tō'kōdī'nəmom'ətər/, an electronic device for monitoring and recording contractions of the uterus in labor. It is made up of an electronic device that is connected to the lower abdomen with a belt, and a machine that records the contractions on graph paper. See also **electronic fetal monitor.**

tocolytic drug /tō'kōlit'ik/, any drug used to suppress premature labor.

tocopherol. See **vitamin E.**

toddler, a child between 12 and 36 months of age. During this period of development the child gets a sense of independence through the mastery of various tasks. Some of these tasks are control of bodily functions, movement and language skills, and learning socially acceptable behavior, especially delayed satisfaction of needs, and acceptance of separation from the mother or parents. The state or condition of being a toddler is called **toddlerhood.**

toe, any one of the digits of the feet.

toeing in, a birth defect of the foot in which the front part points in toward the middle of the body and the heel remains straight. Also called **metatarsus varus.**

toeing out, a birth defect of the foot in which the front part points out away from the middle of the body and the heel remains straight. Also called **metatarsus valgus.**

toenail, one of the heavy nail structures covering the end bones of the toes. Also called **unguis** /ung'gwis/.

Tofranil, a trademark for a tricyclic antidepressant (imipramine hydrochloride).

togaviruses /tō'gə-/, a family of viruses that includes organisms causing infection of the brain (encephalitis), tropic diseases (dengue, yellow fever), and rubella.

toilet training, the process of teaching a child to control the functions of the bladder and bowel. Training often begins between 18 and 24 months of age. At this time voluntary control of the anus and urine tract muscles is achieved by most children. Resistance occurs if the parents try to train the child before the child is physically and mentally ready. Bowel training is usually successful before bladder training because the urge to empty the bowel is stronger than the urge to empty the bladder. Also, the need is less frequent and more regular.

tolazamide, a sulfonylurea drug used to treat diabetes. It is taken by mouth. Unstable diabetes, serious blockage of kidneys, liver, or thyroid function, pregnancy, or known allergy to this drug or to other sulfonylurea drugs prohibits its use. Side effects include lack of glucose in the blood (hypoglycemia), skin reactions, and blood disorders.

tolazoline hydrochloride, a drug for widening the veins in the outer part of the body (peripheral vasodilator). It is given to treat blood flow disorders, including Buerger's disease, Raynaud's disease, and scleroderma. Heart artery disease, brain vessel (cerebrovascular) accident, or known allergy to this drug prohibits its use. Side effects include irregular heart beat, high blood pressure, increase of peptic ulcer, and a poor response in seriously damaged limbs.

tolbutamide, a sulfonylurea drug used against diabetes. It is taken by mouth. Unstable diabetes, serious blockage of kidney, liver, or thyroid function, pregnancy, or known allergy to this drug or to other sulfonylurea drugs prohibits its use. Side effects include lack of glucose in the blood (hypoglycemia), skin reactions, and blood disorders.

tolerance, the ability to live through hardship, pain, or ordinarily injurious substances, as drugs, without apparent body or mental injury.

Toleron, a trademark for a drug that improves the quality of blood (ferrous fumarate).

Tolinase, a trademark for a drug used against diabetes (tolazamide).

tolmetin sodium, a nonsteroid anti-inflammatory drug. It is mainly given to treat different forms of arthritis and osteoarthritis. Blocked kidney function, stomach and intestinal disease, or known allergy to this drug or similar drugs, or to aspirin prohibits its use. Side effects include peptic ulcer, distress of the stomach and intestines, dizziness, skin rash, and ringing in the ears (tinnitus). This drug interacts with many other drugs.

tolnaftate, an antifungal drug given to treat a variety of fungus infections of the skin. Known allergy to this drug prohibits its use. Side effects include allergic reactions and mild irritation of the skin.

tomography /təmog'rəfē/, an x-ray method that makes a film representing a detailed cross section of tissue structure at a predetermined depth. It is a valuable diagnostic tool for space-occupying tumors, as might be found in the brain, liver, pancreas, and gallbladder. One form of this technique is called **positron-emission tomography (PET).** The patient either inhales or is injected with a radioactive substance that is mostly harmless. The computers of the PET device find gamma rays and change them into pictures that show the processes in the tissues being studied. See also **radiation.**

tongue, the main organ for the sense of taste. It also assists in the chewing and swallowing of food. It is located in the floor of the mouth within the curve of the lower jaw (mandible). The front two thirds of the tongue are covered with small nipple-shaped elevations. The back third is smoother and has numerous mucous glands and lymph follicles. The use of the tongue as an organ of speech is learned. Also called **lingua.**

tongue-tie a defect of the mouth in which the membrane under the tongue is too short (lingual frenulum). It limits the movement of the tongue and impairs the speech. It may be corrected. Also called **ankyloglossia.**

tonicity /tōnis'itē/, the quality of possessing muscle contraction (tone or tonus).

tonic neck reflex /ton'ik/, a normal response in newborns to extend the arm and the leg on the side of the body to which the head is quickly turned while the infant is lying with the face upward and to flex the limbs of the opposite side. The reflex prevents the infant from rolling over. See also **crawling reflex.**

tonofibril /ton'əfī'bril/, a bundle of fine fibers found in the cytoplasm of epithelial cells.

tonometer /tōnom'ətər/, an instrument used in measuring tension or pressure, especially within the eye.

tonometry /-trē/, the measuring of pressure in the eyes. It is done by determining the resistance of the eyeball to flattening by an applied force. Several kinds of tonometers are used. The air-puff tonometer, which does not touch the eye, records turning aside of the cornea from a puff of pressurized air. The Schiötz tonometers record the pressure needed to flatten the corneal surface.

tonsil, a small, rounded mass of tissue, especially lymphoid tissue. **Lingual tonsil** refers to a mass of small lymph nodes (nodules) that form part of the mucous membrane near the root of the tongue. The lingual tonsil is part of the body's defense system against infection. The **palatine tonsils** are a pair of almond-shaped masses of spongy (lymphoid) tissue on either side of the soft palate (palatine) arches. They are covered with mucous membrane and contain many lymph sacs (follicles) and many spaces. See also **adenoid.**

tonsillectomy /-ek'-/, the surgical removal of the tonsils (palatine). Tonsillar tissue is cut apart and removed. General anesthesia is usually used. Bleeding areas are stitched or destroyed by heat (cauterized). An airway remains in place until swallowing returns. On recovery from anesthesia, ice chips or clear liquids without a drinking straw may be offered. Tonsillectomy is often combined with removal by surgery of the adenoids.

tonsillitis, an infection or inflammation of a tonsil. Sudden tonsillitis is often caused by a streptococcus infection. It is marked by severe sore throat, fever, headache, malaise, difficulty in swallowing, earache, and large, tender lymph nodes in the neck. Sudden tonsillitis may go along with scarlet fever. A **peritonsillar abscess,** also called **quinsy,** is an infection of tissue between the tonsil and throat, most often after an attack of tonsillitis. The tonsil and soft palate are red and swollen. Treatment of tonsillitis includes antibiotics, painkillers, and warm washes of the throat. Soft foods and fluids are given.

tonus /tō'nəs/, the normal state of balanced tension in the tissues of the body, especially the muscles. Tonus is essen-

T–Z

tial for many normal body functions. For example, holding the spine erect, the eyes open, and the jaw closed. Also called **tone.**

tooth, *pl.* **teeth,** one of numerous dental structures that develop in the jaws as part of the digestive system. They are used to cut, grind, and process food in the mouth for ingestion. Each tooth is made up of a crown above the gum; two to four roots in the sockets; and a neck, stretching between the crown and the root. Each tooth also has a cavity filled with pulp, richly supplied with blood vessels and nerves that enter the cavity through a small opening at the base of each root. The solid portion of the tooth consists of dentin, enamel, and a thin layer of bone on the surface of the root. The dentin comprises the bulk of the tooth. The enamel covers the exposed portion of the crown. **Tooth form** refers to the identifying curves, lines, angles, and contours of a tooth that make it different from other teeth. Two sets of teeth appear at different periods of life. A **deciduous tooth** is any of the 20 teeth that appear normally during infancy, often called baby teeth. A **permanent tooth** is any of the 32 teeth that appear during childhood and early adulthood. An **accessory tooth** is an extra one that does not look like a normal tooth in size, shape, or position. **Drifting tooth** refers to any tooth that migrates from normal position. See also **dentition, teething.**

tooth alignment, the arrangement of the teeth in relation to their supporting bone, adjacent teeth, and opposing teeth. **Avulsed teeth** are those that have been forcibly moved from their normal position.

tooth-borne base, a denture base restoring an area without teeth that has real teeth at each end for support.

tooth germ, a cell in the embryo that is the starting place of a tooth.

tophus /tō′fəs/, *pl.* **tophi,** a stone (urate deposit) that forms in a joint, particularly of a big toe in persons with gout.

topical /top′ikəl/, **1.** referring to the surface of a part of the body. **2.** referring to a drug or treatment applied to the skin.

topical anesthesia, surface pain killing produced by application of a anesthetic in the form of a solution, gel, or ointment to the skin, mucous membrane, or cornea. Also called **surface anesthesia.** See also **anesthesia.**

Topicort, a trademark for a topical drug that raises the concentration of liver glycogen and blood sugar (desoximetasone).

Topsyn, a trademark for a a drug that raises the concentration of liver glycogen and blood sugar (fluocinonide).

TORCH, an abbreviation for *toxoplasmosis, other, rubella virus, cytomegalovirus, and herpes simplex viruses.* This is a group of agents that can infect the fetus or the newborn infant causing a set of infections called the **TORCH syndrome.** A pregnancy with a TORCH agent may lead to abortion or stillbirth, slowed growth within the uterus, or too early childbirth. At birth and during the first days after birth an infant infected with any one of the organisms may have various problems, as fever, weakness, poor feeding, red spots or purplish-brown areas on the skin, pneumonia, large liver and spleen, liver disease (jaundice), and anemias. Other disorders can be brain inflammation, too small head, fluid in the brain (hydrocephalus), calcium formation in the head, hearing damage, and too small eyes. In addition, each of the agents is linked to several other abnormalities involving immune response, cataracts, glaucoma, blisters (vesicles), ulcers, and inborn heart defects. Before pregnancy women may be tested for susceptibility to the rubella virus. They may be vaccinated against it if not immune. There are currently no vaccines that confer immunity to the other TORCH agents. However, the mother may be tested for antibody levels to them.

Torecan Maleate, a trademark for a phenothiazine drug used against nausea and vomiting (thiethylperazine maleate).

torque /tôrk/, **1.** a twisting force produced by contraction of the thigh muscles that tend to rotate the thigh inwards. **2.** (in dentistry) a force applied to a tooth to rotate it.

torsades de pointes /tôrsäd′ dəpô·eNt′/, an abnormal fast beat of the lower heart chambers. It is often drug-induced, but may be the result of low potassium levels in the blood (hypokalemia) or profound slow heart beat (bradycardia). The abnormal rapid beat may be sudden. The patient may be conscious. The treatment is a temporary electronic pacemaker until the offending drug can be processed and released.

torsion /tôr′shən/, **1.** the process of twisting in a positive (clockwise) or negative (counterclockwise) direction. **2.** the state of being turned.

torsion fracture, a spiral broken bone. It is usually caused by a torsion injury.

torsion of the testis, a twisting of the sperm cord that cuts off the blood supply to the testicle, epididymis, and other structures. Complete loss of circulation for 6 hours may result in dying off (gangrene) of the testis. Partial loss may result in wasting away (atrophy). The condition may be caused by injury with severe swelling. Torsion of the testis occurs more often on the left than on the right side. It happens most often in the first year of life and during puberty. Surgical correction is needed in most cases. If surgery is done within 5 hours of the beginning of symptoms, the testis can usually be saved.

torticollis /tôr′tikol′is/. See **wryneck.**

torulopsosis /tôr′yəlop′səsis/,   an infection with the yeast *Torulopsis glabrata*. This yeast is normally found in the throat, the intestinal and stomach tract, and the skin. However, it causes disease in severely weakened patients or in those with blocked immune function.

total body radiation,   radiation that exposes the entire body so that, theoretically, all cells in the body receive the same radiation.

total body water (TBW),   all the water within the body, including water in tissue cells as well as blood and lymph, plus the water in the stomach and intestines and urinary tract.

total lung capacity (TLC),   the volume of air in the lungs at the end of a maximum breathing in.

total nitrogen,   the nitrogen content of the feces. It is measured to detect various disorders, improper functioning of the pancreas, and blocked protein digestion.

total renal blood flow (TRBF),   the total volume of blood that flows into the kidney arteries. The average TRBF in a normal adult is 1200 ml per minute.

touch,   1. the ability to feel objects; the tactile sense. **2.** the ability to note pressure when it is put on the skin or the mucosa of the body. **3.** to examine with the hand.

touch deprivation,   a lack of touch stimulation. It happens especially in early infancy. If it is continued for some length of time, it may lead to serious developmental and emotional disturbances, as slow growth, personality disorders, and social regression. See also **hospitalism.**

tourniquet /toor′nikit, tur′-/,   a device used to control bleeding. It is made up of a wide constricting band applied to the limb between the heart and the site of bleeding. The use of a tourniquet is a drastic measure. It is to be used only if the bleeding is life threatening and if other, safer measures have proved ineffective. **Rotating tourniquet** refers to a method in which three tourniquets are used in a rotating order. This pools blood in the arms and legs to relieve fluid buildup in the lungs. Tourniquets are applied to the upper parts of three of the four arms and legs at one time. Every 15 minutes, in a clockwise pattern, a tourniquet is placed on an arm or leg, and one tourniquet is removed. At the end of the treatment, one tourniquet is removed every 15 minutes in rotation.

tourniquet infusion method,   a technique of regional chemotherapy. It is used to treat a bone tumor (osteogenic sarcoma). The technique uses one or two external tourniquets, which slow or interrupt the blood flow to a limb temporarily while an anticancer drug is infused into the area. The method increases the concentration of the anticancer drug by as much as 100 times as compared with injecting the drug into the circulation.

tourniquet test,   a test of capillary fragility. A blood pressure cuff is applied for 5 minutes to a person's arm. The number of small red spots (petechiae) within a certain area of the skin may be counted.

toxemia /toksē′mē·ə/.   See **blood poisoning.**

toxemia of pregnancy.   See **preeclampsia.**

toxic,   1. referring to a poison. **2.** (of a disease or condition) severe and progressive.

toxic atmosphere,   any area, inside or outside a structure, where the air contains substances harmful to human life or health when inhaled.

toxic dose (TD),   the amount of a substance that may be expected to produce a poisonous effect. A **median toxic dose (TD$_{50}$)** is the dose of a drug that causes side effects in one half of the patients to whom it is given.

toxic epidermal necrolysis (TEN),   a rare skin disease with redness of the outer skin, death of skin cells, and skin erosion. This condition, which affects mainly adults, makes the skin appear scalded, often leaving scars. The cause of TEN is unknown. It may result from airborne poisons, as carbon monoxide, or allergic or drug reactions. Early symptoms include inflammation of the mucous membranes, fever, a burning sensation in eye membranes, and tender skin. As the disease progresses, large blisters develop and rupture, exposing wide expanses of denuded skin. This causes extensive body complications, as fluid pooling in the lungs, bleeding in the digestive tract, poison in the blood (sepsis), shock, and kidney failure. Treatment involves giving fluids in the veins to replace body fluids.

toxic goiter.   See **Graves' disease.**

toxic nodular goiter.   See **goiter.**

toxic products of combustion,   the toxic by-products of the combustion process.

toxicity /toksis′itē/,   **1.** the degree to which something is poisonous. **2.** a condition that results from exposure to a poison or to poisonous amounts of a substance that does not cause side effects in smaller amounts.

toxicity signal words,   indicates the relative degree of acute toxicity of a hazardous material. Located in the center of the front label panel of a container label, it is one of the most important label markings. The three toxic categories are high toxicity, moderate toxicity, and low toxicity.

toxicokinetics /tok′sikōkinet′-/,   the passage through the body of a poisonous substance or its products.

toxicologist /-kol′-/,   a specialist in the scientific study of poisons and the diseases they bring about (toxicology).

toxicology /-kol′-/,   the scientific study of poisons, their detection, their effects, and methods of treatment for conditions they produce.   **–toxicologic, toxicological,** *adj.*

toxic shock syndrome (TSS),   a severe sudden disease caused by infection with strains of *Staphylococcus aureus*. These strains make a unique poison, enterotoxin F. It is

T–Z

most common in menstruating women using high absorbency tampons. However, it has been seen in newborn infants, children, and men. Early symptoms include sudden high fever, headache, sore throat with swelling of the mucous membranes, diarrhea, nausea, and red spots on the skin (erythroderma). Acute kidney failure, abnormal liver function, confusion, and hard-to-treat low blood pressure usually follow. Death may occur. It is probable that mild forms of the syndrome are not reported and, therefore, are not diagnosed. Giving large amounts of fluid in the vein, help with breathing, and giving drugs that contract the muscle tissue of blood veins (vasopressors) may be necessary in treating severe TSS.

toxin, a poison, usually one produced by or occurring in a plant or microorganism. An **endotoxin** is a poison contained in the cell walls of some bacteria. It is released when the germ dies. Fever, chills, shock, and a number of other symptoms result, depending on the condition of the infected person. An **exotoxin** is a poison that is released or excreted by a living microorganism.

toxocariasis /tok'sōkerī'əsis/, infection with the larvae of *Toxocara canis,* the common roundworm of dogs and cats. Ingestion of viable eggs, commonly found in soil, leads to the spread of tiny larvae throughout the body. This results in breathing symptoms, large liver, skin rashes, pooling of white cells the blood (eosinophilia), and delayed eye injury. Children who eat dirt are particularly subject to this disease. Specific drug therapy is not very useful. The outcome is usually good without therapy. Regular worming of pets helps prevent infection. Also called **visceral larva migrans.**

toxoid, a toxin that has been treated with chemicals or with heat to lessen its poisonous effect but keeps its power to stimulate antibody formation. It is given to make immunity by stimulating the creation of antibodies. See also **toxin, vaccine.**

Toxoplasma /-plaz'mə/, a genus of protozoa with only one known species, *Toxoplasma gondii.* It is a parasite of cats and other hosts and causes a nerve disease (toxoplasmosis) in humans.

toxoplasmosis /-plazmō'-/, a common infection with the protozoan parasite *Toxoplasma gondii.* When transmitted to the fetus through the placenta, there is liver and brain involvement with calcium in the brain (cerebral calcification), convulsions, blindness, too small head and fluid on the brain (microcephaly and hydrocephaly), and mental retardation. Symptoms of an acquired form include rash, disease of the lymph nodes (lymphadenopathy), fever, central nervous system disorders, and inflammation of the heart wall and lung tissue. It may be acquired by eating inadequately cooked meat containing the parasite.

trabecula carnea /trəbek'yələ/, *pl.* **trabeculae carneae,** any one of the irregular bands and bundles of muscle that project from the inner surfaces of the lower heart chambers (ventricles). Some of these trabeculae are ridges of muscle along the lower heart chamber walls. Compare **chordae tendineae.** See also **heart, ventricle.**

trabeculectomy /-ek'-/, the removal by surgery of a section of tissue to increase the outflow of eye fluid (aqueous humor) in patients with severe glaucoma.

trace element, an element needed in tiny amounts for nutrition or mental processes.

tracer, a radioactive isotope that is used in diagnostic x-ray techniques to allow a biologic process to be seen. The tracer, which is put into the body, binds with a specific substance and is followed with a scanner or fluoroscope as it passes through many organs or systems in the body. Kinds of tracers include **radioactive iodine (^{131}I)** and **radioactive carbon(^{14}C).** See also **radioisotope scan.**

trachea /trā'kē·ə/, a nearly cylindric tube in the neck. It is made up of cartilage and membrane. It extends from the voice box (larynx) to the top of the lungs, where it divides into two bronchi extending into the lungs. It is covered in the neck by the thyroid gland and various other structures. Also called **windpipe.** –**tracheal,** *adj.*

tracheitis /trā'kē·ī'-/, any inflammation of the windpipe. It may be sudden or long-term. It may result from infection, allergy, or physical irritation.

tracheobronchitis /trā'kē·ōbrongkī'-/, inflammation of the windpipe and bronchi. It is a common form of breathing infection.

tracheoesophageal fistula /-ēsof'əjē'əl/, an abnormal tubelike passage between the windpipe and the esophagus.

tracheostomy /trā'kē·os'-/, an opening through the neck into the windpipe through which a tube may be inserted. After tracheostomy humidified oxygen is given via tent or directly into the tracheostomy tube, and the patient is reassured that the tube is open and that air can pass through it. The tube is suctioned frequently to keep it free from fluids. The patient is taught to cough to move fluids up and out of the bronchi. Pen and paper or a magic slate is kept available for communication because the patient cannot speak. Complications of tracheostomy include air or gas in the lung space (pneumothorax), breathing difficulty, obstruction of the tracheostomy tube or its displacement from the windpipe, and lung infection. Other problems are lung collapse, an abnormal passage between the windpipe and esophagus (tracheoesophageal fistula), and bleeding. If the opening was done as an emergency, the tracheostomy is closed once normal breathing is restored. If the tracheostomy is permanent, as with a removed voice box (larynx), the patient is taught self-care. Compare **tracheotomy.**

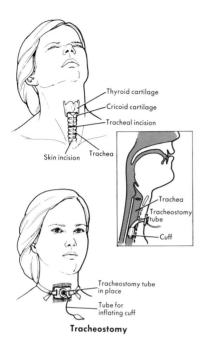

Thyroid cartilage
Cricoid cartilage
Tracheal incision
Skin incision   Trachea

Trachea
Tracheostomy tube
Cuff

Tracheostomy tube in place
Tube for inflating cuff

Tracheostomy

tracheotomy /-ot′-/, a cut made into the windpipe through the neck below the voice box (larynx). It is done to get access to the airway below a blockage with a foreign body, tumor, or fluid pooling in the vocal apparatus (edema of the glottis). The opening may be made as an emergency measure at an accident site, at a hospitalized patient's bedside, or in the operating room. A small hole is made in the fibrous tissue of the windpipe. The opening is then widened to allow the intake of air. In an emergency any available instrument may be used as a widener, even the barrel of a ballpoint pen with the inner portion removed. Compare **tracheostomy.**

trachoma /trəkō′mə/, a long-term, infectious disease of the eye. It is caused by the bacterium *Chlamydia trachomatis.* First symptoms are inflammation, pain, intolerance to light (photophobia), and watery eyes. If untreated, sacs form on the upper eyelids and grow larger until the granulations invade the cornea, eventually causing blindness. Trachoma is a significant cause of blindness. It is present in hot, dry, poverty-ridden areas. Teaching an affected population about the spread of trachoma and having an adequate water supply for washing hands, towels, and handkerchiefs are important factors in getting rid of the disease.

tract, a long group of tissues and structures that function together as a pathway, as the digestive tract or the parts of nerve cells (axons) that are grouped together to form a pathway.

traction, the process of pulling a part of the body along, through, or out of its socket or cavity. An example is **axis-traction,** used during childbirth to pull a baby's head with forceps in a direction of least resistance through the mother's birth canal. See also **orthopedic traction.**

traction frame, an apparatus that supports the pulleys, the ropes, and the weights by which traction is applied to many parts of the body or by which many parts of the body are hung. Traction frames are used to treat bone fractures and dislocations, disease processes of the muscle and skeleton system, to correct many bone defects, and to keep rigid specific areas of the body. The main parts of a traction frame are metal uprights that attach to the bed and support an overhead metal bar. In addition to traction equipment, traction frames are often rigged with trapeze bars that the patient can grasp to help in changing position and to exercise the muscles of the arms and the trunk.

tractor plow, any tracked vehicle with a plow for exposing mineral soil, with transportation and personnel for its operation.

trademark, a word, symbol, or device given to a product by its manufacturer. It is registered as a part of its identity. See also **generic name.**

trait, **1.** a mode of behavior or any mannerism or physical feature that separates one individual or culture from another. **2.** any quality or condition that is inborn. See also **dominance, gene, Mendel's laws, recessive.**

Tral, a trademark for a nerve-blocking drug (hexocyclium methyl sulfate).

trance, **1.** a sleeplike state marked by the complete or partial loss of consciousness and the loss or lack of muscle movement, as seen in hypnosis. **Death trance** refers to a state in which a person appears to be dead but is not. A **hypnotic trance** is an artificially induced sleeplike state, as in hypnosis. A sleep walking state that is a symptom of hysteric neurosis is called **hysteric trance.** An **induced trance** can result from a hysteric neurosis or from hypnotism. **2.** a dazed or confused condition; stupor.

Trancopal, a trademark for a tranquilizer (chlormezanone).

Tranmep, a trademark for a tranquilizer (meprobamate).

tranquilizer, a drug to calm people who are nervous, excited, or anxious. Major tranquilizers are generally used to treat serious mental conditions. Minor tranquilizers are given to treat anxiety, irritability, tension, or failure to deal with unsolved problems. Tranquilizers often bring on drowsiness and can cause addiction to the drug. See also **antipsychotic.**

T–Z

transcondylar fracture /transkon'dilər/, a broken bone near the end of a long bone, as the elbow or ankle.

transcutaneous electric nerve stimulation (TENS) /-kōo-tā'nē·əs/, a method of pain control using electric signals sent to the nerve endings. Electrodes are placed on the skin and joined to a machine by wires. The electric signals are like those of the body, but different enough to block pain signals sent to the brain. It is a fairly safe method with no known side effects. It is not done with patients who have pacemakers.

transdermal delivery system /-dur'məl/, applying a drug to unbroken skin. The drug is absorbed through the skin and enters the blood system. It is used mainly to give a heart drug and a nerve-blocking drug (nitroglycerin and scopolamine).

transect, to sever or cut across, as in doing a cross section of tissue.

transference /trans'fərəns, transfur'əns/, **1.** shifting symptoms from one part of the body to another, as occurs in conversion disorder. **2.** a way of shifting feelings that are linked to earlier events on people in one's life to others, such as a physician or therapist, that are currently in one's life. This is often done without knowing it. **Countertransference** is the conscious or unconscious emotional response of a psychotherapist or analyst to a patient.

transfer factor, a substance made from white blood cells (leukocytes) that transfers a delayed allergy from one person to another. Transfer factor may be used to treat a long-term infection (mucocutaneous candidiasis) and an immune system disease (Wiskott-Aldrich syndrome). It is also used to give immunity against tumors in patients with many types of cancer.

transferrin /transfer'in/, a protein in the blood that is needed to move iron from one place in the body to another.

transfusion. See **blood transfusion.**

transient ischemic attack (TIA) /tran'shənt/, an episode of brain blood vessel damage (stroke). It is caused by a blockage of a vessel, by a blood clot, or a buildup of fats. The symptoms depend on where the blockage is and how much of the brain is affected. Normal vision may be disturbed, and dizziness, weakness, difficulty in swallowing, numbness, or unconsciousness may occur. The attack is most often brief, lasting a few minutes; rarely, symptoms continue for several hours. See also **ischemia, stroke.**

transillumination, shining a light through body tissue to look at its structure.

transitional cell carcinoma, a malignant, nipplelike tumor. It occurs most often in the bladder, urinary tubes, and the kidneys.

transmission, the transfer or carrying of a thing or condition, as a signal from the brain, an infectious or inborn disease, or an inborn trait, from one person or place to another. –**transmissible,** *adj.*

transplacental /-pləsen'təl/, across or through the placenta, especially referring to the exchange of nutrients, waste products, and other material between the growing fetus and the mother.

transplant, 1. also **to graft.** to transfer an organ or tissue from one person to another or from one body part to another in order to replace a diseased structure, to restore function, or to change appearance. This may be temporary, as an emergency skin transplant for burns, or permanent, as the grafted tissue growing to become a part of the body. Skin, bone, cartilage, blood vessel, nerve, muscle, cornea, and whole organs, as the kidney or the heart, may be grafted. Skin and kidneys are the structures most often transplanted. The best donors are identical twins or persons having the same blood type and immune features. Rejection is the major problem. Fever, pain in the graft area, and loss of function 4 to 15 days later are signs that the donor tissue is being rejected by the immune system of the patient. Drugs are given in large doses to prevent antibody production and rejection. The transplanted structure may need several weeks to become established. Late rejection may occur several months or even 1 year later. **2.** a tissue or organ that is transplanted, or the patient who receives donated tissue or an organ or something linked to the procedure. An **allograft** is the transfer of tissue between two beings with unlike genes, as an organ transplant between two humans who are not identical twins. An **autograft** is the transplant by surgery of any tissue from one part of the body to another part in the same patient. Autografts are commonly used to replace skin lost in severe burns. An **isograft** is the transplant of compatible tissue from genetically identical individuals, as between a patient and identical twin. A **xenograft** refers to tissue from another species used as a temporary graft. Its use is in treating a severely burned patient when enough tissue from the patient or from a tissue bank is not available. Although it soon is rejected, it gives a cover for the burn for the first few days. A **zoograft** is the tissue of an animal transplanted to a human, as a heart valve from a pig to replace a damaged heart valve in a human. See also **corneal grafting, skin graft.**

transport index, the number placed on a radioactive materials package label which is indicative of the control required during transport. The transport index is the radiation level, in millirems per hour, at 3 feet from accessible external package surface or, for fissile class II packages, an assigned value based on criticality safety requirements for the package contents.

transposition, 1. an abnormality occuring during growth in the womb in which a part of the body normally on the left is found on the right or vice versa. **2.** the shifting of genetic material from one chromosome to another at some point in the reproductive process, often resulting in a birth defect.

transposition of the great vessels,   a birth defect in which the lung blood vessel (pulmonary artery) arises from the left lower heart chamber (ventricle) and the main heart vessel (aorta) from the right ventricle, the opposite of the normal positions. The primary symptoms are bluish skin and lack of oxygen, especially in infants with small defects. Signs of congestive heart failure develop rapidly, especially in infants with large ventricle defects. Surgical correction of the defect is put off, if possible, until after 6 months of age when the infant can better tolerate the procedure. See also **blue baby.**

transudate /tran'sōōdāt/,   a fluid passed through a membrane or squeezed through a tissue or into the space between the cells of a tissue. It is thin and watery and contains few blood cells or other large proteins. See also **edema.**

transurethral resection (TUR) /-yōōrē'thrəl/,   a surgical process through the urethra, as in a prostate operation.

transverse,   at right angles to the long part of an object, as the planes that cut the long part of the body into upper and lower portions.

transverse fissure,   a crack dividing two surfaces of the brain.

transverse fracture,   a broken bone that occurs at right angles to the long part of the bone involved.

transverse mesocolon,   a broad fold of the bowel connecting the large intestine (transverse colon) to the wall of the abdomen. See also **colon.**

Tranxene,   a trademark for a tranquilizer (chlorazepate dipotassium).

tranylcypromine sulfate,   a monoamine oxidase (MAO) inhibitor that acts as an antidepressant. It is given to treat severe mental depression. Diseases of the heart or brain vessels, paranoid schizophrenia, liver problems, alcoholism, adrenal gland tumors, or known allergy to this drug prohibits its use. It is not given to children under 16 years of age. Among the most serious side effects are severe periods of high blood pressure that can be brought on by eating foods high in tyramine or by being given at the same time many nervous system drugs. Common side effects include headache, dizziness, dry mouth, blurred vision, and fainting when standing up.

trapezius /trəpē'zē·əs/,   a large flat triangular muscle of the shoulder and upper back. It raises the shoulder, and flexes the arm.

trapezoid bone /trap'əzoid/,   the smallest wrist bone.

trauma /trou'mə, trô'mə/,   **1.** physical injury caused by violent or disruptive action, or by a poisonous substance getting into the body. **2.** mental or emotional injury caused by a severe emotional shock.   **–traumatic,** *adj.,* **traumatize,** *v.*

trauma center,   a service that gives emergency and specialized intensive care to very ill and injured patients.

traumatic anesthesia,   a total lack of normal feeling in a part of the body, caused by injury, destruction of nerves, or blocking of nerve pathways.

traumatophilia /trô'mətōfil'yə/,   a mental condition in which the patient gets unknowing pleasure from injuries and surgical operations.

travail /trəvāl'/,   **1.** physical or mental effort, especially when it causes distress. **2.** the effort of labor and childbirth.

Travase,   a trademark for an enzyme that splits proteins (sutilains).

traveler's diarrhea,   any of several diarrheal disorders commonly seen in people visiting regions of the world other than their own. Some strains of *Escherichia coli,* which produce a powerful poison enzyme (exotoxin), are the common cause. Other organisms that cause the condition include *Giardia lamblia* and species of *Salmonella* and *Shigella.* Symptoms last for a few days and include stomach and intestinal cramps, nausea, vomiting, slight fever, and watery stools. Also called **Montezuma's revenge, turista.**

Treacher Collins' syndrome,   an inborn disorder marked by an incomplete form of a head and face birth defect (mandibulofacial dysostosis). See also **Pierre Robin's syndrome.**

treatment,   **1.** the care and overseeing of a patient to fight, reduce, or prevent a disease, disorder, or injury. **2.** a method of fighting, reducing, or preventing a disease, disorder, or injury. Treatment may be pharmacologic, using drugs; surgical, involving surgery; or supportive, building the patient's strength. It may focus on finding a cure for the disorder, or just try to relieve symptoms without bringing about a cure. **Active** or **curative** treatment is designed to cure. **Causal** treatment focuses on the cause of a disorder. **Conservative** treatment avoids drastic measures and procedures. **Definitive** treatment refers to any that is generally accepted as the specific cure of a disease. **Empiric** treatment employs methods shown to work by experience. **Expectant** treatment relieves symptoms as they arise in the course of a disease, rather than treating the cause of the illness itself. An example is amputating a leg with gangrene in a patient with diabetes. **Palliative** treatment is directed to ease pain and distress, but not to cure. Examples are the use of narcotics to relieve pain in late cancer, making a hole in the colon (colostomy) to bypass a tumor of the bowel that cannot be removed by surgery, and the removal of dead tissue in a patient with cancer. **Pre-**

T–Z

ventive treatment is designed to keep a disease from occurring or a mild disorder from getting more severe. **Prophylactic** treatment is for the prevention of a disease or disorder. **Rational** treatment is based on a knowledge of a disease process and the action of the measures used.

treatment room, a room in a patient care unit, usually in a hospital, in which various treatments or procedures that need special equipment are done, as removing stitches, draining a blood blister, packing a wound, or doing a diagnostic test.

Trecator-SC, a trademark for a tuberculosis drug (ethionamide).

Trechona /trikō′nə/, a genus of spiders, family Dipluridae, the bite of which is poisonous and irritating to humans.

trematode /trem′ətōd/. See **fluke.**

tremor /trem′ər, trē′mər/, rhythmic, quivering movements with no purpose caused by the uncontrolled tightening and relaxing of groups of muscles attached to the skeleton. This disorder occurs in some older patients, in certain families, and in patients with different nerve disorders. **Continuous tremor** refers to small, regular, purposeless movements that continue during rest. They may disappear briefly during voluntary movements. The trembling seen in Parkinson's disease is a typical continuous tremor. The tremors of Graves' disease, alcoholism, mercury poisoning, and other disorders caused by poisons are usually less rhythmic. **Essential tremor** is an uncontrollable fine shaking of the hand and head, especially during routine movements of the body. It is an inherited disorder that appears during adolescence or in middle age. **Flapping tremor (asterixis)** often occurs with processing (metabolic) disorders. The tremor is usually seen when the arm is extended and the wrist is flexed backwards. Asterixis is seen often in patients in a coma from liver disease. **Passive tremor** is an undesired trembling occurring when the patient is at rest, one of the signs of Parkinson's disease. **Senile tremor** features fine, quick movements, especially of the hands, rhythmic head nodding, and increased trembling during useful movements.

tremulous /trem′yələs/, referring to tremors, or uncontrolled muscular contractions.

trench fever, an infection that goes away by itself, caused by *Rochalimaea quintana,* an organism in the Rickettsia group of microorganisms, carried by body lice, marked by weakness, fever, rash, and leg pains.

trench mouth. See **gingivitis.**

Trendelenburg's operation /trendel′ənbərgz/, tying off varicose veins whose valves no longer work. It is done to take out weak parts of veins and pockets in which clots might lodge.

Trendelenburg's test, a simple test for nonworking valves in a person who has varicose veins. The person lies down and raises the leg to empty the vein, then stands, and the vein is looked at as it fills. If the valves are not working correctly, the vein fills from above; if the valves are normal, they do not allow backflow of blood, and the vein fills from below.

trephine /trifīn′, trifēn′/, a circular, sawlike instrument used in removing pieces of bone or tissue, usually from the skull. Also called **trepan** /trē′pan/.

treponematosis /trep′ənē′mətō′-/, any disease caused by slender, spiral microorganisms (spirochetes) of the genus *Treponema*. All of these infections are effectively treated with penicillin; often one dose, given in the muscle, results in cure. Examples are syphilis and yaws.

tretinoin, a drug used to treat acne. Known allergy to this drug prohibits its use. Side effects include red, fluid-filled, blistered, or crusted skin.

triacetin, an antifungus drug used to treat surface fungus infections of the skin, including athlete's foot.

triage /trē·äzh′/, a process in which a group of patients is sorted according to their need for care. The kind of illness or injury, the severity of the problem, and the facilities available are the factors used to sort the patients.

triamcinolone, a steroid drug used to treat inflammation, as in many skin diseases. Fungus infections or known allergy to this drug prohibits its systemic use. Viral or fungus infections of the skin, slowed circulation, or known allergy to this drug prohibits its local use. Side effects include stomach and intestinal, endocrine, nervous system, and fluid disturbances. A variety of skin reactions may occur from local use of this drug.

triamterene, a fluid-releasing drug (diuretic) that keeps potassium from being excreted. It is given alone or with another diuretic to treat fluid buildup, high blood pressure, and congestive heart failure. Absence of urine (anuria), severe liver or kidney problems, high levels of potassium in the blood, or known allergy to this drug prohibits its use. Side effects include electrolyte disturbances, especially high levels of potassium in the blood, and stomach and intestinal problems.

triangular bandage, a square of cloth folded or cut into the shape of a triangle. It may be used as a sling, a cover, or a thick pad to control bleeding.

triangular bone, a wrist bone.

Triavil, a trademark for a nervous system drug that has a calming drug (perphenazine) and a drug to control depression (amitriptyline hydrochloride).

triazolam, a sleeping pill. It is given in the short term to treat insomnia. Known allergy to this drug or other drugs like it prohibits its use. It is not given to pregnant women, nursing mothers, or patients younger than 18 years of age.

Side effects include loss of memory, reactions conflicting with the expected, rapid heart beat, depression, confusion or reduced memory, and vision problems.

triceps brachii /trī′seps brak′ē·ī/, a large muscle that runs along the entire length of the back of the upper arm. It extends the forearm and moves the arm toward the body.

triceps reflex. See **deep tendon reflex.**

triceps surae limp, an abnormal action in walking, linked to a weakness in the knee muscle (triceps surae). Such a weakness keeps the triceps surae from raising the pelvis and carrying it forward during the walking cycle. As a result, the pelvis sags below its normal level and lags behind in the walking movement.

trichiasis /trikī′əsis/, an abnormal turning inward of the eyelashes that irritates the eyeball. It usually follows infection. Compare **ectropion.**

trichinosis /trik′inō′-/, an infection caused by the parasitic roundworm *Trichinella spiralis,* acquired by eating raw or undercooked pork or bear meat. Early symptoms of infection include stomach or intestinal pain, nausea, fever, and diarrhea; later, muscle pain, tenderness, fatigue, and a buildup of white blood cells (eosinophilia) are observed.

trichlormethiazide, a fluid-releasing and high blood pressure drug. It is given to treat high blood pressure and fluid buildup. Urine buildup (anuria) or known allergy to this drug or to other drugs like it prohibit its use. Side effects include too little potassium in the blood, high blood sugar levels, high uric acid blood levels, and many allergic reactions.

trichloroethylene /trīklôr′ō·eth′ilēn/, a general anesthetic for dentistry, minor surgery, and the first stages of labor. It is too harmful to the heart for deep anesthesia.

trichoepithelioma /trik′ō·ep′ithē′leō′mə/, a skin tumor that comes from the cells of the sacs (follicles) of fine body hair.

trichologia /-lō′jē·ə/, an abnormal condition in which a person pulls out his or her own hair, usually seen only in a state of severe confusion (delirium).

trichomonacide, a drug that destroys *Trichomonas vaginalis,* a microorganism that causes a stubborn form of irritation of the outer urinary tract and vagina.

trichomoniasis /-mənī′əsis/, a vaginal infection caused by the microorganism *Trichomonas vaginalis,* marked by itching, burning, and frothy, pale yellow to green, bad smelling vaginal discharge. With long-term infection all symptoms may disappear, although the organisms are still present. In men, infection is usually without symptoms but may be shown by irritation of the urethra that continues or comes back. Infection is carried by sexual intercourse or, in newborns, by passage through the birth canal. Reinfec-

tion is common if sexual partners are not treated at the same time.

Trichophyton /trikof′iton/, a genus of fungi that infects skin, hair, and nails. See also **dermatomycosis.**

trichostrongyliasis /-stron′jəlī′əsis/, a condition of being infested with *Trichostrongylus,* a genus of roundworm. Also called **trichostrongylosis.**

trichotillomania /-til′ō-/, an abnormal impulse or desire to pull out one's hair, often seen in cases of severe mental retardation and conditions of severe confusion (delirium). Also called **hair pulling, trichomania.** See also **trichologia.**

trichuriasis /trik′yo͞orī′əsis/. See **whipworm infection.**

Triclos, a trademark for a sleeping pill and calming drug (triclofos sodium).

tricuspid /trīkus′pid/, **1.** referring to three points or points of the crowns of teeth (cusps). **2.** referring to the tricuspid valve of the heart.

tricuspid atresia, a heart birth defect that features a lack of the tricuspid valve between the right upper heart chamber (atrium) and right lower heart chamber (ventricle). Other heart defects are usually present, allowing some flow of blood into the lungs. Symptoms include bluish skin from lack of oxygen, difficulty in breathing, lack of oxygen to tissues, and signs of right-sided heart failure. Treatment includes grafting blood vessels to the lung to increase blood flow to the lungs. Total corrective surgery has been successful in a limited number of older children.

tricuspid valve. See **heart valve.**

tricyclic compound, a chemical substance used in the treatment of depression. It blocks the body's use of an adrenal gland hormone, norepinephrine. Its action is not fully understood.

Tridesilon, a trademark for a steroid drug (desonide).

trifluoperazine hydrochloride, a tranquilizer. It is given to treat anxiety, delusions (schizophrenia), and other mental disorders, and as an antinausea and antivomiting drug. Parkinson's disease, use of central nervous system depressants at the same time, liver or kidney disorders, severe low blood pressure, or known allergy to this drug prohibits its use. Side effects include low blood pressure, liver disease, many movement disorders, a variety of blood diseases, and allergic reactions.

trifluorothymidine, an antivirus drug. Also called **trifluridine.** It is given to treat eye diseases caused by herpes simplex virus. Known allergy to this drug prohibits its use. Poisoning of the eyes may result from being given this drug for more than 21 days. Side effects include allergic reactions, fluid buildup, and increased eye pressure.

triflupromazine hydrochloride, a tranquilizer. It is given to treat severe agitation and other mental disorders and for the control of severe vomiting. Parkinson's disease, use

T–Z

of central nervous system depressants at the same time, liver or kidney disease, severe low blood pressure, or known allergy to this drug or to other similar drugs prohibits its use. Side effects include low blood pressure, many motor problems, blood diseases, and allergic reactions.

trigeminal nerve /trījem′inəl/, either of the largest pair of skull nerves, necessary for the act of chewing and general control of the face. The trigeminal nerves have sensory, motor, and intermediate roots and connect to three areas in the brain. Also called **fifth nerve, trifacial nerve.**

trigeminal neuralgia, a nerve condition of the trigeminal facial nerve. Symptoms include sudden spasms of flashing, stablike pain moving along the course of a branch of the nerve from the angle of the jaw. It is caused by breakdown of the nerve or by pressure on it. Any of the three branches of the nerve may be affected. Severe, sharp pain (neuralgia) of the first branch results in pain around the eyes and over the forehead; of the second branch, in pain in the upper lip, nose, and cheek; of the third branch, in pain on the side of the tongue and the lower lip. Also called **tic douloureux** /tik′doo͞oloorœ′/.

trigeminy /trījem′inē/, **1.** a grouping in threes. **2.** an irregular heart beat of a normal beat followed by two irregular beats that occur quickly after each other.

triglyceride /trīglis′ərīd/, a compound made up of a fatty acid (oleic, palmitic, or stearic) and glycerol. Triglycerides make up most animal and vegetable fats and appear in the blood bound to a protein, forming high- and low-density lipoproteins. See also **lipoprotein.**

trigonitis /trī′gənī′-, trig′-/, inflammation of part (trigone) of the bladder. This often occurs with a bladder tube infection (urethritis).

trihexyphenidyl hydrochloride, a nerve-blocking drug. It is given to treat Parkinson's disease and to control motor problems brought on by the giving of drugs. Narrow-angle eye disease (glaucoma), asthma, blockage of the genitals or urinary tract, or of the stomach and intestinal tract, severe inflammation of the colon with ulcers, or known allergy to this drug prohibits its use. Side effects include blurred vision, central nervous system problems, rapid heart beat, dry mouth, less sweating, and allergic reactions.

triiodothyronine (T₃), a hormone that helps control growth and development, the body's chemical processes, and body temperature. It is used to treat an underactive thyroid gland (hypothyroidism) and an enlarged thyroid gland (goiter). See also **thyroid hormone.**

Trilafon, a trademark for a tranquilizer (perphenazine).

trimeprazine tartrate, an antiitching drug. It is given to treat itching and allergic reactions of the skin. Coma, decrease of the function of bone marrow, producing breast

milk, or known allergy to this drug prohibits its use. It is not given to children under 6 months of age or to patients receiving large amounts of central nervous system depressants. Side effects include confused excitement, parkinson-like problems, inflammation of the liver (hepatitis), and disorders of the stomach and intestines.

trimester /trīmes′tər/, one of the three periods of roughly 3 months into which pregnancy is divided. The first trimester includes the time from the first day of the last menstrual period to the end of 12 weeks. The second trimester, closer to 4 months in length than 3, extends from the twelfth to the twenty-eighth week of pregnancy. The third trimester begins at the twenty-eighth week and extends to the time of childbirth.

trimethadione, an anticonvulsing drug. It is given to prevent seizures in petit mal epilepsy, especially seizures that do not respond to other treatments. Severe kidney or liver conditions, blood diseases, or known allergy to this drug prohibits its use. Side effects include skin disorders, blood diseases, and low red blood cell levels. Sleepiness and poor vision in bright light (hemeralopia) may occur.

trimethaphan camsylate, a nerve-blocking agent. It is given to produce an even low blood pressure during surgery and to lower blood pressure in high blood pressure emergencies. It is not used where low blood pressure places a patient in undue risk or when allergy to this drug prohibits its use. Side effects include severe low blood pressure.

trimethobenzamide hydrochloride, an antivomiting drug. It is given to relieve nausea and vomiting. Disease of the brain and spinal cord (Reye's syndrome) or known allergy to this drug prohibits its use. Side effects with high doses include drowsiness, diarrhea, allergic reactions, and motor problems. Side effects are rare at usual dosages.

trimethoprim, an antibacteria drug. It is given to treat many infections, especially of the urinary tract, middle ear, and breathing tubes. Known allergy to this drug prohibits its use. It should not be used to treat strep throat. Side effects include blood diseases and allergic reactions, stomach and intestinal problems, and central nervous system disorders.

trimipramine maleate, an antidepressant. It is given to treat anxiety, depression, and insomnia. Use at the same time of an MAO antidepressant (monoamine oxidase) within 14 days or known allergy to this drug prohibits its use. It is not given during recovery from heart attack or to patients with a mental disorder (schizophrenia). It should not be given to children. Side effects include rapid heart rate, seizures, parkinson-like disorders, blurred vision, low blood pressure, and making glaucoma worse.

Trimox, a trademark for an antibiotic drug (amoxicillin trihydrate).

Trimpex, a trademark for an antibacterial drug (trimethoprim).

tripelennamine hydrochloride, an antihistamine. It is given to treat stuffy nose and allergic reactions of the skin. Asthma, glaucoma, difficulty in urination, use at the same time of an antidepressant (monoamine oxidase inhibitor), or known allergy to this drug prohibits its use. It is not given to premature or newborn infants or to mothers producing breast milk. Side effects include sleepiness, high heart rate, and stomach and intestinal upset.

triplet, any one of three offspring born of the same gestation period during a single pregnancy.

triploid. See **euploid.**

triprolidine hydrochloride, an antihistamine. It is given to treat many allergic reactions, including stuffy nose, skin rash, and itching. Asthma or known allergy to this drug prohibits its use. It is not given to newborn infants or mothers producing breast milk. Side effects include drowsiness, skin rash, allergic reactions, dry mouth, and fast heart rate.

trismus /triz′məs/, a long-term spasm of the muscles of the jaw. Also called (informal) **lockjaw.** See also **tetanus.**

trisomy /trī′səmē/, a birth defect resulting from the presence of three copies of a particular chromosome, rather than the normal pair. This defect occurs in Down's syndrome.

Trisoralen, a trademark for a skin coloring drug (trioxsalen).

Trobicin, a trademark for an antibacteria drug (spectinomycin hydrochloride).

trocar /trō′kär/, a sharp, pointed rod that fits inside a tube. It is used to pierce the skin and the wall of a cavity or canal in the body to suck in or out fluids, to put in a drug or solution, or to guide the placement of a soft tube (catheter). See also **cannula.**

trochanter /trōkan′tər/, one of the two bony structures that stick out on the end of the thigh. It serves for the attachment of various muscles.

troche /trō′kē/, a small oval, round, or oblong tablet that has a drug mixed in a flavored, sweetened base that dissolves in the mouth, releasing the drug. Also called **lozenge.**

trochlear nerve /trok′lē·ər/, either of the smallest pair of skull nerves, necessary for control of the eye muscles. The trochlear nerves branch to supply the superior oblique muscle and link to the eye (ophthalmic) division of the trigeminal nerve, connecting with two areas in the brain. Also called **fourth cranial nerve.**

trochoid joint /trō′koid/. See **pivot joint.**

Trocinate, a trademark for a nerve-blocking drug (thiphenamil hydrochloride).

troleandomycin, an antibiotic. It is given to treat certain infections, including pneumococcal pneumonia and Group A streptococcal infections of the upper breathing tract. Known allergy to this drug prohibits its use. Side effects include stomach and intestinal disturbances, mild to severe allergic reactions (including anaphylaxis), and poisoning of the liver.

tromethamine, a drug that makes alkaline. It is given to correct excess levels of acid in the body's fluids, especially metabolic acidosis in certain heart conditions. Absence of urine formation or kidney disorder (uremia) prohibits its use. It is not given during pregnancy except in severe life-threatening situations. Side effects include low levels of sugar in the blood (hypoglycemia), shallow breathing, and tissue damage at the site of injection.

Tronothane Hydrochloride, a trademark for a local anesthetic (pramoxine hydrochloride).

trophic action /trof′ik/, the starting of cell reproduction and enlargement by nurturing and causing growth.

trophic fracture, a break in a bone caused by the weakening of bone tissue caused by nutritional disturbances.

trophoblast /trof′əblast/, the layer of tissue that forms the wall of the early embryo (blastocyst) of mammals with placentas in the early stages of the growth of the embryo. –**trophoblastic,** adj.

trophoblastic cancer, a malignant tumor of the uterus that grows from early fetal skin cells. Symptoms include vaginal bleeding and a heavy, foul-smelling discharge; a persistent cough or coughing up of blood signals lung involvement. Removal of the uterus (hysterectomy) should be done in most cases, but does not end the chance of the disease coming back. Chemotherapy is effective in curing a large percentage of patients with trophoblastic tumors. Also called **trophoblastic disease.** See also **choriocarcinoma, hydatid mole.**

tropicamide, a nerve-blocking drug. It is given for diagnostic purposes in eye tests. Glaucoma or known allergy to this drug prohibits its use. Side effects include intolerance of light and fast heart rate.

tropical medicine, the branch of medicine that deals with the diagnosis and treatment of diseases commonly occurring in tropic and subtropic regions of the world.

tropical sprue. See **sprue.**

Trousseau's sign /trōōsōz′/, a test for muscle cramps in which a wrist spasm is brought about by inflating a blood pressure cuff on the upper arm to a pressure higher than normal systolic blood pressure for 3 minutes.

truncus arteriosus, the main artery in the embryo that initially opens from both lower heart chambers (ventricles) and later divides into the aorta and the main lung artery.

T–Z

truss, a device worn to prevent or slow the pushing through of the intestines or other organ through an opening in the abdominal wall.

Trypanosoma /trip′ənōsō′mə/, a genus of one-celled parasites that live in the body. Several species can cause serious diseases in humans. Most *Trypanosoma* organisms live part of their life-cycle in insects and enter humans by insect bites.

trypanosomiasis /-sōmī′əsis/, a parasitic disease caused by protozoal organisms carried to humans by the bite of bloodsucking insects.

trypanosomicide /-sō′misīd/, a drug that destroys trypanosomes, especially the species of the parasite given to humans by various insect carriers common in Africa and Central and South America.

Tryptacin, a trademark for an amino acid (L-tryptophan), used as an antidepressant and to bring on sleep.

tryptophan (Trp) /trip′təfan/, an amino acid necessary for normal growth in infants and for nitrogen balance in adults. Tryptophan is the basis of several substances, including serotonin and niacin. Most of the body's need for tryptophan is acquired from protein in foods, especially legumes, grains, and seeds. See also **amino acid, protein.**

tubal dermoid cyst, a tumor that comes from embryonal tissues that grows in a fallopian tube.

tubal ligation, one of several sterilization methods in which both fallopian tubes are blocked to prevent conception from occurring. Spinal or local anesthesia is used unless the procedure goes along with major surgery. Through a small incision in the abdomen, the fallopian tubes are tied off in two places with suture. The part between the two tied places is then cut out. The operation is less commonly done through the vagina. Problems that result, which are rare but serious, include bleeding, infection, and tubal pregnancy. The requirements for giving one's legal permission to have sterilization operations are different among states and institutions.

tubal pregnancy, a pregnancy in which the embryo is implanted in the fallopian tube. Tubal pregnancy seldom occurs in first pregnancies. The most important factor that might bring on tubal pregnancy is prior tubal injury. Pelvic infection, scarring and healing tissue from surgery, or problems from using an IUD birth control device may cause damage that decreases transport of the ovum through the tube. Most often the tube, which cannot hold the growing fetus for very long, breaks. This causes bleeding in the peritoneal cavity that, if not stopped, can lead rapidly to shock and, often, death. Occasionally, the conceptus does not firmly implant in the tube and is pushed out from the fringed end of the tube as a tubal abortion. Some conceptuses seem to die and are absorbed back into the tube.

Treatment is surgical and involves opening the pelvic area for examination (laparotomy), taking out the conceptus and any blood in the cavity, and the removal or repair of the involved tube. A woman who has had one tubal pregnancy has one chance in five of having another in a following pregnancy. See also **pregnancy.**

tube, a hollow, cylinder-shaped piece of equipment or structure of the body. An example is a **chest tube** inserted into the chest cavity through the skin for removing air or fluid or pus. It is commonly used after chest surgery and lung collapse. An **endotracheal tube** inserts through the mouth or nose and into the throat (trachea). It is used for giving oxygen and for general anesthesia. A **nasogastric tube** passes into the stomach through the nose. A **nasotracheal tube** is put into the windpipe (trachea) through the nose and throat. It is often used to give oxygen and other breathing therapies. A **T tube** is a device in the shape of a T, inserted through the skin into a cavity or wound, used for drainage.

tube feeding. See **nasogastric feeding.**

tubercle /tōō′bərkəl/, **1.** a small group of cells or a bump (nodule), as that on a bone. **2.** a nodule, especially an elevation of the skin that is larger than a pimple. **3.** a small rounded nodule caused by infection with *Mycobacterium tuberculosis,* made up of a gray mass of small round cells.

tubercles of Montgomery, small pimples (papillae) on the surface of nipples and dark circles around the nipples (areolae) that release a fatty lubricating substance.

tuberculin purified protein derivative /tōōbur′kyəlin/, a solution that has a pure protein taken from strains of *Mycobacterium tuberculosis.* It is used as an aid in the diagnosis of tuberculosis, in the Mantoux test, and in multiple puncture skin test devices.

tuberculin test, a test to find past or present tuberculosis infection based on a positive skin reaction, using one of several methods. A purified protein derivative (PPD) of tubercle bacilli, called **tuberculin,** is placed into the skin in various ways. In the **Heaf test** several skin punctures are made. The **Mantoux test** is done with an injection. The tuberculin material is scratched onto the skin in the **Pirquet test.** The **tine test** uses a small disposable disk with multiple prongs to puncture the skin. If a raised, red, or hard zone forms around the tuberculin test site, the person is said to be sensitive to tuberculin, and the test is read as positive. However, a negative tuberculin reaction does not rule out a diagnosis of earlier or active tuberculosis. Bacteria grown from samples taken from saliva and from stomach material, acid-fast staining, and x-ray studies are often needed to make a sure diagnosis of tuberculosis.

tuberculoma /to͞obur′kyəlō′mə/, a tumorlike growth of tuberculous tissue in the central nervous system, marked by symptoms of an expanding brain, or spinal mass.

tuberculosis (TB) /to͞obur′kyəlō′-/, a long-term grainy tumorous infection caused by a bacterium, *Mycobacterium tuberculosis.* Generally exposure is by breathing in or eating infected droplets, and it usually affects the lungs, although infection of other organ systems by other ways of getting the disease occurs. Listlessness, vague chest pain, inflammation of the membranes around the lungs (pleurisy), loss of appetite, fever, and weight loss are early symptoms of lung (pulmonary) tuberculosis. Night sweats, bleeding in the lungs, coughing up of sputum with pus, and shortness of breath (dypsnea) develop as the disease progresses. The lung tissues react to the bacterium by making protective cells that go around the disease organism, forming small groups of cells or bumps (tubercles). Untreated, the tubercles enlarge and merge to form larger tubercles that undergo a change into a grainy mass of tissue (caseation). Eventually the separated dead tissue ends up in the cavities of the lungs, and coughing up of blood occurs. The infecting organism does not produce bacterial poisons (endotoxins) or substances that disrupt red blood cells (hemolysins), but **tuberculin,** a poisonous substance, is released as the bacillus breaks apart. Tuberculin has no effect in people who have never been infected but produces a typical skin reaction when injected in the skin in people who have or have had tuberculosis. X-ray films of the lungs show various signs of tubercular activity. Tuberculosis may spread from the lungs via the lymphatics and blood vessels to the liver, spleen, and other organs.

tuberculosis vaccine. See **BCG vaccine.**

tuberculous spondylitis /to͞obur′kyələs/, a rare, serious form of tuberculosis caused by the invasion of *Mycobacterium tuberculosis* into the spine. The disks between the backbones may be destroyed, causing the collapse, shortening, and angling of the spine. See also **tuberculosis.**

tuberosity /to͞o′bəros′itē/, a bump or raised place, especially of a bone. An example is the **tuberosity of the tibia,** a large oblong elevation at the end of the lower leg bone (tibia) that attaches to the ligament of the kneecap.

tuberous carcinoma /to͞o′bərəs/, a hard, bumpy cancerous tumor of the skin.

tuberous sclerosis, a nervous system and skin disease marked by epilepsy, mental symptoms, calcium deposits on the brain, tumors on the eyes, and tumors of the heart or kidneys. **Adenoma sebaceum** is a skin condition in tuberous sclerosis. There are many, wartlike, yellowish-red, small waxy bumps (papules) on the face. They are not true adenomas but tumors made of fully-grown connective tissue (fibromas). There is no effective treatment.

tubocurarine chloride, a skeletal muscle relaxing drug. It is given as an added drug to anesthesia and electroshock treatment, in the diagnosis of severe muscle weakness (myasthenia gravis), and to aid in the treatment of patients undergoing machine-aided breathing. Asthma or known allergy to this drug prohibits its use. It should not be given to patients who cannot tolerate histamine release. Side effects include low blood pressure, shortage of oxygen, and allergic reactions. Many drugs act to increase the activity of tubocurarine.

tuboplasty /to͞o′bəplas′tē/, an operation in which cut or damaged fallopian tubes are repaired.

tubule /to͞o′byo͞ol/, a small tube, as one of the collecting tubules in the kidneys or the semen-producing tubules of the testicles.

tuft fracture, fracture of any one of the finger or toe bones.

Tuinal, a trademark for a central nervous system drug that has two relaxing and sleep drugs (amobarbital sodium and secobarbital sodium).

tularemia /to͞o′lərē′mē·ə/, an infectious disease of animals caused by the bacillus *Francisella (Pasteurella) tularensis,* which may be passed to humans by insect carriers or direct contact. Symptoms include fever, headache, and an open skin sore with enlarged lymph glands, or by eye infection, stomach and intestinal sores, or pneumonia, depending on the site of entry and the response of the patient. Treatment includes antibiotics. Recovery produces lifelong immunity. A vaccine is available. Also called **deerfly fever, rabbit fever.**

tumor, a new growth of tissue with continuing, uncontrolled spreading of cells. The tumor may be localized or spreading, harmless or cancerous. A tumor may be named foritslocation,foritscellularmakeup,orforthepersonwhofirst identified it. A **mixed tumor** is a growth made up of more than one kind of tumor tissue. Also called **neoplasm.**

tumoricide /to͞omôr′isīd/, a substance that can destroy a tumor. **–tumoricidal,** *adj.*

tumorigenesis /to͞o′mərijen′əsis/, the process of starting and helping the growth of a tumor. See also **carcinogen.** **–tumorigenic,** *adj.*

tumor marker, a substance in the body that is linked to a cancer. Tumor marker molecules found in blood or other tissue samples do not always mean the presence of cancer.

tunica, a covering membrane, such as the **tunica vaginalis testis,** the tissue surrounding the testicle and an attached tube (epididymis).

tuning fork, a small metal instrument consisting of a stem and two prongs that makes a constant pitch when either prong is struck. It is used in tests of hearing.

tunnel vision, a defect in sight in which there is a great loss of side vision, as if looking through a hollow tube or tunnel.Theconditionoccursinadvancedlong-termglaucoma.

T–Z

turban tumor, a noncancerous tumor made up of many pink or maroon bumps that may cover the entire scalp and may also occur on the trunk and arms and legs.

turgid /tur′jid/, swollen, hard, and blocked, usually as a result of a gathering of fluid.

turgor /tur′gər/, the normal strength and tension of the skin caused by the outward pressure of the cells and the fluid that surrounds them. Loss of body water causes decreased skin turgor, which appears as loose skin. Marked fluid gain or too much fluid causes increased turgor that appears as smooth, taut, shiny skin that cannot be grasped and raised.

turnbuckle cast, a deformity-correcting (orthopedic) device used to encase and immobilize the entire trunk, one arm to the elbow, and the opposite leg to the knee. It is made of plaster of paris or fiberglass and uses hinges as part of its design in the treatment of curvature of the spine (scoliosis).

Turner's syndrome, a chromosome disorder seen in about 1 in 3000 live female births, marked by the absence of one X chromosome, inborn ovarian failure, genital tissue defects, heart and circulation problems, dwarfism, short metacarpals, "shield chest," bone growths on the larger bone of the leg, and underdeveloped breasts, uterus, and vagina. See also **Noonan's syndrome.**

Tussionex, a trademark for a drug containing an antitussive (hydrocodone bitartrate) and an antihistamine (phenyltoloxamine citrate).

twin, either of two offspring born of the same pregnancy and developed from either a single egg or from two eggs that were released from the ovary and fertilized at the same time. Twin births occur approximately 1 in 80 pregnancies. **Dizygotic twins,** also called **fraternal twins,** are developed from two eggs that were released from the ovary and fertilized at the same time. They may be of the same or opposite sex. They may differ both physically and in genetic traits, and have two separate placentas and membranes. Dizygotic twins are most common in the black race and when the mother is 35 to 39 years old. **Monozygotic twins,** also called **identical twins,** are grown from one fertilized egg that splits into equal halves. This results in separate fetuses. Such twins are always of the same sex. They have the same genes and have identical blood groups. They closely look like each other. They may have single or separate placentas and membranes. **Interlocked twins** are identical twins so positioned in the uterus that their necks become entwined making vaginal delivery impossible. **Conjoined twins** grow from the same egg and are physically joined at birth. The defect may be mild. A serious defect occurs when the fetuses share a large part of their body. Another is a small, partly formed fetus joined to a more fully formed one. Conjoined twins result when cell division is incomplete during early development. Whether one or both can live depends on the extent of the fusion and the degree of growth of the fetuses. **Siamese twins** are equally developed and produced from the same egg, but have not developed completely, resulting in their being joined together at some part of the body. With modern surgical methods, most Siamese twins can be successfully separated. **Unequal twins** refers to two nonjoined fetuses born of the same pregnancy in which only one of the pair is fully formed, with the other showing developmental defects.

twinning, 1. the development of two or more fetuses during the same pregnancy, either by itself or through outside control for experimental purposes on animals. **2.** the making of two like structures or parts by division.

tybamate, a minor tranquilizer. It is given to reduce worry and tension in mental nerve disorders. Acute intermittent porphyria or known allergy to this or a like drug prohibits its use. Side effects include drowsiness, dizziness, and rashes.

Tylenol, a trademark for a painkiller and fever-reducing drug (acetaminophen).

tympanic /timpan′ik/, referring to a structure that sounds when struck; drumlike, as a **tympanic abdomen** that sounds on percussion because the intestines are enlarged with gas.

tympanic antrum, a relatively large, irregular opening in the upper front part of the mastoid portion of the temporal bone at the base of the skull. It is linked to the mastoid air cells and lined with a mucous membrane. See also **mastoid process.**

tympanic membrane. See **ear.**

tympanic reflex, the reflection of a beam of light shining on the eardrum. In a normal ear a bright, wedge-shaped reflection is seen; its highpoint is at the end of the malleus, and its base is at the front lower edge of the eardrum. In disorders of the middle ear or eardrum, this shape may be distorted. Also called **light reflex.**

tympanoplasty /tim′pənōplas′tē, timpan′-/, any of several operations on the eardrum or small bones of the middle ear, to restore or improve hearing in patients with deafness (conductive). These operations may be used to repair a broken eardrum, increasing deafness (otosclerosis), or dislocation of one of the small bones of the middle ear. See also **myringoplasty.**

Type A packaging, packaging designed to prevent the loss or dispersal of its radioactive contents under normal conditions of transport. This type of packaging carries radioactive materials that, because of their level of radioactivity or physical properties, constitute little hazard.

Type A personality, a behavior pattern of individuals who are highly competitive and work compulsively to meet deadlines. The behavior also goes with a higher than usual rate of coronary heart disease.

Type B packaging, packaging that meets the same criteria as Type A but in addition is designed to meet standards for performance under hypothetical accident conditions. This type of packaging is designed to carry greater quantities of radioactivity than Type A.

Type B personality, a form of behavior that goes with persons who seem not to be passive and who lack an inner need to meet deadlines, are not highly competitive at work and play, and have a lower risk of heart attack.

Type E personality, a term used to describe women who fit neither Type A or Type B personality categories, but who have a high sense of insecurity and try to convince themselves that they are worthwhile. Type E women try to be ''all things to all people.''

type I hyperlipidemia, a rare disease with the gathering of triglycerides in the bloodstream, causing recurring bouts of inflammation of the pancreas (acute pancreatitis). The symptoms begin in childhood. The disease is caused by a low level of activity of an enzyme that normally removes triglycerides from the blood. The buildup of triglycerides is basically in proportion to the amount of fat in the diet. Treatment is mainly dietary; both saturated and unsaturated fats are limited. Also called **exogenous hyperlipemia.**

typhoid fever, a bacterial infection usually caused by *Salmonella typhi,* carried by contaminated milk, water, or food. Symptoms include headache, mental confusion and excitement, cough, watery diarrhea, rash, and a high fever. The period between first being exposed to the bacteria and getting the first symptoms may be as long as 60 days. Patches of rosy spots and pimples are scattered over the skin of the intestinal area. The disease is serious and may be fatal. Further problems are bleeding or holes in the intestines and vein inflammation with blood clotting (thrombophlebitis). Some people who recover from the disease continue to be carriers and spread the disease. Typhoid vaccine gives some protection but requires annual booster doses for best effect.

typhoid vaccine, a bacterial vaccine prepared from an inactivated, dried strain of *Salmonella typhi.* It is given for primary immunization against typhoid fever for adults and children. Acute infection or use of steroids at the same time prohibits its use. Side effects include allergic reaction, and pain and inflammation at the site of injection.

typhus, any of a group of acute infectious diseases caused by various species of *Rickettsia* and usually carried from infected rodents to humans by the bites of lice, fleas, mites, or ticks. These diseases all feature headache, chills, high fever, and red rash that covers much of the body. **Brill-Zinsser disease** is a mild form of typhus that returns in a patient who appears to have completely recovered

from a severe case of the disease. Some rickettsiae remain in the body after the symptoms of the disease are gone, causing the symptoms to return. **Epidemic (classic) typhus** results from the bite of the body louse. The rickettsia is in the feces of the louse and enters the body when the bite is scratched. An intense headache and a fever reaching 104° F begin after a period of 10 days to 2 weeks. The rash follows. Further problems may include collapse of blood vessels, kidney failure, pneumonia, or gangrene. The death rate is high among older patients. **Murine typhus** is carried by the bite of an infected flea. Recovery is usually rapid, but death can occur in elderly or feeble patient. **Scrub typhus** occurs in Asia, India, northern Australia, and the western Pacific islands, and is carried from rats and mice to humans by mites.

typhus vaccine, any one of three vaccines, each of which is made to deal with the different rickettsial organisms that cause epidemic typhus, murine typhus, or Brill-Zinsser disease. Each of the vaccines is given for immunization against a form of typhus. Acute infection, diseases that cause weakness, use of corticosteriods at the same time, or allergy to eggs prohibits its use. Side effects include allergic reactions. Pain at the site of injection also may occur.

typing, the process of finding out the classification of a specimen of blood, tissue, or other substance. See also **blood typing, tissue typing.**

tyramine, an amino acid made in the body from the essential acid tyrosine. Tyramine starts the release of epinephrine and norepinephrine. It is important that people taking MAO (monoamine oxidase) inhibitors avoid eating foods and drinks that have tyramine, especially aged cheeses and meats, bananas, yeast-containing products, and alcoholic beverages. See also **epinephrine, norepinephrine.**

tyrosinemia /tī′rōsinē′mē·ə/, a disorder of the amino acid tyrosine. **Neonatal tyrosinemia** is a harmless, temporary condition of the newborn, especially premature infants, in which too much of the amino acid tyrosine is found in the blood and urine. The defect goes away with treatment, or it may disappear by itself. **Hereditary tyrosinemia** is an inborn disorder that involves a problem of processing the amino acid tyrosine. Treatment consists of a diet low in tyrosine and phenylalanine and high in doses of vitamin C. In severe cases the outlook is extremely poor, and a liver transplant may be needed.

tyrosinurea /-sinŏŏr′ē·ə/, tyrosine in the urine.

Tyzine, a trademark for an alpha-adrenergic drug (tetrahydrozoline hydrochloride).

Tzanck test /tsangk/, a microscopic examination of material from skin sores to help diagnose certain small blister diseases.

T–Z

U

ulcer, a craterlike skin or mucous membrane lesion. The cause may be an inflammation, infection, or malignant process. A **stress ulcer** is one that develops in the stomach or intestine of patients who are under heavy stress. For example, **Curling's ulcer,** an ulcer of the upper small intestine (duodenum), grows in patients who have severe burns on the surface of the body. **Serpent ulcer** refers to an open sore of the skin that heals in one place while growing in another. A **stasis ulcer** is a scaly, craterlike sore on the skin of the lower leg caused by long-term clogging of veins, often from varicose veins. Healing is slow, and care to prevent irritation and infection is essential. A **trophic ulcer** is a pressure sore caused by outer injury to a part of the body that is in poor condition from disease, low levels of blood flow, or loss of nerve fibers. Trophic ulcers may be painless or linked to severe burning pain (causalgia). See also **bedsore, peptic ulcer.**

ulcerative colitis /ul'sərā'tiv/, a chronic, inflammatory disease of the large intestine and rectum, marked by profuse watery diarrhea containing blood, mucus, and pus. Other symptoms include severe intestinal pain, fever, chills, anemia, weight loss, and difficulty in moving the bowel. Children with the disease may have retarded physical growth. Patients with ulcerative colitis often cannot perform the normal activities of daily living. Treatment with steroids or other antiinflammatory drugs may help to control the symptoms. Those with severe disease or life-threatening problems often need surgery. See also **colitis.**

ulocarcinoma /yoo'lōkär'sinō'mə/, cancer of the gums.

Ultracef, a trademark for an antibiotic (cefadroxil monohydrate).

Ultralente Iletin, a trademark for an insulin zinc suspension.

ultrasound imaging, the use of high-frequency sound to make a picture of structures inside the body, such as fetuses, gallstones, heart defects, and tumors. Ultrasound imaging differs from x-ray imaging in that there is no radiation involved. **Cardiac ultrasound** refers to a method used to test heart and blood vessel problems. The device is placed over the chest. Its high-pitched sound wave is bounced off the heart. This makes an image of the heart chambers and valves. **Doppler scanning** is a method used in ultrasound imaging to monitor the behavior of a moving structure, as flowing blood or a beating heart. A shift in frequency of sound waves reflected from a moving surface gives information about the moving structure. Fetal heart detectors work on this principle. **Intraoperative ultrasound** uses a portable ultrasound device to scan the spinal cord during spinal surgery. This helps surgeons locate and see the size of tumors of the central nervous system that may not be found by other methods.

ultraviolet (UV) light, light rays that are beyond the range of human vision. It occurs in sunlight; it burns and tans the skin and converts in the skin to vitamin D. Ultraviolet lamps are used to control infectious, airborne bacteria, and viruses and to treat psoriasis and other skin conditions. Also called **ultraviolet radiation.**

umbilical cord, a flexible structure connecting the umbilicus with the placenta in the pregnant uterus, and giving passage to the umbilical arteries and vein. In the newborn it is about 2 feet long and ½ inch in diameter. It is first formed during the fifth week of pregnancy.

umbilical fistula, an abnormal passage from the umbilicus to the intestine or another internal structure.

umbilical hernia. See **hernia.**

umbilicus. See **navel.**

unconditioned response, a normal, instinctive, unlearned reaction to a stimulus. It is one occurring naturally, not acquired by association and training. Also called **inborn reflex, instinctive reflex, unconditioned reflex.** Compare **conditioned response.**

unconscious, 1. being unaware of the environment; insensible; unable to respond to sensory stimuli. 2. (in psychiatry) the part of mental function in which thoughts, ideas, emotions, or memories are beyond awareness and not subject to ready recall.

unconsciousness, a state of unawareness or lack of response to sense stimuli as a result of a lack of oxygen caused by breathing difficulties or shock. It can also be caused by depressants, as drugs, poisons, ketones or electrolyte imbalance. Other causes are from a brain injury, seizures, stroke, or brain tumor or infection. See also **coma.**

undecylenic acid, an antifungus drug. It is given to treat athlete's foot and ringworm. Known allergy to this drug prohibits its use. It is not used in the eyes or on mucous membranes. Caution is advised when the patient is diabetic. Side effects include skin irritation and allergic reactions.

underwater exercise, any physical activity in a pool or large tub where the buoyancy of the water aids movement of weak or injured muscles. See also **exercise.**

underweight, less than normal body weight given height, body build, and age.

undescended testis, failure of one or both of the testicles to move down into the scrotum. If descent does not occur by 1 year of age, hormones may be given. If not successful, surgery (orchipexy) will likely be done before the boy is 5 years of age. A condition in which only one testicle has come down into the male scrotum is called **monorchism.** Also called **cryptorchidism.**

undisplaced fracture, a bone break in which cracks in the tissue may radiate in several directions without the separation of fragmented sections.

undulant fever /un′dyələnt/. See **brucellosis.**

unengaged head, the head of a fetus before it moves down into the mother's pelvic area. See also **engagement.**

unfinished business, the concerns of a dying patient that need to be resolved before death can be accepted by the patient. Unfinished business may range from money matters to personal relations.

unified command, a method for all agencies or individuals who have jurisdictional responsibility, and in some cases those who have functional responsibility at the incident, to contribute to determining overall objectives for the incident and selection of a strategy to achieve the objectives.

unilateral paralysis /yoo′nēlat′ərəl/. See **hemiplegia.**

uniovular /-ov′yələr/, developing from a single ovum, as in identical twins.

Unipen, a trademark for an antibacterial (nafcillin sodium).

unipolar depressive response, a mental disorder marked by symptoms of depression only.

unit, that organization element having functional responsibility for a specific incident planning, logistic, or finance activity.

United Nations International Children's Emergency Fund (UNICEF), a fund established by the United Nations in 1946 to aid children of the world.

United States Pharmacopeia (USP), a drug encyclopedia with descriptions, uses, strengths, and standards of purity for certain drugs and their dosage.

United States Public Health Service (USPHS), an agency of the federal government responsible for the control of any people, goods, or substances that may affect the health of U.S. citizens. The agency sets standards for domestic handling and processing of food and the manufacture of serums, vaccines, cosmetics, and drugs. It supports and does research, aids localities in times of disaster and epidemics, and provides medical care for certain groups of Americans.

universal antidote, a mixture of 50% activated charcoal, 25% magnesium oxide, and 25% tannic acid, formerly thought useful as an antidote for most types of acid, heavy metal, alkaloid, and glycoside poisons.

universal donor. See **blood donor.**

Unna's paste boot /oo′nəz/, a dressing for varicose ulcers made by putting gelatin-glycerin-zinc oxide paste on the leg and then a spiral bandage that is covered with coats of paste to make a rigid boot.

unsaturated fatty acid. See **fatty acid.**

unsocialized aggressive reaction, a behavior disorder of childhood marked by hostility, disobedience, aggression, vengefulness, quarreling, and destructiveness. It includes lying, stealing, temper tantrums, vandalism, and violence. It is more prevalent in boys than in girls.

urate /yoor′āt/, any salt of uric acid. Urates are found in the urine, blood, and tophi or stonelike deposits in tissues. They may also be deposited as crystals in body joints. See also **gout, uric acid.**

urea /yoor′ē·ə/, **1.** the main nitrogen part of urine made from protein breakdown. **2.** a sterile form of the chemical used as a diuretic given to reduce fluid pressure in the brain and eyes and used on the skin as a drying agent.

Ureaphil, a trademark for a diuretic (urea).

Ureaplasma urealyticum /-plaz′mə/, a sexually spread germ often found in the urogenital systems of men and women. The germ may invade the placenta in pregnancy, causing miscarriage, premature birth, or death of the newborn infant. How the effects on pregnancy occur is not known.

Urecholine, a trademark for a nervous system drug (bethanechol chloride).

uremia /yoor′ē′mē·ə/, the presence of excessive amounts of urea and other waste products in the blood, as occurs in kidney failure.

uremic frost /yoor′ē′mik/, a pale, frostlike deposit of white crystals on the skin caused by kidney failure and uremia. Urea compounds and other waste products that cannot be excreted by the kidneys into the urine are carried

T–Z

through capillaries to the skin, where they collect on the surface.

ureter /yo͞ore͞'tər/, one of a pair of tubes that carry the urine from the kidneys into the bladder. The ureter enters the bladder through a tunnel that also works as a valve to stop the backflow of urine when the bladder contracts. – **ureteral,** *adj.*

ureteritis /yo͞ore͞'tərī'-/, an inflammatory condition of a ureter caused by infection or by a kidney stone.

ureterocele /yo͞ore͞'tərōsēl'/, a slipping out of place (prolapse) of a portion of the ureter into the bladder. The condition may block the flow of urine and lead to loss of kidney function. Compare **cystocele.**

ureterography /yo͞ore͞'tərog'rafē/, the x-ray imaging of a ureter. The examination may involve injection of a radiopaque dye through a urinary catheter or by injection of a dye that filters through the kidneys to the ureters.

ureterosigmoidostomy /yo͞ore͞'tərsig'moidos'-/, surgery in which a ureter is implanted in the intestinal tract.

ureterotomy /yo͞or'ētərot'-/, a cut into a ureter.

urethra /yo͞ore͞'thrə/, a small tubular structure that drains urine from the bladder. In men, the urethra also serves as a passage for semen. See also **ureter.**

urethral /yo͞ore͞'thrəl/, pertaining to the urethra.

urethritis /yo͞or'ēthrī'-/, an inflammation of the urethra, often caused by infection in the bladder or kidneys. **Nongonococcal urethritis (NGU)** is an infection with a mild urination problem and a small to moderate amount of discharge. The discharge may be white or clear, thin or mucuslike, with pus cells. The infection is often caused by a parasite, *Chlamydia trachomatis.* Untreated NGU in males may result in urethral narrowing, and inflammation of the prostate and epididymis. Women may develop wasting of the cervix and pus-filled cervical mucus. An infant passing through the cervix and vagina of an infected mother may develop eye, nose, and throat infections in the first few days after birth and pneumonia at 3 to 4 months of age. Most cases of NGU are successfully treated with antibiotics. Sexual partners should also be treated. Nearly 50% of all cases of an inflamed urethra are nongonococcal. **Nonspecific urethritis (NSU)** is not known to be caused by a specific disease organism, but is often linked to sexual intercourse. A long-term phase is a common urinary tract problem in women. Symptoms include urethral discharge in men and reddening of the urethral mucosa in women. Treatment with antibiotics is not always successful.

urethrocele /yo͞ore͞'thrəsēl'/, (in women) a herniation of the urethra. There is a bulging of a segment of the urethra and the connective tissue surrounding it into the wall of the vagina. The herniation may be slight and high in the vagina, or it may be large and low in the anterior wall with visible bulging at the vaginal entrance. The condition may be congenital or acquired, associated with obesity and poor muscle tone. Surgery is often done.

urethrography /yo͞or'ēthrog'rafē/, the x-ray examination of the urethra after the injection of a radiopaque dye into the urethra, usually through a catheter. It may be done as a part of an x-ray examination of the lower urinary tract.

Urex, a trademark for an antibacterial (methenamine hippurate).

uric acid /yo͞or'ik/, a product of the body's use (metabolism) of protein present in the blood and excreted in the urine. See also **gout, urine.**

uricaciduria /yo͞or'ikas'ido͞or'ē·ə/, a more than normal amount of uric acid in the urine, often linked to kidney stones or gout.

urinalysis /yo͞or'inal'isis/, a physical, microscopic, or chemical examination of urine. The specimen is examined for color, density, acidity, and other conditions. Then it is spun in a device (centrifuge) to allow collection of a sediment. This is examined using a microscope for blood cells, pus, bacteria, and other substances. Chemical analysis may be done to identify any of a large number of substances.

urinary /yo͞or'iner'ē/, pertaining to urine.

urinary bladder, the muscular membranous sac in the pelvis that stores urine for discharge through the urethra. Urine reaches this sac from the kidneys by way of the ureters.

urinary calculus, a mineral deposit (stone) formed in the urinary tract, including the bladder. It may be large enough to block the flow of urine or small enough to be passed with the urine. See also **calculus, kidney stone.**

urinary frequency, a greater than normal number of times of the urge to void without an increase in the total daily volume of urine. It is a sign of inflammation in the bladder or urethra or of diminished bladder capacity or other structural abnormalities. See also **cystitis, cystocele.**

urinary hesitancy, a decrease in the force of the stream of urine, often with difficulty in starting the flow. Hesitancy is usually the result of a blockage or a too narrow place between the bladder and the urethral opening; in men it may indicate a swelling of the prostate gland, in women, a tightening of the urethral opening.

urinary incontinence, involuntary passage of urine, with the failure of voluntary control over bladder and urethral openings (sphincters). Some causes are bladder dysfunction stemming from lesions of the brain and spinal cord, a tumor or stone in the bladder, aging, repeated childbirth in women, or injury. Treatment with drugs, surgery, or psychotherapy is often effective.

urinary output, the total volume of urine excreted daily. Various metabolic and renal diseases may change the normal urinary output. See also **anuria, oliguria, polyuria.**

urinary retention, a high buildup of urine in the bladder. Causes include a loss of muscle tone in the bladder, nerve damage to the bladder, a blocked tube (urethra), or the use of a narcotic painkiller, as morphine.

urinary system assessment, an examination in which the kidneys, bladder, ureters, and urethra are evaluated. A check is made of disorders in the urinary system. The patient is asked about frequency or burning on urination, dribbling, a decreased urinary stream, increased urination, stress incontinence, headache, and back pain, or if increased thirst has occurred. The color, odor, and amount of urine voided are checked. Diagnostic tests may include cystoscopy, excretory and intravenous urography, renal angiography, and x-ray films of the kidneys, ureters, and bladder.

urinary tract, all organs and ducts involved in the release and elimination of urine.

urinary tract infection (UTI), an infection of the urinary tract. Most of these infections are caused by bacteria. Symptoms include urinary frequency, burning, pain with voiding, and, if the infection is severe, visible blood and pus in the urine. The state is more common in women than in men and may lack symptoms. Treatment includes antibacterial, analgesic, and urinary antiseptic drugs. Kinds of urinary tract infections include **cystitis, pyelonephritis, urethritis.**

urination, the act of passing urine. Also called **micturition.**

urine, the fluid secreted by the kidneys, transported by the ureters, stored in the bladder, and voided through the urethra. Normal urine is clear, straw-colored, slightly acid, and odorless. It contains water, urea, sodium and potassium chloride, phosphates, uric acid, organic salts, and pigment. Abnormal substances in urine indicating disease include ketone bodies, protein, bacteria, blood, glucose, pus, and certain crystals. See also **bacteriuria, glycosuria, hematuria, ketoaciduria, proteinuria.**

Urised, a trademark for a urinary fixed-combination drug with an antibacterial (methenamine), an analgesic (phenyl salicylate), anticholinergics (atropine sulfate and hyoscyamine), an antifungal (benzoic acid), and an antiseptic (methylene blue).

Urispas, a trademark for a smooth muscle relaxant (flavoxate hydrochloride).

Urobiotic, a trademark for a urinary drug with antibacterials (oxytetracycline hydrochloride and sulfamethizole) and an analgesic (phenazopyridine hydrochloride).

urogenital system /yŏŏr′ōjen′ətal/, the urinary and genital organs including the kidneys, the ureters, the bladder, the urethra, and the genital structures of the male and female. In women these are the ovaries, the uterine tubes, the uterus, the clitoris, and the vagina. In men these are the testes, the seminal vesicles, the seminal ducts, the prostate, and the penis.

urography /yŏŏrog′rəfē/, x-ray techniques used to check the urinary system. A dye is injected, and x-ray films are taken as the substance is passed through or excreted from the system. In one method, called **intravenous pyelography,** the dye is put in a vein, and x-ray films are taken as the medium is cleared from the blood. Tumors, cysts, stones, and many abnormalities may be seen using this technique. A cathartic or an enema is usually given the day before the procedure. The patient may be asked to void right before injection of the dye. Another method, called **retrograde pyelography,** is useful in finding a blockage in the urinary tract. The dye is injected through a urinary tube (catheter) into the tubes of the kidneys.

urology /-ol′-/, the branch of medicine concerned with the anatomy and physiology, disorders, and care of the urinary tract in men and women and of the male genital tract. A licensed physician who specializes in urology is called a **urologist.**

uropathy /yŏŏrop′əthē/, any disease or abnormal state of the urinary tract. –**uropathic,** adj.

ursodeoxycholic acid, a secondary bile salt. It is used to dissolve gallstones. See also **chenodeoxycholic acid.**

urticaria /ur′tiker′ē·ə/, a skin eruption with temporary wheals of varying shapes and sizes with clear margins and pale centers, caused by capillary dilation. Treatment includes antihistamines and removal of the cause, which may include drugs, food, insect bites, inhalants, emotional stress, exposure to heat or cold, and exercise. **Cholinergic urticaria** is usually linked with sweating in persons exposed to stress, strong exertion, or hot weather. The condition features small, pale, itchy pimples surrounded by reddish areas. Also called **hives.** –**urticarial,** adj.

urushiol /əroo′shē·ôl/, a toxic resin in the sap of certain plants of the genus *Rhus,* as poison ivy, poison oak, and poison sumac, that produces allergic contact dermatitis in many people.

USAN, abbreviation for *United States Adopted Names,* a list of approved drugs.

use effectiveness, (of a contraceptive method) the actual effectiveness of a drug, device, or method to prevent pregnancy. Inconsistent use and human error often reduce the possible effectiveness of a method of contraception.

T–Z

uterine anteflexion /yoo̅′tərin, -īn/, an abnormal position of the uterus in which the uterine body is folded over forward on itself.

uterine anteversion, a position of the uterus in which the body of the uterus is slanted forward. Mild degrees of anteversion are of no significance. On examination of the vagina, a physician may diagnose acute anteversion of the uterus from the location of the cervix in the back of the vaginal vault. Slight anteversion is the most common position of the uterus; on examination the cervix is in the middle of the top of the vaginal vault, and it bulges directly downward toward the vaginal opening.

uterine cancer, any cancer of the uterus. It may be cervical cancer affecting the cervix or endometrial cancer affecting the lining of the body of the uterus. See also **cervical cancer, endometrial cancer.**

uterine retroflexion, a position of the uterus in which the body of the uterus is bent backward on itself. It does not prevent conception or adversely affect pregnancy. On examination of the vagina, the condition may be diagnosed by the location of the cervix in the front of the vaginal vault.

uterine retroversion, a position of the uterus in which the body of the uterus is directed away from the midline, toward the back. Mild degrees of retroversion are common and have no significance. Severe retroversion may be found with vague persistent pelvic discomfort and painful sexual intercourse and may prevent the fitting of a contraceptive diaphragm.

uteroovarian varicocele /yoo̅′təroo̅over′ē·ən/, a swelling of the veins of the female pelvis. Compare **ovarian varicocele, varicocele.**

uterus /yoo̅′tərəs/, the hollow, pear-shaped inner female organ of reproduction in which the fertilized ovum is implanted and the fetus develops, and from which the menses flows. It is composed of three layers: the endometrium, the myometrium, and the parametrium. The endometrium lines the uterus and becomes thicker in pregnancy and during the second half of the menstrual cycle under the influence of the hormone progesterone. The myometrium is the middle muscular layer of the organ. After childbirth the fibers contract, creating natural ligatures that stop the flow of blood from the large blood vessels supplying the placenta. The parametrium is the outermost layer of the uterus. During pregnancy it becomes many times its usual size. The uterus has two parts: a body and a cervix. The cervix has a vaginal portion bulging into the vagina. **Infantile uterus** refers to one that has failed to attain adult form.

Uticillin VK, a trademark for an antibacterial (penicillin V potassium).

uvea /yoo̅′vē·ə/, a layer of the eyeball that includes the iris, the ciliary body, and the choroid of the eye. Also called **uveal tract.** –**uveal,** *adj.*

uveitis /yoo̅′vē·ī′-/, inflammation of the uvea of the eye. Symptoms include an irregularly shaped pupil, redness around the cornea, pus, opaque deposits on the cornea, pain, and tearing. Causes include allergy, infection, injury, diabetes, and skin diseases. A major complication may be glaucoma.

uvula /yoo̅′vyələ/, *pl.* **uvulae,** the small, cone-shaped tissue suspended in the mouth from the middle of the back edge of the soft palate. –**uvular,** *adj.*

uvulitis /yoo̅′vyəlī′-/, inflammation of the uvula. Common causes are allergy and infection.

V

vaccination, any injection of weakened bacteria given to protect against or to reduce the effects of related infectious diseases. The first vaccinations in history were given to protect against smallpox. Vaccinations are now available to protect against many diseases, as typhoid, measles, and mumps. **–vaccinate,** *v.*

vaccine /vak′sēn, vaksēn′/, weakened or dead germs given by mouth, by injection into the muscle or under the skin, or into a muscle to protect against infectious disease. Vaccines may be used one at a time or in combinations. Compare **antiserum.**

vaccinia /vaksin′ē·ə/. See **cowpox.**

vacuole /vak′yoo·ōl/, **1.** a clear or fluid-filled space within a cell, as when a drop of water is taken into the cell. **2.** a small space in the body enclosed by a membrane, usually containing fat or other matter.

vacuum aspiration. See **suction curettage.**

vagal /vā′gəl/, of or concerning the vagus nerve.

vagina, the part of the female genitals that forms a canal from the opening through the passageway to the cervix. It is behind the bladder and in front of the rectum. In the adult woman the front wall of the vagina is about 7 cm long and the back wall is about 9 cm long. The vagina is a canal in which the walls usually touch. The vagina is lined with mucous membrances covering a layer of tissue and muscle.

vaginal bleeding /vaj′inəl/, a problem in which blood flows from the vagina at other times than during menstruation. It may be caused by problems of the uterus or cervix; by an abnormal pregnancy, by glandular problems, by abnormalities of one or both ovaries or one or both fallopian tubes, or by an abnormality of the vagina. The following terms are commonly used in approximating the amount of vaginal bleeding: **heavy,** which is greater than heaviest normal menstrual flow; **moderate,** which is equal to heaviest normal menstrual flow; **light,** which is less than heaviest normal menstrual flow; **staining,** which is a very light flow of blood barely requiring the use of a sanitary napkin or tampon; and **spotting,** which is the passage of a few drops of blood. **Bloody show** refers to an episode of light vaginal bleeding as often occurs in early labor, during labor, and, particularly, at the time of complete widening of the cervix at the end of the first stage of labor. **Breakthrough bleeding** is the escape of blood from the uterus between menstrual periods. This is a side effect some women have who use birth control pills. **Withdrawal bleeding** is blood flow from the uterus caused by the shedding of the lining of the uterus (endometrium) that has been stimulated and maintained by hormonal drugs. It occurs when the drug is no longer given.

vaginal cancer, a cancer of the vagina occurring rarely as a first new growth. More often it accompanies other cancers (vulvar, cervical, endometrial, or ovarian). Most primary vaginal cancers arise in white women over 50 years of age. Symptoms are vaginal bleeding, the discharge of pus, pain, and painful or difficult urination. Depending on the patient's age and condition and place and size of the tumor, treatment may be by radiation or by removal of the vagina or the uterus.

vaginal discharge, any discharge from the vagina. A clear or pearly-white discharge (**leukorrhea**) is normal. A heavy, irritating, foul-smelling, green or yellow discharge may indicate vaginal or uterine infection or other disease. During the course of the menstrual cycle, the amount and nature of the discharge varies in each woman at different times. The amount also varies greatly from woman to woman. A greater than usual amount is normal in pregnancy, and a decrease is to be expected after childbirth and after menopause. The discharge is largely made of fluids from the endocervical glands.

vaginal instillation of medication, the application of a medicated cream, a suppository, or a gel into the vagina, usually done to treat a local infection of the vagina or cervix. The woman voids before the treatment. She then lies back. The nurse, physician, or patient sometimes, wearing gloves, separates the labia majora, exposing the vaginal opening. The medication is put in gently. A cream or gel is squeezed into an applicator from a tube and is then placed in the vagina by depressing the plunger of the applicator while withdrawing the device from the vagina. A tablet or suppository is usually placed in the vagina near the cervix with another style of applicator. The woman remains lying down after the instillation to prevent escape of the medica-

T–Z

tion from the vagina. Most applicators may be washed and reused for the same woman for the next dose. They are thrown away after a course of treatment.

vaginal jelly, a jellylike product that prevents conception by killing sperm on contact. It is usually used along with a contraceptive diaphragm or cervical cap. Some drugs are also supplied in the form of a vaginal jelly.

vaginal sponge, a plastic sponge that contains a sperm-killing chemical. The sponge is shaped like a mushroom and fits into the upper vagina. It is believed to work in three ways: by killing sperm, by absorbing semen, and by blocking the cervical opening. The sponge can be kept in place to provide protection for 24 hours. The vaginal sponge is believed to be about as effective as other vaginal methods.

vaginismus /vaj′iniz′məs/, a mental and physical reaction of women, marked by a strong tightening of the muscles in the pelvic area and the vagina. It is caused by fear of a painful entry before intercourse or a pelvic examination. Vaginismus may be a normal response if painful genital conditions exist or if forcible or premature intercourse is expected. See also **dyspareunia.**

vaginitis /vaj′inī′-/, an inflammation of the vaginal tissues, as in trichomoniasis.

vaginography /vaj′inog′rəfē/, the examination of the vagina by means of x-ray tests after the injection of a dye that shows up well on x-ray films.

Vagisec, a trademark for a vaginal douche used to treat trichomoniasis.

Vagitrol, a trademark for a vaginal drug with an antibacterial (sulfanilamide) and a topical antiinfective (aminacrine hydrochloride).

vagotomy /vāgot′-/, the cutting of certain branches of the vagus nerve, done with stomach surgery, to reduce the amount of gastric acid released and to lessen the chance of a return of an ulcer. See also **gastrectomy, ulcer, vagus nerve.**

vagotonus /vā′gətō′nəs/, an abnormal increase in the activity of the vagus nerve, especially abnormal slowness of the heart beat, causing faintness and a sudden loss of strength. It occurs in some women after surgery or simple manipulation of the cervix.

vagovagal reflex /-vā′gəl/, a stimulation of the vagus nerve by reflex in which irritation of the throat (larynx or the trachea) results in slowing of the pulse rate.

vagus nerve /vā′gəs/, either of the longest pair of cranial nerves essential for speech, swallowing, and the feelings and functions of many parts of the body. Also called **tenth cranial nerve.**

valgus /val′gəs/, an abnormal position in which a part of a limb is bent or twisted outward, away from the middle of the body. Compare **varus.**

valine (Val) /val′in/, an essential amino acid needed for best growth in infants and for nitrogen balance in adults. See also **amino acid.**

Valisone, a trademark for a drug that raises the blood sugar (betamethasone valerate).

Valium, a trademark for a tranquilizer (diazepam), used to assist in achieving anesthesia.

vallecula /vəlek′yələ/, any groove or furrow on the surface of an organ or structure.

Valmid, a trademark for a sedative (ethinamate).

Valpin, a trademark for an anticholinergic (anisotropine).

valproic acid /valprō′ik/, a drug used to stop or prevent convulsions, such as petit mal seizures. It is not recommended for use during pregnancy or lactation. Known allergy to this drug prohibits its use. Side effects include harm to the blood and liver, stomach and intestinal upset, hair loss, rash, headache, and insomnia.

Valsalva's maneuver, any forced effort of the breath against a closed throat as when a person holds the breath and tightens the muscles while making a strong effort to move a heavy object or to change position in bed. Most healthy people perform Valsalva's maneuvers during normal daily activities without any ill effects; but such efforts are dangerous for many patients with diseases of the heart and blood vessels. Persons who may be harmed by performing Valsalva's maneuver are commonly instructed to exhale instead of holding their breath when they move. The exhalation decreases the risk of heart attack.

Valsalva's test, a method for proving that the eustachian tubes are wide open. With mouth and nose kept tightly closed, the person breathes out very forcefully; if the eustachian tubes are open, air will enter into the middle ear cavities and the patient will hear a popping sound. See also **Valsalva's maneuver.**

valve, a structure, either natural or artificial, in a passage that opens to allow fluid to flow in one direction, but closes to prevent it from flowing back in the other direction. Valves in veins are folds of membrane that prevent the backflow of blood. See also **heart valve.** –**valvular,** *adj.*

-valve, a combining form meaning "a thing that controls the flow of."

valvotomy /valvot′-/, the cutting into a valve, especially one in the heart, to correct a defect and allow the valve to open and close properly. Before surgery a tube (catheter) is inserted into the heart through a vein in the arm. The damaged valve is repaired, if possible, or removed, and an artificial valve put in its place.

valvular heart disease /val′vyələr/, a flaw in a heart valve, either present from birth or acquired later. There may be a narrowing of the vessels and blocked blood flow or damage to the valve and a backward blood flow (reflux). This may be caused by defects present at birth, or a disease, such as bacterial endocarditis or, most often, rheumatic fever. Rheumatic fever often affects heart valves, causing them to remain open or to become stiff. Poor action of the valves can result in changes in blood pressure and circulation. Other signs may be weakness, loss of appetite, blood clots and fluid in the lungs. A valve defect may lead to unsteady heart beat, heart failure, and heart attack. See also **stenosis.**

valvulitis /val′vyəlī′-/,   an inflammation of a valve, especially a heart valve. Rheumatic fever is often the cause. Infected valves wear out, or they become stiff and hard, resulting in stenosis and blocked blood flow.

vanadium (V),   a grayish metallic element. Absorption of vanadium results in a condition called **vanadiumism.** Symptoms include anemia, conjunctivitis, pneumonitis, and irritation of the throat and lungs.

Vanceril,   a trademark for a drug to raise blood sugar (beclomethasone dipropionate), used for mouth breathing therapy in asthma.

Vancocin Hydrochloride,   a trademark for a drug that kills bacteria (vancomycin hydrochloride).

vancomycin hydrochloride,   an antibiotic used to treat infections, particularly staphylococcal infections resistant to other antibiotics. Use at the same time as some drugs (neurotoxic, nephrotoxic, or ototoxic) or known allergy to this drug prohibits its use. Side effects include allergic reactions, dizziness, and a ringing or roaring in the ears (tinnitus).

van den Bergh's test,   a test for the presence of a yellow bile pigment (bilirubin) in the blood serum. Blood is obtained from a patient who has fasted overnight.

Vanobid,   a trademark for a drug that kills fungus (candicidin).

Vanoxide,   a trademark for a drug with an antibacterial (benzoyl peroxide) and a drying agent (chlorhydroxyquinoline).

Vaponefrin,   a trademark for an adrenaline-like substance (epinephrine hydrochloride), used to aid in clearing the lungs.

vapor bath,   the exposure of the body to vapor, as steam.

vapor density,   the weight of a pure vapor or gas compared with the weight of an equal volume of dry air at the same temperature and pressure. If the vapor density is less than one, the material is lighter than air and may rise. If the vapor density is greater than one, the material is heavier than air and will stay low to the ground.

vapor pressure,   the pressure exerted by the vapor within the container against the sides of a container. This pressure is temperature dependent; as the temperature increases, so

does the vapor pressure. The lower the boiling point of a liquid, the greater vapor pressure is at a given temperature.

varicella /ver′isel′ə/.   See **chickenpox.**

varicella-zoster virus (VZV),   a member of the herpesvirus family, which causes chickenpox (varicella) and shingles (herpes zoster). The virus is very contagious and may be spread by direct contact or droplets. See also **chickenpox, herpes zoster.**

varicelliform /ver′isel′ifôrm/,   resembling the rash of chickenpox.

varicocele /ver′ikōsēl′/,   a disorder of the spermatic cord. It causes a soft, painful swelling. It is most common in men between 15 and 25 years of age. It is usually more noticeable and painful in the standing position. Compare **ovarian varicocele, uteroovarian varicocele.**

varicose /ver′ikōs/,   abnormally and permanently distended, such as the bulging veins in some individuals.

varicose vein,   a twisted, widened vein with faulty valves. Symptoms include pain and muscle cramps with a feeling of fullness and heaviness in the legs. Causes include inborn defects of the valves or walls of the veins or congestion and increased pressure in the vessels resulting from long standing, poor posture, pregnancy, and obesity. Varicose veins are common, especially in women. The condition, called **varicosis,** usually occurs between 30 and 60 years of age. The veins of the legs are most often affected. Raising the legs and use of elastic stockings are often enough therapy for simple cases. Surgery may be required in severe cases. See also **vein ligation and stripping.**

variola /vərī′ōlə/.   See **smallpox.**

varioloid /ver′ē-əloid′/,   **1.** resembling smallpox. **2.** a mild form of smallpox in a vaccinated person or one who has previously had the disease.

varix /ver′iks/, *pl.* **varices** /ver′isēz/,   a twisted, widened vein, artery, or lymph vessel.

varus /ver′əs/,   an abnormal position in which a part of a limb is turned inward toward the midline. Compare **valgus.**

vas /vas/, *pl.* **vasa** /vā′sə/,   any one of the many vessels of the body, especially those that carry blood, lymph, or sperm.

vascular /vas′kyələr/,   relating to a blood vessel.

vascular insufficiency,   poor blood circulation. Symptoms include pale, bluish, or spotted skin over the affected area. Numbness, tingling, loss of a sense of temperature, muscle pains, and reduced or absent pulses are also seen. In advanced disease, weakness of muscles of the arms or legs occurs. It is caused by cholesterol deposits (atherosclerosis) or clots (emboli), and by damaged, diseased, or weak vessels. Other causes are an abnormal connection between an artery and a vein (fistula), bulging artery walls

T–Z

(aneurysms), clotting problems, or heavy use of tobacco. **Arterial insufficiency** is lack of enough blood flow in arteries. The disorder may be diagnosed by checking pulses, by x-ray tests of blood vessels (angiography), by ultrasound, by blood studies, and by skin temperature tests. Treatment may include a diet low in saturated fats, moderate exercise, sleeping on a firm mattress, avoidance of smoking, and proper standing or sitting posture. The use of drugs to widen the blood vessels and surgery are also done.

vascularization, the process by which body tissue develops small blood vessels, especially capillaries. It may be natural or may be caused by surgical methods. **–vascularize,** *v.*

vasculitis /vas'kyəlī'-/, an inflammation of blood vessels that occurs in certain systemic diseases. It may also be **allergic vasculitis,** which is caused by an allergen. This sometimes occurs in patients treated with drugs, such as iodides, penicillin, and sulfonamides. Symptoms include itching, a slight fever, and rashes, or small ulcers on the skin. With **necrotizing vasculitis,** tissue death occurs and overgrowth of the inner layer of the vessel wall. This may result in blocking the blood flow. Necrotizing vasculitis may occur in rheumatoid arthritis and systemic lupus erythematosus. It is usually treated with adrenal hormone drugs. **Segmented hyalinizing vasculitis** is a long-term, recurring disease with inflammation of the blood vessels of the lower legs linked with bumpy or purple-colored sores on the skin that may leave scars. **Umbilical vasculitis** refers to an inflammation of the umbilical cord and its blood vessels.

vas deferens /def'ərənz/, a tube passing from the testicles through the scrotum and joining the seminal vesicle. Also called **deferent duct, spermatic duct, testicular duct.** See also **testis.**

vasectomy /vasek'-/, an operation that makes a man sterile by cutting out a section of the vas deferens. Vasectomy is most commonly done in the doctor's office using local anesthesia. It is also done routinely before removal of the prostate gland to prevent inflammation of the testicles. Potency is not affected. A signed and witnessed form indicating informed consent is usually required.

vaso-, a combining form meaning "relating to a vessel or duct."

vasoactive /vā'zō·ak'tiv, vas'-/, (of a drug) tending to cause the widening or narrowing of a vessel.

vasoconstriction, a narrowing of any blood vessel, especially the arterioles and the veins in the skin, stomach, and intestines. It is done by many means that together control blood pressure and the distribution of blood throughout the body. Compare **vasodilatation.**

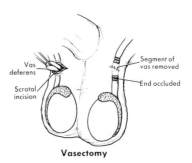
Vasectomy

vasoconstrictor, relating to a process, condition, or substance that causes the narrowing of blood vessels. The hormones epinephrine and norepinephrine produced by the body cause blood vessels to contract. Also called **vasopressor.**

Vasodilan, a trademark for a drug that widens vessels (isoxsuprine hydrochloride).

vasodilatation /-dil'ətā'shən/, widening or enlarging of blood vessels, particularly arterioles, usually caused by nerve impulses or certain drugs that relax smooth muscle in the walls of the blood vessels. Also called **vasodilation** /-dīlā'shən/. Compare **vasoconstriction.**

vasodilator /-dī'lātər/, a nerve or agent that causes widening or relaxation of blood vessel walls. Vasodilators have been used to treat severe heart failure in heart attack, in cases linked to severe mitral valve weakness, and in failure resulting from heart disease.

vasomotor, relating to the nerves and muscles that control the width of the blood vessels. Muscles of arteries can contract, causing constriction, or they can relax, causing dilation.

vasomotor system, the part of the nervous system that controls the narrowing and widening of the blood vessels. See also **vasoconstriction, vasodilatation.**

vasopressin. See **antidiuretic hormone.**

vasospastic /-spas'-/, **1.** relating to irregular narrowing of a blood vessel. **2.** any agent that produces spasms of the blood vessels.

Vasosulf, a trademark for an eye drug with an antibacterial (sulfacetamide sodium) and an adrenergic drug (phenylephrine hydrochloride).

vasovasostomy /-vasos'-/, an operation in which the function of the vas deferens on each side of the testes is restored, having been cut and tied in a preceding vasectomy.

Vasoxyl, a trademark for an alpha-adrenergic drug (methoxamine hydrochloride).

vastus intermedius, one of the four muscles of the quadriceps femoris, situated in the center of the thigh. It functions with the other three muscles of the quadriceps to extend the leg.

vastus lateralis, the largest of the four muscles of the quadriceps femoris, situated on the outside of the thigh. It functions to help extend the leg.

vastus medialis, one of the four muscles of the quadriceps femoris, situated in the inside of the thigh. It functions together with other parts of the quadriceps femoris to extend the leg.

V-Cillin K, a trademark for a drug that kills bacteria (penicillin V potassium).

VD, abbreviation for **venereal disease.**

VDRL test, abbreviation for *Venereal Disease Research Laboratory test,* a test for syphilis. It is also positive in other diseases, as yaws.

vector, a carrier that transmits disease. A **biological vector** is usually a parasite. A **mechanical vector** carries the infecting organism from one host to another. Kinds of vectors include mosquitoes, which transmit malaria, and ticks, which carry Rocky Mountain spotted fever.

Veetids, a trademark for a drug that kills bacteria (penicillin V potassium).

vegetation, an abnormal growth of tissue around a valve, made of protein, platelets, and bacteria.

vehicle warning placard, a sign, displayed on the outside of a carrier of hazardous material, indicating the nature of the cargo. The design and use of placards are specified by DOT regulations.

vein, one of the many vessels that convey blood without oxygen back to the heart from all parts of the body. Veins have thinner walls and are less elastic than arteries and collapse when cut. Examples are the veins that drain the blood from the spinal column, the nearby muscles, and the membrane (meninges) covering the spinal cord. Compare **artery.**

vein ligation and stripping, an operation that ties off the longest (saphenous) vein in the leg and removes it from groin to ankle. It is done to treat phlebitis or varicose veins or for getting a blood vessel to graft in another site, as in a coronary bypass operation. See also **ligation, stripping.**

Velban, a trademark for a drug that prevents new growths, as tumors (vinblastine sulfate).

velopharyngeal closure /vē′lōfərin′jē·əl/, the blocking of any escape of air by the raising of the soft palate and the closing of the throat.

Velosef, a trademark for an antibiotic (cephradine).

Velpeau's bandage /velpōz′/, a roller bandage that stabilizes the elbow and shoulder by holding the arm against the side and the flexed forearm on the chest. The palm of the hand rests on the collarbone (clavicle) of the opposite side.

vena cava /vē′nə kā′və/, *pl.* **venae cavae,** one of two large veins returning blood from outer parts of the body to the right chamber of the heart. The **inferior vena cava** is the large vein that returns blood to the heart from parts of the body below the diaphragm. The **superior vena cava,** the second largest vein of the body, returns blood from the upper half of the body to the the the heart.

venereal /vənir′ē·əl/, relating to or caused by sexual intercourse or genital contact.

venereal disease. See **sexually transmitted disease.**

venereal sore. See **chancre.**

venereal wart, a soft, wartlike growth common on the genitals. It is caused by a virus and is carried by sexual contact. Also called **condyloma acuminatum.**

venereology /vənir′ē·ol′-/, the study of venereal diseases. –**venereologist,** *n*.

venipuncture /ven′ipungk′chər/, a method in which a vein is punctured by a sharp instrument carrying a flexible plastic catheter or by a steel needle attached to a syringe or catheter. The purpose is to take out a specimen of blood, to put in a medication, to start a feeding, or to inject a substance to aid in the x-ray examination of a part or system of the body. See also **intravenous infusion, phlebotomy.**

venom /ven′əm/, a poisonous fluid secreted by some snakes, insects, spiders, and other animals and transmitted by their stings or bites.

venom extract therapy, the giving of antivenin as protection against the poisonous effects of the bite of a specific poisonous snake or spider, or other poisonous animal.

venous /vē′nəs/, relating to a vein.

venous insufficiency, an abnormal circulatory condition with decreased return of vein blood from the legs to the trunk of the body. Fluid buildup (edema) is usually the first sign of the condition; pain, varicose veins, and ulceration may follow.

venous pressure, the pressure of circulating blood on the walls of veins. Symptoms of increased pressure are continued distention of veins on the back of the hand when it is raised above the top of the rib cage and enlarging of the neck veins when the individual is sitting with the head raised 30 to 45 degrees.

venous sinus, one of many sinuses that collect blood from the brain and drain it into the inner jugular vein.

ventilate, 1. to provide the lungs with air from the atmosphere and to get air or oxygen into the blood for the lungs. 2. (in psychiatry) to open discussion of something, as to ventilate feelings.

ventilation, the process by which gases are moved into and out of the lungs. Compare **respiration.** –**ventilatory,** *adj.*

ventilator, any of several devices used in respiratory therapy to provide assisted breathing and intensive positive pressure breathing.

Ventolin a trademark for a bronchodilator (albuterol).

ventral /ven′trəl/,   relating to a position toward the belly of the body; frontward; anterior. Compare **dorsal.**

ventricle /ven′trikəl/,   a small cavity, as one of the cavities filled with cerebrospinal fluid in the brain, or the right and the left ventricles of the heart. In the heart, the **left ventricle** is a thick-walled lower chamber that pumps blood through the aorta, the arteries, and capillaries to the body's tissues. It has walls about three times thicker than those of the right ventricle. The **right ventricle** pumps blood received from the right upper chamber (atrium) into the lung (pulmonary) arteries to the lungs for oxygen. The right ventricle is shorter and rounder than the long, conic left ventricle.

ventricular /ventrik′yələr/,   relating to a ventricle.

ventricular fibrillation.   See **fibrillation.**

ventricular septal defect (VSD).   See **septal defect.**

ventriculocisternostomy   /ventrik′yəlōsis′tərnos′-/,   an operation done to treat water on the brain (hydrocephalus). An opening is created that allows fluid to drain through a shunt from the ventricles of the brain. See also **shunt.**

ventriculography /-log′rəfē/,   **1.** an x-ray examination of the head after air or some other substance has been injected into the brain ventricles. **2.** an x-ray examination of a ventricle of the heart after injection of a substance that allows x-ray films to be made.

ventriculoperitoneostomy   /-per′itō′nē·os′-/,   an operation for temporarily diverting fluid in water on the brain (hydrocephalus), usually in the newborn.

venule /ven′yōōl/,   any one of the small blood vessels that gather blood from the capillary plexuses and join together to form the veins.   −**venular,** *adj.*

verapamil,   a drug given to treat spastic and exercise-related heart diseases. Severe heart problems, low blood pressure, shock, sick sinus syndrome, or heart block prohibits its use. Side effects include low blood pressure, fluid buildup, heart block, heart failure, fluid in the lungs, and dizziness.

Vercyte,   a trademark for a drug used to prevent new growths, as tumors (pipobroman).

vermicide /vur′misīd/,   an agent that kills worms, particularly those in the intestine. Compare **anthelmintic, vermifuge.**

vermiform appendix /vur′mifôrm/.   See **appendix.**

vermifuge /vur′mifyōōj′/,   an agent that causes parasitic worms to be flushed from the body.

vermis /vur′mis/, *pl.* **vermes,   1.** a worm. **2.** a structure resembling a worm.   −**vermiform,** *adj.*

Vermox,   a trademark for a drug used to kill parasitic worms in the intestine (mebendazole).

vernix caseosa /vur′niks kas′ē·ō′sə/,   a grayish-white, cheeselike substance consisting of fatty gland secretions, a kind of woolly down (lanugo), and scaly cells. It covers the skin of the fetus and newborn. It acts as a protection for the fetus while it is in the uterus and is thought to help keep it warm.

verruca /vərōō′kə/.   See **wart.**

verrucous carcinoma /ver′ōōkəs/,   a very distinct scaly growth of soft tissue of the mouth, voicebox (larynx), or genitals. A slow-growing tumor, it does not usually spread.

version,   the changing of the position of the fetus in the uterus, usually done to ease delivery. Version may occur by itself as a result of contractions of the uterus or be caused by action taken by the physician. **External version** is done by manipulating the fetus through the wall of the abdomen. **Podalic version** refers to the shifting of the position of a fetus to bring the feet to the outlet during labor. See also **breech birth.**

vertebra /vur′təbrə/, *pl.* **vertebrae,**   any one of the 33 bones of the spinal column. There are 7 in the neck, 12 in the back, 5 in the lower back, 5 in the pelvic area, and 4 in the tailbone. The **cervical vertebrae** are the first seven segments of the spine at the top. They are smaller than the thoracic and the lumbar vertebrae. The first cervical vertebra (**atlas**) supports the head. The second backbone located in the neck is the **axis.** The atlas rotates on the axis, allowing the head to turn, extend, and flex. The seventh cervical vertebra is above the collarbones. It has a very long, bony extension that is nearly horizontal. It can be felt with the fingers. The 12 bony segments of the spinal column of the upper back are the **thoracic vertebrae.** They are named T1 to T12. T1 is just below the seventh cervical backbone (C7). T12 is just above the first lumbar backbone (L1). The vertebrae become thicker and heavier in descending order from T1 to T12. The chest portion of the spine is flexible and has a rounded and somewhat hollowed out curvature. The vertebrae are separated from each other by intervertebral disks. The five largest segments of the movable part of the spinal column are the **lumbar vertebrae.** They are larger and heavier than verterbrae higher in the spinal column because they must support more weight. The body of each lumbar vertebra is flattened or slightly concave. The bony spine at the back of each is thick, broad, and shorter than vertebrae at the level of the chest. The body of the fifth lumbar vertebra is defective in some individuals, tending to weaken the spinal column. **Sacral vertebrae** are five parts of the vertebral column that join together in the adult to form the **sacrum,** the large, triangle-shaped bone at the top part of the pelvis. It looks like a wedge set between the two hip bones. The sacrum is shorter and wider in women than in men. **Coccygeal vertebrae** are four parts of the spinal column that join to form the adult **coccyx,** the tailbone at the very end of the spine. The coccyx fuses with the sacrum by adulthood.

vertebral artery,   each of two arteries that carry blood to the deep neck muscles, the spine, and parts of the brain.

vertebral body,   the solid central portion of a vertebra that supports the weight of the body.

vertex /vur′teks/,   **1.** the top of the head; crown. **2.** the highest point of any structure.

vertex presentation,   (in the delivery of a baby) a birth in which the fetus is lying in the womb with its head downward. The head will be born first. See also **breech birth.**

vertical transmission,   the transfer of a disease, condition, or trait from a mother to her child, either in the genes or at the time of birth, as the spread of an infection through breast milk or through the placenta.

vertigo /vur′tigō, vərtī′gō/,   a feeling of faintness, dizziness, or an inability to keep normal balance in a standing or seated position. Symptoms may include mental confusion, nausea, and weakness. A person who feels dizziness should be carefully lowered to a safe position on a bed, chair, or floor to avoid injury from falling. **Postural vertigo** is a severe, long-lasting dizziness brought on by moving the head to certain positions. There are many causes, among them ear infection, ear surgery, or injury to the inner ear. In addition to extreme dizziness, symptoms are nausea, vomiting, and muscle imbalance.

very-low-density lipoprotein (VLDL). See **lipoprotein.**

vesicle /ves′ikəl/,   a small sac or blister, as a small, thin-walled, raised bump on the skin containing clear fluid, or a seminal vesicle.   **–vesicular,** *adj.*

vesicle reflex,   the sensation of a need to urinate when the bladder is partly full. See also **micturition reflex.**

vesicoureteral reflux /ves′ikōyŏŏrē′tərəl/,   an abnormal backflow of urine from the bladder to the ureter, resulting from a defect present at birth blocking the outlet of the bladder, or infection of the lower urinary tract. The condition causes pain in the stomach, intestines, or sides, and pus or blood in the urine. Surgery may be necessary to fix the damage.

vesiculitis /vəsik′yəlī′-/,   inflammation of any vesicle, particularly the seminal vesicles. It is usually linked with prostatitis.

vesiculography /-log′rəfē/,   the x-ray examination of the seminal vesicles and nearby structures, with a dye.

Vesprin,   a trademark for a phenothiazine tranquilizer (triflupromazine hydrochloride) for injection into the muscles.

vessel,   any one of the many small tubes throughout the body that convey fluids, as blood and lymph. The main kinds of vessels are the arteries, the veins, and the lymphatic vessels.

vestibular /vestib′yələr/,   relating to a vestibule, as the vestibular part of the mouth, which lies between the cheeks and the teeth.

vestibular gland,   any one of four small glands, two on each side of the opening of the vagina. The vestibular glands secrete a lubricating substance.

vestibule /ves′tibyŏŏl/,   a space that serves as the entrance to a passageway, as the vestibule of the vagina or the vestibule of the ear.

vestige /ves′tij/,   a mainly useless organ or other structure of the body that was important at an earlier stage or in a simpler form of life, as the appendix (vermiform).   **–vestigial,** *adj.*

viable /vī′əbəl/,   capable of developing, growing, and otherwise sustaining life, as a normal human fetus at 28 weeks of pregnancy.   **–viability,** *n.*

Vibramycin Hyclate,   a trademark for a tetracycline antibiotic (doxycycline hyclate).

vibrio /vib′rē·ō/,   any bacterium that is curved and able to move, as those belonging to the genus *Vibrio*. **Vibrio cholerae** is the species of comma-shaped, motile bacillus that is the cause of cholera. **Vibrio fetus** causes sudden infectious diarrhea in newborn infants. Symptoms may also include weight loss, vomiting, fever, poor feeding, and irritability. It is one of many highly contagious types of stomach upset in infants but may be controlled with antibiotics. *Vibrio parahaemolyticus* causes an infectious disease resulting from eating infected seafood. Symptoms include nausea, vomiting, stomach pain, and diarrhea.

vidarabine,   a drug that is used to kill a virus (antiviral). It is used to treat herpes infections of the brain and eyes. It is used in pregnancy only when the benefits are greater than the risk of damage to the baby. Known allergy to this drug prohibits its use. Side effects include severe nausea, various nervous system effects, and bone marrow depression. Irritation, sensitivity to light, and corneal edema may occur when put in the eyes.

villous adenoma /vil′əs/,   a slow-growing, soft, spongy, possibly cancer-causing growth of the mucous membranes of the large intestine.

villous carcinoma,   a tumor with many long, velvety fingerlike growths. Also called **carcinoma villosum.**

villus, *pl.* **villi,**   one of the many tiny projections, barely visible to the naked eye, that cover the whole lining of the small intestine. The villi absorb and carry fluids and nutrients.

vinblastine sulfate,   a drug that prevents the growth of cancer cells. It is used to treat many cancerous diseases, as choriocarcinoma, testicular carcinoma, Hodgkin's disease, and non-Hodgkin's lymphoma.

vincristine sulfate,   a drug that prevents the growth of cancer cells. It is given to treat many cancerous diseases,

T–Z

as leukemia, neuroblastoma, lymphomas, and sarcomas. Pregnancy, white blood cell decrease, neuromuscular disease, or known allergy to this drug prohibits its use. Side effects include poisoning, severe decrease in white blood cells, constipation, pain in the abdomen, and loss of hair.

vindesine sulfate, a drug that prevents the growth of cancer cells. It is used to treat acute lymphoblastic leukemia, breast cancer, cancerous melanoma, lymphosarcoma, and non-small-cell lung carcinoma.

Vioform, a trademark for a drug that kills amebas (antiamebic) and is used to treat skin infections (iodochlorhydroxyquin).

Viokase, a trademark for an enzyme (pancreatin).

violent rupture, associated with chemical reactions having a release rate of less than one second (i.e., deflagration). There is no time to react. This behavior is commonly associated with runaway cracking and overpressures of closed containers.

Vira-A, a trademark for a drug used to fight a virus (vidarabine).

viral hepatitis /vī′rəl/. See **hepatitis.**

viral infection, any of the diseases caused by one of about 200 viruses dangerous to humans. Some are the most dangerous diseases known; some are harmless. Disease exists when the virus damages any cells. Viruses enter the body through breaks in the skin, by being breathed into the lungs, or by entering the stomach when eaten.

viral pneumonia. See **pneumonia.**

viremia /vīrē′mē ·ə/, viruses in the blood. Compare **bacteremia, fungemia, parasitemia.**

virile /vir′əl/, **1.** of, relating to, or typical of, an adult male; masculine; manly. **2.** having masculine strength, vigor, force, or energy. **3.** of or relating to the male sexual functions; capable of making a woman pregnant. Compare **virilism** –**virility,** n.

virilism /vir′ilizm/, **1.** the growth of male secondary sexual characteristics in a female. This state is usually caused by an adrenal gland disorder, hormone drugs, or tumors of the ovary. **2.** early development of masculine traits in the male.

virology /vīrol′-, virol′-/, the study of viruses and viral diseases.

Viroptic, a trademark for a drug that fights viruses in the eyes (trifluridine).

virucide /vī′rəsīd/, any drug that destroys or makes harmless a virus. – **virucidal,** adj.

virulence /vir′yələns/, the power of a microbe to cause disease.

virus, a tiny organism that can only grow in the cells of another animal. More than 200 viruses have been found to cause disease in humans. A **virion** is a simple virus parti-

cle. Some kinds of viruses are **adenovirus, arenavirus, enterovirus, herpesvirus, rhinovirus.** See also specific entry. –**viral,** adj.

viscera /vis′ərə/, sing. **viscus** /vis′kəs/, the internal organs held within a space in the body, mainly the stomach and intestines.

visceral /vis′ərəl/, relating to the viscera, or internal organs in the body cavity.

visceral larva migrans. See **toxocariasis.**

visceral nervous system. See **central nervous system.**

viscosity /viskos′itē/, the quality of a sticky or gummy fluid.

vision, the ability to see.

Visken, a trademark for a heart drug (pindolol).

Vistaril, a trademark for a sedative (hydroxyzine hydrochloride).

visual field defect, one or more spots or defects in the vision that move with the eye, unlike a floater. This fixed defect may be caused by injuries to the eye, by disease, or by damage to the brain.

visual pathway, a pathway over which a visual sensation is carried from the retina to the brain. A pathway consists of an optic nerve and other optic structures.

visual purple. See **rhodopsin.**

vital capacity (VC), a measurement of the amount of air that can be breathed out slowly after the largest possible breath has been taken. This shows the most air that the lungs can hold.

vital signs, the measurements of pulse rate, rate of breathing, and body temperature. Although not strictly a vital sign, blood pressure is also usually included. See also **blood pressure, body temperature, pulse, respiratory rate.**

vital statistics, numeric data on births, deaths, diseases, injuries, and other factors affecting the general health and condition of human populations. Also called **biostatistics.**

vitamin, a natural compound needed in small quantities for normal bodily functions. With few exceptions, vitamins cannot be made by the body and must be gotten from the diet or dietary supplements. No one food contains all the vitamins. See also specific vitamins.

vitamin A, a vitamin needed for the growth of the skeleton, maintaining the mucous membranes, and keen sight. It is present in leafy green vegetables, yellow fruits and vegetables, the liver oils of the cod and other fish, liver, milk, cheese, butter, and egg yolk. Lack of this vitamin causes diseases of the mucous membranes and the eyes. Symptoms of getting too much vitamin A are irritability, fatigue, lethargy, stomach pain, painful joints, severe throbbing headache, insomnia and restlessness. **Oleovitamin A** is an oily mixture, usually fish liver oil, which may be plain or mixed with a vegetable oil that can be eaten, containing the natural or artificial form of vitamin A.

vitamin B$_1$.   See **thiamine.**

vitamin B$_2$.   See **riboflavin.**

vitamin B$_6$.   See **pyridoxine.**

vitamin B$_{12}$.   See **cyanocobalamin.**

vitamin B$_{17}$.   See **amygdalin.**

vitamin B complex,   a group of vitamins differing from each other in structure and their effect on the human body. All of the B vitamins are found in large quantities in liver and yeast, and they are present one at a time or several together in many foods. Heat and prolonged cooking, especially cooking with water, can destroy B vitamins. See also **folic acid,** and see specific B vitamins.

vitamin C,   a water-soluble, white crystalline vitamin. It is in citrus fruits, tomatoes, berries, and potatoes. Fresh, green, leafy vegetables, as broccoli, brussels sprouts, collards, turnip greens, parsley, sweet peppers, and cabbage also contain vitamin C. It is needed by the body to form collagen and fiber for teeth, bone, cartilage, connective tissue, skin, and capillary walls. It helps in fighting bacterial infections. Symptoms of its lack are bleeding gums, tendency to bruising, swollen or painful joints, and nosebleeds. Anemia, lowered resistance to infections, and slow healing of wounds or fractures are other symptoms. Severe lack results in scurvy. An excess may cause a burning sensation during urination, diarrhea, skin rash, and nausea. It may disturb the absorption and processing of vitamin B$_{12}$. Also called **ascorbic acid.**

vitamin D,   a vitamin related to the steroids and needed for the normal growth of bones and teeth and for absorbing calcium and phosphorus from the intestines. The vitamin is present in natural foods in small amounts. Needed amounts are usually gotten from vitamins added to various foods, especially milk and dairy products, and exposure to sunlight. The natural foods containing vitamin D are of animal origin and include saltwater fish, especially salmon, sardines, and herring, organ meats, fish-liver oils, and egg yolk. A lack of the vitamin results in rickets in children, and other bone diseases in adults. Too much vitamin D results in poisoning that causes a loss of appetite, vomiting, headache, drowsiness, diarrhea, and hardening of soft tissues. See also **calciferol, vitamin D$_3$.**

vitamin D$_2$.   See **calciferol.**

vitamin D$_3$,   a vitamin that is needed for calcium and phosphorus metabolism. It is found in most fish-liver oils, butter, brain, and egg yolk and is formed in the skin, fur, and feathers of animals and birds exposed to sunlight or ultraviolet rays. Also called **activated 7-dehydrocholesterol, cholecalciferol.**

vitamin E,   a vitamin needed for muscle development, and various other bodily functions. A lack of this vitamin causes muscle damage, blood disorders (anemia), and liver and kidney damage and is linked with the aging process. The richest dietary sources are wheat germ, soybean, cottonseed, peanut, and corn oils, margarine, whole raw seeds and nuts, soybeans, eggs, butter, liver, sweet potatoes, and the leaves of many vegetables, as turnip greens. Also called **tocopherol.**

vitamin H.   See **biotin.**

vitamin K,   a group of vitamins that are needed to help the liver work properly and to help the blood to clot. The vitamin is widely distributed in foods, especially leafy green vegetables, pork liver, yogurt, egg yolk, kelp, alfalfa, fish-liver oils, and blackstrap molasses and is made by bacteria in the intestines. It can also be made artificially. A lack of this vitamin is marked by blood disorders. It is used to reduce the clotting time in patients with some types of jaundice and in certain kinds of bleeding linked with some diseases of the intestines and liver. It is given to infants to protect against a bleeding disease of the newborn. A form of the vitamin is used to preserve food. Natural vitamin K is stored in the body and produces no poisons. Very large doses of artificial vitamin K may cause anemia in newborn infants and hemolysis in patients with glucose-6-phosphate deficiency.

vitamin P.   See **bioflavonoid.**

vitellin /vītel′in/,   a protein containing lecithin, found in the yolk of eggs. Also called **ovovitellin.**

vitelline circulation,   the flow of blood and nutrients between the developing embryo and the yolk sac by way of the simple (vitelline) arteries and veins. See also **fetal circulation.**

vitellus /vītel′əs/,   the yolk of an egg (ovum).

vitiligo /vit′ili̅′gō, -lē′gō/,   a harmless skin disease of unknown cause, having uneven patches of various sizes totally lacking in color and often having very colorful borders. Exposed areas of skin are most often affected. Waterproof makeup is often used to cover the patches. Compare **albinism, piebald.**   –**vitiliginous,** *adj.*

vitreous cavity /vit′rē·əs/,   the space behind the lens of the eyes that contains the vitreous humor and membrane that lines it.

vitreous hemorrhage,   bleeding into the vitreous humor of the eye.

vitreous humor,   a clear, jellylike substance contained in a thin membrane filling the space behind the crystal-like lens of the eye. Also called **vitreous body.**

Vivactil,   a trademark for a drug used to relieve depression (protriptyline hydrochloride).

Vivonex,   a trademark for a food supplement containing protein, carbohydrate, and fat.

VLDL, abbreviation for **very-low-density lipoprotein.**

vocal cord, either of two strong bands of yellow stretchy tissue in the larynx held by membranes called vocal folds. **False vocal cord** refers to either of two thick folds of mucous membrane in the throat (larynx).

vocal cord nodule, a small swelling or fiberlike growth that develops on the vocal cords of people who always strain their voices. Also called **screamer's nodule, singer's nodule, teacher's nodule.**

voice box. See **larynx.**

void, to empty, as urine from the bladder.

volar /vō′lər/, relating to the palm of the hand or the sole of the foot.

Volkmann's splint, a splint that supports and prevents movement of the lower leg. It has a footpiece attached to two sides that extends from the foot to the knee, allowing the patient to walk.

volume, the amount of space taken up by a body, given in cubic units.

voluntary, referring to an action or thought that is under the person's control.

voluntary muscle. See **striated muscle.**

volvulus /vol′vyələs/, a twisting of the bowel on itself, causing intestinal blockage. If it is not corrected, the blocked bowel becomes damaged, and death may follow. Severe, gripping pain, nausea and vomiting, a lack of bowel sounds, and tense, bloated intestines are symptoms. Compare **intussusception.**

vomit, the act of forcing out the contents of the stomach through the esophagus and out of the mouth. Vomit also refers to the material expelled.

von Gierke's disease /fôngir′kəz/. See **glycogen storage disease.**

Vontrol, a trademark for a drug used to prevent vomiting (diphenidol).

von Willebrand's disease, an inherited disorder with abnormally slow blood clotting, sudden nose bleeds, and bleeding gums. Excessive bleeding is common after giving birth, during menstruation, and after injury or surgery. See also **hemophilia.**

voyeurism /voi′yərizm/, a mental and sexual disorder in which a person gets sexual excitement and satisfaction from looking at the naked bodies and genitals or seeing the sexual acts of others, especially from a hiding place.

vulva /vul′və/, the outer genitals of a woman. This includes the fleshy skin folds (labia), the opening of the vagina, and the various glands.

vulvectomy /vəlvek′-/, removal by surgery of part or all of the tissues of the vulva. This is done most often to treat cancer. **Simple vulvectomy** includes the removal of the skin of the labia outside the vaginal opening and the clitoris. **Radical vulvectomy** involves removing the labia, clitoris, surrounding tissues, and pelvic lymph nodes.

vulvocrural /vul′vōkrŏŏr′əl/, relating to the vulva and the thigh.

vulvovaginitis /-vaj′inī′-/, an inflammation of the vulva and vagina, or their glands.

VZV, abbreviation for **varicella zoster virus.**

W

Wagner-Meissner corpuscle /-mīs′nər/, one of a number of small nerve endings sensitive to pressure. It can be found on the hand and foot, the forearm, the skin of the lips, and the tongue. Also called **tactile corpuscle of Meissner.**

Wagstaffe's fracture, a fracture with separation of the inner malleolus.

waking imagined analgesia (WIA), the pain relief method made up by concentrating on previous pleasant experiences that gave tranquillity, as lying on a beach beside cooling ocean water or drifting down a quiet river in a canoe. This technique is often effective in reducing mild to moderate pain, especially when used with a mild pain reliever. See also **pain intervention.**

walker, a very light, movable apparatus, about waist high, made of metal tubing, used to help a patient in walking. It has four widely placed, sturdy legs. Compare **crutch.**

walking pneumonia. See **pneumonia.**

walking rounds, a hospital tour in which the doctor responsible leads a group of interns and medical students to visit the patients for whom they are all responsible. In some hospitals nurses may join in walking rounds.

wall, a structure within the body that closes a space, as the wall of the stomach or the wall of a cell.

wander, to move about without purpose or to cause to move back and forth in a searching manner.

Wangensteen apparatus, a catheter and a suction apparatus. It is used for constant, gentle drainage and pressure relief of the stomach or first part of the small intestines (duodenum). It may be used to relieve stomach bloating that often occurs after an operation or that may complicate a stomach and intestinal disorder, especially a blocked intestine.

ward, a hospital room made and equipped to house more than four patients.

warfarin poisoning /wôr′fərin/, a toxic condition caused by swallowing warfarin. The poison results in inner bleeding.

warfarin sodium, a drug that acts to prevent clot formation. It is given to prevent and treat thrombosis and embolism. Bleeding or known allergy to this drug prohibits its use. The most serious side effect is bleeding. Many other drugs interact with this drug to increase or decrease its effects.

warm-blooded, having a high and constant body temperature, as the temperatures kept by humans, other mammals, and birds, despite changes in outside temperatures. Heat is made in the warm-blooded human body by the breakdown of foods. About 80% of the body heat that is lost in humans is lost through the skin. The rest is lost through the mucous membranes of the breathing, the digestive, and the urinary systems. The average temperature of the healthy human is 98.6° F (37° C).

warm zone area, forward control area for hazardous materials operations outside the hot zone. Personnel protection is not required. Restricted to operations and support personnel essential to hands-on work performed in the hot zone.

wart, a harmless growth (verruca) on the skin caused by a virus. It has a rough surface. A flat wart (**verruca plana**) is a small, slightly raised, smooth, tan or "flesh"-colored wart, sometimes occurring in large numbers on the face, neck, back of the hands, wrists, and knees, especially in children. A **digitate wart** is a fingerlike, horny bump that grows from a pea-shaped base on the scalp or near the hairline. A **plantar wart** is a painful growth on the sole of the foot. It occurs most often at points of pressure, as on the heel. There is a soft core surrounded by a firm, callus-like ring. Many tiny, black spots on the surface are bits of clotted blood in the wart. **Mosaic wart** describes a group of neighboring warts (plantar) on the sole of the foot. Treatment for warts can be burning off (electrosurgery), freezing (cryotherapy), or using drugs. One way of taking off warts is called **acid therapy.** Plaster patches with a mild acid are placed on the warts.

wasp, a slender, narrow-waisted insect with two pairs of wings that are folded lengthwise when at rest like parts of a fan. Many species of wasps may give painful stings. They may have severe results in allergic persons. Treatment is as for bee stings.

wasting, a process of breakdown marked by weight loss and decreased physical vigor, appetite, and mental activity.

water (H_2O), a chemical compound. A molecule of water has one atom of oxygen and two atoms of hydrogen. Almost three quarters of the earth's surface is covered by water. Water is essential to life as it exists on this planet. It comprises more than 70% of living things. Pure water freezes at 0° C (32° F). It boils at 100° C (212° F) at sea level.

waterborne, carried by water, as a waterborne epidemic of typhoid fever.

Waterhouse-Friderichsen syndrome, a disorder with a large amount of bacteria in the blood (bacteremia). Symptoms are a sudden fever, bluish skin color (cyanosis), small red spots (petechiae), and collapse from massive bleeding. The condition requires immediate emergency treatment, hospitalization, and intensive care.

water intoxication, an increase in the volume of free water in the body. This results in a lack of salt.

water tender, any ground vehicle capable of transporting specified quantities of water.

water-reactive materials, materials that will react and release energy after coming in contact with water.

waxy flexibility, a condition often found in catatonic schizophrenia. The arms and legs stay for an indefinite period of time in the positions in which they are placed.

WBC, abbreviation for **white blood cell.** See **leukocyte.**

W/D, abbreviation for *well developed*. It is often used in the patient record to describe the patient's physical appearance.

wean, **1.** to make a child give up breast feeding and to accept other food. Many children are ready for weaning during the second half of the first year. Some wean themselves. **2.** to take from a patient something on which he or she is dependent.

weaver's bottom. See **bursitis.**

web, a network of fibers forming a tissue or a membrane.

Weber's tuning fork test, a method of testing hearing. The test is done by placing the stem of a vibrating 256 Hz tuning fork in the center of the person's forehead or on the jaw. The loudness of the sound is equal in both ears if hearing is normal.

Wechsler intelligence scales /weks'-lər/, a series of standardized tests made to measure the intelligence at several age levels. It is done by means of questions that examine general information, arrangement of pictures and objects, vocabulary, memory, reasoning, and other abilities.

wedge fracture, a fracture of vertebral structures with frontal pressure.

wedge resection, the surgical removal of part of an organ. The segment taken away may be wedge-shaped.

weeping, **1.** crying. **2.** slow-flowing fluid, as with a sore or rash.

Weil's disease /wīls/. See **leptospirosis.**

well baby care, regular health care for infants and children to promote the best possible physical, emotional, and intellectual growth and development. Such health care measures include routine vaccinations and screening procedures for early detection and treatment of illness. Parental guidance and instruction in proper nutrition, accident prevention, and specific care and rearing of the child at various stages of growth are other measures to be taken. The advised preventive health care schedule for children who are growing normally is monthly for the first 6 months of life, every 2 months until 1 year of age, every 3 months during the second year, and every 6 months during the third year. It must be followed by yearly visits.

well baby clinic, a clinic that specializes in medical supervision and services for healthy infants.

well-being, achievement of a good existence as defined by the individual.

wellness, a dynamic state of health in which an individual grows toward a higher level of functioning, having the best balance between inner and outer environments.

wen, a common, noncancerous swelling (cyst) under the skin. It is lined by packed outer skin cells and filled with oil and dead cells. It may become infected.

Werdnig-Hoffmann disease, a genetic disorder beginning in infancy or young childhood with wasting away of the skeletal muscles. The condition is usually visible at birth. Symptoms include weak muscle tone at birth, lack of stretch reflexes, and paralysis, especially of the trunk and limbs. There is also lack of sucking ability, involuntary movements of the tongue and sometimes of other muscles, and, often, speech problems. Treatment depends on the symptoms. Death generally occurs in early childhood, often from breathing problems.

Wernicke's encephalopathy /wur'nikēz, ver'-/. See **encephalopathy.**

wet dream. See **nocturnal emission.**

wet lung, an abnormal condition of the lungs with a persistent cough. It occurs in workers exposed to lung irritants, as ammonia, chlorine, sulfur dioxide, organic acids that evaporate, dusts, and vapors of corrosive chemicals. Treatment includes removing the person from exposure to the irritant. Compare **pulmonary edema.** See also **pleural effusion, pleurisy.**

wet nurse, a woman who cares for and breast-feeds another's infant.

W/F, symbol for *white female*. It is often used in the first identifying statement in a patient record.

Wharton's jelly, a soft, jellylike substance of the umbilical cord.

wheal, an individual patch of itchy skin, as in hives.

wheelchair, a mobile chair with large wheels and brakes. If long-term use of the chair is expected, a physical therapist may advise certain personalized requirements, as size, left- or right-hand propulsion, type of brakes, height of armrests, and special seat pads.

wheeze, a sound of high-pitched rattling in the throat when breathing. It is caused by a fast flow of air through a narrowed airway. Wheezes are linked to asthma and long-term inflammation of the bronchi. See also **rale, rhonchi.**

whiplash injury, *informal.* an injury to the neck (cervical) vertebrae or their supporting ligaments and muscles. There is pain and stiffness. It usually results from sudden speeding or slowing down, as in a rear-end car collision that causes a violent back and forth movement of the head and neck.

Whipple's disease, a rare intestinal disease. It features severe inability to absorb nutrients, excess fat in feces (steatorrhea), anemia, weight loss, and pain and swelling in joints. See also **malabsorption syndrome.**

whipworm infection, a condition of being infested with the roundworm *Trichuris trichiura.* Heavy infestation may cause nausea, stomach and bowel pain, diarrhea, and anemia. It is common in tropic areas with poor sanitation. Eggs are passed in feces. Contamination of the hands, food, and water results in taking the eggs into the body that hatch in the bowels. The worms may live 15 to 20 years. Treatment is with mebendazole. Prevention includes proper disposal of feces and good personal hygiene. Also called **trichuriasis.**

whirlpool bath, putting the body in a tank of hot water moved by a jet of equal amounts of hot water and air.

white blood cell. See **leukocyte.**

whitehead. See **milia.**

white substance, the tissue surrounding the gray substance of the spinal cord. It is made up mainly of sheathed nerve fibers, but with some unsheathed nerve fibers. It is subdivided in each half of the spinal cord into three parts (funiculi): the anterior, the posterior, and the lateral white column. Compare **gray substance.** See also **spinal cord.**

whitlow, an inflammation of the end of a finger or toe that results in pus. See also **felon.**

WHO, abbreviation for **World Health Organization.**

whole blood, blood that is unchanged except for the presence of a drug that prevents clotting of the blood. It is used for transfusion.

whole-body exposure, an exposure of the body to radiation, where the entire body rather than an isolated part is irradiated. If a radioisotope is uniformly distributed throughout the body tissues, rather than concentrated in certain parts (local exposure), the irradiation can be considered as whole-body exposure.

whooping cough, an acute, contagious disease. It features severe coughing attacks that end with a loud whooping breath taken in. It occurs mainly in children less than four years old who have not been immunized. The disease is spread directly by coughing and sneezing, and indirectly by contact with articles from the patient. Early symptoms are like those of bronchitis or influenza, with a runny nose, sneezing, a dry cough, fever, and lack of appetitie. The cough develops into a series of short, rapid bursts followed by the high pitched whoop. Large amounts of mucus may cause vomiting. The illness lasts 6 to 8 weeks. Hospitalization may be needed for children with a prolonged cough. Antibiotics may be given to control secondary infections. Also called **pertussis.**

whorl, a spiral turn, as one of the turns of ridges that form fingerprints.

Widal's test /vēdals'/, a test used to aid in the diagnosis of salmonella infections, as typhoid fever.

Wigraine, a trademark for a drug with a substance that blocks the passage of impulses through the parasympathetic nerves (belladonna alkaloids) and a painkiller (phenacetin). It also has a substance that contracts the blood vessels (ergotamine tartrate). It is used to treat migraine.

will, 1. the mental faculty that enables one consciously to choose or decide on a course of action. **2.** determination or purpose; willfulness. **3.** (in law) an expression or declaration of a person's wishes as to the use of property, taking effect after death.

Wilms' tumor, a cancerous tumor of the kidney. It occurs in young children, before the fifth year in 75% of the cases. The common early sign is high blood pressure. It is followed by the appearance of a lump that can be felt, pain, and blood in the urine (hematuria). Diagnosis usually can be made by x-rays of the urinary tract and part of the body. The tumor is well enclosed in the early stage. It may later extend into lymph nodes and other sites. Prompt removal of the tumors is recommended. Chemotherapy along with surgery and irradiation is proving highly effective.

Wilson's disease, an inherited disorder in which copper accumulates in the liver. It is then released and taken up in other parts of the body. A gray-green to red-gold colored ring (**Kayser-Fleischer ring**) at the margin of the cornea of the eye is a sign of Wilson's disease. A blood disease (hemolytic anemia) occurs as the copper pools in the red blood cells. Pooling in the brain destroys certain tissues. It may cause tremors, muscle rigidity, speech problems, and dementia. Kidney function is diminished. The liver becomes swollen. Treatment of Wilson's disease includes

T–Z

reducing copper in the diet and giving copper-binding agents and penicillamine.

wind chill, the loss of heat from the body when it is exposed to wind of a given speed at a given temperature and humidity. The **wind chill index** is given in kilocalories per hour per square meter of skin surface. The **wind chill factor** is given in degrees Celsius or Fahrenheit as the real temperature felt by a person exposed to the weather.

window, a surgically created opening in the surface of a structure or an existing opening in the surface or between the chambers of a structure.

windowed, (of an orthopedic cast) having an opening, as to relieve pressure that may irritate the skin.

windpipe See **trachea.**

Winstrol. a trademark for a drug that stimulates male characteristics (stanozolol). It is used as an anabolic drug.

winter cough, *nontechnical.* a long-term condition with a persistent cough caused by cold weather. See also **cough.**

winter itch, itching occurring in cold weather in people who have dry skin, particularly with inflammation. Warmer temperature, increased humidity, and soothing drugs on the skin may offer relief.

wipe sample (smear sample), a sample taken for the purpose of determining the presence of removable radioactive contamination on a surface. It is made by wiping a piece of soft filter paper, with slight pressure, over a representative surface area.

wisdom tooth, either of the last teeth on each side of the upper and lower jaw. These are the last teeth to come out. This usually happens between 17 and 21 years of age. It often causes considerable pain, dental problems, and the need for pulling out the tooth. See also **molar.**

wish fulfillment, the satisfaction of a desire or the release of emotional tension through dreams, daydreams, and neurotic symptoms.

Wiskott-Aldrich syndrome /-ôl′drich/, an inherited disorder with a lack of resistance. It features a blood disease (thrombocytopenia) and a skin disease (eczema). The person is easily affected by infections and cancer. Treatment includes appropriate antibiotics for specific infectious organisms.

witch hazel, a solution with the extract from the shrub *Hamamelis virginiana,* alcohol, and water, used as a contraction drug (astringent).

witch's milk, a milklike substance released from the breast of the newborn. It is caused by a milk-producing hormone from the mother. Also called **hexenmilch** /hek′sənmilsh′/.

withdrawal, a common response to physical danger or severe stress. It is marked by a state of apathy, weakness, depression, and retreat into oneself. See also **schizophrenia.**

withdrawal bleeding. See **vaginal bleeding.**

withdrawal method, a birth control method in which the penis is withdrawn from the vagina before ejaculation. It is not reliable because small amounts of sperm may be released without sensation before full ejaculation. Also called **coitus interruptus.**

withdrawal symptoms, the unpleasant, sometimes life-threatening bodily changes that occur when some drugs are withdrawn after long-term, regular use.

W/M, symbol for *white male.* It is often used in the first identifying statement in a patient record.

W/N, symbol for *well nourished.* It is often used in the first identifying statement in a patient record.

Wolff-Parkinson-White syndrome, a heart disorder with an abnormal early contraction of part of the heart muscle. This condition can be diagnosed by an electrocardiogram.

woman-year, (in statistics) 1 year in the reproductive life of a sexually active woman. It is a unit that represents 12 months of exposure to the risk of pregnancy. Woman-years are used in determining the pregnancy rate of the various methods of family planning.

womb. See **uterus.**

Wood's light, an ultraviolet light used to diagnose some scalp and skin diseases. The light causes hairs infected with a fungus, such as ringworm, to become brilliantly fluorescent. Also called **Wood's lamp.**

word association, a process of releasing repressed ideas. This is done in response to words spoken by a psychoanalyst.

word association test, a technique used in mental or educational evaluation. A person is asked to respond to a word with the first thing that comes to mind. The time taken to respond and the associations made are compared to pretested responses. They are classified for diagnosis.

word salad, a jumble of words and phrases that lacks meaning. It is often seen in seriously confused persons and schizophrenics.

work tolerance, the kind and amount of work that a physically or mentally ill person can or should do.

work-up, the process of making a complete evaluation of a patient, including history, physical examination, laboratory tests, and x-ray or other diagnostic techniques. The purpose is to get the facts on which a diagnosis and treatment plan may be established.

World Health Organization (WHO), an agency of the United Nations. It is mainly concerned with worldwide or regional health problems. Its tasks include offering technical assistance, advancing an investigation of diseases, recommending health regulations, and promoting cooperation among professional health groups.

wormian bone /wur′mē·ən, vôr′-/, any of several tiny, smooth, segmented bones. They are usually found as the sawlike borders of the joints between the skull bones. Wormian bones were named for the Danish anatomist Ole Worm.

wound, **1.** any physical injury involving a break in the skin. It is usually caused by an act or accident rather than by a disease, as a chest wound, gunshot wound, or puncture wound. **2.** to cause an injury, especially one that breaks the skin.

wound irrigation, the cleansing of a wound or the cavity formed by a wound using a solution with drugs, water, or liquid substance that suppresses or kills the growth of microorganisms. Wounds are irrigated to remove fluid and dried blood. Another purpose is to keep the wound surface open to encourage healing from the inside out. When the washing solution returns clear, the wound is clean.

wound repair, restoration of the normal structure after an injury, especially of the skin. See also **healing, intention.**

wrist, the joint area between the forearm and the hand, made up of eight bones arranged in two rows. Also called **carpus.**

writer's cramp, a painful involuntary tightening of the muscles of the hand when attempting to write. It often occurs after long periods of writing.

wrongful death statute, (in law) a statute existing in all states that says that the death of a person allows for legal action against the person whose willful or negligent acts caused the death. Before the existence of these statutes, a civil suit could be brought only if the injured person survived the injury.

wrongful life action, (in law) a civil suit usually brought against a physician or health facility on the basis of negligence that led to wrongful birth or life of an infant. The parents of the unwanted child seek to get payment from the defendant for the medical expenses of pregnancy and birth. They also seek to get payment for pain and suffering, and for the education and upbringing of the child. Wrongful life actions have been brought and won in several situations, including malpractice sterilizations (of both men and women), and abortions.

wryneck an abnormal condition in which the head is inclined to one side as a result of the contraction of the muscles on that side of the neck. Also called **torticollis,** the disorder may be inborn or acquired. Treatment may include surgery, heat, or support, depending on the cause and the severity of the condition. **Spasmodic torticollis** refers to attacks of spasms of the neck muscles. The condition often only lasts a brief while, and examination rarely reveals a physical cause. In some cases, severe stress and muscular spasm may be the cause.

Wyamine, a trademark for an alpha-adrenergic drug (mephentermine).

Wycillin, a trademark for an antibacterial (penicillin G procaine).

Wydase, a trademark for an enzyme (hyaluronidase).

Wymox, a trademark for an antibiotic (amoxicillin).

Wytensin, a trademark for drug used to fight high blood pressure (guanabenz).

T–Z

X

Xanax, a trademark for an antianxiety drug (alprazolam).

xanthelasmatosis /zanˈthilazˈmətōˈ-/, a skin disease with yellowish plaques. It is often linked to a cancer of bone marrow (multiple myeloma).

xanthine /zanˈthēn/, a nitrogen compound normally found in the muscles, liver, spleen, pancreas, and urine.

xanthine derivative, any one of the closely linked alkaloids caffeine, theobromine, or theophylline. They are found in plants in many different areas. They are consumed in beverages, such as coffee, tea, cocoa, and cola drinks. The xanthine derivatives stimulate the central nervous system. They also promote urine release and relax smooth muscles. Theobromine has low potency. It is seldom used as a drug.

xanthinuria /-ŏŏrˈē·ə/, **1.** the presence of excess quantities of xanthine in the urine. **2.** a rare disorder that results in the release of large amounts of xanthine in the urine. It is caused by the lack of an enzyme that is needed in xanthine processing. This inherited lack may cause the development of kidney stones.

xanthogranuloma /zanˈthōgranˈyəlōˈmə/, a tumor or knot of granulated tissue with lipid deposits. **Juvenile xanthogranuloma** is a skin problem with groups of yellow, red, or brown lumps on the arms and legs and in some cases on the eyes, the membranes that cover the brain and spinal cord, and the testes. The lesions often appear in early childhood and disappear in a few years.

xanthoma /zanthōˈmə/, a harmless, fatty, fibrous, yellowish plaque, knot, or tumor that develops in the skin, often around tendons.

xanthomatosis /-mətōˈ-/, an abnormal condition in which there are deposits of yellowish fatty material in the skin, internal organs, and other tissues.

xanthopsia /zanthopˈsē·ə/, an abnormal visual condition in which everything appears to have a yellow hue. It is sometimes linked to liver disease (jaundice) or digitalis poisoning.

xanthosis /zanthōˈ-/, a yellowish discoloration of the skin. It is sometimes seen in the wasting tissues of cancerous diseases. It is commonly caused by eating large amounts of yellow vegetables with carotene pigment. The antimalarial drug quinacrine, if taken over a long period, may produce a similar skin color. Xanthosis can be told apart from liver disease (jaundice) because the white outer coats of the eyeballs (sclerae) are colored yellow in jaundice but are not discolored in xanthosis. See also **carotenemia.**

X chromosome, a sex chromosome that in humans is present in both sexes. It appears singly in the cells of normal males and in duplicate in the cells of normal females. The chromosome is carried as a sex determinant by all of the female gametes and one half of all male gametes. It has many sex-linked genes linked to important disorders, as hemophilia, Duchenne's muscular dystrophy, and Hunter's syndrome. Compare **Y chromosome.**

xenobiotic /zēˈnōbī·otˈik/, referring to organic substances that are foreign to the body, as drugs or organic poisons.

xenogeneic /-jənēˈik/, referring to individuals or cell types from different species and different genotypes.

xenophobia, an anxiety disorder with a strong, irrational fear or uneasiness in the presence of strangers, especially foreigners, or in new surroundings.

xero-, a combining form meaning dryness.

xeroderma /zirˈədurˈmə/, a long-term skin condition with dryness and roughness. **Xeroderma pigmentosum** is a rare, inherited skin disease with extreme sensitivity to ultraviolet light. Exposure to ultraviolet light may result in freckles, horny growths, and harmless or cancerous tumors. Growths and tumors developing on the eyelids and cornea may result in blindness. Exposure to sunlight must be avoided.

xerophthalmia /zirˈofthalˈmē·ə/, a condition of dry and lusterless corneas and areas covering the eyes. It is usually the result of a lack of vitamin A and linked to night blindness.

xeroradiography /-rāˈdē·ogˈrəfē/, a diagnostic x-ray technique in which an image is made electrically rather than chemically. It allows lower exposure times and radiation of lower energy than that of ordinary x-rays. Xeroradiography is used mainly for radiography of the breasts.

xerostomia /-stō′mē·ə/,   dryness of the mouth. The condition is a symptom of many diseases, as diabetes, acute infections, and hysteria. It is also a common side effect of drugs.

xiphoid process /zī′foid, zif′-/,   the smallest of three parts of the breastbone near the seventh rib.

X-linked,   referring to genes or to the traits or conditions they transmit that are carried on the X chromosome. Most X-linked traits and conditions, as hemophilia, are recessive and therefore occur mostly in males, because they have only one X chromosome. Compare **Y-linked.**

X-linked dominant inheritance,   a pattern of inheritance in which the carrying of a dominant gene on the X chromosome causes a trait to be revealed. Affected individuals all have an affected parent. All of the daughters of an affected male are affected but none of the sons. One half of the sons and one half of the daughters of an affected female are affected. Normal children of an affected parent have normal offspring. The inheritance shows a clear positive family history. X-linked dominant inheritance closely looks like non-sex-linked (autosomal) inheritance. Compare **X-linked recessive inheritance.**

X-linked recessive inheritance,   a pattern of inheritance in which the carrying of an abnormal recessive gene on the X chromosome results in a carrier state in females and traits of the condition in males. Affected people have unaffected parents (except for the rare situation in which the father is affected and the mother is a carrier). One half of the female siblings of an affected male carry the trait. Unaffected male siblings do not carry the trait. Sons of affected males are unaffected. Daughters of affected males are carriers. Unaffected male children of a carrier female do not carry the trait. Compare **X-linked dominant inheritance.**

XO,   (in genetics) the designation for the presence of only one sex chromosome. Either the X or Y chromosome is missing. Each cell has a total of 45 chromosomes. See also **Turner's syndrome.**

x-ray,   electromagnetic radiation of wavelengths shorter than visible light. X-rays are made when electrons, traveling at high speed, strike certain materials, particularly heavy metals, as tungsten. They can go through most substances. They are used to investigate the integrity of certain structures and to destroy diseased tissue. They are also used to make photographic images for diagnostic purposes, as in radiography and fluoroscopy. Also called **roentgen ray.**

x-ray film,   a radiograph made by projecting x-rays through organs or structures of the body onto a photograph-

ic plate. A **localization film** is an x-ray film taken to confirm a treatment effect or to view the position of a radioactive implant, especially for the purpose of computing the dose delivered. Because some tissue, as bone, allows fewer x-rays to pass through (radiopaque) than other tissue, like skin or fat, a shadow is created on the plate that is the image of a bone or of a cavity filled with a radiopaque substance. See also **radiopaque.**

x-ray fluoroscopy,   an examination that uses an x-ray source that projects through the patient onto a fluorescent screen or image intensifier.

x-ray therapy,   the use of x-rays in treatment. **Deep x-ray therapy** describes the use of x-rays to treat internal cancers, as Wilms' tumor of the kidney and Hodgkin's disease. **External radiation therapy (ERT)** refers to x-ray-therapy with a beam outside the body. ERT is used most often to treat cancer. It is also used in the therapy of keloids and other skin conditions.

XX,   the designation for the normal sex chromosome complement in the human female. See also **X chromosome.**

XXX syndrome,   a human sex chromosomal disorder with the presence of three X chromosomes. The condition occurs about once in every 1000 live female births. Individuals with the disorder show no significant symptoms. However, there is usually some degree of mental retardation. Also called **triple X syndrome.**

XXXX, XXXXX,   an abnormal sex chromosome complement in the human female in which there are four or five instead of the normal two X chromosomes. The risk of abnormalities and mental retardation increases with the increase in the number of X chromosomes.

XXXY, XXXXY, XXYY,   an abnormal sex chromosome complement in the human male in which there are more than the normal one X chromosome. The more X chromosomes there are, the greater the number of inborn defects and the severity of mental retardation in the affected individual. See also **Klinefelter's syndrome.**

XY,   the normal sex chromosome complement in the human male.

xylitol /zī′litôl/,   a sweet, crystal-like alcohol. It is used as an artificial sweetener.

Xylocaine,   a trademark for a local anesthetic (lidocaine).

xylometazoline hydrochloride,   a drug that is given to treat nasal congestion in colds, hay fever, sinusitis, and other upper breathing allergies. Glaucoma or known allergy to this drug or similar drugs prohibits its use. It is used carefully in patients with heart and blood vessel disease. Side effects include irritation to the mucosa, returning nasal congestion, and effects linked to systemic absorp-

T–Z

tion, including sedation and changes in the function of heart and blood vessels.

XYY syndrome, having an extra Y chromosome. It tends to have a positive effect on height. It may have a negative effect on mental and psychologic development. However, the extra Y chromosome also occurs in normal males. See also **trisomy.**

Y

yaws /yôs/, a nonvenereal infection caused by a spiral-shaped germ (*Treponema pertenue*). It is transmitted by direct contact. It features long-term ulcerlike sores anywhere on the body with eventual tissue and bone destruction. It leads to crippling if untreated. It is a disease of unsanitary tropic living conditions.

Y chromosome, a sex chromosome that in humans is present only in the male. It is present singly in the normal male. It is carried as a sex determinant by one half of the male gametes and none of the female gametes. It has genes linked to triggering the development of male characteristics. Compare **X chromosome.**

yeast /yēst/, a fungus that reproduces by budding. *Candida albicans* is a kind of disease producing yeast.

yellow fever, an infection carried by mosquitoes. It features headache, fever, liver disease (jaundice), vomiting, and bleeding. There is no specific treatment. Recovery is followed by lifelong immunity. Vaccination for travelers to risk areas is advised.

yellow fever vaccine, a vaccine made from live yellow fever virus grown in chick embryos. It is given for vaccination against yellow fever. Among the more serious side effects are fever, discomfort, and allergic reactions.

Yersinia arthritis /yursin′ē·ə/, an inflammation of many joints. It occurs a few days to 1 month after the beginning of infection caused by either of two bacteria (*Yersinia enterocolitica* or *Y. pseudotuberculosis*). Knees, ankles, toes, fingers, and wrists are most often affected. It may look like juvenile rheumatoid arthritis, rheumatic fever, or Reiter's syndrome. It may be linked to allergies that cause redness of the skin. Treatment is with antibiotics.

Y fracture, a **Y**-shaped fracture between the rounded bumps (condyles) at the ends of bones.

Y-linked, referring to genes or to the traits or conditions they transmit that are carried on the Y chromosome. Compare **X-linked.**

Yodoxin, a trademark for a drug that destroys amebas (diiodohydroxyquin).

yogurt, a slightly acid, semisolid, curdled milk preparation. It is rich in vitamins of the B complex group and a good source of protein.

yolk, the material, rich in fats and proteins, in the egg (ovum) to supply nourishment to the developing embryo. The amount of the yolk within the egg depends on the species of animal. In humans and most mammals the yolk is absent or greatly spread through the cell. The reason is that embryos absorb nutrients directly from the mother through the placenta.

yolk sac, a structure that develops in the inner cell mass of the embryo and expands into a sac. After supplying the nourishment for the embryo, the yolk sac usually disappears during the seventh week of pregnancy. The **yolk stalk** is the narrow duct connecting the yolk sac with the embryo during the early stages of prenatal development.

Y-plasty, a method of surgical revision of a scar. It uses a **Y**-shaped incision to reduce scar contractures. See also **Z-plasty.**

Yutopar, a trademark for a drug used to stop premature labor (ritodrine hydrochloride).

T–Z

487

Z

Zahorsky's disease. See **roseola infantum.**

Zanosar, a trademark for a drug that prevents the formation of cancerous cells (streptozocin).

Zarontin, a trademark for a drug that prevents convulsions (ethosuximide).

Zaroxolyn, a trademark for a drug that lowers the blood pressure and increases urine release (metolazone).

Zenker's diverticulum, a bulging of part of the mucous membrane of the throat where it joins the esophagus. Food may become trapped in the bulge (diverticulum) and be breathed into the lungs. In most cases it is small, causes no problem, and requires no treatment.

Zentron, a trademark for a drug that improves the quality of blood. It has iron and vitamins.

Zephiran Chloride, a trademark for a disinfectant (benzalkonium chloride).

Zetar, a trademark for a drug used against eczema.

Zinacef, a trademark for a cephalosporin antibiotic (cefuroxime sodium).

zinc (Zn), a bluish-white crystal-like metal. It is an essential nutrient in the body and is used in numerous drugs, as zinc acetate, zinc oxide, zinc permanganate, and zinc stearate. Zinc acetate is used as a drug that causes vomiting and stops bleeding. Zinc oxide is used as a drug that prevents spasms. It is also used as a skin protective in ointments. Zinc permanganate is used to treat an inflammation of the urethra (urethritis). Zinc stearate is used to treat acne, eczema, and other skin diseases.

zinc deficiency, a condition resulting from a lack of zinc in the diet. It features abnormal weakness, decreased alertness, a decrease in taste and odor sensitivity, poor appetite, slowed growth, delayed sexual maturity, lengthy healing of wounds, and risk of infection and injury. Prevention and treatment are made up of a diet of foods high in protein that are also rich in zinc, including meats, eggs, liver, seafood, vegetables with pods, nuts, peanut butter, milk, and whole-grain cereals.

zinc gelatin, a protectant gel used for varicose veins and other lesions of the lower limbs.

zinc salt poisoning, a poisonous condition caused by eating or breathing a zinc salt. Symptoms include a burning sensation of the mouth and throat, vomiting, diarrhea, stomach and chest pain, and, in severe cases, shock and coma. Treatment includes washing out the stomach, followed by giving an oily drug. A drug is also given that binds zinc (calcium edetate). Fluid therapy is also given.

zinc sulfate, an eye drug that causes contractions. It is given in drops for nasal congestion or irritation of the eye. It is put on the skin in deodorants. It is given by mouth in tablets to promote healing and as a diet supplement.

zoanthropy /zō·an′thrəpē/, the false belief that one has the form and characteristics of an animal. −**zoanthropic,** *adj.*

Zollinger-Ellison syndrome, a condition marked by severe ulcers of the esophagus, stomach, or small intestines (duodenum), too much release of gastric juice, and a tumor of the pancreas or of the small intestine (duodenum). The disorder may occur in early childhood. However, it is seen more often in patients between 20 and 50 years of age. Two thirds of the tumors are cancerous. Total removal of the stomach (gastrectomy) may be necessary. See also **ulcer.**

zona pellucida /pəloo′sidə/, the thick, transparent membrane that encloses the egg (ovum). It is released by the ovum during its development in the ovary. It is kept until near the time of implantation. Also called **oolemma** /ō′əlem′ə/.

zone, an area with specific boundaries and traits, as the epigastric, the mesogastric, or the hypogastric zones of the stomach.

zonesthesia /zō′nesthē′zhə/, a painful sensation of constriction, as of a bandage bound too tightly. Also called **girdle sensation.**

zone therapy, the treatment of a disorder by stimulation and irritation of a body area in the same zone as the affected organ or region.

zonography /zōnog′rəfē/, an x-ray imaging technique. It is used to produce films of body sections similar to those made by tomography.

zonula ciliaris /zōn′yələ sil′ē·er′is/, a series of fibers connecting the ciliary body of the eye with the lens. It holds the lens in place. It relaxes by the contraction of the ciliary muscle. This allows the lens to become more rounded. See also **ciliary body, eye.**

zoology, the study of animal life.

zoonosis /zō′ənō′-, zō·on′əsis/, a disease of animals that can be carried to humans. Some kinds of zoonoses are **equine encephalitis, leptospirosis, rabies, yellow fever.**

zooparasite /zō′əper′əsīt/, any parasitic animal organism. Kinds of zooparasites are **arthropods, protozoa, worms.** –**zooparasitic,** *adj.*

zoophilia /zō′əfil′y·ə/, **1.** an abnormal fondness for animals. **2.** (in psychiatry) a sexual disorder in which sexual excitement and satisfaction come from fondling animals or from the fantasy or act of having sexual activity with animals.

zoophobia /zō′ə-/, an anxiety disorder. It is marked by a persistent, irrational fear of animals, particularly dogs, snakes, insects, and mice.

zoopsia /zō·op′sē·ə/, hallucination of seeing insects or other animals. This often occurs in mental disturbance with trembling linked to alcohol withdrawal (delirium tremens).

zootoxin /zō′ətok′sin/, a poisonous substance from an animal, such as the venom of snakes, spiders, and scorpions. –**zootoxic,** *adj.*

zoster. See **herpes zoster.**

zoster immune globulin (ZIG), a passive vaccinating drug for preventing or weakening herpes zoster virus infection in less resistant (immunosuppressed) persons who are at great risk of severe herpes zoster virus infection.

Zovirax, a trademark for an antiviral drug (acyclovir).

Z-plasty, a method of surgical revision of a scar or closure of a wound using a **Z**-shaped cut. This lessens abnormal shortening of muscle tissue of the nearby skin. See also Y-plasty.

zygoma /zīgō′mə, zig-/, **1.** a long slender projection from the temporal bone of the skull. **2.** the cheekbone (zygomatic bone).

zygomatic bone, one of the pair of bones that forms the area of the cheek.

zygomaticus major /-mat′ikəs/, one of the 12 muscles of the mouth. It is used to smile or laugh.

zygomaticus minor, one of the 12 muscles of the mouth. It is used in making a frown.

zygomycosis /-mīkō′-/, a serious, and sometimes deadly, fungal infection. It is caused by certain water molds. It is seen mainly in patients with long-term wasting diseases, especially uncontrolled diabetes mellitus. It often begins with fever and with pain and discharge from the nose. The fungus may invade the eye and the lower breathing tract, enter blood vessels, and spread to the brain and other organs. Treatment includes improved control of diabetes mellitus, extensive removal of tumors on the face and head, and drugs. Also called **mucormycosis.** Compare **phycomycosis.**

zygote /zī′gōt/, (in embryology) the developing egg (ovum) from the time it is fertilized until, as a blastocyst, it is implanted in the uterus.

Zyloprim, a trademark for a a drug that prevents xanthine oxidase (allopurinol).

-zyme, a combining form meaning a ferment or enzyme.

T–Z

APPENDIXES

1 *EMERGENCY MEDICAL SERVICES REFERENCE GUIDE*

1-1/MEDICAL TERMINOLOGY

STANDARD TERMS

Abduction .... Movement away from the body's midline

Adduction .... Movement toward the body's midline

Anterior or ventral .... The front surface of the body

Anterior to....................Situated infront of

Caudad .... Toward the tail end

Cephalad .... Toward the head

Circumduction...........Circular movement of a part, as an eye or limb

Craniad .... Toward the cranium

Deep .... Situated remote from the surface

Depression....................Lowering a body part

Distal .... Situated away from the point of origin

Dorsiflexion..... Bending backward, as the hand or foot

Elevation .... Raising a body part

Eversion ..... A turning outward of the soles of the feet

Extension...... Stretching, or moving jointed parts away from each other

External..........................Situated outside

Flexion .Bending, or moving jointed parts closer together

Inferior .... Situated below

Internal ....Situated inside

Inversion ...... A turning inward of the soles of the feet

Laterad .... Toward the side of the body

Lateral .... Situated away from the body's midline

Lateral rotation .... Rotating outward away from the body's midline

Left laterally recumbent .... Lying horizontal on the left side

Mediad .... Toward the midline of the body

Medial .... Situated toward the body's midline

Medial rotation .... Rotating inward toward the body's midline

Palmar .... The inner surface of the hand

Peripheral .... Away from a central structure

Plantar .... The sole of the foot

Plantar flexion.................... Extending the foot

Posterior or dorsal .... The back surface of the body

Posterior to .... Situated behind

Pronation .... Turning the hand so the palm faces downward or backward

Prone .... Lying horizontal, face down and flat

Protraction........ A pushing forward, as the mandible

Proximal .... Situated nearest the point of origin

Recumbent .... Lying horizontal, generally speaking

Retraction .... A drawing back, as the tongue

Right laterally recumbent .... Lying horizontal on the right side

Rotation.................... Turning around an axis

Superficial .... Situated near the surface

Superior.........................Situated above

Supination .... Turning the hand so the palm faces forward or upward

Supine ....Lying horizontal, flat on the back and face up

From Rescue Training Associates, Ltd, ACTION GUIDE FOR EMERGENCY SERVICE PERSONNEL, © 1985, pp 442–443 (A Brady Book). Reprinted by permission of Prentice-Hall, Inc, Englewood Cliffs, NJ.

1-2/MEDICAL PREFIXES AND SUFFIXES

Prefixes

A- .... No; not; without
A-; Ab- .... Away from
Ab- .... Deviating from normal
Ac- .... Pertaining to
Ac-; Ad-; Af-; Ag- .... Toward
Acu- .... A needle
Ambi- .... Both
Amph-; Amphi- .... Both
An- .... No; not; without
Ana- .... Up; again; backward
Anis- .... Unequal
Ant-; ante-; anter- .... Before; forward
Anti- .... Against
Ap- .... Toward
Apo- .... Upon
Ap-; at- .... Toward

Bi- .... Two
Brady- .... Slow
Brachy- .... Short

Cac-; caco- .... Bad; poor
Cat-; cata-; cath- .... Down; downward
Circum- .... Around
Co-; com-; con-; cor- .... With; together
Contra- .... Against

De- .... Lack of
Dec-; deca- .... Ten
Deci- .... Tenth
Demi- .... Half
Dextr- .... Right
Di- .... Two
Di- .... Double
Di-; dia- .... Complete; through
Di-; dia-; dis- .... Apart, away from
Dipl- .... Double
Dys- .... Bad; poor

E-; ec- .... Out; outside
Ect-; ecto- .... Outer; outside
Em- .... In

Prefixes

End- .... Inner; inside
Endo- .... Within
Ep-; epi- .... Over; upon
Eso- .... Inward
Eu- .... Good
Ex- .... From; out of
Ex-; Exo- .... Outside of; in addition to
Extra- .... Outside of; in addition to
Hect- .... One hundred
Hemi- .... Half
Hen- .... One
Hept- .... Seven
Heter-; hetero- .... Different
Hex- .... Six
Holo- .... All
Hyper- .... More than normal
Hypo- .... Less than normal

Il- .... Not
Im- .... Not
In- .... Not
Infra- .... Beneath, below; inferior
Inter- .... Between
Intra-; intro- .... Within
Ir- .... Not
Iso- .... Equal

Kil-; kilo- .... One thousand

Macro- .... Large
Mal- .... Bad; poor
Meso- .... Middle
Meta- .... After, beyond; change
Micro- .... Small
Multi- .... Much; many

Neo- .... New
Non- .... Nine
Nulli- .... None

Ob-; oc- .... Against; toward
Oct- .... Eight

From Rescue Training Associates, Ltd, ACTION GUIDE FOR EMERGENCY SERVICE PERSONNEL, © 1985, pp 443–445 (A Brady Book).
Reprinted by permission of Prentice-Hall, Inc, Englewood Cliffs, NJ.

Continued.

1-2/Medical Prefixes and Suffixes — cont'd

Prefixes

Para-	Beside; near
Pent-	Five
Per-	Through
Peri-	Around
Poly-	Much; many
Post-	After; behind
Pre-	In front of; before
Pro-	Before
Quadri-	Four
Quinque-	Five
Re-	Back
Retro-	Behind
Semi-	Half
Sub-	Under; below
Suf-	Under; below
Sup-	Under; below
Supa-	Above
Sym-; syn-	Joined together
Tachy-	Fast
Tetra-	Four
Trans-	Across; over
Tri-	Three
Uni-	One
Ultra-	Beyond

Suffixes

-Ac	Pertaining to
-Agogue	Leading; introducing
-Agra	Excessive pain
-Al	Pertaining to
-Algesia	Oversensitivity to pain
-Algia	Painful condition
-Ar	Pertaining to
-Arche	Beginning
-Ary	Pertaining to
-Ase	Enzyme
-Asthenia	Weakness
-Blast	Embryonic; immature

Suffixes

-Capnia	Carbon dioxide
-Cele	Herniation; tumor; cyst
-Centesis	Surgical puncture
-Chalasis	Relaxation
-Cidal	Killing
-Cide	Destruction; killing
-Cipient	Receiver
-Cise	Cut
-Clasis; -clast	Break
-Clysis	Irrigation; washing
-Coccus	Berry-shaped
-Crescent	Grow
-Crine	Secrete; separate
-Crit	Separate
-Cusis	Hearing
-Cyesis	Pregnancy
-Cyte	Cell
-Cytosis	Condition of cells
-Desis	Binding together
-Drome	Run
-Dynia	Painful condition
-Dys	Bad; painful; difficult
-Eal	Pertaining to
-Ectasia	Dilation
-Ectomy	Surgical removal
-Emesis	Vomiting
-Emia	Condition of the blood
-Er	One who
-Ferent	Bearing
-Ferous	Bearing
-Form	Shape
-Fugal; -fuge	Driving away
-Fusion	Pour
-Genic	Produced by or in
-Globin; globulin	Protein
-Grade	Go
-Gram	A recording
-Graph	Device for recording
-Graphy	Procedure for recording
-Ia; -iasis	Condition; process
-Iac; -ic	Pertaining to
-Ion	Process

Continued.

1-2/Medical Prefixes and Suffixes—cont'd

Suffixes		Suffixes	
-Ior	Pertaining to	-Phonia	Voice; sound
-Ism	Process	-Phoresis	Transmission
-Ist	Specialist	-Phoria	Feeling (mental state)
-Itis	Irritation; inflammation	-Phylaxis	Prevention
-Ium	Structure; tissue	-Physis	Grow; growth
		-Phyte	Plant
-Llema	Sheath; covering	-Plasia	Growth
-Logist	One who studies	-Plasty	Surgical repair
-Logy	Study	-Plegia	Paralysis
-Lysis	Destruction; killing	-Pnea	Respiration
-Lytic	Reduce; destroy	-Poesis	Formation
		-Porosis	Passage
-Malacia	Softening	-Prandial	Meal
-Mania	Obsessive preoccupation	-Praxia	Action
-Megaly	Enlargement	-Ptosis	Prolapse
-Meter	Measure	-Ptysis	Spitting
-Metry	Procedure for measuring		
-Mimetic	Mimic; copy	-Rrhage; -rrhagia	Profuse flow of blood
-Mittent	Sending	-Rrhaphy	Suture
		-Rrhea	Profuse flow
-Oid	Resembling	-Rrhexis	Rupture
-Ole	Little; small		
-Oma	Tumor	-Salpinx	Fallopian tubes
-Opia	Vision	-Schisis	Split
-Opsy	View	-Sclerosis	Hardening
-Or	One who	-Scope	Device for examining visually
-Ose	Pertaining to	-Scopy	Visual examination
-Osis	Abnormal condition	-Sect	Cut
-Osmia	Smell	-Sis	Condition
-Ostomy	Creation of a new opening	-Somnia	Sleep
-Otomy	Surgical incision	-Spasm	Contraction of muscles
-Ous	Pertaining to	-Sphyxia	Pulse
		-Stalsis	Contraction
-Para	Births (viable offspring)	-Stasis	Maintenance of a constant level
-Paresis	Slight paralysis	-Stenosis	Tightening; Stricture
-Partum	Birth; labor	-Sthenia	Strength
-Pathy	Disease process	-Stomy	New opening
-Paresis	Weakness		
-Pellent	Drive	-Therapy	Treatment
-Penia	Deficiency	-Thorax	Chest
-Pepsia	Digestion	-Thymia	Mind
-Pexy	Surgical fixation	-Tic	Pertaining to
-Phagia	Eating; swallowing	-Tocia	Labor; birth
-Pheresis	Removal	-Tocin	Labor; birth
-Philia	Affinity for	-Tome	Instrument for cutting
-Phobia	Abnormal fear	-Tomy	Process of cutting

Continued.

1-2/Medical Prefixes and Suffixes — cont'd

Suffixes

-Tresia . . . . Opening
-Tripsy . . . . Surgical crushing
-Trophy . . . . Development; nourishment
-Tropia . . . . Turn
-Tropin . . . . Nourish; develop; stimulate

Suffixes

-Ule . . . . Small; little
-Um . . . . Structure; tissue
-Uresis . . . . Urinary excretion
-Uria . . . . Condition of urine

-Version . . . . Turn

1-3/METRIC CONVERSIONS

Mass (Weight)

When you know . . .	Multiply by . . .	To find . . .
Ounces (oz)	28.0	Grams (g)
Pounds (lb)	0.45	Kilograms (kg)
Short tons (2000 lb)	0.9	Metric ton (t)
Grams (g)	0.035	Ounces (oz)
Kilograms (kg)	2.2	Pounds (lb)
Metric ton (1000 kg)	1.1	Short tons

Volume

When you know . . .	Multiply by . . .	To find . . .
Teaspoon (tsp)	5.0	Milliliters (mL)
Tablespoons (Tbsp)	15.0	Milliliters (mL)
Cubic inches (in^3)	16.0	Milliliters (mL)
Fluid ounces (fl oz)	30.0	Milliliters (mL)
Cups (c)	0.24	Liters (L)
Pints (pt)	0.47	Liters (L)
Quarts (qt)	0.95	Liters (L)
Gallons (gal)	3.8	Liters (L)
Cubic feet (ft^3)	0.03	Cubic meters (m^3)
Cubic yards (yd^3)	0.76	Cubic meters (m^3)
Milliliters (mL)	0.03	Fluid ounces (fl oz)
Milliliters (mL)	0.06	Cubic inches (in^3)
Liters (L)	2.1	Pints (pt)
Liters (L)	1.06	Quarts (qt)
Liters (L)	0.26	Gallons (gal)
Cubic meters (m^3)	35.0	Cubic feet (ft^3)
Cubic meters (m^3)	1.3	Cubic yards (yd^3)

Temperature

When you know . . .	Multiply by . . .	To find . . .
Degrees Fahrenheit (°F)	5/9 (after subtracting 32)	Degrees Celsius (°C)
Degrees Celsius (°C)	9/5 (then add 32)	Degrees Fahrenheit (°F)

From Rescue Training Associates, Ltd, ACTION GUIDE FOR EMERGENCY SERVICE PERSONNEL, © 1985, pp 453–454 (A Brady Book). Reprinted by permission of Prentice-Hall, Inc, Englewood Cliffs, NJ.

1-4/ADULT SKELETON—FRONT

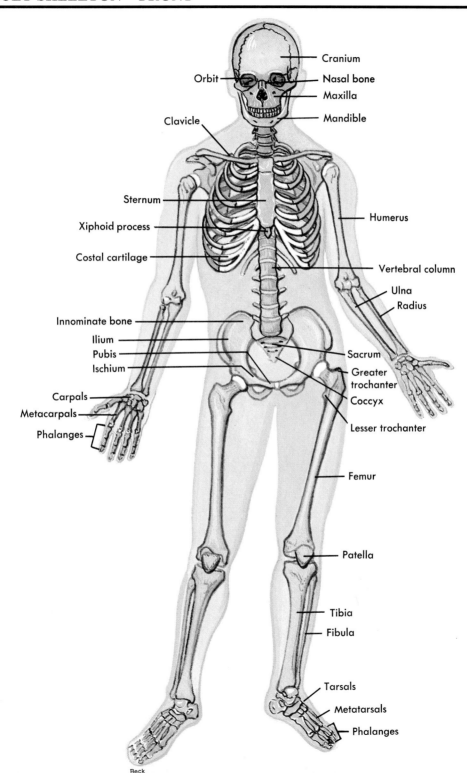

Cranium

Orbit

Nasal bone

Maxilla

Mandible

Clavicle

Sternum

Humerus

Xiphoid process

Costal cartilage

Vertebral column

Ulna

Radius

Innominate bone

Ilium

Pubis

Sacrum

Ischium

Greater trochanter

Carpals

Coccyx

Metacarpals

Lesser trochanter

Phalanges

Femur

Patella

Tibia

Fibula

Tarsals

Metatarsals

Phalanges

Beck

1-5/ADULT SKELETON—REAR

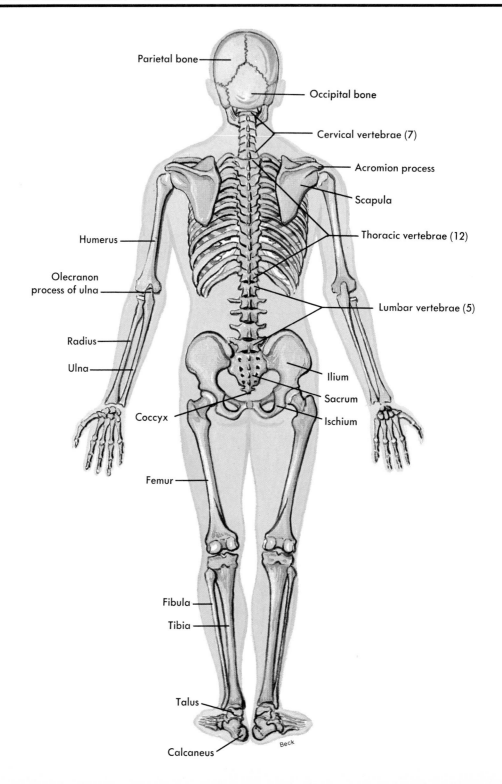

Parietal bone

Occipital bone

Cervical vertebrae (7)

Acromion process

Scapula

Thoracic vertebrae (12)

Humerus

Olecranon
process of ulna

Lumbar vertebrae (5)

Radius

Ulna

Ilium

Sacrum

Coccyx

Ischium

Femur

Fibula

Tibia

Talus

Calcaneus

Beck

1-6/FRONT AND SIDE VIEW OF SKULL

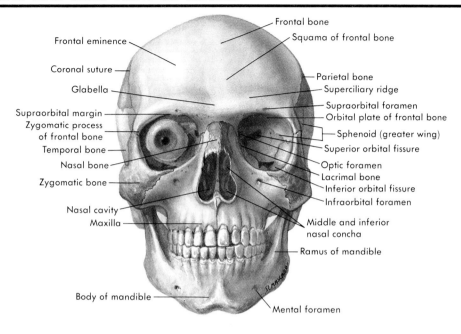

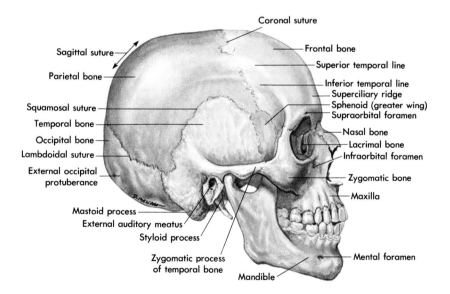

1-7/THORAX, RIBS, AND PELVIS

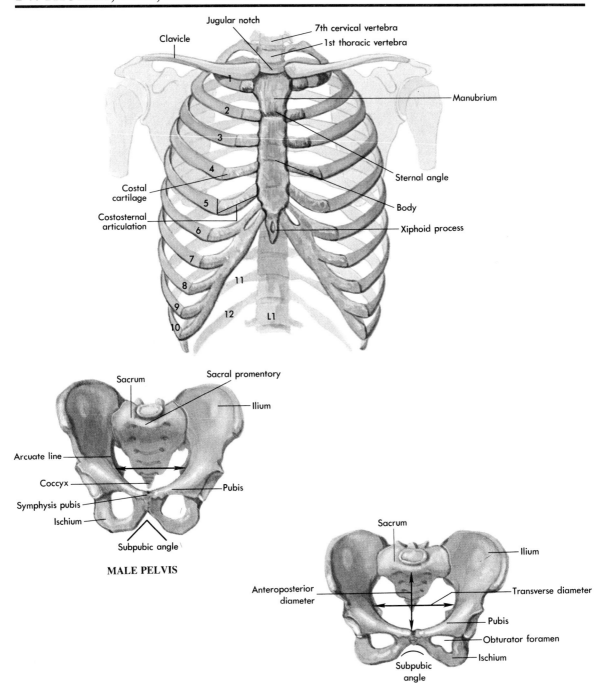

MALE PELVIS

FEMALE PELVIS

1-8/PRINCIPAL VEINS AND ARTERIES

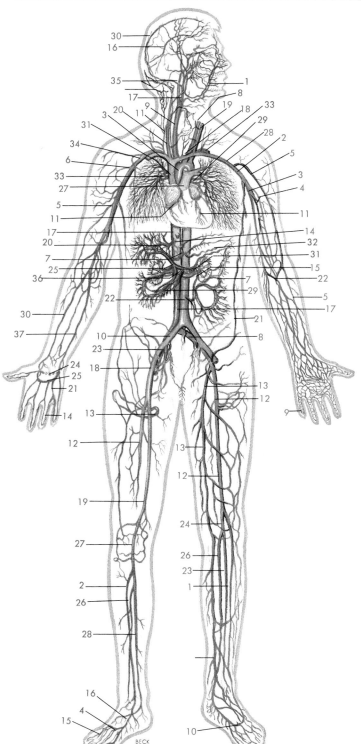

PRINCIPAL VEINS AND ARTERIES

Principal arteries

1 Angular
2 Anterior tibial
3 Aorta
4 Arcuate
5 Axillary
6 Brachial
7 Celiac
8 Common carotid, left
9 Common carotid, right
10 Common iliac, right
11 Coronary, left
12 Deep femoral
13 Deep medial
  circumflex femoral
14 Digital
15 Dorsal metatarsal
16 Dorsalis pedis
17 External carotid
18 External iliac
19 Femoral
20 Hepatic
21 Metacarpal
22 Inferior mesenteric
23 Internal iliac
  (hypogastric)
24 Palmar arch, deep
25 Palmar arch, superficial
26 Peroneal
27 Popliteal
28 Posterior tibial
29 Pulmonary
30 Radial
31 Renal
32 Splenic
33 Subclavian, left (cut)
34 Subclavian, right
35 Superficial temporal
36 Superior mesenteric
37 Ulnar

Principal veins

1 Anterior tibial
2 Axillary
3 Basilic
4 Brachial
5 Cephalic
6 Cervical plexus
7 Colic
8 Common iliac, left
9 Digital
10 Dorsal venous arch
11 External jugular
12 Femoral
13 Great saphenous
14 Hepatic
15 Inferior mesenteric
16 Inferior sagittal sinus
17 Inferior vena cava
18 Brachiocephalic, left
19 Internal jugular, left
20 Internal jugular, right
21 Lateral thoracic
22 Median cubital
23 Peroneal
24 Popliteal
25 Portal
26 Posterior tibial
27 Pulmonary
28 Subclavian, left
29 Superior mesenteric
30 Superior sagittal sinus
31 Superior vena cava

APPEN-DIX

1-9/CORONARY VESSELS—FRONTAL

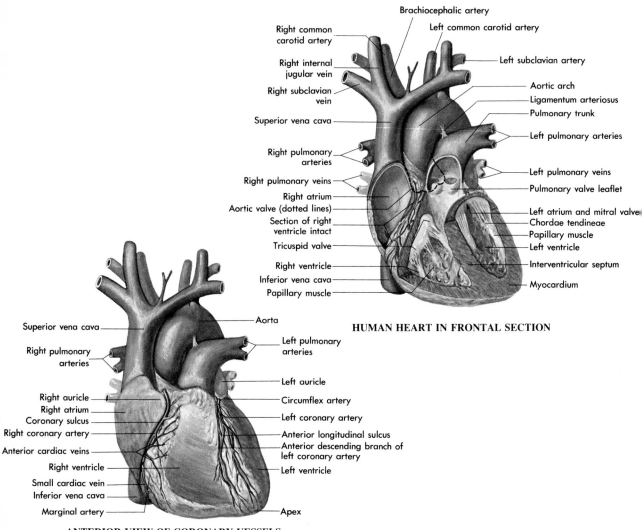

HUMAN HEART IN FRONTAL SECTION

ANTERIOR VIEW OF CORONARY VESSELS

1-10/LYMPHATIC SYSTEM

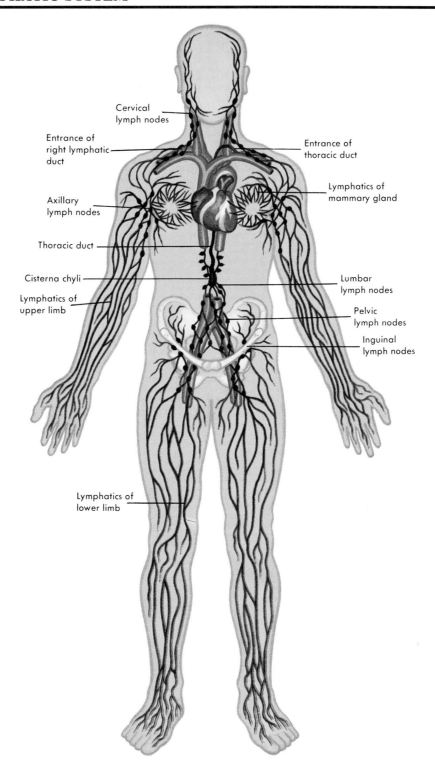

Cervical
lymph nodes

Entrance of
right lymphatic
duct

Entrance of
thoracic duct

Axillary
lymph nodes

Lymphatics of
mammary gland

Thoracic duct

Cisterna chyli

Lumbar
lymph nodes

Lymphatics of
upper limb

Pelvic
lymph nodes

Inguinal
lymph nodes

Lymphatics of
lower limb

1-11/RESPIRATORY SYSTEM

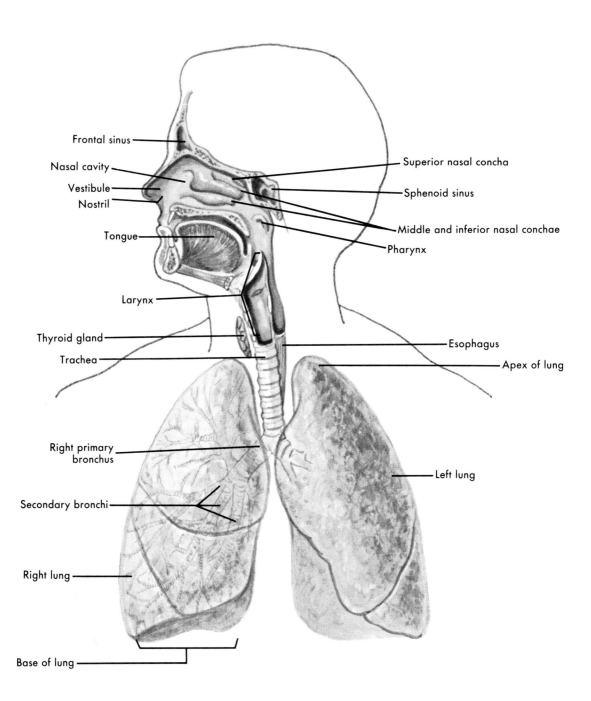

Frontal sinus

Nasal cavity

Vestibule

Nostril

Tongue

Larynx

Thyroid gland

Trachea

Right primary bronchus

Secondary bronchi

Right lung

Base of lung

Superior nasal concha

Sphenoid sinus

Middle and inferior nasal conchae

Pharynx

Esophagus

Apex of lung

Left lung

1-12/STRUCTURES OF THE LARYNX AND UPPER TRACHEA

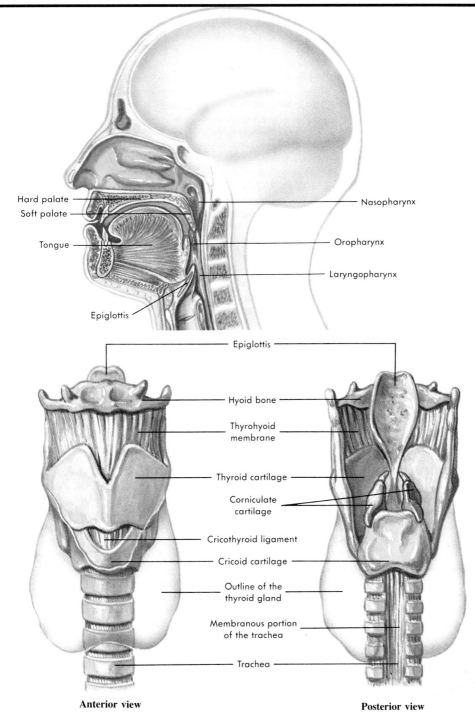

Hard palate
Soft palate
Tongue
Epiglottis
Nasopharynx
Oropharynx
Laryngopharynx

Epiglottis
Hyoid bone
Thyrohyoid membrane
Thyroid cartilage
Corniculate cartilage
Cricothyroid ligament
Cricoid cartilage
Outline of the thyroid gland
Membranous portion of the trachea
Trachea

Anterior view

Posterior view

1-13/DIGESTIVE SYSTEM

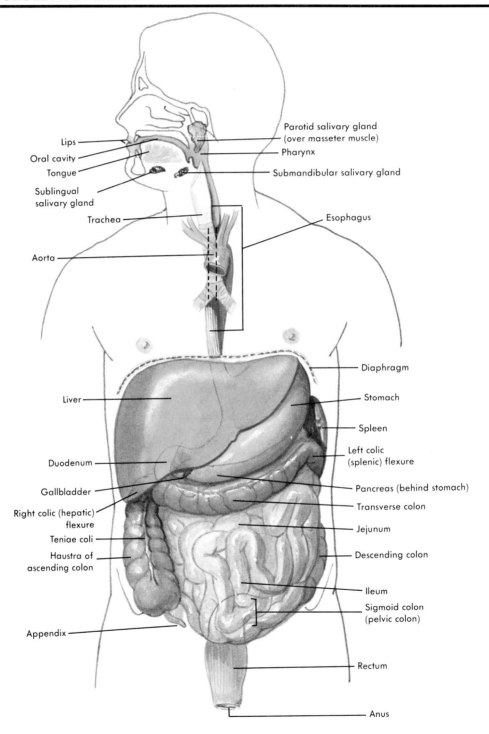

1-14/URINARY SYSTEM

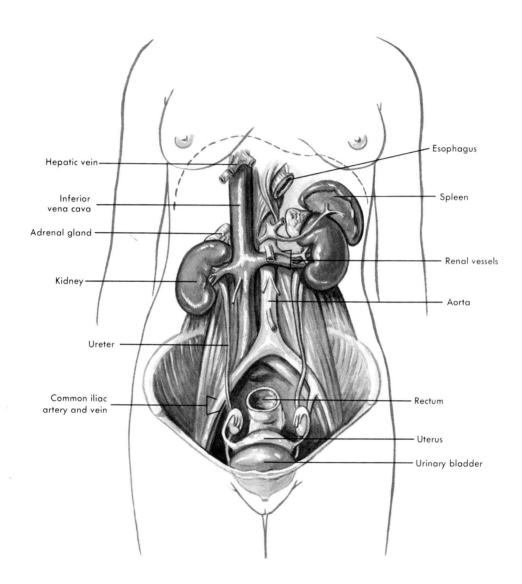

Hepatic vein

Inferior vena cava

Adrenal gland

Kidney

Ureter

Common iliac artery and vein

Esophagus

Spleen

Renal vessels

Aorta

Rectum

Uterus

Urinary bladder

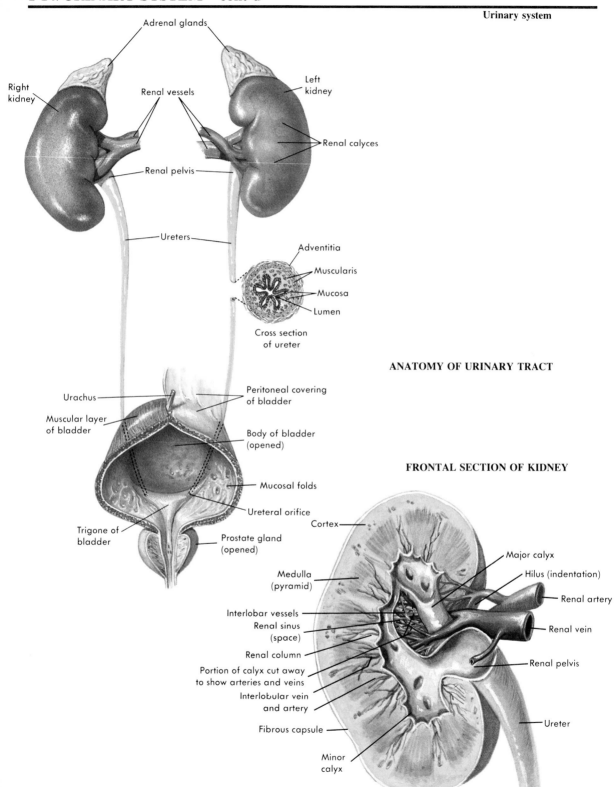

Adrenal glands

Right kidney

Renal vessels

Left kidney

Renal calyces

Renal pelvis

Ureters

Adventitia

Muscularis

Mucosa

Lumen

Cross section of ureter

ANATOMY OF URINARY TRACT

Urachus

Peritoneal covering of bladder

Muscular layer of bladder

Body of bladder (opened)

FRONTAL SECTION OF KIDNEY

Mucosal folds

Ureteral orifice

Trigone of bladder

Prostate gland (opened)

Cortex

Major calyx

Hilus (indentation)

Renal artery

Medulla (pyramid)

Renal vein

Interlobar vessels

Renal sinus (space)

Renal pelvis

Renal column

Portion of calyx cut away to show arteries and veins

Interlobular vein and artery

Ureter

Fibrous capsule

Minor calyx

1-15/GROSS ANATOMY OF THE EAR—FRONTAL

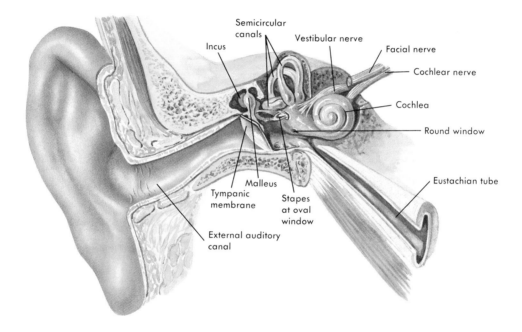

1-16/CROSS-SECTIONAL VIEW OF THE EYE

Sight

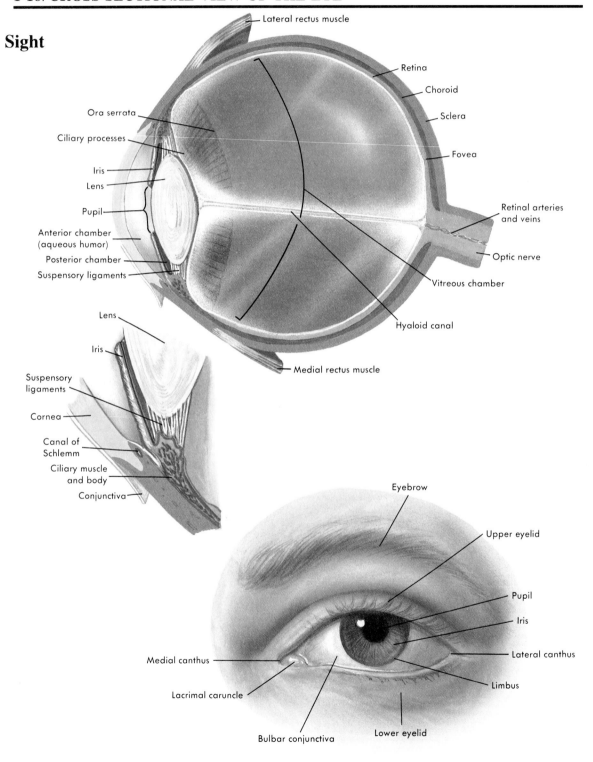

1-17/SKIN PROTECTION AND TOUCH

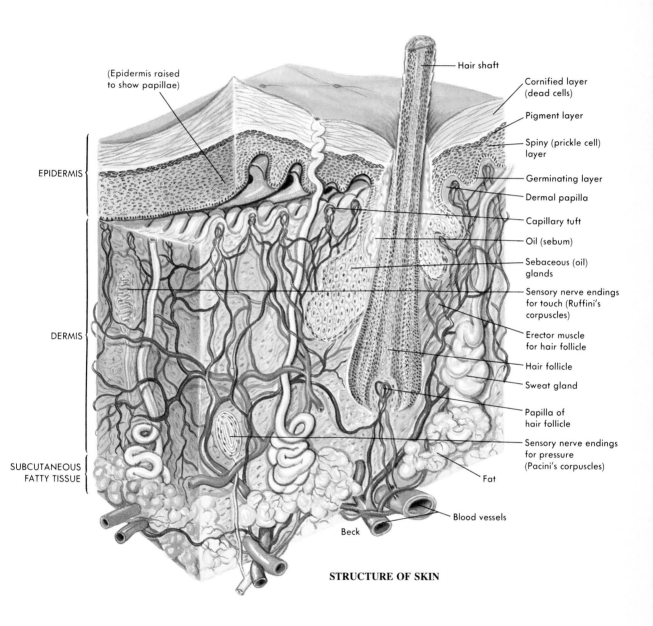

(Epidermis raised
to show papillae)

Hair shaft

Cornified layer
(dead cells)

Pigment layer

Spiny (prickle cell)
layer

EPIDERMIS

Germinating layer

Dermal papilla

Capillary tuft

Oil (sebum)

Sebaceous (oil)
glands

Sensory nerve endings
for touch (Ruffini's
corpuscles)

DERMIS

Erector muscle
for hair follicle

Hair follicle

Sweat gland

Papilla of
hair follicle

Sensory nerve endings
for pressure
(Pacini's corpuscles)

SUBCUTANEOUS
FATTY TISSUE

Fat

Blood vessels

Beck

STRUCTURE OF SKIN

1-18/USA POISON CONTROL CENTERS

UNITED STATES*
Poison control centers and state coordinators

The location and telephone numbers of poison control centers operating in the United States as of October 1982 and state poison control coordinators are listed in alphabetic order of city or town within state. The listing was compiled from information supplied to the Poisoning Surveillance and Epidemiology Branch (HFN 720) (United States Food and Drug Administration, National Center for Drugs and Biologics, Office of Drugs) by poison control centers, organizations representing them, and state public health agencies. Before they were listed in the Directory, each of the institutions identified as a poison control center was contacted by the Division of Poison Control to verify that it was active. The first poison control center began operating in Chicago in 1953 with the number increasing to over 600 nationwide in

*Provided by U.S. Department of Health and Human Services, Food and Drug Administration, Office of Drugs, Poisoning Surveillance and Epidemiology Branch, 5600 Fishers Lane, Rockville, MD 20857.

health professionals in cases of known or suspected poisoning by providing information on the appropriate first aid and clinical management. They may also offer specialized poisoning treatment and consultative services, professional training, and poisoning prevention education for consumers. In recent years, the number of small centers, most of them based in local hospital emergency rooms, has been declining due to their replacement with large regional poison control centers that serve populations of several million and provide more comprehensive services.

Organizations and agencies

A listing of private, professional, and public service organizations and federal agencies dealing in prevention, treatment, and control of poisoning.

Poison prevention materials

A listing of sources of poison prevention educational materials and resources compiled by the Poison Prevention Week Council.

Directory of centers

State coordinators and cities	Address	Telephone	Comments
ALABAMA			
State Coordinator	Department of Public Health Montgomery, AL 36117	(205) 832-3194 832-3935	
Birmingham	The Children's Hospital of Birmingham 1601 6th Ave., S. Birmingham, AL 35233	(205) 933-4050 (800) 292-6678 (statewide)	
Tuscaloosa	The Alabama Poison Control Center Druid City Hospital 809 University Blvd., E. Tuscaloosa, AL 34501	(205) 345-0600 (800) 462-0800 (statewide)	
ALASKA			
State Coordinator	Department of Health and Social Services Juneau, AK 99811	(907) 465-3100	
Anchorage	Anchorage Poison Center Providence Hospital 3200 Providence Dr. Anchorage, AK 99504	(907) 274-6535	

A, Center meets the American Association of Poison Control Centers' criteria for designation as a Regional Poison Control Center. This is a voluntary program, and negative inferences about the quality and level of service offered by a center should not be drawn from the absence of regional center designation. *x,* Calls to center go through hospital switchboard.

State coordinators and cities	Address	Telephone	Comments
Fairbanks	Fairbanks Poison Center Fairbanks Memorial Hospital 1650 Cowles Fairbanks, AK 99701	(907) 456-7182	
ARIZONA			
State Coordinator	Arizona Poison Control System University of Arizona College of Pharmacy Tucson, AZ 85724	(602) 626-6016 (800) 362-0101 (statewide)	
Flagstaff	Flagstaff Hospital and Medical Center of N. Arizona 1215 N. Beaver St. Flagstaff, AZ 86001	(602) 779-0555	
Phoenix	St. Lukes Hospital and Medical Center 525 N. 18th St. Phoenix, AZ 85006	(602) 253-3334	
Tucson	Arizona Poison and Drug Information Center Arizona Health Sciences Center University of Arizona Tucson, AZ 85724	(602) 626-6016 (800) 362-0101 (statewide)	A
ARKANSAS			
State Coordinator	Division of Environmental Health Protection Arkansas Department of Health Little Rock, AR 72201	(501) 661-2301	
El Dorado	Warner Brown Hospital Emergency Room 460 W. Oak St. El Dorado, AR 71730	(501) 863-2266	
Fort Smith	St. Edward Mercy Medical Center Emergency Room 7301 Rogers Ave. Fort Smith, AR 72904	(501) 452-5100 ext. 2401	x
	Sparks Regional Medical Center Emergency Room 1311 S. "I" St. Fort Smith, AR 72902	(501) 441-5011	
Harrison	Boone County Hospital Emergency Room 620 N. Willow St. Harrison, AR 72601	(501) 741-6141 ext. 275	x
Helena	Helena Hospital Emergency Room Hi-way 49 By Pass Helena, AR 72342	(501) 338-6411 ext. 340	x
Little Rock	University of Arkansas Medical Center Emergency Room 4301 W. Markham St. Little Rock, AR 72201	(501) 661-6161	
	Statewide Poison Control Drug Info. Ctr. U.A.M. Sc. College of Pharmacy Slot 522 4301 W. Markham St. Little Rock, AR 72205 Pulaski Co.	(800) 428-8948	
Osceola	Osceola Memorial Hospital Emergency Room 611 Lee Ave., W. Osceola, AR 72370	(501) 563-7182 or (501) 563-3174	

Continued.

Directory of centers — cont'd

State coordinators and cities	Address	Telephone	Comments
Pine Bluff	Jefferson Regional Medical Center Emergency Department 1515 W. 42nd Ave. Pine Bluff, AR 71601	(501) 541-7111 or (501) 541-7100 ext. 5350	
CALIFORNIA			
State Coordinator	Emergency Medical Services Authority 1600 Ninth St., Room 460 Sacramento, CA 95814	(916) 322-4336	
Fresno	Central Valley Regional Poison Control Center Fresno Community Hospital Fresno & R Sts. Fresno, CA 93715	(209) 445-1222	
Los Angeles	Los Angeles County Medical Association Regional Poison Information Center 1925 Wilshire Blvd. Los Angeles, CA 90057	(213) 484-5151	
Oakland	Children's Hospital Medical Center of N. California 51st & Grove Sts. Oakland, CA 94609	(415) 428-3248	
Orange	University of California Irvine Medical Center 101 City Dr., Route 32 Orange, CA 92688	(714) 634-5988	
Sacramento	Sacramento Medical Ctr. Univ. California at Davis Poison Control Center 2315 Stockton Blvd. Sacramento, CA 95817	(916) 453-3692 (800) 852-7221 (N. CA)	A
San Diego	San Diego Regional Poison Center Univ. California at San Diego Medical Center 225 W. Dickinson St. San Diego, CA 92103	(619) 294-6000	A
San Francisco	San Francisco Bay Area Regional Poison Control Center Room 1E 86 San Francisco General Hospital 1001 Potrero Ave. San Francisco, CA 94110	(415) 666-2845 (800) 792-0720 (N. CA)	A
San Jose	Central-Coast Counties Regional Poison Control Center Santa Clara Valley Medical Center 751 S. Bascom Ave. San Jose, Ca 95128	(408) 279-5112 (800) 662-9886 (statewide)	
COLORADO			
State Coordinator	Department of Health Emergency Medical Services Division 4210 E. 11th Ave. Denver, CO 80220	(303) 320-8476	
Denver	Rocky Mountain Poison Center Denver General Hospital W. 8th Ave. & Cherokee Sts. Denver, CO 80204	(303) 629-1123 (800) 332-3073	A
CONNECTICUT			
State Coordinator	University of Connecticut Health Center Farmington, CT 06032	(203) 674-3456	

State coordinators and cities	Address	Telephone	Comments
Bridgeport	Bridgeport Hospital 267 Grant St. Bridgeport, CT 06602	(203) 384-3566	
	St. Vincent's Medical Center 2800 Main St. Bridgeport, CT 06606	(203) 576-5178	
Danbury	Danbury Hospital 95 Locust Ave. Danbury, CT 06810	(203) 797-7300	
Farmington	Connecticut Poison Control Center University of Connecticut Health Center Farmington, CT 06032	(203) 674-3456	
Middletown	Middlesex Memorial Hospital 28 Crescent St. Middletown, CT 06457	(203) 344-6684	
New Haven	The Hospital of St. Raphael 1450 Chapel St. New Haven, CT 06511	(203) 789-3464	
	Yale–New Haven Hospital Emergency Service 20 York St. New Haven, CT 06510	(203) 785-8958	
Norwalk	Department of Emergency Medicine Norwalk Hospital Maple St. Norwalk, CT 06856	(203) 852-2160	
Waterbury	St. Mary's Hospital Emergency Room 56 Franklin St. Waterbury, CT 06702	(203) 574-6011	

DELAWARE

State Coordinator	Wilmington Medical Center Delaware Division Wilmington, DE 19801	(302) 655-3389	
Wilmington	Wilmington Medical Center Delaware Division 501 W. 14th St. Wilmington, DE 19899	(302) 655-3389	

DISTRICT OF COLUMBIA

Washington	National Capitol Poison Center Georgetown University Hospital 3800 Reservoir Rd. Washington, DC 20007	(202) 625-3333	A

FLORIDA

State Coordinator	Department of Health and Rehabilitative Services Office of Emergency Medical Services Tallahassee, FL 32301	(904) 487-1566	
Bradenton	Manatee Memorial Hospital 206 Second St., E. Bradenton, FL 33505	(813) 748-2121	
Daytona Beach	Halifax Hospital Emergency Department P.O. Box 1990 Daytona Beach, FL 32014	(904) 258-1513	

Continued.

Directory of Centers—cont'd

State coordinators and cities	Address	Telephone	Comments
Ft. Lauderdale	Broward General Medical Center Poison Control Center 1600 S. Andrews Ave. Ft. Lauderdale, FL 33316	(305) 463-3131 ext. 1955/6	x
Fort Myers	Lee Memorial Hospital 2776 Cleveland Ave. P.O. Drawer 2218 Fort Myers, FL 33902	(813) 334-5287	
Ft. Walton Beach	General Hospital of Ft. Walton Beach 1000 Mar-Walt Dr. Ft. Walton Beach, FL 32548	(904) 862-1111 ext. 106	x
Gainesville	Shands Teaching Hospital and Clinics University of Florida Gainesville, FL 32610	(904) 392-3389	
Inverness	Citrus Memorial Hospital 502 Highland Blvd. Inverness, FL 32650	(904) 726-2800	
Jacksonville	St. Vincent's Medical Ctr. P.O. Box 2982 Jacksonville, FL 32203	(904) 387-7500 387-7499 (TTY)	
Lakeland	Lakeland Regional Medical Center Lakeland General Hospital Lakeland Hills Blvd. Lakeland, FL 33802	(813) 687-1137	
Leesburg	Leesburg Regional Medical Center 600 E. Dixie Leesburg, FL 32748	(904) 787-9900	
Melbourne	James E. Holmes Regional Medical Center Emergency Department 1350 S. Hickory St. Melbourne, FL 32901	(305) 727-7000 ext. 675	x
Naples	Naples Community Hospital 350 7th St., N. Naples, FL 33940	(813) 262-3131	x
Ocala	Munroe Regional Medical Center 131 S.W. 15th St. Ocala, FL 32670	(904) 351-7607	
Orlando	Orlando Regional Medical Center Orange Memorial Division 1414 S. Kuhl Ave. Orlando, FL 32806	(305) 841-5222	
Pensacola	Gulf Region Poison Center Baptist Hospital P.O. Box 17500 Pensacola, FL 32522	(904) 434-4611 (800) 874-1555 (out of state) (800) 342-3222 (statewide)	
Punta Gorda	Medical Center Hospital 809 E. Marion Ave. Punta Gorda, FL 33950	(813) 637-2529	
Rockledge	Wuesthoff Memorial Hospital 110 Longwood Ave. Rockledge, FL 32955	(305) 636-4357	
St. Petersburg	Bay Front Medical Center, Inc. 701 6th St., S. St. Petersburg, FL 33701	(800) 282-3171 (statewide)	
Sarasota	Memorial Hospital 1901 Arlington St. Sarasota, FL 33579	(813) 953-1332	

State coordinators and cities	Address	Telephone	Comments
Tallahassee	Tallahassee Memorial Regional Medical Center 1300 Miccosukee Rd. Tallahassee, FL 32304	(904) 681-5411	
Tampa	Tampa Bay Regional Poison Control Center Tampa General Hospital Davis Island Tampa, FL 33606	(813) 251-6995 (800) 282-3171 (statewide)	
Titusville	Jess Parrish Memorial Hospital 951 N. Washington Ave. P.O. Drawer W Titusville, FL 32780	(305) 268-6260	
West Palm Beach	Good Samaritan Hospital Palm Beach Lakes Blvd. West Palm Beach, FL 33402	(305) 655-5511 ext. 4250	x
Winter Haven	Poison Control Center Winter Haven Hospital, Inc. 200 Avenue F., N.E. Winter Haven, FL 33880	(813) 299-9701	

GEORGIA

State coordinators and cities	Address	Telephone	Comments
State Coordinator	Department of Human Resources Emergency Health Section Atlanta, GA 30303	(404) 894-5170	
Albany	Phoebe Putney Memorial Hospital 417 Third Ave. Albany, GA 31705	(912) 888-4150	
Athens	Athens General Hospital 1199 Prince Ave. Athens, GA 30613	(404) 543-5215	
Atlanta	Georgia Poison Control Center Grady Memorial Hospital Box 26066 80 Butler St., S.E. Atlanta, GA 30305	(404) 588-4400 (800) 282-5846 (statewide) (404) 525-3323 (TTY)	A
Augusta	University Hospital 1350 Walton Way Augusta, GA 30902	(404) 724-5050	
Columbus	The Medical Center 710 Center St. Columbus, GA 31902	(404) 571-1080	
Macon	Medical Center of Central Georgia Regional Poison Control Center 777 Hemlock St. Macon, GA 31201	(912) 744-1427	
Rome	Floyd Hospital Turner McCall Blvd. Rome, GA 31061	(404) 295-5500	x
Savannah	Savannah Regional EMS Poison Center Dept. of Emergency Medicine Memorial Medical Center P.O. Box 23089 Savannah, GA 31403	(912) 355-5228	
Thomasville	John D. Archbold Memorial Hospital 900 Gordon Ave. Thomasville, GA 31792	(912) 226-4121 ext. 169	x
Valdosta	South Georgia Medical Center P.O. Box 1727 Valdosta, GA 31603	(912) 333-1110	

Continued.

Directory of Centers — cont'd

State coordinators and cities	Address	Telephone	Comments
Waycross	Memorial Hospital 410 Darling Ave. Waycross, GA 31501	(912) 283-3030	x
GUAM			
State Coordinator	Guam Memorial Hospital P.O. Box AX Agana, Guam 96910	646-5801	
Agana	Pharmacy Service, Box 7667 U.S. Naval Regional Medical Center (Guam) FPO San Francisco, CA 96630	344-9265 9354	
HAWAII			
State Coordinator	Department of Health Honolulu, HI 96801	(808) 531-7776	
Honolulu	Kapiolani-Children's Medical Center 1319 Punahou St. Honolulu, HI 96826	(808) 941-4411 (808) 362-3585	
IDAHO			
State Coordinator	Department of Health & Welfare Boise, ID 83720	(208) 334-4245	
Boise	Idaho Emergency Medical Poison Center 1055 N. Curtis Rd. Boise, ID 83706	(208) 334-2241 (800) 632-8000 (statewide)	
Idaho Falls	Consolidated Hospitals Emergency Department 900 Memorial Dr. Idaho Falls, ID 83401	(208) 522-3600	
Pocatello	Idaho Drug Information Service and Poison Control Center Pocatello Regional Medical Center 777 Hospital Way Pocatello, ID 83202	(208) 234-0777 ext. 2019 (800) 632-9490 (statewide)	x
ILLINOIS			
State Coordinator	Division of Emergency Medical Services and High- way Safety Springfield, IL 62761	(217) 785-2080	
Chicago	Rush Presbyterian-St. Luke's Poison Center Rush Presbyterian-St. Luke's Medical Center 1753 W. Congress Pkwy. Chicago, IL 60612	(312) 942-5969 (800) 942-5969 (Chicago and N.E. Illinois)	
Peoria	Peoria Poison Center St. Francis Hospital and Medical Center 530 N.E. Glen Oak Ave. Peoria, IL 61637	(309) 672-2334 (800) 322-5330 (Northern and Central Illi- nois)	
Springfield	Central & Southern Illinois Poison Resource Center St. John's Hospital 800 E. Carpenter Springfield, IL 62769	(217) 753-3330 (800) 252-2022 (statewide)	A
INDIANA			
State Coordinator	Indiana State Board of Health Hazardous Products Section and Division of Drug Control P.O. Box 1964 Indianapolis, IN 46206	(317) 633-0332	

State coordinators and cities	Address	Telephone	Comments
Anderson	Community Hospital 1515 N. Madison Ave. Anderson, IN 46012	(317) 646-5143	
	St. John's Hickey Memorial Hospital 2015 Jackson St. Anderson, IN 46014	(317) 646-8222	
Angola	Cameron Memorial Hospital, Inc. 416 E. Maumee St. Angola, IN 46703	(219) 665-2141 ext. 146	x
Crown Point	St. Anthony Medical Center Main at Franciscan Rd. Crown Point, IN 46307	(219) 738-2100 ext. 1311	x
Evansville	Poison Control Center Deaconess Hospital, Inc. 600 Mary St. Evansville, IN 47710	(812) 426-3333	
	Welborn Memorial Baptist Hospital 401 S.E. 6th St. Evansville, IN 47713	(812) 426-8336	
Fort Wayne	Emergency Department Lutheran Hospital 3024 Fairfield Ave. Fort Wayne, IN 46807	(219) 458-2211	
	Parkview Memorial Hospital 2200 Randalia Dr. Fort Wayne, IN 46805	(219) 484-9711	
	St. Joseph's Hospital 700 Broadway Fort Wayne, IN 46802	(219) 426-8280	
Gary	Methodist Hospital of Gary, Inc. 600 Grant St. Gary, IN 46402	(219) 886-4710	
Hammond	Poison Control Center St. Margaret's Hospital 25 Douglas St. Hammond, IN 46320	(219) 931-4477	
Indianapolis	Indiana Poison Center 1001 W. Tenth St. Indianapolis, IN 46202	(317) 630-7351 (800) 382-9097	A
Kokomo	Howard Community Hospital 3500 S. LaFountain St. Kokomo, IN 46901	(317) 453-8444	
Lafayette	Lafayette Home Hospital 2400 South St. Lafayette, IN 47902	(317) 447-6811	x
	Poison Control Center St. Elizabeth Hospital 1501 Hartford St. Lafayette, IN 47904	(317) 423-6699	
Lebanon	Witham Memorial Hospital 1124 N. Lebanon St. Lebanon, IN 46052	(317) 482-2700 ext. 241	x
Madison	King's Daughter's Hospital 112 Presbyterian Ave. Madison, IN 47250	(812) 265-5211 ext. 131	x

APPEN-DIX

Continued.

Directory of Centers — cont'd

State coordinators and cities	Address	Telephone	Comments
Marion	Marion General Hospital Wabash and Euclid Aves. Marion, IN 46952	(317) 662-4693	x
Muncie	Ball Memorial Hospital 2401 University Ave. Muncie, IN 47303	(317) 747-4321	
Richmond	Reid Memorial Hospital 1401 Chester Blvd. Richmond, IN 47374	(317) 983-3148	
Shelbyville	William S. Major Hospital 150 W. Washington St. Shelbyville, IN 46176	(317) 392-3211 ext. 252	x
South Bend	St. Joseph's Medical Center 811 E. Madison St. South Bend, IN 46622	(219) 237-7264	
Terre Haute	Union Hospital, Inc. 1606 N. Seventh St. Terre Haute, IN 47804	(812) 238-7000 ext. 7523	x
Valparaiso	Porter Memorial Hospital 814 LaPorte Ave. Valparaiso, IN 46383	(219) 464-8611 ext. 301	x
Vincennes	The Good Samaritan Hospital 520 S. 7th St. Vincennes, IN 47591	(812) 885-3348	
IOWA			
State Coordinator	Department of Health Des Moines, IA 50319	(515) 281-4964	
Des Moines	Variety Club Poison and Drug Information Center Iowa Methodist Medical Center 1200 Pleasant St. Des Moines, IA 50308	(515) 283-6254 (800) 362-2327 (statewide)	
Dubuque	Mercy Health Center Mercy Dr. Dubuque, IA 52001	(319) 589-9099	
Fort Dodge	Trinity Regional Hospital Kenyon Rd. Fort Dodge, IA 50501	(515) 573-3101	x
Iowa City	University of Iowa Hospitals and Clinics Poison Control Center Iowa City, IA 52242	(319) 356-2922 (800) 272-6477 (statewide)	A
Waterloo	Allen Memorial Hospital Emergency Department 1825 Logan Ave. Waterloo, IA 50703	(319) 235-3893	
KANSAS			
State Coordinator	Kansas Department of Health and Environment Bureau of Food and Drugs Forbes Field Topeka, KS 66620	(913) 862-9360 ext. 541	
Atchison	Atchison Hospital 1301 N. 2nd St. Atchison, KS 66002	(913) 367-2131 ext. 111	x
Dodge City	Dodge City Regional Hospital Ross & Ave., "A" Dodge City, KS 67801	(316) 225-9050 ext. 381	x

State coordinators and cities	Address	Telephone	Comments
Emporia	Newman Memorial Hospital 12th and Chestnut Sts. Emporia, KS 66801	(316) 343-6800 ext. 545	x
Fort Riley	Irwin Army Hospital Emergency Room Fort Riley, KS 66442	(913) 239-7776	
Fort Scott	Mercy Hospital 821 Burke St. Fort Scott, KS 66701	(316) 223-2200 ext. 136	x
Great Bend	Central Kansas Medical Center 3515 Broadway Great Bend, KS 67530	(316) 792-2511 ext. 115	x
Hays	Hadley Regional Medical Center 201 E. 7th St. Hays, KS 67601	(913) 628-8251 ext. 145	x
Kansas City	Mid-America Poison Center University of Kansas 39th and Rainbow Blvd. Kansas City, KS 66103	(913) 588-6633 (800) 332-6633 (statewide)	
Lawrence	Lawrence Memorial Hospital 325 Maine St. Lawrence, KS 66044	(913) 843-3680 ext. 162	x
Salina	St. John's Hospital 139 N. Penn St. Salina, KS 67401	(913) 827-3187	
Topeka	Stormont-Vail Regional Medical Center 10th & Washburn Sts. Topeka, KS 66606	(913) 354-6100	
	Northeast Kansas Poison Center St. Francis Hospital and Medical Center 1700 W. 7th St. Topeka, KS 66606	(913) 295-8094	
Wichita	Wesley Medical Center 550 N. Hillside Ave. Wichita, KS 67214	(316) 688-2277	
KENTUCKY			
State Coordinator	Department for Human Resources Frankfort, KY 40601	(502) 564-3970	
Fort Thomas	St. Lukes Hospital 85 N. Grand Ave. Fort Thomas, KY 41075	(606) 572-3215 (800) 352-9900 (statewide)	
Lexington	Central Baptist Hospital 1740 S. Limestone St. Lexington, KY 40503	(606) 278-3411 ext. 363	x
	Drug Information Center University of Kentucky Medical Center Lexington, KY 40536	(606) 233-5320	
Louisville	Kentucky Regional Poison Center of Kosair- Children's Hospital NKC, INC. P.O. Box 35070 Louisville, KY 40232	(502) 589-8222 (800) 722-5725 (statewide)	
Murray	Murray-Calloway County Hospital 803 Popular Murray, KY 420701	(502) 753-7588	
Owensboro	Owensboro-Daviess County Hospital 811 Hospital Ct. Owensboro, KY 42301	(502) 926-3030 ext. 180	x

Continued.

Directory of Centers — cont'd

State coordinators and cities	Address	Telephone	Comments
Paducah	Western Baptist Hospital 2501 Kentucky Ave. Paducah, KY 42001	(502) 444-5180	
Prestonburg	Poison Control Center Highlands Regional Medical Center Prestonburg, KY 41653	(606) 886-8511 ext. 132	x
LOUISIANA			
State Coordinator	LSU Poison Control and Drug Abuse Information Center Louisiana State University P.O. Box 33932 Shreveport, LA 71130	(318) 425-1524	
Alexandria	Rapides General Hospital Poison Control Center P.O. Box 7146 Alexandria, LA 71301	(318) 445-4665	
Layfayette	Our Lady of Lourdes Hospital 611 St. Landry St. Lafayette, LA 70501	(318) 234-7381	x
Lake Charles	Lake Charles Memorial Hospital P.O. Drawer M Lake Charles, LA 70601	(318) 478-6800	
Monroe	School of Pharmacy Northeast Louisiana University 700 University Ave. Monroe, LA 71209	(318) 342-3008	
	St. Francis Hospital P.O. Box 1901 Monroe, LA 71301	(318) 325-6454	
New Orleans	Charity Hospital 1532 Tulane Ave. New Orleans, LA 70140	(504) 568-5222	
Shreveport	Louisiana State University Poison Control and Drug Abuse Information Center LSU Medical Center P.O. Box 33932 Shreveport, LA 71130	(318) 425-1524	
MAINE			
State Coordinator	Maine Poison Control Center Portland, ME 04102	(207) 871-2950	
Portland	Maine Medical Center Emergency Division 22 Bramhall St. Portland, ME 04102	(207) 871-2381 (800) 442-6305 (statewide)	
MARYLAND			
State Coordinator	Maryland Poison Center University of Maryland School of Pharmacy Baltimore, MD 21201	(301) 528-7604 (statewide)	
Baltimore	Maryland Poison Center University of Maryland School of Pharmacy 636 W. Lombard St. Baltimore, MD 21201	(301) 528-7701 (800) 492-2414 (statewide)	A
Cumberland	Tri-State Poison Center Sacred Heart Hospital 900 Seton Dr. Cumberland, MD 21502	(301) 722-6677	

State coordinators and cities	Address	Telephone	Comments
MASSACHUSETTS			
State Coordinator	Department of Public Health Boston, MA 02111	(617) 727-2700	
Boston	Massachusetts Poison Control System 300 Longwood Ave. Boston, MA 02115	(617) 232-2120 (800) 682-9211 (statewide) (617) 277-3323 TTY (MA only)	A
MICHIGAN			
State Coordinator	Department of Public Health Emergency Medical Services Lansing, MI 48909	(517) 373-1406	
Adrian	Poison Control Center Emma L. Bixby Hospital 818 Riverside Ave. Adrian, MI 49221	(517) 263-2412	
Ann Arbor	Poison Control Center University Hospital 1405 E. Ann St. Ann Arbor, MI 48104	(313) 764-7667	
Battle Creek	Community Hospital Pharmacy Department 183 West St. Battle Creek, MI 49016	(616) 963-5521	x
Bay City	Bay Medical Center 1900 Columbus Ave. Bay City, MI 48706	(517) 894-3131	
Coldwater	Community Health Center of Branch County 274 E. Chicago St. Coldwater, MI 49036	(517) 278-7361	
Detroit	Children's Hospital Poison Center Children's Hospital 3901 Beaubien Detroit, MI 48201	(313) 494-5711 (800) 572-1655 (statewide)	A
Flint	Poison Information Center Hurley Medical Center One Hurley Plaza Flint, MI 48502	(313) 257-9111 (800) 572-5396 (statewide)	
Grand Rapids	Western Michigan Regional Poison Center Blodgett Memorial Medical Center 1840 Wealthy, S.E. Grand Rapids, MI 49506	(616) 774-7854 (800) 632-2727 (statewide)	A
Kalamazoo	Midwest Poison Center Borgess Medical Center 1521 Gull Rd. Kalamazoo, MI 49001	(616) 383-7104 (800) 632-4177 (statewide)	
	Great Lakes Poison Center Bronson Methodist Hospital 252 E. Lovell St. Kalamazoo, MI 49006	(616) 383-6409 (800) 442-4112 (statewide)	
Lansing	St. Lawrence Hospital 1210 W. Saginaw St. Lansing, MI 48914	(517) 372-5112	

Directory of Centers—cont'd

State coordinators and cities	Address	Telephone	Comments
Marquette	Upper Peninsula Regional Poison Center Marquette General Hospital 420 W. Magnetic Dr. Marquette, MI 49855	(906) 228-9440 (800) 562-9781 (N. MI only)	
Pontiac	Poison Information Center St. Joseph Mercy Hospital 900 S. Woodward Ave. Pontiac, MI 48053	(313) 858-7373	
Port Huron	Port Huron Hospital Poison Control Center 1001 Kearney St. Port Huron, MI 48060	(313) 987-5555	
Saginaw	Saginaw Region Poison Center Saginaw General Hospital 1447 N. Harrison Saginaw, MI 48602	(517) 755-1111	
Traverse City	Munson Medical Center Sixth and Madison Streets Traverse City, MI 49684	(616) 947-6140 ext. 303	
MINNESOTA			
State Coordinator	EMS Section Minnesota Dept. of Health 717 S.E. Delaware St. Minneapolis, MN 55404	(612) 623-5284	
Duluth	St. Luke's Hospital Poison Control Center 915 E. First St. Duluth, MN 55805	(218) 726-5466	
	St. Mary's Hospital 407 E. 3rd St. Duluth, MN 55805	(218) 726-4500	
Fridley	Unity Medical Center 550 Osborne Rd. Fridley, MN 55432	(612) 786-2200 ext. 6844	x
Mankato	Immanuel-St. Joseph's Hospital Poison Control Center 325 Garden Blvd. Mankato, MN 56001	(507) 625-4031 ext. 2760	x
Minneapolis	Hennepin Poison Center Hennepin County Medical Center 701 Park Ave. Minneapolis, MN 55415	(612) 347-3141	A
Morris	Stevens County Memorial Hospital Morris, MN 56267	(612) 589-1313 ext. 231	x
Rochester	Southeastern Minnesota Poison Control Center St. Mary's Hospital 1216 Second St., S.W. Rochester, MN 55901	(507) 285-6162	x
St. Cloud	St. Cloud Hospital 1406 6th Ave., N. St. Cloud, MN 56301	(612) 255-5617	
St. Paul	St. John's Hospital 403 Maria Ave. St. Paul, MN 55106	(612) 228-3132	
	United and Children's Hospital 333 N. Smith St. Paul, MN 55102	(612) 298-8402	

State coordinators and cities	Address	Telephone	Comments
	Minnesota Poison Information Center St. Paul-Ramsey Medical Center 640 Jackson St. St. Paul, MN 55101	(612) 221-2113	
Worthington	Worthington Regional Hospital 1016 6th Ave. Worthington, MN 56187	(507) 372-2941 ext. 109	x
MISSISSIPPI			
State Coordinator	State Board of Health Jackson, MS 39205	(601) 354-7660	
Biloxi	Gulf Coast Community Hospital 4642 W. Beach Blvd. Buloxi, MS 39531	(601) 388-1919	
	USAF Hospital Keesler Keesler Air Force Base Biloxi, MS 39534	(601) 377-6555	
Brandon	Rankin General Hospital Emergency Department 350 Crossgates Blvd. Brandon, MS 39042	(601) 825-2811 ext. 405	x
Columbia	Marion County General Hospital Sumrall Rd. Columbia, MS 39429	(601) 736-6303 ext. 1020	x
Greenwood	Greenwood-Leflore Hospital River Rd. Greenwood, MS 38930	(601) 459-2790	
Hattiesburg	Forrest County General Hospital 400 S. 28th Ave. Hattiesburg, MS 39401	(601) 264-4235	
Jackson	St. Dominic-Jackson Memorial Hospital 969 Lakeland Dr. Jackson, MS 39216	(601) 982-0121 ext. 2345	x
	University Medical Center 2500 N. State St. Jackson, MS 39216	(601) 354-7660	
Laurel	Jones County Community Hospital Jefferson St. at 13th Ave. Laurel, MS 39440	(601) 649-4000 ext. 630	x
Meridian	Meridian Regional Hospital Highway 39, N. Meridian, MS 39301	(601) 483-6211 ext. 440	x
Pascagoula	Singing River Hospital Emergency Department 2609 Denny Ave. Pascagoula, MS 39567	(601) 938-5162	
University	University of Mississippi School of Pharmacy Poison Information Center University, MS 38677	(601) 234-1522	
MISSOURI			
State Coordinator	Bureau of EMS Missouri Division of Health Jefferson City, MO 65102	(314) 751-2713	
Cape Girardeau	St. Francis Medical Center St. Francis Dr. Cape Girardeau, MO 63701	(314) 651-6235	

Continued.

Directory of Centers—cont'd

State coordinators and cities	Address	Telephone	Comments
Columbia	University of Missouri Hospital and Clinics 807 Stadium Rd. Columbia, MO 65212	(314) 882-8091	
Hannibal	St. Elizabeth's Hospital 109 Virginia St. Hannibal, MO 63401	(314) 221-0414 ext. 264	x
Jefferson City	Charles E. Still Osteopathic Hospital 1125 Madison Jefferson City, MO 65101	(314) 635-7141 ext. 215	x
Joplin	St. John's Medical Center 2727 McClelland Blvd. Joplin, MO 64801	(417) 781-2727 ext. 2305	x
Kansas City	Children's Mercy Hospital 24th at Gillham Rd. Kansas City, MO 64108	(816) 234-3000	A
Kirksville	Kirksville Osteopathic Health Center #1 Osteopathy Ave. Kirksville, MO 63501	(816) 626-2266	x
Poplar Bluff	Lucy Lee Hospital 2620 N. Westwood Blvd. Poplar Bluff, MO 63901	(314) 785-7721 ext. 264	x
Rolla	Phelps County Regional Medical Center 1000 W. 10th St. Rolla, MO 65401	(314) 364-3100 ext. 287	x
St. Joseph	Methodist Medical Center Seventh to Ninth on Faron St. St. Joseph, MO 64501	(816) 271-7580 232-8481	
St. Louis	St. Louis Regional Poison Center Cardinal Glennon Memorial Hospital for Children 1465 S. Grand Ave. St. Louis, MO 63104	(314) 772-5200	A
	St. Louis Children's Hospital 500 S. Kingshighway St. Louis, MO 63110	(314) 454-6099	
Springfield	Ozark Poison Center Lester E. Cox Medical Center 1423 N. Jefferson St. Springfield, MO 65802	(417) 831-9746	
MONTANA			
State Coordinator	Department of Health and Environmental Sciences Helena, MT 59620	(406) 449-3895	
Helena	Montana Poison Control System Cogswell Bldg. Helena, MT 59620	(406) 442-2480 (800) 525-5042	
NEBRASKA			
State Coordinator	Department of Health Lincoln, NE 68502	(402) 471-2122	
Omaha	Mid-Plains Regional Poison Center Children's Memorial Hospital 8301 Dodge Omaha, NE 68114	(402) 390-5400 (800) 642-9999 (statewide) (800) 228-9515 (surrounding states)	

State coordinators and cities	Address	Telephone	Comments
NEVADA			
State Coordinator	Department of Human Resources Carson City, NV 89710	(702) 885-4750	
Las Vegas	Southern Nevada Memorial Hospital 1800 W. Charleston Blvd. Las Vegas, NV 89102	(702) 385-1277	
	Sunrise Hospital Medical Center 3186 S. Maryland Pkwy. Las Vegas, NV 89109	(702) 732-4989	
Reno	St. Mary's Hospital 235 W. 6th Reno, NV 89520	(702) 789-3013	
	Washoe Medical Center 77 Pringle Way Reno, NV 89520	(702) 785-4129	
NEW HAMPSHIRE			
State Coordinator	New Hampshire Poison Center NH - Dartmouth Hitchcock Medical Center 2 Maynard St. Hanover, NH 03756	(603) 646-5000 (800) 562-8236 (statewide)	
Hanover	New Hampshire Poison Center Mary Hitchcock Hospital 2 Maynard St. Hanover, NH 03756	(603) 646-5000 (800) 562-8236 (statewide)	x
NEW JERSEY			
State Coordinator	Department of Health Accident Prevention and Poison Control Program Trenton, NJ 08625	(609) 292-5666	
Atlantic City	Atlantic City Medical Center 1925 Pacific Ave. Atlantic City, NJ 08401	(609) 344-4081 ext. 2359	x
Belleville	Clara Maass Medical Center 1A Franklin Ave. Belleville, NJ 07109	(201) 450-2000 ext. 781	x
Berlin	West Jersey Hospital South Division Berlin, NJ 08009	(609) 768-6666	
Boonton	Riverside Hospital Powerville Rd. Boonton, NJ 07055	(201) 334-5000 ext. 186	x
Bridgeton	Bridgeton Hospital Irving Ave. Bridgeton, NJ 08302	(609) 451-6600 ext. 251	x
Denville	St. Clare's Hospital Pocono Rd. Denville, NJ 07834	(201) 625-6065 ext. 6063	x
East Orange	East Orange General Hospital 300 Central Ave. E. Orange, NJ 07019	(201) 672-8400 ext. 223	x
Elizabeth	St. Elizabeth's Hospital 225 Williams St. Elizabeth, NJ 07207	(201) 527-5059	
Englewood	Englewood Hospital 350 Engle St. Englewood, NJ 07631	(201) 894-3262	

Directory of Centers—cont'd

State coordinators and cities	Address	Telephone	Comments
Flemington	Hunterdon Medical Center Route 31 Flemington, NJ 08822	(201) 782-2121 ext. 369	x
Livingston	St. Barnabas Medical Center Old Short Hills Rd. Livingston, NJ 07039	(201) 992-5161	
Long Branch	Monmouth Medical Center Emergency Department Dunbar and 2nd Ave. Long Branch, NJ 07740	(201) 222-2210	
Montclair	Mountainside Hospital Bay and Highland Aves. Montclair, NJ 07042	(201) 429-6202	
Mount Holly	Burlington County Memorial Hospital 175 Madison Ave. Mt. Holly, NJ 08060	(609) 267-7877	
Neptune	Jersey Shore Medical Center Fitkin Hospital 1945 Corlies Ave. Neptune, NJ 07753	(201) 775-5500 (800) 822-9761 (statewide)	
Newark	Newark Beth Israel Medical Center 201 Lyons Ave. Newark, NJ 07112	(201) 926-7240	
New Brunswick	Middlesex General Hospital 180 Somerset St. New Brunswick, NJ 08903	(201) 937-8583	
	St. Peter's Medical Center 245 Easton Ave. New Brunswick, NJ 08903	(201) 745-8527	
Newton	Newton Memorial Hospital 175 High St. Newton, NJ 07860	(201) 383-2121 ext. 270	x
Orange	Hospital Center at Orange Emergency Department 188 S. Essex Ave. Orange, NJ 07051	(201) 266-2120	
Passaic	St. Mary's Hospital 211 Pennington Ave. Passaic, NJ 07055	(201) 473-1000 ext. 441	x
Perth Amboy	Perth Amboy General Hospital 530 New Brunswick Ave. Perth Amboy, NJ 08861	(201) 442-3700 ext. 2501	x
Phillipsburg	Warren Hospital 185 Roseberry St. Phillipsburg, NJ 08865	(201) 859-1500 ext. 222	x
Point Pleasant	Point Pleasant Hospital Osborn Ave. & River Front Point Pleasant, NJ 08742	(201) 892-1100 ext. 383	x
Princeton	The Medical Center at Princeton 253 Witherspoon St. Princeton, NJ 08540	(609) 734-4554	
Saddle Brook	Saddle Brook General Hospital 300 Market St. Saddle Brook, NJ 07662	(201) 368-6025	
Somers Point	Shore Memorial Hospital Brighton & Sunny Aves. Somers Point, NJ 08244	(609) 653-3515	

State coordinators and cities	Address	Telephone	Comments
Somerville	Somerset Medical Center Rehill Ave. Somerville, NJ 08876	(201) 725-4000 ext. 436	x
Summit	Overlook Hospital 193 Morris Ave. Summit, NJ 07901	(201) 522-2232	
Teaneck	Holy Name Hospital 718 Teaneck Rd. Teaneck, NJ 07666	(201) 833-3242	
Trenton	Helene Fuld Medical Center 750 Brunswick Ave. Trenton, NJ 08638	(609) 396-1077	
Union	Memorial General Hospital 1000 Galloping Hill Rd. Union, NJ 07083	(201) 687-1900 ext. 3710	x
Wayne	Greater Paterson General Hospital 224 Hamburg Turnpike Wayne, NJ 07470	(201) 942-6900 ext. 224	x
NEW MEXICO			

State Coordinator	New Mexico Poison Drug Information & Medical
	   Center
	University of New Mexico
	Albuquerque, NM 87131
		(505) 843-2551
		(800) 432-6866
		  (statewide)
			A

NEW YORK			
State Coordinator	Department of Health Albany, NY 12237	(518) 474-3785	
Binghamton	Southern Tier Poison Center United Health Services Binghamton General Hospital Binghamton, NY 13903	(607) 723-8929	
	Our Lady of Lourdes Memorial Hospital 169 Riverside Dr. Binghamton, NY 13905	(607) 798-5231	
Buffalo	Western New York Poison Control Center Children's Hospital of Buffalo 219 Bryant St. Buffalo, NY 14222	(716) 878-7654	
Dunkirk	Brooks Memorial Hospital 10 W. 6th St. Dunkirk, NY 14048	(716) 366-1111 ext. 414	x
East Meadow	Long Island Regional Poison Control Center Nassau County Medical Center 2201 Hempstead Turnpike E. Meadow, NY 11554	(516) 542-2324 (516) 542-2323 (TTY)	A
Elmira	Arnot Ogden Memorial Hospital Roe Ave. & Grove St. Elmira, NY 14901	(607) 737-4194	
	St. Joseph's Hospital Health Center 555 E. Market St. Elmira, NY 14901	(607) 734-2662	
Endicott	Ideal Hospital 600 High Ave. Endicott, NY 13760	(607) 754-7171	x
Glens Falls	Glens Falls Hospital 100 Park St. Glens Falls, NY 12801	(518) 761-5261	

Continued.

Directory of Centers—cont'd

State coordinators and cities	Address	Telephone	Comments
Jamestown	W.C.A. Hospital 207 Foote Ave. Jamestown, NY 14701	(716) 484-8648	
Johnson City	Wilson Memorial Hospital 33 Harrison St. Johnson City, NY 13790	(607) 773-6611	
Kingston	Kingston Hospital 396 Broadway Kingston, NY 12401	(914) 331-3313	
New York City	New York City Poison Center Department of Health Bureau of Laboratories 455 First Ave. New York City, NY 10016	(212) 340-4494 (212) 764-7667	A
Nyack	Hudson Valley Poison Center Nyack Hospital N. Midland Ave. Nyack, NY 10960	(914) 353-1000	
Rochester	Finger Lakes Poison Center LIFELINE University of Rochester Medical Center Rochester, NY 14642	(716) 275-5151 275-2700 (TTY)	A
Schenectady	Ellis Hospital Poison Control 1101 Nott St. Schenectady, NY 12308	(518) 382-4039 382-4121	
Syracuse	Syracuse Poison Information Center 750 E. Adams St. Syracuse, NY 13210	(315) 476-7529	
Troy	St. Mary's Hospital Poison Control Center 1300 Massachusetts Ave. Troy, NY 12180	(518) 272-5792	
Utica	St. Lukes Memorial Hospital Center P.O. Box 479 Utica, NY 13502	(315) 798-6200	
Watertown	House of the Good Samaritan Hospital Washington & Pratt Sts. Watertown, NY 13602	(315) 788-8700	
NORTH CAROLINA			
State Coordinator	Duke University Medical Center Durham, NC 27710	(919) 684-8111 (800) 672-1697 (statewide)	
Asheville	Western North Carolina Poison Control Center Memorial Mission Hospital 509 Biltimore Ave. Asheville, NC 28801	(704) 255-4490	
Charlotte	Mercy Hospital 2001 Vail Ave. Charlotte, NC 28207	(704) 379-5827	
Durham	Duke University Medical Center Poison Control Center P.O. Box 3007 Durham, NC 27710	(919) 684-8111	
Greensboro	Triad Poison Center Moses H. Cone Memorial Hospital 1200 N. Elm St. Greensboro, NC 27401	(919) 379-4105	

State coordinators and cities	Address	Telephone	Comments
Hendersonville	Margaret R. Pardee Memorial Hospital Fleming St. Hendersonville, NC 28739	(704) 693-6522 ext. 555	x
Hickory	Catawba Memorial Hospital Fairgrove-Church Rd. Hickory, NC 28601	(704) 322-6649	
Jacksonville	Onslow Memorial Hospital Western Blvd. Jacksonville, NC 28540	(919) 577-2555	
Wilmington	New Hanover Memorial Hospital 2131 S. 17th St. Wilmington, NC 28401	(919) 343-7046	
Winston-Salem	Wake Forest University Medical Center North Carolina Baptist Hospital 300 S. Hawthorne Road Winston-Salem, NC 27103	(919) 748-4991	
NORTH DAKOTA			
State Coordinator	Department of Health Bismarck, ND 58505	(701) 224-2388	
Bismarck	Bismarck Hospital Emergency Department 300 N. 7th St. Bismarck, ND 58501	(701) 223-4357	
Fargo	St. Luke's Poison Center St. Luke's Hospitals Fifth St. at Mills Ave. Fargo, ND 58122	(701) 280-5575	
Grand Forks	United Hospital 1200 S. Columbia Rd. Grand Forks, ND 58201	(701) 780-5282	x
Minot	St. Joseph's Hospital Third St. & Fourth Ave., S.E. Minot, ND 58701	(701) 857-2553	
Williston	Mercy Hospital 1301 15th Ave., W. Williston, ND 58801	(701) 572-7661	x
OHIO			
State Coordinator	Department of Health Columbus, OH 43216	(614) 466-5190	
Akron	Children's Hospital Medical Center of Akron 281 Locust St. Akron, OH 44308	(216) 379-8562 (800) 362-9922 (statewide)	
Canton	Aultman Hospital Emergency Room 2600 Sixth St., S.W. Canton, OH 44710	(216) 438-6203 452-9911	
Cincinnati	Drug & Poison Information Center Bridge Medical Science Bldg. Room 7701 231 Bethesda Ave. Cincinnati, OH 45267	(513) 872-5111	
Cleveland	Greater Cleveland Poison Control Center 2119 Abington Rd. Cleveland, OH 44106	(216) 231-4455	

Directory of Centers—cont'd

State coordinators and cities	Address	Telephone	Comments
Columbus	Central Ohio Poison Center Children's Hospital of Ohio 700 Children's Dr. Columbus, OH 43205	(614) 228-1323	
Dayton	Children's Medical Center One Children's Plaza Dayton, OH 45404	(513) 222-2227 (800) 762-0727 (statewide)	
Lorain	Lorain Community Hospital 3700 Kolbe Rd. Lorain, OH 44053	(216) 282-2220	
Mansfield	Mansfield General Hospital 335 Glessner Ave. Mansfield, OH 44903	(419) 522-3411 ext. 2545	x
Springfield	Community Hospital 2615 E. High St. Springfield, OH 44505	(513) 325-1255	
Toledo	Poison Information Center Medical College Hospital P.O. Box 6190 Toledo, OH 43679	(419) 381-3897	
Youngstown	Mahoning Valley Poison Center St. Elizabeth Hospital Medical Center 1044 Belmont Ave. Youngstown, OH 44501	(216) 746-2222 (216) 746-5510 (TTY)	
Zanesville	Bethesda Poison Control Center Bethesda Hospital 2951 Maple Ave. Zanesville, OH 43701	(614) 454-4221	
OKLAHOMA			
State Coordinator	Oklahoma Poison Control Center Oklahoma Children's Memorial Hospital P.O. Box 26307 Oklahoma City, OK 73126	(405) 271-5454 (800) 522-4611 (statewide)	
Ada	Valley View Hospital 1300 E. 6th St. Ada, OK 74820	(405) 332-2323 ext. 200	x
Lawton	Comanche County Memorial Hospital 3401 Gore Blvd. Lawton, OK 73501	(405) 355-8620 ext. 296	x
McAlester	McAlester General Hospital Inc., W. P.O. Box 669 McAlester, OK 74501	(918) 426-1800 ext. 240	x
Oklahoma City	Oklahoma Poison Control Center Oklahoma Children's Memorial Center P.O. Box 26307 Oklahoma City, OK 73126	(405) 271-5454 (800) 522-4611 (statewide)	
Ponca City	St. Joseph Medical Center 14th and Hartford Ponca City, OK 74601	(405) 765-0584	x
Tulsa	Hillcrest Medical Center 1120 S. Utica Tulsa, OK 74104	(918) 560-5755	
OREGON			
State Coordinator	Oregon Poison Control and Drug Information Center University of Oregon Health Sciences Center Portland, OR 97201	(503) 225-8968 (800) 452-7165 (statewide)	

State coordinators and cities	Address	Telephone	Comments
PANAMA			
Ancon	U.S.A. MEDDAC Panama Gorgas U.S. Army Hospital Ancon, Panama APO Miami 34004	252-7500	x
PENNSYLVANIA			
State Coordinator	Director, Division of Drugs, Devices and Cosmetics Department of Health P.O. Box 90 Harrisburg, PA 17108	(717) 787-2307	
Allentown	Lehigh Valley Poison Center Allentown General Hospital 17th and Chew Sts. Allentown, PA 18102	(215) 433-2311	
Altoona	Keystone Region Poison Center Mercy Hospital 2500 Seventh Ave. Altoona, PA 16603	(814) 946-3711	
Bloomsburg	The Bloomsburg Hospital 549 E. Fair St. Bloomsburg, PA 17815	(717) 784-4241	
Chester	Sacred Heart General Hospital Ninth and Wilson Sts. Chester, PA 19013	(215) 494-4400	
Danville	Susquehanna Poison Center Geisinger Medical Center N. Academy Ave. Danville, PA 17821	(717) 275-6116	
Erie	Doctors Osteopathic Hospital 252 W. 11th St. Erie, PA 16502	(814) 454-2120	
	Millcreek Community Hospital 5515 Peach St. Erie, PA 16509	(814) 864-4031	x
	Hamot Medical Center 201 State St. Erie, PA 16550	(814) 452-4242	
	Saint Vincent's Health Center 232 W. 25th St. Erie, PA 16544	(814) 452-3232	
Gettysburg	Annie M. Warner Hospital S. Washington St. Gettysburg, PA 17325	(717) 334-9155	x
Hanover	Hanover General Hospital 300 Highland Ave. Hanover, PA 17331	(717) 637-3711	
Hershey	Capital Area Poison Center The Milton S. Hershey Medical Center University Dr. Hershey, PA 17033	(717) 534-6111 (treatment)	
Jersey Shore	Jersey Shore Hospital ER - Poison Center Thompson St. Jersey Shore, PA 17740	(717) 398-0100	x
Johnstown	Conemaugh Valley Memorial Hospital Poison Control Center 1086 Franklin St. Johnstown, PA 15905	(814) 535-5351	

APPEN DIX

Continued.

Directory of Centers — cont'd

State coordinators and cities	Address	Telephone	Comments
	Laurel Highlands Poison Center 320 Main St. Johnstown, PA 15901	(814) 535-8255	
	Mercy Hospital Poison Control Center 1020 Franklin St. Johnstown, PA 15905	(814) 535-5353	
Lancaster	Lancaster General Hospital ER - Poison Control Center 555 N. Duke St. Lancaster, PA 17604	(717) 295-8322	
	St. Joseph's Hospital Poison Control Center 250 College Ave. Lancaster, PA 17604	(717) 299-4546	
Lehighton	Gnaden-Huetten Memorial Hospital 11th & Hamilton Sts. Lehighton, PA 18235	(215) 377-1300	x
Lewistown	Lewistown Hospital Poison Control Center Highland Ave. Lewistown, PA 17044	(717) 248-5411	x
Nanticoke	Nanticoke State Hospital N. Washington St. Nanticoke, PA 18634	(717) 735-5000	x
Paoli	Paoli Memorial Hospital Emergency Room Paoli, PA 19301	(215) 648-1043	
Philadelphia	Philadelphia Poison Information 321 University Ave. Philadelphia, PA 19104	(215) 922-5523 922-5524	
Philipsburg	Philipsburg State General Hospital Loch Lomond Rd. Philipsburg, PA 16866	(814) 342-3320	x
Pittsburgh	Pittsburgh Poison Center Children's Hospital 125 DeSoto St. Pittsburgh, PA 15214	(412) 681-6669 647-5600	
Reading	Community General Hospital 145 N. 6th St. Reading, PA 19601	(215) 375-9115	
Sayre	The Robert Packer Hospital Guthrie Square Sayre, PA 18840	(717) 888-6666	x
Sellersville	Grandview Hospital Lawn Ave. Sellersville, PA 18960	(215) 257-3611	x
State College	Centre Community Hospital Orchard Rd. State College, PA 16801	(814) 238-4351	x
York	Memorial Osteopathic Hospital 325 S. Belmont St. York, PA 17403	(717) 843-8623 ext. 123	x
	York Hospital 1001 S. George St. York, PA 17405	(717) 771-2311	

State coordinators and cities	Address	Telephone	Comments
PUERTO RICO			
State Coordinator	University of Puerto Rico Rio Piedras, PR	(809) 765-4880 765-0615	
Arecibo	District Hospital of Arecibo Arecibo, PR 00613	(809) 878-3535 ext. 707 (809) 878-8212	x
Fajardo	District Hospital of Fajardo Fajardo, PR 00649	(809) 863-0505	
Mayaguez	Mayaguez Medical Center Department of Health P.O. Box 1868 Mayaguez, PR 00709	(809) 832-8686 ext. 1816 1514	x
Ponce	District Hospital of Ponce Ponce, PR 00731	(809) 842-2550	
Rio Piedras	Childrens Hospital Center of Puerto Rico Rio Piedras, PR 00936	(809) 754-8535	
San Juan	Pharmacy School Medical Sciences Campus San Juan, PR 00936	(809) 753-4849	
RHODE ISLAND			
State Coordinator	Rhode Island Poison Center Rhode Island Hospital 593 Eddy St. Providence, RI 02902	(401) 277-5727	
Providence	Rhode Island Poison Center Rhode Island Hospital Annex Bldg. 422 593 Eddy St. Providence, RI 02902	(401) 277-5727	
SOUTH CAROLINA			
State Coordinator	Department of Health and Environmental Control Columbia, SC 29201	(803) 758-5654	
Charleston	National Pesticide Telecommunications Network Medical University of South Carolina 171 Ashley Ave. Charleston, SC 29403	(803) 792-4201 (800) 845-7633 (outside SC)	
Columbia	Palmetto Poison Center University of South Carolina College of Pharmacy Columbia, SC 29208	(803) 765-7359 (800) 922-1117	
SOUTH DAKOTA			
State Coordinator	Department of Health Pierre, SD 57501	(605) 773-3361	
Aberdeen	The Dakota Midland Poison Control Center Dakota Midland Hospital 1400 15th Ave., N.W. Aberdeen, SD 57401	(605) 225-1880 (800) 592-1889	
Rapid City	Rapid City Regional Poison Control Center 353 Fairmont Blvd. P.O. Box 6000 Rapid City, SD 57709	(605) 341-3333 (800) 742-8925	
Sioux Falls	McKennan Poison Center McKennan Hospital 800 E. 21st St. Sioux Falls, SD 57101	(605) 336-3894 (800) 952-0123 (statewide) (800) 843-0505 (NE, MN, IA)	

Continued.

Directory of Centers — cont'd

State coordinators and cities	Address	Telephone	Comments
TENNESSEE			
State Coordinator	Department of Public Health Division of Emergency Services Nashville, TN 37216	(615) 741-2407	
Chattanooga	T.C. Thompson Children's Hospital 910 Blackford St. Chattanooga, TN 37403	(615) 755-6100	
Columbia	Maury County Hospital 1224 Trotwood Ave. Columbia, TN 38401	(615) 778-4500 ext. 110	x
Cookeville	Cookeville General Hospital 142 W. 5th St. Cookeville, TN 38501	(615) 526-4818	
Jackson	Jackson-Madison General Hospital 708 W. Forest Jackson, TN 38301	(901) 424-0424 ext. 525	x
Johnson City	Johnson City Medical Center Hospital Emergency Department 400 State of Franklin Rd. Johnson City, TN 37601	(615) 461-6572	
Knoxville	Memorial Research Center Hospital 1924 Alcoa Hwy. Knoxville, TN 37920	(615) 971-3261	
Memphis	Southern Poison Center LeBonheur Children's Medical Center 848 Adams Ave. Memphis, TN 38103	(901) 528-6048	
Nashville	Vanderbilt University Hospital 21st and Garland Nashville, TN 37232	(615) 322-6435	
TEXAS			
State Coordinator	Texas Department of Health Div. of Occupational Health Austin, TX 78756	(512) 458-7254	
Abilene	Hendrick Hospital 19th & Hickory Sts. Abilene, TX 79601	(915) 677-7762	
Amarillo	Amarillo Emergency Receiving Center Amarillo Hospital District P.O. Box 1110 1501 Coulter Dr. Amarillo, TX 79175	(806) 376-4292	
Austin	Brackenridge Hospital 14th & Sabine Sts. Austin, TX 78701	(512) 478-4490	
Beaumont	Baptist Hospital of Southeast Texas P.O. Box 1591 College & 11th St. Beaumont, TX 77701	(713) 833-7409	
Corpus Christi	Memorial Medical Center P.O. Box 5280 2606 Hospital Blvd. Corpus Christi, TX 78405	(512) 881-4559	
El Paso	El Paso Poison Control Center R.E. Thomason General Hospital 4815 Alameda Ave. El Paso, TX 79905	(915) 533-1244	

State coordinators and cities	Address	Telephone	Comments
Fort Worth	W.I. Cook Children's Hospital Cook Poison Center-Fort Worth 1212 W. Lancaster St. Fort Worth, TX 76102	(817) 336-6611	
Galveston	Southeast Texas Poison Center The University of Texas Medical Branch Eighth & Mechanic Sts. Galveston, TX 77550	(713) 765-1420	A
Harlingen	Valley Baptist Hospital P.O. Box 2588 2101 S. Commerce St. Harlingen, TX 78550	(512) 421-1859	
Houston	Southeast Texas Poison Control Center Eighth & Mechanic Sts. Galveston, TX 77550	(713) 654-1701	A
Laredo	Mercy Hospital 1515 Logan St. Laredo, TX 78040	(512) 724-6247	
Lubbock	Methodist Hospital 3615 19th St. Lubbock, TX 79410	(806) 793-4366	
Odessa	Medical Center Hospital Poison Control Center P.O. Box 7239 Odessa, TX 79760	(915) 333-1231	
Plainview	Central Plains Regional Hospital 2601 Dimmitt Rd. Plainview, TX 79072	(806) 296-9601	
San Angelo	Shannon West Texas Memorial Hospital 120 E. Harris San Angelo, TX 76901	(915) 653-6741 ext. 318	x
San Antonio	Department of Pediatrics University of Texas Health Science Center at San Antonio 7703 Floyd Curl Dr. San Antonio, TX 78284	(512) 223-6361 ext. 473	x
Tyler	Medical Center Hospital 1000 S. Becham St. Tyler, TX 75701	(214) 597-0351	x
Waco	Hillcrest Baptist Hospital 3000 Herring Ave. Waco, TX 76708	(817) 753-1412	x
Wichita Falls	Wichita General Hospital 1600 8th St. Wichita Falls, TX 76301	(817) 322-6771	
UTAH			
State Coordinator	Utah Department of Health Division of Family Health Services Salt Lake City, UT 84113	(801) 533-6161	
Salt Lake City	Intermountain Regional Poison Control Center 50 N. Medical Dr. Salt Lake City, UT 84132	(801) 581-2151	A
VERMONT			
State Coordinator	Department of Health Burlington, VT 05401	(802) 862-5701	

APPEN-
DIX

Continued.

Directory of Centers—cont'd

State coordinators and cities	Address	Telephone	Comments
Burlington	Vermont Poison Center Medical Center Hospital of Vermont Burlington, VT 05401	(802) 658-3456	
VIRGINIA			
State Coordinator	Division of Emergency Medical Services Room 1102 109 Governor St. Richmond, VA 23219	(804) 786-5188	
Alexandria	Alexandria Hospital 4320 Seminary Rd. Alexandria, VA 22314	(703) 379-3070	
Arlington	Arlington Hospital 5129 N. 16th St. Arlington, VA 22205	(703) 558-6161	
Blacksburg	Montgomery County Community Hospital Rt. 460, S. Blacksburg, VA 24060	(703) 951-1111 ext. 140	x
Charlottesville	Blue Ridge Poison Center University of Virginia Hospital Charlottesville, VA 22903	(804) 924-5543 (800) 446-9876 (TTY) (out of state) (800) 552-3723 (TTY) (statewide)	
Falls Church	Fairfax Hospital 3300 Gallows Rd. Falls Church, VA 22046	(703) 698-3600	
Hampton	Hampton General Hospital 3120 Victoria Blvd. Hampton, VA 23661	(804) 722-1131	
Harrisonburg	Rockingham Memorial Hospital Emergency Room 235 Cantrell Harrisonburg, VA 22801	(703) 433-8311	
Lexington	Stonewall Jackson Hospital Lexington, VA 22043	(703) 463-9141 ext. 219	x
Lynchburg	Lynchburg General Marshall Lodge Hospital, Inc. Tate Springs Rd. Lynchburg, VA 24504	(804) 528-2066	
Nassawadox	Northampton-Accomack Memorial Hospital Nassawadox, VA 23413	(804) 442-8700	
Newport News	Riverside Hospital 500 J. Clyde Morris Blvd. Newport News, VA 23601	(804) 599-2050	
Norfolk	DePaul Hospital Granby St. at Kingsley La. Norfolk, VA 23505	(804) 489-5288	
Portsmouth	U.S. Naval Hospital Portsmouth, VA 23708	(804) 398-5898	
Richmond	Central Virginia Poison Center Medical College of Virginia Virginia Commonwealth University P.O. Box 522, MCV Station Richmond, VA 23298	(804) 786-9123	
Roanoke	Southwest Virginia Poison Center Roanoke Memorial Hospital Belleview at Jefferson St. P.O. Box 13367 Roanoke, VA 24033	(703) 981-7336	

State coordinators and cities	Address	Telephone	Comments
Staunton	King's Daughter's Hospital P.O. Box 3000 Staunton, VA 24401	(703) 885-6848	x
Waynesboro	Waynesboro Community Hospital 501 Oak Ave. Waynesboro, VA 22980	(703) 942-4096	x
Williamsburg	Williamsburg Community Hospital 1238 Mr. Vernon Ave. P.O. Drawer H Williamsburg, VA 23185	(804) 253-6005	

VIRGIN ISLANDS

State Coordinator	Department of Health St. Thomas, VI 00801	(809) 774-6097 774-0117	
St. Croix	Charles Harwood Memorial Hospital Christiansted St. Croix, VI 00820	(809) 773-8331	
St. John	Morris F. DeCastro Clinic Cruz Bay St. John, VI 00830	(809) 776-6252	
St. Thomas	Knud-Hansen Memorial Hospital St. Thomas, VI 00801	(809) 774-9000 ext. 224/5 (809) 774-1212	x

WASHINGTON

State Coordinator	Department of Social and Health Services Emergency Medical Services Olympia, WA 98504	(206) 522-7478	
Seattle	Seattle Poison Center Children's Orthopedic Hospital and Medical Center 4800 Sand Point Way, NE Seattle, WA 98105	(206) 634-5252 (800) 732-6985	A
Spokane	Spokane Poison Center Deaconess Hospital 800 W. 5th Ave. Spokane, WA 99210	(509) 747-1077 (800) 572-5842 (statewide) (509) 747-1077 (TTY)	A
Tacoma	Mary Bridge Poison Information Center Mary Bridge Children's Hospital South L St. Tacoma, WA 98405	(206) 272-1281 (800) 542-6319 (statewide)	x
Yakima	Central Washington Poison Center Yakima Valley Memorial Hospital 2811 Tieton Dr. Yakima, WA 98902	(509) 248-4400 (800) 572-9176 (statewide)	

WEST VIRGINIA

State Coordinator	The West Virginia Poison System West Virginia University School of Pharmacy 3110 Mac Corkle Ave., S.E. Charleston, WV 25304	(304) 348-4211 (800) 642-3625 (statewide)	

APPEN-DIX

Continued.

Directory of Centers — cont'd

State coordinators and cities	Address	Telephone	Comments
WISCONSIN			
State Coordinator	Department of Health and Social Services Division of Health Madison, WI 53701	(608) 267-7174	
Eau Claire	Eau Claire Poison Center Luther Hospital 1225 Whipple Eau Claire, WI 54701	(715) 835-1515	
Green Bay	Green Bay Poison Center St. Vincent Hospital 835 S. Van Buren St. Green Bay, WI 54305	(414) 433-8100	
LaCrosse	St. Francis Medical Center 700 West Ave., N. LaCrosse, WI 54601	(608) 784-3971	
Madison	Madison Area Poison Center University Hospital & Clinic 600 Highland Ave. Madison, WI 53792	(608) 262-3702	
Milwaukee	Milwaukee Poison Center Milwaukee Children's Hospital 1700 W. Wisconsin Ave. Milwaukee, WI 53233	(414) 931-4114	
WYOMING			
State Coordinator	Office of Emergency Medical Services Department of Health and Social Services Cheyenne, WY 82002	(307) 777-7955	
Cheyenne	Wyoming Poison Center DePaul Hospital 2600 E. 18th St. Cheyenne, WY 82001	(307) 635-9256 (800) 442-2704	

1-19/GENERAL SIGNS AND SYMPTOMS OF POISONING

Sign or symptom	Poison
EYES	
Dilation of pupil (mydriasis)	Belladonna group, meperidine, alcohols, chloroform, papaverine, sympathomimetics (amphetamine, cocaine), parasympatholytics, antihistamines; gelsemium, cocaine, camphor, aconitine, benzene, barium, thallium, botulinus toxin, cyanide, carbon monoxide
Constriction of pupil (miosis)	Opium, morphine group, sympatholytics, parasympathomimetics, dibenamine, cholinesterase inhibitors, choloral hydrate, picrotoxin, nicotine, caffeine, barbiturates
Purple-yellow vision	Digitalis, santonin
Blurred vision	Belladonna group, methyl alcohol, ethyl alcohol, ergot, carbon tetrachloride, cholinesterase inhibitors, vesicant war gases (mustard gas), camphor
Partial or total blindness	Methyl alcohol
Photophobia, lacrimation, pain	Vesicant war gases (mustard gas), Mace, tear gases (bromacetone, etc.)
FACE AND SCALP	
Dull and masklike expression	Barbiturates, bromides, gelsemine, manganese, thallium
Facial twitchings	Lead, mercury, phenothiazines, butyrophenones
Alopecia	Thallium, arsenic, ergot, hypervitaminosis A, gold, lead, boric acid, thiocyanates
SKIN AND MUCOUS MEMBRANES	
Pallor	Aniline derivatives, colchicine, sympathomimetics, insulin, pilocarpine
Livid, ashy coloration	Dinitrocresol, dinitrophenol, ergot, lead, phenacetin
Cyanosis	Nitrobenzene, chlorates, acetanilid, carbon monoxide, methane, nitrous oxide, aniline derivatives, nitrites, morphine, sulfides, ergot, amyl nitrite, and well over 100 other drugs and chemicals
Yellow	Atabrine, jaundice from hepatic injury (chlorinated compounds, arsenic and other heavy metals, chromates, mushrooms, and many drugs); jaundice from hemolytic anemias (aniline, nitrobenzene, quinine derivatives, arsine, fava beans, and many drugs)
Sweating	Pilocarpine, nicotine, physostigmine, picrotoxin
Dry, hot skin	Belladonna group, botulinus toxin
Blue-gray	Silver salts
Brown, black	Iodine, silver nitrate
Deep brown	Bromine
White	Phenol derivatives
Gray	Mercuric chloride
NERVOUS SYSTEM	
Coma	Morphine derivatives and analogs, all hypnotics, sedatives, and general anesthetics, barbiturates, chloral hydrate, sulfonal, trional, paraldehyde, chloroform, ethers, alcohols; lead, cyanide, carbon monoxide, carbon dioxide, nicotine, benzene, atropine, phenols, scopolamine, xylene, cholinesterase inhibitors, insulin, aniline derivatives, mushrooms, salicylates, copper salts, and numerous others
Delirium, mental disturbances	Belladonna group, cocaine, alcohol, lead, marijuana, arsenic, ergot, amphetamines and derivatives, antihistamines, camphor, benzene, barbiturates, DDT, aniline derivatives, physostigmine, veratrine, nerve gases, PCP, LSD

From: Arena, JM: Poisoning, ed 4, 1979. Courtesy of Charles C Thomas, Publisher, Springfield, Illinois.   *Continued.*

APPEN-
DIX

1-19/General Signs and Symptoms of Poisoning—cont'd

Sign or symptom	Poison
Convulsions	Strychnine, picrotoxin, camphor, santonin, cocaine, belladonna group (atropine), veratrine, aconite, cholinesterase inhibitors, pentylenetetrazol, amphetamine and derivatives, ergot, nicotine, lead, antipyrine, barium, sodium fluoroacetate, mushrooms, caffeine, carbon monoxide, cyanides, salicylates, copper salts, PCP
Headache	Carbon monoxide, phenol, benzene, nitrobenzene, nitrates, nitrites, aniline, lead, indomethacin
Muscle spasms	Atropine, cadmium, strychnine, copper salts, bites of black widow spider, scorpion, and sting ray
GASTRIONTESTINAL TRACT	
Nausea, vomiting, diarrhea, dehydration, abdominal pain	Heavy metal salts, corrosive acids and alkalis, halogens, cathartics (croton oil, castor oil), ergot, nicotine, aconitine, cantharides, solanine, acetanilid and derivatives, phosphorus, phenols, cresol, methy alcohol, muscarine, cardioactive glycosides (digitalis), fluorides, morphine and analogs, DDT, cholinesterase inhibitors, pilocarpine, veratrine, colchicine, botulinus toxin, mushrooms, boric acid and sodium borate, cocaine, procaine and local anesthetics, salicylates.

1-20/GENERAL SIGNS AND SYMPTOMS OF TOXIC INHALATION

CNS	Dizziness, headache, confusion, seizures, hallucinations, coma
Respiratory	Tachypnea, cough, hoarseness, stridor, dyspnea, retractions, wheezing, chest pain/tightness, rales/rhonchi, sooty sputum
Facial	Singed nasal hairs, soot in oropharynx, facial burns
Cardiac	Arrhythmias

From Bayer, M, Rumack, B, and Wanke, L: TOXICOLOGIC EMERGENICES, © 1984, p. 13 (A Brady Book). Reprinted by permission of Prentice-Hall Inc, Englewood Cliffs, New Jersey.

1-21/ADSORPTION CHARACTERISTICS OF COMPOUNDS TO ACTIVATED CHARCOAL

COMPOUNDS WITH SIGNIFICANT ADSORPTION

Acetaminophen	Glutethimide	Phenothiazines
Aconitine	Hexachlorophene	Phenytoin
Amphetamines	Iodine	Phosphorus
Antimony	Ipecac	Phenylpropanolamine
Antipyrine	Isoniazid	Potassium permanganate
Atropine	Kerosene	Primaquine
Arsenic	Malathion	Probenecid
Barbiturates	Mefenamic acid	Propantheline
Camphor	Meprobamate	Propoxyphene
Cantharides	Mercuric chloride	Quinacrine
Chlordane	Methyl salicylate	Quinidine
Chloroquine	Methylene blue	Quinine
Chlorpheniramine	Muscarine	Salicylamide
Cocaine	Narcotics	Salicylates
Colchicine	Nicotine	Selenium
2,4-D	Oxalates	Silver
Digitalis	Parathion	Stramonium
Digitoxin	Penicillin	Strychnine
Ergotamine	Phenol	Sulfonamides
Ethchlorvynol	Phenolphthalein	Tricyclic antidepressants

COMPOUNDS WITH LITTLE OR NO ADSORPTION

Alcohol	Cyanide	Mineral acids
Alkali	Ferrous sulfate	N-methyl carbamate
Boric acid	Methanol	

From Bayer, M, Rumack, R, and Wanke, L: TOXICOLOGIC EMERGENCIES, Bowie, Maryland, 1984, Brady Communications Co Inc. Reprinted by permission of Prentice-Hall, Inc, Englewood Cliffs, NJ.

APPEN-
DIX

1-22/POISON ANTIDOTES

Specific agent	Symptoms requiring treatment	Antidote	Dosage
Acetaminophen (Tylenol®, Nebs®)	Hepatotoxicity (hepatocellular necrosis)	N-acetylcysteine	*Oral:* 140 mg/kg initial dose followed by 70 mg/kg every 8 hours for 17 doses.
Anticholinergic agents	Central and/or peripheral anticholinergic symptoms and at least one of the following: Hypertension Hallucinations Convulsions Coma Arrhythmias	Physostigmine	*Adults:* 1 or 2 mg IV slowly (1 mg/minute). Repeat in 20 minutes if no reversal. Then 1 to 2 mg IV for recurrent symptoms. *Children:* 0.5 mg IV (0.5 mg/minute). Readminister at 5-minute intervals to maximum of 2 mg if symptoms persist. Repeat with lowest effective trial dose if life-threatening symptoms recur.
Cholinergic agents Physostigmine Neostigmine Pyridostigmine Pilocarpine Bethanechol Methacholine	Cholinergic crisis Diaphoresis Lacrimation Bronchial secretions Excessive urination and defecation Convulsions Fasciculations	Atropine sulfate	*Adults:* 2 mg IV. *Children:* 0.05 mg/kg IV. Repeat until cessation of secretions.
Cyanide (potassium cyanide, hydrocyanic acid, laetrile, nitroprusside sodium)	Cyanosis Cardiopulmonary arrest Convulsions Coma	Sodium nitrite then Sodium thiosulfate	*Adults:* 300 mg IV (10 ml of 3% solution). *Children:* Dose based on serum hemoglobin. *Adults:* 12.5 grams IV (50ml of 25% solution)
Ethylene glycol	Acidosis Oxalate crystals in urine	Ethanol	*Loading dose:* 600 mg/kg (1 ml absolute alcohol × 790 mg) IV in D$_5$W over 15 minutes. *Maintenance dose:* To maintain blood level of 100 mg percent. Varies depending on drinking history of patient.
Neuroleptic agents Haloperidol (Haldol®) Loxapine succinate (Loxitane®) Molindone (Moban®) Phenothiazines Chlorpromazine (Thorazine®) Fluphenazine (Prolixin®)	Extrapyramidal symptoms: Dystonia Dyskinesia Oculogyric crisis Parkinsonian symptoms	Diphenhydramine or Benztropine	25 to 50 mg IV, IM, or 1 to 2 mg IV, IM.

From Conner, CS, et al: Rational use of emergency antidotes. In Bayer, MJ and Rumack, BH: Poisoning and overdose, Aspen Systems, Rockville, Maryland, 1983, pp 28–29. Reprinted with permission of Aspen Publishers, Inc, © 1983.

Specific agent	Symptoms requiring treatment	Antidote	Dosage
Thioridazine (Mellaril®)			
Iron salts (ferrous sulfate, ferrous gluconate)	Hypotension Shock Coma (free serum iron present)	Deferoxamine	*Shock and/or coma:* 15 mg/kg/hour IV for 8 hours. *Absence of shock or coma but SI > TIBC:* 90 mg/kg IM every 8 hours × 3 doses.
Methanol	Acidosis Methanol blood level exceeding 20 mg%	Ethanol	*Loading dose:* 600 mg/kg (1 ml absolute alcohol = 790 mg) IV in D_5W over 15 minutes. *Maintenance dose:* To maintain blood level of 100 mg percent. Varies depending on drinking history of the patient.
Methemoglobin-producing agents Nitrates/nitrites Phenazopyridine Phenacetin	Methemoglobinemia (> 30%)	Methylene blue	1 to 2mg/kg IV (0.1 to 0.2 ml/kg) of 1 percent solution. NOTE: Contraindicated in methemoglobinemia secondary to sodium nitrite in cyanide poisoning.
Narcotic analgesics and related agents	Respiratory depression Hypotension Coma	Naloxone	*Adults:* 0.8 mg IV, IM, SC. *Children:* 0.01 mg/kg IV, IM, SC. Repeat at 10 × (times) original dose if no response.
Organophosphate insecticides Malathion Parathion	Cholinergic crisis Diaphoresis Lacrimation Bronchial secretions Excessive urination and defecation Convulsions Fasciculations Profound weakness Muscular twitching	Atropine sulfate	*Adults:* 2 to 4 mg IV slowly; repeat every 10 to 30 minutes to attain and maintain atropinization (decreased bronchial secretions). *Children:* 0.05 mg/kg IV. Slowly repeat every 10 to 30 minutes to attain and maintain atropinization (decreased bronchial secretions).
		Pralidoxime	*After atropine:* *Adults:* 1 g IV (500 mg/minute). Repeat × 3 at 8- to 12-hour intervals if muscle weakness not relieved. *Children:* 25 to 50 mg/kg IV. Repeat × 3 at 8- to 12-hour intervals if muscle weakness not relieved.

*See text specific dosages and precautions.
**Investigational.

1-23/OVER-THE-COUNTER DRUG REACTIONS

This chart deals strictly with products that can be bought over the counter and points out the potentially hazardous reactions that may occur.

As described in the chart, the combination of alcohol-containing products can increase the damage to the stomach lining and possibly cause blood loss.

Also described in this chart is the combination of alcohol-containing OTC products that, when combined with other OTC antihistamine-containing products, may cause drowsiness. Although some cough and cold remedies cause drowsiness when taken alone, combination compounds the decrease in alertness.

When selecting a product in the OTC category it is always advisable to evaluate the ingredients to avoid any further complications with other OTC products or prescription medications, as pointed out in this and following charts.

The OTC products that interact with other prescription medications are described in the following charts.

Any of these OTC drugs may interact with	any of these OTC/food items as described in introductory material.	
Alcoholic beverages	A.P.C. and A.P.C. Compound	PAC
Beer	A.S.A., A.S.A. Compound	Pamprin
Cheracol, Cheracol D	Alka-Seltzer	Phensal
Cosanyl-DM	Alka-2	Pyrilamine
Creo-Terpin	Allerest	Robitussin-AC
Demazin Syrup	Anacin products	Sinutab
Dristan Cough Formula	A.R.M.	Sleep-Eze
Histadyl E.C.	Arthritis Strength Bufferin	Sodium salicylate
Neo-Synephrine Tablets	Ascriptin	Sominex
Novahistine-DH and Novahistine Expectorant	Aspergum	Sudafed Plus
	Aspirin	Triaminic liquids
Nyquil	Bayer products	Triaminicin
Pertussin	Bufferin	Triaminicol
Robitussin, Robitussin-AC, Robitussin DM	Cama	Vanquish
	Chlorpheniramine products	Vicks Formula 44
Triaminic Expectorant	Chlor-Trimeton	Cough Mixture
Valadol Liquid	Compoz	
Vicks Formula 44 Cough Mixture	Comtrex	
	Conar	
	Contac	
	Coricidin products	
	Coryban-D Capsules	
	Demazin	
	Dormin	
	Ecotrin	
	Empirin compound	
	Excedrin	
	4-Way Cold Tablets	
	Histadyl E.C.	
	Measurin	
	Midol	
	Neo-Synephrine Tablets	
	Novahistine products	
	Nyquil	
	Nytol	

Continued.

Antihistamine Interactions

Any of these prescription drugs* may interact with	any of these prescription drug groups	and result in this interaction	OTC/food items
Azatadine (Optimine) Brompheniramine (Dimetane) Chlorpheniramine (Chlor-Trimeton, Teldrin) Clemastine (Tavist) Cyproheptadine (Periactin) Dexchlorpheniramine (Polaramine) Dimetapp Diphenhydramine (Benadryl) Disophrol Drixoral Naldecon Nolamine Novafed-A Ornade Promethazine (Phenergan) Pyribenzamine Tripelennamine (PBZ) Triprolidine (Actidil)	Acenocoumarol (Sintrom) Anisindione (Miradon) Bishydroxy-coumarin (Dicumarol) Griseofulvin (Fulvicin, Grifulvin) Oral contraceptives Oxyphenbutazone (Tandearil) Phenindione (Hedulin) Phenprocoumon (Liquamar) Phenylbutazone (Azolid, Butazolidin) Phenytoin (Dilantin) Warfarin (Coumadin)	This interaction can cause a decrease in the effectiveness of the prescription drugs listed in column 2.	A.R.M. Alcoholic products Allerest Bayer Decongestant Cold Tablets Beer Cheracol, Cheracol D Coldene Compoz Comtrex Conar Contac Coricidin Coryban-D Cosanyl-DM Demazin Dormin Dristan Dristan Cough Formula Histadyl E.C. Neo-Synephrine Novahistine Nyquil Nytol Pertussin Pyrilamine Robitussin-AC & Robitussin DM Sinutab Sleep-Eze Sominex Super Anahist Triaminicin Triaminicol Vicks Formula 44 products Vicks Sinex products
	Atropine products Belladonna products (Donnatal) Dicyclomine (Bentyl) Furazolidone (Furoxone) Glycopyrrolate (Robinul) Isocarboxazid (Marplan) Pargyline (Eutonyl) Phenelzine (Nardil) Procarbazine (Matulane) Propantheline (Pro-Banthine) Tranylcypromine	The combination of these medications may cause constipation, dry mouth, blurred vision, urine retention, and possible increased heart rate. Also a possibility of decreased mental alertness may occur. See below for additional prescription drug–prescription drug interactions involving antihistamines listed in column 1.	

The drugs listed in here, column 1, are antihistamines and antihistamine combinations. The combinations listed usually contain a decongestant such as pseudoephedrine or phenylpropanolamine.

Indications, depending on the type of antihistamine, include allergies, nasal congestion and drainage, and watery eyes. Antihistamines are commonly employed to aid in the treatment of nausea, vomiting, dizziness, vertigo, and insomnia.

Hydroxyzine (Atarax, Vistaril) is an antihistamine but is also indicated to be useful in the management of pruritus resulting from allergic conditions and contact dermatoses.

Antihistamines can potentiate other central nervous system–acting drugs, so special precautions should be exercised when these are used in conjunction, especially with narcotics, barbiturates, and alcohol.

Antihistamines may cause anticholinergic effects, such as dry mouth, which could be relieved by chewing gum. Smoking tends to cause further irritation and should be avoided. If nausea or upset stomach is a problem, the medication should be taken with food or milk.

The interactions denoted here between antihistamines and OTC drugs should be

Antihistamine Interactions—cont'd

avoided since an increased potential for severe drowsiness or decrease in mental alertness may occur.

Any of these prescription drugs* may interact with	any of these prescription drug groups	and result in this interaction	OTC/food items
	(Parnate) Trihexphenidyl (Artane)		

Azatadine (Optimine)
Brompheniramine (Dimetane)
Chlorpheniramine (Chlor-Trimeton, Teldrin)
Clemastine (Tavist)
Cyproheptadine (Periactin)
Dexchlor-pheniramine (Polaramine)
Dimetapp
Diphenhydramine (Benadryl)
Disophrol
Drixoral
Naldecon
Nolamine
Novafed-A
Ornade
Promethazine (Phenergan)
Pyribenzamine
Tripelennamine (PBZ)
Triprolidine (Actidil)
	Amobarbital (Amytal)
	Chloral hydrate (Noctec)
	Chlordiazepoxide (Librium)
	Chlorpromazine (Thorazine)
	Clonazepam (Clonopin)
	Clorazepate (Tranxene, Azene)
	Codeine-containing products
	Cyclobenzaprine (Flexeril)
	Diazepam (Valium)
	Esgic
	Ethchlorvynol (Placidyl)
	Fiorinal
	Fluphenazine (Prolixin)
	Flurazepam (Dalmane)
	Glutethimide (Doriden)
	Hydroxyzine (Atarax, Vistaril)
	Librax
	Limbitrol
	Lorazepam (Ativan)
	Meprobamate (Equanil, Miltown)
	Oxazepam (Serax)
	Oxybutynin (Ditropan)
	Pentobarbital (Nembutal)
	Perphenazine (Trilafon)
	Phenobarbital (Luminal)
	Prazepam (Centrax)
	Prochlorperazine (Compazine)
	Promazine (Sparine)
	Propoxyphene (Darvon, Darvocet)
		The combination of the medications listed in column 2 with the drugs in column 1 could cause an increase in the likelihood of central nervous system depression.
		    Such a combination could result in drowsiness, dizziness, blurred vision, loss of appetite, and a decrease in mental alertness.
		    Caution must be exercised if operating any type of machinery or driving. It is not advisable to drink alcoholic beverages while taking any of these medications as this may compound the problem of adverse side effects.	

Secobarbital (Seconal)
Thioridazine (Mellaril)
Thiothixene (Navane)
Triclofos (Triclos)
Trifluoperazine
  (Stelazine)
Tuinal

*Some prescription drugs listed or their active ingredients may be available OTC.

1-24/CROSS-REFERENCE GUIDE TO DRUGS (GENERIC AND BRAND NAMES)

Drugs or drug type	Brand names	Generic name
Acetaminophen (systemic)	Algophen* Atasol* Atasol Forte* Campain* Datril Empracet* Exdol* Liquiprin Phenaphen Robigesic* Rounox* SK-APAP Tempra Tivrin* Tylenol Tylenol Extra Strength Valadol	Acetaminophen
Acetaminophen and codeine (systemic)	Aceta with Codeine Capital with Codeine Empracet with Codeine Papa-Deine Pavadon Phenaphen with Codeine Proval SK-APAP with Codeine Tylenol with Codeine	
Acrisorcin (topical)	Akrinol	Acrisorcin
Adrenocorticoids (dental)	Orabase HCA	Hydrocortisone
	Kenalog in Orabase	Triamcinolone
Adrenocorticoids (ophthalmic)	Decadron Maxidex Novadex*	Dexamethasone
	FML Liqui-film	Fluorometholone
	Cortamed* Cortisol Hydrocortone	Hydrocortisone

Drugs or drug type	Brand names	Generic name
HMS Liquifilm Prednisone	Optef Medrysone AK-Tate Econopred Hydeltrasol Inflamase Metreton Pred Forte Pred Mild Predulose	AK-Pred
Adrenocorticoids (otic)	Decadron Maxidex	Dexamethasone
	Hydeltrasol Metreton	Prednisolone
Adrenocorticoids (topical)	Cyclocort	Amcinonide
	Benisone Betacort* Betaderm* Betnovate* Celestoderm* Celestone Valisone	Betamethasone
	Tridesilon	Desonide
	Topicort	Desoximetasone
	Aeroseb-Dex Decaderm Decadron Decaspray Hexadrol	Dexamethasone
	Florone	Diflorasone
	Locacorten* Locorten	Flumethasone
	Dermalar* Fluoderm* Fluonid Flurosyn Synalar	Fluocinolone
	Lidemol* Lidex Topsyn	Fluocinonide
	Oxylone	Fluorometholone
	Cordran Drenison*	Flurandrenolide
	Halciderm Halog	Halcinonide
	Cortaid Cort-Dome	Hydrocortisone

*Not available in the United States.

Drugs or drug type	Brand names	Generic name	Drugs or drug type	Brand names	Generic name
Adrenocroticoids (systemic)	Cortef			Doca	Desoxycorticoste-rone
	Corticreme*			Percorten	
	Cortisol			Florinef	Fludrocortisone
	Cortril		Alcohol and acetone (topical)	Seba-Nil	
	Dermacort			Sebasum	
	Hyderm*			Tyrosum	
	Hydrocortone		Alcohol and sulfur (topical)	Acne Aid	
	Hytone			Acnomead	
	Texacort			Epi-Clear	
	Medrol	Methylprednisolone		Liquimat	
	Meti-Derm	Prednisolone		Postacne	
	Aristocort	Triamcinolone		Transact	
	Aristogel			Xerac	
	Kenalog		Allopurinol (systemic)	Lopurin	Allopurinol
	Kenalog-E*			Purinol*	
	Spencort			Zyloprim	
	Triacet		Amantadine (systemic)	Symmetrel	Amantadine
	Triaderm*		Aminocaproic acid (systemic)	Amicar	Aminocaproic acid
	Triamalone*				
	Trimacort*		Aminoglycosides (systemic)	Amikin	Amikacin
	Betnelan*	Betamethasone			
	Betnesol*			Apogen	Gentamicin
	Celestone			Bristagen	
	Cortone	Cortisone		Cidomycin*	
	Decadron	Dexamethasone		Garamycin	
	Dexasone			U-Gencin	
	Hexadrol			Kantrex	Kanamycin
	Alphadrol	Fluprednisolone		Klebcil	
	A-Hydrocort	Hydrocortisone		Mycifradin	Neomycin
	Cortef				Streptomycin
	Cortenema			Nebcin	Tobramycin
	Hydrocortone		4-Aminoquinolones (systemic)	Camoquin	Amodiaquine
	Solu-Cortef			Aralen	Chloroquine
	Betapar	Meprednisone		Plaquenil	Hydroxychloroquine
	A-MethaPred	Methylprednisolone			
	Duralone		Aminosalicylates (systemic)	Nemasol*	Aminosalicylic acid
	Medralone			P.A.S.	
	Medrol			Parasal	
	Methylone			Teebacin	
	Haldrone	Paramethasone	Amphetamines (systemic)	Benzedrine	Amphetamine
	Delta-Cortef	Prednisolone		Dexampex	Dextroamphet-amine
	Hydeltrasol			Dexedrine	
	Meticortelone			Diphylets	
	Sterone			Ferndex	
	Predoxine	Prednisolone, Buffered		Obotan	
				Oxydess	
	Colisone*	Prednisone		Spancap	
	Deltasone			Desoxyn	Methamphetamine
	Meticorten			Methampex	
	Orasone		Amphotericin B (systemic)	Fungizone	Amphotericin B
	Sterapred				
	Winpred*		Amphotericin B (topical)	Fungizone	Amphotericin B
	Aristocort	Triamcinolone			
	Aristospan		Anthralin (topical)	Anthra-Derm	Anthralin
	Cinonide			Lasan	
	Kenacort		Anticoagulants (systemic)	Miradon	Anisindione
	Kenalog			Dufalone*	Dicumarol
	Tramacort				

*Not available in the United States.

Continued.

APPEN-DIX

1-24/Cross-Reference Guide to Drugs (Generic and Brand Names)—cont'd

Drugs or drug type	Brand names	Generic name
	Danilone*	Phenindione
	Hedulin	
	Liquamar	Phenprocoumon
	Marcumar*	
	Athrombin-K	Warfarin Potassium
	Coumadin	Warfarin Sodium
	Panwarfin	
	Warfilone*	
	Warnerin*	
Antidiabetics, oral (systemic)	Dimelor*	Acetohexamide
	Dymelor	
	Chloromide*	Chlorpropamide
	Chloronase*	
	Diabinese	
	Tolinase	Tolazamide
	Mobenol*	Tolbutamide
	Neo-Dibetic*	
	Novobutamide*	
	Oramide*	
	Orinase	
	Tolbutone*	
Antidyskinetics—anticholinergic agents used to treat Parkinson's disease (systemic)	Bensylate*	Benztropine
	Cogentin	
	Akineton	Biperiden
	Pagitane	Cycrimine
	Parsidol	Ethopropazine
	Parsitan*	
	Kemadrin	Procyclidine
	Aparkane*	Trihexyphenidyl
	Artane	
	Tremin	
Antiglaucoma agents, cholinergic—long-acting cholinesterase inhibitors (ophthalmic)	Humorsol	Demecarium
	Echodide	Echothiophate
	Phospholine Iodide	Isoflurophate
	Floropryl	
Antihistamines (systemic)	Idulian*	Azatadine
	Optimine	
	Ambodryl	Bromodiphenhydramine
	Deserol*	
	Bromphen	Brompheniramine
	Dimetane	
	Ilvin*	
	Puretane	
	Symptom 3	
	Allergefon*	Carbinoxamine
	Clistin	
	Chloramate	Chlorpheniramine
	Chlor-Trimeton	
	Histalon*	
	Histaspan	
	Ibioton*	

Drugs or drug type	Brand names	Generic name
	Novopheniram*	
	Phenetron	
	Piriton*	
	Teldrin	
	Tavegil*	Clemastine
	Tavist	
	Cyprodine	Cyproheptadine
	Nuran*	
	Periactin	
	Vimicon*	
	Polaramine	Dexchlorpheniramine
	Dramamine	Dimenhydrinate
	Eldodram	
	Gravol*	
	Novodimenate*	
	Travamine*	
	Dimethpyrindene	Dimethindene
	Forhistal	
	Triten	
	Benadryl	Diphenhydramine
	Bendylate	
	Eldadryl	
	Insomnal*	
	Nautamine*	
	Valdrene	
	Diafen	Diphenylpyraline
	Hispril	
	Decapryn	Doxylamine
	Allertoc	Pyrilamine
	Mepyramine	
	Neo-Antergan*	
	Thylogen	
	Benzoxal*	Tripelennamine
	PBZ	
	Pyribenzamine	
	Pyrizil*	
	Actidil	Triprolidine
	Actidilon*	
	Pro-Actidil*	
Antipyrine, benzocaine, and glycerin (otic)	Auralgan	
	Aurasol	
Antithyroid agents (systemic)	Tapazole	Methimazole
	Thiamazole	
	Propacil	Propylthiouracil
	Propyl-Thyracil	
APC (Aspirin, phenacetin, and caffeine) (systemic)	Acetophen	
	Aidant	
	APAC	
	A.S.A. Compound	

*Not available in the United States.

Drugs or drug type	Brand names	Generic name	Drugs or drug type	Brand names	Generic name
APC and codeine (systemic)	Asalco No. 1			Butisol	
	Asphac-G			Sombulex	Hexobarbital
	P-A-C Compound			Mebaral	Mephobarbital
	Phencaset			Gemonil	Metharbital
	Sal-Fayne			Nembutal	Pentobarbital
	Salphenine			Nova-Rectal*	
	Tabloid APC			Pentogen*	
	Empirin Compound with Codeine			Eskabarb*	Phenobarbital
	A.S.A. and Codeine Compound			Gardenal*	
				Nova-Pheno*	
	P-A-C Compound with Codeine			Sedadrops	
	Salatin with Codeine			SK-Phenobarbital	
	Tabloid APC with Codeine			Solfoton	
				Secogen*	Secobarbital
				Seconal	
				Seral*	
				Tuinal	Secobarbital and Amobarbital
Appetite suppressants (systemic)	Didrex	Benzphetamine		Lotusate	Talbutal
	Pre-State	Chlorphentermine	Beclomethasone (inhalation)	Beclovent	Beclomethasone
				Vanceril	
	Voranil	Clortermine	Belladonna alkaloids and barbiturates (systemic)	Minabel	Atropine, hyoscyamine, scopolamine, and butabarbital
	Dietec*	Diethylpropion		Omnibel	
	Regibon*			Palbar	
	Tenuate				
	Tepanil			Cyclo-Bell	Atropine, hyoscyamine, scopolamine, butabarbital, pentobarbital, and phenobarbital
	Sanorex	Mazindol			
	Bontril PDM	Phendimetrazine			
	Phendiet				
	Plegine			Barbidonna	Atropine, hyoscyamine, scopolamine, and phenobarbital
	Preludin	Phenmetrazine		Donna-Sed	
	Fastin	Phentermine		Donnatal	
	Ionamin			Donphen	
Asparaginase (systemic)	Elspar			Hasp	
				Hybephen	
Atropine (anticholinergics) (ophthalmic)	Atropisol	Atropine		Hyosophen	
	BufOpto Atropine			Kinesed	
	Isopto Atropine			Sedralex	
	Homatrocel	Homatropine		Setamine	
	Isopto Homatropine			Spalix	
				Spasmolin	
				Spasmophen	
	Isopto Hyoscine	Scopolamine		Spasmorel	
				Tri-Spas	
Azathioprine (systemic)	Imuran	Azathioprine		Alised	Atropine and phenobarbital
				Antrocol	
Baclofen (systemic)	Lioresal	Baclofen		Atrobarb	
				Amobell	Belladonna and amobarbital
Barbiturates (systemic)	Amytal	Amobarbital			
	Isobec*			Butibel	Belladonna and butabarbital
	Buticaps	Butabarbital		Belap	Belladonna and phenobarbital
				Bellophen	
				Bello-Phen	
				Chardonna	

*Not available in the United States.

Continued.

APPEN-DIX

1-24/Cross-Reference Guide to Drugs (Generic and Brand Names) — cont'd

Drugs or drug type	Brand names	Generic name	Drugs or drug type	Brand names	Generic name
	Donabarb		Bleomycin (systemic)	Blenoxane	Bleomycin
	Donnabarb		Bromocriptine (systemic)	Parlodel	Bromocriptine
	Oxoids		Brompheniramine, giuaifenesin, phenylephrine, and phenylpropanolamine (systemic)	Dimatane expectorant	
	Phenobel			Midatane expectorant	
	Phenobella			Normatene expectorant	
	Sedajen			Puretane expectorant	
	Valaspas			Spentane expectorant	
	Hybar	Hyoscyamine, scopolamine, and phenobarbital	Brompheniramine, guaifenesin, phenylephrine, phenylpropanolamine, and codeine (systemic)	Dimatane expectorant-DC	
	Cystospaz-SR	Hyoscyamine and butabarbital		Midatane DC expectorant	
	Anaspaz PB	Hyoscyamine and phenobarbital		Normatane DC expectorant	
	Levsin-PB			Puretane Expectorant DC	
	Levsin w/Phenobarbital			Spentane DC expectorant	
	Levsinex w/Phenobarbital		Brompheniramine, phenylephrine, and phenylpropanolamine (systemic)	Brompheniramine Compound	
Benzodiazepines (systemic)	A-poxide	Chlordiazepoxide		Bromatapp	
	C-Tran*			Dimetapp	
	Librium			Eldatapp	
	Nack*			Puretapp	
	Novopoxide*		Busulfan (systemic)	Myleran	Busulfan
	Relaxil*		Butalbital and APC (systemic)	Fiorinal	
	SK-Lygen		Butalbital, APC, and codeine (systemic)	Fiorinal with codeine	
	Tranxene	Clorazepate			
	D-Tran*	Diazepam	Butorphanol (systemic)	Stadol	Butorphanol
	E-Pam*		Calcitonin (systemic)	Calcimar	Calcitonin
	Novodipam*		Capreomycin (systemic)	Capastat	Capreomycin
	Valium		Carbachol (ophthalmic)	Carbacel	Carbachol
	Vivol*			Isopto Carbachol	
	Dalmane	Flurazepam		Miostat	
	Ativan	Lorazepam		Murocarb	
	Serax	Oxazepam	Carboprost (systemic)	Prostin/15 M	Carboprost
	Verstran	Prazepam	Carisoprodol (systemic)	Rela	Carisoprodol
Benzoyl peroxide (topical)	Benoxyl	Benzoyl peroxide		Soma	
	Benzac			Soprodol	
	Benzagel		Carmustine (systemic)	BiCNU	Carmustine
	Clear By Design		Cephalosporins (systemic)	Ceclor	Cefaclor
	Dermodex			Duricef	Cefadroxil
	Desquam-X				
	Epi-Clear				
	Fostex BPO				
	Panoxyl				
	Persadox				
	Persa-Gel				
	Porox 7				
	Teen				
	Topex				
	Xerac BP				
Beta-adrenergic blocking agents (systemic)	Lopressor	Metoprolol			
	Corgard	Nadolol			
	Inderal	Propranolol			
Bethanechol (systemic)	Duvoid				
	Myotonachol				
	Urecholine				

*Not available in the United States.

Drugs or drug type	Brand names	Generic name	Drugs or drug type	Brand names	Generic name
	Ultracef		Chlorpheniramine, phenylpropano-lamine, and iso-propamide (systemic)	Allernade Capade Ornade	
	Mandol	Cefamandole			
	Ancef	Cefazolin			
	Kefzol				
	Mefoxin	Cefoxitin	Chlorzoxazone (systemic)	Paraflex	Chlorzoxazone
	Ceporex*	Cephalexin			
	Keflex		Chlorzoxazone and acetamino-phen (systemic)	Chlorofon-F	
	Kafocin	Cephaloglycin		Chlorzone Forte	
	Ceporan*	Cephaloridine			
	Loridine			Lobac	
	Ceporacin*	Cephalothin		Miflex	
	Keflin Neu-tral			Parachlor	
				Parafon Forte	
	Cefadyl	Cephapirin		Tuzon	
	Anspor	Cephradine			
	Velosef		Cholestyramine (oral)	Questran	Cholestyramine
Charcoal, activated (oral)	Charcocaps Charcodote Charcotabs		Cimetidine (systemic)	Tagamet	Cimetidine
Chloral hydrate (systemic)	Aquachloral Chloralex* Chloralvan* Cohidrate Noctec Novochlorhy-drate* Oradrate		Cisplatin (systemic)	Platinol	Cisplatin
			Clindamycin (topical)	Cleocin T	Clindamycin
			Clofibrate (systemic)	Atromid-S	Clofibrate
			Clomiphene (systemic)	Clomid	Clomiphene
Chlorambucil (systemic)	Leukeran	Chlorambucil	Clonidine (systemic)	Catapres	Clonidine
Chloramphenicol (ophthalmic)	Chloromyce-tin Chloroptic Econochlor Fenicol* Ophthochlor Pentamyce-tin* Sopamycetin*	Chloramphenicol	Clonidine and chlorthalidone (systemic)	Combipres	
			Clotrimazole (topical)	Lotrimin Mycelex	Clotrimazole
			Clotrimazole (vaginal)	Gyne-Lotrim-in	Clotrimazole
			Coal tar (topical)	DHS tar Estar Medotar Pentrax Tar Pso-Rite Supertah Tar Dak Tarbonis Tarpaste Tersa-Tar Ul-Tar Zetar	
Chloramphenicol (otic)	Chloromyce-tin	Chloramphenicol			
Chloramphenicol (systemic)	Amphicol Chloromyce-tin Novochloro-cap* Pentamyce-tin*	Chloramphenicol			
Chloramphenicol (topical)	Chloromyce-tin	Chloramphenicol	Colchicine (systemic)	Colsalide Im-proved	Colchicine
Chlordiazepoxide and amitriptyline (systemic)	Limbitrol		Colestipol (systemic)	Colestid	Colestipol
Chlordiazepoxide and clidinium (systemic)	Librax		Colistin, neomy-cin, and hydro-cortisone (otic)	Coly-Mycin S	
Chloroxine (topical)	Capitrol	Chloroxine	Cromolyn (inhalation)	Intal	Cromolyn

APPEN DIX

1-24/Cross-Reference Guide to Drugs (Generic and Brand Names) — cont'd

Drugs or drug type	Brand names	Generic name	Drugs or drug type	Brand names	Generic name
Cyclandelate (systemic)	Cyclospasmol	Cyclandelate	Diphenoxylate and atropine (systemic)	Colonil Lomotil SK-Diphe-noxylate	
Cyclobenzaprine (systemic)	Flexeril	Cyclobenzaprine	Dipivefrin (ophthalmic)	Propine	Dipivefrin
Cyclopentolate (ophthalmic)	Cyclogyl Mydplegic*	Cyclopentolate	Dipyridamole (systemic)	Persantine	Dipyridamole
Cyclophosphamide (systemic)	Cytoxan Procytox*	Cyclophosphamide	Disopyramide (systemic)	Norpace Rythmodan*	Disopyramide
Cycloserine (systemic)	Seromycin	Cycloserine	Disulfiram (systemic)	Antabuse	Disulfiram
Cytarabine (systemic)	Cytosar-U	Cytarabine	Doxapram (systemic)	Dopram	Doxapram
Dacarbazine (systemic)	DTIC-Dome	Dacarbazine	Doxylamine and pyridoxine (systemic)	Bendectin	
Dactinomycin (systemic)	Cosmegen	Dactinomycin	Drocode, prome-thazine, and APC (systemic)	Synalgos-DC	
Danazol (systemic)	Cyclomen* Danocrine	Danazol	Ephedrine (systemic)	Ectasule Mi-nus Ephedsol	
Dantrolene (systemic)	Dantrium	Dantrolene	Epinephrine (ophthalmic)	Epifrin Epitrate Glaucon Murocoll Mytrate Epinal Eppy/N	Epinephrine Epinephryl Borate
Dapsone (systemic)	Avlosulfon	Dapsone			
Desonide and ace-tic acid (otic)	Tridesilon				
Dexamethasone (nasal)	Decadron	Dexamethasone	Epinephrine (systemic)	Adrenalin AsthmaHaler Bronitin Bronkaid Medihaler-Epi Primatene	Epinephrine
Dexbrompheniram-ine and pseudoe-phedrine (systemic)	Disophrol Drixoral				
Diazoxide (oral)	Proglycem	Diazoxide		AsthmaNefrin microNE-FRIN Vaponefrin	Racepinephrine
Dicyclomine (systemic)	Bentyl Bentylol* Cyclobec* Dyspas	Dicyclomine	Ergoloid mesy-lates (systemic)	Hydergine	
Digitalis medicines (systemic)	Cedilanid-D	Deslanoside	Ergonovine (systemic)	Ergotrate	Ergonovine
	Digifortis Pil-Digis	Digitalis		Methergine	Methylergonovine
	Crystodigin Purodigin	Digitoxin	Ergotamine (systemic)	Ergomar Ergostat Gynergen Medihaler Er-gotamine	Ergotamine tartrate
	Lanoxin	Digoxin			
	Gitaligin	Gitalin	Ergotamine, bella-donna alka-loids, and phe-nobarbital (systemic)	Bellergal Bellergal-S	
	Cedilanid	Lanatoside C			
	Strophanthin-G	Ouabain			
Dimethyl sulfoxide (topical)	Rimso-50	Dimethyl sulfoxide			
Dinoprost (intra-amniotic)	Prostin F$_2$ Al-pha	Dinoprost			
Dinoprostone (vaginal)	Prostin E$_2$	Dinoprostone			
Dione-type anti-convulsants (systemic)	Paradione Tridione	Paramethadione Trimethadione			

*Not available in the United States.

Drugs or drug type	Brand names	Generic name	Drugs or drug type	Brand names	Generic name
Ergotamine and caffeine (systemic)	Cafergot Cafermine Cafetrate Ergocaf Ergocaffeine Lanatrate Migrastat			Premarin	Conjugated estrogens
Ergotamine, caffeine, belladonna alkaloids, and phenobarbital (systemic)	Cafergot-PB			Ogen Piperazine Estrone Sulfate	Estropipate
Erythromycin (ophthalmic)	Ilotycin	Erythromycin	Estrogens and progestins — oral contraceptives (systemic)	Demulen	Ethynodiol diacetate and ethinyl estradiol
Erythromycin (topical)	Ilotycin	Erythromycin		Ovulen	Ethynodiol diacetate and mestranol
Erythromycin (systemic)	E-Mycin Erythromid* Ilotycin Novorythro* Robimycin RP-Mycin	Erythromycin		Ovcon Brevicon Modicon	Norethindrone and ethinyl estradiol
	Ilosone	Erythromycin estolate		Norinyl Ortho-Novum	Norethindrone and mestranol
	E.E.S. E-Mycin E Pediamycin Wyamycin E	Erythromycin ethylsuccinate		Norlestrin Loestrin	Norethindrone acetate and ethinyl estradiol
	Ilotycin	Erythromycin gluceptate		Enovid	Norethynodrel and mestranol
	Erythrocin	Erythromycin lactobionate		Ovral Lo-Ovral	Norgestrel and ethinyl estradiol
	Bristamycin Erypar Erythrocin Ethril Pfizer-E SK-Erythromycin Wyamycin S	Erythromycin stearate	Ethacrynic acid (systemic)	Edecrin	Ethacrynic acid
Estrogens (systemic)	TACE DES	Chlorotrianisene Diethylstilbestrol	Ethambutol (systemic)	Etibi* Myambutol	Ethambutol
	Stilphostrol Delestrogen	Estradiol	Ethchlorvynol (systemic)	Placidyl	Ethchlorvynol
	Estrace Progynon		Ethinamate (systemic)	Valmid	Ethinamate
	Premarin	Conjugated estrogens	Ethionamide (systemic)	Trecator-SC	Ethionamide
	Amnestrogen Theelin Ogen Piperazine Estrone Sulfate	Esterified estrogens Estrone Estropipate	Ethylnorepinephrine (systemic)	Bronkephrine	Ethylnorepinephrine
	Estinyl Feminone	Ethinyl estradiol	Fenfluramine (systemic)	Pondimin	Fenfluramine
	Estrovis	Quinestrol	Fenoprofen (systemic)	Nalfon	Fenoprofen
Estrogens (vaginal)	DV Cream DES	Dienestrol Diethylstilbestrol	Flucytosine (systemic)	Ancobon Ancotil*	Flucytosine
			Fluorouracil (systemic)	Adrucil	Fluorouracil
			Fluorouracil (topical)	Efudex Fluoroplex	Fluorouracil
			Furosemide (systemic)	Furoside* Lasix Neo-renal Novosemide* Uritol*	Furosemide
			Gentamicin (ophthalmic-otic)	Garamycin Genoptic	Gentamicin
			Gentamicin (topical)	Garamycin	Gentamicin

*Not available in the United States.

Continued.

1-24/Cross-Reference Guide to Drugs (Generic and Brand Names) — cont'd

Drugs or drug type	Brand names	Generic name	Drugs or drug type	Brand names	Generic name
Gentian violet (vaginal)	Genapax Hyva	Gentian violet	Haloprogin (topical)	Halotex	Haloprogin
Glutethimide (systemic)	Doriden Dormtabs	Glutethimide	Heparin (systemic)	Hepalean* Heprinar	Heparin
Glycerin (systemic)	Glyrol Osmoglyn			Lipo-Hepin Liquaemin	
Gold compounds (systemic)	Solganal Myochrysine	Aurothioglucose Gold sodium thio-	Hydantoin-type anticonvulsants	Panheprin Peganone	Ethotoin
		malate	(systemic)	Mesantoin Methoin*	Mephenytoin
Griseofulvin (systemic)	Fulvicin P/G Fulvicin-U/F	Griseofulvin		Dantoin* Dilantin	Phenytoin
	Grifulvin V Grisactin			Di-Phen Diphenylan	
	Grisovin-FP* grisOwen Gris-PEG			Diphenylhy- dantoin	
Guaifenesin (systemic)	2/G Anti-Tuss	Guaifenesin	Hydralazine (systemic)	Apresoline Rolazine*	Hydralazine
	Breonesin Genetuss		Hydrocodone (systemic)	Codone Corutol DH*	Hydrocodone
	Glycotuss Glytuss			Dicodid Robidone*	
	Hytuss Malotuss		Hydrocodone and hematropine	Hycodan	
	Nortussin Proco		(systemic) Hydrocodone and	Tussionex	
	Robitussin		phenyltolox- amine resin		
Guaifenesin and codeine	Cheracol Nortussin w/		complexes (systemic)		
(systemic)	Codeine Robitussin A-		Hydrocodone and pseudoephe-	Tussend	
	C Tolu-Sed		drine (systemic)		
Guaifenesin and dextromethorpan	Anti-Tuss DM		Hydrocodone, pseudoephe-	Tussend expectorant	
(systemic)	Cheracol D Dextro-Tuss		drine, and guai- fenesin		
	GG 2-G-DM		(systemic) Hydrocortisone	Cortifoam	Hydrocortisone
	G-Tuss DM Guaiadex		(rectal)	Cort-Dome Proctocort	
	Neo-Vadrin Queltuss		Hydrocortisone and acetic acid	Vōsol HC	
	Robitussin- DM		(otic) Hydrocortisone,	Wyanoids HC	
	Silexin Tolu-Sed DM		belladonna, ephedrine, zinc		
	Trocal Unproco		oxide, boric acid, bismuth,		
Guanethidine (systemic)	Ismelin	Guanethidine	and peruvian balsam (rectal)		
Guanethidine and hydrochlorothia-	Esimil		Hydrocortisone, bismuth, benzyl	Anusol-HC	
zide (systemic)			benzoate, peru- vian balsam,		
Haloperidol (systemic)	Haldol	Haloperidol	and zinc oxide (rectal)		

*Not available in the United States.

Drugs or drug type	Brand names	Generic name	Drugs or drug type	Brand names	Generic name
Hydroxyurea (systemic)	Hydrea	Hydroxyurea	Isoniazid (systemic)	INH Isotamine* Nydrazid Rimifon*	Isoniazid
Hydroxyzine (systemic)	Atarax Vistaril	Hydroxyzine			
Ibuprofen (systemic)	Motrin	Ibuprofen	Isoproterenol (systemic)	Aerolone Iprenol	Isoproterenol
Idoxuridine (ophthalmic)	Dendrid Herplex Stoxil	Idoxuridine		Isuprel Medihaler-Iso Norisodrine Aerotrol Proternol Vapo-Iso	
Indomethacin (systemic)	Indocid* Indocin	Indomethacin			
Insulin (systemic)	Actrapid Regular Insulin Regular Iletin II (new)	Insulin injection	Isoproterenol and phenylephrine (systemic)	Duo-Medihaler	
	Velosulin		Isoxsuprine (systemic)	Vasodilan Vasoprine	Isoxsurpine
	Globin Insulin	Globin zinc insulin injection	Kanamycin (oral)	Kantrex	Kanamycin
	insulatard	Isophane insulin suspension	Kaolin and pectin (oral)	Kaomead Kaopectate Pargel	
	NPH NPH Iletin II				
	Mixtard	Isophane insulin suspension and insulin injection	Kaolin, pectin, belladonna alkaloids, and opium (systemic)	Donnagel-PG	
	Lentard Lente Insulin Lente Iletin II	Insulin zinc suspension	Kaolin, pectin, and paregoric (systemic)	Parepectolin	
	Monotard Ultralente Ultralente Iletin Ultratard	Extended insulin zinc suspension	Laxatives, bulk-forming (oral)	Maltsupex	Malt soup extract
	Semilente Semilente Iletin Semitard	Prompt insulin zinc suspension		Cellothyl Cologel Hydrolose	Methylcellulose
	Protamine Zinc & Iletin II PZI	Protamine zinc insulin suspension		Mitrolan	Polycarbophil Polycarbophil Calcium
Iodochlorhydroxyquin (topical)	Vioform	Iodochlorhydroxyquin		Effersyllium Konsyl L.A. Formula Metamucil Modane Bulk Mucilose Plova Serutan Siblin	Psyllium muciloid Psyllium seed Psyllium
Iodochlorhydroxyquin and hydrocortisone (topical)	Dek-Quin Domeform-HC HCV Mity-Quin Racet Vioform-HC				
Iodoquinol (systemic)	Moebiquin Yodoxin	Iodoquinol	Laxatives, emollient (oral)	Surfak	Docusate calcium
Isoetharine (systemic)	Bronkometer Bronkosol	Isoetharine		Kasof	Docusate potassium
Isometheptene, dichloralphenazone, and acetaminophen (systemic)	Midrin			Afko-Lube Colace Colax Comfolax	Docusate sodium

*Not available in the United States.

Continued.

1-24/Cross-Reference Guide to Drugs (Generic and Brand Names) — cont'd

Drugs or drug type	Brand names	Generic name	Drugs or drug type	Brand names	Generic name
	Dioctyl Sodi-um Sulfo-succinate			Bendopa	Levodopa
				Dopar	
				Larodopa	
	Alaxin	Poloxamer 188		Levopa*	
	Magcyl		Lime, sulfurated	Vlem-Dome	
Laxatives, hyperos-motic-lactulose and saline (oral)	Chronulac	Magnesium citrate	(topical)	Vleminckx's solution	
	Citrate of Magnesia		Lincomycins (systemic)	Cleocin	Clindamycin
				Dalacin C*	
	Adlerika	Magnesium sulfate		Lincocin	Lincomycin
	Epsom Salts		Lindane	GBH*	Lindane
	Phospho-Soda	Sodium phosphate	(topical)	Kwell	
	Sal hepatica	(or phosphates)		Kwellada*	
		Effervescent sodi-um phosphate	Lithium (systemic)	Eskalith	Lithium carbonate
				Lithonate	
Laxatives, lubricant (oral)	Liquid petro-latum	Mineral oil		Lithobid	
				Lithonate-S	
	Nujol			Lithane	
	Neo-Cultol	Mineral oil (jel-lied)	Lomustine (systemic)	Cee Nu	Lomustine
Laxatives, stimu-lant (oral)	Cenalax	Bisacodyl	Loperamide (systemic)	Imodium	Loperamide
	Codylax				
	Dulcolax		Loxapine (systemic)	Daxolin	Loxapine
	Theralax			Loxitane	
	Cascara Sa-grada	Cascara	Magnesia, milk of (oral)	Magnesia	
	Cas-Evac			Magnesium hydroxide	
	Alphanmul	Castor oil	Mannitol (systemic)	Osmitrol	Mannitol
	Neoloid				
	Dorbane	Danthron	Mecamylamine (systemic)	Inversine	Mecamylamine
	Modane				
	Cholan-DH	Dehydrocholic acid	Mechlorethamine (systemic)	Mustargen	Mechlorethamine
	Decholin				
	Neocholan		Meclizine	Bucladin-S	Buclizine
	Alophen	Phenolphthalein	(systemic)	Marezine	Cyclizine
	Espotabs			Antivert	Meclizine
	Evac-U-Gen			Bonine	
	Evac-U-Lax		Meclofenamate (systemic)	Meclomen	Meclofenamate
	Ex-Lax				
	Feen-A-Mint		Melphalan (systemic)	Alkeran	Melphalan
	Phenolax				
	Prulet		Meperidine (systemic)	Demerol	Meperidine
	Black Draught	Senna		Demer-Idine*	
	Casa Fru			Pethadol	
	Dr. Cald-well's Senna Laxative		Meprobamate (systemic)	Equanil	Meprobamate
				Lan-Dol*	
				Medi-Tran*	
	Fletcher's Castoria			Mep-E*	
	Senokot			Meprospan	
	Swiss Kriss			Miltown	
	X-Prep			Neo-Tran*	
	Glysennid	Sennosides A and B		Novo-Mepro*	
	Senokot			Quietal*	
	X-Prep			SK-Bamate	
Levodopa (systemic)	Sinemet	Carbidopa and le-vodopa		Tranmap	

*Not available in the United States.

Drugs or drug type	Brand names	Generic name	Drugs or drug type	Brand names	Generic name
Meprobamate, ethoheptazine, and aspirin (systemic)	Equagesic Heptogesic Mepro Compound Meprogesic		Metyrosine (systemic)	Demser	Metyrosine
			Miconazole (systemic)	Monistat	Miconazole
Mercaptopurine (systemic)	Purinethol	Mercaptopurine	Miconazole (topical)	Micatin	Miconazole
Metaproterenol (systemic)	Alupent Metaprel	Metaproterenol	Miconazole (vaginal)	Monistat	Miconazole
Methadone (systemic)	Dolophine Westadone	Methadone	Minoxidil (systemic)	Loniten	Minoxidil
Methaqualone (systemic)	Mequelon* Mequin Parest Quaalude Sedalone* Sopor Triador* Tualone*	Methaqualone	Mithramycin (systemic)	Mithracin	Mithramycin
			Mitomycin (systemic)	Mutamycin	Mitomycin
			Mitotane (systemic)	Lysodren	Mitotane
			Monoamine oxidase (MAO) inhibitors (systemic)	Marplan Nardil Parnate	Isocarboxazid Phenelzine Tranylcypromine
Methenamine (systemic)	Hiprex Urex Mandelamine Methandine* Prov-U-Sep Sterine*	Methenamine hippurate Methenamine mandelate	Nalbuphine (systemic)	Nubain	Nalbuphine
			Nalidixic acid (systemic)	Neg Gram	Nalidixic acid
			Naproxen (systemic)	Anaprox Naprosyn	Naproxen
Methocarbamol (systemic)	Delaxin Forbaxin Marbaxin-750 Metho-500 Robamol Robaxin Spinaxin Tumol	Methocarbamol	Natamycin (opthalmic)	Natacyn	Natamycin
			Neomycin (ophthalmic)	Myciguent	Neomycin
			Neomycin (oral)	Mycifradin Neobiotic	Neomycin
			Neomycin (topical)	Herisan Antibiotic* Myciguent	
Methotrexate (systemic)	Mexate	Methotrexate	Neomycin, polymyxin B, and bacitracin (ophthalmic)	Mycitracin Neo-Polycin Neosporin Polyspectrin Pyocidin	
Methoxsalen (systemic)	Oxsoralen	Methoxsalen			
Methyldopa (systemic)	Aldomet Dopamet* Medimet-250* Novomedopa*	Methyldopa	Neomycin, polymyxin B, and bacitracin (topical)	Mycitracin Neo-Polycin Neosporin	
Methyldopa and thiazide diuretics (systemic)	Aldoclor Aldoril	Methyldopa and chlorothiazide Methyldopa and hydrochlorothiazide	Neomycin, polymyxin B, and gramicidin (ophthalmic)	Neo-Polycin Neosporin	
Methylphenidate (systemic)	Methidate* Ritalin	Methylpenidate	Neomycin, polymyxin B, and hydrocortisone (ophthalmic)	Cortisporin	
Methyprylon (systemic)	Noludar	Methyprylon	Neomycin, polymyxin B, and hydrocortisone (otic)	Cortisporin Otobione	
Methysergide (systemic)	Sansert	Methysergide			
Metronidazole (systemic)	Flagyl Neo-Tric* Novonidazole* Trikacide*	Metronidazole	Nicotinyl alcohol (systemic)	Roniacol	Nicotinyl alcohol

APPENDIX

1-24/Cross-Reference Guide to Drugs (Generic and Brand Names) — cont'd

Drugs or drug type	Brand names	Generic name	Drugs or drug type	Brand names	Generic name
Organic nitrates (other than nitro-glycerin) (systemic)	Cardilate	Erythrityl tetrani-trate	Oxolinic acid (systemic)	Utibid	Oxolinic acid
	Coronex*	Isosorbide dinitrate	Oxtriphylline and guaifenesin (systemic)	Brondecon	
	Dilatrate-SR			Brondelate	
	Iso-Bid	Duotrate	Oxycodone and acetaminophen (systemic)	Percocet-5	
	Isordil	Kaytrate		Tylox	
	Isotrate	Pentraspan			
	Sorate	Pentritol	Oxycodone and aspirin (systemic)	Percodan	
	Sorbide	Peritrate		Percodan-Demi	
	Sorbitrate		Oxymetazoline (nasal)	Afrin	Oxymetazoline
	Pentaerythri-tol tetrani-trate			Duration	
				Nafrine*	
Nitrofurantoin (systemic)	Cyantin			St. Joseph Deconges-tant for Children	
	Furadantin				
	Furatine*				
	Macrodantin				
	Nephronex*		Papaverine (systemic)	Cerebid	Papaverine
	Nifuran*			Cerespan	
	Novofuran*			Dipav	
Nitroglycerin (systemic)	Glyceryl tri-nitrate	Nitroglycerin		Dylate	
	Nitro-Bid			Hyobid	
	Nitroglyn			Kavrin	
	Nitrol			Myobid	
	Nitrong			Orapav	
	Nitrospan			P-A-V	
	Nitrostat			Pavabid	
Nylidrin (systemic)	Arlidin	Nylidrin		Pavacap	
				Pavacon	
Nystatin (oral)	Mycostatin	Nystatin		Pavadur	
	Nadostine*			Pavakey	
	Nilstat			Pavased	
Nystatin (topical)	Candex	Nystatin		Pavasule	
	Mycostatin			Pavatest	
	Nadostine*			Pavatran	
	Nilstat			Paverolan	
	Nyaderm*			Ro-Papav	
Nystatin (vaginal)	Korostatin	Nystatin		Sustaverine	
	Mycostatin			Vasal	
	Nadostine*			Vasospan	
	Nilstat		Paraldehyde (systemic)	Paral	
Nystatin, neomy-cin, gramicidin, and triamcino-lone (topical)	Mycolog		Pargyline (systemic)	Eutonyl	
	Myco Triacet				
	Mytrex		Pemoline (systemic)	Cylert	
	Triamcino-lone NNG		Penicillamine (systemic)	Cuprimine	
Orphenadrine (systemic)	Flexojet			Depen	
	Flexon		Penicillins (systemic)	Amoxil	Amoxicillin
	Marflex			Larotid	
	Myolin			Novamoxin*	
	Neocyten			Penamox*	
	Norflex			Polymox	
	Ro-Orphena			Robamox	
	Tega-Flex			Sumox	
	X-Otag			Trimox	
Orphenadrine and APC (systemic)	Norgesic			Utimox	
	Norgesic Forte			Wymox	
				Amcill	Ampicillin

*Not available in the United States.

Drugs or drug type	Brand names	Generic name	Drugs or drug type	Brand names	Generic name
	Ampicin*		Phenazopyridine	Azo-100	Phenazopyridine
	Omnipen		(systemic)	Azodine	
	Penbritin			Azo-Standard	
	Pensyn			Di-Azo	
	Polycillin			Phen-Azo	
	Principen			Phenazodine	
	Supen			Pyridiate	
	Totacillin			Pyridium	
	Geocillin	Carbenicillin		Pyrodine	
	Geopen		Phenothiazines	Tindal	Acetophenazine
	Pyopen		(systemic)	Repoise	Butaperizine
	Bactopen*	Cloxacillin		Proketazine	Carphenazine
	Cloxapen			Chloramead	Chlorpromazine
	Novocloxin*			Chlor-Proma-nyl*	
	Tegopen			Chlorprom*	
	Cyclapen-W	Cyclacillin		Promapar	
	Dycill	Dicloxacillin		Promosol*	
	Dynapen			Largactil*	
	Pathocil	Hetacillin		Thorazine	
	Veracillin			Modecate*	Fluphenazine
	Versapen			Moditen*	
	Versapen-K	Methicillin		Permitil	
	Azapen			Prolixin	
	Celbenin	Nafcillin		Serentil	Mesoridazine
	Staphcillin			Phenazine*	Perphenazine
	Nafcil			Trilafon	
	Unipen			Quide	Piperacetazine
	Bactocil	Oxacillin		Compazine	Prochlorperazine
	Prostaphlin			Stemetil	
	Bicillin	Penicillin G		Norzine*	Promazine
	Crystapen*			Promanyl*	
	Crysticillin			Sparine	
	Duracillin			Mellaril	Thioridazine
	Megacillin*			Novorida-zine*	
	Penioral*			Thioril*	
	Pentids			Clinazine*	Trifluoperazine
	Permapen			Novoflura-zine*	
	Wycillin			Pentazine*	
	Betapen-VK	Penicillin V		Solazine*	
	Novopen-V*			Stelazine*	
	Penapar VK			Terfluzine*	
	Pen-Vee K			Triflurin*	
	Uticillin VK			Tripazine*	
	V-Cillin			Psyquil*	Triflupromazine
	Veetids			Vesprin	
	Ticar	Ticarcillin	Phenoxyben-zamine	Dibenzyline	
Pentazocine (systemic)	Talwin	Pentazocine	Phenylbutazone (systemic)	Oxalid	Oxyphenbutazone
Pentazocine and aspirin (systemic)	Talwin Compound			Tandearil	
				Algoverine*	Phenylbutazone
Pentobarbital and carbromal (systemic)	Carbrital			Azolid	
				Butagesic*	
Perphenazine and amitriptyline (systemic)	Etrafon Triavil			Butazolidin	
				Intrabuta-zone*	

*Not available in the United States.

Continued.

APPEN-DIX

1-24/Cross-Reference Guide to Drugs (Generic and Brand Names) — cont'd

Drugs or drug type	Brand names	Generic name	Drugs or drug type	Brand names	Generic name
	Malgesic* Nadozone* Neo-Zoline* Novobuta- zone* Phenbuta- zone* Azolid-A Butazolidin Alka Phenylzone- A	Buffered phenylbutazone		Isopto Car- pine Miocarpine* Ocusert Pilo Pilocar Pilomiotin P. V. Car- pine	
			Potassium iodide (systemic)	Kl-N Pima	Potassium iodide
Phenylephrine (nasal)	Alcon-Efrin Allerest Contac Coricidin Isophrin Neo-Mist Neo-Syneph- rine Pyracort-D Rhinall Sinarest Super Ana- hist Synasal Vacon		Potassium phos- phates (systemic)	K-Phos Orig- inal Neutra-Phos- K	Monobasic potassi- um phosphates Potassium phos- phates
			Potassium and so- dium phos- phates (system- ic)	Uro-KP-Neu- tral K-Phos M. F. K-Phos Neu- tral K-Phos No. 2 Neutra-Phos	Dibasic potassium and sodium phosphates Monobasic potassi- um and sodium phosphates Potassium and so- dium phosphates
Phenylephrine (ophthalmic)	Efricel Isopto Frin Mydfrin Neo-Syneph- rine Ocusol Phenoptic Prefrin Soothe Eye Tear-Efrin		Potassium supple- ments (sysemic)	Potassium Triplex Tri-K Trikates K-Lyte KEFF	Potassium acetate, potassium bicar- bonate, and po- tassium citrate Potassium bicar- bonate and citric acid Potassium bicar- bonate, potassi- um carbonate, and potassium chloride
Phenylpropanol- amine (systemic)	Coffee-Break Control Delcopro Diadax Dietac Obestat Pro-Dax 21 Propadrine Rhindecon			Klorvess K-Lyte/Cl	Potassium bicar- bonate and po- tassium chloride Potassium bicar- bonate, potassi- um chloride, and citric acid
Phenylpropanol- amine, phenyl- ephrine, phenyl- toloxamine, and chlorpheniramine (systemic)	Naldecon			Kaochlor-Eff Kaochlor	Potassium bicar- bonate, potassi- um chloride, and potassium citrate Potassium chloride
Physostigmine (ophthalmic)	Eserine Isopto Eser- ine	Physostigmine		Kaon-Cl Kato Kay-Ciel	
Pilocarpine (ophthalmic)	Adsorbocar- pine Almocarpine	Pilocarpine		K-Lor KLOR-10% KLOR-CON	

*Not available in the United States.

Drugs or drug type	Brand names	Generic name	Drugs or drug type	Brand names	Generic name
	Klorvess			Novopropox-	
	Klotrix			yn*	
	K-Lyte/Cl			Pargesic 65	
	Slow-K			Pro-65*	
	Kolyum	Potassium chloride		Proxagesic	
		and potassium		Proxene	
		gluconate		SK-65	
	Twin-K	Potassium citrate		642*	
		and potassium	Propoxyphene and	Darvocet-N	
		gluconate	acetaminophen	Dolacet	
	Kaon	Potassium gluco-	(systemic)	Dolene AP-	
		nate		65	
Prazosin	Minipress	Prazosin		SK-65-APAP	
(systemic)				Wygesic	
Primidone	Mysoline	Primidone	Propoxyphene and	Darvon	
(systemic)			APC	Compound	
Probenecid	Benemid	Probenecid	(systemic)	Dolene Com-	
(systemic)	Benuryl*			pound-65	
	Probalan			SK-65 Com-	
Probucol	Lorelco	Probucol		pound	
(systemic)					
Procainamide	Procamide	Procainamide	Propoxyphene and	Darvon with	
(systemic)	Procan		aspirin	A.S.A.	
	Procan SR		(systemic)	Darvon-N	
	Procopan			with	
	Pronestyl			A.S.A.	
	Sub-Quin		Pseudoephedrine	Afrinol	Pseudoephedrine
Procarbazine	Matulane	Procarbazine	(systemic)	D-Feda	
(systemic)	Natulan*			Eltor*	
Prochlorperazine	Combid			Neobid	
and isoprop-				Novafed	
amide				Pseudofrin*	
(systemic)				Robindrine*	
Progestins	Duphaston	Dydrogesterone		Ro-Fedrin	
(systemic)	Delalutin	Hydroxyprogeste-		Sudafed	
		rone		Sudrin	
	Provera	Medroxyprogeste-	Pyrilamine and	Eme-Nil	
		rone	pentobarbital	Wans	
	Megace	Megestrol	(systemic)		
	Micronor	Norethindrone	Pyrithione zinc	Danex	
	Nor-Q.D.		(topical)	Head and	
	Norlutin			Shoulders	
	Norlutate	Norethindrone ace-		Zincon	
		tate	Pyrvinium	Pamovin*	Pyrvinium
	Ovrette	Norgestrel	(systemic)	Povan	
	Proluton	Progesterone		Pyr-Pam*	
	Lipo-Lutin			Vanquin*	
Promethazine	Historest	Promethazine	Quinidine	Cardioquin	
(systemic)	Phenergan		(systemic)	Cin-Quin	
	Remsed			Duraquin	
Propantheline	Pro-Banthine	Propantheline		Quinaglute	
(systemic)				Dura-Tabs	
Propoxyphene	Algodex*	Propoxyphene		Quinate*	
(systemic)	Darvon			Quinidex Ex-	
	Depronal-			tentabs	
	SA*			Quinora	
	Dolene		Quinine	Coco-Qui-	Quinine
			(systemic)	nine	

*Not available in the United States.

APPEN
DIX

Continued.

1-24/Cross-Reference Guide to Drugs (Generic and Brand Names) — cont'd

Drugs or drug type	Brand names	Generic name	Drugs or drug type	Brand names	Generic name
	Kinine*		Rifampin	Rifadin	Rifampin
	Quine		(systemic)	Rimactane	
Quinine and ami-	Quinamm			Rofact*	
nophylline	Quinite		Rifampin and iso-	Rifamate	
(systemic)	Strema		niazid		
Rauwolfia alkaloids	Harmonyl	Deserpidine	(systemic)		
(systemic)	Raunormine*	Rauwolfia serpenti-	Salicyclates	Bayer Aspi-	Aspirin
	Raudixin	na	(systemic)	rin	
	Raulfia			Ecotrin	
	Raupoid			Empirin An-	
	Rauserpa			algesic	
	Rau-Sed	Reserpine		Measurin	
	Reserpoid			St. Joseph	
	Sandril			Aspirin	
	Serpasil			Ascriptin	Buffered aspirin
Rauwolfia alkaloids	Oreticyl	Deserpidine and		Bufferin	
and thiazide di-	Oreticyl	hydrochlorothia-		CAMA In-	
uretics	Forte	zide		lay-Tabs	
(systemic)	Enduronyl	Deserpidine and		Calurin	Carbaspirin
		methyclothiazide		Arthropan	Choline salicylate
	Rauzide	Rauwolfia serpenti-		Parbocyl	Sodium salicylate
		na and bendro-		Uracel	
		flumethiazide	Salicylic acid	Calicylic	
	Exna-R	Reserpine and	(topical)	Domerine	
		benzthiazide		Fomac	
	Diupres	Reserpine and		Hydrisalic	
		chlorothiazide		Ionil	
	Demi-	Reserpine and		Keralyt	
	Regroton	chlorthalidone		Mediplast	
	Regroton			Saligel	
	Hydropres	Reserpine and hy-		Sebisol	
	Reserpazide	drochlorothiazide		Xseb	
	Serpasil-		Salicylic acid and	Acne-Dome	
	Esidrix		sulfur	Acno	
	Salutensin	Reserpine and hy-	(topical)	Antiseb	
	Salutensin-	droflumethiazide		BUF	
	Demi			Exzit	
	Diutensen-R	Reserpine and me-		Fostex	
		thyclothiazide		Klaron	
	Renese-R	Reserpine and po-		Meted	
		lythiazide		Pernox	
	Hydromox-R	Reserpine and qui-		Rezamid	
		nethazone		SAStid	
	Metatensin	Reserpine and tri-		Sebex	
	Naquival	chlormethiazide		Sebulex	
Reserpine and hy-	Serpasil-			Therac	
dralazine	Apresoline			Vanseb	
(systemic)			Salicylic acid, sul-	Antiseb-T	
Reserpine, hydral-	Ser-Ap-Es		fur, and coal tar	Sebex-T	
azine, and hy-	Tri-Hydro-		(topical)	Sebutone	
drochlorothiazide	serpine			Vanseb-T	
(systemic)			Selenium sulfide	Exsel	
Resorcinol and	Acne-Dome		(topical)	Iosel	
Sulfur	Acnomel			Selsun	
(topical)	Cenac			Selsun Blue	
	Exzit			Sul-Blue	
	pHisoAc		Sodium fluoride	Denta-Fl	
	Sulforcin		(systemic)	Flo-Tab	

*Not available in the United States.

Drugs or drug type	Brand names	Generic name	Drugs or drug type	Brand names	Generic name
	Fluorident			Vagidine	
	Fluoritab			Vagimine	
	Fluorodex			Vagitrol	
	Flura			Sultrin	Sulfathiazole, sul-
	Karidium			Trysul	facetamide, and
	Luride				sulfabenzamide
	Luride-SF			Koro-Sulf	Sulfisoxazole
	Nafeen			Vagilia	Sulfisoxazole, ami-
	Pedi-Dent				nacrine, and al-
	Pediaflor				lantoin
	Stay-Flo		Sulfonamides and	Azo Ganta-	Sulfamethoxazole
	Studaflor		phenazopyridine	nol	and phenazopy-
Spironolactone	Aldactone	Spironolactone	(systemic)		ridine
(systemic)				Azo Gantri-	Sulfisoxazole and
Spironolactone and	Aldactazide			sin	phenazopyridine
hydrochlorothia-				Azo-Soxa-	
zide				zole	
(systemic)				Azosul	
Succinimide-type	Zarontin			Azo-Sulfizin	
anticonvulsants	Celontin			Suldiazo	
(systemic)	Milontin		Sulindac	Clinoril	Sulindac
	Ethosuximide		(systemic)		
	Methsux-		Tamoxifen	Nolvadex	Tamoxifen
	imide		(systemic)		
	Phensux-		Terbutaline	Brethine	Terbutaline
	imide		(systemic)	Bricanyl	
Sulfasalazine	Azulfidine	Sulfasalazine	Terpin hydrate	Cortussis	
(systemic)	S.A.S.-500		and codeine		
	Salazopyrin*		(systemic)		
Sulfinpyrazone	Anturan*	Sulfinpyrazone	Testolactone	Teslac	Testolactone
(systemic)	Anturane		(systemic)		
	Zynol		Tetracyclines	Aureomycin	Chlortetracycline
Sulfonamides	Bleph	Sulfacetamide	(ophthamic)	Achromycin	tetracycline
(ophthalmic)	Cetamide		Tetracyclines	Declomycin	Demeclocycline
	Isopto		(systemic)	Doxychel	doxycycline
	Cetamide			Doxy-Tabs	
	Optosulfex*			Vibramycin	
	Sulamyd			Vibra-Tabs	
	Sulf-10			Rondomycin	Methacycline
	Gantrisin	Sulfisoxazole		Minocin	Minocycline
Sulfonamides	Renoquid	Sulfacytine		Ultramycin*	
(systemic)	Gantanol	Sulfamethoxazole		Oxlopar	Oxytetracycline
	Methoxal			Oxy-Kesso-	
	Methoxanol			Tetra	
	Bactrim	Sulfamethoxazole		Terramycin	
	Septra	and trimethoprim		Tetramine	
	Gantrisin	Sulfisoxazole		Achromycin	Tetracycline
	Lipo			Bio-Tetra*	
	Gantrisin			Bristacycline	
	Novosoxa-			Cyclopar	
	zole*			Medicycline*	
	Sosol			Neo-Tetrine*	
	Sulfalar			Novotetra*	
	Sulfizin			Panmycin	
	Sulfizole*			Retet	
Sulfonamides (vag-	AVC	Sulfanilamide, am-		Robitet	
inal)	Femguard	inacrine, and al-		Sumycin	
	Nil	lantoin		Tetracrine*	
	Tricholan			Tetracyn	

*Not available in the United States.

Continued.

1-24/Cross-Reference Guide to Drugs (Generic and Brand Names) — cont'd

Drug or drug type	Brand names	Generic name	Drug or drug type	Brand names	Generic name
Tetracyclines (topical)	Aureomycin	Chlortetracycline		Uridon	
	Achromycin	Tetracycline		Anhydron	Cyclothiazide
	Topicycline			Esidrix	Hydrochlorothia-
Theophylline, ephedrine, and barbiturates (systemic)	Asminyl			Hydro-Aquil	zide
	Asma-lief			HydroDIU-RIL	
	Phedral			Novohydra-zide*	
	Tedfern			Oretic	
	Tedral			Diucardin	Hydroflumethiazide
	Thalfed			Saluron	
	Thedrizem			Aquatensen	Methyclothiazide
	Theodrine			Duretic	
	Theofed			Enduron	
	Theofenal			Diulo	Metolazone
	Theoral			Zaroxolyn	
	Theotabs			Renese	Polythiazide
Theophylline, ephedrine, guai-fenesin, and bar-biturates (systemic)	Broncholate			Hydromox	Quinethazone
	Bronkolixir			Metahydrin	Trichlormethiazide
	Bronkotabs			Naqua	
	Duovent		Thioxanthenes (systemic)	Taractan	Chlorprothixene
	Luftodil			Tarasan*	
	Mudrane GG			Navane	Thiothixene
	Quibron Plus		Thyroid hormones (systemic)	Levothroid	Levothyroxine
	Verequad			L-T-S	
Theophylline, ephedrine, and hydroxyzine (systemic)	Asminorel			Ro-Thyrox-ine	
	E.T.H. Com-pound			Synthroid	
	Hydrophed			Cytomel	Liothyronine
	Marax			Ro-Thy-ronine	Liotrix
	Theophozine			Tertroxin	
	Theozine			Euthroid	
Theophylline and guaifenesin (systemic)	Asbron G			Proloid	Thyroglobulin
	Asma			S-P-T	Thyroid
	Cerylin			Thyrar	
	Dialixir			Thyrocrine	
	Glybron		Thyrotropin (systemic)	Thyrotron	Thyrotropin
	Glyceryl T			Thytropar	
	Hylate		Timolol (ophthalmic)	Timoptic	Timolol
	Lanophyllin-GG		Tolmetin (systemic)	Tolectin	Tolmetin
	Quibron		Tolnaftate (topical)	Aftate	Tolnaftate
	Slo-Phyllin GG			Tinactin	
	Synophylate-GG		Tretinoin (topical)	Retin-A	Tretinoin
	Theo-Col		Triamterene (systemic)	Dyrenium	Triamterene
	Theo-Guaia		Triamterene and hydrochlorothi-azide (systemic)	Dyazide	
Thiazide diuretics (systemic)	Naturetin	Bendroflumethia-zide			
	Aquastat	Benzthiazide	Tricyclic antide-pressants (systemic)	Amitid	Amitriptyline
	Aquatag			Amitil	
	Exna			Elavil	
	Hydrex			Endep	
	Diuril	Chlorothiazide		Norpramin	
	SK-Chloro-thiazide				
	Hygroton	Chlorthalidone			
	Novothali-done*				

*Not available in the United States.

Drug or drug type	Brand names	Generic name	Drug or drug type	Brand names	Generic name
	Desipramine		(methyl)-Xan-thines	Aminodur	Aminophylline
	Pertofrane		(systemic)	Aminophyl*	
	Adapin	Doxepin		Amphylline*	
	Sinequan			Corophyllin*	
	Imavate	Imipramine		Lixaminol	
	Janimine			Mini-Lix	
	SK-Pramine			Somophyllin	
	Tofranil			Aerophyl-	Dilin
	Aventyl	Nortriptyline		line*	Dilor
	Pamelor			Airet	
	Vivactil	Protiptyline		Lufyllin	Dyphylline
	Surmontil	Trimipramine		Neothylline	
Trifluridine	Viroptic	Trifluridine		Protophyl-	
(ophthalmic)				line*	
Trimethobenzamide	Tigan	Trimethobenzamide		Choledyl	Oxtriphylline
(systemic)				Accurbron	Theophylline
Triprolidine and	Actifed			Aerolate	
pseudoephedrine	Allerphed			Asthmophyl-	
(systemic)	Tagafed			line*	
Tropicamide	Mydriacyl	Tropicamide		Bronkodyl	
(ophthalmic)				Elixicon	
Undecylenic acid₁	Decylenes			Elixophyllin	
compound	Desenex			Physpan	
(topical)	Medaped			Slophyllin	
	Quinsana			Somophyllin-	
	Plus			T	
Urea	Ureaphil			Theobid	
(systemic)				Theoclear	
Valproic acid	Depakene	Valproic acid		Theodur	
(systemic)				Theolair	
Vidarabine	Vira-A	Vidarabine		Theolixir	
(ophthalmic)				Theophyl	
Vinblastine	Velban	Vinblastine		Theospan	
(systemic)	Velbe*		Xylometazoline	4-Way Long	
Vincristine	Oncovin	Vincristine	(nasal)	Acting	
(systemic)				Neo-syneph-	
Vitamins and fluo-	Vita-Flor	Multiple vitamins		rine II	
ride	Adeflor	and fluoride		Otrivin	
(systemic)	Mulvidren-F			Rhinall Long	
	Novacebrin			Acting	
	with Fluo-			Sine-Off	
	ride			Once-A-	
	Vi-Penta F			Day	
	Poly-Vi-Flor			Sinex Long-	
	V-Daylin			Acting	
	with Fluo-			Sinutab Long	
	ride			Acting Si-	
	Cari-Tab	Vitamins A, D,		nus Spray	
	Tri-Vi-Flor	and C, and fluo-			
		ride			

*Not available in the United States.

1-25/COMMUNICABLE AND INFECTIOUS DISEASES

Name	Synopsis of symptoms	Incubation period	Mode of transmission	Period of communicability
Actinomycosis	Chronic disease most frequently localized in jaw, thorax, or abdomen; septicemic spread with generalized disease may occur. Lesions are firmly indurated areas of purulence and fibrosis.	Irregular; probably years after colonization in oral tissues, plus days or months after precipitating trauma and actual penetration of tissues.	Contact from person to person as part of normal oral flora.	Time and manner in which *A. israelii* becomes part of normal flora is unknown.
Amebiasis	Infection with a protozoan parasite that exists in two forms: the hardy, infective cyst and the more fragile, potentially invasive trophozoite. Parasite may act as a commensal or invade tissues, giving rise to intestinal or extraintestinal disease.	Variation—from a few days to several months or years. Commonly 2 to 4 weeks.	Contaminated water or food containing cysts from feces of infected persons, often as complication of another infection such as shigellosis.	During period of cyst passing, which may continue for years.
Ancylostomiasis (hookworm disease, uncinariasis, necatoriasis)	Chronic, debilitating disease with a variety of vague symptoms varying greatly, usually in proportion to degree of anemia and hypoproteinemia.	Symptoms may develop after a few weeks to many months.	Eggs in feces are deposited on ground, and under favorable environmental conditions, hatch; larvae develop to third stage, becoming infective in 7 to 10 days. Human infection occurs when infected larvae penetrate skin, usually foot.	Not transmitted from person to person, but infected persons can contaminate soil for several years in absence of treatment.
Arenaviral hemorrhagic fever	Acute febrile illnesses, duration 7 to 15 days. Onset is gradual with malaise, headache, retroorbital pain, conjunctival injection, sustained fever, and sweats, followed by prostration. An exanthem appears on thorax and flanks 3 to 5 days after onset.	Commonly 7 to 16 days.	Saliva and excreta of infected rodents contain virus. May be air-borne transmission by dust contaminated by infected rodent excreta.	Probably not often directly transmitted from person to person (although this has occurred in the Bolivia disease).
A. Arthropod-borne viral diseases (arboviral diseases)				

1. Arthropod-borne viral arthritis and rash	Acute self-limited disease characterized by arthritis, primarily in small joints of extremities that lasts from 2 days to 8 months.	10 to 11 days.	Culicine mosquitoes.	No evidence of transmission from person to person.
2. Arthropod-borne viral encephalitides a. Mosquito-borne	Group of acute inflammatory diseases of short duration. Mild cases often occur as aseptic meningitis. Severe infections are usually marked by acute onset, headache, high fever, meningeal signs, stupor, disorientation, coma, tremors, occasionally convulsions, and spastic paralysis.	Usually 5 to 15 days.	Infective mosquitoes.	Not directly transmitted from person to person. Virus is not usually demonstrable in blood of humans after onset of disease. Mosquitoes remain infective for life.
b. Tick-borne	Group of diseases resembling mosquito-borne encephalitides, except Russian spring-summer type often is associated with flaccid paralysis, particularly of the shoulder girdle.	Usually 7 to 14 days.	By infective ticks or by consuming milk from certain infected animals.	Not directly transmitted from person to person. Tick infected at any stage remains infective for life.
Angiostrongyliasis (eosinophilic meningoencephalitis, eosinophilic meningitis)	Disease of central nervous system caused by a nematode. Invasion may be asymptomatic or mildly symptomatic; more commonly characterized by severe headache, stiffness of neck and back, and various paresthesias. Temporary facial paralysis and low-grade fever may be present.	Usually 1 to 3 weeks.	Ingestion of raw or insufficiently cooked snails, slugs, or land planaarians, which are intermediate or transport hosts harboring infective larvae.	Not transmitted from person to person.
Anisakiasis	Disease of human gastrointestinal tract manifested by intestinal colic, fever, and eosinophilic abscesses resulting from ingesting uncooked fish containing larval nematodes of the family Anisakidae.	Stomach involvement may develop within a few hours of ingestion.	Infective larvae live in organs of fish until its death when they invade somatic muscles. When ingested by humans and liberated by digestion in stomach they penetrate gastric or intestinal mucosa.	No direct transmission from person to person.
Anthrax	Acute bacterial disease usually affecting skin but may rarely involve mediastinum or intestinal tract.	Within 7 days, usually 2 to 5 days.	Infection of skin is by contact with tissues of animals dying of the disease or with contaminated animal by-products (e.g., wool or hides).	No evidence of transmission from person to person. Articles and soil contaminated with spores may remain infective for years.

Continued.

APPEN-DIX

1-25/Communicable and Infectious Diseases — cont'd

Name	Synopsis of symptoms	Incubation period	Mode of transmission	Period of communicability
B. Arthropod-borne viral fevers				
1. Mosquito-borne a. Yellow fever	Acute infectious disease of short duration and varying severity. Mildest cases are clinically indeterminate; typical attacks are characterized by denguelike illness, i.e., sudden onset, fever, headache, backache, prostration, nausea, and vomiting.	3 to 6 days.	In urban and certain rural areas transmitted by infective *Aedes aegypti* mosquitoes.	Blood is infective for mosquitoes shortly before onset of fever and for first 3 to 5 days of illness. Highly communicable where many susceptible persons and abundant vector mosquitoes coexist.
b. Dengue (breakbone fever)	Characterized by sudden onset, fever for about 5 days and intense headache, retroorbital pains, joint and muscle pains, and rash.	3 to 15 days, commonly 5 to 6 days.	Infective mosquitoes.	Not directly transmitted from person to person.
c. Venezuelan equine fever	Clinical manifestations of infection are influenza-like, with abrupt onset of severe headache, chills, fever, myalgia, retroorbital pain, nausea, and vomiting.	Usually 2 to 6 days, can be as short as 1 day.	Infected mosquitoes.	Person-to-person transmission may occur but has not been demonstrated.
2. Tick-borne a. Colorado tick fever and other tick-borne fevers	Acute febrile, diphasic, denguelike disease with infrequent rash. Brief remission is usual, followed by second bout of fever lasting 2 or 3 days; neutropenia almost always occurs on fourth or fifth day of fever.	Usually 4 to 5 days.	Infective vector ticks.	Not directly transmitted from person to person except by transfusion. Virus is present during course of fever and, in Colordo tick fever, from 2 to 16 weeks or more after onset.
Ascariasis (roundworm infection)	Helminthic infection of small intestine. Symptoms are variable, often vague or absent, and ordinarily mild; live worms, passed in stools or regurgitated, are frequently first recognized sign of infection.	Worms reach maturity about 2 months after ingestion of embryonated eggs.	By ingestion of infective eggs from soil contaminated with human feces containing eggs, but not directly from person to person.	As long as mature female worms live in intestine. Maximum lifespan of adult worms is under 18 months; however, female produces up to 200,000 eggs a day that can remain viable in soil for months or years.
Aspergillosis	Variety of clinical syndromes can be produced by several *Aspergillus* species.	Probably a few days.	Inhalation of air-borne spores.	Not directly transmitted from person to person.
Babesiosis	Fever, fatigue, and hemolytic anemia lasting several days to a few months.	1 to 12 months.	During the summer months by bite of nymphal *Ixodes* ticks carried by voles or deer mice. Adult tick is normally found on deer.	Transmission from person to person is unlikely except by blood transfusion.

Disease	Clinical features	Incubation period	Mode of transmission	Period of communicability
Balantidiasis	Disease of colon characteristically producing diarrhea or dysentery accompanied by abdominal colic, tenesmus, nausea, and vomiting.	Unknown; may be only a few days.	By ingestion of cysts from feces of infected hosts; in epidemics, mainly by fecally contaminated water.	As long as infection persists.
Blastomycosis	Chronic granulomatous mycosis primarily of lungs or skin. *Acute pulmonary blastomycosis* begins with fever and symptoms of respiratory infection and can progress gradually with fever, weight loss, cachexia, cough, and purulent sputum.	Indefinite; probably a few weeks or less to months.	Conidia, typical of the mold or saprophytic growth form, probably are inhaled in sporeladen dust.	Not transmitted directly from humans or from animals to humans.
Botulism, infant	Illness typically begins with constipation followed by lethargy, listlessness, poor feeding, ptosis, difficulty in swallowing, loss of head control, hypotonia, generalized weakness, and in some cases, respiratory insufficiency and arrest. Wide spectrum of clinical severity ranging from mild illness to sudden infant death.	Usually unknown, because it cannot be determined precisely when the infant ingested the botulinal spores.	By ingestion of botulinal spores. Sources of spores for infants probably are multiple.	Excretion of *C. botulinum* toxin and organisms. Continues at high levels in patient's feces for weeks to months. No instances of secondary person-to-person transmission have been documented.
Brucellosis (undulant fever)	Systemic disease with acute or insidious onset characterized by continued, intermittent, or irregular fever of variable duration, headache, weakness, profuse sweating, chills, arthralgia, depression, and generalized aching.	Highly variable — usually 5 to 30 days; sometimes several months.	By contact with tissues, blood, urine, vaginal discharges, aborted fetuses and especially placentas, and by ingestion of raw milk or dairy products from infected animals. Air-borne infection occurs in humans in laboratories and slaughterhouses.	No evidence of communicability from person to person.
Candidiasis (moniliasis, thrush, candidosis)	Mycosis usually confined to superficial layers of skin or mucous membranes with patient have oral thrush, intertrigo, vulvovaginitis, paronychia, or onychomycosis.	Variable, 2 to 5 days in thrush of infants.	Through contact with excretions of mouth, skin, vagina, and especially feces from patients or carriers from mother to infant during childbirth; and by indogenous spread.	Presumably for duration of lesions.
Capillariasis A. Intestinal capillariasis	Enteropathy with massive protein loss and a malabsorption syndrome that lead to progressive weight loss and extreme emaciation.	Unknown in humans.	Uncertain. Often obtain history of ingesting raw or inadequately cooked fish.	Not transmitted directly from person to person.

Continued.

1-25/Communicable and Infectious Diseases—cont'd

Name	Synopsis of symptoms	Incubation period	Mode of transmission	Period of communicability
B. Hepatic capillariasis (also a pulmonary capillariasis—but only 10 documented cases of human infection recorded).	Uncommon and occasionally fatal disease in humans caused by presence of adult *Capillaria hepatica* in liver. Acute or subacute hepatitis with marked eosinophilia resembling visceral larva migrans.	3 to 4 weeks.	Ingesting liver of infected animal.	Not transmitted directly from person to person.
Carditis, Coxsackie (viral carditis, enteroviral carditis)	Acute or subacute myocarditis or pericarditis, which occurs as the only manifestation, or may occasionally be associated with other manifestations.	Usually 3 to 5 days.	Fecal-oral or respiratory droplet contact with infected person.	Apparently during acute stage of disease.
Cat-scratch disease	Subacute, self-limited infectious disease characterized by malaise, granulomatous lymphadenitis, and variable patterns of fever.	Variable; usually 3 to 14 days from innoculation to primary lesions.	90% of patients report history of scratch, bite, lick, or other exposure to healthy cat or kitten.	Unknown. Not directly transmitted from person to person.
Chancroid (ulcus molle, soft chancre)	Acute, localized, genital infection characterized by single or multiple painful necrotizing ulcers at site of innoculation, frequently accompanied by painful inflammatory swelling and suppuration of regional lymph nodes. Extragenital lesions have been reported.	From 3 to 5 days, up to 14 days.	By direct sexual contact with discharges from open lesions and pus from buboes; suggestive evidence of asymptomatic infections in women. Multiple sexual partners and uncleanliness favor transmission.	As long as infectious agent persists in original lesion or discharging regional lymph nodes; usually until healed—a matter of weeks.
Chickenpox, herpes zoster (varicella shingles)	Acute generalized viral disease with sudden onset of slight fever, mild constitutional symptoms, and a skin eruption that is maculopapular for a few hours, vesicular for 3 to 4 days, and leaves a granular scab.	From 2 to 3 weeks; commonly 13 to 17 days.	From person to person by direct contact, droplet, or airborne spread of secretion of respiratory tract of chickenpox cases or of vesicle fluid of patients with herpes zoster.	As long as 5 days but usually 1 to 2 days before onset of rash, and not more than 6 days after appearance of first crop of vesicles.
Cholera	Acute intestinal disease with sudden onset, profuse watery stools, occasional vomiting, rapid dehydration, acidosis, and circulatory collapse. Death may occur within a few hours.	From a few hours to 5 days, usually 2 to 3 days.	Through ingestion of food or water contaminated with feces or vomitus of infected persons or with feces of carriers.	Thought to be for duration of stool-positive stage, usually only a few days after recovery. Carrier stage may last for several months.

Disease	Clinical features	Incubation period	Mode of transmission	Period of communicability
Chromoblastomycosis (chromomycosis, dermatitis verrucosa)	Chronic spreading mycosis of skin and subcutaneous tissues, usually of a lower extremity. Hematogenous spread to brain has been reported.	Unknown; probably months.	Traumatic contact with contaminated wood or other materials.	Not directly transmitted from person to person.
Clonorchiasis (Chinese or oriental liver fluke disease)	Symptoms result from local irritation of bile ducts by flukes, from toxemia and possibly from secondary bacterial invaders. Loss of appetite, diarrhea, and sensation of abdominal pressure are early common symptoms.	Unpredictable, varies with the number of worms present; flukes reach maturity within 1 month after encysted larvae are ingested.	Humans infected by eating freshwater fish containing encysted larvae (*Clonorchis sinensis*).	Not directly transmitted from person to person, but infected individual may pass viable eggs for as long as 30 years.
Coccidioidomycosis (valley fever, desert fever, desert rheumatism, coccidiodal granuloma).	Internal mycosis that begins as respiratory infection. *Primary infection* may be entirely asymptomatic or resemble acute influenza illness with fever, chills, cough, and pleural pain.	1 to 4 weeks in primary infection.	Inhalation of spores from soil and in laboratory accidents from cultures.	Not directly transmitted from humans or animals to humans.
Conjunctivitis, acute bacterial	Clinical syndrome beginning with lacrimation, irritation, and hyperemia of the palpebral and bulbar conjunctivae of one or both eyes, followed by edema of lids, photophobia. and mucopurulent discharge.	Usually 24 to 72 hours.	Contact with discharges from conjunctivae or upper respiratory tract of infected persons through contaminated fingers, clothing, or other articles.	During course of active infection.
Conjunctivitis, epidemic hemorrhagic (Apollo 11 disease)	Virus infection with sudden onset of pain or sensation of a foreign body in eye. Disease rapidly progresses)1 to 2 days) to full case of swollen eyelids, hyperemia of the conjunctivae, often with a circumcorneal distribution, seromucous discharge, and frequent subconjunctival hemorrhages.	1 to 2 days or even shorter.	Through direct or indirect contact with discharge from infected eyes and possibly by droplet infection from those with virus in throat.	Unknown, but assumed to be for period of active disease, usually 1 to 2 weeks.
Conjunctivitis, inclusion (swimming pool conjunctivitis, paratrachoma)	In the newborn, acute papillary conjunctivitis with abundant mucopurulent discharge. In children and adults, acute follicular conjunctivitis with preauricular lymphadenopathy, often with superficial corneal involvement.	5 to 12 days.	During sexual intercourse; genital discharges of infected persons are infectious.	While genital infection persists; can be longer than 1 year in female.

Continued.

1-25/Communicable and Infectious Diseases—cont'd

Name	Synopsis of symptoms	Incubation period	Mode of transmission	Period of communicability
Contagious pustular dermatitis	Primarily a proliferative cutaneous disease of sheep and goats transmissible to humans and usually a solitary lesion located on hands, arms, or face that is maculo-papular or pustular.	Generally 3 to 6 days.	By direct contact with mucous membranes of infected animals.	Unknown. Human lesions show a decrease in number of virus particles as disease progresses.
Cryptococcosis (torulosis, European blastomycosis	Mycosis, usually subacute or chronic meningoencephalitis. Infection of lung, kidney, prostate, bone, or liver.	Unknown. Pulmonary disease may precede brain infection by months or years.	Presumably by inhalation.	Not directory transmitted from humans or animals to humans.
Cutaneous larva migrans caused by *Ancylostoma braziliense* resulting from *Ancylostoma caninum*	Infective larvae of dog and cat hookworm that causes dermatitis in humans.	Each larva causes serpiginous track, advancing several mm to a few cm a day.	Larva, which enter skin from contact with contaminated soil, migrate intracutaneously for long periods, but eventually penetrate to deeper tissues.	Disease is self-limited, with spontaneous cure after several weeks or months.
Cytomegalovirus infections Congenital cytomegalovirus infection Cytomegalic inclusion disease	Most severe form of disease occurs in perinatal period, following congenital infection, with signs and symptoms of severe generalized infection especially involving central nervous system and liver.	Information inexact. 3 to 8 weeks following transfusion with infected blood. 3 to 12 weeks after birth.	Intimate exposure to infectious secretions or excretions. Virus is excreted in urine, saliva, cervical secretions, breast milk, and semen.	Virus is excreted in urine or saliva for months and may persist for several years following primary infection.
Dermatophytosis A. Ringworm of scalp and beard (tinea capitis, tinea kerion, favus)	Begins as small papule and spreads peripherally, leaving scaly patches of temporary baldness. Infected hairs become brittle and break off easily. Kerions sometimes develop.	10 to 14 days	Direct or indirect contact with articles infected with hair from humans or infected animals.	As long as lesions are present and viable fungus persists on contaminated materials.
B. Ringworm of nails (tinea unguium, onychomycosis)	Chronic infectious disease involving one or more nails of hands or feet. Nail thickens becoming discolored and brittle with an accumulation of caseous-appearing material beneath nail.	Unknown.	Presumably by direct extension from skin or nail lesions of infected persons. Low rate of transmission.	Possibly as long as infected lesion is present.
C. Ringworm of groin and perianal region (dhobie itch, tinea cruris)	Characteristically appears as flat, spreading, ring-shaped lesions. Periphery is usually reddish, vesicular, or pustular and may be dry and scaly	4 to 10 days.	Direct or indirect contact with skin and scalp lesions of infected persons or animals.	As long as lesions are present and viable fungus persists on contaminated materials.

Disease	Characteristics/Symptoms	Incubation Period	Mode of Transmission	Period of Communicability
D. Ringworm of the body (tinea corporis)	or moist and crusted.			
E. Ringworm of the foot (tinea pedis, athlete's foot)	Scaling or cracking of skin, especially between toes, or blisters containing this watery fluid are characteristic. In severe cases vesicular lesions appear on various parts of body.	Unknown.	Direct or indirect contact with skin lesions of infected persons or contaminated floors or shower stalls.	As long as lesions are present and viable spores persist on contaminated materials.
Diarrhea, acute A. Diarrhea caused by *Escherichia coli*	May be invasive, enterotoxigenic, and enteropathogenic. *Invasive* — fever and mucoid and occasionally bloody diarrhea occur. *enterotoxigenic* — profuse watery diarrhea without blood or mucous. *enteropathogenic* — associated with outbreaks of acute diarrhea disease in newborn nurseries.	12 to 72 hours.	Fecal contamination of food, water, or fomites. Persons with diarrhea excrete large numbers of organisms and constitute greatest hazard.	Not known; presumably for duration of fecal excretion, which may be several weeks or longer.
B. Diarrhea caused by *Campylobacter* (vibriosis, vibrionic enteritis)	Acute enteric disease characterized by diarrhea, abdominal pain, malaise, fever, nausea, vomiting, and constitutional complaints	Range is 1 to 10 days with a usual period of 3 to 5 days.	By ingestion of organisms in food or contaminated water; contact with contaminated animals; drinking unpasteurized milk.	Throughout course of infection from several days to several weeks.
Diphtheria	Characteristic lesion marked by patch or patches of grayish membrane with surrounding dull red inflammatory zone. Throat is moderately sore in faucial diphtheria, with cervical lymph nodes enlarged and tender; occasionally swelling and edema of neck.	2 to 5 days, sometimes longer.	Contact with patient or carrier; more rarely with articles soiled with discharges from lesions of infected persons. Raw milk has been a vehicle.	Variable, until virulent bacilli have disappeared from discharge and lesions. Usual period is 2 to 4 weeks but chronic carriers may shed organisms for 6 months or more.
Diphyllobothriasis	Symptoms commonly are trivial or absent; depending on severity, vitamin B$_{12}$ deficiency anemia, diarrhea, and toxic symptoms may be present.	From 3 to 6 weeks from ingestion to passage of eggs in stool.	From eating raw or inadequately cooked fish.	Not directly transmitted from person to person.
Dracontiasis	Infection of subcutaneous and deeper tissues by large nematode. Blister appears, usually on a lower extremity, as gravid, meter-long adult female prepares to discharge her larvae.	About 12 months.	Humans swallow infected copepods by drinking water from contaminated stepwells and ponds.	Not directly transmitted from person to person.

Continued.

1-25/Communicable and Infectious Diseases—cont'd

Name	Synopsis of symptoms	Incubation period	Mode of transmission	Period of communicability
Echinococcosis multilocularis infection (alveolar hydatid disease)	Disease primarily of liver caused by poorly circumscribed microvesicular larval masses of *Echinococcus multilocularis*; may be found also in lungs and other organs.	Variable from months to years, depending on number and location of cysts and how rapidly they grow.	By ingestion of infective eggs or by fecally soiled dog fur, harnesses, and environmental fomites.	Not directly transmitted from person to person or from one intermediate host to another.
Enterobiasis (pinworm disease, oxyuriasis)	Intestinal infection with mild or nonspecific symptoms, if any. May be anal itching, disturbed sleep, irritability, and local irritation with secondary infection of scratched skin.	Life cycle of *Enterobius vermicularis* is 4 to 6 weeks.	Direct transfer of infective eggs by hand from anus to mouth of the same or new host, or indirectly through materials contaminated with eggs of parasite. Dust-borne infection by inhalation is possible.	As long as gravid females are discharging eggs on perianal skin. Continuous reinfection occurs by ano-oral transfer of eggs from self-or infected others.
Food poisoning A. Staphylococcal food poisoning	Intoxication (not infection) of abrupt and sometimes violent onset, with severe nausea, cramps, vomiting, usually diarrhea, and prostration; sometimes with subnormal temperature and lowered blood pressure.	Interval between eating food and onset of symptoms is 1 to 6 hours, but usually 2 to 4 hours.	By ingesting of food contacted by food-handler's hands without subsequent cooking or inadequately heated, such as pastries, custards, salads, and meat products.	Not applicable.
B. Botulism	Severe intoxication (not infection as in infant botulism) characterized by clinical manifestations relating primarily to the nervous system. Ptosis, visual difficulty, dry mouth, and sore throat are often first complaints.	Symptoms usually appear within 12 to 36 hours, sometimes several days, after eating contaminated food.	By ingestion of food in which toxin had been formed, primarily from jars or cans inadequately heated during canning, and eaten without subsequent adequate cooking.	Not applicable.
C. Clostridial food poisoning (*C. welchii*)	Intestinal disorder characterized by sudden onset of abdominal colic followed by diarrhea. Nausea is common but vomiting and fever are usually absent.	From 6 to 24 hours, usually 10 to 12 hours.	Ingestion of food contaminated by soil or feces in which conditions have permitted multiplication of organism.	Not applicable.
D. *Vibrio parahaemolyticus* food poisoning	Intestinal disorder characterized by watery diarrhea and abdominal cramps; nausea, vomiting, fever, and headache are variably present.	Usually 12 to 24 hours, but can range from 4 to 96 hours.	Ingestion of raw or inadequately cooked seafood.	Not communicable from person to person.

Disease	Clinical features	Incubation period	Mode of transmission	Period of communicability
E. *Bacillus cereus* food poisoning	Gastrointestinal disorder characterized in some cases by sudden onset of nausea and vomiting and in others by intense abdominal colic and diarrhea.	From 1 to 5 hours in cases when vomiting is predominant symptom; from 6 to 16 hours when diarrhea is predominant.	Ingestion of food that has been kept at ambient temperatures after cooking, permitting multiplication of organisms.	Not communicable from person to person.
Gastroenteritis, viral A. Epidemic viral gastroenteritis	Usually self-limited mild disease that often occurs in outbreaks with clinical symptoms of nausea, vomiting, diarrhea, abdominal pain, myalgia, headache, malaise, low grade fever, or a combination thereof.	24 to 48 hours; in volunteer studies with Norwalk agent range was 10 to 51 hours.	Unknown; probably by fecal-oral route. Several recent outbreaks strongly suggest food-borne and water-borne transmission.	During acute stage of disease and shortly thereafter.
B. Rotavirus gastroenteritis (sporadic viral gastroenteritis of infants and children)	Sporadic severe gastroenteritis of infants and young children characterized by diarrhea and vomiting, often with severe dehydration and occasional deaths.	Approximately 48 hours.	Probably fecal-oral and possibly respiratory routes.	During acute stage of disease and later while virus shedding continues. Virus is not usually detectable after eighth day of illness.
Giardiasis (*Giardia* enteritis, lambliasis)	Protozoan infection principally of upper small bowel; often asymptomatic, it may also be associated with a variety of intestinal symptoms such as chronic diarrhea, steatorrhea, abdominal cramps, bloating, frequent loose and pale, greasy, malodorus stools, fatigue, and weight loss.	In a water-borne epidemic in United States, clinical illnesses occurred 1 to 4 weeks after exposure; average 2 weeks.	Localized outbreaks occur from contaminated water supplies. By ingestion of cysts in fecally contaminated water and occasionally by fecally contaminated food.	Entire period of infection.
Gonococcal infections A. Gonococcal infection of genitourinary tract (gonorrhea, gonococcal urethritis)	*Males* — purulent discharge from anterior urethra with dysuria appears 2 to 7 days after infecting exposure. *Females* — few days after exposure initial urethritis or cervicitis occurs, frequently so mild as to pass unnoticed. About 20% of patients have uterine invasion at the first, second, or later menstrual period with symptoms of endometritis, salpingitis, or pelvic peritonitis.	Usually 2 to 7 days, sometimes longer.	By contact with exudates from mucous membranes of infected persons, almost always result of sexual activity.	May extend for months if untreated, especially in females who frequently are asymptomatic. Specific therapy usually ends communicability within hours except with penicillin-resistant strains.
B. Gonococcal conjunctivitis neonatorum (gonorrheal ophthalmia neonatorum)	Acute redness and swelling of conjunctiva of one or both eyes, with mucopurulent or purulent discharge in which gonococci are identifiable by microscopic and cultural methods.	Usually 1 to 5 days.	Contact with infected birth canal during childbirth.	While discharge persists if untreated; for 24 hours following initiation of specific treatment.

Continued.

1-25/Communicable and Infectious Diseases—cont'd

Name	Synopsis of symptoms	Incubation period	Mode of transmission	Period of communicability
Granuloma inguinale (donovanosis)	Mildly communicable, nonfatal, chronic and progressive, autoinoculable bacterial disease of skin and mucous membranes of external genitalia, inguinal, and anal region. Small nodule, vesicle, or papule is present.	Unknown; probably 8 to 80 days.	Presumably by direct contact with lesions during sexual activity.	Unknown and probably for duration of open lesions on skin or mucous membranes.
Hemorrhagic nephrosonephritis	Acute infectious disease characterized by abrupt onset of fever of 3 to 8 day duration, conjunctival injection, prostration, anorexia, and vomiting.	Usually 12 to 16 days, but varying from 9 to 35 days.	Unknown; transmission from rodent excreta is presumed.	Apparently not directly transmitted from person to person.
Hepatitis, viral				
A. Viral hepatitis A (infectious hepatitis, epidemic hepatitis, epidemic jaundice, catarrhal jaundice, Type A hepatitis)	Onset is usually abrupt with fever, malaise, anorexia, nausea, and abdominal discomfort, followed within a few days by jaundice.	From 15 to 50 days, depending on dose; average 28-30 days.	Person to person by fecal-oral route. Common-vehicle outbreaks have been related to contaminated water and food.	Studies indicate maximum infectivity during latter half of incubation period, continuing for a few days, after onset of jaundice.
B. Viral hepatitis B (Type B hepatitis, serum hepatitis)	Onset is usually insidious with anorexia, vague abdominal discomfort, nausea, and vomiting, sometimes arthralgias and rash, often progressing to jaundice. Fever may be absent or mild.	Usually 45 to 160 days, average 60 to 90 days. Variation is related in part to amount of virus in inoculum, mode of transmission, and host factors.	HB$_s$AG, the infectious agent, has been found in virtually all body secretions, but only blood, saliva, and semen have been shown to be infectious. Transmission usually be percutaneous inoculation of infected blood and blood products; contaminated needles, syringes, and IV equipment.	From several weeks before onset of symptoms through clinical course of disease; carrier state can last for years.
C. Hepatitis, non-A, non-B (non-B transfusion-associated hepatitis, hepatitis C)	Chronic infection may be symptomatic or asymptomatic. Differential diagnosis depends on exclusion of hepatitis types A and B.	2 weeks to 6 months, model 6 to 8 weeks.	Most common posttransfusion hepatitis in United States and is more common when paid donors are used. Percutaneous transmission documented and other modes similar to those of hepatitis B virus are suspected.	Degree of immunity following infection is not known.

Disease	Clinical characteristics	Incubation period	Mode of transmission	Period of communicability
Herpangina; hand-foot-and-mouth disease, acute lymphonodular pharyngitis	*Herpangina* — grayish papulovesicular pharyngeal lesions on an erythematous base. *Hand-foot-and-mouth disease* — more diffuse oral lesions on buccal surfaces of cheeks, gums, and tongue. *Acute lymphonodular pharyngitis* — lesions are firm, raised, discrete, whitish to yellowish nodules.	3 to 5 days for herpangina and hand-foot-and-mouth disease. 5 days for acute lymphonodular pharyngitis.	Direct contact with nose and throat discharges and feces of infected (possibly asymptomatic) persons and by droplet spread.	During acute stage of illness and longer because virus persists in stools for as long as several weeks.
Herpes simplex	Viral infection characterized by localized primary lesion, latency, and a tendency to localized recurrence. In perhaps 10% of primary infections overt disease may appear as illness of varying severity marked by fever and malaise lasting 1 week or more.	2 to 12 days.	HSV Type 1: Direct contact with virus in saliva of carriers. HSV Type 2: Sexual contact.	Secretion of virus in saliva has been reported for as long as 7 weeks after recovery from stomatitis. Patients with primary lesions are infective for about 7 to 12 days, with recurrent disease for 4 days to 1 week.
Histoplasmosis, histoplasma capsulatum (Darling's disease, American histoplasmosis)	Systemic mycosis of varying severity with primary lesion, usually in lung. Whereas infection is common, overt clinical disease is not. Five clinical forms are recognized.	Symptoms appear within 5 to 18 days after exposure, commonly 10 days.	Inhalation of air-borne spores.	Not transmitted from person to person.
Influenza	Acute viral disease of respiratory tract characterized by fever, chilliness, headache, myalgia, prostration, coryza, and mild sore throat. Cough is often severe and protracted.	Usually 24 to 72 hours.	By direct contact through droplet infection; probably air-borne among crowded populations in enclosed spaces.	Probably limited to 3 days from clinical onset.
Keratoconjunctivitis, epidemic	Acute viral disease of eye. Onset is sudden with pain, photophobia, blurred vision, occasionally low grade fever, headache, malaise, and tender preauricular lymphadenopathy.	Probably 5 to 12 days.	Direct contact with eye secretions of infected person or indirectly through contaminated instruments or solutions.	From late in incubation period to 14 days after onset.
Lassa fever	Acute viral illness with duration of 7 to 31 days. Onset is gradual with malaise, fever, headache, sore throat, cough, nausea, vomiting, diarrhea, myalgia, and chest and abdominal pain; fever is persistent or intermittent-spiking.	Commonly 7 to 21 days.	Primarily through direct or indirect contact with urine of infected rodents in dust or on food.	Person-to-person infections occur during acute febrile phase when virus is present in throat. Virus may be excreted in urine of patients for 3 weeks or as long as 60 days.

Continued.

APPENDIX

1-25/Communicable and Infectious Diseases—cont'd

Name	Synopsis of symptoms	Incubation period	Mode of transmission	Period of communicability
Legionellosis (legionnaire's disease, legionnaire's pneumonia, Pontiac fever)	Characterized initially by anorexia, malaise, myalgia, and headache. Within 1 day is usually rapidly rising fever associated with chills. Nonproductive cough, abdominal pain, and diarrhea often occur.	Legionnaire's disease: 2 to 10 days; most often 5 to 6 days. Pontiac fever: 5 to 66 hours; most often 24 to 48 hours.	Evidence supports air-borne transmission.	Person-to-person transmission has not been documented.
Leishmaniasis, cutaneous	Polymorphic disease of skin and mucous membranes characterized by ulcerating lesions that may be single or multiple and self-limited or indolent, or multiple nodular lesions.	From a few days to many months.	Bite of infective sandfly.	As long as parasites remain in lesions; in untreated cases, 1 year or more.
Leishmaniasis, visceral	Chronic systemic infectious disease characterized by fever, hepatosplenomegaly, lymphadenopathy, anemia with leukopenia, and progressive emaciation and weakness.	Generally 2 to 4 months; range is 10 days to 2 years.	Bite of infective sandfly.	As long as parasites persist in circulating blood or skin. Transmission from person to person, and by blood transfusion, sexual contact, and bites of infected laboratory animals have been reported.
Leprosy (Hansen's disease)	Chronic bacterial disease characterized by lesions of skin and mucous membranes, by involvement and often palpable enlargement of peripheral nerves with consequent anesthesia, muscle weakness, paralysis, and trophic changes in skin, muscle, and bone.	Shortest known is 7 months. Average is probably 3 to 6 years.	Not clearly established, but household and prolonged intimate contact are important. Organisms may gain entrance through broken skin and respiratory tract.	As long as morphologically normal bacilli are demonstrable, infectiousness should be considered possible.
Listeriosis	Bacterial disease usually manifested as acute meningoencephalitis with or without associated septicemia, less frequently septicemia only; very often neonatal. Onset of meningoencephalitis is usually sudden with fever intense headache, nausea, vomiting, and signs of meningeal irritation.	Unknown; probably 4 days to 3 weeks. Fetus is usually infected within several days after maternal disease.	Largely neonatal; infection is transmitted from mother to unborn infant in utero during its passage through infected birth canal.	Mothers of infected newborn infants may shed infectious agent in vaginal discharges or urine for 7 to 10 days after delivery. Period of person-to-person communicability unknown.
Lyme disease	Characterized by distinctive skin lesion (ECM), systemic symptoms, polyarthritis, and neurological and cardiac involvement in varying combination.	From 3 to 21 days after tick exposure.	Presumably tick-borne.	No evidence of transmission from person to person.

Lymphocytic chorio-meningitis (LCM, benign or serous lymphocytic meningitis)	Viral disease of animals, especially mice, transmissible to man with marked diversity of clinical manifestations. At times it begins with influenza-like attack followed by complete recovery; or after 1 to 2 weeks or remission, meningeal symptoms suddenly appear.	Probably 8 to 13 days; 15 to 20 days to meningeal symptoms.	Virus is excreted in urine, saliva, and feces of infected animals, usually mice transmission to humans, usually through contaminated food or dust.	Not known to be directly transmitted from person to person.
Lymphogranuloma venereum (lymphogranuloma inguinale, esthiomene, climatic bubo, tropical bubo)	Venerally acquired infection, beginning with painless evanescent erosion, papule, nodule, or herpetiform lesion on penis or vulva, frequently unnoticed. Regional lymph nodes undergo suppuration followed by extension of inflammatory process to adjacent tissues.	Usually 7 to 12 days, with a range of 4 to 21 days to primary lesion. If bubo is first manifestation, 10 to 30 days, sometimes several months.	Direct contact with open lesions of infected persons usually during sexual intercourse.	Variable, from weeks to years, during presence of active lesions.
Malaria	Fever, chills, sweats, and headache that may progress to icterus coagulation defects, shock, renal and liver failure, acute encephalitis, and coma are symptoms of most serious form (falciparum malaria). Symptoms difficult to differentiate in the four human malarias so laboratory confirmation is needed by demonstration of malaria parasites in blood films.	Average 12 days for *P. falciparum*, 12 days for *P. vivax* and *P. ovale*, and 30 days for *P. malariae*.	By infective female anopheline mosquito.	For infection of mosquitoes, as long as infective gametocytes are present in blood of patients; varies with species and strain of parasite and with response to therapy.
Measles (rubeola, hard measles, red measles, morbilli)	Acute, highly communicable viral disease with prodromal fever, conjunctivitis, coryza, bronchitis, and Koplik's spots on the buccal mucosa. A characteristic red blotchy rash appears on third to seventh day, beginning on face, becoming generalized, lasting 4 to 7 days and sometimes ending in branny desquamation. Leukopenia is common.	About 10 days varying from 8 to 13 days from exposure to onset of fever; about 14 days until rash appears; uncommonly longer or shorter human normal immune globulin (IG), given later than third day of incubation period for passive protection, may extend the incubation period to 21 days instead of preventing disease.	By droplet spread or direct contact with nasal or throat secretions of infected persons. Measles is one of most readily transmitted communicable diseases.	From slightly before beginning of prodromal period of 4 days after appearance of rash; communicability is minimal after second day of rash.

Continued.

APPEN-DIX

1-25/Communicable and Infectious Diseases — cont'd

Name	Synopsis of symptoms	Incubation period	Mode of transmission	Period of communicability
Melioidosis	Range of clinical manifestations from apparent infection or asymptomatic pulmonary consolidation to rapidly fatal septicemia. May simulate typhoid fever or even tuberculosis.	As short as 2 days; however, several months or years may elapse between presumed exposure and appearance of clinical disease.	Usually by contact with contaminated soil or water through overt or inapparent skin wounds, by aspiration or ingestion of contaminated water or by inhalation of dust from soil.	Person-to-person transmission and laboratory acquired infections are uncommon.
Meningitis, aseptic (viral meningitis, serous meningitis, nonbacterial or abacterial meningitis)	Common, rarely fatal, clinical syndrome with multiple causes, most commonly viral, characterized by sudden onset of febrile illness with signs and symptoms of meningeal involvement. Spinal fluid findings of pleocytosis (usually mononuclear but may be polymorphonuclear in early stages), increased protein, normal sugar, and absence of bacteria. Active illness seldom exceeds 10 days.	Varies with specific infectious agent (refer to specific diseases).	Varies with specific infectious agent (refer to specific diseases).	
Meningitis, bacterial	Clinical signs and symptoms may be indistinguishable from those caused by meningococci including rash. Differentiation is based on smears and bacteriological studies.			
Meningitis, meningococcal (cerebrospinal fever, meningococcemia)	Characterized by sudden onset of fever, intense headache, nausea and often vomiting, stiff neck, and frequently a petechial rash with pink macules or, very rarely, vesicles. Delirium and coma often appear; occasional fulminating cases exhibit sudden prostration, ecchymoses, and shock at onset.	Varies from 2 to 10 days, commonly 3 to 4 days.	By direct contact, including droplets and discharges from nose and throat of infected persons, more often carriers than cases.	Until meningococci are no longer present in discharges from nose and throat. If organisms are sensitive to sulfonamides, meningococci usually disappear from nasopharynx within 24 hours after institution of treatment. They are not fully eradicated from oronasopharynx by penicillin.
Meningitis, hemophilus (meningitis caused by Heamophilus influenzae)	Most common bacterial meningitis in children 2 months to 3 years old in U.S. Otitis media or sinusitis may be precursor. Almost always associated with bacteremia.	Probably short — within 2 to 4 days.	By droplet infection and discharges from nose and throat during infectious period. May be purulent rhinitis. Portal of entry is most commonly nasopharyngeal.	As long as organisms are present, which may be for prolonged period even without nasal discharge.

Disease	Clinical features	Incubation period	Transmission / Comments
Meningitis, pneumococcal	Onset is sudden with symptoms of fever, vomiting, lethargy, and meningeal irritation. High fatality rate is associated with this disease. Usually fulminant and occurs with bacteremia but not necessarily with another focus; although there may be otitis media or mastoiditis. Symptoms of high fever, lethargy or coma, and signs of meningeal irritation usually signal onset.		
Meningitis, neonatal	Patients exhibit symptoms of lethargy, seizures, apneic episodes, poor feeding, hypothermia or hyperthermia, and sometimes respiratory distress in first week of life.		Acquired from birth canal. For prevention of early onset form, ampicillin treatment at onset of labor has been recommended for mothers known to be infected with Group B *Streptococcus*.
Meningoencephalitis caused by *Naegleria* and *Acanthamoeba*	*Naegleria:* Disease organisms cause a typical syndrome of fulminating pyogenic meningoencephalitis with severe frontal headache, occasional olfactory hallucinations, nausea, vomiting, high fever, nuchal rigidity, and somnolence. *Acanthamoeba:* Disease organisms invade the brain and meninges, usually without involvement of nasal and olfactory tissues, causing disease characterized by insidious onset and prolonged course.	*Naegleria:* 3 to 7 days in documented cases. *Acanthamoeba:* Much longer than in *Naegleria.*	*Naegleria:* Infection acquired by forcing infected water into nasal passages. *Naegleria* trophozoites colonize nasal tissues, then invade brain and meninges by extension along olfactory nerves. *Acanthamoebae* trophozoites reach central nervous system by metastasis from skin lesion or other site of primary colonization. No person-to-person transmission has been observed.
Acanthamebiasis of eye, skin, and vagina	Lesions of conjunctiva, cornea, and inner structures of eye. Granulomatous lesions of the skin have been recorded. Also secondary invasion of central nervous system and occasionally of vagina.		

Continued.

APPENDIX

1-25/Communicable and Infectious Diseases—cont'd

Name	Synopsis of symptoms	Incubation period	Mode of transmission	Period of communicability
Molluscum contagiosum	Viral disease of skin that results in pearly pink to white papules with prominent central area in adults; may occur anywhere in children. Eruption usually clears spontaneously in 6 to 9 months.	2 to 7 weeks.	Usually by direct contact, but transmission by fomites is possible. Sexual transmission occurs.	Unknown, but probably as long as lesions persist.
Mononucleosis, infectious (glandular fever, EBV mononucleosis)	Characterized by fever, sore throat (often with exudative pharyngotonsillitis), and lymphadenopathy (especially posterior cervical). Jaundice occurs in about 4% of infected young adults and splenomegaly in 50%. Duration is from 1 to several weeks.	From 4 to 6 weeks.	Person-to-person spread by oropharyngeal route via saliva. Spread may also occur via blood transfusion to susceptible recipients.	Prolonged; pharyngeal excretion may persist for 1 year after infection; 15% to 20% of healthy adults are oropharyngeal carriers.
Mumps (infectious parotitis)	Acute viral disease characterized by fever, swelling, and tenderness of one or more salivary glands, usually parotid and sometimes sublingual or submaxillary glands.	About 2 to 3 weeks, commonly 18 days.	By droplet spread and by direct contact with saliva of an infected person.	Virus has been isolated from saliva from 6 days before salivary gland involvement to as long as 9 days thereafter; but height of infectiousness occurs about 48 hours before swelling begins. Urine may be positive for as long as 14 days after onset of illness.
Mycetoma, actinomycotic (mycetomia, mycotic)	Characterized by swelling and suppuration of subcutaneous tissues, and formation of sinus tracts with visible granules in pus draining from sinus tracts. Lesions usually are on foot or lower leg.	Usually months.	Subcutaneous implantation of spores or hyphal elements from a saprophytic source by penetrating wounds (thorns, splinters).	Not transmitted from person to person.
Nocardiosis	Chronic disease often originating in lungs, with hematogenous spread to produce abscesses of brain, subcutaneous tissue and other organs; high fatality rate.	Unknown; probably weeks.	Nocardia are presumed to enter body principally by inhalation of contaminated dust into lung.	Not directly transmitted from humans or animals to humans.
Onchocerciasis	Chronic, nonfatal filarial disease with fibrous nodules in subcutaneous tissues, particularly head and shoulders.	Microflariae are found in skin usually about 1 year or more after infection.	By infected female blackflies.	Not directly transmitted from person to person; however, humans infect flies as long as living microfilariae occur in skin; i.e., for 10 to 15 years if untreated.

Disease	Clinical characteristics	Incubation period	Mode of transmission	Communicability
Ornithosis (psittacosis, parrot fever)	Acute generalized infectious disease with variable clinical presentations; fever, headache, myalgia, chills, and upper or lower respiratory tract disease are commonly present.	From 4 to 15 days, commonly 10 days.	Infection is usually acquired by inhaling agent from desiccated droppings of infected birds. Turkeys are usually involved but ducks and pigeons are occasionally responsible for human disease. Household birds are frequent source.	Person-to-person transmission is rare but can occur, especially with paroxysmal coughing.
Paracoccidioidomycosis	Chronic mycosis characterized by patchy pulmonary infiltrates or ulcerative lesions of mucosa (oral, nasal, gastrointestinal) and of skin. Lymphadenopathy is frequent. In disseminated cases all viscera may be affected; adrenal gland is especially susceptible.	Highly variable, from 1 month to many years.	Presumably acquired through inhalation of contaminated soil and dust.	Not known to be transmitted directly from person to person.
Paragonimiasis (pulmonary distomiasis, lung fluke disease)	Clinical signs depend on path of migration and organs parasitized. Lungs are most frequently involved; symptoms are cough and hemoptysis.	Flukes mature and begin to lay eggs approximately 6 weeks after humans ingest infective larvae. Interval until symptoms appear is long and variable depending on organ invaded and number of worms involved.	Infection occurs when raw or partially cooked flesh of freshwater crabs or crayfish containing infective larvae (metacercariae) are eaten.	Not directly transmitted from person to person, but eggs may be discharged by the human host for 20 years or more.
Paratyphoid fever	Frequently generalized bacterial enteric infection, often with abrupt onset, continued fever, enlargement of spleen, sometimes rose spots on trunk, usually diarrhea, and involvement of lymphoid tissues of mesentery and intestines.	1 to 3 weeks for enteric fever; 1 to 10 days for gastroenteritis.	Direct or indirect contact with feces or urine of patient or carrier. Spread is by food, especially milk, milk products, and shellfish. Flies may be vectors.	As long as infectious agent persists in excreta, which is from appearance of prodromal symptoms, throughout illness, and for periods up to several weeks or months. Commonly 1 to 2 weeks after recovery.
Pediculosis (lousiness)	Infestation of head, hairy parts of body, or clothing with adult lice, larvae, or nits (eggs), which results in severe itching and excoriation of scalp or scratch marks of body.	Under optimum conditions, eggs of lice hatch in 1 week, reach sexual maturity in approximately 2 weeks.	Direct contact with infected person and indirectly by contact with personal belongings, especially clothing and headgear. Crab lice are usually transmitted through sexual contact.	Communicable as long as lice remain alive on infested person or in clothing, and until eggs in hair and clothing have been destroyed.

Continued.

1-25/Communicable and Infectious Diseases—cont'd

Name	Synopsis of symptoms	Incubation period	Mode of transmission	Period of communicability
Pinta (carate)	Scaling papule with satellite lymphadenopathy appears within 1 to 8 weeks after infection, usually on hands, legs, or dorsum of feet. In 3 to 12 months, a maculopapular, erythematous secondary rash appears and may evolve into tertiary dyschromic macules of variable size. Organ systems are not involved.	3 to 60 days	Presumably person-to-person transmission by direct and prolonged contact with initial and early dyschromic skin lesions; location of primary lesions suggests that trauma provides portal of entry.	Unknown; potentially communicable while dyschromic skin lesions are active, sometimes for many years.
Plague (pest)	Specific zoonosis involving rodents and their fleas that transfer infection to various animals including humans. Initial response is commonly lymphadenitis in node receiving drainage from site of fleabite. Nodes become swollen and tender and fever is often present. Secondary involvement of lungs may result in severe pneumonia with mediastinitis and pleural effusion.	From 2 to 6 days; may be longer in vaccinated individuals.	Plague in humans occurs as result of intrusion into zoonotic transmission cycle or by entry of sylvatic infected animals and their infected fleas into human's habitat.	Fleas may remain infected for days, weeks, or months under suitable conditions of temperature and humidity.
Pleurodynia, epidemic	Acute viral disease characterized by sudden onset of severe pain localized in chest or abdomen that may be intensified by movement, usually accompanied by fever and frequently by headache.	Usually 3 to 5 days.	Probably fecal-oral or respiratory droplet contact with infected person or with articles freshly soiled with feces or throat discharges of infected person who may or may not have symptoms.	Apparently during acute stage of disease.
The pneumonias A. Pneumococcal pneumonia	Acute bacterial infection characterized by sudden onset with single shaking chill, fever, pleural pain, dyspnea, cough productive of "rusty" sputum and leukocytosis.	Not well determined; believed to be 1 to 3 days.	By droplet spread; by direct oral contact or indirectly, through articles freshly soiled with respiratory antisms is common.	Presumably until discharges of mouth and nose no longer contain virulent pneumococci in significant numbers. Penicillin will render patient noninfectious within 24 to 48 hours.
B. Mycoplasmal pneumonia (primary atypical pneumonia)	Predominantly afebrile lower respiratory infection. Onset is gradual with headache, malaise, cough often paroxysmal, and usually substernal pain (not pleuritic). Sputum, scant at first, may increase later.	14 to 21 days.	Probably by droplet inhalation, direct contact with infected person or with articles freshly soiled with discharges of nose and throat from acutely ill and coughing patient.	Probably less than 10 days; occasionally longer with persisting febrile illness or persistence of the organisms in convalescence (as long as 13 weeks is known).

Disease	Identification	Incubation period	Mode of transmission	Period of communicability
C. Pneumocystis pneumonia (interstitial plasmacell pneumonia)	Acute pulmonary disease occurring early in life, especially in malnourished, chronically ill, or premature infants. Characterized by progressive dyspnea, tachypnea, and cyanosis; fever may not be present.	Analysis of data from institutional outbreaks among infants indicates 1 to 2 months.	Unknown.	Unknown.
D. Chlamydial pneumonia (pertussoid eosinophilic pneumonia)	Subacute pulmonary disease occurring in early infancy, primarily in infants of mothers with infection of uterine cervix with causative organism. Characterized by insidious onset, cough, lack of fever, patchy infiltrates on chest x-ray with hyperinflation; eosinophilia, elevated IgM and IgG.	Not known, but pneumonia may occur in infants from 1 to 18 weeks of age (more commonly between 4 and 12 weeks). Nasopharyngeal infection is usually not present before 2 weeks of age.	Presumed to be vertically transmitted from infected cervix to infant during birth, with resultant nasopharyngeal infection (and occasionally conjunctival infection as inclusion conjunctivitis). Direct contact or respiratory transmission has not been established.	Unknown, but length of nasopharyngeal excretion can be at least 2 months.
Poliomyelitis (infantile paralysis)	Acute viral infection whose symptoms include fever, malaise, headache, nausea, vomiting, and stiffness of neck and back with or without paralysis.	Commonly 7 to 14 days for paralytic cases, with a range from 3 to possibly 35 days.	Direct contact through close association. In rare instances milk, foodstuffs, and other fecally-contaminated materials have been incriminated as vehicles. Fecal-oral is major route when sanitation is poor, but during epidemics and when sanitation is good, pharyngeal spread becomes relatively more important.	Not accurately known. Cases are probably most infectious during first few days after onset of symptoms.
Q fever (query fever)	Acute febrile rickettsial disease; onset may be sudden with chills, retrobulbar headache, weakness, malaise, and severe sweats. Pneumonitis occurs in many cases with cough, scanty expectoration, chest pain, and minimal physical findings. Chronic endocarditis, pericarditis, hepatitis, and generalized infections have been reported.	Depends on size of the infecting dose; usually 2 to 3 weeks.	Commonly by air-borne dissemination of rickettsiae in dust from premises contaminated by placental tissues, birth fluids, and excreta of infected animals.	Direct transmission from person to person is very rare, but may occur in cases of pneumonia.

Continued.

APPEN-
DIX

1-25/Communicable and Infectious Diseases—cont'd

Name	Synopsis of symptoms	Incubation period	Mode of transmission	Period of communicability
Rabies (hydrophobia, lyssa)	Almost invariably fatal acute encephalomyelitis; onset is with sense of apprehension, headache, fever, malaise, and indefintie sensory changes often referred to site of preceding animal bite wound. Disease progresses to paresis or paralysis; spasm of deglutition muscles on attempts to swallow, fear of water, and convulsions.	Usually 2 to 8 weeks, occasionally as short as 10 days or as long as 1 year or more depending on severity and site of wound.	Virus-laden saliva of a rabid animal is introduced by bite or, very rarely, through intact mucous membranes.	In dogs and most other biting animals, for 3 to 5 days before onset of clinical signs and during course of disease.
Rat-bite fever				
A. Streptobacillary fever	Abrupt onset with chills and fever, headache, and muscle pain is shortly followed by maculopapular or sometimes petechial rash. One or more joints may be swollen, red, and painful. Bacterial endocarditis and focal abscesses may occur late in untreated cases.	3 to 10 days, rarely longer.	Infection is transmitted by secretions of mouth, nose or conjunctival sac of infected animal, most frequently introduced by biting.	Not directly transmitted from person to person.
B. Spirillum fever	Symptoms rarely include arthritic symptoms, but distinctive rash of reddish or purplish plaques is evident.	1 to 3 weeks.		
Relapsing fever	Systemic spirochetal disease in which periods of fever lasting 2 to 9 days alternate with afebrile periods of 2 to 4 days; number of relapses varies from 1 to 10 or more.	5 to 15 days; usually 8 days.	Not directly transmitted from person to person.	Louse becomes infective 4 to 5 days after ingestion of blood from infected person and remains so for life (20 to 40 days).
Respiratory disease (excluding influenza)				
A. Acute febrile respiratory disease	Viral diseases of respiratory tract are characterized by fever and one or more constitutional reactions such as chills or chilliness, headache, general aching, malaise, and anorexia; in infants by occasional gastrointestinal disturbances.	From a few days to 1 week or more.	Directly by oral contact or by droplet spread, indirectly by hands or other materials soiled by respiratory discharges of infected person.	For duration of active disease; little is known about subclinical or latent infections.

	Description	Incubation	Mode of transmission	Communicability
B. Common cold (acute coryza)	Acute catarrhal infections of upper respiratory tract characterized by coryza, sneezing, lacrimation, irritated nasopharynx, chilliness, and malaise lasting 2 to 7 days. Fever is uncommon in children and rare in adults.		Presumably by direct oral contact or by droplet spread; indirectly by hands and articles freshly soiled by discharges of nose and throat of infected person.	
Rickettsioses, tick-borne (spotted fever group) A. Rocky Mountain spotted fever	Characterized by sudden onset with moderate to high fever that ordinarily persists for 2 to 3 weeks, significant malaise, deep muscle pain, severe headache, chills, and conjunctival injection. A maculopapular rash appears about the third day. Petechiae and hemorrhages are common.	From 3 to about 14 days.	Ordinarily by infected tick.	Not directly transmitted from person to person. Tick remains infective for life; commonly as long as 18 months.
B. Boutonneuse fever	Mild to moderately severe febrile illness of a few days to 2 weeks; characterized by primary lesion at site of tick bite. Lesion (tache noire), usually present at onset of fever, is small ulcer 2 mm to 5 mm in diameter with black center and red areola; regional lymph nodes are enlarged.	Usually 5 to 7 days.	By infected ticks.	Same as in Rocky Mountain spotted fever.

Also: (1) Queensland tick typhus, (2) North Asian tick fever, (3) Rickettsial pox

Rubella (German measles)

	Description	Incubation	Mode of transmission	Communicability
A. Congenital rubella	Mild febrile infectious disease with diffuse punctate and macular rash. Sometimes resembling that of measles, scarlet fever, or both. May be few or no constitutional symptoms in children but adults may experience 1 to 5 day prodrome characterized by low-grade fever, headache, malaise, mild coryza, and conjunctivitis. As many as 20% to 50% of infections may occur without evident rash; overall 50% are not recognized.	From 16 to 18 days with a range of 14 to 21 days.	Contact with nasopharyngeal secretions of infected person. Infection is by droplet spread or direct contact with patients and indirect contact.	For about 1 week before and at least 4 days after onset of rash. Highly communicable. Infants with congenital rubella syndrome may shed virus for months after birth.

Continued.

APPEN-DIX

1-25/Communicable and Infectious Diseases—cont'd

Name	Synopsis of symptoms	Incubation period	Mode of transmission	Period of communicability
B. Erythema infectiosum (fifth disease)	Mild nonfebrile erythematous eruption occurring as epidemics among children. Characterized by striking erythema of cheeks, reddening of skin, and lacelike serpiginous rash of body.			
C. Exanthema subitum (roseola infantum)	Acute illness of probable viral cause characterized by high fever that suddenly appears and lasts 3 to 5 days. A maculopapular rash on trunk and later on rest of body ordinarily follows lysis of fever.			
Salmonellosis	Commonly manifested by acute gastroenteritis. Acute infectious disease with sudden onset of abdominal pain, diarrhea, nausea, and sometimes vomiting. Dehydration may be severe. Fever is nearly always present.	6 to 72 hours, usually about 12 to 36 hours.	By ingestion of organisms in food contaminated by feces of infected person or animal.	Throughout course of infection—extremely variable.
Scabies (sarcoptic acariasis)	Infectious disease of skin caused by mite whose penetration is visible as papules or vesicles, or as tiny linear burrows containing mites and their eggs.	2 to 6 weeks before onset of itching in persons without previous exposure. Persons who have been previously infested develop symptoms 1 to 4 days after reexposure.	Transfer of parasites is by direct skin-to-skin contact and to limited extent from undergarments or soiled bedclothes freshly contaminated by infected persons; frequently acquired during sexual contact.	Until mites and eggs are destroyed by treatment, ordinarily after one or occasionally two courses of treatment 1 week apart.
Shigellosis (bacillary dysentery)	Acute bacterial disease primarily involving large intestine, characterized by diarrhea, accompanied by fever, nausea, sometimes vomiting, cramps, and tenesmus. In severe cases stools contain blood, mucous, and pus.	1 to 7 days, usually 1 to 3 days.	By direct or indirect fecal-oral transmission from patient or carrier. Infection may occur after ingestion of very few organisms.	During acute infection and until infectious agent is no longer present in feces, usually within 4 weeks of illness.
Slow virus infections of central nervous system A. Kuru	Signs include cerebellar ataxia, temors, rigidity, progressive wasting, and variable cranial nerve signs in patients 4 years of age or older.	8 to 9 years in childhood cases; range is 4 to more than 30 years.	Exact route of transmission not firmly established. Principally by traditional mortuary practices with intimate contact with infected tissues.	CNS tissues are infectious throughout symptomatic illness.

Disease	Clinical features	Incubation	Transmission	Communicability
B. Jakob-Creutzfeldt disease	Insidious onset of confusion, progressive dementia, and variable ataxia in patients 25 years of age or older.	Unknown in most cases.	Unknown.	Same.
Smallpox	Systemic disease with usually characteristic exanthem. Onset is sudden, with fever, malaise, headache, severe backache, prostration, and occasionally abdominal pain. Rash appears after 2 to 4 days and goes through stages of macules, papules, vesicles, pustules, and finally scabs.	From 7 to 17 days; commonly 10 to 12 days to onset of illness and 2 to 4 days more to onset of rash.	Transmission normally through close contact with respiratory discharges and skin lesions of patients, and material they had recently contaminated. Air-borne spread occurs infrequently.	From a few days before development of earliest lesions to disappearance of all scabs; about 3 weeks. Most communicable during first week.
Sporotrichosis	Fungal disease, usually of skin, which begins as nodule. As nodule grows, lymphatics draining area become firm and cordlike and form series of nodules, which in turn may soften and ulcerate.	Lymphatic form may develop 1 week to 3 months after injury.	Introduction of fungus through skin following pricks by thorns or barbs, handling of sphagnum moss or by slivers from wood or lumber.	Not transmitted from person to person. Environment presumably may be contaminated for duration of active lesion.
Staphylococcal disease A. Staphylococcal disease in community; Boils, carbuncles, furuncles; Impetigo	Staphylococci produce variety of syndromes with clinical manifestations that range from single pustule to impetigo to septicemia to death.	Variable and indefinite. Commonly 4 to 10 days.	Major site of colonization is anterior nares. Autoinfection is responsible for at least one third of infections.	As long as purulent lesions continue to drain or carrier state persists.
Cellulitis, abscesses; Staphylococcal septicemia; Staphylococcal pneumonia; Osteomyelitis; Endocarditis	Lesion or lesions containing pus is primary clinical finding, abscess formation is typical.		Person with draining lesion or any purulent lesion or who is asymptomatic (usually nasal) carrier of pathogenic strain. Air-borne spread is rare.	
B. Staphylococcal disease in hospital nurseries; Impetigo; Abscess of breast	Characteristic lesions develop secondary to colonization of nose or umbilicus, conjunction, circumcision site, or rectum of infants with pathogenic strain.	Commonly 4 to 10 days but may occur several months after colonization.	Spread by hands of hospital personnel is primary mode of transmission within hospitals; to a lesser extent, air-borne.	Same.

Continued.

1-25/Communicable and Infectious Diseases—cont'd

Name	Synopsis of symptoms	Incubation period	Mode of transmission	Period of communicability
C. Staphylococcal disease in medical and surgical wards of hospitals	Lesions vary from simple furuncles or stitch abscesses to extensively infected bedsores or surgical wounds, septic phlebitis, chronic osteomyelitis, fulminating pneumonia, endocarditis, or septicemia.	Variable and indefinite. Commonly 4 to 10 days.	Major site of colonization is anterior nares. Autoinfection is responsible for at least one third of infections. Person with a draining lesion or any purulent lesion or who is an asymptomatic (usually nasal) carrier of a pathogenic strain. Air-borne spread is rare.	As long as purulent lesions continue to drain or carrier state persists.
D. Toxic shock syndrome	Characterized by sudden onset of fever, vomiting, profuse watery diarrhea, and myalgia, followed by hypotension, and in severe cases, shock. An erythematous "sunburnlike" rash is present during acute phase.	Thought to be related to use of tampons; however, mode of transmission is still under investigation.		
Streptococcal diseases caused by group A (beta hemolytic) streptococci				
A. Streptococcal sore throat	Fever, sore throat, exudative tonsillitis or pharyngitis, and tender anterior cervical lymph nodes	Short, usually 1 to 3 days, rarely longer.	Transmission results from direct or intimate contact with patient or carrier, rarely by indirect contact through objects or hands. Nasal carriers are particularly likely to transmit diseases.	In untreated uncomplicated cases 10 to 21 days; in untreated conditions with purulent discharges, weeks or months.
B. Streptococcal skin infections	Usually superficial, may proceed through vesicular, pustular, and encrusted stages			
C. Scarlet fever	Skin rash and symptoms similar to streptococcal sore throat, enanthem, strawberry tongue, and exanthem. Rash is usually fine erythema.			
D. Erysipelas	Acute cellulitis characterized by fever, constitutional symptoms, leukocytosis, and red, tender, edematous, spreading lesion of skin with definite raised border.			

E. Streptococcal puerperal fever	Acute disease, usually febrile accompanied by local and general symptoms and signs of bacterial invasion of genital tract and sometimes bloodstream in postpartum or postabortion patient.		
Streptococcal (group B) disease of the newborn	Produces diseases of newborn infants including cases of septicemia, evidence of pulmonary involvement, and meningeal involvement.	Acquired during passage through birth canal. Some cases are acquired through environment.	
Strongyloidiasis	Helminthic infection of duodenum and upper jejunum, asymptomatic in majority of cases. Clinical manifestations include dermatitis, cough, rales, and abdominal symptoms.	Infective larvae that develop in moist soil contaminated with feces penetrate skin, enter venous circulation, and are carried to lungs.	As long as living worms remain in intestine; up to 35 years.
Syphilis, venereal (lues)	Acute and chronic treponematosis characterized clinically by primary lesion, secondary eruption involving skin and mucous membranes, long periods of latency, and late lesions of skin, bone, viscerae, and central nervous and cardiovascular systems. Papule appears 3 weeks after exposure at site of initial invasion; after erosion, most common form is indurated chancre.	By direct contact with infectious exudates form obvious or concealed moist early lesions of skin and mucous membrane, body fluids, and secretions of infected persons during sexual contact.	Variable and indefinite during primary and secondary stages and also in mucocutaneous recurrences; some cases may be intermittently communicable for 2 to 4 years.
From penetration of skin by filariform larvae until rhabitiform larvae appear in feces is about 2 to 3 weeks; period until symptoms appear is variable.			
10 days to 10 weeks, usually 3 weeks.			
Syphilis, nonvenereal endemic	Acute disease of limited geographical distribution, characterized clinically by eruption of skin and mucous membrane, usually without evident primary sore.	Direct or indirect contact with infectious early lesions of skin and mucous membranes. Congenital transmission does not occur.	Until moist eruptions of skin and mucous patches disappear — sometimes several weeks or months.
2 weeks to 3 months.			

Continued.

1-25/Communicable and Infectious Diseases—cont'd

Name	Synopsis of symptoms	Incubation period	Mode of transmission	Period of communicability
Taeniasis and cysticercosis *Taenia solium* infection, intesinal form (pork tapeworm) Cysticercosis (cysticerciasis, infection by *Cysticercus cellulosae*) *Taenia saginata* infection (beef tapeworm)	Taeniasis is intestinal infection with adult stage of large tapeworms. Cysticercosis is somatic infection with larvae stage of one species, *Taenia solium*. Clinical manifestations of infection with adult worm are variable and may include nervousness, insomnia, anorexia, weight loss, abdominal pain, and digestive disturbance. Cysticercosis is serious somatic disease that may involve many different organs. Eggs of tapeworm, when swallowed, hatch in small intestines and larvae migrate throughout body.	For adult tapeworm, from 8 to 14 weeks.	Ova of *Taenia saginata* passed in stool of infected person are infectious only to cattle. Infection of man follows ingestion of raw or inadequately cooked beef containing cysticerci. Ova of *Taenia solium* are infectious to both man and pigs. Human infection occurs by direct transfer of eggs in feces of person harboring adult worm to own or another's mouth, or indirectly through ingestion of food or water contaminated with eggs, resulting in somatic cysticercosis. Intestional infection of humans (taeniasis) follows ingestion of raw or inadequately cooked infected pork.	*Taenia saginata* is not directly transmitted from person to person but *Taenia solium* may be; eggs of both species are disseminated into environment as long as worm remains in intestines, sometimes more than 30 years; eggs may remain viable for months.
Tetanus (tetanus neonatorum, lockjaw)	Acute disease induced by tetanus bacillus that grows anaerobically at site of injury and produces neurotoxin. Characterized by painful muscular contractions, abdominal rigidity, and generalized spasms. Symptoms usually appear between fifth and twelfth day, most frequently about seventh day.	4 to 21 days, dependent on character, extent, and location of wound; average 10 days. Most cases occur within 14 days.	Tetanus spores introduced into body during injury, usually puncture wound contaminated with soil, street dust, or animal or human feces, but also through lacerations, burns, and trivial or unnoticed wounds.	Not directly transmitted from person to person
Toxocariasis (larva migrans visceralis, *Toxocara* [Canis] [Cati] infection, visceral larva migrans syndrome)	Chronic and usually mild disease of young children caused by migration of certain nematode larvae in organs and tissues. Characterized by eosinophilia of variable duration, hepatomegaly, hyperglobulinemia, pulmonary symptoms, and fever.	Probably weeks or months, depending on intensity of infection and sensitivity of patient.	By direct or indirect transmission of infectious *Toxocara* eggs from contaminated soil to mouth; directly related to eating of dirt by young children. Eggs reach soil in feces from infected cats and dogs.	Not directly transmitted from person to person.

Disease	Description	Incubation period	Mode of transmission	Period of communicability
Toxoplasmosis (congenital toxoplasmosis)	Systemic protozoal disease. Primary infection is frequently asymptomatic; acute disease may occur with fever, lymphadenopathy, and lymphocytosis persisting for days or weeks. Rare severe manifestations include cerebral signs, pneumonitis, generalized muscle involvement, and death.	Unknown; 10 to 23 days in one outbreak larva vehicle was undercooked meat and 5 to 20 days in an outbreak associated with infected cats.	Transplacental infection may occur in women with primary infection. Postnatal infections might be acquired by eating raw or undercooked infected meat or more often by ingesting infective oocysts. Drinking water contaminated with feces of *Felidae* has been incriminated.	Not directly transmitted from person to person except in utero.
Trachoma	Communicable keratoconjunctivitis characterized by conjunctival inflammation with papillary hyperplasia, associated with ascular invasion of cornea, and in later stages by conjunctival scarring that may eventually lead to blindness.	5 to 12 days (based on volunteer studies).	By direct contact with ocular discharges and possibly mucoid or purulent discharges of nasal mucous membranes of infected persons or materials. Flies (*Musca sorbens*) may contribute to spread of disease.	As long as active lesions are present in the conjunctivae and adnexal mucous membranes.
Trench fever (Wolhynian fever, quintan fever)	Nonfatal, febrile disease of protean manifestations characterized by headache, malaise, pain, and tenderness especially in shins; onset either sudden or slow with fever, which may be relapsing, typhoidlike, or limited to single short febrile episode lasting several days.	Generally 7 to 30 days.	Not directly transmitted from person to person. Humans infected by inoculation of organism in louse feces through a skin break from either bite of louse or other means.	Organisms may circulate in blood (by which lice can be infected) for weeks, months, or years and may recur with or without symptoms. History of trench fever is permanent contraindication to blood donation.
Trichinosis (trichiniasis, trichinellosis)	Disease caused by larvae of *Trichinella spiralis* that migrate to and become encapsulated in muscles. Clinical manifestations usually include mild febrile disease, but can range from inapparent infection to fulminating, fatal disease.	Usually about 10 to 14 days after ingestion by humans of infective meat; varies between 1 and 45 days.	Eating raw or insufficiently cooked flesh of animals containing viable encysted trichinae, chiefly pork and pork products.	Not transmitted directly from person to person. Animal hosts remain infective for months as does meat from such animals for appreciable periods unless processed to kill larvae.
Trichomoniasis	Common disease of genitourinary tract, characterized in women by vaginitis, with small petechial or sometimes punctate hemorrhagic lesions and profuse, thin, foamy, yellowish discharge with foul odor; frequently asymptomatic. In men, infectious agent 4 to 20 days, average 7 days.	By contact with vaginal and urethral discharges of infected persons during sexual intercourse and possibly by contact with contaminated articles.	For duration of infection.	

Continued.

1-25/Communicable and Infectious Diseases—cont'd

Name	Synopsis of symptoms	Incubation period	Mode of transmission	Period of communicability
Trichuriasis (trichocephaliasis)	invades and persists in prostate, urethra, or seminal vesicles, but rarely produces symptoms or demonstrable lesions. Nematode infection of large intestine, often asymptomatic. Heavy infections result in bloody stools and diarrhea. Rectal prolapse may occur in very heavily infected children.			
Trypanosomiasis, (African sleeping sickness)	In early stages chancre usually appears at primary tsetse fly bite site with fever, intense headache, insomnia, lymph node enlargement, anemia, local edema, and rash. In late stage is body wasting, somnolence, and signs referable to central nervous system.	In *T. rhodesiense* infection usually 2 to 3 weeks; in *T. gambiense* infection, usually longer and extremely variable—months or even years.	By bite of infective *Glossina*, the tsetse fly. Congenital transmission can occur in humans, as well as direct mechanical transmission by blood on proboscis of *Glossina* and other human-biting flies, or in laboratory accidents.	To tsetse fly, as long as parasite is present in blood of infected person or animal. Parasitemia is extremely variable in untreated cases and occurs in late and early stages of disease.
Trypanosomiasis, American (Chagas' disease)	Acute disease usually occurs in children; chronic manifestations generally appear later in life. Acute disease is characterized by variable fever, malaise, lymphadenopathy and hepatosplenomegaly. Inflammatory response at site of infection (chagoma) may last up to 8 weeks. Unilateral bipalpebral edema occurs in significant percentage of acute cases. Life-threatening or fatal manifestations include myocarditis and meningoencephalitis.	About 5 to 14 days after bite of insect vector; 30 to 40 days if infected by blood transfusion.	By fecal material passed while biting by infected vectors. Infection is through contamination of conjunctiva, mucous membranes, abrasions, or skin wounds by fresh infected bug feces. Transmission also may occur by blood transfusion and organisms may pass through placenta to cause congenital infection.	Organisms are present regularly in blood during acute period and may persist in very small numbers throughout life in symptomatic and asymptomatic persons. Vector becomes infective 10 to 30 days after biting an infective host and remains so for life (as long as 2 years).
Tuberculosis	Mycobacterial disease. Initial infection usually goes unnoticed; tuberculin sensitivity appears within a few weeks; lesions commonly heal, leaving no residual changes except pulmonary or tracheobraonchial lymph node calci-	From infection to demonstrable primary lesion, about 4 to 12 weeks. Whereas subsequent risk of progressive pulmonary or extrapulmonary tuberculosis is greatest within 1 or 2 years after infection, it may persist for	Exposure to bacilli in airborne droplet nuclei from sputum of persons with infectious tuberculosis. Bovine tuberculosis results from exposure to tubercular cattle and ingestion of unpasteurized dairy products.	As long as infectious tubercle bacilli are being discharged.

Disease	Clinical description	Incubation period	Mode of transmission	Period of communicability
	...fication. May progress to pulmonary tuberculosis or, by lymphohematogenous dissemination of bacilli, to produce miliary, meningeal, or other extrapulmonary involvement.	a lifetime as latent infection.		
Tularemia (rabbit fever, deerfly fever, Ohara's disease)	Clinical manifestations related to route of introduction and virulence of strain. Most often ulcer, often on hand, accompanied by swelling of regional lymph nodes. May be no apparent primary ulcer but only enlarged and painful lymph nodes that may suppurate.	Related to virulence of infecting strain and to size of inoculum; 2 to 10 days, usually 3 days.	Inoculation of skin, conjunctival sac, or oropharyngeal mucosa with blood or tissue while handling infected animals; or by fluids from infected flies, ticks, or other animals; or through bite of arthropods.	Not directly transmitted from person to person. Unless treated, infectious agent may be found in blood during first 2 weeks of disease, and in lesions for 1 month from onset—sometimes longer.
Typhoid fever (enteric fever, typhus abdominalis)	Systemic infectious disease characterized by sustained fever, headache, malaise, anorexia, relative bradycardia, enlargement of spleen, rose spots on trunk, nonproductive cough, constipation more commonly than diarrhea, and involvement of lymphoid tissues.	Depends on size of infecting dose; usual range 1 to 3 weeks.	By food or water contaminated by feces or urine of patient or carrier.	As long as typhoid bacilli appear in excreta; usually first week throughout convalescence; variable thereafter. About 10% of untreated patients will discharge bacilli for 3 months after onset of symptoms; 2 to 5% become permanent carriers.
Typhus fever, epidemic louse-borne (exanthematic typhus, classical typhus fever)	Onset is variable, often sudden and marked by headache, chills, prostration, fever, and general pains. Macular eruptions appears on fifth or sixth day, initially on upper trunk followed by spread to entire body but usually not to face, palms, or soles. Toxemia is usually pronounced and disease terminates by rapid lysis after about 2 weeks of fever.	From 1 to 2 weeks, commonly 12 days.	The body louse, *Pediculus humanis corporis*, is infected by feeding on blood of patient with acute typhus fever. Humans are infected by rubbing feces or crushed lice into bites of louse or other superficial abrasions. Inhalation of infective louse feces as dust may account for some infections.	Disease is not directly transmitted from person to person. Patients are infective for lice during febrile illness and possibly for 2 or 3 days after temperature returns to normal.
Typhus fever, flea-borne (murine typhus, endemic typhus fever, shop typhus)	Course of flea-borne typhus fever resembles that of epidemic louse-borne typhus, but is milder. Fatality rate for all ages is about 2%; it increases with age.	From 1 to 2 weeks, commonly 12 days.	Infective rat fleas (usually *Xenopsylla cheopis*) defecate rickettsiae while sucking blood and contaminate bite site and other fresh skin wounds. Occasional case may follow inhalation of dried infective flea feces.	Not directly transmitted from person to person. Once infected, fleas remain so for life.

Continued.

APPENDIX

1-25/Communicable and Infectious Diseases — cont'd

Name	Synopsis of symptoms	Incubation period	Mode of transmission	Period of communicability
Typhus, scrub (tsutsu-gamushi disease, mite-borne typhus fever)	Often characterized by primary skin ulcer (eschar) corresponding to site of attachment of infected mite. Acute febrile onset follows within several days, along with headache, profuse sweating, conjunctival injection, and lymphadenopathy.	Usually 10 to 12 days; varies from 6 to 21 days.	By infected larval mites; nymphs and adults do not feed on vertebrate hosts.	Not directly transmitted from person to person.
Urethritis, chlamydial Urethritis, nongonorrheal and nonspecific	Sexually transmitted urethritis of males caused by chlamydial agent. Clinical manifestations are usually indistinguishable from gonorrhea but are often milder and include opaque discharge of moderate or scanty quantity, urethral itching, and burning on urination. Infection of women results in cervicitis and salpingitis; infections are often asymptomatic.	5 to 7 days or longer.	Sexual contact.	Unknown.
Verruca vulgaris (warts)	Viral disease manifested by a variety of skin and mucous membrane lesions. Include the common wart, a circumscribed, hyperkeratotic, rough textured, painless papule varying in size from pinhead to large masses; also filiform warts, venereal warts, and plantar warts.	About 4 months; range is 1 to 20 months.	Usually by direct contact, but contaminated floors and fomites are frequently implicated. Warts may be autoinoculated. *Condyloma acuminatum* is usually sexually transmitted.	Unknown, but probably as long as visible lesions persist.
Whooping cough (pertussis)	Acute bacterial disease involving tracheobronchial tree. Initial catarrhal stage has insidious onset with irritating cough that gradually becomes paroxysmal, usually within 1 to 2 weeks, and lasts for 1 to 2 months.	Commonly 7 days; almost uniformly within 10 days, and not exceeding 21 days.	Primarily by direct contact with discharges from respiratory mucous membranes of infected persons by airborne route, probably by droplets. Frequently brought into home by older sibling.	Highly communicable in early catarrhal stage before paroxysmal cough stage. For control purposes, communicable stage extends from 7 days after exposure to 3 weeks after onset of typical paroxysms in patients not treated with antibiotics; in patients treated with erythromycin, period of infectiousness extends only 5 to 7 days after onset of therapy.

Yaws (frambesia, pian, bouba, parang)	Chronic relapsing nonvenereal treponematosis characterized by early cutaneous lesions and noncontagious late, destructive lesions. Typical initial lesion (mother yaw) is papilloma on face or extremities that persists for several weeks or months.	From 2 weeks to 3 months.	Principally by direct contact with exudates of early skin lesions of infected persons. Indirect transmission by contamination from scratching, skin piercing articles, and by flies on open wounds is probable but of undetermined importance.	Variable; may extend intermittently over several years while moist lesions are present. Infectious agent is not usually found in late ulcerative lesions.
Yersinia (pseudotuberculosis)	Acute enteric disease manifested by diarrhea, enterocolitis, acute mesenteric lymphadenitis mimicking appendicitis, low-grade fever, headache, pharyngitis, anorexia, vomiting, erythema nodosum, arthritis, cutaneous ulceration, abscesses, and septicemia.	Probably 3 to 7 days, generally less than 10 days.	Fecal-oral transmission takes place by contact with infected persons or animals (hand-to-mouth), or by eating and drinking contaminated food and water.	Fecal shedding as long as symptoms exist. Chronic carrier state probably exists.
Zygomycosis (mucormycosis, phycomycosis)	Group of mycoses usually caused by fungi of the family Mucoraceae of the class Zygomycetes. These fungi have affinity for blood vessels, causing thrombosis and infarction. In its craniofacial form is usually nasal or paranasal sinus infections, most often during ketoacidotic episodes of diabetes mellitus.	Unknown. Fungus spreads rapidly in susceptible tissues.	By inhalation or ingestion of fungus by susceptible individuals. Direct inoculation by minor trauma, intravenous catheters, and cutaneous burns are occasionally implicated.	Not directly transmitted from human or animal to human.

APPEN-DIX

1-26/STATE DIRECTORS OF EMERGENCY MEDICAL SERVICES

Alabama

Arthur Harman, Director
Alabama Dept. of Health
EMS Division
State Office Bldg., Rm. 644
Montgomery, AL 36130-1701
205/261-5261

Alaska

Mark S. Johnson, Chief
EMS Section
Dept. of Health and Social Services
P.O. Box H-06C
Juneau, AK 99811-0600
907/465-3027

American Samoa

Fuapopo Avegalio
Coordinator/Trainer
Emergency Medical Services
American Samoa Government
LBJ Tropical Medical Center
Pago Pago, AS 96799

Arizona

Forrest C. Wood Jr., Office Chief
Div. of EMS
AZ Dept. of Health Services
3008 North 3rd Street
Phoenix, AZ 85012
602/220-6400

Irene Conlan, Asst. Dir.
Div. of EMS and Health Care Facilities
AZ Dept. of Health Services
3008 North 3rd Street
Phoenix, AZ 85012
602/220-6400

Arkansas

Carolyn R. Schmidt, Dir.
Office of EMS
Arkansas Dept. of Health
4815 W. Markham Street
Little Rock, AR 72205-3867
501/661-2262

California

Bruce E. Haynes, MD, Dir.
EMS Authority
1030 15th Street, Suite 302
Sacramento, CA 95814
916/322-4336

Colorado

William R. Metcalf, Dir.
EMS Division
Colorado Dept. of Health
4210 E. 11th Avenue
Denver, CO 80220
303/331-8630

Connecticut

(Mr.) Chris A. Gentile, Dir.
Office of EMS
Department of Health
150 Washington St.
Hartford, CT 06106
203/566-7336

Delaware

Charles E. Nabb, Director
EMS, Capitol Square
Jesse S. Cooper Mem. Bldg.
Dover, DE 19901
302/736-4710

District of Columbia

Mary Berkeley, Exec. Dir.
Emergency Health and Medical Svces.
1875 Connecticut Ave. NW,
Rm. 833D
Washington, DC 20009
202/673-6744

Florida

Larry S. Jordan, Admin.
EMS Dept. of Health and Rehabilitation
1317 Winewood Blvd., PDHIM
PDHEMS
Tallahassee, FL 32399-0700
904/487-1911

Georgia

(Ms.) Dallas Jankowski, JD,
Director, EMS Office
878 Peachtree St. N.E.,
Room 207
Atlanta, GA 30309
404/894-6505

Guam

Angelina G. Mummert,
EMS Administrator
Office of EMS
Dept. of Public Health and Social Svces.
P.O. Box 2816
Agana, Guam 96910
617/472-8507

Hawaii

Donna Maiava, Acting Chief
EMSS BR. State of Hawaii
Dept. of Health
3627 Kilauea Ave., Rm. 102
Honolulu, HI 96816
808/735-5267

Dr. Gregory Gifford
Medical Director
EMSS Branch, State of Hawaii
P.O. Box 1225
Kailua, HI 96734
808/735-5267

Idaho

Paul B. Anderson, Chief
EMS Bureau
Dept. of Health & Welfare
450 W. State St.
Boise, ID 83720
208/334-5994

Illinois

Leslee Stein-Spencer, RN, MS,
Chief, Div. of EMS
Dept. of Public Health
525 W. Jefferson Street,
Room 450
Springfield, IL 62761
217/785-2080

Indiana

Daniel A. Garman, Director
Indiana EMS Commission
State Office Bldg., Rm. 315
100 N. Senate Ave.
Indianapolis, IN 46204
317/232-3980

Addresses provided by the National Association of State EMS Directors

Iowa

Donald E. Kerns, Prog. Mgr.
EMS, IA Dept. of Health
Lucas State Office Building
Des Moines, IA 50319-0075
515/281-3239

Kansas

Lyle E. Eckhart, Dir.
Bureau of EMS
111 West 6th St.
Topeka, KS 66603-3805
913/296-7296

Kentucky

(Mrs.) Pat Loar Jones,
EMS Mgr.
Cabinet for Human Resources
272 East Main St.
Frankfort, KY 40621
502/564-8963

Louisiana

Albert Heck
Bureau of EMS
4550 North Boulevard, 2nd floor
P.O. Box 44215
Baton Rouge, LA 70804
504/922-1300

Maine

Kevin K. McGinnis, Dir.
Maine EMS
295 Water Street
Augusta, ME 04330
207/289-3953

Maryland

Ameen Ramzy, MD, Dir.
EMS - MIEMSS
22 S. Greene St.
Baltimore, MD 21201
301/328-5074

Massachusetts

Frank Keslof, Dir.
Office of EMS
Dept. of Public Health
80 Boylston St., Suite 1040
Boston, MA 02116
617/451-3433

Michigan

Director
Div. of EMS
3500 N. Logan
P.O. Box 30035
Lansing, MI 48909
517/335-8503

Minnesota

Norm Hanson, Chief
EMS, MN Dept. of Health
393 N. Dunlap Street
P.O. Box 64900
Minneapolis, MN 55164-0900
612/643-2164

Mississippi

Wade N. Spruill, Jr., Dir.
Office of EMS
State Board of Health
P.O. Box 1700
Jackson, MS 39205-1700
601/987-3880

Missouri

Kenneth E. Cole, Jr., Dir.
Bureau of EMS
Missouri Dept. of Health
P.O. Box 570, 1730 East Elm
Jefferson City, MO 65102
314/751-6356

Montana

Drew E. Dawson, Chief
EMS Bureau
Dept. of Health and Env. Sciences
Cogswell Building
Helena, MT 59620
406/444-3895

Nebraska

Robert Leopold, Director
Div. of EMS
301 Centennial Mall S.,
3rd Floor, Box 95007
Box 95007
Lincoln, NE 68509-5007
402/471-2158

Nevada

Sheryl Yount, Dir. EMS
505 E. King Street
Capitol Complex, Kinkead
Building
Carson City, NV 89710
702/885-3065

New Hampshire

Marcia E. Houck, Bureau Chief
Emergency Medical Svces.
Health & Welfare Building
Hazen Drive
Concord, NH 03301
603/271-4569

New Jersey

George Leggett, Chief Administrator
EMS State Dept. of Health
CN 364
Trenton, NJ 08625
609/984-1348

New Mexico

Barak Wolff, EMS Chief
Primary Care and EMS Bureau
Health Services Division
Health and Environment Dept.
P.O. Box 968
Santa Fe, NM 87504-0968
505/827-2509

New York

Michael Gilbertson, Director
EMS Development Program
Corning Tower Building, Rm. 729
Albany, NY 12237
518/474-2219

North Carolina

Bob W. Bailey, Chief
Office of EMS
701 Barbour Drive
Raleigh, NC 27603
919/733-2285

North Dakota

Timothy W. Wiedrich, Acting Dir.
Emerg. Health Svces. Div.
Department of Health
State Capitol Bldg.
Bismarck, ND 58505
701/224-2388

Continued.

1-26/State EMS Directors/Addresses Provided by the National Association of State EMS Directors—cont'd

Ohio

James E. Bartholomew, DDS
Administrator, EMS Agency
Public Safety Services
65 S. Front St., Rm. 916
Columbus, OH 43266-0308
614/466-9447

Oklahoma

John E. Ward, Dir., EMS
1000 N.E. 10th, Rm. 407.3
P.O. Box 53551
Oklahoma City, OK 73152
405/271-5104

Oregon

Nancy Clarke, EMS Mgr.
State Health Dept.
P.O. Box 231
Portland, OR 97201
503/229-6365

Pennsylvania

Kum S. Ham, Ph.D., Acting Dir.
Div. of EMS
Health & Welfare Bldg.
Room 1033
P.O. Box 90
Harrisburg, PA 17108
717/787-8741

Puerto Rico

Benito Colon, MD, Dir.
EMS
G.P.O. Box 71423
San Juan, PR 00936
809/765-1594

Rhode Island

Harold A. Pace, Dir.
Div. of EMS
Dept. of Health
75 Davis St.
Providence, RI 02908
401/277-2401

South Carolina

Albert M. Futrell Jr., Dir.
Div. of EMS
Dept. of Health and Environ. Control
2600 Bull Street
Columbia, SC 29201
803/737-7009

South Dakota

Robert Graff, Dir. EMS
Dept. of Health
Foss Bldg.,
523 E. Capitol St.
Pierre, SD 57501
605/773-3737

Tennessee

Joseph B. Phillips, Dir.
Div. of EMS
TN Dept. of Health and Environ.
283 Plus Park Blvd.
Nashville, TN 37217
615/367-6278

Texas

Pam West, Dir., EMS
Texas Dept. of Health
1100 W. 49th St.
Austin, TX 78756
512/465-2601

Utah

Richard L. Warburton, Dir.
Bureau of EMS
P.O. Box 16660
Salt Lake City, UT
84116-0660
801/538-6435

Vermont

Dan Manz, Director
EMS Division
Box 70, 60 Main Street
Burlington, VT 05402
802/863-7310

Virgin Islands

Kirk Grybowski, Dir. EMS
Dept. of Health
Knud Hansen Health Facility
Charlotte Amalie, VI 00802
809/774-9000, ext. 236

Virginia

Susan D. McHenry, Dir.
Mary Kemp, Asst.
Bureau of EMS
State Dept. of Health
109 Governor Street,
Room 1001
Richmond, VA 23219
804/786-5188

Washington

Howard Farley, Sect. Head
EMS, Division of Health
DSHS Mail Stop ET-34
Olympia, WA 98504
206/753-5898/2095

West Virginia

Frederick Cooley, MD, Dir.
EMS, Dept. of Health
Building 3, Room 426
1800 Washington St., East
East Charleston, WV 25305
304/348-3956

Wisconsin

Michael F. French, Chief
EMS, Div. of Health
P.O. Box 309
Madison, WI 53701
608/266-7743

Wyoming

Jimm Murray, Chief
EMS Program
Hathaway Bldg., Rm. 527
Cheyenne, WY 82002
307/777-7955

National Assoc. of State EMS Directors Association Staff

Ellen J. Hume, Assoc. Dir.
The National EMS Clearinghouse
The Council of State Governments
P.O. Box 11910, Iron Works Pike
Lexington, KY 40578
606/252-2291

1-27/RULE OF NINES — ADULT

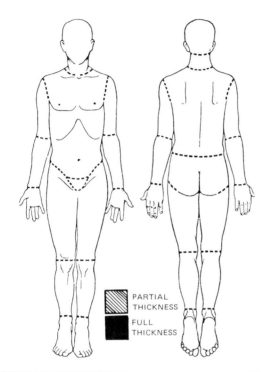

Date:_____

Height:_____ Weight: _____

$2°$_____ + $3°$_____ = _____ %

PARTIAL THICKNESS

FULL THICKNESS

Percent Surface Area Burned
(Berkow Formula)

AREA	1 YEAR	1-4 YEARS	5-9 YEARS	10-14 YEARS	Y 15 YEARS	ADULT	2°	3°
Head	19	17	13	11	9	7		
Neck	2	2	2	2	2	2		
Ant. Trunk	13	13	13	13	13	13		
Post Trunk	13	13	13	13	13	13		
R. Buttock	2½	2½	2½	2½	2½	2½		
L. Buttock	2½	2½	2½	2½	2½	2½		
Genitalia	1	1	1	1	1	1		
R. U. Arm	4	4	4	4	4	4		
L. U. Arm	4	4	4	4	4	4		
R. L. Arm	3	3	3	3	3	3		
L. L. Arm	3	3	3	3	3	3		
R. Hand	2½	2½	2½	2½	2½	2½		
L. Hand	2½	2½	2½	2½	2½	2½		
R. Thigh	5½	6½	8	8½	9	9½		
L. Thigh	5½	6½	8	8½	9	9½		
R. Leg	5	5	5½	6	6½	7		
L. Leg	5	5	5½	6	6½	7		
R. Foot	3½	3½	3½	3½	3½	3½		
L. Foot	3½	3½	3½	3½	3½	3½		
TOTAL								

Reproduced with permission from Artz, CP and Moncrief, JA: The treatment of burns, ed 2, Philadelphia, 1969, WB Saunders Co.

1-28/BURN CENTERS IN THE UNITED STATES AND CANADA

State	City	Hospital	Zip code	Telephone number for patient referral	Burn unit bed capacity or burn service capability*	Burn service medical director or M.D.'s most active in burn treatment
Alabama	Birmingham	Children's Hospital	35233	205/933-4000	12	Marshall Pitts
		U. of Alabama Hospitals	35233	205/934-3411	13	Alan R. Dimick
	Mobile	U. of So. Alabama Medical Center Hospital	36617	205/471-7000	7	Arnold Luterman
Alaska	Anchorage	Providence Hospital	99504	907/562-2211	10	Mary Finn/Clifford Dasco; Paul Steer; W. J. Mills (hypothermia)
	Fairbanks	Fairbanks Memorial Hospital	99701	907/452-8181	5*	William Wennen
Arizona	Phoenix	Maricopa Medical Center	85008	602/267-5700	20	Richard Parry; John M. Stein
	Tucson	St. Mary's Hospital	85703	602/795-8700	9	Philip Fleishman
Arkansas	Little Rock	Arkansas Children's Hospital	72201	501/370-1100 ext. 149	14	Fred T. Caldwell; John Crabtree
		Univ. Hospital/U. of Arkansas Medical Science Campus	72205	501/661-5000	6*	Fred T. Caldwell
California	Baldwin Park	Terrace Plaza Medical Center	91706	213/338-1101 ext. 260	9*	William T. Choctaw
	Berkeley	Alta Bates Hospital	94705	415/540-1573	6	Jerold Z. Kaplan
	Castro Valley	Eden Hospital	94546	415/537-1234	6	Eleanor Kohn; Eric Bachelor; Stanley Hegg; Ronald Iverson
	Chico	Chico Community Hospital	95926	916/345-2411 or 916/342-7513	6	Donald J. Mangus; Stanley Korock
	Culver City	Brotman Medical Center	90239	213/836-7000 ext. 3340 or 2510	17/23*	Stanley Frileck; Arthur Kahn
	Downey	Rancho Los Amigos Hospital	90242	213/922-7454	24*	G. Brody et al (reconstructive only)
	Eureka	St. Joseph's Hospital	95501	707/443-8051	*	Russel Pardoe
	Fresno	Valley Medical Center	93702	209/453-4220	6	Steven N. Parks
	Los Angeles	LAC/USC Medical Center	90033	213/226-7991	26/37*	Bruce E. Zawacki
	Orange	U. of Calif. Irvine Medical Center	92668	714/634-5304	8	Bruce M. Achauer
	Sacramento	U. of Calif. Davis Medical Center	95817	916/453-3636	8	F. William Blaisdell (Acting Director)

Continued.

State	City	Hospital	Zip	Phone	No.	Contact
	San Bernardino	San Bernardino Community Hospital	92411	714/887-7047 ext. 405 or 444	6*	David Hess
		San Bernardino County Medical Center	92404	714/383-3142	9	Appannagari Gnanavez
	San Diego	Univ. Hospital/U. of Calif. Medical Center	92103	619/294-6502	14	Hugh Frank (Acting Director)
	San Francisco	San Francisco General Hospital	94110	415/821-8197	6	Anthony A. Meyer Guy Trengove-Jones
	San Jose	St. Francis Memorial Hospital	94109	415/775-4321	10	Edward Falces
		Santa Clara Valley Medical Center	95128	408/279-5242	6	Ronald M. Sato
	San Pablo	Brookside Hospital	94806	415/235-7000	6	Robert L. Shapiro
	Sherman Oaks	Sherman Oaks Community Hospital	91403	213/981-7111	30	A. Richard Grossman
	Stockton	Dameron Hospital	95203	209/944-5550	7	Genest de L'Arbre
	Torrance	Torrance Memorial Hospital	90505	213/325-9110	10	William D. Davies
Colorado	Colorado Springs	Penrose Hospital	80917	303/630-5770	8	Ian G. Walker
	Denver	Children's Hospital	80218	303/861-6517	8*	Claude Poliakoff William Carl Bailey
		University Colorado Health Science Center	80262	303/394-8052	10	John Hansbrough
	Grand Junction	St. Mary's Hospital	81502	303/242-9127	2*	William Merkel
	Greeley	N. Colorado Medical Center	80631	303/352-4121	4*	James R. Wheeler
	Pueblo	St. Mary-Corwin Hospital	81004	303/560-4000	4*	Donald Leubke
Connecticut	Bridgeport	Bridgeport Hospital	06610	203/384-3728	22	Michael L. D'Aiuto
	Hartford	Hartford Hospital	06114	203/524-2840	5*	Philip E. Trowbridge and others
	New Haven	Yale–New Haven Hospital	06504	203/785-2573 or 203/785-2574	4*	Stephen Ariyan Charles Cuono Zeno Chicarilli Richard Stahl
District of Columbia	Washington	Children's Hospital National Medical Center	20010	202/745-5116 or 202/745-5152	12	Judson G. Randolph
		Washington Hospital Center	20010	202/541-7241 or 202/541-6662	23	Marion Jordan
Florida	Gainesville	Shands Teaching Hospital	32610	904/392-3054 or 904/392-3055	6	Hal G. Bingham
	Miami	U. of Miami Jackson Memorial Hospital	33136	305/325-7085	8	C. Gillon Ward Jeffrey Hammond Donald Buckner
	Orlando	Orlando Regional Medical Center	32806	305/841-5176	5	Juan Sauer
	Tampa	Tampa General Hospital	33606	813/253-0711 or 813/251-7617	17	C. Wayne Cruse
Georgia	Atlanta	Grady Memorial Hospital	30335	404/588-4307	30	Roger Sherman
	Augusta	Doctor's Hospital of Augusta	30910	404/863-3232	10	Alton Garrison
		Eugene Talmadge Memorial Hospital, Medical College of Georgia	30912	404/828-3893	6	Joseph Still Richard C. Treat Edward Hall

APPENDIX

1-28/Burn Centers in the United States and Canada—cont'd

State	City	Hospital	Zip code	Telephone number for patient referral	Burn unit bed capacity or burn service capability*	Burn service medical director or M.D.'s most active in burn treatment
	Columbus	Medical Center	31902	404/571-1336	6*	Robert K. Worman
Hawaii	Honolulu	Straub Clinic & Hospital	96813	808/523-2311	3*	James H. Penoff / Robert W. Schulz
Illinois	Chicago	Children's Memorial Hospital	60614	312/880-4094	*	Victor E. Lewis
		Cook County Hospital	60612	312/633-6564 or 312/633-6570	30	Takayoshi Matsuda / Marella Hanumadass / Richard Kagan
		Edgewater Hospital	60660	312/878-6000	4*	Ramesh Kharwadkar
		U. of Chicago Hospitals	60637	312/962-6112	20	Robert Parsons (Acting Director)
	Evanston	Evanston Hospital	60201	312/492-7720	8*	Charles Drueck
	Maywood	Foster G. McGaw Hospital, Loyola U. of Chicago	60153	312/531-3988	14	Raymond Warpeha
	Rock Island	Franciscan Medical Center	61202	309/793-3173	14	Frank E. Miller
	Rockford	St. Anthony's Hospital Medical Center	61101	815/226-2000	8	Raymond Hoffman
	Springfield	Memorial Medical Center	62708	217/788-3325	10	Elof Eriksson
Indiana	Fort Wayne	St. Joseph's Hospital	46802	219/425-3431	7	Jack Patterson
	Indianapolis	J. W. Riley Hospital	46223	317/264-3927	8	A. Michael Sadove (children)
	Indianapolis	Methodist Hospital of Indiana	46202	317/929-8056	10*	Wally Zollman / Stephen Olvey
	Indianapolis	W. N. Wishard Memorial Hospital	46202	317/630-6471	8	David J. Smith, Jr.
Iowa	Iowa City	U. of Iowa Hospitals & Clinics	52242	319/356-2496	13	Albert E. Cram
		St. Luke's Reg. Medical Center	51104	712/279-3440	8	Larry D. Foster
Kansas	Kansas City	U. of Kansas Medical Center	66103	913/588-6540	10	Mani M. Mani / David W. Robinson
	Wichita	St. Francis Hospital	67201	316/268-5388	11	Thomas E. Kendall and others
	Wichita	Wesley Medical Center	67214	316/688-2688	2*	Richard C. Shaw and others
Kentucky	Lexington	University Hospital	40536	606/233-5260	4	Edward Luce
	Louisville	Humana Hospital University	40217	502/562-3000	5	Hiram C. Polk, Jr.
		Kosair-Children's Hospital	40202	502/895-5466	8	John M. Whetter
Louisiana	Baton Rouge	Baton Rouge General Hospital	70821	504/387-7716	14	D. V. Cacioppo
	Marrero	West Jefferson Hospital	70072	504/347-5511	14	Frank C. DiVincenti
	Shreveport	L.S.U. Medical Center Hospital	33932	318/674-6133	16	Edwin Deitch
Maine	Portland	Maine Medical Center	04102	207/871-2991	4	Joel Johnson (Acting Director)
Maryland	Baltimore	Baltimore City Hospital	21224	301/396-8765	21	Andrew Munster

State	City	Hospital	ZIP	Phone	No.	Director(s)
Massachusetts	Boston	Boston City Hospital	02118	617/424-5204	2*	Erwin Hirsch
		Brigham & Women's Hospital	02115	617/732-7712	10	Robert H. Demling
		Massachusetts General Hospital	02114	617/726-3354	10	John F. Burke
		Shriner's Burns Institute	02114	617/722-3000	30	John P. Remensnyder
	Worcester	Worcester City Hospital	01610	617/799-8110	4*	Felix Cataldo
Michigan	Ann Arbor	Michigan Burn Center University Hospital	48109	313/995-BURN	29	Irving Feller, Jai K. Prasad
		Chelsea Community Hospital				
	Detroit	Children's Hospital of Michigan	48201	313/494-5678	15	James R. Lloyd
		Detroit Receiving Hospital & Univ. Health Center	48201	313/494-3216 or 313/494-3218	18	Martin C. Robson, David J. Smith, Jr.
	Flint	Hurley Medical Center	48502	313/257-9188	13	M.S. Haffajee
	Grand Rapids	Blodgett Memorial Medical Center	49506	616/774-7670	8	William Simpson
	Kalamazoo	Bronson Methodist Hospital	49007	616/383-6485 or 1-800/632-3403	12	Richard A. Wehrenberg, Frank J. Newman, Paul Fierke, Michael Nave
	Lansing	Edward R. Sparrow Hospital	48909	517/483-2677	6	Errikos Constant, Jorge Gomez, Preecha Supanwanid, William Blackburn
	Marquette	Marquette General Hospital	49855	906/228-9440	*	James Kelinger, Constance N. Arnold
	Saginaw	St. Mary's Hospital	48601	517/790-5055	6	Syed Akhtar
Minnesota	Duluth	Miller-Dwan Hospital & Medical Center	55805	218/727-8762	12	John W. Wolfe
	Minneapolis	Hennepin Co. Medical Center	55415	612/347-2915	10	John Twomey
	Rochester	St. Mary's Hospital	55901	507/285-5123/5591, 507/285-6691	6*	George B. Irons (adults), Robert Telander (children)
	St. Paul	St. Paul-Ramsey Medical Center	55101	612/221-3351	24	Lynn D. Solem
Mississippi	Greenville	Delta Medical Center	38701	601/378-3783	16	Robert Love
Missouri	Columbia	U. of Missouri Health Sciences Center	65212	314/882-7994	7	Boyd E. Terry
	Kansas City	Children's Mercy Hospital	64108	816/234-3520	6	Ronald J. Sharp
	St. Louis	Barnes Hospital	63110	314/362-5370	6	William W. Monafo
		St. John's Mercy Medical Center	63141	314/569-6055	17	Vatche H. Ayvazian, Thomas Vitale
	Springfield	St. John's Reg. Health Center	65802	417/885-2876	9	Marc Wittmer
Montana	Billings	St. Vincent Hospital	59101	406/245-2458	4*	David F. Sloan
	Lincoln	St. Elizabeth Community Health Center	68510	402/489-7181 or 402/483-9206	10	Robert W. Gillespie
Nevada	Las Vegas	Southern Nevada Memorial	89102	702/383-2268	12	Charles A. Buerk

Continued.

APPEN-DIX

1-28/Burn Centers in the United States and Canada — cont'd

State	City	Hospital	Zip code	Telephone number for patient referral	Burn unit bed capacity or burn service capability*	Burn service medical director or M.D.'s most active in burn treatment
New Jersey	Hackensack	Hackensack Hospital	07601	201/441-2020	9*	Anthony Barbara, Frederick Fuller, Esber Mansour, Sylvia Petrone
	Livingston	Saint Barnabas Medical Center	07039	201/533-5920	12	John L. Coon
New Mexico	Albuquerque	St. Joseph's Hospital	87102	505/247-2449 or 1-800/221-3664	*	John O. Kucan
		U. of New Mexico Hospital	87106	505/843-2111	10	
New York	Albany	Albany Medical Center	12208	518/445-3010	8	Dhiraj M. Shah
	Buffalo	Children's Hospital	14222	716/878-7301 or 716/878-7435	*	Theodore Jewett, Donald R. Cooney, Melvyn P. Karp
		Millard Fillmore Hospital	14209	716/887-4776 or 716/887-4649	4	Evan J. Evans
		Sheehan Emergency Hospital	14203	716/842-2200	10	Louis C. Cloutier
	East Meadow	Nassau Co. Medical Center	11554	516/542-3207	18	Roger L. Simpson
	Elmira	St. Joseph's Hospital	14902	607/733-6541	4*	James Marshall, James Sonsire
	New York City Bronx	Bronx Municipal Health Center	10461	212/430-8065	11*	Stanley Levenson, Mahendra Patel, Steven May
	Brooklyn	Kings County Hospital	11203	212/735-3131	5	Winston Mitchell
	Manhattan	Harlem Hospital Center	10037	212/491-1335	5	James E. C. Norris
		N.Y. Hospital—Cornell Medical Center	10021	212/472-5132	24	Cleon W. Goodwin
		St. Vincent's Hospital	10011	212/790-8941 or 212/790-8940	6	Ronald N. Ollstein
	Rochester	Strong Memorial Hospital	14642	716/275-5475	9	R. Christie Wray, Jr.
	Syracuse	Upstate Medical Center	13210	315/473-6083	6	William Clark
	Valhalla	Westchester Co. Medical Center	10595	914/347-4909	10	Roger E. Salisbury, Jane A. Petro
	West Islip	Good Samaritan Hospital	11795	516/957-4000	*	Richard A. Giery
North Carolina	Chapel Hill	No. Carolina Memorial Hospital	27514	919/966-4131	23	H. D. Peterson
	Charlotte	Charlotte Memorial Medical Center	28203	704/331-2525	4	Harold F. Hamit
	Durham	Duke University Hospital	27710	919/681-2404	7	Gregory Georgiade, Joseph Moylan
	Winston-Salem	North Carolina Baptist Hospital	27103	919/748-7766	6	Jesse H. Meredith, Connell Shearin
North Dakota	Fargo	St. Luke's General Hospital	58122	701/280-5504	4*	David W. Todd

State	City	Hospital	ZIP	Phone	No.	Contact
Ohio	Akron	Children's Hospital Medical Center Akron Reg. Burn Center (admits adults with burns)	44308	216/379-8224	12	C. R. Boeckman, R. L. Klein
	Cincinnati	U. of Cincinnati Hospital	45267	513/872-3100	10	Robert P. Hummel
		Shriner's Burns Institute	45219	513/751-3900	30	Bruce G. MacMillan
	Cleveland	Cleveland Metro General Hospital	44109	216/459-5627	16	Richard Fratianne
	Columbus	Children's Hospital	43205	614/461-2000	14	E. Thomas Boles
		Ohio State Univ. Hospital	43210	614/422-4516	6	Robert Ruberg
	Dayton	Children's Medical Center	45404	513/226-8300	6	Charles D. Goodwin
		Miami Valley Hospital	45409	513/223-6192	8	R. K. Finley, Sidney Miller, Larry Jones
	Toledo	St. Vincent's Medical Center	43608	419/259-4734	12	Michael Yanik, Paul Silverstein
Oklahoma	Oklahoma City	Baptist Medical Center	73112	405/949-3345 or 405/949-3311	32	
		Okla. Children's Memorial Hospital	73104	405/271-4733	12	William P. Tunell
	Tulsa	Hillcrest Medical Center	74104	918/584-1351	20	Bernard Swartz
Oregon	Portland	Oregon Burn Center (at Emanuel Hospital)	97227	503/280-4233	12	Philip Parshley
Pennsylvania	Allentown	Lehigh Valley Hospital Center	18103	215/821-2058	6	Walter J. Okunski
	Chester	Crozer-Chester Medical Center	19013	215/876-0356	19	Charles E. Hartford
	Danville	Geisinger Medical Center	17821	717/271-6353 or 717/271-6591	6*	Philip C. Breen
	Erie	Hamot Medical Center	16550	814/459-0344	8	Charles R. Bales, Forrest C. Mischler
	Hershey	Hershey Medical Center	17033	717/534-8521	*	William P. Graham
	Philadelphia	Saint Agnes Medical Center	19145	215/339-4339	11/20*	Frederick A. DeClement
		St. Christopher's Hospital for Children	19133	215/427-5000	4	Stuart J. Hulnick
	Pittsburgh	Mercy Hospital	15219	412/232-8225	7	Thomas Layton
		Western Penna. Hospital	15224	412/363-2876	18	John Gaisford
		York Hospital	17405	717/771-2345	6*	Robert Davis, Richard W. Dabb
Rhode Island	Providence	Rhode Island Hospital	02902	401/277-4000	4*	Lawrence Bowen
South Carolina	Charleston	Medical University Hospital	29425	803/792-3681 or 803/792-3851	12	Dabney R. Yarborough (adults), H. Biemann Othersen, Jr. (children)
Tennessee	Chattanooga	Baroness Erlanger Hospital	37403	615/778-7881	6	Phil D. Craft
	Memphis	Regional Medical Center	38103	901/528-5500	*	William Hickerson, Gary Reynolds
	Nashville	Vanderbilt Univ. Hospital	38232	615/322-7311	20	John B. Lynch
Texas	Austin	Brackenridge Hospital	78701	512/476-6461	*	Robert A. Ersek and others
	Beaumont	Baptist Hospital of Southeast Texas	77701	409/835-3781	10	Duane Larson, Wesley Washburn
	Corpus Christi	Memorial Medical Center	78405	512/881-4360	9	Robert H. Balme

Continued.

APPEN-DIX

1-28/Burn Centers in the United States and Canada—cont'd

State	City	Hospital	Zip code	Telephone number for patient referral	Burn unit bed capacity or burn service capability*	Burn service medical director or M.D.'s most active in burn treatment
	Dallas	Parkland Memorial Hospital	75235	214/637-8546 or 211/688-2152	30	John Hunt
	El Paso	Sun Towers Hospital	79902	915/532-6281	12	Charles Lyon and others
	Ft. Sam Houston	Brooke Army Medical Center	78234	512/221-4604 or 512/221-2943	40	Basil A. Pruitt, Jr.
	Fort Worth	John Peter Smith Hospital	76104	817/921-3431	*	Charles Crenshaw and others
	Galveston	U. of Texas Medical Branch Hospitals	77550	713/761-2277	16	Sally Abston
	Houston	Shriner's Burns Institute	77550	713/761-2516	30	David N. Herndon
		Ben Taub General Hospital	77030	713/791-7000	8*	Frank Gerow
		Hermann Hospital	77030	713/797-4350	15	Donald H. Parks
	Lubbock	Lubbock General Hospital	79424	806/743-3406	6*	Richard Baker / Timothy Harnar
	Pasadena	Humana Hospital Southmore	77502	713/477-0411	12	David Katrana
	San Antonio	Medical Center Hospital	78284	512/696-3030 or 512/691-6151/7473	*	A.B. Cruz, Jr.
Utah	Salt Lake City	U. of Utah Hospital	84121	801/581-2700	12	Glenn Warden / Jeffrey Saffle
Vermont	Burlington	Medical Center Hospital of Vermont	05401	802/656-4545	6*	John Davis / Richard Gamelli
Virginia	Charlottesville	U. of Virginia Medical Center	22908	804/924-5520	6	Richard Edlich
	Norfolk	Norfolk General Hospital	23507	804/628-3117	8	William Bethea
	Richmond	Medical College of Virginia Hospital	23298	804/786-9240	12	Boyd W. Haynes
Washington	Bellingham	St. Joseph's Hospital	98225	206/734-5400 ext. 2501	2*	James Hines
	Seattle	Children's Orthopedic Hospital	98105	206/526-2042	8*	Robert T. Schaller, Jr.
		Harborview Medical Center	98104	206/223-3127	40	David Heimbach / Loren Engrav
	Spokane	Sacred Heart Medical Center	99220	509/455-3344	4*	Charles Miller
	Tacoma	St. Joseph's Hospital	98405	206/591-6677	10	Martin Schaeferle
West Virginia	Huntington	Cabell-Huntington Hospital	25701	304/526-2390	4	James A. Coil, Jr.
Wisconsin	Madison	U. of Wisconsin Hospital & Clinics	53792	608/263-1490/1387	7	Richard Helgerson
	Milwaukee	St. Mary's Hospital	53201	414/225-8000	20	George Collentine
Alberta	Calgary	Foothills Provincial General Hospital	T2N 2T9	403/270-1110	8	D.C. Birdsell / R.L. Lindsay / E. Magi
	Edmonton	U. of Alberta Hospital	T6G 2B7	403/432-6149	5	Gerald Moysa
British Columbia	Vancouver	Vancouver General Hospital	V5Z 1M9	604/875-4111	22	Charles F.T. Snelling and others

Province	City	Hospital	Postal Code	Phone	No.	Contacts
	Victoria	Royal Jubilee Hospital	V8R 1J8	604/595-9200	2	D.A. Baird; H.R. Hollis; T.A. McQueen; P. Gareau; D. Naysmith
Manitoba	Winnipeg	Health Sciences Center	R3A 1M4	204/787-3776	8*	G.A. Robertson
New Brunswick	Fredericton	Dr. Everett Chalmers Hospital	E3B 5N5	506/452-5400	2	W. Cook
	Moncton	The Moncton Hospital	E1C 6Z8	506/855-1600	3	D. Trueman; Douglas Inglis; G.I. Curry
	Saint John	Saint John General Hospital	E2L 4L2	506/648-2200	6*	G.L. Sparkes
Nova Scotia	Halifax	Victoria General Hospital	B3H 2Y9	902/428-2525	4	Winston Parkhill
	Halifax	I.W. Killam Hospital for Children	B3J 3G9	902/424-6111	3	James Ross and others
Ontario	Hamilton	Hamilton General Hospital	L8L 2X2	416/527-0271	10	Darryl G. Truscott
	Kingston	Hotel Dieu Hospital	K7L 3H6	613/548-8871	2	A. Kenneth Wylie
	London	Victoria Hospital Corporation	N6A 4G5	519/432-5241 ext. 4171	6	Robert B. Colcleugh; R. McFarlane
	Ottawa	Children's Hospital of Eastern Ontario	K1H 8L1	613/737-7600	8*	Paul Benoit
	Ottawa	Ottawa General Hospital	K1H 8L6	613/737-8222	5*	Paul Benoit
	Scarborough	Scarborough General Hospital	M1P 2V5	416/438-2911	4	N. Poy; M. Bederman; L. Carlsen; N. Shammas; W. Carman
	Toronto	Hospital for Sick Children	M5G 1X8	416/597-1500	11	Ronald M. Zuker; Hugh G. Thomson
	Toronto	The Wellesley Hospital	M4Y 1J3	416/966-6600	10	Walter Peters
	Windsor	Metropolitan General Hospital	N8W 1L9	519/254-1661	6	Chosen lau, Director; Stuart Young; Howard Adams
Quebec	Montreal	Montreal Children's Hospital	H3H 1P3	514/937-8511	4*	H. Bruce Williams
	Montreal	Montreal General Hospital	H3G 1A4	514/937-6011	22*	H. Bruce Williams
	Montreal	Hotel Dieu de Montreal	H2W 1T8	514/844-0161	10	Jacques Papillon
Saskatchewan	Regina	Regina General Hospital	S4P 0W5	306/359-4256	4	G.P. Holden
	Saskatoon	University Hospital	S7N 0X0	306/343-3759	5*	Leslie R. Chasmar; D.J. Classen; J.H. Zondervan

APPEN-DIX

1-29/ALPHABET FOR THE DEAF

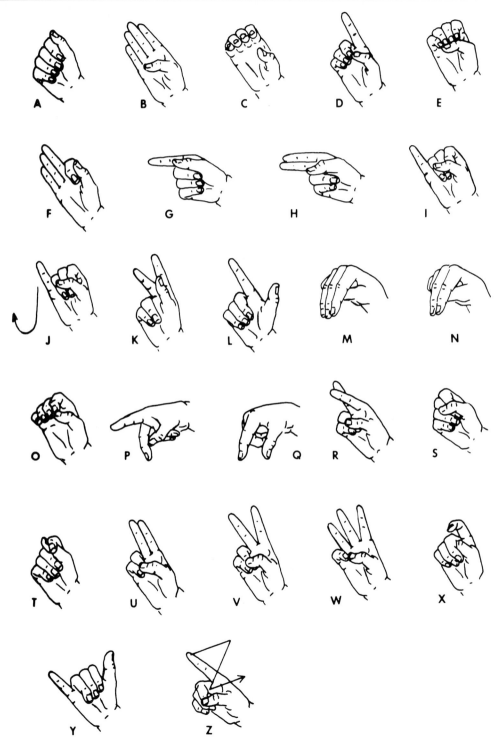

From Clark, PN, and Allen, AS: Occupational therapy for children, St Louis, 1985, The CV Mosby Co.

2 BASIC AND ADVANCED CARDIAC LIFE SUPPORT STANDARDS (AHA)

APPEN-DIX

2-1/ONE RESCUER CPR: ADULT—PERFORMANCE SHEET

BLS Performance Sheet
Adult One-Rescuer CPR

Name _____ Date _____

Step	Objective	Critical Performance	S	U
1. **A**IRWAY	Assessment: Determine unresponsiveness.	Tap or gently shake shoulder.		
		Shout "Are you OK?"		
	Call for help.	Call out "Help!"		
	Position the victim.	Turn on back as unit, if necessary, supporting head and neck (4–10 sec).		
	Open the airway.	Use head-tilt/chin-lift maneuver.		
2. **B**REATHING	Assessment: Determine breathlessness.	Maintain open airway.		
		Ear over mouth, observe chest: look, listen, feel for breathing (3–5 sec).		
	Ventilate twice.	Maintain open airway.		
		Seal mouth and nose properly.		
		Ventilate 2 times at 1–1.5 sec/inspiration.		
		Observe chest rise (adequate ventilation volume.)		
		Allow deflation between breaths.		
3. **C**IRCULATION	Assessment: Determine pulselessness.	Feel for carotid pulse on near side of victim (5–10 sec).		
		Maintain head-tilt with other hand.		
	Activate EMS system.	If someone responded to call for help, send him/her to activate EMS system.		
		Total time, Step 1—Activate EMS system: 15–35 sec.		
	Begin chest compressions.	Rescuer kneels by victim's shoulders.		
		Landmark check prior to hand placement.		
		Proper hand position throughout.		
		Rescuer's shoulders over victim's sternum.		
		Equal compression–relaxation.		
		Compress 1½ to 2 inches.		
		Keep hands on sternum during upstroke.		
		Complete chest relaxation on upstroke.		
		Say any helpful mnemonic.		
		Compression rate: 80–100/min (15 per 9–11 sec).		
4. Compression/Ventilation Cycles	Do 4 cycles of 15 compressions and 2 ventilations.	Proper compression/ventilation ratio: 15 compressions to 2 ventilations per cycle.		
		Observe chest rise: 1–1.5 sec/inspiration; 4 cycles/52–73 sec.		
5. Reassessment*	Determine pulselessness.	Feel for carotid pulse (5 sec).† If there is no pulse, go to Step 6.		
6. Continue CPR	Ventilate twice.	Ventilate 2 times.		
		Observe chest rise: 1–1.5 sec/inspiration.		
	Resume compression/ventilation cycles.	Feel for carotid pulse every few minutes.		

* If 2nd rescuer arrives to replace 1st rescuer: (a) 2nd rescuer identifies self by saying "I know CPR. Can I help?" (b) 2nd rescuer then does pulse check in Step 5 and continues with Step 6. (During practice and testing only one rescuer actually ventilates the manikin. The 2nd rescuer simulates ventilation.) (c) 1st rescuer assesses the adequacy of 2nd rescuer's CPR by observing chest rise during ventilations and by checking the pulse during chest compressions.

† If pulse is present, open airway and check for spontaneous breathing: (a) If breathing is present, maintain open airway and monitor pulse and breathing. (b) If breathing is absent, perform rescue breathing at 12 times/min and monitor pulse.

Instructor _____ Check: Satisfactory _____ Unsatisfactory _____

Reproduced with permission. © INSTRUCTOR'S MANUAL FOR BASIC LIFE SUPPORT, American Heart Association.

2-2/TWO RESCUER CPR: ADULT — PERFORMANCE SHEET

BLS Performance Sheet

Adult Two-Rescuer CPR*

Name _____   Date _____

Step	Objective	Critical Performance	S	U
1. **A**IRWAY	**One rescuer (ventilator):** Assessment: Determine unresponsiveness.	Tap or gently shake shoulder.		
		Shout "Are you OK?"		
	Position the victim.	Turn on back if necessary (4–10 sec).		
	Open the airway.	Use a proper technique to open airway.		
2. **B**REATHING	Assessment: Determine breathlessness.	Look, listen, and feel (3–5 sec).		
	Ventilate twice.	Observe chest rise: 1–1.5 sec/inspiration.		
3. **C**IRCULATION	Assessment: Determine pulselessness.	Feel for carotid pulse (5–10 sec).		
	State assessment results.	Say "No pulse."		
	Other rescuer (compressor): Get into position for compressions.	Hands, shoulders in correct position.		
	Locate landmark notch.	Landmark check.		
4. Compression/Ventilation Cycles	**Compressor:** Begin chest compressions.	Correct ratio compressions/ventilations: 5/1.		
		Compression rate: 80–100/min (5 compressions/3–4 sec).		
		Say any helpful mnemonic.		
		Stop compressing for each ventilation.		
	Ventilator: Ventilate after every 5th compression and check compression effectiveness.	Ventilate 1 time (1–1.5 sec/inspiration).		
		Check pulse occasionally to assess compressions.		
	(Minimum of 10 cycles.)	Time for 10 cycles: 40–53 sec.		
5. Call for Switch	**Compressor:** Call for switch when fatigued.	Give clear signal to change.		
		Compressor completes 5th compression.		
		Ventilator completes ventilation after 5th compression.		
6. Switch	Simultaneously switch:			
	Ventilator: Move to chest.	Move to chest.		
		Become compressor.		
		Get into position for compressions.		
		Locate landmark notch.		
	Compressor: Move to head.	Move to head.		
		Become ventilator.		
		Check carotid pulse (5 sec).		
		Say "No pulse."		
		Ventilate once (1–1.5 sec/inspiration).†		
7. Continue CPR	Resume compression/ventilation cycles.	Resume Step 4.		

* (a) If CPR is in progress with one rescuer (lay person), the entrance of the two rescuers occurs after the completion of one rescuer's cycle of 15 compressions and 2 ventilations. The EMS should be activated first. The two new rescuers start with Step 6. (b) If CPR is in progress with one healthcare provider, the entrance of a second healthcare provider is at the end of a cycle after check for pulse by first rescuer. The new cycle starts with one ventilation by the first rescuer, and the second rescuer becomes the compressor.

† During practice and testing only one rescuer actually ventilates the manikin. The other rescuer simulates ventilation.

Instructor _____   Check: Satisfactory _____ Unsatisfactory _____

2-3/OBSTRUCTED AIRWAY: CONSCIOUS ADULT — PERFORMANCE SHEET

BLS Performance Sheet
Adult FBAO Management: Conscious

Name _____ Date _____

Step	Objective	Critical Performance	S	U
1. Assessment	Determine airway obstruction.	Ask "Are you choking?"		
		Determine if victim can cough or speak.		
2. Heimlich Maneuver	Perform abdominal thrusts.	Stand behind the victim.		
		Wrap arms around victim's waist.		
		Make a fist with one hand and place the thumb side against victim's abdomen in the midline slightly above the navel and well below the tip of the xiphoid.		
		Grasp fist with the other hand.		
		Press into the victim's abdomen with quick upward thrusts.		
		Each thrust should be distinct and delivered with the intent of relieving the airway obstruction.		
		Repeat thrusts until either the foreign body is expelled or the victim becomes unconscious (see below).		

Victim with Obstructed Airway Becomes Unconscious (Optional Testing Sequence)

Step	Objective	Critical Performance	S	U
3. Positioning	Position the victim.	Turn on back as unit.		
		Place face up, arms by side.		
	Call for help.	Call out "Help!" or, if others respond, activate EMS system.		
4. Foreign Body Check	Perform finger sweep.*	Keep victim's face up.		
		Use tongue–jaw lift to open mouth.		
		Sweep deeply into mouth to remove foreign body.		
5. Breathing Attempt	Ventilate.	Open airway with head-tilt/chin-lift.		
		Seal mouth and nose properly.		
		Attempt to ventilate.		
6. Heimlich Maneuver	(Airway is obstructed.) Perform abdominal thrusts.	Straddle victim's thighs.		
		Place heel of one hand against victim's abdomen, in the midline slightly above the navel and well below the tip of the xiphoid.		
		Place second hand directly on top of first hand.		
		Press into the abdomen with quick upward thrusts.		
		Perform 6–10 abdominal thrusts.		
7. Foreign Body Check	(Airway remains obstructed.) Perform finger sweep.*	Keep victim's face up.		
		Use tongue–jaw lift to open mouth.		
		Sweep deeply into mouth to remove foreign body.		
8. Breathing Attempt	Ventilate.	Open airway with head-tilt/chin-lift.		
		Seal mouth and nose properly.		
		Attempt to ventilate.		
9. Sequencing	(Airway remains obstructed.) Repeat sequence.	Repeat Steps 6–8 until successful.†		

* During practice and testing, simulate finger sweeps.

† After airway obstruction is cleared, ventilate twice and proceed with CPR as indicated.

Instructor _____ Check: Satisfactory _____ Unsatisfactory _____

Reproduced with permission. © INSTRUCTOR'S MANUAL FOR BASIC LIFE SUPPORT, American Heart Association.

2-4/OBSTRUCTED AIRWAY: UNCONSCIOUS ADULT—PERFORMANCE SHEET

BLS Performance Sheet
Adult FBAO Management: Unconscious

Name _____ Date _____

Step	Objective	Critical Performance	S	U
1. Assessment	Determine unresponsiveness.	Tap or gently shake shoulder. Shout "Are you OK?"		
	Call for help.	Call out "Help!"		
	Position the victim.	Turn on back as unit, if necessary, supporting head and neck (4–10 sec).		
	Open the airway.	Use head-tilt/chin-lift maneuver.		
	Determine breathlessness.	Maintain open airway.		
		Ear over mouth, observe chest: look, listen, feel for breathing (3–5 sec).		
2. Breathing Attempt	Ventilate.	Maintain open airway.		
		Seal mouth and nose properly.		
		Attempt to ventilate.		
	(Airway is obstructed.) Ventilate.	Reposition victim's head.		
		Seal mouth and nose properly.		
		Reattempt to ventilate.		
	(Airway remains obstructed.) Activate EMS system.	If someone responded to call for help, send him/her to activate EMS system.		
3. Heimlich Maneuver	Perform abdominal thrusts.	Straddle victim's thighs.		
		Place heel of one hand against victim's abdomen in the midline slightly above the navel and well below the tip of the xiphoid.		
		Place second hand directly on top of first hand.		
		Press into the abdomen with quick upward thrusts.		
		Each thrust should be distinct and delivered with the intent of relieving the airway obstruction.		
		Perform 6–10 abdominal thrusts.		
4. Foreign Body Check	Perform finger sweep.*	Keep victim's face up.		
		Use tongue–jaw lift to open mouth.		
		Sweep deeply into mouth to remove foreign body.		
5. Breathing Attempt	Ventilate.	Open airway with head-tilt/chin-lift maneuver.		
		Seal mouth and nose properly.		
		Reattempt to ventilate.		
6. Sequencing	Repeat sequence.	Repeat Steps 3–5 until successful.†		

* During practice and testing simulate finger sweeps.

† After airway obstruction is cleared, ventilate twice and proceed with CPR as indicated.

Instructor _____ Check: Satisfactory _____ Unsatisfactory _____

APPEN
DIX

2-5/ONE RESCUER CPR: CHILD—PERFORMANCE SHEET

BLS Performance Sheet
Child One-Rescuer CPR*

Name _____ Date _____

Step	Objective	Critical Performance	S	U
1. AIRWAY	Assessment: Determine unresponsiveness.	Tap or gently shake shoulder.		
		Shout "Are you OK?"		
	Call for help.	Call out "Help!"		
	Position the victim.	Turn on back as unit, if necessary, supporting head and neck (4–10 sec).		
	Open the airway.	Use head-tilt/chin-lift maneuver.		
2. BREATHING	Assessment: Determine breathlessness.	Maintain open airway.		
		Ear over mouth, observe chest: look, listen, feel for breathing (3–5 sec).		
	Ventilate twice.	Maintain open airway.		
		Seal mouth and nose properly.		
		Ventilate 2 times at 1–1.5 sec/inspiration.		
		Observe chest rise.		
		Allow deflation between breaths.		
3. CIRCULATION	Assessment: Determine pulselessness.	Feel for carotid pulse on near side of victim (5–10 sec).		
		Maintain head-tilt with other hand.		
	Activate EMS system.	If someone responded to call for help, send him/her to activate EMS system.		
		Total time, Step 1—Activate EMS system: 15–35 sec.		
	Begin chest compressions.	Rescuer kneels by victim's shoulders.		
		Landmark check prior to initial hand placement.§		
		Proper hand position throughout.		
		Rescuer's shoulders over victim's sternum.		
		Equal compression–relaxation.		
		Compress 1 to 1½ inches.		
		Keep hand on sternum during upstroke.		
		Complete chest relaxation on upstroke.		
		Say any helpful mnemonic.		
		Compression rate: 80–100/min (5 per 3–4 sec).		
4. Compression/Ventilation Cycles	Do 10 cycles of 5 compressions and 1 ventilation.	Proper compression/ventilation ratio: 5 compressions to 1 slow ventilation per cycle.		
		Observe chest rise: 1–1.5 sec/inspiration (10 cycles/60–87 sec).		
5. Reassessment†	Determine pulselessness.	Feel for carotid pulse (5 sec).‡ If there is no pulse, go to Step 6.		
6. Continue CPR	Ventilate once.	Ventilate one time.		
		Observe chest rise: 1–1.5 sec/inspiration.		
	Resume compression/ventilation cycles	Feel for carotid pulse every few minutes.		

* If child is above age of approximately 8 years, the method for adults should be used.

† 2nd rescuer arrives to replace 1st rescuer: (a) 2nd rescuer identifies self by saying "I know CPR. Can I help?" (b) 2nd rescuer then does pulse check in Step 5 and continues with Step 6. (During practice and testing only one rescuer actually ventilates the manikin. The 2nd rescuer simulates ventilation.) (c) 1st rescuer assesses the adequacy of 2nd rescuer's CPR by observing chest rise during ventilations and by checking the pulse during chest compressions.

‡ If pulse is present, open airway and check for spontaneous breathing. (a) If breathing is present, maintain open airway and monitor breathing and pulse. (b) If breathing is absent, perform rescue breathing at 15 times/min and monitor pulse.

§ Thereafter, check hand position visually.

Instructor _____ Check: Satisfactory _____ Unsatisfactory _____

2-6/TWO RESCUER CPR: CHILD—PERFORMANCE SHEET

BLS Performance Sheet
Child Two-Rescuer CPR*

Name _____   Date _____

Step	Objective	Critical Performance	S	U
1. **A**IRWAY	**One rescuer (ventilator):** Assessment: Determine unresponsiveness.	Tap or gently shake shoulder.		
		Shout ''Are you OK?''		
	Position the victim.	Turn on back if necessary (4–10 sec).		
	Open the airway.	Use a proper technique to open airway.		
2. **B**REATHING	Assessment: Determine breathlessness.	Look, listen, and feel (3–5 sec).		
	Ventilate twice.	Observe chest rise: 1–1.5 sec/inspiration.		
3. **C**IRCULATION	Assessment: Determine pulselessness.	Feel for carotid pulse (5–10 sec).		
	State assessment results.	Say ''No pulse.''		
	Other rescuer (compressor): Get into position for compressions.	Hand, shoulders in correct position.		
	Locate landmark notch.	Landmark check.		
4. Compression/Ventilation Cycles	**Compressor:** Begin chest compressions.	Correct ratio compressions/ventilations: 5/1.		
		Compression rate: 80–100/min (5 compressions/3–4 sec).		
		Say any helpful mnemonic.		
		Stop compressing for each ventilation.		
	Ventilator: Ventilate after every 5th compression and check compression effectiveness.	Ventilate 1 time (1–1.5 sec/inspiration).		
		Check pulse occasionally to assess compressions.		
	(Minimum of 10 cycles.)	Time for 10 cycles: 40–53 sec.		
5. Call for Switch	**Compressor:** Call for switch when fatigued.	Give clear signal to change.		
		Compressor completes 5th compression.		
		Ventilator completes ventilation after 5th compression.		
6. Switch	Simultaneously switch:			
	Ventilator: Move to chest.	Move to chest.		
		Become compressor.		
		Get into position for compressions.		
		Locate landmark notch.		
	Compressor: Move to head.	Move to head.		
		Become ventilator.		
		Check carotid pulse (5 sec).		
		Say ''No pulse.''		
		Ventilate once (1–1.5 sec/inspiration).†		
7. Continue CPR	Resume compression/ventilation cycles.	Resume Step 4.		

* (a) If CPR is in progress with one rescuer (layperson), the entrance of the two rescuers occurs after the completion of one rescuer's cycle of 5 compressions and 1 ventilation. The EMS should be activated first. The two new rescuers start with Step 6. (b) If CPR is in progress with one healthcare provider, the entrance of a second healthcare provider is at the end of a cycle after check for pulse by first rescuer. The new cycle starts with one ventilation by the first rescuer, and the second rescuer becomes the compressor.

† During practice and testing only one rescuer actually ventilates the manikin. The other rescuer simulates ventilation.

Instructor _____   Check: Satisfactory _____ Unsatisfactory _____

APPEN DIX

2-7/OBSTRUCTED AIRWAY: CONSCIOUS CHILD—PERFORMANCE SHEET

BLS Performance Sheet
Child FBAO Management: Conscious*

Name _____ Date _____

Step	Objective	Critical Performance	S	U
1. Assessment	Determine airway obstruction.*	Ask "Are you choking?"		
		Determine if victim can cough or speak.		
2. Heimlich Maneuver	Perform abdominal thrusts (only if victim's cough is ineffective and there is increasing respiratory difficulty).	Stand behind the victim.		
		Wrap arms around victim's waist.		
		Make a fist with one hand and place the thumb side against victim's abdomen, in the midline slightly above the navel and well below the tip of the xiphoid.		
		Grasp fist with the other hand.		
		Press into the victim's abdomen with quick upward thrusts.		
		Each thrust should be distinct and delivered with the intent of relieving the airway obstruction.		
		Repeat thrusts until either the foreign body is expelled or the victim becomes unconscious (see below).		

Victim with Obstructed Airway Becomes Unconscious (Optional Testing Sequence)

Step	Objective	Critical Performance	S	U
3. Positioning	Position the victim.	Turn on back as unit.		
		Place face up, arms by side.		
	Call for help.	Call out "Help!" or if others respond, activate EMS system.		
4. Foreign Body Check	Manual removal of foreign body if one is found. DO NOT perform blind finger sweep.	Keep victim's face up.		
		Use tongue–jaw lift to open mouth.		
		Look into mouth; remove foreign body ONLY IF VISUALIZED.		
5. Breathing Attempt	Ventilate.	Open airway with head-tilt/chin-lift.		
		Seal mouth and nose properly.		
		Attempt to ventilate.		
6. Heimlich Maneuver	(Airway is obstructed.) Perform abdominal thrusts.	Kneel at victim's feet if on the floor, or stand at victim's feet if on a table.		
		Place heel of one hand against victim's abdomen, in the midline slightly above navel and well below tip of xiphoid.		
		Place second hand directly on top of first hand.		
		Press into the abdomen with quick upward thrusts.		
		Perform 6–10 abdominal thrusts.		
7. Foreign Body Check	(Airway remains obstructed.) Manual removal of foreign body if one is found. DO NOT perform blind finger sweep.	Keep victim's face up.		
		Use tongue–jaw lift to open mouth.		
		Look into mouth; remove foreign body ONLY IF VISUALIZED.		
8. Breathing Attempt	Ventilate.	Open airway with head-tilt/chin-lift.		
		Seal mouth and nose properly.		
		Reattempt to ventilate.		
9. Sequencing	(Airway remains obstructed.) Repeat sequence.	Repeat Steps 6–8 until successful.†		

* This procedure should be initiated in a conscious child only if the airway obstruction is due to a witnessed or strongly suspected aspiration and if respiratory difficulty is increasing and the cough is ineffective. If obstruction is caused by airway swelling due to infection such as epiglottitis or croup, these procedures may be harmful; the child should be rushed to the nearest ALS facility, allowing the child to maintain the position of maximum comfort.

† After airway obstruction is cleared, ventilate twice and proceed with CPR as indicated.

Instructor _____ Check: Satisfactory _____ Unsatisfactory _____

2-8/OBSTRUCTED AIRWAY: UNCONSCIOUS CHILD—PERFORMANCE SHEET

BLS Performance Sheet
Child FBAO Management: Unconscious

Name _____ Date _____

Step	Objective	Critical Performance	S	U
1. Assessment	Determine unresponsiveness.	Tap or gently shake shoulder.		
		Shout "Are you OK?"		
	Call for help.	Call out "Help!"		
	Position the victim.	Turn on back as unit, if necessary, supporting head and neck (4–10 sec).		
	Open the airway.	Use head-tilt/chin-lift maneuver.		
	Determine breathlessness.	Maintain open airway.		
		Ear over mouth, observe chest: look, listen, feel for breathing (3–5 sec).		
2. Breathing Attempt	Ventilate.	Maintain open airway.		
		Seal mouth and nose properly.		
		Attempt to ventilate.		
	(Airway is obstructed.) Ventilate.	Reposition victim's head.		
		Seal mouth and nose properly.		
		Reattempt to ventilate.		
	(Airway remains obstructed.) Activate EMS system.	If someone responded to call for help, send him/her to activate EMS system.		
3. Heimlich Maneuver	Perform abdominal thrusts.	Kneel at victim's feet if on the floor, or stand at victim's feet if on a table.		
		Place heel of one hand against victim's abdomen in the midline slightly above navel and well below tip of xiphoid.		
		Place second hand directly on top of first hand.		
		Press into the abdomen with quick upward thrusts.		
		Each thrust should be distinct and delivered with the intent of relieving the airway.		
		Perform 6–10 abdominal thrusts.		
4. Foreign Body Check	(Airway remains obstructed.) Manual removal of foreign body if one is found. DO NOT perform blind finger sweep.	Keep victim's face up.		
		Use tongue-jaw lift to open mouth.		
		Look into mouth; remove foreign body ONLY IF VISUALIZED.		
5. Breathing Attempt	Ventilate.	Open airway with head-tilt/chin-lift maneuver.		
		Seal mouth and nose properly.		
		Reattempt to ventilate.		
6. Sequencing	Repeat sequence.	Repeat Steps 3–5 until successful.*		

* After airway obstruction is cleared, ventilate twice and proceed with CPR as indicated.

Instructor _____ Check: Satisfactory _____ Unsatisfactory _____

APPEN DIX

2-9/ONE RESCUER CPR: INFANT—PERFORMANCE SHEET

BLS Performance Sheet
Infant CPR

Name _____ Date _____

Step	Objective	Critical Performance	S	U
1. AIRWAY	Assessment: Determine unresponsiveness.	Tap or gently shake shoulder.		
	Call for help.	Call out "Help!"		
	Position the infant.	Turn on back as unit, supporting head and neck.		
		Place on firm, hard surface.		
	Open the airway.	Use head-tilt/chin-lift maneuver to sniffing or neutral position.		
		Do not overextend the head.		
2. BREATHING	Assessment: Determine breathlessness.	Maintain open airway.		
		Ear over mouth, observe chest: look, listen, feel for breathing (3–5 sec).		
	Ventilate twice.	Maintain open airway.		
		Make tight seal on infant's mouth and nose with rescuer's mouth.		
		Ventilate 2 times at 1–1.5 sec/inspiration.		
		Observe chest rise.		
		Allow deflation between breaths.		
3. CIRCULATION	Assessment: Determine pulselessness.	Feel for brachial pulse (5–10 sec).		
		Maintain head-tilt with other hand.		
	Activate EMS system.	If someone responded to call for help, send him/her to activate EMS system.		
		Total time, Step 1—Activate EMS system: 15–35 sec.		
	Begin chest compressions.	Imagine line between nipples (intermammary line).		
		Place 2–3 fingers on sternum, 1 finger's width below intermammary line.		
		Equal compression–relaxation.		
		Compress vertically, ½ to 1 inches.		
		Keep fingers on sternum during upstroke.		
		Complete chest relaxation on upstroke.		
		Say any helpful mnemonic.		
		Compression rate: at least 100/min (5 in 3 sec or less).		
4. Compression/Ventilation Cycles	Do 10 cycles of 5 compressions and 1 ventilation.	Proper compression/ventilation ratio: 5 compressions to 1 slow ventilation per cycle.		
		Pause for ventilation.		
		Observe chest rise: 1–1.5 sec/inspiration; 10 cycles/45 sec or less.		
5. Reassessment	Determine pulselessness.	Feel for brachial pulse (5 sec).* If there is no pulse, go to Step 6.		
6. Continue CPR	Ventilate once.	Ventilate 1 time.		
		Observe chest rise: 1–1.5 sec/inspiration.		
	Resume compression/ ventilation cycles.	Feel for brachial pulse every few minutes.		

* If pulse is present, open airway and check for spontaneous breathing. (a) If breathing is present, maintain open airway and monitor breathing and pulse. (b) If breathing is absent, perform rescue breathing at 20 times/min and monitor pulse.

Instructor _____ Check: Satisfactory _____ Unsatisfactory _____

2-10/OBSTRUCTED AIRWAY: CONSCIOUS INFANT—PERFORMANCE SHEET

BLS Performance Sheet

Infant FBAO Management: Conscious*

Name _____ Date _____

Step	Objective	Critical Performance	S	U
1. Assessment	Determine airway obstruction.*	Observe breathing difficulties.*		
2. Back Blows	Deliver 4 back blows.	Supporting head and neck with one hand, straddle infant face down, head lower than trunk, over your forearm supported on your thigh.		
		Deliver 4 back blows, forcefully, between the shoulder blades with the heel of the hand (3–5 sec).		
3. Chest Thrusts	Deliver 4 chest thrusts.	While supporting the head, sandwich infant between your hands and turn on back, with head lower than trunk.		
		Deliver 4 thrusts in the midsternal region in the same manner as external chest compressions, but at a slower rate (3–5 sec).		
4. Sequencing	Repeat sequence.	Repeat Steps 2 and 3 until either the foreign body is expelled or the infant becomes unconscious (see below).		

Infant with Obstructed Airway Becomes Unconscious (Optional Testing Sequence)

5. Call for Help.	Call for help.	Call out "Help!" or, if others respond, activate EMS system.		
6. Foreign Body Check	Manual removal of foreign body if one is found (tongue–jaw lift, NOT blind finger sweep).	Keep victim's face up.		
		Place thumb in infant's mouth, over tongue. Lift tongue and jaw forward with fingers wrapped around lower jaw.		
		Look into mouth; remove foreign body ONLY IF VISUALIZED.		
7. Breathing Attempt	Ventilate.	Open airway with head-tilt/chin-lift.		
		Seal mouth and nose properly.		
		Attempt to ventilate.		
8. Back Blows	(Airway is obstructed.) Deliver 4 back blows.	Supporting head and neck with one hand, straddle infant face down, head lower than trunk, over your forearm supported on your thigh.		
		Deliver 4 back blows, forcefully, between the shoulder blades with the heel of the hand (3–5 sec).		
9. Chest Thrusts	Deliver 4 chest thrusts.	While supporting the head and neck, sandwich infant between your hands and turn on back, with head lower than trunk.		
		Deliver 4 thrusts in the midsternal region in the same manner as external chest compressions, but at a slower rate (3–5 sec).		
10. Foreign Body Check	(Airway remains obstructed.) Manual removal of foreign body if one is found.	Keep victim's face up.		
		Do tongue–jaw lift, but NOT blind finger sweep.		
		Look into mouth, remove foreign body ONLY IF VISUALIZED.		
11. Breathing Attempt	Ventilate.	Open airway with head-tilt/chin-lift.		
		Seal mouth and nose properly.		
		Reattempt to ventilate.		
12. Sequencing	(Airway remains obstructed.) Repeat sequence.	Repeat Steps 8–11 until successful.†		

* This procedure should be initiated in a conscious infant only if the airway obstruction is due to a witnessed or strongly suspected aspiration and if respiratory difficulty is increasing and the cough is ineffective. If the obstruction is caused by airway swelling due to infections, such as epiglottitis or croup, these procedures may be harmful; the infant should be rushed to the nearest ALS facility, allowing the infant to maintain the position of maximum comfort.

† After airway obstruction is cleared, ventilate twice and proceed with CPR as indicated.

Instructor _____ Check: Satisfactory _____ Unsatisfactory _____

APPEN DIX

Reproduced with permission. © INSTRUCTOR'S MANUAL FOR BASIC LIFE SUPPORT, American Heart Association.

2-11/OBSTRUCTED AIRWAY: UNCONSCIOUS INFANT—PERFORMANCE SHEET

BLS Performance Sheet

Infant FBAO Management: Unconscious

Name _____ Date _____

Step	Objective	Critical Performance	S	U
1. Assessment	Determine unresponsiveness.	Tap or gently shake shoulder.		
	Call for help.	Call out "Help!"		
	Position the infant.	Turn on back as unit, if necessary, supporting head and neck.		
		Place on firm, hard surface.		
	Open the airway.	Use head-tilt/chin-lift maneuver to sniffing or neutral position.		
		Do not overextend the head.		
	Determine breathlessness.	Maintain open airway.		
		Ear over mouth, observe chest: look, listen, feel for breathing (3–5 sec).		
2. Breathing Attempt	Ventilate.	Maintain open airway.		
		Make tight seal on mouth and nose of infant with rescuer's mouth.		
		Attempt to ventilate.		
	(Airway is obstructed.) Ventilate.	Reposition infant's head.		
		Seal mouth and nose properly.		
		Reattempt to ventilate.		
	(Airway remains obstructed.) Activate EMS system	If someone responded to call for help, send him/her to activate EMS system.		
3. Back Blows	Deliver 4 back blows.	Supporting head and neck with one hand, straddle infant face down, head lower than trunk, over your forearm supported on your thigh.		
		Deliver 4 back blows, forcefully, between the shoulder blades with the heel of the hand (3–5 sec).		
4. Chest Thrusts	Deliver 4 chest thrusts.	While supporting the head and neck, sandwich infant between your hands and turn on back, with head lower than trunk.		
		Deliver 4 thrusts in the midsternal region in the same manner as external chest compressions, but at a slower rate (3–5 sec).		
5. Foreign Body Check	(Airway remains obstructed.) Manual removal of foreign body if one is found (tongue–jaw lift, NOT blind finger sweep).	Keep victim's face up.		
		Place thumb in infant's mouth, over tongue. Lift tongue and jaw forward with fingers wrapped around lower jaw.		
		Look into mouth; remove foreign body ONLY IF VISUALIZED.		
6. Breathing Attempt	Ventilate.	Open airway with head-tilt/chin-lift.		
		Seal mouth and nose properly.		
		Reattempt to ventilate.		
7. Sequencing	Repeat sequence.	Repeat Steps 3–6 until successful.*		

* After airway obstruction is cleared, ventilate twice and proceed with CPR as indicated.

Instructor _____ Check: Satisfactory _____ Unsatisfactory _____

2-12/ACLS ALGORITHM—VENTRICULAR FIBRILLATION[a] AND PULSELESS VENTRICULAR TACHYCARDIA

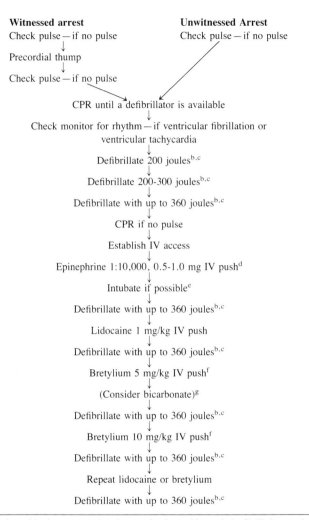

Witnessed arrest
Check pulse — if no pulse
↓
Precordial thump
↓
Check pulse — if no pulse

Unwitnessed Arrest
Check pulse — if no pulse

CPR until a defibrillator is available
↓
Check monitor for rhythm — if ventricular fibrillation or ventricular tachycardia
↓
Defibrillate 200 joules[b,c]
↓
Defibrillate 200-300 joules[b,c]
↓
Defibrillate with up to 360 joules[b,c]
↓
CPR if no pulse
↓
Establish IV access
↓
Epinephrine 1:10,000, 0.5-1.0 mg IV push[d]
↓
Intubate if possible[e]
↓
Defibrillate with up to 360 joules[b,c]
↓
Lidocaine 1 mg/kg IV push
↓
Defibrillate with up to 360 joules[b,c]
↓
Bretylium 5 mg/kg IV push[f]
↓
(Consider bicarbonate)[g]
↓
Defibrillate with up to 360 joules[b,c]
↓
Bretylium 10 mg/kg IV push[f]
↓
Defibrillate with up to 360 joules[b,c]
↓
Repeat lidocaine or bretylium
↓
Defibrillate with up to 360 joules[b,c]

[a]This sequence was developed to assist in teaching how to treat a broad range of patients with ventricular fibrillation or pulseless ventricular tachycardia. Some patients may require care not specified herein. This algorithm should not be construed as prohibiting such flexibility. The flow of the algorithym presumes that ventricular fibrillation is continuing.

[b]Check pulse and rhythm after each shock.

[c]If ventricular fibrillation recurs after transiently converting (rather than persists without ever converting), only 200 joules is necessary for the subsequent shock.

[d]Epinephrine should be repeated every 5 minutes.

[e]Intubation is preferable. If it can be accomplished simultaneously with other techniques, then the earlier the better. However, defibrillation and epinephrine are more important initially if the patient can be ventilated without intubation.

[f]Some may prefer repeated doses of lidocaine, which may be given in 0.5 mg/kg boluses every 8 minutes to a total dose of 3 mg/kg.

[g]The value of sodium bicarbonate is highly questionable during cardiac arrest, and it may be harmful. Consideration of its use in a dose of 1 mEq/kg is appropriate at this point. If it is used, one half of the original dose may be repeated every 10 minutes.

Reproduced with permission. © TEXTBOOK OF ADVANCED CARDIAC LIFE SUPPORT, American Heart Association.

APPEN DIX

2-13/ACLS ALGORITHM — SUSTAINED VENTRICULAR TACHYCARDIA[a]

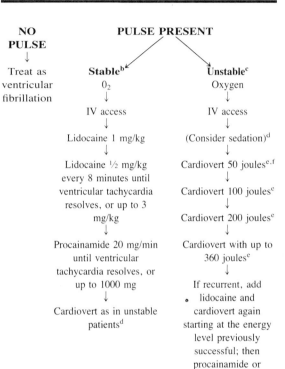

NO PULSE	**PULSE PRESENT**	
↓	**Stable[b]**	**Unstable[c]**
Treat as ventricular fibrillation	0_2	Oxygen
	↓	↓
	IV access	IV access
	↓	↓
	Lidocaine 1 mg/kg	(Consider sedation)[d]
	↓	↓
	Lidocaine ½ mg/kg every 8 minutes until ventricular tachycardia resolves, or up to 3 mg/kg	Cardiovert 50 joules[e,f]
	↓	↓
		Cardiovert 100 joules[e]
		↓
	Procainamide 20 mg/min until ventricular tachycardia resolves, or up to 1000 mg	Cardiovert 200 joules[e]
	↓	↓
	Cardiovert as in unstable patients[d]	Cardiovert with up to 360 joules[e]
		↓
		If recurrent, add lidocaine and cardiovert again starting at the energy level previously successful; then procainamide or bretylium[g,h]

[a]This sequence was developed to assist in teaching how to treat a broad range of patients with sustained ventricular tachycardia. Some patients may require care not specified herein. This algorithm should not be construed as prohibiting such flexibility. The flow of the algorithm presumes that ventricular tachycardia is continuing.

[b]If the patient becomes unstable (see footnote "c" for definition) at any time, move to the unstable arm of the algorithm.

[c]Unstable is defined as symptoms (e.g., chest pain, dyspnea), hypotension (systlolic <90 mm Hg), congestive heart failure, ischemia, or infarction.

[d]Sedation should be considered for all patients, including those defined as unstable, except those who are hemodyamically unstable (e.g., hypotensive, in pulmonary edema, or unconscious).

[e]If the patient is hypotensive, in pulmonary edema, or unconscious, unsynchronized cardioversion should be done to avoid the delay associated with synchronization.

[f]In the absence of hypotension, pulmonary edema, or unconsciousness, a precordial thump may be employed prior to cardioversion.

[g]Once ventricular tachycardia has resolved, begin an IV infusion of the antiarrhythmic agent that has aided the resolution of the ventricular tachycardia.

[h]If the patient is hypotensive, in pulmonary edema, or unconscious, use lidocaine if cardioversion alone is unsuccessful, followed by bretylium. In all other patients, the recommended order of therapy is lidocaine, procainamide, and then bretylium.

2-14/ACLS ALGORITHM — ASYSTOLE[a]

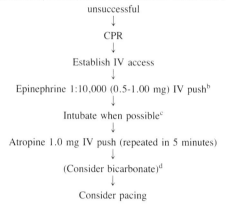

If the rhythm is unclear and possibly low amplitude ventricular fibrillation, defibrillate as for ventricular fibrillation. If unsuccessful

↓

CPR

↓

Establish IV access

↓

Epinephrine 1:10,000 (0.5-1.00 mg) IV push[b]

↓

Intubate when possible[c]

↓

Atropine 1.0 mg IV push (repeated in 5 minutes)

↓

(Consider bicarbonate)[d]

↓

Consider pacing

[a]This sequence was developed to assist in teaching how to treat a broad range of patients with asystole. Some patients may require care not specified herein. This algorithm should not be construed to prohibit such flexibility. The flow of the algorithm presumes asystole is continuing.

[b]Epinephrine should be repeated every 5 minutes.

[c]Intubation is preferable, if it can be accomplished simultaneously with other techniques, then the earlier the better. However, CPR and the use of epinephrine are more important initially if the patient can be ventilated without intubation.

[d]The value of sodium bicarbonate is highly questionable during cardiac arrest, and it may be harmful. Consideration of its use in a dose of 1 mEq/kg is appropriate at this point. If it is used, one half of the original dose may be repeated every 10 minutes.

2-15/ACLS ALGORITHM — ELECTROMECHANICAL DISSOCIATION (EMD)[a]

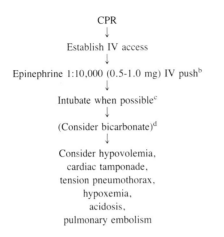

CPR
↓
Establish IV access
↓
Epinephrine 1:10,000 (0.5-1.0 mg) IV push[b]
↓
Intubate when possible[c]
↓
(Consider bicarbonate)[d]
↓
Consider hypovolemia,
cardiac tamponade,
tension pneumothorax,
hypoxemia,
acidosis,
pulmonary embolism

---

[a]This sequence was developed to assist in teaching how to treat a broad range of patients with electromechanical dissociation. Some patients may require care not specified herein. This algorithm should not be construed to prohibit such flexibility. The flow of the algorithm presumes that electromechanical dissociation is continuing.

[b]Epinephrine should be repeated every 5 minutes.

[c]Intubation is preferable. If it can be accomplished simultaneously with other techniques, then the earlier the better. However, epinephrine is more important initially if the patient can be ventilated without intubation.

[d]The value of sodium bicarbonate is highly questionable during cardiac arrest, and it may be harmful. Consideration of its use in a dose of 1 mEq/kg is appropriate at this point. If it is used, one half of the original dose may be repeated every 10 minutes.

Reproduced with permission. © TEXTBOOK OF ADVANCED CARDIAC LIFE SUPPORT, American Heart Association.

2-16/ACLS ALGORITHM — PAROXYSMAL SUPRAVENTRICULAR TACHYCARDIA (PSVT)[a]

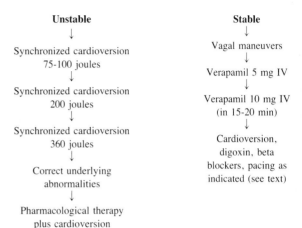

Unstable
↓
Synchronized cardioversion
75-100 joules
↓
Synchronized cardioversion
200 joules
↓
Synchronized cardioversion
360 joules
↓
Correct underlying
abnormalities
↓
Pharmacological therapy
plus cardioversion

Stable
↓
Vagal maneuvers
↓
Verapamil 5 mg IV
↓
Verapamil 10 mg IV
(in 15-20 min)
↓
Cardioversion,
digoxin, beta
blockers, pacing as
indicated (see text)

If conversion occurs but paroxysmal supraventricular tachycardia recurs, repeated electrical cardioversion is *not* indicated. Sedation should be used as time permits.

---

[a]This sequence was developed to assist in teaching how to treat a broad range of patients with sustained paroxysmal supraventricular tachycardia. Some patients may require care not specified herein. This algorithm should be not construed as prohibiting such flexibility. The flow of the algorithm presumes paroxysmal supraventricular tachycardia is continuing.

Reproduced with permission. © TEXTBOOK OF ADVANCED CARDIAC LIFE SUPPORT, American Heart Association.

APPEN DIX

2-17/ACLS ALGORITHM— BRADYCARDIA

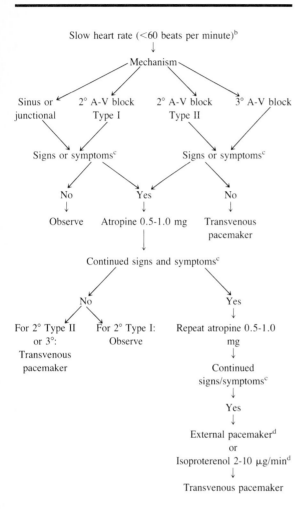

Slow heart rate (<60 beats per minute)[b]
↓
Mechanism

Sinus or junctional   2° A-V block Type I   2° A-V block Type II   3° A-V block

Signs or symptoms[c]   Signs or symptoms[c]

No → Observe
Yes → Atropine 0.5-1.0 mg
No → Transvenous pacemaker

Continued signs and symptoms[c]

No → For 2° Type II or 3°: Transvenous pacemaker
No → For 2° Type I: Observe
Yes → Repeat atropine 0.5-1.0 mg
↓
Continued signs/symptoms[c]
↓
Yes
↓
External pacemaker[d]
or
Isoproterenol 2-10 μg/min[d]
↓
Transvenous pacemaker

---

[a]This sequence was developed to assist in teaching how to treat a broad range of patients with bradycardia. Some patients may require care not specified herein. This algorithm should not be construed to prohibit such flexibility.
[b]A chest thump or a cough may stimulate cardiac electrical activity and result in improved cardiac output and may be used at this point.
[c]Hypotension (BP <90 mm Hg), premature ventricular contractions, altered mental status or symptoms (e.g., chest pain, dyspnea), ischemia, or infarction.
[d]Temporizing therapy.

Reproduced with permission. © TEXTBOOK OF ADVANCED CARDIAC LIFE SUPPORT, American Heart Association.

2-18/ACLS ALGORITHM—ACUTE SUPPRESSIVE THERAPY[a] FOR VENTRICULAR ECTOPY

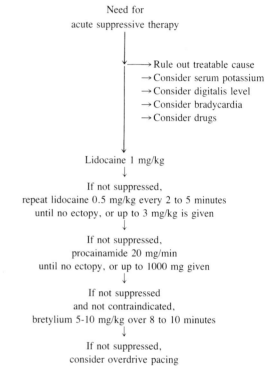

Need for
acute suppressive therapy

→ Rule out treatable cause
→ Consider serum potassium
→ Consider digitalis level
→ Consider bradycardia
→ Consider drugs

Lidocaine 1 mg/kg
↓
If not suppressed,
repeat lidocaine 0.5 mg/kg every 2 to 5 minutes
until no ectopy, or up to 3 mg/kg is given
↓
If not suppressed,
procainamide 20 mg/min
until no ectopy, or up to 1000 mg given
↓
If not suppressed
and not contraindicated,
bretylium 5-10 mg/kg over 8 to 10 minutes
↓
If not suppressed,
consider overdrive pacing

Once ectopy is resolved, maintain as follows:
     after lidocaine 1 mg/kg . . . lidocaine drip 2 mg/min
     after lidocaine 1-2 mg/kg . . . lidocaine drip 3 mg/min
     after lidocaine 2-3 mg/kg . . . lidocaine drip 4 mg/min
     after procainamide . . . procainamide drip 1-4 mg/min (check blood level)
     after bretylium . . . bretylium drip 2 mg/min

---

[a]This sequence was developed to assist in teaching how to treat a broad range of patients with ventricular ectopy. Some patients may require therapy not specified herein. This algorithm should not be construed as prohibiting such flexibility.

Reproduced with permission. © TEXTBOOK OF ADVANCED CARDIAC LIFE SUPPORT, American Heart Association.

3 *PEDIATRICS*

APPE
DIX

3-1/INFANT SKELETON

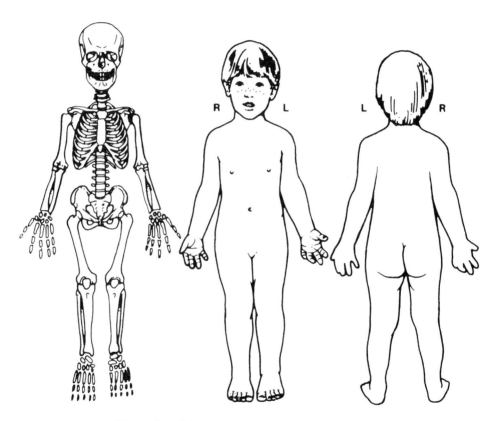

Courtesy Scottish Rites Children's Hospital, Atlanta Georgia.

3-2/MAJOR PEDIATRIC TRIAGE CATEGORIES

Emergent				Urgent*
Abnormal vital signs				Abuse, child
	BP (sys)	*Pulse*	*Resp*	Abuse, sexual
0-2 yr	<60	<80	<10 or >40	Acute symptoms in child <3 mo
2-5 yr	<70	<60	<10 or >30	Behavioral alteration
>5 yr	<90	<50	<5 or >25	Bite, poisonous snake
Respirations				Bleeding, moderate
Irregular				Dehydration
Apneic				Drowning (near)
Labored				Eye: alkali, acid, or chemical burn
Pulse				Fever ≥40° C
Irregular				GI hemorrhage
Arrhythmic				Headache: acute and severe
Coma				Hypertension
Cyanosis				Hyperthermia
Status epilepticus				Hypothermia
Multiple or major trauma				Neck pain or stiffness
Head				Pain: acute and severe
Loss of consciousness				Poisoning
Altered mental status				**Rash** (isolate patient)
Changing neurologic or asymmetric neurologic findings				**SIDS** (near)
CSF leak				
Depressed fracture				
Neck or spinal injury				
Chest				
Abdomen				
Orthopedic				
Two or more long bone fractures				
Pelvic fracture				
Potential neurovascular compromise				
Amputation				
Major burn				
Bleeding: acute and significant				

From Barkin, RM, and Rosen, P: Emergency pediatrics, ed 2, St Louis, 1986, The CV Mosby Co.

If none of these emergent or urgent conditions are present, the patient should be appropriately screened and treated according to normal facility flow patterns unless there is a complicating condition.

*May be emergent, depending on patient's condition.

3-3/DIAGNOSIS OF UNKNOWN POISONS

Vital sign changes

DYSRHYTHMIAS

Amphetamines
Anticholinergics
Beta-blockers (propranolol, etc.)
Carbon monoxide
Chloral hydrate
Digitalis
Phenothiazines
Sympathomimetics (cocaine, etc.)
Tricyclic antidepressants, theophylline

CYANOSIS (secondary to methemoglobinemia; does not respond to oxygen)

Anesthetics, local
Nitrates
Nitrites
Phenacetin
Sulfonamides

Increased	Decreased
BLOOD PRESSURE	
Amphetamines	Cyanide
Anticholinergics	Narcotics
Sympathomimetics	Sedative/hypnotics
HEART RATE	
Alcohol	Barbiturates
Amphetamines	Digitalis
Anticholinergics	Narcotics
Sympathomimetics (caffeine, cocaine, etc.)	Sedatives/hypnotics
Theophylline	
RESPIRATORY RATE	
Amphetamines	Alcohols, (ethanol, isopropyl, methanol)
Anticholinergics	Barbiturates
Hydrocarbons	Narcotics
Secondary to metabolic acidosis (''MUDPIES'')	Sedatives/hypnotics
Secondary to noncardiogenic pulnonary edema	
Carbon monoxide	
Hydrocarbons	
Narcotics	
Organophosphates	
Salicylates	
Sedatives/hypnotics	
TEMPERATURE	
Amphetamines	Alcohol (ethanol)
Anticholinergics	Anesthetic, general
Atropine	Barbiturates
Beta-blockers	Carbon monoxide
Phenothiazines	Narcotics
Salicylates	Phenothiazines
Sympathomimetics (cocaine. etc.)	Sedatives/hypnotics
Tricyclic antidepressants	Tricyclic antidepressants

Neurologic alterations

	Findings associated with coma		
COMA	**Seizures, myoclonus, hyperreflexia**	**Hyporeflexia, hypotension**	**Pulmonary edema, hypotension**
Amphetamines	+		
Anticholinergics	+		
Barbiturates		+	+
Benzodiazepines		+	
Carbamazepine	+		
Carbon monoxide	+		+
Chloral hydrate		+	
Cocaine	+		
Ethanol, isopropyl		+	+
Haloperidol	+		
Narcotics		+	+
Phencyclidine (PCP)	+		
Phenothiazines	+		
Phenytoin	+		
Salicylates			+
Sedative/hypnotics			+
Tricyclic antidepressants	+		

SEIZURES ("CAP")

Camphor	Aminophylline	Pesticides (organophosphates)
Carbon monoxide	Amphetamines and sympathomimetics	Phencyclidine (PCP)
Cocaine	Anticholinergics	Phenol
Cyanide	Aspirin	Propoxyphene

Also lead, isoniazid, drug withdrawal, carbamazepine (Tegretol), lithium, strychnine, tricyclic antidepressants, sympathomimetics and many others

BEHAVIOR DISORDERS

Toxic psychosis: hallucinogens (LSD, phencyclidine), sympathomimetics (cocaine, amphetamines), anticholinergics, heavy metals
Paranoid, violent reactions: phencyclidine
Depression, paranoid hallucinations, emotional lability: sympathomimetics (cocaine, amphetamines)
Hallucinations, delirium, anxiety: anticholinergics, hallucinogens

MOVEMENT DISORDERS

Choreoathetosis, orofacial dyskinesis, nystagmus, ataxia: phenytoin
Extrapyramidal: anticholinergics, phenothiazines, haloperidol
Choreoathetoid movements: tricyclic antidepressants
Ataxia, choreiform movements: heavy metals
Ataxia, tremors: lithium
Nystagmus: phenytoin, carbamazepine, primidone, phencyclidine, carbon monoxide

PUPILS

Pinpoint (miosis)	**Dilated** (mydriasis)	
Barbiturates (late)	Alcohol	Meperidine
Cholinergics	Anticholinergics	Phenytoin
Narcotics (except meperidine)	Antihistamines	Sympathomimetics (i.e., amphetamines, cocaine, ephedrine, LSD, PCP, etc.)
Organophosphates	Barbiturates	

From Barkin, RM, and Rosen, P: Emergency pediatrics, ed 2, St Louis, 1986, The CV Mosby Co.

APPEN-
DIX

3-4/SPINAL CORD INJURIES

Level of lesion	Motor function lost	Sensation lost at and below	Reflex
C2	Breathing	Occiput	
C3	Spontaneous breathing and trapezius	Thyroid cartilage	
C4	function	Suprasternal notch	
C5	Shoulder flexion and abduction	Infraclavicular +/− lateral arm sparing	Biceps brachialis*
C6		Infraclavicular +/− lateral arm, forearm sparing	Brachioradialis*
C7	Elbow and wrist extension	Infraclavicular with sparing as above to middle finger	Triceps*
C8	Small muscles of hand (lumbricales and interossei)	Infraclavicular with sparing as above to little finger	
T1		Infraclavicular with upper extremity sparing to axilla	
T4		Nipple line	
T7	Intercostal and abdominal musculature	Inferior costal margin	Upper abdominal†
T10		Umbilicus	
T12			Lower abdominal†
L1	Hip flexion	Groin	
L2		Anteromedial thigh	
L3	Hip adduction and knee extension	Medial knee	Knee/patellar*
L4	Hip abduction and knee extension	Anterior knee and medial calf	
L5	Foot and great toe dorsiflexion	Lateral dorsum foot and lateral sole foot	
S1	Foot and great toe plantar flexion	Lateral dorsum foot and lateral sole foot	Ankle/Achilles*
S2			
S3	Perianal and rectal sphincter tone	Perianal and rectal sensation	
S4			

From Barkin, RM, and Rosen, P: Emergency pediatrics, ed 2, St Louis, 1986, The CV Mosby Co.

*Deep tendon.

†Superficial.

3-5/RULE OF NINES — INFANT

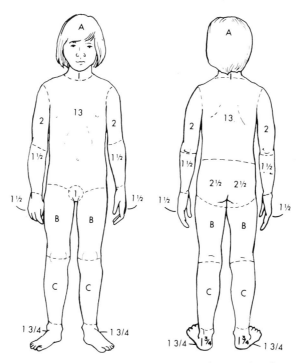

FIG. 46-1. Calculation of burn surface area. (After Lund and Browder.)

				Age		
Area percentage	<1 yr	1 yr	5 yr	10 yr	15 yr	Adult
A, ½ of head	9½	8½	6½	5½	4½	3½
B, ½ of one thigh	2¾	3¼	4	4¼	4½	4¾
C, ½ of one leg	2½	2½	2¾	3	3¼	3½

From Barkin, RM, and Rosen, P: Emergency pediatrics, ed 2, St Louis, 1986, The CV Mosby Co.

4 *HAZARDOUS MATERIALS*

4-1/704 MARKING SYSTEM

THE NFPA 704 MARKING SYSTEM

 THE NFPA 704 MARKING SYSTEM DISTINCTIVELY INDICATES THE PROPERTIES AND POTENTIAL DANGERS OF HAZARDOUS MATERIALS. THE FOLLOWING IS AN EXPLANATION OF THE MEANINGS OF THE QUADRANT NUMERICAL CODES:

HEALTH

IN GENERAL, HEALTH HAZARD IN FIREFIGHTING IS THAT OF A SINGLE EXPOSURE WHICH MAY VARY FROM A FEW SECONDS UP TO AN HOUR. THE PHYSICAL EXERTION DEMANDED IN FIREFIGHTING OR OTHER EMERGENCY CONDITIONS MAY BE EXPECTED TO INTENSIFY THE EFFECTS OF ANY EXPOSURE. ONLY HAZARDS ARISING OUT OF AN INHERENT PROPERTY OF THE MATERIAL ARE CONSIDERED. THE FOLLOWING EXPLANATION IS BASED UPON PROTECTIVE EQUIPMENT NORMALLY USED BY FIREFIGHTERS:

4 MATERIALS TOO DANGEROUS TO HEALTH TO EXPOSE FIREFIGHTERS. A FEW WHIFFS OF THE VAPOR COULD CAUSE DEATH OR THE VAPOR OF LIQUID COULD BE FATAL ON PENETRATING THE FIREFIGHTER'S NORMAL FULL PROTECTIVE CLOTHING. THE NORMAL, FULL-PROTECTIVE CLOTHING AND BREATHING APPARATUS AVAILABLE TO THE AVERAGE FIRE DEPARTMENT WILL NOT PROVIDE ADEQUATE PROTECTION AGAINST INHALATION OR SKIN CONTACT WITH THESE MATERIALS.

3 MATERIALS EXTREMELY HAZARDOUS TO HEALTH, BUT AREAS MAY BE ENTERED WITH EXTREME CARE. FULL-PROTECTIVE CLOTHING INCLUDING SELF-CONTAINED BREATHING APPARATUS, COAT, PANTS, GLOVES, BOOTS AND BANDS AROUND LEGS, ARMS AND WAIST SHOULD BE PROVIDED. NO SKIN SURFACE SHOULD BE EXPOSED.

2 MATERIALS HAZARDOUS TO HEALTH, BUT AREAS MAY BE ENTERED FREELY WITH FULL-FACE MASK AND SELF-CONTAINED BREATHING APPARATUS WHICH PROVIDES EYE PROTECTION.

1 MATERIALS ONLY SLIGHTLY HAZARDOUS TO HEALTH. IT MAY BE DESIRABLE TO WEAR SELF-CONTAINED BREATHING APPARATUS.

0 MATERIALS WHICH WOULD OFFER NO HAZARD BEYOND THAT OF ORDINARY COMBUSTIBLE MATERIAL UPON EXPOSURE UNDER FIRE CONDITIONS.

FLAMMABILITY

SUSCEPTIBILITY TO BURNING IS THE BASIS FOR ASSIGNING DEGREES WITHIN THIS CATEGORY. THE METHOD OF ATTACKING THE FIRE IS INFLUENCED BY THIS SUSCEPTIBILITY FACTOR.

4 VERY FLAMMABLE GASES OR VERY VOLATILE FLAMMABLE LIQUIDS. SHUT OFF FLOW AND KEEP COOLING WATER STREAMS ON EXPOSED TANKS OR CONTAINERS.

3 MATERIALS WHICH CAN BE IGNITED UNDER ALMOST ALL NORMAL TEMPERATURE CONDITIONS. WATER MAY BE INEFFECTIVE BECAUSE OF THE LOW FLASH POINT.

2 MATERIALS WHICH MUST BE MODERATELY HEATED BEFORE IGNITION WILL OCCUR. WATER SPRAY MUST BE USED TO EXTINGUISH THE FIRE BECAUSE THE MATERIAL CAN BE COOLED BELOW ITS FLASH POINT.

1 MATERIALS THAT MUST BE PREHEATED BEFORE IGNITION CAN OCCUR. WATER MAY CAUSE FROTHING IF IT GETS BELOW THE SURFACE OF THE LIQUID AND TURNS TO STEAM. HOWEVER, WATER FOG GENTLY APPLIED TO THE SURFACE WILL CAUSE A FROTHING WHICH WILL EXTINGUISH THE FIRE.

0 MATERIALS THAT WILL NOT BURN.

REACTIVITY (STABILITY)

THE ASSIGNMENT OF DEGREES IN THE REACTIVITY CATEGORY IS BASED UPON THE SUSCEPTIBILITY OF MATERIALS TO RELEASE ENERGY EITHER BY THEMSELVES OR IN COMBINATION WITH WATER. FIRE EXPOSURE WAS ONE OF THE FACTORS CONSIDERED ALONG WITH CONDITIONS OF SHOCK AND PRESSURE.

4 MATERIALS WHICH (IN THEMSELVES) ARE READILY CAPABLE OF DETONATION OR OF EXPLOSIVE DECOMPOSITION OR EXPLOSIVE REACTION AT NORMAL TEMPERATURES AND PRESSURES. INCLUDES MATERIALS WHICH ARE SENSITIVE TO MECHANICAL OR LOCALIZED THERMAL SHOCK. IF A CHEMCIAL WITH THIS HAZARD RATING IS IN AN ADVANCED OR MASSIVE FIRE, THE AREA SHOULD BE EVACUATED.

3 MATERIALS WHICH (IN THEMSELVES) ARE CAPABLE OF DETONATION OR OF EXPLOSIVE DECOMPOSITION OR EXPLOSIVE REACTION BUT WHICH REQUIRE A STRONG INITIATING SOURCE OR WHICH MUST BE HEATED UNDER CONFINEMENT BEFORE INITIATION. INCLUDES MATERIALS WHICH ARE SENSITIVE TO THERMAL OR MECHANICAL SHOCK AT ELEVATED TEMPERATURES AND PRESSURES OF WHICH REACT EXPLOSIVELY WITH WATER WITHOUT REQUIRING HEAT OR CONFINEMENT. FIREFIGHTING SHOULD BE DONE FORM AN EXPLOSIVE-RESISTANT LOCATION.

2 MATERIALS WHICH (IN THEMSELVES) ARE NORMALLY UNSTABLE AND RAPIDLY UNDERGO VIOLENT CHEMICAL CHANGE BUT DO NOT DETONATE. INCLUDES MATERIALS WHICH CAN UNDERGO CHEMICAL CHANGE WITH RAPID RELEASE OF ENERGY AT NORMAL TEMPERATURES AND PRESSURES OR WHICH CAN UNDERGO VIOLENT CHEMICAL CHANGE AT ELEVATED TEMPERATURES AND PRESSURES. ALSO INCLUDES THOSE MATERIALS WHICH MAY REACT VIOLENTLY WITH WATER OR WHICH MAY FORM POTENTIALLY EXPLOSIVE MIXTURES WITH WATER. IN ADVANCE OR MASSIVE FIRES, FIREFIGHTING SHOULD BE DONE FROM A SAFE DISTANCE OR FROM A PROTECTED LOCATION.

1 MATERIALS WHICH (IN THEMSELVES) ARE NORMALLY STABLE BUT WHICH MAY BECOME UNSTABLE AT ELEVATED TEMPERATURES AND PRESSURES OR WHICH MAY REACT WITH WATER WITH SOME RELEASE OF ENERGY BUT NOT VIOLENTLY. CAUTION MUST BE USED IN APPROACHING THE FIRE AND APPLYING WATER.

0 MATERIALS WHICH (IN THEMSELVES) ARE NORMALLY STABLE EVEN UNDER FIRE EXPOSURE CONDITIONS AND WHICH ARE NOT REACTIVE WITH WATER. NORMAL FIREFIGHTING PROCEDURES MAY BE USED.

SPECIAL INFORMATION (WHITE)

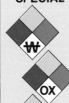

MATERIALS WHICH DEMONSTRATE UNUSUAL REACTIVITY WITH WATER SHALL BE IDENTIFIED WITH THE LETTER W WITH A HORIZONTAL LINE THROUGH THE CENTER (W̶).

MATERIALS WHICH POSSESS OXIDIZING PROPERTIES SHALL BE IDENTIFIED BY THE LETTERS OX.

MATERIALS POSSESSING RADIOACTIVITY HAZARDS SHALL BE IDENTIFIED BY THE STANDARD RADIOCTIVITY SYMBOL.

4-2/GENERAL HAZARD RECOGNITION

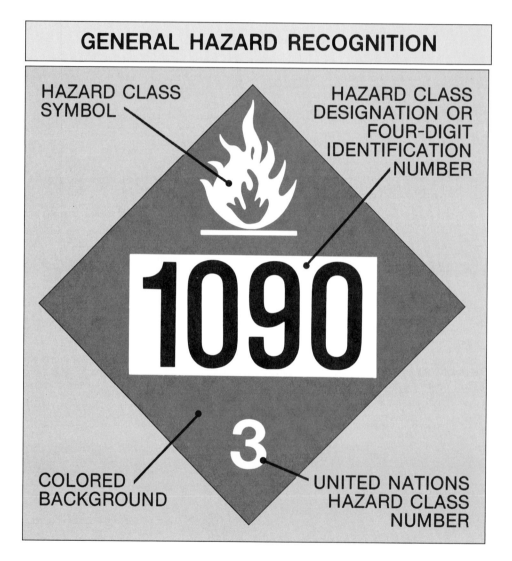

4-3/LABELS VS. PLACARDS

COMPARISON BETWEEN LABELS AND PLACARDS

4-4/PLACARD RECOGNITION INFORMATION

PLACARD RECOGNITION INFORMATION

HAZARD CLASS	SYMBOL	COLORED BACKGROUND	UNITED NATIONS HAZARD CLASS NUMBER
EXPLOSIVES	BURSTING BALL	ORANGE	1
GASES (COMPRESSED, LIQUEFIED OR DISSOLVED UNDER PRESSURE)	FLAMMABLE		2
	FLAME	RED	
	NON-FLAMMABLE		
	CYLINDER	GREEN	
FLAMMABLE LIQUIDS	FLAMMABLE		3
	FLAME	RED	
	COMBUSTIBLE		
	FLAME	RED	
FLAMMABLE SOLIDS OR SUBSTANCES	FLAMMABLE SOLID		4
	FLAME	RED AND WHITE VERTICAL STRIPES	
	WATER REACTIVE MATERIALS		
	SLASHED W (W)	RED AND WHITE VERTICAL STRIPES WITH BLUE TOP QUADRANT	
OXIDIZING SUBSTANCES	CIRCLE WITH FLAME	YELLOW	5 DIVISION 5-1 OXIDIZING SUBSTANCES OR AGENTS DIVISION 5-2 ORGANIC PEROXIDES
POISONOUS AND INFECTIOUS SUBSTANCES	SKULL AND CROSSBONES	WHITE	6
RADIOACTIVE MATERIALS	PROPELLER	YELLOW OVER WHITE	7
CORROSIVES	TEST TUBE OVER HAND/ TEST TUBE OVER METAL	WHITE OVER BLACK	8
MISCELLANEOUS DANGEROUS SUBSTANCES			9

4-5/SPECIAL LABELS

NAME	LABEL	APPLICATION
CARGO AIRCRAFT ONLY	DANGER — DO NOT LOAD IN PASSENGER AIRCRAFT	MATERIALS NOT ACCEPTED FOR PASSENGER-CARRYING AIRCRAFT.
MAGNETIZED MATERIALS	MAGNETIZED MATERIAL	ARTICLES THAT CONTAIN MAGNETS WHICH MAY CAUSE DEVIATIONS IN AIRCRAFT COMPASSES.
SPONTANEOUSLY COMBUSTIBLE		EXPORT SHIPMENTS OF SPONTANEOUSLY COMBUSTIBLE MATERIALS.
POISONOUS SUBSTANCES	HARMFUL	EXPORT SHIPMENTS OF POISONOUS SUBSTANCES. THE TEXT MAY BE IN THE LANGUAGE OF THE COUNTRY OF ORIGIN.
INFECTIOUS SUBSTANCES	INFECTIOUS SUBSTANCE	EXPORT SHIPMENTS OF POISONOUS SUBSTANCES. THE TEXT MAY BE IN THE LANGUAGE OF THE COUNTRY OF ORIGIN.
POISON-INHALATION HAZARD	ORGANIC PEROXIDE / POISON	CHEMICALS WHICH HAVE A POISON-INHALATION HAZARD AND ARE FLAMMABLE, OXIDIZABLE, OR AN ORGANIC PEROXIDE. WHEN SHIPPED IN CONTAINERS WITH A VOLUME GREATER THAN 1 LITER BUT LESS THAN 110 GALLONS, THE LABEL "POISON", AS WELL AS THE LABEL FOR ANY OTHER HAZARD MUST ALSO BE ON THE CONTAINER.
RADIOACTIVE MATERIALS	RADIOACTIVE	LABELS WILL CARRY ADDITIONAL INFORMATION (CONTENTS-NAME OF RADIONUCLICIDE, RADIOACTIVE ACTIVITY, TRANSPORT INDEX). ALL LABELS WILL SHOW VERTICAL BARS INDICATING RADIOACTIVE LEVELS (I, II, OR III) OVERPRINTED IN RED ON LOWER HALF OF EACH LABEL.

 APPEN-DIX

4-6/SPECIAL LABELS

SPECIAL PLACARDS		
NAME	LABEL	APPLICATION
RESIDUAL		EMPTY TANK CARS WHICH LAST CONTAINED HAZMATS AND ITS CONTENTS HAVE BEEN UNLOADED TO THE MAXIMUM EXTENT POSSIBLE, EXCEPT FOR EXPLOSIVES, POISON GAS AND RADIOACTIVE MATERIALS. NOT REQUIRED FOR THOROUGHLY CLEANED OR PURGED TANK CARS. TANK TRUCKS DISPLAY APPROPRIATE PLACARD WHETHER EMPTY OR FULL.
WHITE BACKGROUND		RAIL SHIPMENTS THAT REQUIRE SPECIAL HANDLING. EACH CAR PLACARDED AS EXPLOSIVE A, POISON GAS OR POISON GAS-EMPTY MUST HAVE A PLACARD MOUNTED ON A 15-INCH SQUARE WHITE BACKGROUND.
DANGEROUS		EXPLOSIVES C, IRRITATING MATERIALS AND MIXED LOADS OF 1,000 LBS. OR MORE TOTAL WEIGHT WHERE TWO OR MORE MATERIALS WOULD REQUIRE DIFFERENT PLACARDS.
POISON-INHALATION HAZARD		FOUND ON CHEMICALS WHICH HAVE A POISON INHALATION HAZARD AND ARE FLAMMABLE, CORROSIVE, OXIDIZABLE OR AN ORGANIC PEROXIDE. FREIGHT CONTAINERS WITH A CAPACITY GREATER THAN 110 GALLONS MUST SHOW "POISON" PLACARD AS WELL AS THE REQUIRED PLACARD. THE FOUR-DIGIT ID NUMBER MUST ALSO APPEAR.

4-7/HAZARDOUS MATERIALS IDENTIFICATION NUMBERS

ID no.	Name of material
0004	Ammonium picrate, dry or wetted with less than 10% water
0222	Ammonium nitrate fertilizer, with not more likely 2% of combustible material
0223	Ammonium nitrate fertilizer, which is more likely to explode than UN0222
0357	Substances, explosive
0358	Substances, explosive
0359	Substances, explosive
0402	Ammonium perchlorate, average particle size of less than 45 microns
1001	Acetylene
1001	Acetylene, dissolved
1002	Air, compressed
1003	Air, refrigerated liquid (cryogenic liquid)
1005	Ammonia
1005	Ammonia, anhydrous, liquefied
1005	Anhydrous ammonia
1006	Argon, compressed
1008	Boron trifluoride
1009	Bromotrifluoromethane
1010	Butadiene, inhibited
1011	Butane or butane mixture
1012	Butene
1012	Butylene
1013	Carbon dioxide
1014	Carbon dioxide-oxygen mixture
1015	Carbon dioxide-nitrous oxide mixture
1016	Carbon monoxide
1017	Chlorine
1018	Chlorodifluoromethane
1020	Chloropentafluoroethane
1021	Chlorotetrafluoroethane
1022	Chlorotrifluoromethane
1022	Trifluorochloromethane
1023	Coal gas
1026	Cyanogen
1026	Cyanogen, liquefied
1027	Cyclopropane
1027	Cyclopropane, liquefied
1028	Dichlorodifluoromethane
1029	Dichlorofluoromethane
1029	Dichloromonofluoromethane
1030	Difluoroethane
1032	Dimethylamine, anhydrous
1033	Dimethyl ether
1035	Ethane, compressed
1036	Ethylamine
1036	Monoethylamine
1037	Ethyl chloride
1038	Ethylene, cryogenic liquid
1038	Ethylene, liquid (refrigerated)

ID no.	Name of material
1039	Ethyl methyl ether
1039	Methyl ethyl ether
1040	Ethylene oxide
1041	Carbon dioxide-ethylene oxide mixture, with more than 6% ethylene oxide
1041	Ethylene oxide-carbon dioxide mixture, with more than 6% ethylene oxide
1043	Fertilizer ammoniating solution, with more than 35% free ammonia
1044	Fire extinguisher, with compressed or liquefied gas
1045	Fluorine, compressed
1046	Helium, compressed
1048	Hydrogen bromide, anhydrous
1049	Hydrogen, compressed
1050	Hydrochloric acid, anhydrous
1050	Hydrogen chloride, anhydrous
1051	Hydrocyanic acid
1051	Hydrogen cyanide, anhydrous, stabilized
1052	Hydrofluoric acid, anhydrous
1052	Hydrogen fluoride, anhydrous
1053	Hydrogen sulfide
1055	Isobutylene
1056	Krypton, compressed
1057	Cigarette lighter, with flammable gas
1057	Flammable gas in lighter for cigars, cigarettes, etc.
1057	Lighter, for cigars, cigarettes, etc., with flammable gas
1058	Liquefied gas, nonflammable, charged with nitrogen, carbon dioxide or air
1058	Liquefied nonflammable gas charged with nitrogen, carbon dioxide or air
1060	Methyl acetylene and propadiene mixture, stabilized
1061	Methylamine, anhydrous
1061	Monomethylamine, anhydrous
1062	Methyl bromide
1063	Methyl chloride
1064	Methyl mercaptan
1065	Neon, compressed
1066	Nitrogen, compressed
1067	Nitrogen dioxide
1067	Nitrogen peroxide
1067	Nitrogen tetroxide
1069	Nitrosyl chloride
1070	Nitrous oxide, compressed
1071	Oil gas
1072	Oxygen, compressed
1073	Oxygen, refrigerated liquid (cryogenic liquid)
1075	Liquefied petroleum gas
1075	LPG, liquefied petroleum gas
1075	Petroleum gas, liquefied
1076	Carbonyl chloride
1076	Phosgene

Continued.

4-7/Hazardous Materials Identification Numbers — cont'd

ID no.	Name of material	ID no.	Name of material
1077	Propylene	1127	Chlorobutane
1078	Chlorodifluoromethane and chloropentafluoroethane mixture	1128	Butyl formate
1078	Chlorotrifluoromethane and trifluoromethane mixture	1129	Buyraldehyde
1078	Dichlorodifluoromethane and chlorodifluoromethane mixture	1130	Camphor oil
		1131	Carbon bisulfide
1078	Dichlorodifluoromethane and dichlorotetrafluoroethane mixture	1131	Carbon disulfide
		1132	Carbon remover, liquid
1078	Dichlorodifluoromethane and difluoroethane mixture	1133	Adhesive, containing flammable liquid
		1133	Adhesive
1078	Dichlorodifluoromethane, trichlorofluoromethane and chlorodifluoromethane mixture	1133	Cement, containing flammable liquid
		1133	Cement, liquid, n.o.s.
1078	Dichlorodifluoromethane and trichlorofluoromethane mixture	1134	Chlorobenzene
		1135	Ethylene chlorohydrin
1078	Dichlorodifluoromethane and trichlorotrifluoroethane mixture	1136	Coal tar distillate
		1136	Coal tar oil
1078	Dispersant gas, n.o.s.	1137	Coal tar distille
1078	Refrigerant gas, n.o.s.	1137	Coal tar oil
1078	Trifluoromethane and chlorotrifluoromethane mixture	1139	Coating solution
1079	Sulfur dioxide	1142	Anti-freeze
1080	Sulfur hexafluoride	1142	Cleaning compound
1081	Tetrafluoroethylene, inhibited	1142	Compound, polishing, liquid, etc. (combustible or flammable)
1082	Trifluorochloroethylene		
1083	Trimethylamine, anhydrous	1142	Flammable liquid preparations, n.o.s.
1085	Vinyl bromide	1142	Reducing liquid
1086	Monochloroethylene	1142	Removing liquid
1086	Vinyl chloride	1143	Crotonaldehyde, inhibited
1087	Vinyl methyl ether	1144	Crotonylene
1088	Acetal	1145	Cyclohexane
1089	Acetaldehyde	1146	Cyclopentane
1090	Acetone	1147	Decahydronaphthalene
1091	Acetone oil	1148	Diacetone alcohol
1092	Acrolein, inhibited	1149	Butyl ether
1093	Acrylonitrile, inhibited	1149	Dibutyl ether
1098	Allyl alcohol	1150	1,2-Dichloroethylene
1099	Allyl bromide	1152	Dichloropentane
1100	Allyl chloride	1153	Diethoxyethane
1103	Trimethyl aluminum	1153	Diethyl cellosolve
1104	Amyl acetate	1153	Ethylene glycol diethyl ether
1105	Amyl alcohol	1154	Diethylamine
1105	Isoamyl alcohol	1155	Diethyl ether
1106	Amylamine	1155	Ether
1107	Amyl chloride	1155	Ethyl ether
1108	Amylene	1156	Diethyl ketone
1109	Amyl formate	1157	Di-isobutyl ketone
1110	Amyl methyl ketone	1158	Di-isopropylamine
1110	Methyl amyl ketone	1159	Di-isopropyl ether
1111	Amyl mercaptan	1159	Isopropyl ether
1112	Amyl nitrate	1160	Dimethylamine solution
1113	Amyl nitrite	1161	Dimethyl carbonate
1114	Benzene	1162	Dimethyldichlorosilane
1115	Benzine	1163	Dimethylhydrazine, unsymmetrical
1118	Brake fluid, hydraulic	1164	Dimethyl sulfide
1120	Butanol	1164	Methyl sulfide
1120	Butyl alcohol	1165	Dioxane
1123	Butyl acetate	1166	Dioxolane
1125	Butylamine	1167	Divinyl ether, inhibited
1126	Butyl bromide	1168	Drier, paint or varnish, liquid, n.o.s.
1127	Butyl chloride	1169	Extract, aromatic, liquid

4-7/Hazardous Materials Identification Numbers—cont'd

ID no.	Name of material	ID no.	Name of material
1170	Alcohol (beverage)	1220	Isopropyl acetate
1170	Alcohol (ethyl)	1221	Isopropylamine
1170	Alcoholic beverage	1222	Isopropyl nitrate
1170	Ethanol, and solutions	1223	Kerosene
1170	Ethyl alcohol	1224	Ketone, liquid, n.o.s.
1171	Ethoxyethanol	1226	Cigarette lighter, with flammable liquid
1171	Ethylene glycol monoethyl ether	1226	Lighter, for cigars, cigarettes, etc., with flammable liquid
1172	Ethoxyethyl acetate		
1172	Ethylene glycol monoethyl ether acetate	1226	Lighter fluid
1173	Ethyl acetate	1228	Mercaptan mixture, aliphatic
1175	Ethylbenzene	1228	Mercaptans and mixtures, liquid, n.o.s.
1176	Ethyl borate	1229	Mesityl oxide
1177	Ethylbutyl acetate	1230	Methanol
1178	Ethylbutyraldehyde	1230	Methyl alcohol
1179	Ethyl butyl ether	1230	Wood alcohol
1180	Ethyl butyrate	1231	Methyl acetate
1181	Ethyl chloroacetate	1232	Methyl acetone
1182	Ethyl chloroformate	1233	Methyl amyl acetate
1183	Ethyl dichlorosilane	1234	methylal
1184	Ethylene dichloride	1235	Methylamine, aqueous solution
1185	Ethylene imine, inhibited	1235	Monomethylamine, aqueous solution
1188	Ethylene glycol monomethyl ether	1237	Methyl butyrate
1189	Ethylene glycol monomethyl ether acetate	1238	Methyl chlorocarbonate
1190	Ethyl formate	1238	Methyl chloroformate
1191	Ethyl hexaldehyde	1239	Methyl chloromethyl ether
1191	Octyl aldehyde	1242	Methyl dichlorosilane
1192	Ethyl lactate	1243	Methyl formate
1193	Ethyl methyl ketone	1244	Methylhydrazine
1193	Methyl ethyl ketone	1244	Monomethyl hydrazine
1194	Ethyl nitrite	1245	Methyl isobutyl ketone
1195	Ethyl propionate	1246	Methyl isopropenyl ketone, inhibited
1196	Ethyltrichlorosilane	1246	Methylpropenyl ketone, inhibited
1197	Extract, flavoring, liquid	1247	Methyl methacrylate, monomer, inhibited
1198	Formaldehyde solution (Formalin)	1248	Methyl propionate
1199	Furfural	1249	Methyl propyl ketone
1201	Fusel oil	1250	Methyl trichlorosilane
1202	Gas oil	1251	Methyl vinyl ketone
1203	Gasohol	1255	Naphtha, petroleum
1203	Gasoline	1255	Petroleum naphtha
1203	Motor fuel, n.o.s.	1256	Naphtha, solvent
1203	Motor spirit	1257	Casinghead gasoline
1203	Petrol	1257	Natural gasoline
1204	Glyceryl trinitrate solution	1259	Nickel carbonyl
1204	Spirits of nitroglycerine	1261	Nitromethane
1205	Gutta-percha solution	1262	Isooctane
1206	Heptane	1262	Octane
1207	Hexaldehyde	1263	Enamel
1208	Hexane	1263	Lacquer
1208	Neohexane	1263	Lacquer base, liquid
1210	Ink	1263	Paint, etc., flammable liquid
1212	Isobutanol	1263	Paint related material, flammable liquid
1212	Isobutyl alcohol	1263	Polish, liquid
1213	Isobutyl acetate	1263	Shellac
1214	Isobutylamine	1263	Stain
1216	Isooctene	1263	Thinner
1218	Isoprene, inhibited	1263	Varnish
1219	Isopropanol	1263	Wood filler, liquid
1219	Isopropyl alcohol	1264	Paraldehyde

APPEN-
DIX

Continued.

4-7/Hazardous Materials Identification Numbers — cont'd

ID no.	Name of material	ID no.	Name of material
1265	Isopentane	1325	Flammable solid, n.o.s.
1265	Pentane	1325	Pyroxylin plastic, rod sheet, roll, tube, or scrap
1266	Perfumery products, with flammable solvent	1325	Smokeless powder, small arms
1267	Petroleum crude oil	1326	Hafnium metal, powder, wet
1268	Petroleum distillate, n.o.s.	1327	Bhusa
1270	Oil, petroleum, n.o.s.	1327	Hay
1270	Petroleum oil	1327	Straw
1271	Petroleum ether	1328	Hexamine
1271	Petroleum spirit	1330	Manganese resinate
1272	Pine oil	1331	Matches, strike anywhere
1274	Propanol	1332	Metaldehyde
1274	Propyl alcohol	1333	Cerium, crude
1275	Propionaldehyde	1333	Mischmetal, powder
1276	Propyl acetate	1334	Creosote salts
1277	Monopropylamine	1334	Naphthalene, crude or refined
1277	Propylamine	1336	Nitroguanidine, wet with not less than 20% of water
1278	Propyl chloride	1336	Picrite, wet with not less than 20% water
1279	Dichloropropane	1337	Nitrostarch, wet with not less than 30% solvent
1279	Propylene dichloride	1337	Nitrostarch, wet with not less than 20% water
1280	Propylene oxide	1338	Phosphorus, amorphous, red
1281	Propyl formate	1338	Red phosphorus
1282	Pyridine	1339	Phosphorus heptasulfide, free from yellow or white phosphorus
1286	Rosin oil		
1287	Rubber solution	1340	Phosphorus pentasulfide, free from yellow or white phosphorus
1288	Shale oil		
1289	Sodium methylate, solutions in alcohol	1341	Phosphorus sesquisulfide, free from yellow or white phosphorus
1292	Ethyl silicate		
1292	Tetraethyl silicate	1343	Phosphorus trisulfide, free from yellow or white phosphorus
1293	Tincture, medicinal		
1294	Toluene	1344	Picric acid, wet with not less than 10% water
1295	Trichlorosilane	1344	Trinitrophenol, wet
1296	Triethylamine	1345	Rubber scrap, powdered or granulated
1297	Trimethylamine, aqueous solution	1346	Silicon powder, amorphous
1298	Trimethylchlorosilane	1347	Silver picrate, wet with not less than 30% water
1299	Turpentine	1348	Sodium dinitro-orthocresolate, wet with not less than 15% water
1300	Turpentine substitute		
1301	Vinyl acetate	1349	Sodium picramate, wet, with not less than 20% water
1302	Vinyl ethyl ether		
1303	Vinylidene chloride	1350	Sulfur
1304	Vinyl butyl ether	1352	Titanium, metal, powder, wet with not less than 20% water
1304	Vinyl isobutyl ether		
1305	Vinyl trichlorosilane	1353	Toe puffs, nitrocellulose base
1306	Wood preservative, liquid	1354	Trinitrobenzene, wet
1307	Xylene, (Xylol)	1355	Trinitrobenzoic acid, wet
1308	Zirconium metal, liquid suspension	1356	Trinitrotolune, wet
1309	Aluminum powder, coated	1357	Urea nitrate, wet
1310	Ammonium picrate, wetted with more than 10% water	1358	Zirconium metal, powder, wet
		1360	Calcium phosphide
1312	Borneol	1361	Carbon, animal or vegetable origin
1313	Calcium resinate	1361	Charcoal
1314	Calcium resinate, fused	1361	Coal, ground bituminous, sea coal, etc.
1318	Cobalt resinate, precipitated	1361	Coal facings
1320	Dinitrophenol, wet, with not less than 15% water	1361	Sea coal
1321	Dinitrophenolate, wet, with not less than 15% water	1362	Activated carbon
1322	Dinitroresorcinol, wet, with not less than 15% water	1362	Carbon, activated
1323	Ferrocerium	1363	Copra
1324	Film, motion picture, nitrocellulose base	1364	Cotton waste, oily
1325	Cosmetics, flammable solid, n.o.s.	1365	Cotton, wet

4-7/Hazardous Materials Identification Numbers—cont'd

ID no.	Name of material	ID no.	Name of material
1366	Diethylzinc	1407	Caesium, metal
1367	Diethylmagnesium	1407	Cesium metal
1368	Dimethylmagnesium	1408	Ferrosilicon
1369	Dimethyl-p-nitrosopaniline	1409	Hydride, metal, n.o.s.
1369	Nitrosodimethylaniline	1410	Lithium aluminum hydride
1370	Dimethylzinc	1411	Lithium aluminum hydride, ether solution
1371	Drier, paint or varnish, solid, n.o.s.	1412	Lithium amide
1371	Drier, paint solid, n.o.s.	1413	Lithium borohydride
1372	Fiber, animal or vegetable, burnt, wet or damp, n.o.s.	1414	Lithium hydride
1373	Fabric, animal or vegetable, with oil, n.o.s.	1415	Lithium metal
1373	Fiber, animal or vegetable, with oil, n.o.s.	1417	Lithium silicon
1374	Fish meal and scrap, unstabilized	1418	Magnesium, powder
1375	Fuel, pyrophoric, n.o.s.	1418	Magnesium allow, with more than 50% magnesium, powder
1375	Pyrophoric fuel, n.o.s.	1419	Magnesium aluminum phosphide
1376	Iron oxide, spent	1420	Potassium, metal, liquid alloy
1376	Iron sponge, spent	1420	Potassium metal, liquid alloy
1378	Nickel catalyst, finely divided, activated or spent, wet with not less than 40% of water or other suitable liquid	1421	Alkali metal, liquid alloy
		1421	Alkali metal alloy, liquid, n.o.s.
		1421	Sodium, metal, liquid alloy
1379	Paper, treated with unsaturated oil	1422	Potassium-sodium alloy
1380	Pentaborane	1422	Sodium-potassium alloy
1381	Phosphorus, white or yellow, dry or under water or in solution	1423	Rubidium metal
		1424	Sodium amalgam
1381	White phosphorus, dry	1425	Sodium amide
1381	White phosphorus, wet	1426	Sodium borohydride
1382	Potassium sulfide, anhydrous or with less than 30% water of hydration	1427	Sodium hydride
		1428	Sodium
1383	Aluminum, powder, pyrophoric	1428	Sodium metal
1383	Pyrophoric metal and alloy, n.o.s.	1429	Sodium, metal, dispersion in organic liquids
1383	Zinc powder or dust, pyrophoric	1431	Sodium methylate, dry
1384	Sodium dithionite	1432	Sodium phosphide
1384	Sodium hydrosulfite	1433	Stannic phosphide
1385	Sodium sulfide, anhydrous or with less than 30% water of crystalization	1434	Strontium alloy
		1435	Zinc ashes
1386	Seed cake, with more than 1.5% oil and not more than 11% moisture	1436	Zinc Metal, powder or dust
		1436	Zinc powder or dust, nonpyrophoric
1387	Wool waste, wet	1437	Zirconium hydride
1389	Alkali metal amalgam, n.o.s.	1438	Aluminum nitrate
1390	Alkali metal amide, n.o.s.	1439	Ammonium dichromate
1391	Alkali metal dispersion, n.o.s.	1442	Ammonium perchlorate
1392	Alkaline earth metal amalgam, n.o.s.	1444	Ammonium persulfate
1392	Alkaline earth metal dispersion, n.o.s.	1445	Barium chlorate
1393	Alkaline earth metal, alloy	1446	Barium nitrate
1394	Aluminum carbide	1447	Barium perchlorate
1395	Aluminum ferrosilicon, powder	1448	Barium permanganate
1396	Aluminum powder, uncoated	1449	Barium peroxide
1397	Aluminum phosphide	1450	Bromate, n.o.s.
1398	Aluminum silicon, powder	1451	Caesium nitrate
1399	Barium alloy	1451	Cesium nitrate
1400	Barium	1452	Calcium chlorate
1400	Barium metal	1453	Calcium chlorite
1401	Calcium, metal and alloys	1454	Calcium nitrate
1402	Calcium carbide	1455	Calcium perchlorate
1403	Calcium cyanamide, with more than 0.1% calcium carbide	1456	Calcium permanganate
		1457	Calcium peroxide
1404	Calcium hydride	1458	Borate and chlorate mixture
1405	Calcium silicide	1458	Chlorate and borate mixture
1406	Calcium silicon		

Continued.

4-7/Hazardous Materials Identification Numbers — cont'd

ID no.	Name of material	ID no.	Name of material
1459	Chlorate and magnesium chloride mixture	1509	Strontium peroxide
1461	Chlorate, inorganic, n.o.s.	1510	Tetranitromethane
1462	Chlorite, inorganic, n.o.s.	1511	Urea hydrogen peroxide
1463	Chromic acid, solid	1511	Urea peroxide
1463	Chromic anhydride	1512	Zinc ammonium nitrite
1463	Chromium trioxide, anhydrous	1513	Zinc chlorate
1465	Didymium nitrate	1514	Zinc nitrate
1466	Ferric nitrate	1515	Zinc permanganate
1467	Guanidine nitrate	1516	Zinc peroxide
1469	Lead nitrate	1517	Zirconium picramate, wet
1470	Lead perchlorate	1541	Acetone cyanohydrin
1471	Lithium hypochlorite, dry, with more than 39% available chlorine	1544	Alkaloid, n.o.s.
		1544	Alkaloid salt, n.o.s.
1472	Lithium peroxide	1545	Allyl isothiocyanate, inhibited
1473	Magnesium bromate	1545	Allyl isothiocyanate, stabilized
1474	Magnesium nitrate	1546	Ammonium arsenate
1475	Magnesium perchlorate	1547	Aniline
1476	Magnesium peroxide	1548	Aniline hydrochloride
1477	Nitrate, n.o.s.	1549	Antimony compound, n.o.s.
1478	Nitrate of sodium and potash mixture	1549	Antimony tribromide
1478	Sodium nitrate and potash mixture	1549	Antimony tribromide solution
1479	Cosmetics, oxidizer, n.o.s.	1549	Antimony trifluoride
1479	Cupric nitrate	1549	Antimony trifluoride solution
1479	Oxidizer, n.o.s.	1550	Antimony lactate
1479	Oxidizing material, n.o.s.	1551	Antimony potassium tartrate
1479	Oxidizing substance, n.o.s.	1553	Arsenic acid, liquid
1479	Potassium dichromate	1554	Arsenic acid, solid
1479	Sodium dichromate	1555	Arsenic bromide
1481	Perchlorate, n.o.s.	1556	Arsenic compound, liquid, n.o.s.
1482	Permanganate, inorganic, n.o.s.	1556	Methyl dichloroarsine
1483	Peroxide, inorganic, n.o.s.	1556	Organic compound of arsenic, liquid, n.o.s.
1484	Potassium bromate	1556	Phenyldichloroarsine
1485	Chlorate of potash	1557	Arsenic compound, solid, n.o.s.
1485	Potassium chlorate	1557	Arsenic disulfide
1486	Potassium nitrite	1557	Arsenic iodide, solid
1486	Saltpeter	1557	Arsenic trisulfide
1487	Potassium nitrate and sodium nitrite mixture	1558	Arsenic metal
1487	Sodium nitrite and potassium nitrate mixture	1559	Arsenic pentoxide
1488	Potassium nitrite	1560	Arsenic chloride
1489	Potassium perchlorate	1560	Arsenic trichloride
1490	Potassium permanganate	1561	Arsenic, white, solid
1491	Potassium peroxide	1561	Arsenic trioxide
1492	Potassium persulfate	1562	Arsenical dust
1493	Silver nitrate	1562	Arsenical flue dust
1494	Sodium bromate	1564	Barium compound, n.o.s.
1495	Chlorate of soda	1565	Barium cyanide
1495	Sodium chlorate	1566	Beryllium chloride
1496	Sodium chlorite	1566	Beryllium compound, n.o.s.
1498	Sodium nitrate	1566	Beryllium flouride
1499	Sodium nitrate and potassium nitrate mixture	1567	Beryllium, powder
1500	Sodium nitrite	1569	Bromoacetone
1502	Sodium perchlorate	1570	Brucine
1503	Sodium permanganate	1571	Barium azide, with not less than 50% water or alcohol
1504	Sodium peroxide		
1505	Sodium persulfate	1572	Cacodylic acid
1506	Strontium chlorate	1573	Calcium arsenate
1507	Strontium nitrate	1574	Calcium arsenate and calcium arsenite mixture, solid
1508	Stronthium perchlorate	1574	Calcium arsenite

4-7/Hazardous Materials Identification Numbers — cont'd

ID no.	Name of material	ID no.	Name of material
1575	Calcium cyanide	1622	Magnesium arsenate
1577	Chlorodinitrobenzene	1623	Mercuric arsenate
1577	Dinitrochlorobenzene	1624	Mercuric chloride
1578	Chloronitrobenzene	1625	Mercuric nitrate
1578	Nitrochlorobenzene, liquid	1626	Mercuric potassium cyanide
1578	Nitrochlorobenzene, solid	1627	Mercurous nitrate
1579	4-chloro-o-toluidine hydrochloride	1628	Mercurous sulfate
1580	Chloropicrin	1629	Mercuric acetate
1581	Chloropicrin and methyl bromide mixture	1629	Mercurous acetate
1581	Methyl bromide and chloropicrin mixture	1629	Mercury acetate
1582	Chloropicrin and methyl chloride mixture	1630	Mercury ammonium chloride
1582	Methyl chloride and chloropicrin mixture	1631	Mercury benzoate
1583	Chloropicrin mixture, n.o.s.	1633	Mercury bisulfate
1584	Cocculus, solid	1634	Mercuric bromide
1585	Copper acetoarsenite	1634	Mercurous bromide
1586	Copper arsenite	1634	Mercury bromide
1587	Copper cyanide	1636	Mercuric cyanide
1588	Cyanide, inorganic, n.o.s.	1636	Mercury cyanide
1588	Cyanide or cyanide mixture, dry	1637	Mercury gluconate
1589	Cyanogen chloride, inhibited	1638	Mercury iodide
1590	Dichloroaniline	1639	Mercurol
1591	o-Dichlorobenzene	1639	Mercury nucleate
1592	p-dichlorobenzene	1640	Mercury oleate
1592	Paradichlorobenzene	1641	Mercury oxide
1593	Dichloromethane	1642	Mercuric oxycyanide
1593	Methylene chloride	1642	Mercury oxycyanide
1594	Diethyl sulfate	1643	Mercury potassium iodide
1594	Ethyl sulfate	1644	Mercury salicylate
1595	Dimethyl sulfate	1645	Mercuric sulfate
1595	Methyl sulfate	1646	Mercury thiocyanate
1596	Dinitroaniline	1647	Methyl bromide and ethylene dibromide mixture, liquid
1597	Dinitrobenzene		
1597	Dinitrobenzene solution	1648	Acetonitrile
1598	Dinitro-o-cresol	1648	Methyl cyanide
1599	Dinitrophenol solution, in water or flammable liquid	1649	Anti-knock compound
1600	Dinitrotoluene, liquid	1649	Ethyl fluid
1601	Disinfectant, poisonous, n.o.s.	1649	Lead tetraethyl
1602	Dye, n.o.s. (poisonous)	1649	Lead tetramethyl
1602	Dye intermediate, n.o.s. (poisonous)	1649	Motor fuel anti-knock compound
1603	Ethyl bromoacetate	1649	Tetraethyl lead
1604	Ethylenediamine	1649	Tetramethyl lead
1605	Dibromoethane	1650	Naphthylamine (beta)
1605	Ethylene dibromide	1651	Naphthylthiourea
1606	Ferric arsenate	1652	Naphthylurea
1607	Ferric arsenite	1653	Nickel cyanide
1608	Ferrous arsenate	1654	Nicotine
1610	Halogenated irritating liquid, n.o.s.	1655	Nicotine, compounds and preparations, n.o.s.
1611	Hexaethyl tetraphosphate	1656	Nicotine hydrochloride, and solutions
1612	Hexaethyl tetraphosphate and compressed gas mixture	1657	Nicotine salicylate
		1658	Nicotine sulfate, liquid
1613	Hydrocyanic acid, aqueous solution, with not less than 5% hydrocyanic acid	1658	Nicotine sulfate, solid
		1659	Nicotine tartrate
1614	Hydrogen cyanide, absorbed	1660	Nitric oxide
1616	Lead acetate	1661	Nitroaniline
1617	Lead arsenate	1662	Nitrobenzene
1618	Lead arsenite	1663	Nitrophenol
1620	Lead cyanide	1664	Nitrotoluene
1621	London purple	1665	Nitroxylene

Continued.

APPEN DIX

4-7/Hazardous Materials Identification Numbers — cont'd

ID no.	Name of material	ID no.	Name of material
1665	Nitroxylol	1716	Acetyl bromide
1669	Pentachloroethane	1717	Acetyl chloride
1670	Perchloromethylmercaptan	1718	Acid butyl phosphate
1671	Carbolic acid	1718	Butyl acid phosphate
1671	Phenol, solid	1718	Butyl phosphoric acid
1672	Phenylcarbylamine chloride	1719	Alkaline corrosive liquid, n.o.s.
1673	Paradiaminobenzene	1719	Caustic alkali liquids, n.o.s.
1673	Phenylenediamine	1722	Allyl chlorocarbonate
1674	Phenylmercuric acetate, liquid	1722	Allyl chloroformate
1677	Potassium arsenate	1723	Allyl iodide
1678	Potassium arsenite	1724	Allyl trichlorosilane, stabilized
1679	Potassium cuprocyanide	1725	Aluminum bromide, anhydrous
1680	Potassium cyanide, solid	1726	Aluminum chloride, anhydrous
1680	Potassium cyanide solution	1727	Ammonium bifluoride, solid
1681	Rodenticides, n.o.s.	1727	Ammonium hydrogen fluoride, solid
1683	Silver arsenite	1728	Amyltrichlorosilane
1684	Silver cyanide	1729	Anisoyl chloride
1685	Sodium arsenate	1730	Antimony pentachloride, liquid
1686	Sodium arsenite solution	1731	Antimony pentachloride solution
1687	Sodium azide	1732	Antimony pentafluoride
1688	Sodium cacodylate	1733	Antimony chloride
1689	Sodium cyanide	1733	Antimony trichloride
1690	Sodium fluoride, solid	1733	Antimony trichloride solution
1690	Sodium fluoride solution	1736	Benzoyl chloride
1691	Strontium arsenite	1737	Benzyl bromide
1692	Strychnine, and salts	1738	Benzyl chloride
1693	Irritating agent, n.o.s.	1739	Benzyl chloroformate
1693	Orm-a, n.o.s.	1740	Bifluoride, n.o.s.
1693	Tear gas	1741	Boron trichloride
1693	Tear gas devices, with more than 2% Tear gas substances	1742	Boron trifluoride acetic acid complex
1694	Bromobenzyl, cyanide	1743	Boron trifluoride propionic acid complex
1695	Chloroacetone, stabilized	1744	Bromine
1697	Chloroacetophenone	1744	Bromine solution
1698	Diphenylaminechloroarsine	1745	Bromine pentafluoride
1699	Diphenylchloroarsine	1746	Bromine trifluoride
1700	Tear gas candle	1747	Butyl trichlorosilane
1701	Xylyl bromide	1748	Calcium hypochlorite, dry, including mixtures with more than 39% available chlorine (8.8% available oxygen)
1702	Tetrachloroethane		
1703	Tetraethyl, dithiopyrophosphate, and compressed gas mixture	1749	Chlorine trifluoride
1704	Tetraethyl, dithiopyrophosphate, dry, liquid or mixture	1750	Chloroacetic acid, liquid
		1750	Monochloroacetic acid, liquid
1705	Tetraethyl pyrophosphate and compressed gas mixture	1751	Chloroacetic acid, solid
		1752	Chloroacetyl chloride
1707	Thallium compound, n.o.s.	1753	Chlorophenyl trichlorosilane
1707	Thallium salt, n.o.s.	1754	Chlorosulphonic acid
1707	Thallium sulfate, solid	1754	Chlorosulphonic acid and sulfur trioxide mixture
1708	Toluidines (o-, m-, and p-)	1755	Chromic acid solution
1709	Toluylenediamine	1756	Chromic fluoride, solid
1710	Trichloroethylene	1757	Chromic fluoride solution
1711	Xylidine	1758	Chromium oxychloride
1712	Zinc arsenate, solid	1759	Corrosive solid, n.o.s.
1712	Zinc arsenate and zinc arsenite mixture	1759	Cosmetics, corrosive solid, n.o.s.
1712	Zinc arsenite, solid	1759	Ferrous chloride, solid
1713	Zinc cyanide	1759	Fungicide, corrosive, n.o.s.
1714	Zinc phosphide	1759	Stannous chloride, solid
1715	Acetic anhydride	1760	Acid, liquid, n.o.s.
		1760	Aluminum phosphate solution

4-7/Hazardous Materials Identification Numbers — cont'd

ID no.	Name of material	ID no.	Name of material
1760	Aluminum sulfate solution	1786	Acid mixture, hydrofluoric and sulfuric acids
1760	Aminoethoxyethanol	1786	Hydrofluoric and sulfuric acid mixture
1760	Aminopropyldi-ethanolamine	1786	Sulfuric and hydrofluoric acid mixture
1760	Aminopropylmorpholine	1787	Hydriodic acid
1760	Aminopropylpiperazine	1787	Hydrogen iodide solution
1760	Bis(aminopropyl)amine	1788	Hydrobromic acid
1760	Caproic acid (hexanoic acid)	1788	Hydrogen bromide solution
1760	Chemical kit	1789	Hydrochloric acid solution
1760	Cleaning compound, liquid, corrosive	1789	Hydrogen chloride solution
1760	Compound, tree or weed killing, liquid (corrosive)	1789	Muriatic acid
1760	Corrosive liquid, n.o.s.	1790	Etching acid, liquid
1760	Cosmetics, corrosive liquid, n.o.s.	1790	Fluoric acid
1760	Dichloropropionic acid	1790	Hydrofluoric acid solution
1760	2,2-Dichloropropionic acid	1790	Hydrogen fluoride solution
1760	Ethylphosphonothioic-dichloride, anhydrous	1791	Hypochlorite solution with more than 5% available chlorine
1760	Ethyl phosphoro-dichloridate	1791	Potassium hypochlorite solution
1760	Ferrous chloride solution	1791	Sodium hypochlorite solution
1760	Hexanoic acid	1792	Iodine monochloride
1760	Isopentanoic acid	1793	Isopropyl acid phosphate
1760	Methyl phosphonothioic dichloride	1794	Lead sulfate, with more than 3% free acid
1760	Morpholine, aqueous, mixture	1796	Acid mixture, nitrating
1760	Nitric acid, other than fuming, with not more than 40% acid	1796	Mixed acid
		1796	Nitrating acid
1760	Orm-B, n.o.s.	1796	Nitrating acid, mixture
1760	Paint, etc., corrosive liquid	1798	Nitrohydrochloric acid
1760	Paint related material, corrosive liquid	1798	Nitromuriatic acid
1760	Pentanoic acid	1799	Nonyl trichlorosilane
1760	Textile treating compound	1800	Octadecyl trichlorosilane
1760	Titanium sulfate solution	1801	Octyl trichlorosilane
1760	Valeric acid, (n-pentanoic acid)	1802	Perchloric acid, not more than 50% acid, by weight
1761	Cupriethylenediamine solution	1803	Phenolsulphonic acid, liquid
1762	Cyclohexenyl trichlorosilane	1804	Phenyl trichlorosilane
1763	Cyclohexyl trichlorosilane	1805	Phosphoric acid
1764	Dichloroacetic acid	1806	Phosphorus pentachloride
1765	Dichloroacetyl chloride	1807	Phosphoric anhydride
1766	Dichlorophenyl trichlorosilane	1807	Phosphorus pentoxide
1767	Diethyl dichlorosilane	1808	Phosphorus tribromide
1768	Difluorophosphoric acid, anhydrous	1809	Chloride of phosphorus
1769	Diphenyl dichlorosilane	1809	Phosphorus trichloride
1770	Diphenylmethyl bromide	1810	Phosphorus oxychloride
1771	Dodecyl trichlorosilane	1810	Phosphoryl chloride
1773	Ferric chloride, anhydrous	1811	Potassium bifluoride
1773	Iron chloride, solid	1811	Potassium hydrogen fluoride
1774	Fire extinguisher charge, corrosive liquid	1812	Potassium fluoride
1775	Fluoboric acid	1813	Battery, electric, storage, dry, containing potassium hydroxide
1776	Fluorophosphoric acid, anhydrous	1813	Caustic potash, dry, solid
1776	Monofluorophosphoric acid	1813	Potassium hydroxide, dry, solid
1777	Fluorosulphonic acid	1814	Caustic potash solution
1778	Fluosilicic acid	1814	Potash liquor
1778	Hydrofluosolicic acid	1814	Potassium hydroxide solution
1778	Hydrosilicofluoric acid	1815	Propionyl chloride
1778	Silicofluoric acid	1816	Propyl trichlorosilane
1779	Formic acid	1817	Pyrosulfuryl chloride
1780	Fumaryl chloride	1818	Silicon chloride
1781	Hexadecyl trichlorosilane	1818	Silicon tetrachloride
1782	Hexafluorophosphoric acid	1819	Sodium aluminate solution
1783	Hexamethylene diamine solution		
1784	Hexyl trichlorosilane		

Continued.

APPEN-DIX

4-7/Hazardous Materials Identification Numbers — cont'd

ID no.	Name of material	ID no.	Name of material
1821	Sodium bisulfate, solid	1859	Silicon tetrafluoride
1821	Sodium hydrogen sulfate, solid	1860	Vinyl fluoride
1823	Caustic soda, dry, solid	1862	Ethyl crotonate
1823	Lye, dry, solid	1863	Fuel, aviation, turbine engine
1823	Sodium hydroxide, dry, solid	1864	Gas drips, hydrocarbon
1824	Caustic soda, solution	1865	Propyl nitrate
1824	Caustic soda solution	1866	Resin compound liquid, flammable
1824	Lye solution	1866	Resin solution, flammable
1824	Sodium hydrate	1866	Resin solution (resin compound), liquid
1824	Sodium hydroxide solution	1867	Cigarette, self-lighting
1825	Sodium monoxide	1868	Decaborane
1826	Acid mixture, spent, nitrating	1869	Magnesium, pellets, turnings or ribbon
1826	Mixed acid, spent	1869	Magnesium alloy, with more than 50% magnesium, pellets, turnings or ribbon
1826	Nitrating acid mixture, spent		
1826	Spent mixed acid	1870	Potassium borohydride
1827	Stannic chloride, anhydrous	1871	Titanium hydride
1827	Tin chloride, fuming	1872	Lead dioxide
1827	Tin tetrachloride	1872	Lead peroxide
1828	Chloride of sulfur	1873	Perchloric acid, more than 50% but not more than 72% acid, by weight
1828	Sulfur chloride		
1829	Sulfuric anhydride	1884	Barium oxide
1829	Sulfuric trioxide	1885	Benzidine
1829	Sulfur trioxide, inhibited	1886	Benzylidene chloride
1829	Sulfur trioxide, stabilized	1887	Bromochloromethane
1830	Sulfuric acid, with more than 51% but not more than 95% acid	1888	Chloroform
		1889	Cyanogen bromide
1830	Sulfuric acid, with not more than 51% acid	1891	Ethyl bromide
1831	Oleum	1892	Ethyl dichloroarsine
1831	Sulfuric acid, fuming	1894	Phenylmercuric hydroxide
1832	Sulfuric acid, spent	1895	Phenylmercuric nitrate
1833	Sulfurous acid	1896	Resin solution, poisonous
1834	Sulfuryl chloride	1897	Perchloroethylene
1835	Tetramethyl ammonium hydroxide	1897	Tetrachloroethylene
1836	Thionyl chloride	1898	Acetyl iodide
1837	Thiophosphoryl chloride	1902	Di(2-ethylhexyl) phosphoric acid
1838	Titanium tetrachloride	1902	Di-isooctyl acid phosphate
1839	Trichloroacetic acid	1903	Disinfectant, corrosive, liquid, n.o.s.
1840	Zinc chloride solution	1905	Selenic acid
1841	Acetaldehyde ammonia	1906	Sludge acid
1842	Acetic acid solution	1907	Soda lime
1843	Ammonium dinitro-o-cresolate	1908	Sodium chlorite solution with more than 5% available chlorine
1845	Carbon dioxide, solid		
1845	Dry ice	1910	Calcium oxide
1846	Carbon tetrachloride	1911	Diborane or diborane mixture
1847	Potassium sulfide, hydrated, with not less than 30% water of hydration	1912	Methyl chloride and methylene chloride mixture
		1913	Neon, refrigerated liquid, (cryogenic liquid)
1848	Propanoic acid	1914	Butyl propionate
1848	Propionic acid, solution with not less than 80% acid	1915	Cyclohexanone
		1916	Dichloroethyl ether
1849	Sodium sulfide, hydrated, with not less than 30% water	1917	Ethyl acrylate, inhibited
		1918	Cumene
1849	Sodium sulfide solution	1918	Isopropylbenzene
1850	Eradicator, paint or grease, flammable liquid	1919	Methyacrylate, inhibited
1851	Drugs, n.o.s.	1920	Nonane
1851	Medicines, n.o.s.	1921	Propyleneimine, inhibited
1854	Barium alloy, pyrophoric	1922	Pyrrolidine
1855	Calcium, metal and alloys, pyrophoric	1923	Calcium dithionite
1857	Textile waste, wet, n.o.s.	1923	Calcium hydrosulfite
1858	Hexafluoropropylene		

4-7/Hazardous Materials Identification Numbers—cont'd

ID no.	Name of material	ID no.	Name of material
1924	Ethyl aluminum dichloride	1961	Ethane-propane mixture, liquid (refrigerated)
1925	Ethyl aluminum sesquichloride	1962	Ethylene, compressed
1926	Methyl aluminum sesquibromide	1963	Helium, refrigerated liquid (cryogenic liquid)
1927	Methyl aluminum sesquichloride	1964	Hydrocarbon gas, compressed, n.o.s.
1928	Methyl magnesium bromide, in ethyl ether	1965	Hydrocarbon gas, liquefied, n.o.s.
1929	Potassium dithionite	1966	Hydrogen, cryogenic liquid
1929	Potassium hydrosulfite	1966	Hydrogen, liquefied
1930	Tributyl aluminum	1966	Hydrogen, refrigerated liquid (cryogenic liquid)
1930	Triisobutyl aluminum	1967	Insecticide gas, poisonous n.o.s.
1931	Zinc dithionite	1967	Parathion and compressed gas mixture
1931	Zinc hydrosulfite	1968	Insecticide gas, n.o.s.
1932	Zirconium, scrap	1969	Isobutane or isobutane mixture
1935	Cyanide solution, n.o.s.	1970	Krypton, refrigerated liquid (cryogenic liquid)
1938	Bromoacetic acid, solid	1971	Methane, compressed
1938	Bromoacetic acid solution	1971	Natural gas, compressed, with a high methane content
1939	Phosphorus oxybromide, solid		
1940	Thioglycolic acid	1971	Natural gas with a high methane content, compressed
1941	Dibromodifluoromethane	1972	Liquefied natural gas
1942	Ammonium nitrate, with not more than 0.2% of combustible material	1972	LNG, liquefied natural gas
		1972	Methane, refrigerated liquid (cryogenic liquid)
1942	Ammonium nitrate, with organic coating	1972	Natural gas, refrigerated liquid (cryogenic liquid) with a high methane content
1944	Matches, safety		
1945	Matches, wax (Vesta)	1972	Natural gas, liquid (refrigerated) with a high methane content
1950	Aerosols		
1951	Argon, refrigerated liquid (cryogenic liquid)	1973	Chlorodifluoromethane and chloropentafluoroethane mixture
1952	Carbon dioxide-ethylene oxide mixture with not more than 6% ethylene oxide		
		1974	Bromochlorodifluoromethane
1952	Ethylene oxide-carbon dioxide mixture, with not more than 6% ethylene oxide	1974	Chlorodifluorobromomethane
		1975	Nitric oxide and nitrogen tetroxide mixture
1953	Compressed gas, flammable, poisonous, n.o.s.	1976	Octafluorocyclobutane
1953	Poisonous liquid or gas, flammable, n.o.s.	1977	Nitrogen, refrigerated liquid (cryogenic liquid)
1954	Compressed gas, flammable, n.o.s.	1978	Propane
1954	Dispersant gas, flammable, n.o.s.	1979	Rare gas mixture
1954	Flammable gas, n.o.s.	1980	Helium-oxygen mixture
1954	Refrigerant gas, flammable, n.o.s.	1980	Rare gas-oxygen mixture
1954	Refrigerating machine, containing flammable, non-poisonous, liquefied gas	1981	Rare gas-nitrogen mixture
		1982	Tetrafluoromethane
1955	Chloropicrin and non-flammable gas mixture	1983	Chlorotrifluoroethane
1955	Compressed gas, poisonous, n.o.s.	1984	Trifluoromethane
1955	Methyl bromide and non-flammable compressed gas mixture	1986	Alcohol, denatured (toxic)
		1986	Alcohol, poisonous, n.o.s.
1955	Organic phosphorus compound, mixed with compressed gas	1986	Alcohol, toxic, n.o.s.
		1986	Propargyl alcohol
1955	Perchlorylfluoride	1987	Alcohol, denatured
1955	Phosphorus trifluoride	1987	Alcohol, nontoxic, n.o.s.
1955	Poisonous liquid or gas, n.o.s.	1987	Alcohol, n.o.s.
1955	Tetrafluorohydrazine	1988	Aldehyde, poisonous, n.o.s.
1956	Accumulators, pressurized	1988	Aldehyde, toxic, n.o.s.
1956	Compressed gas, n.o.s.	1989	Aldehyde, n.o.s.
1956	Hexafluoropropylene oxide	1989	Benzaldehyde
1956	Nonflammable gas, n.o.s.	1991	Chloroprene, inhibited
1957	Deuterium	1992	Flammable liquid, poisonous, n.o.s.
1958	Dichlorotetrafluoroethane	1993	Combustible liquid, n.o.s.
1959	Difluoroethylene	1993	Compound, tree or weed killing, liquid (combustible or flammable)
1959	1,1-Difluoroethylene		
1959	Vinylidene fluoride	1993	Cosmetics, flammable liquid, n.o.s.
1960	Engine starting fluid	1993	Creosote, coal tar
1961	Ethane, liquid (refrigerated)		

Continued.

4-7/Hazardous Materials Identification Numbers — cont'd

ID no.	Name of material	ID no.	Name of material
1993	Ethyl nitrate	2030	Hydrazine aqueous solution, with not more than 64% hydrazine by weight
1993	Flammable liquid, n.o.s.		
1993	Fuel oil	2030	Hydrazine hydrate
1993	Insecticide, liquid, n.o.s.	2030	Hydrazine solution, with not more than 64% hydrazine by weight
1993	Organic peroxide, liquid or solution, n.o.s.		
1993	Wax, liquid	2031	Nitric acid, other than fuming, with more than 40% acid
1994	Iron pentacarbonyl		
1999	Asphalt	2032	Nitric acid, fuming
1999	Road asphalt, liquid	2032	Nitric acid, red fuming
1999	Tar, liquid	2033	Potassium monoxide
2000	Celluloid, in blocks, rods, rolls, sheets, tubes, etc., except celluloid scrap	2033	Potassium oxide
		2034	Hydrogen and methane mixture
2001	Cobalt naphthenate, powder	2035	Trifluoroethane
2002	Celluloid scrap	2036	Xenon
2003	Aluminum alkyl	2037	Receptacles, small, with flammable compressed gas
2203	Aluminum tributyl	2038	Dinitrotoluene, solid
2003	Metal alkyl, n.o.s.	2044	Dimethylpropane
2004	Magnesium diamide	2044	Neopentane
2005	Magnesium diphenyl	2045	Butyl aldehyde
2006	Plastics, nitrocellulose-based, spontaneously combustible, n.o.s.	2045	Isobutyl aldehyde
		2045	Isobutyraldehyde
2008	Zirconium metal, powder, dry	2046	Cymene
2009	Zirconium metal, wire, sheet, or strips (thinner than 18 microns)	2046	Methyl propyl benzene
		2047	Dichloropropene
2010	Magnesium hydride	2047	Dichloropropene and propylene dichloride mixture
2011	Magnesium phosphide	2048	Dicyclopentadiene
2012	Potassium phosphide	2049	Diethylbenzene
2013	Strontium phosphide	2050	Di-isobutylene
2014	Hydrogen peroxide solution, with not less than 20% but not more than 52% peroxide	2051	Dimethylaminoethanol
		2051	Dimethylethanolamine
2015	Hydrogen peroxide, stabilized, with more than 52% peroxide	2052	Dipentene
		2053	Methyl amyl alcohol
2016	Ammunition, toxic, non-explosive	2053	Methyl isobutyl carbinol
2016	Chemical ammunition, nonexplosive, with poisonous material	2054	Morpholine
		2055	Styrene monomer, inhibited
2016	Grenade, without bursting charge, with poisonous gas	2056	Tetrahydrofuran
		2057	Tripropylene
2017	Ammunition, tear-producing, non-explosive	2058	Amyl aldehyde
2017	Chemical ammunition, nonexplosive, with irritant	2058	Valeraldehyde
2017	Grenade, tear gas	2059	Collodion
2018	Chloroaniline, solid	2059	Nitrocellulose, solution in a flammable liquid
2019	Chloroaniline, liquid	2059	Nitrocellulose, wet with more than 40% flammable liquid by weight
2020	Chlorophenol, solid		
2020	Pentachlorophenol	2059	Pyroxylin solution
2020	Trichlorophenol	2060	Nitrocellulose, solution in a flammable liquid
2021	Chlorophenol, liquid	2067	Ammonium nitrate fertilizer
2022	Cresylic acid	2068	Ammonium nitrate fertilizer, with calcium carbonate
2022	Mining reagent, liquid	2069	Ammonium nitrate fertilizer, with ammonium sulfate
2023	Epichlorohydrin	2069	Ammonium nitrate-sulfate mixture
2024	Mercury compound, liquid, n.o.s.	2070	Ammonium nitrate fertilizer, with phosphate or potash
2025	Mercury compound, solid, n.o.s.		
2026	Phenylmercuric compound, solid, n.o.s.	2071	Ammonium nitrate fertilizer, containing not more than 45% ammonium nitrate
2027	Sodium arsenite, solid		
2028	Bomb, smoke, nonexplosive, with corrosive liquid, without initiating device	2071	Ammonium nitrate fertilizer, with not more than 0.4% of combustible material
		2072	Ammonium nitrate fertilizer, n.o.s.
2029	Hydrazine anhydrous	2073	Ammonia solution, with more than 44% ammonia
2029	Hydrazine aqueous solution, with more than 64% hydrazine, by weight	2074	Acrylamide

4-7/Hazardous Materials Identification Numbers—cont'd

ID no.	Name of material	ID no.	Name of material
2075	Chloral, anhydrous, inhibited	2118	Cyclohexanone peroxide, not more than 72% in solution
2076	Cresol (o-, m-, and p-)		
2077	Naphthylamine (alpha)	2118	1-Hydroxy-1'-hydroperoxy dicyclohexyl peroxide
2078	Toluene di-isocyanate (T.D.I.)	2119	Cyclohexanone peroxide, not more than 90%, with not less than 10% water
2079	Diethylenetriamine		
2080	Acetyl acetone peroxide	2119	1-hydroxy-1'hydroperoxy dicyclohexyl peroxide
2081	Acetyl benzoyl peroxide	2120	Decanoyl peroxide, technical pure
2082	Acetyl cyclohexane sulfonyl peroxide	2120	Didecanoyl peroxide, technical pure
2083	Acetyl cyclohexane sulfonyl peroxide	2121	Dicumyl peroxide
2084	Acetyl peroxide	2122	Di(2-ethylhexyl)peroxydicarbonate
2084	Diacetyl peroxide	2123	Di(2-ethylhexyl)peroxydicarbonate
2085	Benzoyl peroxide	2124	Dilauroyl peroxide, technical pure
2086	Benzoyl peroxide	2124	Lauroyl peroxide, technical pure
2087	Benzoyl peroxide	2125	Menthane hydroperoxide, para, technical pure
2088	Benzoyl peroxide	2125	Menthyl hydroperoxide, para, technical pure
2089	Benzoyl peroxide	2125	Paramenthane hydroperoxide
2090	Benzoyl peroxide	2126	Isobutyl methyl ketone peroxide
2091	tert-Butyl cumene peroxide	2126	Methyl isobutyl ketone peroxide
2091	tert-Butyl cumyl peroxide	2127	Ethyl methyl ketone peroxide, with not more than 60%, in solution
2091	tert-Butyl isopropyl benzene hydroperoxide		
2092	tert-Butyl hydroperoxide, not more than 80% in Di-tert-butyl peroxide and/or solvent	2127	Methyl ethyl ketone peroxide, with not more than 60% peroxide
2093	tert-Butyl hydroperoxide	2128	Di(3,5,5-trimethylhexanoyl) peroxide
2094	tert-Butyl hydroperoxide	2128	Isononanoyl peroxide, technical pure or in solution
2095	tert-Butyl peroxyacetate	2129	Caprylyl peroxide
2096	tert-Butyl peroxyacetate	2129	Di-n-octanoyl peroxide
2097	tert-Butyl peroxybenzoate	2129	Octanoyl peroxide
2098	tert-Butyl peroxybenzoate	2130	Di-n-nonanoyl peroxide
2099	tert-Butyl monoperoxymaleate, technical pure	2130	Pelargonyl peroxide
2099	tert-Butyl peroxymaleate, technical pure	2131	Peracetic acid, solution
2100	tert-Butyl monoperoxymaleate, solution or paste	2131	Peroxyacetic acid solution
2100	tert-Butyl peroxymaleate, solution or paste	2132	Dipropionyl peroxide
2101	tert-Butyl monoperoxymaleate	2132	Propionyl peroxide
2101	tert-Butyl peroxymaleate	2133	Di-isopropyl peroxydicarbonate, technical pure
2102	tert-Butyl peroxide	2133	Isopropyl peroxydicarbonate
2102	Di-tert-butyl peroxide, technical pure	2133	Propyl peroxydicarbonate
2103	tert-Butyl peroxyisopropyl carbonate, technical pure	2134	Di-isopropyl peroxydicarbonate
2104	tert-Butyl peroxyisononanoate	2134	Isopropyl peroxydicarbonate
2104	tert-Butyl peroxy-3,5,5-trimethylhexanoate	2135	Disuccinic acid peroxide, technical pure
2105	tert-Butyl monoperoxyphthalate	2135	Succinic acid peroxide, technical pure
2105	tert-Butyl peroxyphthalate	2136	Tetralin hydroperoxide, technical pure
2106	Di-tert-butylperoxyphthalate	2137	2,4-Dichlorobenzoyl peroxide
2107	Di-tert-butylperoxyphthalate	2137	Di-2,4-Dichlorobenzoyl peroxide, not more than 75% in water
2108	Di-tert-butylperoxyphthalate		
2110	tert-Butyl peroxypivalate	2138	2,4-Dichlorobenzoyl peroxide
2111	2,2-Di(tert-butylperoxy)-butane	2138	Di-2,4-Dichlorobenzoyl peroxide, not more than 52% as paste
2112	1,4-Di(2-tert-butylperoxyisopropyl)benzene, and 1,3-Di(2-tert-butylperoxyisopropyl)benzene		
		2139	2,4-Dichlorobenzoyl peroxide
2113	p-Chlorobenzoyl peroxide	2139	Di-2,4-Dichlorobenzoyl peroxide, not more than 52% in solution
2113	Di-(4-chlorobenzoyl) peroxide		
2114	p-Chlorobenzoyl peroxide	2140	n-Butyl-4,4-di(tert-butylperoxy)valerate
2114	Di-(4-chlorobenzoyl) peroxide	2141	n-Butyl-4,4-di(tert-butylperoxy)valerate
2115	p-Chlorobenzoyl peroxide	2142	tert-Butyl peroxyisobutyrate
2115	Di-(4-chlorobenzoyl) peroxide	2143	tert-Butyl peroxy-2-ethylhexanoate, technical pure
2116	Cumene Hydroperoxide, technical pure	2144	tert-Butyl peroxydiethylacetate
2117	Cyclohexanone peroxide, more than 90%, with less than 10% water	2145	1,1-Di(tert-butylperoxy)-3,3,5-trimethylcyclohexane
		2146	1,1-Di(tert-butylperoxy)-3,3,5-trimethylcyclohexane
2117	1-Hydroxy-1'-hydroperoxy dicyclohexyl peroxide, more than 90% with less than 10% water	2147	1,1-Di(tert-butylperoxy)-3,3,5-trimethylcyclohexane
		2148	Di(1-hydroxycyclohexyl) peroxide

Continued.

4-7/Hazardous Materials Identification Numbers — cont'd

ID no.	Name of material	ID no.	Name of material
2149	Dibenzyl peroxydicarbonate	2191	Sulfuryl fluoride
2150	Di-sec-butyl peroxydicarbonate	2192	Germane, germanium hydride
2151	Di-sec-butyl peroxydicarbonate	2193	Hexafluoroethane
2152	Dicyclohexyl peroxydicarbonate	2194	Selenium hexafluoride
2153	Dicyclohexyl peroxydicarbonate	2195	Tellurium hexafluoride
2154	Di(4-tert-butylcyclohexyl)peroxydicarbonate	2196	Tungsten hexafluoride
2155	2,5-Dimethyl-2,5-di(tert-butylperoxy)hexane, technical pure	2197	Hydrogen iodide, anhydrous
2156	2,5-Dimethyl-2,5-di(tert-butylperoxy)hexane	2198	Phosphorus pentafluoride
2157	2,5-Dimethyl-2,5-di(2-ethylhexanoylperoxy)hexane, technical pure	2199	Phosphine
		2200	Allene
2158	2,5-Dimethyl-2,5-di(tert-butylperoxy)hexyne-3, technical pure	2200	Propadiene
		2200	Propadiene, inhibited
2159	2,5-Dimethyl-2,5-di(tert-butylperoxy)hexyne-3, with not more than 52% peroxide in inert solid	2201	Nitrous oxide, refrigerated liquid (cryogenic liquid)
2160	tert-Octyl hydroperoxide	2202	Hydrogen selenide anhydrous
2160	1,1,3,3-Tetramethylbutyl hydroperoxide, technical pure	2202	Hydroselenic acid
		2203	Silane
2161	tert-Octyl peroxy-2-ethylhexanoate	2204	Carbonyl sulfide
2161	1,1,3,3-Tetramethylbutylperoxy-2-ethyl hexanoate, technical pure	2205	Adiponitrile
		2206	Isocyanates and solutions, n.o.s. (flammable, poisonous)
2162	Pinane hydroperoxide, technical pure	2207	Isocyanates, n.o.s., b.p. not less than 300 C
2162	Pinanyl hydroperoxide, technical pure	2208	Bleaching powder
2162	Trimethyl norpinanyl hydroperoxide, technical pure	2208	Calcium hypochlorite mixture, dry, with more than 10% but not more than 39% available chlorine
2163	Diacetone alcohol peroxide	2209	Formaldehyde solution (Formalin)
2164	Dicetyl peroxydicarbonate, technical pure	2210	Maneb, or maneb preparation(s) with 60% or more maneb
2165	3,3,6,6,9,9-Hexamethyl-1,2,4,5-tetraoxocyclononane, technical pure	2211	Plastic moulding material, evolving flammable vapor
2166	3,3,6,6,9,9-Hexamethyl-1,2,4,5-tetraoxocyclononane	2211	Polystyrene beads, expanded, mixture with flammable liquid
2167	3,3,6,6,9,9-Hexamethyl-1,2,4,5-tetraoxocyclononane	2212	Asbestos, blue
2168	2,2-Di(4,4-di-tert-butylperoxy cyclohexyl)propane	2212	Blue asbestos
2169	Butyl peroxydicarbonate	2213	Paraformaldehyde
2169	Di-n-butyl peroxydicarbonate	2214	Phthalic anhydride
2170	Butyl peroxydicarbonate	2215	Maleic acid
2170	Di-n-butyl peroxydicarbonate	2215	Maleic anhydride
2171	Di-isopropylbenzene hydroperoxide	2216	Fish meal and scrap, stabilized
2171	Isopropylcumyl hydroperoxide	2217	Seed cake, with not more than 1.5% oil and not more than 11% moisture
2172	2,5-Dimethyl-2,5-di(benzoylperoxy)hexane, technical pure	2218	Acrylic acid
2173	2,5-dimethyl-2,5-di(benzoylperoxy)hexane	2219	Allyl glycidyl ether
2174	2,5-dimethyl-2,5-dihydroperoxyhexane	2220	Aluminum alkyl halide solution
2175	Diethyl peroxydicarbonate	2221	Aluminum alkyl chloride
2176	Di-n-propyl peroxydicarbonate, technical pure	2221	Aluminum alkyl halide
2177	tert-Butyl peroxyneodecanoate	2222	Anisole
2178	2,2-Dihydroperoxy propane	2224	Benzonitrile
2179	1,1-Di(tert-butylperoxy)cyclohexane	2225	Benzene sulfonyl chloride
2180	1,1-Di(tert-butylperoxy)cyclohexane	2226	Benzotrichloride
2182	Di-isobutyryl peroxide	2227	Butyl methacrylate
2183	tert-Butyl peroxycrotonate	2228	Butyl phenol, liquid
2184	Ethyl-3,3-di(tert-butylperoxy)butyrate	2229	Butyl phenol, solid
2185	Ethyl-3,3-di(tert-butylperoxy)butyrate, not more than 77%	2232	Chloroacetaldehyde
		2233	Chloroanisidine
2186	Hydrogen chloride, refrigerated liquid (cryogenic liquid)	2234	Chlorobenzotrifluoride
		2235	Chlorobenzyl chloride
2187	Carbon dioxide, refrigerated liquid (cryogenic liquid)	2236	Chloromethylphenylisocyanate
2188	Arsine	2237	Chloronitroaniline
2189	Dichlorosilane	2238	Chlorotoluene
2190	Oxygen difluoride		

4-7/Hazardous Materials Identification Numbers — cont'd

ID no.	Name of material	ID no.	Name of material
2239	Chlorotoluidine, liquid or solid	2291	Lead compound, soluble, n.o.s.
2240	Chromosulfuric acid	2291	Lead fluoborate
2241	Cycloheptane	2291	Lead thiocyanate
2242	Cycloheptene	2293	Methoxymethylpentanone
2243	Cyclohexyl acetate	2294	Methylaniline
2244	Cyclopentanol	2295	Methyl chloroacetate
2245	Cyclopentanone	2296	Methyl cyclohexane
2246	Cyclopentene	2297	Methyl cyclohexanone
2247	Decane	2298	Methyl cyclopentane
2248	Dibutylamine	2299	Methyl dichloroacetate
2249	Dichlorodimethyl ether	2300	Methyl ethyl pyridine
2250	Dichlorophenylisocyanate	2301	Methylfuran
2251	Dicycloheptadiene	2302	Methylhexanone
2252	Dimethoxyethane	2303	Isopropenyl benzene
2253	Dimethylaniline	2304	Naphthalene, molten
2254	Matches, fusee	2305	Nitrobenzenesulfonic acid
2255	Organic peroxide, sample, n.o.s.	2306	Nitrobenzotrifluoride
2255	Polyester resin kits	2307	Nitrochlorobenzotri-fluoride
2256	Cyclohexene	2308	Nitrosylsulfuric acid
2257	Potassium	2309	Octadiene
2257	Potassium metal	2310	Pentane-2,4-dione
2258	Propylenediamine	2311	Phenetidine
2259	Triethylene tetramine	2312	Phenol, molten
2260	Tripropylamine	2313	Picoline
2261	Xylenol	2315	PCBs
2262	Dimethylcarbamoyl chloride	2315	Polychlorinated, biphenyl
2263	Dimethylcyclohexane	2316	Sodium cuprocyanide, solid
2264	2,3-Dimethylcyclohexyl amine	2317	Sodium cuprocyanide solution
2265	Dimethylformamide	2318	Sodium hydrosulfide, solid, with less than 25% water of crystallization
2265	N,N-Dimethylformamide		
2266	Dimethyl-N-propylamine	2319	Terpene hydrocarbons, n.o.s.
2267	Dimethyl thiophosphoryl chloride	2320	Tetraethylenepentamine
2269	Dipropylene triamine	2321	Trichlorobenzene, liquid
2269	Iminobispropylamine	2322	Trichlorobutene
2270	Ethylamine solution	2323	Triethyl phosphite
2271	Ethyl amyl ketone	2324	Triisobutylene
2272	Ethylaniline	2325	Mesitylene
2272	N-Ethylaniline	2325	Trimethylbenzene
2273	2-Ethylaniline	2326	Trimethylcyclohexylamine
2274	Ethylbenzylaniline	2327	Trimethylhexamethyl-enediamine
2275	Ethylbutanol	2328	Trimethylhexamethylenedi-isocyanate
2276	Ethyl hexylamine	2329	Trimethyl phosphite
2277	Ethyl methacrylate	2330	Hendecane
2278	Heptene	2330	Undecane
2279	Hexachlorobutadiene	2331	Zinc chloride, anhydrous
2280	Hexamethylene diamine, solid	2332	Acetaldehyde oxime
2281	Hexamethylene di-isocyanate	2333	Allyl acetate
2282	Hexanol	2334	Allyl amine
2283	Isobutyl methacrylate	2335	Allyl ethyl ether
2284	Isobutyronitrile	2336	Allyl formate
2285	Isocyanatobenzotrifluoride	2337	Phenyl mercaptan
2286	Isododecane	2338	Benzotrifluoride
2286	Pentamethyl heptane	2339	2-bromobutane
2287	Isoheptene	2340	Bromoethyl ethyl ether
2288	Isohexene	2341	Bromomethylbutane
2289	Isophoronediamine	2342	Bromomethylpropane
2290	Isophorone di-isocyanate	2343	Bromopentane
2291	Lead chloride	2344	Bromopropane

Continued.

4-7/Hazardous Materials Identification Numbers — cont'd

ID no.	Name of material	ID no.	Name of material
2345	Bromopropyne	2402	Isopropyl mercaptan
2346	Butanedione	2402	Propanethiol
2346	Diacetyl	2402	Propyl mercaptan
2347	Butanethiol	2403	Isopropenyl acetate
2347	Butyl mercaptan	2404	Propionitrile
2348	Butyl acrylate	2405	Isopropyl butyrate
2350	Butyl methyl ether	2406	Isopropyl isobutyrate
2351˙	Butyl nitrite	2407	Isopropyl chloroformate
2352	Butyl vinyl ether	2408	Isopropyl formate
2353	Butyryl chloride	2409	Isopropyl propionate
2354	Chloromethyl ethyl ether	2410	Tetrahydropyridine
2356	Chloropropane	2411	Butyronitrile
2357	Cyclohexylamine	2412	Tetrahydrothiophene
2358	Cyclooctatetraene	2413	Tetrapropyl-ortho-titanate
2359	Diallylamine	2414	Thiophene
2360	Diallylether	2416	Trimethylborate
2361	Di-isobutylamine	2417	Carbonyl fluoride
2362	1,1-Dichloroethane	2418	Sulfur tetrafluoride
2362	Ethylidene chloride	2419	Bromotrifluoroethylene
2363	Ethyl mercaptan	2420	Hexafluoroacetone
2364	Propyl benzene	2421	Nitrogen trioxide
2366	Diethyl carbonate	2422	Octafluorobutene
2367	Methyl valeraldehyde	2424	Octafluoropropane
2368	Pinene	2424	Perfluoropropane
2369	Ethylene glycol monobutyl ether	2426	Ammonium nitrate, liquid (hot concentrated solution)
2370	Hexene	2426	Ammonium nitrate solution, with not less than 15% water
2371	Isopentene		
2372	Bis(dimethylamino)ethane	2427	Potassium chlorate solution
2372	1,2-Di(dimethylamino)ethane	2428	Sodium chlorate solution
2373	Diethoxymethane	2429	Calcium chlorate solution
2374	Diethoxypropene	2430	Alkyl phenol, n.o.s.
2375	Diethyl sulfide	2431	Anisidine
2376	Dihydropyran	2432	Diethyl aniline
2377	Dimethoxyethane	2433	Chloronitrotoluene
2378	Dimethylaminoaceto-nitrile	2434	Dibenzyldichlorosilane
2379	1,3-Dimethylbutylamine	2435	Ethyl phenyl dichlorosilane
2380	Dimethyldiethoxysilane	2436	Thioacetic acid
2381	Dimethyldisulfide	2437	Methylphenyldichlorosilane
2382	Dimethylhydrazine, symmetrical	2438	Pivaloyl chloride
2383	Dipropylamine	2438	Trimethylacetylchloride
2384	Dipropyl ether	2439	Sodium bifluoride, solid
2385	Ethyl isobutyrate	2439	Sodium bifluoride solution
2386	Ethyl piperidine	2439	Sodium hydrogen fluoride
2387	Fluorobenzene	2440	Stannic chloride, hydrated
2388	Fluorotoluene	2441	Titanium trichloride, pyrophoric
2389	Furan	2441	Titanium trichloride mixture, pyrophoric
2390	Iodobutane	2442	Trichloroacetyl chloride
2391	Iodomethylpropane	2443	Vanadium oxytrichloride
2392	Iodopropane	2443	Vanadium oxytrichloride and titanium tetrachloride mixture
2393	Isobutyl formate		
2394	Isobutyl propionate	2444	Vanadium tetrachloride
2395	Isobutyryl chloride	2445	Butyl lithium
2396	Methacrylaldehyde	2445	Lithium alkyl
2397	Methyl butanone	2446	Nitrocresol
2398	Methyl butyl ether	2447	Phosphorus, white, molten
2399	Methylpiperidine	2448	Sulfur, molten
2400	Methyl isovalerate	2449	Ammonium oxalate
2401	Piperidine	2449	Cupric oxalate

4-7/Hazardous Materials Identification Numbers — cont'd

ID no.	Name of material	ID no.	Name of material
2449	Oxalates, n.o.s.	2504	Acetylene tetrabromide
2451	Nitrogen trifluoride	2504	Tetrabromoethane
2452	Ethyl acetylene, inhibited	2505	Ammonium fluoride
2453	Ethyl fluoride	2506	Ammonium hydrogen sulfate
2454	Methyl fluoride	2507	Chloroplatinic acid, solid
2455	Methyl nitrite	2508	Molybdenum pentachloride
2456	Chloropropene	2509	Potassium bisulfate
2457	Dimethylbutane	2509	Potassium hydrogen sulfate
2458	Hexadiene	2511	Chloropropionic acid
2459	Methylbutene	2512	Aminophenol
2460	Methylbutene	2513	Bromoacetyl bromide
2461	Methylpentadiene	2514	Bromobenzene
2462	Methylpentane	2515	Bromoform
2463	Aluminum hydride	2516	Carbon tetrabromide
2464	Beryllium nitrate	2517	Chlorodifluoroethane
2465	Dichloroisocyanuric acid, and its salts, dry	2517	Difluorochloroethane
2465	Dichlorotriazinetrione and its salts	2518	Cyclododecatriene
2465	Potassium dichloroisocyanurate	2520	Cyclooctadiene
2465	Sodium dichloro-isocyanate	2521	Diketene
2465	Sodium dichloro-S-triazinetrione	2522	Dimethylaminoethyl methacrylate
2466	Potassium superoxide	2524	Ethyl orthoformate
2467	Sodium percarbonate	2525	Ethyl oxalate
2468	Trichloroisocyanuric acid, dry	2526	Furfurylamine
2468	Trichlorotriazine-trione and its salts, dry	2527	Isobutyl acrylate
2469	Zinc bromate	2528	Isobutyl isobutyrate
2470	Phenylacetonitrile	2529	Isobutyric acid
2471	Osmium tetroxide	2530	Isobutyric anhydride
2472	Pindone	2531	Methacrylic acid
2473	Sodium arsanilate	2533	Methyl trichloroacetate
2474	Thiophosgene	2534	Methyl chlorosilane
2475	Vanadium trichloride	2535	Methylmorpholine
2477	Methyl isothiocyanate	2536	Methyl tetrahydrofuran
2478	Isocyanates and solutions, n.o.s. (flammable)	2538	Nitronaphthalene
2480	Methyl isocyanate, and solutions	2541	Terpinolene
2481	Ethyl isocyanate	2542	Tributylamine
2482	Propyl isocyanate	2545	Hafnium metal, powder, dry
2483	Isopropyl isocyanate	2546	Titanium, metal, powder, dry
2484	t-Butyl iso-cyanate	2547	Sodium superoxide
2485	n-Butyl isocyanate	2548	Chlorine pentafluoride
2486	Isobutyl isocyanate	2550	Ethyl methyl ketone peroxide
2487	Phenyl isocyanate	2550	Methyl ethyl ketone peroxide
2488	Cyclohexyl isocyanate	2551	tert-Butyl peroxydiethyl-acetate with tert-Butyl peroxybenzoate
2489	Diphenylmethyl di-isocyanate (M.D.I.)		
2489	methylene-diphenylene di-isocyanate (M.D.I.)	2552	Hexafluoroacetone hydrate
2490	Dichloroisopropyl ether	2553	Coal tar naphtha
2491	Ethanolamine, and solutions	2553	Naphtha
2491	Monoethanolamine	2554	Methyl allyl chloride
2493	Hexamethyleneimine	2555	Nitrocellulose, wet with not less than 20% water
2495	Iodine pentafluoride	2556	Nitrocellulose, wet with not less than 25% alcohol
2496	Propionic anhydride	2557	Lacquer base, dry
2497	Sodium phenolate, solid	2557	Nitrocellulose, with plasticizer
2498	Tetrahydrobenzaldehyde	2558	Epibromohydrin
2501	1-Aziridinyl phoshine oxide (TRIS)	2560	Methylpentanol
2501	Phosphoric acid triethyleneimine	2561	Methylbutene
2501	Tri(1-aziridinyl) phosphine oxide	2561	3-Methyl-1-butene
2501	Tris(1-aziridinyl)phosphine oxide	2562	tert-Butyl peroxyisobutyrate
2502	Valeryl chloride	2563	Methyl ethyl ketone peroxide, with not more than 50% peroxide
2503	Zirconium tetrachloride		

Continued.

APPEN
DIX

4-7/Hazardous Materials Identification Numbers — cont'd

ID no.	Name of material	ID no.	Name of material
2564	Trichloroacetic acid solution	2609	Triallyl borate
2565	Dicyclohexylamine	2610	Triallylamine
2567	Sodium pentachlorophenate	2611	Chloropropanol
2570	Cadmium acetate	2611	2-Chloro-1-propanol
2570	Cadmium bromide	2611	Propylene chlorohydrin
2570	Cadmium chloride	2612	Methyl propyl ether
2570	Cadmium compound	2614	Methallyl alcohol
2571	Ethyl sulfuric acid	2615	Ethoxypropane
2572	Phenylhydrazine	2615	Ethyl propyl ether
2573	Thallium chlorate	2616	Triisopropyl borate
2574	Tricresylphosphate	2617	Hexahydrocresol
2576	Phosphorus oxybroide, molten	2617	Methyl cyclohexanol
2577	Phenylacetyl chloride	2618	Vinyl toluene
2578	Phosphorus trioxide	2619	Benzyl dimethylamine
2579	Piperazine	2620	Amyl butyrate
2580	Aluminum bromide solution	2621	Acetyl methyl carbinol
2581	Aluminum chloride solution	2622	Glycidaldehyde
2582	Ferric chloride solution	2623	Fire lighter, solid with flammable liquid
2582	Iron chloride solution	2624	Magnesium silicide
2583	Alkyl sulfonic acid, solid	2626	Chloric acid solution
2583	Aryl sulfonic acid, solid	2627	Nitrite, n.o.s.
2583	Toluene sulfonic acid, solid	2628	Potassium fluoroacetate
2584	Alkyl sulfonic acid, liquid	2629	Sodium fluoroacetate
2584	Aryl sulfonic acid, liquid	2630	Barium selenate
2584	Dodecylbenzene-sulfonic acid	2630	Barium selenite
2584	Toluene sulfonic acid, liquid	2630	Calcium selenate
2585	Alkyl sulfonic acid, solid	2630	Copper selenate
2585	Aryl sulfonic acid, solid	2630	Copper selenite
2585	Tuluene sulfonic acid, solid	2630	Potassium selenate
2586	Alkyl sulfonic acid, liquid	2630	Potassium selenite
2586	Toluene sulfonic acid, liquid	2630	Selenates and selenites
2587	Benzoquinone	2630	Sodium selenate
2588	Insecticide, dry, n.o.s.	2630	Sodium selenite
2588	Pesticide, solid, n.o.s.	2630	Zinc selenate
2589	Vinyl chloroacetate	2630	Zinc selenite
2590	Asbestos, white	2642	Fluoroacetic acid
2590	White asbestos	2643	Methyl bromoacetate
2591	Xenon, refrigerated liquid (cryogenic liquid)	2644	Methyl iodide
2592	Distearyl peroxidydicarbonate	2645	Phenacyl bromide
2593	Di(2-methylbenzoyl) peroxide	2646	Hexachlorocyclopentadiene
2594	tert-Butyl peroxyneodecanoate	2647	Malonic dinitrile
2595	Dimyristyl peroxydicarbonate	2647	Malononitrile
2596	tert-Butyl peroxy-3-phenylphthalide	2648	Dibromobutanone
2597	Di(3,5,5-trimethyl-1,2-dioxolanyl-3)peroxide	2649	1,3-Dichloroacetone
2598	Ethyl-3,3-Di(tert-butylperoxy)butyrate	2649	Dichloropropanone
2599	Chlorotrifluoromethane and trifluoromethane mixture	2650	Dichloronitroethane
2599	Trifluoromethane and chlorotrifluoromethane mixture	2651	Diaminodiphenyl methane
2600	Carbon monoxide-hydrogen mixture	2653	Benzyl iodide
2601	Cyclobutane	2655	Potassium fluorosilicate, solid
2602	Dichlorodifluoromethane and difluoroethane azeotropic mixture	2655	Potassium silicofluoride, solid
		2656	Quinoline
2603	Cycloheptatriene	2657	Selenium disulfide
2604	Boron trifluoride diethyl etherate	2658	Selenium metal, powder
2605	Methoxymethyl isocyanate	2659	Sodium chloroacetate
2606	Methyl orthosilicate	2660	Nitrotoluidine (mono)
2606	Tetramethoxy silane	2661	Hexachloroacetone
2607	Acrolein dimer, stabilized	2662	Hydroquinone
2608	Nitropropane	2664	Dibromomethane

4-7/Hazardous Materials Identification Numbers — cont'd

ID no.	Name of material	ID no.	Name of material
2664	Methylene bromide	2717	Camphor, synthetic
2666	Ethyl cyanoacetate	2718	Tripropylaluminum
2666	Malonic ethyl ester nitrile	2719	Barium bromate
2667	Butyl toluene	2720	Chromium nitrate
2668	Chloroacetonitrile	2721	Copper chlorate
2669	Chlorocresol	2722	Lithium nitrate
2670	Cyanuric chloride	2723	Magnesium chlorate
2671	Aminopyridine	2724	Manganese nitrate
2672	Ammonia solution with not less than 12% and not more than 44% ammonia	2725	Nickel nitrate
		2726	Nickel nitrite
2672	Ammonium hydroxide	2727	Thallium nitrate
2673	Aminochlorophenol	2728	Zirconium nitrate
2674	Sodium fluorosilicate	2729	Hexachlorobenzene
2674	Sodium silicofluoride, solid	2730	Nitroanisole
2676	Stibine	2732	Nitrobromobenzene
2677	Rubidium hydroxide solution	2733	Alkylamine, n.o.s.
2678	Rubidium hydroxide, solid	2733	Alkylamines or polyalkylamines, n.o.s.
2679	Lithium hyroxide solution	2733	Polyalkylamine, n.o.s.
2680	Lithium hydroxide monohydrate	2734	Alkylamine, n.o.s.
2681	Caesium hydroxide solution	2734	Alkylamines or polyalkylamines, n.o.s.
2681	Cesium hydroxide solution	2734	Polyalkylamine, n.o.s.
2682	Caesium hydroxide	2735	Alkylamine, n.o.s. (corrosive)
2682	Cesium hydroxide	2735	Alkylamines or polyalkylamines, n.o.s. (corrosive)
2683	Ammonium hydrosulfide solution	2735	Polyalkylamine, n.o.s. (corrosive)
2683	Ammonium sulfide solution	2738	Butylaniline
2684	Diethylaminopropylamine	2739	Butyric anhydride
2685	Diethylethylene diamine	2740	n-Propylchloroformate
2686	Diethylaminoethanol	2741	Barium hypochlorite
2687	Dicyclohexylammonium nitrite	2742	Chloroformate, n.o.s.
2688	Chlorobromopropane	2743	Butylchloroformate
2689	Glycerol-alpha-monochlorohydrin	2744	Cyclobutylchloroformate
2690	Butyl imidazole	2745	Chloromethylchloroformate
2691	Phosphorus pentabromide	2746	Phenylchloroformate
2692	Boron tribromide	2747	tert-Butylcyclohexyl-chloroformate
2693	Ammonium bisulfite, solid	2748	Ethyl hexylchloroformate
2693	Ammonium bisulfite solution	2749	Tetramethhyl silane
2693	Bisulfite, aqueous solution, n.o.s.	2750	Dichloropropanol
2693	Calcium bisulfite solution	2751	Diethylthiophosphoryl chloride
2693	Calcium hydrogen sulfite solution	2752	Epoxyethoxypropane
2693	Magnesium bisulfite solution	2752	1,2-Epoxy-3-ethyloxypropane
2693	Potassium bisulfite solution	2753	Ethylbenzyl toluidine
2693	Sodium bisulfite solution	2754	Ethyl toluidine
2693	Zinc bisulfite solution	2755	3-Chloroperoxybenzoic acid
2698	Tetrahydrophthalic anhydride	2756	Organic peroxide mixture
2699	Trifluoroacetic acid	2757	Aldicarb
2703	Isopropyl mercaptan	2757	Carbamate pesticde, solid, n.o.s.
2705	Pentol	2757	Carbaryl
2707	Dimethyldioxane	2757	Carbofuran
2708	Butoxyl	2757	Mercaptodimethur
2709	Butyl benzene	2757	Mexacarbate
2710	Butyrone	2758	Carbamate pesticide, flammable liquid, n.o.s.
2710	Dipropyl ketone	2759	Arsenical pesticide, n.o.s.
2711	Dibromobenzene	2759	Bordeaux arsenite, liquid or solid
2713	Acridine	2760	Arsenical pesticide, flammable liquid, n.o.s.
2714	Zinc resinate	2761	Aldrin and its mixtures
2715	Aluminum resinate	2761	DDT
2716	Butynediol	2761	Dichlone
2717	Camphor	2761	Dichlorodiphenbyltrichloroethane, DDT

Continued.

4-7/Hazardous Materials Identification Numbers — cont'd

ID no.	Name of material	ID no.	Name of material
2761	Dieldrin	2783	Diazinon
2761	Endosulfan	2783	Dichlorvos
2761	Endrin mixture, dry or liquid	2783	Disulfoton
2761	Heptachlor	2783	Ethion
2761	Kelthane	2783	Guthion
2761	Kepone	2783	Hexaethyl tetraphosphate mixture
2761	Lindane	2783	Malathion
2761	Methoxychlor	2783	Methyl parathion, liquid
2761	Organochlorine pesticide, n.o.s.	2783	Methyl parathion mixture, dry
2761	TDE (1,1-dichloro-2,2-bis-(p-chlorophenyl)ethane)	2783	Mevinphos
2761	Toxaphene	2783	Naled
2762	Chlordane, flammable liquid	2783	Organic phosphate compound, liquid (Poison B)
2762	Organochlorine pesticide, flammable liquid, n.o.s.	2783	Organic phosphate compound, solid (Poison B)
2763	Triazine pesticide, solid, n.o.s.	2783	Organophosphorus pesticide, n.o.s.
2764	Triazine pesticide, flammable liquid, n.o.s.	2783	Parathion mixture, liquid or dry
2765	2,4-D	2783	Tetraethyl pyrophosphate mixture, dry
2765	2,4-D Ester	2783	Trichlorfon
2765	Dichlorophenoxyacetic acid ester	2784	Organophosphorus pesticide, flammable liquid, n.o.s.
2765	Dichlorophenoxyacetic acid salt		
2765	Phenoxy pesticide, n.o.s.	2784	Parathion, flammable liquid
2765	Propargite	2784	Tetraethyl pyrophosphate, flammable liquid
2765	2,4,5-T	2785	Thiapentanal
2765	2,4,5-T Amine, ester, or salt	2786	Organotin pesticide, n.o.s.
2765	2,4,5-TP	2787	Organotin pesticide, flammable liquid, n.o.s.
2765	2,4,5-TP Ester	2789	Acetic acid, glacial
2765	Trichlorophenoxyacetic acid amino	2789	Acetic acid solution, more than 80% acid
2765	2,4,5-Trichlorophenoxyacetic acid ester or salt	2790	Acetic acid solution, more than 10% but not more than 80% acid
2765	Trichlorophenoxypropionic acid		
2765	Trichlorophenoxypropionic acid ester	2792	Igniter for aircraft thrust device
2766	Phenoxy pesticide, flammable liquid, n.o.s.	2793	Ferrous metal, borings, cuttings, shavings, or turnings
2767	Diuron		
2767	Phenyl urea pesticide, n.o.s.	2793	Iron swarf
2768	Phenyl urea pesticide, flammable liquid, n.o.s.	2793	Steel swarf
2769	Benzoic derivative pesticide, solid, n.o.s.	2794	Battery, electric, storage, wet, filled with acid
2769	Dicamba	2794	Battery, wet, filled with acid (electric storage)
2769	Dichlobenil	2795	Battery, electric, storage, wet, filled with alkali
2770	Benzoic derivative pesticide, flammable liquid, n.o.s.	2795	Battery, wet filled with alkali (electric storage)
		2796	Battery fluid, acid
2771	Dithiocarbamate pesticide, n.o.s.	2796	Electrolyte, battery fluid, acid
2771	Thiram	2797	Battery, electric, storage, wet, filled with alkali
2772	Dithiocarbamate pesticide, flammable liquid, n.o.s.	2797	Battery fluid, alkali
2773	Phthalimide derivative pesticide, n.o.s.	2798	Benzene phosphorus dichloride
2774	Phthalimide derivative pesticide, flammable liquid, n.o.s.	2798	Phenyl phosphorus dichloride
		2799	Benzene phsophorus thiodichloride
2775	Copper-based pesticide, solid, n.o.s.	2799	Phenyl phosphorus thiodichloride
2776	Copper-based pesticide, flammable liquid, poison, n.o.s.	2800	Battery, electric, storage wet, nonspillable
		2800	Battery, wet, nonspillable (electric storage)
2777	Mercury-based pesticide, n.o.s.	2801	Dye, n.o.s. (corrosive)
2778	Mercury-based pesticide, flammable liquid, n.o.s.	2801	Dye intermediate, n.o.s. (corrosive)
2779	Substituted nitrophenol pesticide, solid, n.o.s.	2802	Copper chloride
2780	Substituted nitrophenol pesticide, flammable liquid, n.o.s.	2803	Gallium, metal
		2805	Lithium hydride, fused, solid
2781	Bipyridilium pesticide, n.o.s.	2806	Lithium nitride
2781	Diquat	2809	Mercury
2782	Bipyridilium pesticide, flammable liquid, n.o.s.	2809	Mercury metal
2783	Azinphos methyl (Guthion)	2810	3,5-Dichloro-2,4,6-trifluoropyridine
2783	Chlorpyrifos	2810	Poison B liquid, n.o.s.
2783	Coumaphos	2810	Poisonous liquid, n.o.s. (Poison B)

4-7/Hazardous Materials Identification Numbers — cont'd

ID no.	Name of material	ID no.	Name of material
2811	Flue dust, poisonous	2856	Silicofluoride, solid, n.o.s.
2811	Lead fluoride	2857	Refrigerating machine, containing nonflammable,
2811	Lead iodide		nonpoiisonous, liquefied gas
2811	Lead stearate	2858	Zirconium metal, wire, sheet, or strips (thinner than
2811	Lead sulfide		254 microns but not thinner than 18 microns)
2811	Poisonous solid, n.o.s.	2859	Ammonium metavanadate
2811	Selenium oxide	2860	Vanadium trioxide
2811	Sodium vanadate	2861	Ammonium polyvanadate
2812	Sodium aluminate, solid	2862	Vanadium pentoxide
2813	Lithium acetylide-ethyl-enediamine complex	2863	Sodium ammonium vanadate
2813	Substances, which, when in contact with water, emit	2864	Potassium metavanadate
	flammable gases, n.o.s.	2865	Hydroxylamine sulfate
2813	Water reactive solid, n.o.s.	2867	Ink
2814	Etiologic agent, n.o.s.	2869	Titanium trichloride mixture
2814	Infectious substance, human, n.o.s.	2870	Aluminum borohydride
2815	Aminoethylpiperazine	2870	Aluminum borohydride in devices
2817	Ammonium bifluoride, solution	2871	Antimony, powder
2817	Ammonium hydrogen fluoride solution	2871	Antimony powder
2818	Ammonium polysulfide solution	2872	Dibromochloropropane
2819	Amyl acid phosphate	2873	Dibutylaminoethanol
2820	Butyric acid	2874	Furfuryl alcohol
2821	Phenol solution	2875	Hexachlorophene
2822	Chloropyridine	2876	Resorcinol
2823	Crotonic acid	2877	Thiourea
2825	Di-isopropylethanolamine	2878	Titanium sponge, granules or powder
2826	Ethyl chlorothioformate	2879	Selenium oxychloride
2829	Caproic acid	2880	Calcium hypochlorite, hydrated, including mixtures
2830	Lithium ferrosilicon		with not less than 5.5% but not more than 10%
2831	Methyl chloroform		water
2831	Trichloroethane	2881	Nickel catalyst, dry
2834	Phosphorous acid (ortho)	2883	2,2-Di(tert-butylperoxy)-propane
2835	Sodium aluminum hydride	2884	2,2-Di(tert-butylperoxy)-propane
2837	Sodium bisulfate solution	2885	1,1-Di(tert-butylperoxy)-cyclohexane
2837	Sodium hydrogen sulfate solution	2886	tert-Butyl peroxy-2-ethyl-hexanoate, with 2,2Di-(tert-
2838	Vinyl butyrate		butyl peroxy)-butane
2839	Aldol	2887	tert-Butyl peroxy-2-ethyl-hexanoate, with 2,2-di-(t-
2840	Butyraldoxime		butylperoxy)4butane
2841	Diamylamine	2888	tert-Butyl peroxy-2-ethyl-hexanoate, with more than
2842	Nitroethane		50%, with phlegmatizer
2844	Calcium manganese silicon	2889	Di-isotridecyl-peroxydicarbonate
2845	Ethyl phosphonous dichloride, anhydrous	2890	tert-Butyl peroxy-benzoate
2845	Methyl phosphonous dichloride	2891	tert-Amylperoxy-neodecanoate
2845	Pyrophoric liquid, n.o.s.	2892	Dimyristyl peroxydi-carbonate, not more than 42%,
2846	Pyrophoric solid, n.o.s.		in water
2849	3-Chloropropanol	2893	Dilauroyl peroxide, not more than 42%, in water
2849	3-Chloropropanol-1	2893	Lauroyl peroxide, not more than 42%
2849	Trimethylene chlorohydrin	2894	Di(4-tert-butylcyclohexyl)-peroxydicarbonate
2850	Propylene tetramer	2895	Dicetyl peroxydicarbonate, not more than 42%
2851	Boron trifluoride dihydrate	2896	Cyclohexanone peroxide, not more than 72% as a
2852	Dipicryl sulfide, wet with not less than 10%		paste
	water	2897	1,1-Di(tert-butylperoxy)-cyclohexane
2853	Magnesium fluorosilicate	2898	tert-Amylperoxy-2-ethyl-hexanoate
2853	Magnesium silicofluoride, solid	2899	Organic peroxide, trial quantity, n.o.s.
2854	Ammonium fluorosilicate	2900	Infectious substance, nonhuman, n.o.s.
2854	Ammonium silicoflurodie, solid	2901	Bromine chloride
2855	Zinc fluorosilicate	2902	Allethrin
2855	Zinc silicofluoride, solid	2902	Fungicide, poisonous, n.o.s.
2856	Fluorosilicates, n.o.s.	2902	Insecticide, liquid, poisonous, n.o.s.

Continued.

4-7/Hazardous Materials Identification Numbers — cont'd

ID no.	Name of material	ID no.	Name of material
2902	Pesticide, liquid, poisonous, n.o.s.	2955	2,2′-Azodi(2,4-dimethyl-4-methoxyvaleronitrile)
2903	Pesticide, poison, flammable liquid, n.o.s.	2956	tert-Butyl-2,4,6-trinitro-m-xylene
2904	Chlorophenate, liquid	2956	Musk xylene
2905	Chlorophenate, solid	2957	tert-Amylperoxypivalate
2906	Triisocyanatoisocyanurate of isophoronediisocyanate, 70% solution	2958	Diperoxy azelaic acid
		2959	2,5-Dimethyl-2,5-Di-(benzoylperoxy)hexane
2907	Isosorbide dinitrate mixture	2960	Di(2-ethylhexyl)peroxydicarbonate
2908	Radioactive material, empty packages	2961	2,4,4-Trimethylpentyl-2-peroxyphenoxyacetate
2909	Radioactive material, articles manufactured from natural or depleted uranium or natural thorium	2962	Disuccinic acid peroxide, not more than 72%, in water
2910	Radioactive material, limited quantity, n.o.s.	2963	Cumyl peroxy-neodecanoate
2911	Radioactive material, instruments and articles	2964	Cumyl peroxypivalate
2912	Radioactive material, low specific activity (LSA), n.o.s.	2965	Boron trifluoride dimethyl etherate
		2966	Thioglycol
2918	Radioactive material, fissile, n.o.s.	2967	Sulfamic acid
2920	Corrosive liquid, flammable, n.o.s.	2968	Maneb, or maneb preparation(s), stabilized against self-heating
2921	Corrosive solid, flammable, n.o.s.		
2922	Corrosive liquid, poisonous, n.o.s.	2969	Castor beans, meal, pomace or flake
2922	Dimethyl chlorothiophosphate	2970	Benzene sulfohydrazide
2922	Dimethyl phosphorochloridothioate	2971	Benzene-1,3-disulfohydrazide
2922	Sodium hydrosulfide solution	2972	Dinitrosopentamethylene tetramine
2923	Corrosive solid, poisonous, n.o.s.	2973	Dinitroso-dimethyl terephthalamide
2923	Sodium hydrosulfide, solid, with not less than 25% water of crystallization	2974	Radioactive material, special form, n.o.s.
		2975	Thorium metal, pyrophoric
2924	Dichlorobutene	2976	Thorium nitrate, solid
2924	Flammable liquid, corrosive, n.o.s.	2977	Uranium hexafluoride, fissile (containing more than 0.7% U-235)
2925	Flammable solid, corrosive, n.o.s.		
2926	Flammable solid, poisonous, n.o.s.	2978	Uranium hexafluoride, low specific activity (containing not more than 0.7% U-235)
2927	Poison, corrosive liquid, n.o.s.		
2928	Poison, corrosive solid, n.o.s.	2979	Uranium metal, pyrophoric
2929	Chloropicrin mixture, flammable	2980	Uranium nitrate hexahydrate solution
2929	Poison, flammable liquid, n.o.s.	2981	Uranyl nitrate, solid
2930	Poison, flammable solid, n.o.s.	2982	Radioactive material, n.o.s.
2931	Vanadyl sulfate	2983	Ethylene oxide-propylene oxide mixture
2933	Methyl chloropropionate	2984	Hydrogen peroxide solution with not less than 8% but less than 20% peroxide
2934	Isopropyl chloropropionate		
2935	Ethyl chloropropionate	2985	Chlorosilane, n.o.s. (flammable, corrosive)
2936	Thiolactic acid	2986	Chlorosilane, n.o.s. (flammable, corrosive)
2937	Methylbenzyl alcohol (alpha)	2987	Chlorosilane, n.o.s. (corrosive)
2938	Methylbenzoate	2988	Chlorosilane, n.o.s. (emits flammable gas when wet, corrosive)
2940	Cyclooctadiene phosphine		
2940	Phosphabicyclononane	2989	Lead phosphite, dibasic
2941	Fluoroaniline	2990	Aircraft evacuation slide
2942	2-Trifluoromethylaniline	2990	Aircraft survival kit
2943	Tetrahydrofurfurylamine	2990	Life raft
2944	Fluoroaniline	2990	Life-saving appliances, self-inflating
2945	Methylbutylamine	2991	Carbamate pesticide, flammable liquid, n.o.s.
2946	2-amino-5-diethylaminopentane	2992	Carbamate pesticide, liquid, n.o.s.
2947	Isopropyl chloroacetate	2993	Arsenical pesticide, flammable liquid, n.o.s.
2948	3-Trifluoromethylaniline	2994	Arsenical pesticide, liquid, n.o.s.
2949	Sodium hydrosulfide, with not less than 25% water of crystallization	2995	Organochlorine pesticide, flammable liquid, n.o.s.
		2996	Organochlorine pesticide, liquid, n.o.s.
2949	Sodium hydrosulfide solution	2997	Triazine pesticide, flammable liquid, n.o.s.
2950	Magnesium granules, coated	2998	Triazine pesticide, liquid, n.o.s.
2951	Diphenyloxide-4,4′-Di-sulfohydrazide	2999	Phenoxy pesticide, flammable liquid, n.o.s.
2952	Azodi(isobutyronitrile)	3000	Phenoxy pesticide, liquid, n.o.s.
2953	2,2′-Azodi(2,4-dimethyl-valeronitrile)	3001	Phenyl urea pesticide, flammable liquid, n.o.s.
2954	Azodi(1,1′-hexahydrobenzonitrile)	3002	Phenyl urea pesticide, liquid, n.o.s.

4-7/Hazardous Materials Identification Numbers — cont'd

ID no.	Name of material
3003	Benzoic derivative pesticide, flammable liquid, n.o.s.
3004	Benzoic derivative pesticide, liquid, n.o.s.
3005	Dithiocarbamate pesticide, flammable liquid, n.o.s.
3006	Dithiocarbamate pesticide, liquid, n.o.s.
3007	Phthalimide derivative pesticide, flammable liquid, n.o.s.
3008	Phthalimide derivative pesticide, liquid, n.o.s.
3009	Copper-based pesticide, poison, flammable liquid, n.o.s.
3010	Copper-based pesticide, liquid, n.o.s.
3011	Mercury-based pesticide, flammable liquid, n.o.s.
3012	Mercury-based pesticide, liquid, n.o.s.
3013	Substituted nitrophenol pesticide, flammable liquid, n.o.s.
3014	Substituted nitrophenol pesticide, liquid, n.o.s.
3015	Bipyridilium pesticide, flammable liquid, n.o.s.
3016	Bipyridilium pesticide, liquid, n.o.s.
3017	Organophosphorus pesticide, flammable liquid, n.o.s.
3018	Organophosphorus pesticide, liquid, n.o.s.
3019	Organotin pesticide, flammable liquid, n.o.s.
3020	Organotin pesticide, liquid, n.o.s.
3021	Pesticide, flammable liquid, poison, n.o.s.
3022	Butylene oxide, stabilized
3022	1.2-Butyleneoxide, stabilized
3023	t-Octyl mercaptan
3024	Coumarin derivative pesticide, flammable liquid, n.o.s.
3025	Coumarin derivative pesticide, flammable liquid, n.o.s.
3026	Coumarin derivative pesticide, liquid, n.o.s.
3027	Coumarin derivative pesticide, solid, n.o.s.
3028	Battery, electric, storage, dry, containing potassium hydroxide
3030	Azodi(2-methyl-butyronitrile)
3031	Self-reactive substances, samples, n.o.s.
3032	Self-reactive substances, trial quantities, n.o.s.
3033	3-Chloro-4-diethylamino-benzenediazonium zinc chloride
3034	4-Dipropylaminobenzene-diazonium zinc chloride
3035	3-(2-Hydroxyethoxy)-4-pyrrolidin-1-ylbenzene-di-azonium zinc chloride
3036	2,5-Diethoxy-4-morpholinobenzenediazonium zinc chloride
3037	4-(Benzyl(ethyl)amino)-3-ethoxybenzenediazonium zinc chloride
3038	4-(Benzyl(methyl)amino)-3-ethoxybenzenediazonium zinc chloride
3039	4-Dimethylamino-6-(2-dimethylaminoethoxy) toluene-2 diazonium zinc chloride
3040	Sodium 2-diazo-1-naphthol-4-sulfonate
3041	Sodium 2-diazo-1-naphthol-5-sulfonate
3042	2-Diazo-1-naphthol-4-sulfochloride
3043	2-Diazo-1-naphthol-5-sulfochloride
3044	tert-Amylperoxybenzoate
3045	Peroxyacetic acid solution
3046	Methyl cyclohexanone peroxide

ID no.	Name of material
3047	tert-Butyl peroxypivalate
3048	Aluminum phosphide pesticide
3049	Metal alkyl halide, n.o.s.
3050	Metal alkyl hydride, n.o.s.
3051	Aluminum alkyl
3052	Aluminum alkyl halide
3053	Magnesium alkyl
3054	Cyclohexyl mercaptan
3055	Aminoethoxyethanol
3056	n-Heptaldehyde
3057	Trifluoroacetyl chloride
3058	Di-(2-phenoxyethyl)-peroxydicarbonate, technically pure
3059	D-(2-Phenoxyethyl)-peroxydicarbonate, not more than 85% with water
3060	2,5-Dimethyl-2,5-Di-(iso-nonanoylperoxy)hexane not more than 77% in solution
3060	2,5-Dimethyl-2,5-Di-(3,5,5-trimethylhexanoylperoxy)-hexane, not more than 77% in solution
3061	Acetyl acetone peroxide, not more than 32% as a paste
3062	tert-Butyl peroxy-stearyl carbonate, technical pure
3063	Diperoxydodecane diacid, not more than 42% with not less than 56% sodium sulfate
3064	Nitroglycerin, solution in alcohol, with more than 1% but not more than 5% nitroglycerin
3065	Alcoholic beverage
3066	Paint, etc., corrosive liquid
3066	Paint related material, corrosive liquid
3067	tert-Amyl hydroperoxide, not more than 88%
3068	Methyl ethyl ketone peroxide, with not more than 40% peroxide
3069	1,1-Di-(tert-butylperoxy)-cyclohexane
3070	Dichlorodifluoromethane and ethylene oxide mixture
3070	Ethylene oxide-dichloro difluoromethane mixture, with not more than 12% ethylene oxide
3071	Mercaptan, liquid, n.o.s.
3071	Mercaptan mixture, liquid, n.o.s.
3072	Life-saving appliances not self inflating
3073	Vinyl methyl pyridine
3073	Vinyl pyridine, inhibited
3074	Benzoyl peroxide, not more than 62%, with not less than 28% inert solid and not less than 10% water
3075	tert-Butyl hydroperoxide, not more than 82%, with not less than 7% water and not less than 9% Di-tert-butyl peroxide
3076	Aluminum alkyl hydride
3077	Environmentally hazardous substance, solid, n.o.s.
3078	Cerium, turnings or gritty powder
3079	Methacrylonitrile, inhibited
3080	Isocyanates, n.o.s. or isocyanate solutions, n.o.s., flash point not less than 23°C and not more than 60.5°C
3081	3-Chloroperoxybenzoic acid, not more than 57% with water and 3-chlorobenzoic acid
3082	Environmentally hazardous substance, liquid, n.o.s.
3083	Perchloryfluoride
3084	Corrosive solid, oxidizing, n.o.s.

APPEN-DIX

Continued.

4-7/Hazardous Materials Identification Numbers — cont'd

ID no.	Name of material	ID no.	Name of material
3085	Oxidizing substance, solid, corrosive, n.o.s.	9138	Nickel ammonium sulfate
3086	Poisonous, solid, oxidizing, n.o.s.	9139	Nickel chloride
3087	Oxidizing substance, solid, poisonous, n.o.s.	9140	Nickel hydroxide
3088	Self-heating substances, solid, n.o.s.	9141	Nickel sulfate
	Space Reserved	9142	Potassium chromate
	Begin ID No. 9000 Series	9145	Sodium chromate
9011	Camphene	9146	Sodium dodecylbenzene sulfonate
9018	Dichlorodifluoroethylene	9147	Sodium phosphate, dibasic
9026	Dinitrocyclohexyl phenol	9148	Sodium phosphate, tribasic
9035	Gas identification set	9149	Strontium chromate
9037	Hexachloroethane	9151	Triethanolamine dodecylbenzene-sulfonate
9069	Tetramethylmethylenediamine	9152	Vanadyl sulfate
9077	Adipic acid	9153	Zinc acetate
9078	Aluminum sulfate, solid	9154	Zinc ammonium chloride
9079	Ammonium acetate	9156	Zinc bromide
9080	Ammonium benzoate	9157	Zinc carbonate
9081	Ammonium bicarbonate	9158	Zinc fluoride
9083	Ammonium carbamate	9159	Zinc formate
9084	Ammonium carbonate	9160	Zinc phenolsulfonate
9085	Ammonium chloride	9161	Zinc sulfate
9086	Ammonium chromate	9162	Zirconium potassium fluoride
9087	Ammonium citrate	9163	Zirconium sulfate
9088	Ammonium fluoroborate	9170	Thorium metal, pyrophoric
9089	Ammonium sulfamate	9171	Thorium nitrate, solid
9090	Ammonium sulfite	9173	Uranium hexafluoride, fissile (more than 0.7% of U-235)
9091	Ammonium tartrate		
9092	Ammonium thiocyanate	9174	Uranium hexafluoride, low specific activity (0.7% or less U-235)
9093	Ammonium thiosulfate		
9094	Benzoic acid	9175	Uranium metal, pyrophoric
9095	Butyl phthalate	9177	Uranyl nitrate, solid
9096	Calcium chromate	9178	Uranyl nitrate hexahydrate solution
9097	Calcium dodecylbenzene sulfonate	9180	Uranium acetate
9099	Captan	9180	Uranyl acetate
9100	Chromic sulfate	9183	Organic peroxide, liquid or solution, n.o.s.
9101	Chromic acetate	9184	Pyrethrins
9102	Chromous chloride	9187	Organic peroxide, solid, n.o.s.
9103	Cobaltous bromide	9188	Hazardous substance, liquid or solid, n.o.s.
9104	Cobaltous formate	9188	ORM-E, liquid or solid, n.o.s.
9105	Cobaltous sulfamate	9189	Hazardous waste, liquid or solid, n.o.s.
9106	Cupric acetate	9190	Ammonium permanganate
9109	Cupric sulfate	9191	Chlorine dioxide hydrate, frozen
9110	Cupric sulfate, ammoniated	9192	Fluorine, refrigerated liquid (cryogenic liquid)
9111	Cupric tartrate	9193	Oxidizer, corrosive liquid, n.o.s.
9117	EDTA	9194	Oxidizer, corrosive solid, n.o.s.
9117	Ethylenediamine tetraacetic acid	9195	Metal alkyl solution, n.o.s.
9118	Ferric ammonium citrate	9199	Oxidizer, poisonous liquid, n.o.s.
9119	Ferric ammonium oxalate	9200	Oxidizer, poisonous solid, n.o.s.
9120	Ferric fluoride	9201	Antimony trioxide
9121	Ferric sulfate	9202	Carbon monoxide, cryogenic liquid
9122	Ferrous ammonium sulfate	9205	Lithium battery
9125	Ferrous sulfate	9206	Methyl phosphonic dichloride
9126	Fumaric acid	9207	Acetophenone
9127	Isopropanolamine dodecylbenzenesulfonate	9255	m-Dichlorobenzene
9134	Lithium chromate		
9137	Napthenic acid		

4-8/EVACUATION DISTANCES

Name of material spilling or leaking (ID no.)	Initial isolation for a spill or leak from a drum or small container (or small leak from tank) isolate in all directions (feet)	Initial evacuation for a large spill from a tank (or from many containers or drums) First, isolate in all directions (feet)	Then evacuate in a downward direction Width (miles)	Length (miles)
Acetone cyanohydrin (1541)	50	150	0.2	0.2
Acrolein (1092)	300	600	1.5	3.0+
Acrylonitrile (1093)	75	150	0.2	0.4
Allyl alcohol (1098)				
Allyl bromide (1099)	50	150	0.2	0.2
Allyl chloride (1100)				
Allylamine (2334)	75	150	0.2	0.4
Ammonia (1005)				
Ammonia, anhydrous, liquefied (1005)	150	300	0.4	0.8
Ammonia solution, with more than 44% (2073)	75	150	0.2	0.4
Anhydrous ammonia (1005)	150	300	0.4	0.8
Arsine (2188)	150	N/A	N/A	N/A
Boron tribromide (2692)	50	150	0.2	0.2
Boron trifluoride (1008)	600	900	1.5	3.0+
Bromine (1744)	300	600	0.8	1.5
Bromine trifluoride (1746)	50	150	0.2	0.2
n-Butyl isocyanate (2485)				
t-Butyl isocyanate (2484)	50	150	0.2	0.2
Carbon bisulfide (1131)				
Carbon disulfide (1131)	75	150	0.2	0.4
Carbon monoxide, cryogenic liquid (9202)	300	600	0.8	1.5
Carbonyl chloride (1076)	600	N/A	N/A	N/A
Chloride of phosphorus (1809)	150	300	0.4	0.8
Chlorine (1017)	150	300	0.8	1.5
Chlorine pentafluoride (2548)	50	N/A	N/A	N/A
Chlorine tirfluoride (1749)	75	150	0.2	0.4
Chloroacetic acid, liquid (1750)	75	150	0.2	0.4
Chloroacetonitrile (2668)	50	150	0.2	0.2
Chloropicrin (1580)				
Chloropicrin and Methyl bromide mixture (1581)	50	150	0.2	0.2
Chloropicrin and Methyl chloride mixture (1582)				
Chlorosulfonic acid (1754)	50	150	0.2	0.2
Crotonaldehyde (1143)	50	150	0.2	0.2
Cyanogen, liquefied (1026)				
Cyanogen chloride (1589)	150	300	0.8	1.5
Cyclohexyl isocyanate (2488)	50	150	0.2	0.2
Diamylamine (2841)	50	150	0.2	0.2
Diketene (2521)	50	150	0.2	0.2
Dimethylamine, anhydrous (1032)	150	300	0.8	1.5
Dimethyl hydrazine, symmetrical, (2382) or unsymmetrical (1163)	75	150	0.2	0.4
Dimethyl sulfate (1595)	150	300	1.5	3.0
Epichlorohydrin (2023)	75	150	0.2	0.4

Continued.

4-8/Evacuation Distances — cont'd

Name of material spilling or leaking (ID no.)	Initial isolation for a spill or leak from a drum or small container (or small leak from tank) isolate in all directions (feet)	Initial evacuation for a large spill from a tank (or from many containers or drums) First, isolate in all directions (feet)	Then evacuate in a downward direction Width (miles)	Length (miles)
Ethyl chloroformate (1182)	50	150	0.2	0.2
Ethylene chlorohydrin (1135)	50	150	0.2	0.2
Ethylene imine (1185)	300	600	1.5	3.0
Ethylene oxide (1040)	150	300	0.4	0.8
Ethyl isocyanate (2481)	50	150	0.2	0.2
Fluorine, refrigerated liquid (cryogenic liquid) (9192)	300	900	3.0	3.0+
Hydrochloric acid, anhydrous (1050)	300	600	0.8	1.5
Hydrocyanic acid	150	300	0.8	1.5
Hydrofluoric acid, anhydrous (1052)	150	300	0.8	1.5
Hydrogen chloride, anhydrous (1050) or refrigerated liquid, (cryogenic liquid) (2186)	300	600	0.8	1.5
Hydrogen cyanide, absorbed, (1614) or anhydrous (1051)	150	300	0.8	1.5
Hydrogen fluoride, anhydrous (1052)	150	300	0.8	1.5
Hydrogen selenide (2202)	300	N/A	N/A	N/A
Hydrogen sulfide (1053)	150	300	0.8	1.5
Iron pentacarbonyl (1994)	300	N/A	N/A	N/A
Isobutyl isocyanate (2486)	50	150	0.2	0.2
Isopropyl chloroformate (2407)	50	150	0.2	0.2
Methoxymethyl isocyanate (2605)	50	150	0.2	0.2
Methylamine, anhydrous (1061)	150	300	0.4	0.8
Methyl bromide (1062)	75	150	0.2	0.4
Methyl bromide and Chloropicrin mixture (1581)	75	150	0.2	0.4
Methyl chloride (1063) Methyl chloride and Chloropicrin mixture (1582) Methyl chloroformate (1238)	50	150	0.2	0.2
Methyl chloromethyl ether (1239)	75	150	0.2	0.4
Methyl hydrazine (1244)	75	150	0.2	0.4
Methyl isocyanate (2480)	75	150	0.2	0.4
Methyl mercaptan (1064)	300	900	1.5	3.0+
Methyl orthosilicate (2606)	50	150	0.2	0.2
Methyl sulfate (1595)	150	300	1.5	3.0
Monochloroacetic acid, liquid (1750)	75	150	0.2	0.4
Monomethylamine, anhydrous (1061)	150	300	0.4	0.8
Monomethyl hydrazine (1244)	75	150	0.2	0.4
Nickel carbonyl (1259)	300	N/A	N/A	N/A
Nitric acid, fuming (2032) or red fuming (2032) Nitric oxide (1660)	150	300	0.4	0.8
Nitric oxide and Nitrogen tetroxide mixture (1975) Nitrogen dioxide (1067) Nitrogen peroxide (1067) Nitrogen tetroxide (1067) Nitrogen trifluoride (2451)	150	300	0.4	0.8
Nitrogen trioxide (2421)	150	N/A	N/A	N/A
t-Octylmercaptan (3023)	50	150	0.2	0.2
Oleum (1831)	300	600	1.5	3.0+
Oxygen difluoride (2190)	300	N/A	N/A	N/A
Pentaborane (1380)	150	N/A	N/A	N/A

4-8/Evacuation Distances — cont'd

Name of material spilling or leaking (ID no.)	Initial isolation for a spill or leak from a drum or small container (or small leak from tank) isolate in all directions (feet)	Initial evacuation for a large spill from a tank (or from many containers or drums)		
		First, isolate in all directions (feet)	Then evacuate in a downward direction Width (miles)	Length (miles)
Perchloromethylmercaptan (1670)	300	600	1.5	3.0
Phosgene (1076)	600	1200	3.0	3.0+
Phosphorus oxychloride (1810)				
Phosphorus pentafluoride (2198)	150	300	0.4	0.8
Phosphorus trichloride (1809)				
n-Propyl chloroformate (2740)	50	150	0.2	0.2
Selenium hexafluoride (2194)	150	N/A	N/A	N/A
Sulfur dioxide (1079)	150	300	0.8	1.5
Sulfuric acid, fuming (1831)				
Sulfuric anhydride (1829)	300	600	1.5	3.0+
Sulfur trioxide (1829)				
Tetramethoxy silane (2606)	50	150	0.2	0.2
Tetranitromethane (1510)	50	N/A	N/A	N/A
Titanium tetrachloride (1838)	50	150	0.2	0.2
Trimethoxy silane (----)	50	150	0.2	0.2
Trimethylamine, anhydrous (1083)	75	150	0.2	0.4

APPEN-
DIX

4-9/EMERGENCY RESPONSE GUIDEBOOKS

GENERAL INFORMATION	SPECIALIZED INFORMATION
EMERGENCY RESPONSE GUIDEBOOK FOR HAZARDOUS MATERIALS OFFICE OF HAZARDOUS MATERIALS RESEARCH AND SPECIAL PROGRAMS ADMINISTRATION, U.S. DEPARTMENT OF TRANSPORTATION WASHINGTON, DC 20036	**FARM CHEMICAL BOOK** MEISTER PUBLISHING COMPANY 37841 EUCLID AVENUE WILLOUGHBY, OH 44094 SUBJECT AREA: PESTICIDES AND AGRICULTURAL CHEMICALS
FIRE PROTECTION GUIDE ON HAZARDOUS MATERIALS NATIONAL FIRE PROTECTION ASSOC. BATTERYMARCH PARK QUINCY, MA 02269	**RECOGNITION AND MANAGEMENT OF PESTICIDE POISONINGS (ORDER # 055-044-0013-7)** SUPERINTENDENT OF DOCUMENTS GOVERNMENT PRINTING OFFICE WASHINGTON, DC 20402 SUBJECT AREA: PESTICIDES AND AGRICULTURAL CHEMICALS
EMERGENCY HANDLING OF HAZARDOUS MATERIALS IN SURFACE TRANSPORTATION HAZARDOUS MATERIALS SYSTEMS ASSOCIATION OF AMERICAN RAILROADS 50 F STREET, NW WASHINGTON, DC 20001	**THE PESTICIDE HANDBOOK** THE ENTOMOLOGICAL SOCIETY OF AMERICA (ENTOMA) 603 CALVERT ROAD BOX AJ COLLEGE PARK, MD 20741 SUBJECT AREA: PESTICIDES
EMERGENCY ACTION GUIDESHEETS HAZARDOUS MATERIALS SYSTEMS ASSOCIATION OF AMERICAN RAILROADS 50 F STREET, NW WASHINGTON, DC 20001	**GATX TANK CAR MANUAL** GENERAL AMERICAN TRANSPORTATION CORPORATION 120 SOUTH RIVERSIDE PLAZA CHICAGO, IL 60606 SUBJECT AREA: RAILROAD TANK CARS
CHRIS (CHEMICAL HAZARDS RESPONSE INFORMATION SYSTEM) SUPERINTENDENT OF DOCUMENTS U.S. GOVERNMENT PRINTING OFFICE WASHINGTON, DC 20402 NOTE: ALTHOUGH CHRIS IS COMPOSED OF FOUR SEPARATE DOCUMENTS, ONLY MANUAL 2-HAZARDOUS CHEMICAL DATA IS NORMALLY USED BY RESPONDERS.	**GUIDELINES FOR THE SELECTION OF CHEMICAL PROTECTIVE CLOTHING, VOLUMES I AND II (REPORT CG-D-7-87)** NATIONAL TECHNICAL INFORMATION SERVICE SPRINGFIELD, VA 22161 SUBJECT AREA: CHEMICAL PROTECTIVE CLOTHING
NIOSH/OSHA POCKET GUIDE TO CHEMICAL HAZARDS (ORDER # 017-33-00418) SUPERINTENDENT OF DOCUMENTS U.S. GOVERNMENT PRINTING OFFICE WASHINGTON, D.C. 20402	**HAZARDOUS MATERIALS INJURIES: A HANDBOOK FOR PRE-HOSPITAL CARE** BRADFORD COMMUNICATIONS CORP. 7500 GREENWAY CENTER DRIVE GREENBELT, MD 20770 SUBJECT AREA: EMERGENCY MEDICAL CARE
THE FIREFIGHTER'S HANDBOOK OF HAZARDOUS MATERIALS MALTESE ENTERPRISES, INC. P.O. BOX 34048 INDIANAPOLIS, IN 46234	
DANGEROUS PROPERTIES OF INDUSTRIAL MATERIALS (SAX) LAB SAFETY SUPPLY COMPANY P.O. BOX 1368 JANESVILLE, WI 53547	
MANUAL FOR SPILL OF HAZARDOUS MATERIALS (ENVIRONMENT CANADA-ORDER # EN40-320-1948E) CANADIAN GOVERNMENT PUBLICATION CENTER OTTOWA, ONTARIO KIA OS9 CANADA	

4-10/HAZARDOUS MATERIALS ELECTRONIC DATABASES

HAZARDOUS MATERIALS ELECTRONIC DATABASES

DATABASE	HAZARDOUS SUBSTANCES DATABANK (HSDB) TOXICOLOGY DATABANK (TDB) TOXLINE REGISTRY OF TOXIC EFFECTS OF CHEMICAL SUBSTANCES (RTECS) MEDLINE
SOURCE	NATIONAL LIBRARY OF MEDICINE MEDLARS MANAGEMENT SECTION 8600 ROCKVILLE PIKE BETHESDA, MD. 20209 (301) 496-6193
DATABASE	OVER THIRTY DIFFERENT DATABASES WITH BOTH SCIENTIFIC AND REGULATORY CHEMICAL-RELATED INFORMATION. IT INCLUDES OHM-TADS (OIL AND HAZARDOUS MATERIALS TECHNICAL ASSISTANCE DATA SYSTEM) AND CHRIS (CHEMICAL HAZARDS RESPONSE INFORMATION SYSTEM).
SOURCE	CHEMICAL INFORMATION SYSTEMS, INC. 7215 YORK RD. BALTIMORE, MD. 21212 (301) 321-8440
DATABASE	HAZARDLINE
SOURCE	OCCUPATIONAL HEALTH SERVICES 400 PLAZA DRIVE P.O. BOX 1505 SECAUCUS, NJ. 07094 (201) 865-7500
DATABASE	OVER TWENTY-FIVE SEPARATE CHEMICAL– RELATED INFORMATION DATABASES UNDER THE TITLE OF INTEGRATED CHEMICAL INFORMATION SYSTEMS (ICIF)
SOURCE	INFORMATION CONSULTANTS, INC. 1133 15TH STREET, NW SUITE 301 WASHINGTON, D.C. 20005 (202) 822-5200
DATABASE	COMPUTER–AIDED MANAGEMENT OF EMERGENCY OPERATIONS (CAMEO)
SOURCE	U.S. DEPARTMENT OF COMMERCE NATIONAL OCEANOGRAPHIC AND ATMOSPHERIC AGENCY (NOAA) HAZARDOUS MATERIALS RESPONSE BRANCH 7600 SAND POINT WAY, NE SEATTLE, WA 98115 (206) 526-6317
DATABASE	EMERGENCY/HAZMAT INFORMATION SYSTEM
SOURCE	MANAGEMENT LOGISTICS INTERNATIONAL, LTD. 1401 WILSON BLVD. ARLINGTON, VA. 22209 (703) 522-4550

APPEN-
DIX

4-11/EPA LEVELS OF PROTECTION

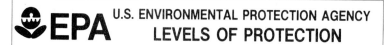

EPA U.S. ENVIRONMENTAL PROTECTION AGENCY
LEVELS OF PROTECTION

LEVEL A PROTECTION SHOULD BE WORN WHEN THE HIGHEST LEVEL OF RESPIRATORY, SKIN, EYE, AND MUCOUS MEMBRANE PROTECTION IS NEEDED.

- PERSONAL PROTECTIVE EQUIPMENT
  - ☐ POSITIVE-PRESSURE (PRESSURE-DEMAND), SELF-CONTAINED BREATHING APPARATUS (MSHA/NIOSH APPROVED).
  - ☐ FULLY-ENCAPSULATING CHEMICAL RESISTANT SUIT.
  - ☐ GLOVES, INNER, CHEMICAL RESISTANT.
  - ☐ GLOVES, OUTER, CHEMICAL RESISTANT.
  - ☐ BOOTS, CHEMICAL RESISTANT, STEEL TOE AND SHANK; (DEPENDING ON SUIT BOOT CONSTRUCTION, WORN OVER OR UNDER SUIT BOOT.)
  - ☐ UNDERWEAR, COTTON, LONG-JOHN TYPE.*
  - ☐ HARD HAT (UNDER SUIT).*
  - ☐ COVERALLS (UNDER SUIT).*
  - ☐ TWO-WAY RADIO COMMUNICATIONS (INTRINSICALLY SAFE).

LEVEL B PROTECTION SHOULD BE SELECTED WHEN THE HIGHEST LEVEL OF RESPIRATORY PROTECTION IS NEEDED, BUT A LESSER LEVEL OF SKIN AND EYE PROTECTION. LEVEL B PROTECTION IS THE MINIMUM LEVEL RECOMMENDED ON INITIAL SITE ENTRIES UNTIL THE HAZARDS HAVE BEEN FURTHER IDENTIFIED AND DEFINED BY MONITORING, SAMPLING, AND OTHER RELIABLE METHODS OF ANALYSIS, AND PERSONNEL EQUIPMENT CORRESPONDING WITH THOSE FINDINGS UTILIZED.

- PERSONAL PROTECTIVE EQUIPMENT
  - ☐ POSITIVE-PRESSURE (PRESSURE-DEMAND), SELF-CONTAINED BREATHING APPARATUS (MSHA/NIOSH APPROVED).
  - ☐ CHEMICAL RESISTANT CLOTHING (OVERALLS AND LONG SLEEVED JACKET, COVERALLS, HOODED TWO PIECE CHEMICAL SPLASH SUIT, DISPOSABLE CHEMICAL RESISTANT COVERALLS.)
  - ☐ COVERALLS (UNDER SPLASH SUIT).*
  - ☐ GLOVES, OUTER, CHEMICAL RESISTANT.
  - ☐ GLOVES, INNER, CHEMICAL RESISTANT.
  - ☐ BOOTS, OUTER, CHEMICAL RESISTANT, STEEL TOE AND SHANK.
  - ☐ BOOTS, OUTER, CHEMICAL RESISTANT.*
  - ☐ TWO-WAY RADIO COMMUNICATIONS (INTRINSICALLY SAFE).
  - ☐ HARD HAT.*

LEVEL C PROTECTION SHOULD BE SELECTED WHEN THE TYPE OF AIRBORNE SUBSTANCE IS KNOWN, CONCENTRATION MEASURED, CRITERIA FOR USING AIR-PURIFYING RESPIRATORS MET, AND SKIN AND EYE EXPOSURE IS UNLIKELY. PERIODIC MONITORING OF THE AIR MUST BE PERFORMED.

- PERSONAL PROTECTIVE EQUIPMENT
  - ☐ FULL-FACE, AIR-PURIFYING RESPIRATOR (MSHA/NIOSH APPROVED).
  - ☐ CHEMICAL RESISTANT CLOTHING (ONE PIECE COVERALL, HOODED TWO PIECE CHEMICAL SPLASH SUIT, CHEMICAL RESISTANT HOOD AND APRON, DISPOSABLE CHEMICAL RESISTANT COVERALLS.)
  - ☐ GLOVES, OUTER, CHEMICAL RESISTANT.
  - ☐ GLOVES, INNER, CHEMICAL RESISTANT.*
  - ☐ BOOTS, STEEL TOE AND SHANK, CHEMICAL RESISTANT.
  - ☐ CLOTH COVERALLS (INSIDE CHEMICAL PROTECTIVE CLOTHING.)*
  - ☐ TWO-WAY RADIO COMMUNICATIONS (INTRINSICALLY SAFE).*
  - ☐ HARD HAT.*
  - ☐ ESCAPE MASK.*

LEVEL D IS PRIMARILY A WORK UNIFORM. IT SHOULD NOT BE WORN ON ANY SITE WHERE RESPIRATORY OR SKIN HAZARDS EXIST.

*Optional

4-12/CHEMICAL ELEMENTS AND SYMBOLS

Element	Symbol	Element	Symbol
Actinium	Ac	Molybdenum	Mo
Aluminum	Al	Neodymium	Nd
Americium	Am	Neon	Ne
Antimony	Sb	Neptunium	Np
Argon	Ar	Nickel	Ni
Arsenic	As	Niobium (Columbium)	Nb
Astatine	At	Nitrogen	N
Barium	Ba	Nobelium	No
Berkelium	Bk	Osmium	Os
Beryllium	Be	Oxygen	O
Bismuth	Bi	Palladium	Pd
Boron	B	Phosphorus	P
Bromine	Br	Platinum	Pt
Cadmium	Cd	Plutonium	Pu
Calcium	Ca	Polonium	Po
Californium	Cf	Potassium	K
Carbon	C	Praseodymium	Pr
Cerium	Ce	Promethium	Pm
Cesium	Cs	Protactinium	Pa
Chlorine	Cl	Radium	Ra
Chromium	Cr	Radon	Rn
Cobalt	Co	Rhenium	Re
Columbium	Cb	Rhodium	Rh
Copper	Cu	Rubidium	Rb
Curium	Cm	Ruthenium	Ru
Dysprosium	Dy	Samarium	Sm
Einsteinium	Es or E	Scandium	Sc
Erbium	Er	Selenium	Se
Europium	Eu	Silicon	Si
Fermium	Fm	Silver	Ag
Fluorine	F	Sodium	Na
Francium	Fr	Strontium	Sr
Gadolinium	Gd	Sulfur	S
Gallium	Ga	Tantalum	Ta
Germanium	Ge	Technetium	Tc
Gold	Au	Tellurium	Te
Hafnium	Hf	Terbium	Tb
Helium	He	Thallium	Tl
Holmium	Ho	Thorium	Th
Hydrogen	H	Thulium	Tm
Indium	In	Tin	Sn
Iodine	I	Titanium	Ti
Iridium	Ir	Tungsten (Wolfram)	W
Iron	Fe	Uranium	U
Krypton	Kr	Vanadium	V
Lanthanum	La	Wolfram (Tungsten)	W
Lawrencium	Lr	Xenon	Xe
Lead	Pb	Ytterbium	Yb
Lithium	Li	Yttrium	Y
Lutetium	Lu	Zinc	Zn
Magnesium	Mg	Zirconium	Zr
Manganese	Mn		
Mendelevium	Md		
Mercury	Hg		

APPEN-
DIX

4-13/COMPRESSED GAS CYLINDER SIZES AND VOLUMES

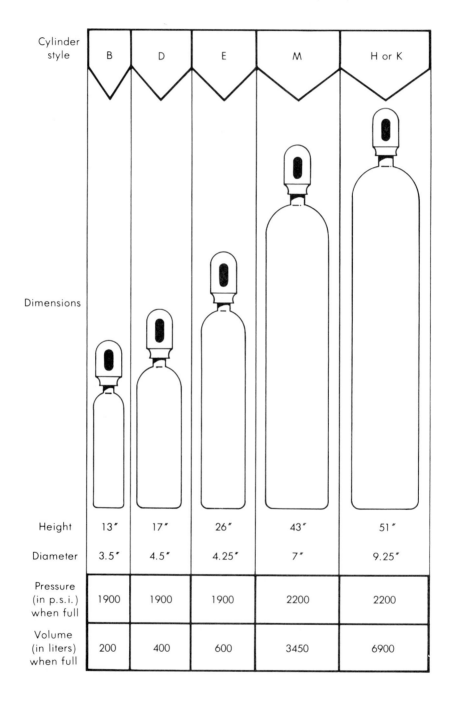

	B	D	E	M	H or K
Cylinder style	B	D	E	M	H or K
Height	13″	17″	26″	43″	51″
Diameter	3.5″	4.5″	4.25″	7″	9.25″
Pressure (in p.s.i.) when full	1900	1900	1900	2200	2200
Volume (in liters) when full	200	400	600	3450	6900

Redrawn from Rescue Training Associates, Ltd, ACTION GUIDE FOR EMERGENCY SERVICES PERSONNEL, © 1985, p 336, (A Brady Book). Reprinted with permission of Prentice-Hall, Inc, Englewood Cliffs, New Jersey.

4-14/CRYOGENIC FLUID EXPLOSION AND HEALTH PROPERTIES

Symbol	Oxygen (O_2)	Nitrogen (N_2)	Argon (Ar)	Helium (Ne)	Krypton (Kr)	Xenon (Xe)	Neon (Ne)	Methane (CH_4)	Hydrogen (H_2)	Carbon monoxide (CO)
Explosion hazard										
With combustible materials	Yes	No	No	No	No	No	No	No	No	No
With oxygen or air	—	No	No	No	No	No	No	Yes	Yes	Yes
									(Within flammable units)	
Pressure rupture if liquid or cold vapor is trapped	Yes	Yes	Yes	Yes	Yes	Yes	Yes	Yes	Yes	Yes
Fire hazard										
Combustible	Nil	Nil	Nil	Nil	Nil	Nil	Nil	Yes	Yes	Yes
Promotes ignition	Yes	No	No	No	No	No	No	Yes	Yes	Yes
Condenses air and expands flammable range	No	Yes	No	Yes	No	No	Yes	No	Yes	Yes
Flammable limits in air (percent by volume)	—	—	—	—	—	—	—	5-15	4-74	13-74

From Rescue Training Associates, Ltd, ACTION GUIDE FOR EMERGENCY SERVICES PERSONNEL, © 1985, p 363-364, (A Brady Book). Reprinted with permission of Prentice-Hall, Inc, Englewood Cliffs, New Jersey.

APPEN-DIX

4-15/CRYOGENIC FLUID HEALTH HAZARDS

Symbol	Oxygen (O$_2$)	Nitrogen (N$_2$)	Argon (Ar)	Helium (Ne)	Krypton (Kr)	Xenon (Xe)	Neon (Ne)	Methane (CH$_4$)	Hydrogen (H$_2$)	Carbon monoxide (CO)
Local effects										
Cold contact injuries result from skin contact with liquid, impinging vapors, or surfaces at liquid temperature.	Yes	Yes	Yes	Yes	Yes	Yes	Yes	Yes	Yes	Yes
General effects										
Inhalation of vapor or cold gas produces respiratory discomfort or difficulty.	Yes	Yes	Yes	Yes	Yes	Yes	Yes	Yes	Yes	Yes
Exposure to vapor or cold gas produces frostbite or hypothermia.	Yes	Yes	Yes	Yes	Yes	Yes	Yes	Yes	Yes	Yes
Inhalation of the gas can cause asphyxiation	No	Yes	Yes	Yes	Yes	Yes	Yes	Yes	Yes	Yes
Toxic.	No	No	No	No	No	No	No	No	No	Yes

From Rescue Training Associates, Ltd, ACTION GUIDE FOR EMERGENCY SERVICES PERSONNEL, © 1985, p 364-365, (A Brady Book). Reprinted with permission of Prentice-Hall, Inc, Englewood Cliffs, New Jersey.

4-16/DECONTAMINATION PROCEDURE

ACTIONS		ENTER● PROCEDURES
PERSONNEL ENTER DECON AREA AND DROP TOOLS ON CONTAMINATED SIDE. MOVE TO STEP 2.	**1**	DIRECTION OF TRAVEL — 1 TOOLS
REMOVE AS MUCH CONTAMINATION AS POSSIBLE. DILUTION IS CONDUCTED INSIDE DIKED AREA. PERSONNEL ARE IN SCBA. MOVE TO STEP 3.	**2**	2 RUN-OFF CONTROL — DIKE — 3 SCBA AREA
REMOVE SCBA TO CONTAMINATED SIDE AND MOVE TO STEP 4 OR DON NEW SCBA FROM CLEAN SIDE AND RE-ENTER WORK AREA. MOVE TO STEP 4.	**3**	4 PROTECTIVE CLOTHING AREA
REMOVE PROTECTIVE CLOTHING AND PLACE ON CONTAMINATED SIDE. MOVE TO STEP 5 OR TRANSPORT PERSONNEL TO FIXED DECON FACILITY.	**4**	5 PERSONAL CLOTHING AREA
REMOVE ALL PERSONAL CLOTHING AND ISOLATE ITEMS ON CONTAMINATED SIDE. BAG PERSONAL ITEMS. MOVE TO STEP 6.	**5**	6 SHOWER AREA
PERSONAL SHOWERING USING SOAP AND SPONGES. BAG CLEANING ITEMS FOR DISPOSAL. MOVE TO STEP 7.	**6**	7 DRY-OFF AREA
PERSONNEL DRY OFF. BAG TOWELS. PUT ON CLEAN CLOTHING. MOVE TO STEP 8.	**7**	8 MEDICAL EVALUATION
PERSONNEL RECEIVE MEDICAL EVALUATION AND TREATMENT AS NECESSARY. MOVE TO STEP 9.	**8**	9 TRANSPORT AREA
IDENTIFY PERSONNEL. COMPLETE FIELD RECORDS. TRANSPORT PERSONNEL TO HOSPITAL OR TO A FIXED DECON FACILITY FOR STEPS 5-8.	**9**	NOTE: STEPS 5-9 MAY BE DONE OFF SITE

CLEAN SIDE   CONTAMINATED SIDE

EXIT

APPEN-DIX

4-17/DOE REGIONAL RADIOLOGICAL OFFICES

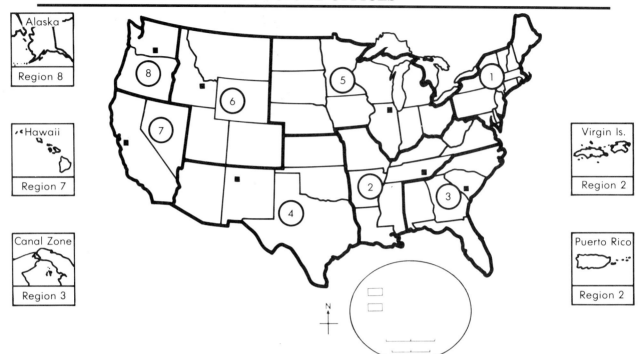

Regional Coordinating Office	Post Office Address	Telephone
1 Brookhaven Area Office	Upton, L.I., New York 11973	(516) 345-2200
2 Oak Ridge Operations Office	P.O. Box E, Oak Ridge, Tennessee 37830	(615) 576-1005
		or
		(615) 525-7885
3 Savannah River Operations Office	P.O. Box A, Aiken, S.C. 29801	(803) 725-3333
4 Albuquerque Operations Office	P.O. Box 5400, Albuquerque, N.M. 87115	(505) 844-4667
5 Chicago Operations Office	9800 S. Cass Ave., Argonne, Illinois 60439	(312) 972-4800
		Off Duty Hrs.
		(312) 972-5731
6 Idaho Operations Office	P.O. Box 2108, Idaho Falls, Idaho 83401	(208) 526-1515
7 San Francisco Operations Office	1333 Broadway, Oakland, California 94612	(415) 273-4237
8 Richland Operations Office	P.O. Box 550, Richland, Washington 99352	(509) 376-7381

4-18/RADIOLOGICAL UNITS CHART

Multiple	Decimal equivalent	Prefix	Symbol
10^6	1,000,000	mega-	M
10^3	1,000	kilo-	k
10^2	100	hecto-	h
10	10	deka-	da
10^{-1}	0.1	deci-	d
10^{-2}	0.01	centi-	c
10^{-3}	0.001	milli-	m
10^{-6}	0.000001	micro-	μ

5

THE INCIDENT COMMAND SYSTEM

5-1/COMMAND SECTION

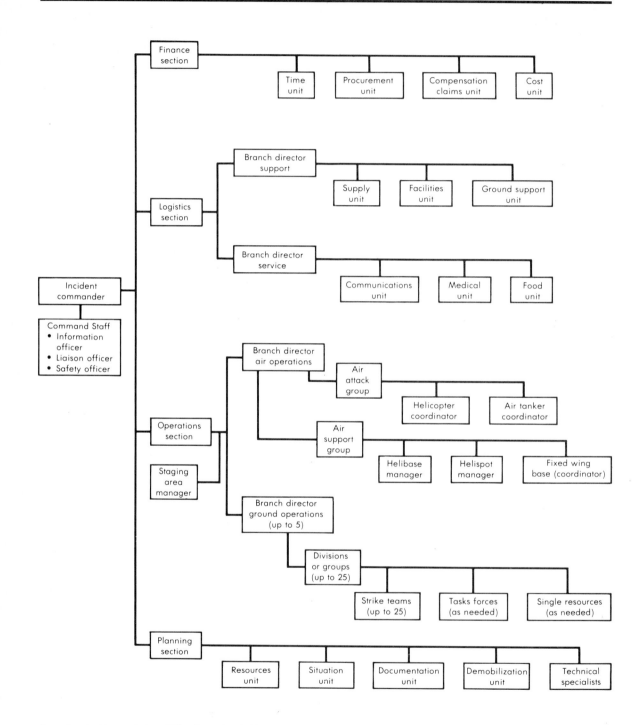

Reproduced with permission of Fire Protection Publications, Oklahoma State University, Stillwater, Oklahoma, 1983.